RUSSELL AND RUBINSTEIN'S
Pathology of Tumors of the Nervous System

NOTICE

The publishers wish to draw attention to some minor imperfections in artwork reproduction in this printing.

A small number of black-and-white images have Moiré interference patterns in the background which the Publishers believe will not interfere with interpretation of their content. Many of these are unique illustrations from the collection of Lucien Rubinstein that – while perfect in their original form – had to be re-originated for this edition. All illustrations for this edition have been recorded in digital format for future electronic delivery; unfortunately, it was during this process of digitisation that the interference patterns were introduced.

In addition, some of the color balance is different to that on the original slides provided by the Editors due to the printer's need to make compromises across many color illustrations in each 32 page section.

Both these factors occurred post-proof and were therefore outside the control of the Editors and contributors.

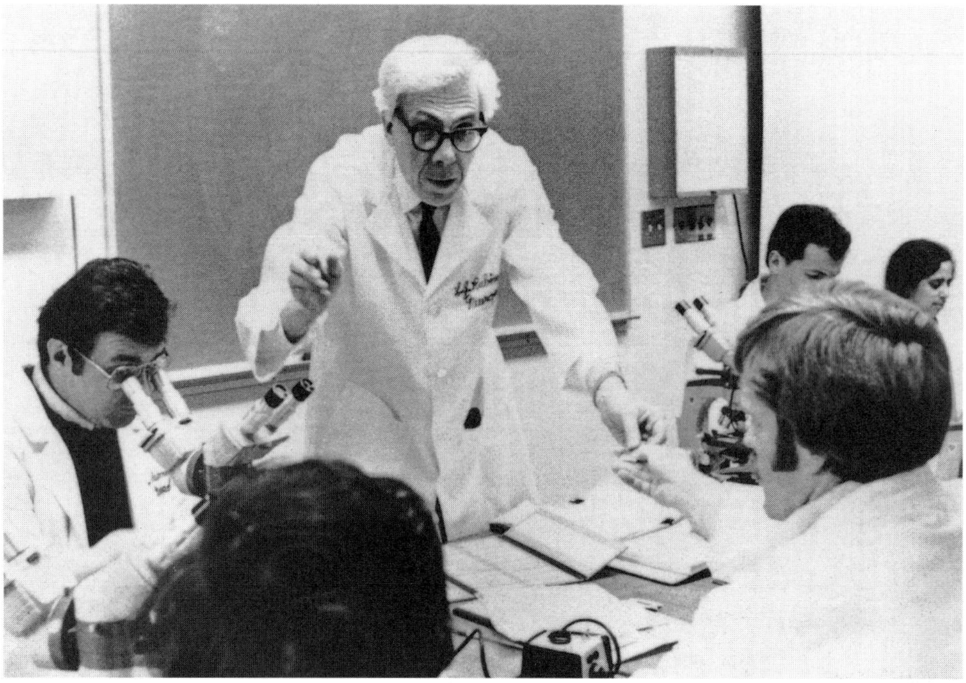

Lucien J Rubinstein, 1924–1990

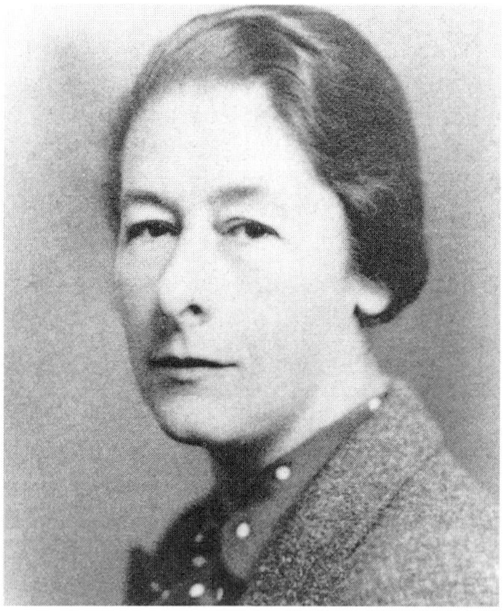

Dorothy S Russell, 1895–1983

Dorothy S. Russell occupied a unique position in the development of neuropathology in Britain. She was most justly famous for her work on brain tumors, which culminated in the publication in 1959 of the first edition of *Pathology of Tumours of the Nervous System* (with Lucien J. Rubinstein) and subsequent editions in 1963, 1971, 1977 and, posthumously, 1989. Her interests were remarkably wide ranging and included hydrocephalus, head injuries, non-metastatic effects of cancer in the nervous system and many other topics. Professor Russell's dedication and the standard she set of honesty and accuracy in scientific work have laid a sure foundation for those who succeeded her in neuropathology.

RUSSELL AND RUBINSTEIN'S
Pathology of Tumors of the Nervous System

SIXTH EDITION

Edited by

Darell D Bigner MD PhD

Edwin L Jones Jr and Lucille Finch Jones Cancer Research Professor of Pathology (Neuropathology); Vice Chairman for Investigative Pathology, Department of Pathology; Deputy Director, Duke Comprehensive Cancer Center; Duke University Medical Center, Durham, North Carolina, USA

Roger E McLendon MD

Assistant Professor of Pathology; Chief, Section of Neuropathology, Department of Pathology, Duke University Medical Center, Durham, North Carolina, USA; Associate Professor of Pathology, Mercer University School of Medicine, Macon, Georgia, USA

Janet M Bruner MD

Professor of Pathology and Neuro-Oncology; Chief, Section of Neuropathology, Department of Pathology, The University of Texas MD Anderson Cancer Center, Houston, Texas, USA

With editorial and administrative assistance from **Ann S. Tamariz**, ELS, Assistant Editor, Duke Brain Tumor Research Program

ARNOLD

A member of the Hodder Headline Group

LONDON • SYDNEY • AUCKLAND

Co-published in the USA by Oxford University Press, Inc., New York

First published in 1959
Fifth edition published in 1989
Sixth edition published in Great Britain 1998 by
Arnold, a member of the Hodder Headline Group,
338 Euston Road, London NW1 3BH

Co-published in the United States of America by
Oxford University Press, Inc.,
198 Madison Avenue, New York, NY10016
Oxford is a registered trademark of Oxford University Press

British Library Cataloguing in Publication Data
A catalogue record for this book is available from the British Library

Library of Congress Cataloging-in-Publication Data
A catalog record for this book is available from the Library of Congress

Publisher: Georgina Bentliff
Project Manager: Mairwen Lloyd-Williams
Project Editor: Sophie Oliver
Production Controller: Rose James
Cover Designer: Terry Griffiths

ISBN 0340 58113 1 (hb)

Phototypeset in 10/11 Times New Roman
by Scribe Design, Gillingham, Kent
Printed and bound in Great Britain by the Bath Press

Contents of Volume 1

Contents of Volume 2

Contributors

David M Ashley MD PhD
Formerly: Clinical Associate, Department of Pediatrics, Duke University Medical Center, Durham, North Carolina, USA
Now: Oncologist, Royal Children's Hospital, Parkville, Victoria, Australia

Surinder K Batra PhD
Formerly: Assistant Professor of Pathology (Molecular Biology), Department of Pathology, Duke University Medical Center, Durham, North Carolina, USA
Now: Associate Professor, Department of Biochemistry and Molecular Biology, University of Nebraska Medical Center, Omaha, Nebraska, USA

Darell D Bigner MD PhD
Edwin L Jones Jr and Lucille Finch Jones Cancer Research Professor of Pathology (Neuropathology); Vice Chairman for Investigative Pathology, Department of Pathology; Deputy Director, Duke Comprehensive Cancer Center; Duke University Medical Center, Durham, North Carolina, USA

Sandra H Bigner MD
Professor of Pathology, Department of Pathology, Duke University Medical Center, Durham, North Carolina, USA

Garrett M Brodeur MD
Professor of Pediatric Oncology, Children's Hospital of Philadelphia and the University of Pennsylvania, Philadelphia, Pennsylvania, USA

Janet M Bruner MD
Professor of Pathology and Neuro-Oncology; Chief, Section of Neuropathology, Department of Pathology, The University of Texas MD Anderson Cancer Center, Houston, Texas, USA

Faith G Davis PhD
Professor and Director, Division of Epidemiology and Biostatistics, School of Public Health, University of Illinois at Chicago, Chicago, Illinois, USA

David S Enterline MD
Assistant Professor of Radiology, Department of Radiology, Neuroradiology Section, Duke University Medical Center, Durham, North Carolina, USA

Kar-Ming Fung MD PhD
Department of Pathology and Laboratory Medicine, University of Pennsylvania School of Medicine, Hospital of the University of Pennsylvania, Philadelphia, Pennsylvania, USA

Laura P Hale MD PhD
Assistant Professor of Pathology, Department of Pathology, Duke University Medical Center, Durham, North Carolina, USA

Kalman Kovacs MD PhD DSc FRCP(C) FCAP FRCPath
Professor of Pathology, Department of Pathology, University of Toronto, St Michael's Hospital, Toronto, Ontario, Canada

Ole Didrik Laerum MD PhD
Professor of Experimental Pathology and Oncology, Department of Pathology, The Gade Institute, University of Bergen, Haukeland Hospital, Bergen, Norway

Roger E McLendon MD, FCAP
Assistant Professor of Pathology; Chief, Section of Neuropathology, Department of Pathology, Duke University Medical Center, Durham, North Carolina, USA; Associate Professor of Pathology, Mercer University School of Medicine, Macon, Georgia, USA

Sverre J Mørk MD PhD
Professor of Medicine (Neuropathology), Department of Pathology, The Gade Institute, University of Bergen, Haukeland Hospital, Bergen, Norway

Monica Nistér MD PhD
Associate Professor of Experimental Pathology, Department of Pathology, University Hospital, University of Uppsala, Uppsala, Sweden

Susan Preston-Martin PhD
Professor of Preventive Medicine, University of Southern California, USC/Norris Comprehensive Cancer Center, Los Angeles, California, USA

B K Ahmed Rasheed PhD
Research Assistant Professor of Pathology, Department of Pathology, Duke University Medical Center, Durham, North Carolina, USA

John H Sampson MD PhD
Chief Resident (Neurosurgery Service), Department of Surgery; Research Associate, Department of Pathology, Duke University Medical Center, Durham, North Carolina, USA

Hiroyuki Shimada MD PhD
Director, Electron Microscopy Laboratory, Department of Pathology and Laboratory Medicine, Children's Hospital of Los Angeles, Los Angeles, California, USA

James A Swenberg DVM PhD
Director of Toxicology Curriculum; Professor of Environmental Sciences and Engineering; Professor of Nutrition and Pathology, University of North Carolina, Chapel Hill, North Carolina, USA

Kamal Thapar MD PhD
Resident, Division of Neurosurgery, Department of Surgery, University of Toronto, St Michael's Hospital, Toronto, Ontario, Canada

Wade L Thorstad MD
Radiation Oncologist, Fellow in Nuclear Medicine, Department of Radiology, Division of Nuclear Medicine, Duke University Medical Center, Durham, North Carolina, USA

Robert D Tien MD MPH
Formerly: Associate Professor of Radiology, Department of Radiology, Duke University Medical Center, Durham, North Carolina, USA
Now: Department of Diagnostic Imaging, Tan Tock Seng Hospital, Singapore

S Thomas Traweek MD
Associate Professor of Pathology; Director of Hematopathology, Department of Pathology, Duke University Medical Center, Durham, North Carolina, USA

John Q Trojanowski MD PhD
Department of Pathology and Laboratory Medicine, University of Pennsylvania School of Medicine, Hospital of the University of Pennsylvania, Philadelphia, Pennsylvania, USA

Henry Urich MD FRCP FRCPath
Professor Emeritus of Neuropathology, University of London, The London Hospital Medical College, London, UK

Dale M Walker DVM
Research Scientist, Wadsworth Center for Laboratories and Research, New York State Department of Health, Albany, New York, USA

Vernon E Walker DVM PhD
Research Scientist, Wadsworth Center for Laboratories and Research, New York State Department of Health, Albany, New York, USA

Bengt Westermark PhD
Professor of Tumor Biology, Department of Pathology, University Hospital, University of Uppsala, Uppsala, Sweden

Carol J Wikstrand PhD
Associate Research Professor, Department of Pathology, Duke University Medical Center, Durham, North Carolina, USA

Preface

This sixth edition of Russell and Rubinstein's *Pathology of Tumors of the Nervous System* is dedicated to the memory and life work of Professor Lucien J. Rubinstein (1924–1990). The most appropriate way to introduce the preface, we thought, was to begin with a quotation from the memorial tribute to Lucien Rubinstein that appeared in the *Journal of Neuro-Oncology*.[1]

> Lucien J. Rubinstein (B.S., M.R.C.S., L.R.C.P., M.B., M.D. [Pathology]), Professor of Neuropathology at the University of Virginia, died at his home near Charlottesville, Virginia, on January 22, 1990. His loss will be deeply felt world-wide, for in the subject of brain tumors, his eminence had long been recognized. It was usual for any truly remarkable specimens to be sent to him for consultation from every part of the world. His fame was derived in part from his publications, which were numerous and encompassed a period of 35 years. Of these, the most important are a textbook and a monograph, mentioned further in these paragraphs.
>
> Rubinstein was born in Antwerp on October 15, 1924, and so was not yet 16 when the German army swept through Belgium. Over the next two years he managed, with his young sister, to cross occupied France and eventually reach London. After a year at Queen Mary College, he was admitted to the medical college of London Hospital, the Dean being clearly impressed by his determination in escaping across Europe. He qualified in 1948.
>
> Joining the staff of the Pathology Institute at London Hospital, after military service, he fell under the spell of Professor Dorothy S. Russell. Dr Russell, successor to the chair of Professor H.M. Turnbull, was determined to maintain the highest standards of morbid anatomy and histology. She brought her own special powers of observation and description to the study of diseases of the brain, especially tumors. Rubinstein became her star pupil, and a fruitful period of collaboration culminated in their co-authorship of the textbook *Pathology of Tumours of The Nervous System*, published in 1959. This book, based so much on personal observation and experience and derived from collected material, quickly established its position as a standard work with its lucid, authoritative view of a complex subject and formed an ideal companion volume to *Greenfield's Neuropathology*. Five new editions were published, the latest in 1989.
>
> The death of Professor Dorothy Russell in 1983 left Rubinstein a free hand to accomplish a most formidable task. There had now been four editions of the textbook, with continuous updating; but nearly 25 years had passed since the first typescript, and recent progress had been rapid. Much new subject matter, such as the impact of molecular biology, had to be included if the book was to retain its pre-eminent position. Many new illustrations were needed; some chapters were overlaid with obsolete controversies and needed revision. It would have been tempting to invite specialists from various related fields to contribute. However, realizing that multi-author textbooks invariably suffer from the loss of the 'single voice' and tend to become burdened with statements derived from the literature rather than personal experience, Rubinstein set out on a marathon, like his beloved Proust, and single-handedly wrote a book whose size and scope would nowadays be associated with a team of writers. This substantial volume, the fifth edition of Russell and Rubinstein's *Pathology of Tumours of The Nervous System*, appeared in 1989 and will be his most fitting memorial.
>
> In addition to *Pathology of Tumours of the Nervous System* and the widely acclaimed *AFIP*

[1] Barnard, R. and Bigner, D.D. (1990) In memoriam, Lucien J. Rubinstein, M.D. (1924–1990). *Journal of Neuro-Oncology* **9**, III–VI. Reprinted with kind permission of Kluwer Academic Publishers.

[Armed Forces Institute of Pathology] *Atlas on Tumors of the Central Nervous System*, his work in neuropathology comprises over 139 articles in the scientific literature, 14 book chapters, over 50 published papers presented to national and international meetings, and the translation of the *Manual of Basic Neuropathology* by Escourolle and Poirier. He had major editorial responsibilities for eight journals and fostered scientific literature of the highest standards. In his own publications, he applied uniformly high and exacting standards to himself and his collaborators. His numerous contributions include: 1) early descriptions of mixed gliomas-sarcomas and the importance of stromal and neural cell interactions in CNS tumors; 2) early morphologic characterization of the causative viruses of PML and SSPE; 3) definitive description of numerous tumor entities (true polar spongioblastomas, ependymoblastoma, pleomorphic xanthoastrocytoma and infantile desmoplastic ganglioglioma); 4) definitive analyses of desmoplastic medulloblastomas, cerebral neuroblastomas, a number of important astrocytoma variants, pineal parenchymal tumors, ependymal neoplasms, and meningeal mesenchymal chondrosarcomas; 5) complications of CNS tumor radiation; 6) a conceptual framework for understanding cytogenesis and differentiation of CNS tumors; 7) pioneering work in the application of glial fibrillary acid protein to neuro-oncology; 8) further immunohistochemical characterization of numerous CNS and peripheral nervous system tumors; and 9) growth kinetics of gliomas and medulloblastomas in matrix culture. His research in the primary matrix culture of brain tumors with Dr Mary Herman and the use of the neuroepithelial cell component of the experimental OTT-6050 teratoma with Dr Scott Vandenberg provided new and important information on the differentiation potential of CNS tumors *in vivo* and *in vitro*.

Lucien Jules Rubinstein was, in any company, outstanding. His whole personality was sufficiently unusual and memorable to stand out. He was tall, and in middle age stooping, with an expressive, sensitive face. He could convey meaning with his stance and with his hands as well as with his voice, which was always distinctive, at times strident, but more often gentle and purring. His French retained the cadences and rhythms which are now seldom heard; he complained once of being 'only 75 per cent' in two languages, but few attain his standards in any one language. His mastery of English prose style was itself remarkable and now rare amongst scientific writers. He loved music, books, classical theater and the tapestries of Lurçat; his collections, like his study, were always the epitome of tidiness and order. One may regret that he did not have time to enjoy more leisure in his spacious house with its tranquil views of distant blue hills; but, for a man who loved his work intensely and greatly feared the possibility of any decline in his mental powers, there is perhaps some consolation in departing life with a magnum opus completed and a reputation at its peak.

Lucien expressed his wishes to Darell Bigner about the sixth edition of *Pathology of Tumors of the Nervous System* several times. He invited Darell to his home in Charlottesville and, anticipating the remarkable progress in the field that has occurred since 1989, he indicated that in the sixth edition there would have to be multiple authors. He clearly recognized that he could not do the sixth edition alone, nor would any single author have the breadth to cover sufficiently all the now highly specialized areas in pathology of the nervous system.

In 1991, Dr Mary Herman, Lucien's wife, and the staff at Edward Arnold Publishing discussed the next edition of this book and decided that the three of us—Darell, Roger and Janet—would undertake the sixth edition, enlisting internationally recognized coauthors with the necessary knowledge of their respective areas. Much reorganization has taken place in this edition. It has 23 chapters and is in two volumes, increased from 15 chapters in the fifth edition. There are over 8500 references, many of them new. To retain the historical aspects of the book, however, we have also retained references from previous editions. The introductory and basic science chapters on incidence and epidemiology, molecular genetics and cytogenetics, growth factors, DNA damage and repair, experimental tumors and immunology are all new. In addition, these chapters address the growing data on brain tumor etiology and progression and provide a foundation for causation issues, which neuropathologists are being called upon by regulatory and judicial bodies to address. With the advent of molecular biologic techniques, the genetic bases of many of the tumor syndromes have now been characterized. Molecular genetics and cytogenetics are covered specifically in Chapter 2, but are also woven into the text throughout the book. Similarly, epidemiology is covered fully in Chapter 1 and briefly reconsidered under each tumor type where appropriate. The generous information on tissue and organ culture presented in the previous editions has been supplanted by data on cell cultures and tumor xenografts, also throughout the book. New full-length chapters on pituitary and other neoplasms of the sellar region (Chapter 21) and on cerebrospinal fluid cytology (Chapter 22) have been added, as has a chapter on flow cytometry (Chapter 23). A significant transition from black-and-white to color figures and the addition of imaging studies have been important inclusions. Wherever possible, Rubinstein's style and content have been maintained, but since 1989 there has been an enormous new literature about brain tumors that had to be incorporated.

The literary and photographic archives of Lucien Rubinstein and Dorothy Russell that are found in the previous edition of this book clearly represented a unique treasury of neuropathologic material. Therefore, we borrowed heavily from that edition, both literally and figuratively. A very pleasant surprise was to find that many of the figures in the fifth edition were originally taken in color, and they are published in that format herein, along with the new material.

The first of the anatomic pathology chapters, 'Tumors of central neuroepithelial origin' (Chapter 9), has been totally reorganized and streamlined to discuss the various types of gliomas and neuronal/neuronal–glial tumors according to tumor histologic type and the 1993 WHO classification, then by individual site-specific types as required. Information regarding contemporary grading schemes and cell kinetic measures, along with additional or updated immunohistology, has been added. The literature for each individual type has been updated. The polar spongioblastoma was omitted as a distinct histologic type of tumor and is now recognized as a growth pattern that can occur in diverse glioma types. The discussion of 'special variants' of astrocytomas has been enlarged with circumscribed and more benign tumors now being emphasized. The section on oligodendrogliomas has been updated to a contemporary classification with discussion of grading and prognosis. Astroblastomas have been moved into the group of tumors of presumed tanycytic, or ependymal, origin as a result of one of Lucien Rubinstein's last papers. The section on spread and metastasis of gliomas has been incorporated into Chapter 9 rather than keeping it as a separate chapter.

The chapter on 'Tumors of the meninges and related tissues' (Chapter 11) also has been revised and reorganized. The classification has been aligned with the 1993 WHO classification, eliminating the term 'angioblastic meningioma' and reclassifying these neoplasms as hemangiopericytomas of the meninges. The information on epidemiology and association with steroid hormone receptors has been revised and supporting molecular genetic data have been included. Also added was information on cell kinetics; newly described variants, such as clear-cell tumors; and the recently described solitary fibrous tumor of the meninges.

Other major revisions include 'Tumors of the cranial, spinal and peripheral nerve sheaths' (Chapter 12), which has been extensively revised and updated, and 'Nervous system involvement by lymphoma, leukemia and other hematopoietic cell proliferations' (Chapter 13), which has been entirely revised and reorganized.

In 'Tumors of vascular origin' (Chapter 14), we reverted to the organization imposed in editions one through four, presenting all vascular diseases under one heading. Admittedly, this presentation is arbitrary in that diseases such as Sturge-Weber could just as easily have been reorganized and discussed in the chapter 'Tumors and tumor-like lesions of maldevelopmental origin' (Chapter 15). In order to recognize the genetic basis of many syndromes, we reorganized the presentation of the phakomatoses. Therefore, the chapter entitled 'Genetic syndromes associated with tumors and/or hamartomas' (Chapter 16) includes only those inherited diseases associated with neuroectodermal neoplasms, and the subject of neurocutaneous melanosis has been moved to Chapter 15 in order to present a complete discussion of this lesion alongside meningeal melanosis and malignant melanoma.

'Tumors of peripheral neuroblasts and ganglion cells' (Chapter 19) and 'Pheochromocytomas and paragangliomas' (Chapter 20) have been completely rewritten, emphasizing the new advances in classification and molecular biology.

Although the pituitary is clearly a specialized tissue of central neuroepithelial origin, the recent breadth and depth of information that has become available on this region has resulted in the pituitary meriting a chapter of its own, Chapter 21. Conveniently included in this chapter are tumors of parasellar and Rathke's cleft origin, having been moved from the chapter on tumors and tumor-like lesions of maldevelopmental origin in the last edition, as well as pituitary adenomas, which appeared heretofore in the chapter on secondary tumors. The chapter on 'Structural changes produced by intracranial tumors and by various forms of antineoplastic therapy' (Chapter 18) contains an updated discussion of cerebral edema; updated literature on the effects of therapy, especially radiation therapy; and a newly added section on radiology.

It was a daunting task to undertake revising and updating the fifth edition of this work of Dorothy Russell and Lucien Rubinstein. Remarkably, the task was accomplished in our original schedule set for completion, thanks to the cooperation of the authors.

A number of people need to be acknowledged for their considerable time and effort in reviewing the present manuscript and making suggestions for clarity and content. In particular, we would like to thank Drs Sandra Bigner, Christine Hulette, Allan Friedman and Gordon Klintworth for their input into these pages. However, we must reserve blame for any errors that have crept into the text entirely for ourselves.

The timely completion of this book would not have been possible without the dedicated work of Ann Tamariz, Assistant Editor in the Duke Brain Tumor Research Program. She contributed in many ways, both editorially and administratively. She edited chapters, checking for proper style and word usage and insisting on clarity and consistency from the authors; she checked standardization of the gene nomenclature with the GDB™ genome database (<http://gdbwww.gdb.com>); she supervised students in checking every cited reference that it was reasonably possible to check; and she compiled lists and reports for the editors and the publisher. In addition to these responsibilities, she acted as our communications coordinator, dispensing hundreds of letters, faxes, e-mail notes and telephone calls to inform and synchronize the work of the authors and editors with that of the publisher.

We also thank Nancy Hall, Marjorie Penny, Andrea Faulkner-Pollard, Norma Martin and, at Arnold Publishing, Sophie Oliver, Georgina Bentliff and Richard Stileman for their help and friendly cooperation. We are indebted to Steve Conlon and Susan Reeves for their expert advice and assistance with reproduction of the figures.

Ultimately, we thank our families in supporting us in what has proven to be a 3-year endeavor to bring this edition to fruition.

Darell D Bigner MD PhD
Roger E McLendon MD
Janet M Bruner MD
1998

Abbreviations

aa	amino acid
ACE	angiotensin 1-converting enzyme
ACNU	1-(4-amino-2-methyl-5-pyrimidinyl)methyl-3-(2-chloroethyl)-3-nitrosourea
ACTH	adrenocorticotropic hormone
AFP	α-fetoprotein
AgNOR	nucleolar organizer region
AI	apoptotic index
AIDS	acquired immunodeficiency syndrome
AILD	angioimmunoblastic T-cell lymphoma
ALL	acute lymphocytic leukemia
ANLL	acute nonlymphocytic leukemia
AP	apurinic/apyrimidinic
APC	adenomatosis polyposis coli [gene]
APE	human AP endonuclease 1
APEX	apurinic/apyrimidinic endonuclease
ASV	avian sarcoma virus
BCNU	1,3-bis(2-chloroethyl)-1-nitrosourea
BDNF	brain-derived neurotrophic factor
BMP	bone morphogenetic protein
bp	base pair
BRAG	brain-related apoptosis gene
BrdU	bromodeoxyuridine
cAMP	cyclic adenosine monophosphate
CBTRUS	Central Brain Tumor Registry of the United States
CCNU	*N*-2(chlorethyl)-*N*'-cyclohexyl-*N*-nitrosourea (lomustine)
CD	cluster designation/cluster of differentiation
CDK	cyclin-dependent kinase
CDKI	cyclin-dependent kinase inhibitor
CEA	carcinoembryonic antigen
CENU	choloroethylnitrosourea
CGH	comparative genomic hybridization
CHO	Chinese hamster ovary [cell]
CI	confidence interval
CK	cytokeratin
CLSM	confocal laser scanning microscopy
cM	centimorgan
CMV	cytomegalovirus
CNS	central nervous system
CRALBP	cellular retinaldehyde-binding protein
CRH	corticotropin-releasing hormone
CSF	cerebrospinal fluid
CSF-R	colony-stimulating factor receptor
CT	computed tomography
CTL	cytotoxic T lymphocyte
D2	dopamine type 2
dBcAMP	dibutyryl cyclic adenosine monophosphate
DI	DNA index
DMBA	dimethylbenz[a]anthracene
Dmin	double-minute chromosome/chromatin body
DMNU	*N,N*-dimethyl-*N*-nitrosourea
DNL	disseminated necrotizing leukoencephalopathy
DNT	dysembryoplastic neuroepithelial tumor
DOPA	3,4-dihydroxy-phenylalanine
EBV	Epstein-Barr virus
ECM	extracellular matrix [molecule]
EGF	epidermal growth factor
EGFR	epidermal growth factor receptor
ELISA	enzyme-linked immunosorbent assay
EMA	epithelial membrane antigen
EMF	electromagnetic field
ENU	ethylnitrosourea
EPA	Environmental Protection Agency
ERCC	excision repair cross complementing
FAL	fractional allelic loss
FDG	18-fluoro-deoxyglucose
FDG-PET	18-fluoro-deoxyglucose-positron emission tomography
FGF	fibroblast growth factor
FGFR	fibroblast growth factor receptor
FHF	fibroblast growth factor homologous factor
FISH	fluorescence *in situ* hybridization
FITC	fluorescein isothiocyanate
FMTC	familial medullary thyroid carcinoma
FN	fibronectin

FSH	follicle-stimulating hormone
GalC	galactocerebroside
GAP	GTPase-associated protein
GBM	glioblastoma multiforme
GFAP	glial fibrillary acidic protein
GFOC	gliofibillary oligodendrocyte
GH	growth hormone
GHRH	growth hormone-releasing hormone
GM-CSF	granulocyte-macrophage colony-stimulating factor
GnRH	gonadotropin-releasing hormone
GRP	gastrin-releasing peptide
GST	glutathione-*S*-transferase
GST-pi	glutathione-*S*-transferase placental type [enzyme]
H&E	hematoxylin and eosin
HCG	human chorionic gonadotropin
HGF	hepatocyte growth factor
HGFR	hepatocyte growth factor receptor
HIOMT	hydroxyindole-*O*-methyltransferase
HIV	human immunodeficiency virus
HMA	homovanillic acid
HNK-1	human natural killer cell antigen 1
HPRT	hypoxanthine-guanine phosphoribosyltransferase
HPTLC	high-performance thin-layer chromatography
HSR	homogeneously staining region
HTLV-1	human T-cell lymphotrophic virus type 1
IADSRCT	intra-abdominal desmoplastic small round-cell tumor
IARC	International Agency for Research on Cancer
ICAM	intracellular adhesion molecule
ICD	International Classification of Diseases
ICDO	International Classification of Diseases for Oncology
IdU	iododeoxyuridine
IFN	interferon
IFP	intermediate filament protein
IGF	insulin-like growth factor
IGFR	insulin-like growth factor receptor
IgSF	immunoglobulin supergene family
IL	interleukin
insulinR	insulin receptor
IRBP	interphotoreceptor retinoid-binding protein
IRS1	insulin receptor substrate 1
ISEL	*in situ* end labeling
JA	juvenile astrocytoma
JAA	juvenile anaplastic astrocytoma
JPA	juvenile pilocytic astrocytoma
kb	kilobase
kDa	kilodalton
L&H cells	lymphocytic and histiocytic cells
LAK cell	lymphokine-activated killer cell
LDH	lactate dehydrogenase
LFA	lymphocyte function-associated antigen
LH	luteinizing hormone
LI	labeling index
LOH	loss of heterozygosity
LTR	long terminal repeat
MAb	monoclonal antibody
MAG	myelin-associated glycoprotein
MALToma	mucosal-associated lymphoid tissue lymphoma
MAP	microtubule-associated protein
MAPK	mitogen-activated protein kinase
MBP	myelin basic protein
MCA	methylcholanthrene
MCSF	macrophage stimulatory factor
MDM2	murine double-minute 2
3MeA	3-methyladenine
MEN	multiple endocrine neoplasia
MGMT	O^6-methylguanine-DNA methyltransferase
MHC	major histocompatibility complex
MI	mitotic index
$[^{131}I]$MIBG	$[^{131}]$meta-iodobenzylguanidine
MKI	mitotic-karyorrhectic index
MMR	mismatch repair
MNU	*N*-methyl-*N*-nitrosourea
MPNST	malignant peripheral nerve sheath tumor
MRI	magnetic resonance image(ing)
mRNA	messenger RNA
MRP	multidrug-resistance protein
MST	mean survival time
MSV	Moloney murine sarcoma virus
MTD	maximum tolerated dose
MW	molecular weight
NBF	neutral buffered formalin
NCAM	neural cell adhesion molecule
NER	nucleotide excision repair
NF	neurofibromatosis
NFP	neurofilament protein
NFP-H	high-molecular-weight neurofilament protein
NFP-L	low-molecular-weight neurofilament protein
NFP-M	medium-molecular-weight neurofilament protein
NG-CAM	neurite-glia cell adhesion molecule
NGF	nerve growth factor
NGFR	nerve growth factor receptor
NHL	non-Hodgkin's lymphoma
NK cell	natural killer cell
NLPHD	nodular lymphocyte predominance Hodgkin's disease
NMR	nuclear magnetic resonance [imaging]
NOC	*N*-nitrosourea compound
NOS	not otherwise specified
NSE	neuron-specific enolase
NT	neurotrophin
NTP	National Toxicology Program
O-2A	oligodendrocyte type-2 astrocyte (progenitor cells)
OR	odds ratio
PAH	polycyclic aromatic hydrocarbon
PANCH	adenoma–adenohypophyseal neuronal choristoma
PAS	periodic acid–Schiff [stain]
PBL	peripheral blood leukocyte
PCNA	proliferating cell nuclear antigen

PCNSL	primary central nervous system lymphoma
PCR	polymerase chain reaction
PCV	procarbazine, lomustine (CCNU) and vincristine
PDGF	platelet-derived growth factor
PDGFR	platelet-derived growth factor receptor
PET	positron emission tomography
P-gp	P-glycoprotein
PGP	protein gene product
PHA	phytohemagglutinin
PKC	protein kinase C
PLAP	placental alkaline phosphatase
PLP	periodonate-lysine-paraformaldehyde
PML	progressive multifocal leukoencephalopathy
PNET	primitive neuroectodermal tumor
PNMT	phenylethanolamine *N*-methyltransferase
PNS	peripheral nervous system
POMC	proopiomelanocortin
pPNET	peripheral primitive neuroectodermal tumor
PRL	prolactin
PTAH	[Mallory's] phosphotungstic acid–hematoxylin [stain]
PTB	phosphotyrosine binding [domain]
PTK	protein tyrosine kinase
PTLD	posttransplant lymphoproliferative disorder
PVA	polyvinyl alcohol
PVP	polyvinylpyrrolidone
REAL classification	Revised European and American Lymphoma classification
RER	rough endoplasmic reticulum
RF	radiofrequency
RFLP	restriction fragment length polymorphism
RR	relative risk
RT	reverse transcriptase
RT-PCR	reverse transcriptase-polymerase chain reaction
SAS	sarcoma amplified sequence
SCF	stem-cell factor
SCID mice	severe combined immunodeficient mice
SDS-PAGE	sodium dodecyl sulfate polyacrylamide gel electrophoresis
SE	standard error
SEER Program	Surveillance, Epidemiology and End Results Program
SER	smooth endoplasmic reticulum
SF	scatter factor
SGC cell	small-granule-containing cell
SH2	Src homology 2 [domain]
SIF cell	small, intensely fluorescent cell
SIR	standardized incidence ratio
SMR	standardized mortality ratio
SPF	S-phase fraction
SSCP	single-strand conformation polymorphism [analysis]
SSV	simian sarcoma virus
SV40 virus	simian [vacuolating] virus 40
SYN	synaptophysin
TCR	T-cell receptor
TGF	transforming growth factor
T_H1 response	cellular immune response
T_H2 response	humoral, antibody-mediated immune response
TIL	tumor-infiltrating lymphocyte
TNF	tumor necrosis factor
TRH	thyrotropin-releasing hormone
TRK	tyrosine kinase receptor [gene]
TSH	thyroid-stimulating hormone
UEA-1	*Ulex europaeus* agglutinin-1 [lectin]
VC	vinyl chloride
VEGF	vascular endothelial growth factor
VEGFR	vascular endothelial growth factor receptor
VHL	von Hippel-Lindau [disease]
VIP	vasoactive intestinal [poly]peptide
VMA	vanillylmandelic acid
VPF	vascular permeability factor
WHO	World Health Organization
XP	xeroderma pigmentosum

This edition is dedicated to the memory and life work of
Lucien J Rubinstein.

Darell D Bigner
Roger E McLendon
Janet M Bruner

Volume 1

PART I

Pathogenesis

CHAPTER 1

Epidemiology

Incidence and survival

FAITH G. DAVIS AND SUSAN PRESTON-MARTIN

Introduction

The epidemiologic study of brain tumors is challenging. These tumors have been the subject of increasing controversy, both with respect to patterns of occurrence and with respect to potential causes. While rapid progress is being made in understanding the biology of these tumors, collaboration of epidemiologists, neuropathologists, and clinical and basic science researchers is necessary to resolve definitional and etiologic questions and to develop ways to prevent and/or intervene in the disease process. This chapter reviews both the descriptive and analytic epidemiology of brain tumors with the objective of fostering this collaboration.

The epidemiologic study of brain tumors has been limited by a number of factors unique to these diseases. First, it is necessary to separate out primary from metastatic brain tumors, as these are distinctly different disease processes. Second, the histopathology of these tumors is complex. While a general consensus on the classification of these tumors has emerged in the last decade, it has not been incorporated into standard disease codes. As such, estimation of incidence and survival rates for major histologic groups is limited in population-based data resources. Third, while data are generally available on malignant tumors, several tumor types have both malignant and benign variants, and the lack of data on these and other benign tumors limits our understanding of the full spectrum of disease. Fourth, relative to lung, breast and colon cancers, brain tumors are rare tumors. This makes obtaining an adequate number of cases for studies logistically difficult, often requiring collaboration across clinical and regional groups. While this is true, an estimated 28 600 new cases of primary malignant and benign brain tumors were expected in 1995, a development which would make a significant impact on personal and health care resources (CBTRUS, 1996). If progress in the epidemiology of brain tumors is to be made, future studies must address these limitations.

Classification

A pathologic classification scheme for the most common astrocytic brain tumors was developed by Bailey and Cushing in the early 1920s and, as it was complex to use in the clinical setting, it was eventually superseded by a system with four 'grades' proposed by Kernohan in the 1940s. A system of three grades proposed by Ringertz in the 1950s was revised and eventually incorporated into the first World Health Organization (WHO) classification in 1979 (Zulch, 1979). In the late 1980s, Daumas-Duport described a four-level system for which the three highest grades correspond to the approach now being used in the first revision to the WHO classification (Kleihues, Burger and Scheithauer, 1993; see also Daumas-Duport *et al.*, 1988; Coons and Johnson, 1991; Burger, 1995). Immunohistochemical and molecular diagnostic techniques are emerging that will increase diagnostic accuracy and improve the precision of epidemiologic studies by increasing the biologic homogeneity of tumor groups. This continuing evolution of disease classification has provided a 'moving target' for clinicians and researchers, impeding the ability to identify changing patterns of disease over time and limiting the ability to identify risk factors (Vick, 1994).

Cancer registry reporting has been based on the use of the International Classification of Diseases (ICD) system, which began in the late 1800s and has been revised periodically (Percy, 1985). This system described tumors by their location (topography) and behavior (benign versus malignant). Some variation in estimates of overall brain and central nervous system (CNS) tumors results from differences in the site codes used to describe these tumors, as spinal cord, pituitary and pineal tumors are frequently excluded. A description of intracranial and extracranial tumor sites that could be translated into the International Classification of Diseases for Oncology (ICDO) site codes, and used as a basis for standard reporting, has been put forth (Walker, Robins and Weinfeld, 1985).

Tumor nomenclature describing histology was developed by pathologists and incorporated into the ICDO system as a morphology code in 1976 (WHO, 1976). However, only 67 of the morphology codes in the version of ICDO in current use are consistent with the recent WHO brain tumor codes, and 44 ICDO codes have no direct counterpart in the WHO system (WHO, 1990; Kleihues, Burger and Scheithauer, 1993). The lack of a standard definition of site codes and the lack of comparable histology codes limit the use of standard cancer reports for describing brain and CNS tumors, and a practical approach, focused on the most common subtypes, is presented in Table 1.1 in an effort to integrate these systems.

Sources of data

Mortality and incidence reports are frequently restricted to primary malignant CNS tumors, simply because the traditional mandate of cancer registries is limited to malignant tumors. In the early 1970s, Schoenberg recognized the fallacy of limiting databases to brain cancer when he pointed out that some benign brain tumors have a worse prognosis than some malignant brain tumors because of the region of the brain in which they occur; conversely, some malignant tumors have a relatively benign course of disease due to their histopathologic characteristics (Schoenberg, Christine and Whisnant, 1976). With the recent neuropathology consensus on classification and with efforts to standardize coding systems, we can look forward to improvements in brain tumor data.

In the United States, data on the incidence of cancer is routinely collected by two organizations: the Surveillance, Epidemiology and End Results Program and the North American Association of Central Cancer Registries. Currently, these programs report malignant tumors of the brain and CNS in their standard incidence reports (Reis *et al.*, 1994; Howe, Lihner and Derrick, 1996). The Central Brain Tumor Registry of the United States (CBTRUS) has begun to centralize data from population-based registries that collect data on both benign and malignant tumors and to report site and histologic specific estimates (CBTRUS, 1996; 1997). It has conservatively estimated that standard cancer incidence reports may underestimate the occurrence of all brain tumors by about 50% (Davis *et al.*, 1996).

Qualified regional registries around the world routinely report data on the incidence of malignant CNS tumors to the International Agency for Research on Cancer (IARC) for inclusion in *Cancer Incidence in Five Continents* reports, which are published approximately every 5 years (Parkin *et al.*, 1992). It is interesting to note that a recent IARC publication of cancer trends did not include brain tumors because of a perceived lack of data accuracy over time (Coleman *et al.*, 1993).

Currently, variation in definitions of disease by site and behavior, in addition to other issues of data quality, could explain much of the variation in the rates reported. Some issues of data quality that affect mortality rates include unrecognized brain tumor deaths being classified as stroke (Dobkin,

Table 1.1 Brain tumor histology groupings using ICDO morphology codes

WHO histology groupings	ICDO morphology code
Tumors of neuroepithelial tissue	
Diffuse astrocytoma (protoplasmic, fibrillary)	9410/3, 9420/3
Anaplastic astrocytoma	9401/3, 9411/3
Glioblastoma	9440/3, 9441/3, 9442/3
Pilocytic astrocytoma	9421/3
Unique astrocytoma variants	9383/1, 9384/1, 9424
Oligodendroglioma	9450
Anaplastic oligodendroglioma	9451, 9460
Ependymoma/anaplastic ependymoma	9391, 9392, 9393
Ependymoma variants	9394
Mixed glioma	9382/3
Astrocytoma, NOS[a]	9400/3
Glioma, malignant, NOS[a]	9380
Choroid plexus	9390
Neuroepithelial	9381, 9423, 9430/3
Benign neuronal/glial, neuronal and mixed	8680/1, 8693/1, 9490/0, 9505/1, 9506/0
Malignant neuronal/glial, neuronal and mixed	8680/3, 9364/3, 9490/3, 9500/3
Pineal parenchymal	9360, 9361, 9362
Embryonal/primitive/medulloblastoma	8963/3, 9470/3, 9471/3, 9472/3, 9473/3, 9501, 9502/3, 9503/3 9510/3
Tumors of cranial and spinal nerves	
Nerve sheath, benign and malignant	9540, 9550, 9560, 9570
Tumors of the meninges	
Meningioma	9530, 9531, 9532, 9533, 9534, 9537, 9538
Other mesenchymal, benign and malignant	8800/3, 8801/3, 8802/3, 8803/3, 8810/3, 8830, 8850, 8861/0, 8900, 8910/3, 8990/3, 9133/3, 9150/0, 9150/1, 9150/3, 9240/3, 9480/3, 9481/3, 9536/0, 9539/3
Hemangioblastoma	9161, 9535/0
Lymphomas and hemopoietic neoplasms	
Lymphoma	9590/3, 9591/3, 9593/3, 9594/3, 9595/3, 9630/3, 9650/3, 9652/3, 9663/3, 9670, 9671, 9672, 9674, 9675, 9680, 9681/3, 9682, 9684, 9685/3, 9686, 9687/3, 9690/3, 9691/3, 9693/3, 9695/3, 9696, 9698/3, 9702/3, 9714/3, 9723/3, 9731/3, 9766/1, 9970/1
Germ-cell tumors	
Germ cell	8020/3, 9060/3, 9064/3, 9070, 9071, 9080/0, 9080/1, 9080/3, 9084/3, 9085/3, 9100/3
Cysts and tumor-like lesions	
Cysts and heterotopias	9084/0
Tumors of the sellar region	
Pituitary	8040/0, 8140/0, 8140/3, 8146, 8260/0, 8270, 8271/0, 8280, 8281/0, 8290/0, 8300/0, 8323, 8330/0, 8333/0
Craniopharyngioma	9350
Local extensions from regional tumors	
Chordoma/chondrosarcoma	9370/3
Unclassified tumors	
Hemangioma	9120, 9121, 9130/1, 9131/0
Neoplasm, benign	8000/0, 8010/0
Neoplasm, uncertain behavior	8000/1, 8001/1
Neoplasm, malignant	8000/3, 8001/3, 8002/3, 8003/3
All other	8720/3, 9580

[a] NOS, not otherwise specified.

1985), geographic variation in autopsy rates (Codd and Kurland, 1985) and improving survival rates for some tumor types so that mortality rates do not as closely reflect incidence rates. Because tumors that are not clinically apparent can be first diagnosed at autopsy, a high autopsy rate artificially inflates a population-based incidence rate that usually measures clinically relevant disease. This suggests that cases identified by autopsy should be tagged for inclusion/exclusion in the estimation of incidence rates when comparisons are being made across regions. Other issues directly affecting incidence rates are variation in the percent of histologically confirmed cases, variation in the availability of diagnostic techniques across medical systems and variation in strategies for case ascertainment. Improving the accuracy and standardization of descriptive data will increase the likelihood that rates relate consistently to disease rather than to artifactual differences and that hypotheses based on variations in rates are reasonable to consider.

Measurement of disease

Rates are a basic measure of the amount of disease in a defined population. They are estimated by counting the observed number of cases with disease in a defined population during a specified time period and dividing by the total population at risk of disease using the same criteria. Rates are expressed in a standard unit of person-time (usually 100 000 person-years for cancers), which allows rates from different populations to be compared with one another. Incidence rates measure new occurrence of disease, while mortality rates estimate deaths from disease. Adjustment of rates by sex, race, age and use of standard population weighting procedures further refine rate estimates by removing differences in the distribution of these factors across populations.

In order to estimate rates, accurate data on disease must be available on a population basis – data that are lacking for many subtypes of CNS tumors. In this situation, the best measure of disease occurrence that may be available is a proportion: simply the number of specific cases observed divided by the total number of cases observed in a defined case series (Elandt-Johnson, 1975). Proportions of a specific subtype of disease may not be comparable across groups. For example, glioblastomas make up 40% of all malignant brain tumors (Polednak and Flannery, 1995), but 21% of all primary brain tumors (Table 1.2), estimates that are not comparable because the total is specified differently. Given that rate estimates are frequently not available for many of the tumor types discussed in this text, proportions are reported and care has been taken to specify the universe they are based on to assist in their interpretation.

Descriptive epidemiology

Descriptive epidemiology, the process of describing patterns of disease by person (age, gender, ethnicity, etc.), place and time, has proved effective in providing clues for the identification of risk factors. A 'risk factor' refers to any factor that identifies variation in the rate of disease and does not necessarily indicate a causal relationship. Risk factors may be inherent or preventable. Clearly, age and sex cannot be modified while behaviors such as smoking and diet can be. Age is often a risk factor that is helpful in recognizing disease and in selecting target populations at high risk of disease for intervention. Variations in patterns of disease often raise questions that are further addressed in analytic studies.

Population-based incidence and mortality rates for brain tumors by gender are available for many regions, but incidence rates by age, race and histology are less commonly available. Incidence rates for all primary brain tumors from 10 U.S. regions, as compiled by CBTRUS, are shown by gender and histology in Table 1.2, by age and histology in Figs 1.1 through 1.4 and by race and histology in Table 1.3. Rates are based on a 4-year period, 1990–93, and are age-standardized to the 1970 U.S. population to allow for comparison with other incidence reports (CBTRUS, 1997). Tumor groupings as shown in Table 1.1 are broadly based on the distribution of diagnostic codes and an interface of codes from ICDO and WHO (WHO, 1990; Kleihues, Burger and Scheithauer, 1993).

In the United States, the most common brain tumors reported are meningiomas, glioblastomas and astrocytomas (Table 1.2), and patterns by age, sex and race are discussed below.

AGE

The overall age pattern of malignant brain tumors includes a peak incidence at under age 5 years, which declines to about age 20 years (Fig. 1.4) and then increases at older ages (Fig. 1.1). Age patterns vary considerably by tumor type (Figs 1.1 through 1.4), and the rate of increase, as measured by the slope on a log–log scale in previous data, has been shown to be statistically significant (Velema and Percy, 1987). The incidence rates for the most

Table 1.2 Numbers and annual incidence rates per 100 000 person-years of brain tumors by histology grouping and sex[a]

	Male		Female			Total	
Histology grouping	No.	Rate	No.	Rate	M/F ratio	No.	Rate
Tumors of neuroepithelial tissues							
Diffuse astrocytoma (protoplasmic, fibrillary)	95	0.2	92	0.2	1.1	187	0.2
Anaplastic astrocytoma	318	0.6	247	0.4	1.4	565	0.5
Glioblastoma	1693	3.2	1275	2.0	1.6	2968	2.6
Pilocytic astrocytoma	135	0.3	111	0.2	1.2	246	0.3
Unique astrocytoma variants	39	0.1	23	0.0	1.6	62	0.1
Oligodendroglioma	196	0.3	154	0.3	1.3	350	0.3
Anaplastic oligodendroglioma	38	0.1	30	0.0	1.5	68	0.1
Ependymoma/anaplastic ependymoma	150	0.3	124	0.2	1.3	274	0.2
Ependymoma variants	29	0.1	18	0.0	1.6	47	0.0
Mixed glioma	80	0.1	46	0.1	1.9	126	0.1
Astrocytoma, NOS[b]	561	1.0	487	0.8	1.3	1048	0.9
Glioma, malignant, NOS[b]	165	0.3	174	0.3	1.1	339	0.3
Choroid plexus	22	0.0	23	0.0	0.9	45	0.0
Neuroepithelial	8	0.0	8	0.0	1.0	16	0.0
Benign neuronal/glial, neuronal and mixed	68	0.1	48	0.1	1.4	116	0.1
Malignant neuronal/glial, neuronal and mixed	17	0.0	10	0.0	1.6	27	0.0
Pineal parenchymal	13	0.0	18	0.0	0.9	31	0.0
Embryonal/primitive/medulloblastoma	143	0.3	94	0.2	1.5	237	0.2
Tumors of cranial and spinal nerves							
Nerve sheath, benign and malignant	461	0.8	531	0.9	0.9	992	0.9
Tumors of the meninges							
Meningioma	1031	1.9	2411	3.6	0.5	3442	2.8
Other mesenchymal, benign and malignant	27	0.0	27	0.0	1.0	54	0.0
Hemangioblastoma	78	0.1	72	0.1	1.1	150	0.1
Lymphomas and hemopoietic neoplasms							
Lymphoma	310	0.5	166	0.3	2.0	476	0.4
Germ-cell tumors							
Germ-cell	60	0.1	14	0.0	4.3	74	0.1
Cysts and tumor-like lesions							
Cysts and heterotopias	7	0.0	8	0.0	0.9	15	0.0
Tumors of the sellar region							
Pituitary	632	1.1	697	1.1	1.0	1329	1.1
Craniopharyngioma	68	0.1	67	0.1	1.0	135	0.1
Local extension from regional tumors							
Chordoma/chondrosarcoma	12	0.0	17	0.0	1.0	29	0.0
Unclassified tumors							
Hemangioma	19	0.0	22	0.0	1.1	41	0.0
Neoplasm, benign	16	0.0	22	0.0	1.0	38	0.0
Neoplasm, uncertain behavior	53	0.1	38	0.0	1.7	91	0.1
Neoplasm, malignant	95	0.2	94	0.1	1.4	189	0.1
All other	2	0.0	5	0.0	0.4	7	0.0
TOTAL	6641	12.3	7173	11.5	1.1	13814	11.8

[a] Table compiled from CBTRUS data for 1990–93 on 10 states (CBTRUS, 1997); ratios were age-adjusted to 1970 standard U.S. population.
[b] NOS, not otherwise specified.

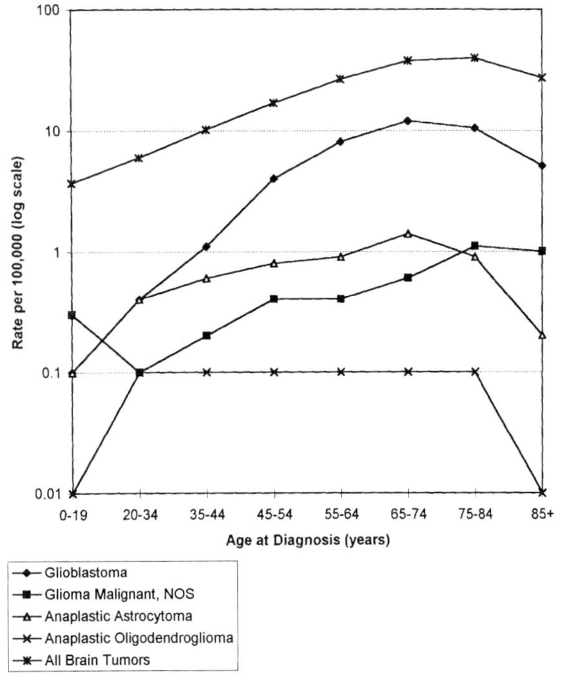

Fig. 1.1 Annual age-specific incidence rates for high-grade gliomas by age at diagnosis; CBTRUS data for 1990–93.

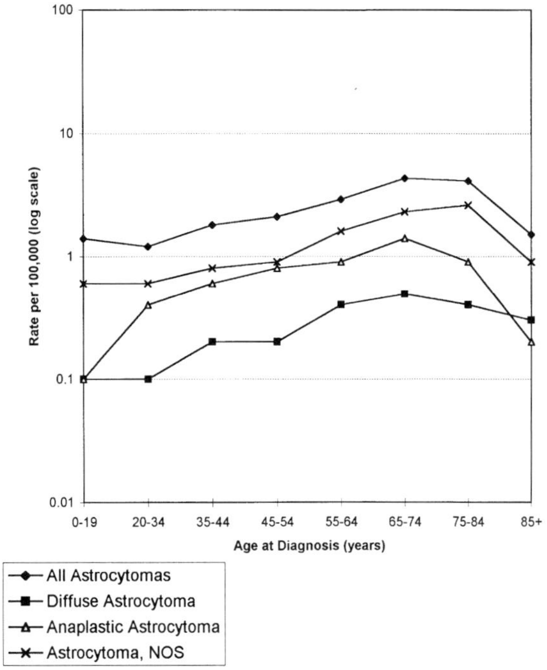

Fig. 1.2 Annual age-specific incidence rates for astrocytomas by age at diagnosis; CBTRUS data for 1990–93.

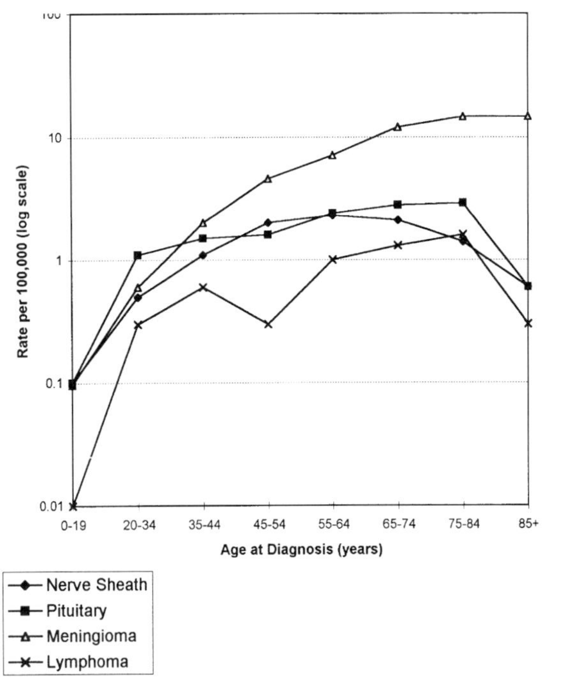

Fig. 1.3 Annual age-specific incidence rates for selected tumors by age at diagnosis; CBTRUS data for 1990–93.

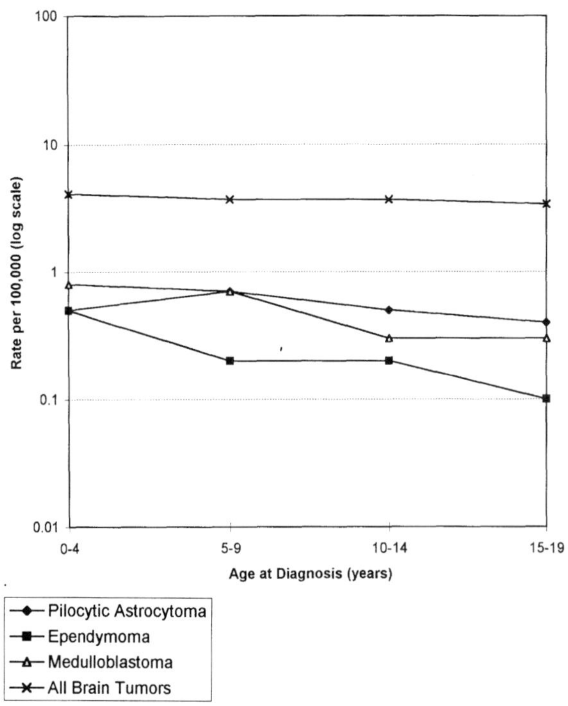

Fig. 1.4 Annual age-specific incidence rates for pediatric brain tumors (age 0–19 years); CBTRUS data for 1990–93.

Table 1.3 Numbers and annual incidence rates per 100 000 person-years of brain tumors by histology groupings and race[a]

Histology grouping	White No.	White Rate	Black No.	Black Rate
Tumors of neuroepithelial tissue				
Diffuse astrocytoma (protoplasmic, fibrillary)	146	0.1	3	0.0
Anaplastic astrocytoma	525	0.5	15	0.2
Glioblastoma	2818	2.6	78	1.0
Pilocytic astrocytoma	200	0.3	24	0.2
Unique astrocytoma variants	56	0.1	3	0.0
Oligodendroglioma	303	0.3	14	0.2
Anaplastic oligodendroglioma	67	0.1	0	0.0
Ependymoma/anaplastic ependymoma	234	0.2	16	0.2
Ependymoma variants	44	0.0	1	0.0
Mixed glioma	115	0.1	2	0.0
Astrocytoma, NOS[b]	961	0.9	40	0.4
Glioma, malignant, NOS[b]	299	0.3	30	0.3
Choroid plexus	38	0.0	4	0.0
Neuroepithelial	13	0.0	1	0.0
Benign neuronal/glial, neuronal and mixed	101	0.1	3	0.0
Malignant neuronal/glial, neuronal and mixed	25	0.0	2	0.0
Pineal parenchymal	23	0.0	5	0.0
Embryonal/primitive/medulloblastoma	206	0.3	16	0.2
Tumors of cranial and spinal nerves				
Nerve sheath, benign and malignant	842	0.8	26	0.3
Tumors of the meninges				
Meningioma	3021	2.7	226	3.0
Other mesenchymal, benign and malignant	50	0.0	3	0.0
Hemangioblastoma	134	0.1	6	0.1
Lymphomas and hemopoietic neoplasms				
Lymphoma	412	0.4	42	0.4
Germ-cell tumors				
Germ-cell	60	0.1	5	0.1
Cysts and tumor-like lesions				
Cysts and heterotopias	13	0.0	0	0.0
Tumors of the sellar region				
Pituitary	1098	1.0	98	1.2
Craniopharyngioma	109	0.1	11	0.1
Local extension from regional tumors				
Chordoma/chondrosarcoma	27	0.0	0	0.0
Unclassified tumors				
Hemangioma	35	0.0	2	0.0
Neoplasm, benign	31	0.0	6	0.1
Neoplasm, uncertain behavior	84	0.1	7	0.1
Neoplasm, malignant	178	0.1	7	0.1
All other	5	0.0	1	0.0
TOTAL	12273	11.6	697	8.5

[a] Table compiled from CBTRUS data for 1990–93 on 10 states (CBTRUS, 1997); data were age-adjusted to 1970 standard U.S. population.
[b] NOS, not otherwise specified.

common malignant tumors—glioblastoma and astrocytoma—peak in the 65- to 74-year-olds (Figs 1.1 and 1.2). It is possible that the leveling off in the over-75-year-olds reflects an underascertainment of cases. The incidence rate of meningioma continues to increase as adult age increases (Fig. 1.3).

About 10% of primary brain tumors occur in the pediatric population, with the most frequent pediatric tumors being astrocytomas, medulloblastomas and pilocytic astrocytomas. The peak age for ependymoma and medulloblastoma is in the 0- to 4-year age group and the peak age for pilocytic astrocytoma is in the 5- to 9-year-old group (Fig. 1.4).

GENDER

More males than females develop brain tumors, with overall male/female ratios ranging from 1.1 to 1.6 (Cohen and Modan, 1968; Kurland *et al.*, 1982; Walker, Robins and Weinfeld, 1985; Sant *et al.*, 1988; Preston-Martin, 1989; Kallio, 1993; Preston-Martin *et al.*, 1993) across countries and for most histologic subtypes of tumors (Table 1.2). The one clear exception to this is meningioma, with ratios ranging from 0.4 to 0.8 (Heshmat *et al.*, 1976; Schoenberg, Christine and Whisnant, 1976; Annegers *et al.*, 1981; Helseth, Langmark and Mørk, 1988; Preston-Martin, 1989; Kallio, 1993; Preston-Martin *et al.*, 1993).

RACE

In the United States, mortality and incidence rates for primary malignant brain tumors have been consistently higher in whites than in blacks (Annegers and Paleologos, 1994). Histologic specific data by race are sparse, but reports from the Washington, D.C., metropolitan area (1960–69), Los Angeles County (1972–85) and, more recently, from CBTRUS (Table 1.3) suggest that this may be true for all adult tumor types except for meningiomas (Heshmat *et al.*, 1976; Preston-Martin, 1989). Another exception may be pediatric craniopharyngiomas, where incidence rates appear to be higher among blacks than whites (Stiller and Nectoux, 1994; CBTRUS, 1996).

PATTERNS OVER TIME

In the United States, brain cancer incidence and mortality rates have been modestly increasing since data collection efforts began (Devesa and Silverman, 1978; Garfinkel and Sarokhan, 1982; Flannery *et al.*, 1985; Bahemuka, Massey and Schoenberg, 1988). These increases were interpreted as primarily reflecting improvements in the diagnosis and reporting of brain tumors. Reports of twofold increases in age-adjusted mortality (Davis and Schwartz, 1988; Davis *et al.*, 1991) and incidence rates (Greig *et al.*, 1990) for brain cancers in the 1960s and 1970s raised the question of whether increases were due to changing environmental factors. Changes in rates were reported for all ages, although the largest increases were in the oldest age groups. Increasing incidence rates were observed for brain cancers (Boyle *et al.*, 1990; Mao *et al.*, 1991) and all primary brain tumors (Helseth, Langmark and Mørk, 1988; Ben-Shlomo and Smith, 1989; D'Alessandro *et al.*, 1995; Radhakrishnan *et al.*, 1995) for some regions, but not for all (Ahlbom and Rodvall, 1989; Levi, La Vecchia and Te, 1990). These increased rates were difficult to interpret as they occurred simultaneously with the expanded use of new diagnostic procedures. They also occurred most frequently in age groups in which metastases to the brain from other tumor sites are common and in which the proportion of histologically verified cases declines.

Numerous reports have argued that the increase in brain tumor rates is largely artifactual (Boyle *et al.*, 1990; Frelick, Huang and Topham, 1992; Modan *et al.*, 1992; Helseth, 1993). Increasing incidence rates were shown to be correlated with increases in several diagnostic practices (Modan *et al.*, 1992). In one analysis, rates of intraspinal tumors were stable over time, while rates of intracranial tumors increased; as intracranial tumors are more difficult to diagnose and are more likely to be diagnosed with imaging techniques, this suggests the increase is due to diagnostic imaging (Helseth, 1993). A very small, but realistic, misclassification of metastatic lung tumors could also explain increases in the United States (Boyle *et al.*, 1990; Frelick, Huang and Topham, 1992).

The amount of increase due to changing diagnostic and reporting practices is unclear. A Canadian review of a random sample of all neurologic records with and without computed tomography (CT) scans or magnetic resonance imaging (MRI) reports concluded that a neurologist would have relied on these newer technologies for about 20% of the increase in diagnosed brain tumors in the late 1970s (Desmeules, Mikkelsen and Mao, 1992). This estimate is not generalizable to the population, because in previous decades, general practitioners, not neurologists, were often making the diagnosis and are likely to have missed brain tumors in patients whose symptoms were compatible with diagnosis such as stroke. A comparison of 1985–89 CBTRUS data with pre-1970 Connecticut data indicates that the increases in rates are specific to histologies that may have gone undetected, particularly meningiomas and nerve sheath tumors (Davis *et al.*, 1996). In Minnesota, a relatively stable population with uniform ascertainment and classification of brain tumors since the 1930s, a modest increase in brain tumors has been attributed to an increase in neuroimaging (Radhakrishnan *et al.*, 1995). A recent comparison of the incidence of brain tumors diagnosed post-CT use versus pre-CT use, by decade, in Norway shows a 15-fold increase in the diagnosis of older cases with use of imaging, and demonstrates that imaging increases the detection of benign tumors more frequently than malignant tumors (Helseth, 1995). Helseth concludes that most of the increase in incidence in the elderly in Norway can be attributed to improved tumor detection.

In Connecticut, rising incidence rates for nonelderly age groups in older cohorts and declines in recent cohorts were observed (Polednak, 1991, 1994). Polednak argues that potential viral or dietary influences, rather than diagnostic influences, could explain these patterns. Using data from the 1980s, Werner argues that the continued increase in incidence rates among the elderly a decade after the diagnostic changes is likely to reflect a real increase (Werner, Phuphanich and Lyman, 1995), but this conclusion assumes a rapid and widespread introduction of diagnostic improvements which, while documented in Norway, seem unlikely in the United States.

At this point it appears that much of the increase observed in the 1980s was due to diagnostic and underreporting bias, but the above data, and the fact that the increase began before the 1970s and continues today, suggest that some portion of the increase may be real. The magnitude of the true increase in rates is unmeasurable from past data, although the pattern is consistent with the general increase in cancer rates in this century and does not point to an emerging epidemic of brain cancer.

Increasing incidence rates have been noted in children in Finland, Sweden, Scotland, Italy *and the United States* (Teppo, Salonen and Hakulinen, 1975; Ericsson, Karnstrom and Mattsson, 1978; Mosso *et al.*, 1992; McKinney *et al.*, 1994; Devesa *et al.*, 1995). In the United States, incidence rates for malignant brain tumors in 0- to 14-year-olds have increased 24.1% in white males and 19.2% in white females from 1975–79 to 1987–91 (Devesa *et al.*, 1995). This increase was most apparent in children under 5 years of age and was seen in astroglial tumors and ependymomas, not primitive neuroectodermal tumors (PNETs) (Gurney *et al.*, 1996a). A decline in the incidence rate of medulloblastoma in children has been reported in the county of Avon, England, from 1976–84 to 1985–91 and also noted in Japan (Thorne *et al.*, 1994; Kuratsu and Ushio, 1996). Further exploration of patterns in children is needed as changes in incidence rates at young ages may reflect recent changes in the prevalence of a carcinogenic agent or in behaviors affecting the younger age groups (Doll, 1991; Cole and Sateren, 1995). For example, the decrease in incidence rates of medulloblastoma in Great Britain has been indirectly attributed to a recent policy of folate supplementation, which has improved the nutritional status of pregnant women (Thorne *et al.*, 1994).

The one secular trend that has been clearly established for brain tumors is an increase in the incidence rate of primary brain lymphomas, which has occurred in all age and gender groups (Eby *et al.*, 1988; Lutz and Coleman, 1994; Werner, Phuphanich and Lyman, 1995; Cote *et al.*, 1996). This increase is not likely to be due to changes in classification or diagnosis (Eby *et al.*, 1988; Lutz and Coleman, 1994). In the 1980s, the overall rate of brain lymphoma increased ninefold. A large portion of this increase is acquired immunodeficiency syndrome (AIDS) related, with the incidence rate of brain lymphoma in AIDS patients, 4.7/1000 person-years, being much higher than that observed in the general population. A substantial increase in incidence rates in persons without AIDS has also occurred, from 0.04/100 000 in 1982 to 0.28/100 000 in 1989 (Cote *et al.*, 1996). This increase in the non-AIDS population is, at present, unexplained.

One secular trend that has not been documented is the pattern of metastatic brain tumors. Age-adjusted incidence rates of secondary intracranial neoplasms in the United States are available for 1973 and 1974: 10.0/100 000 for males and 6.7/100 000 for females (Walker, Robins and Weinfeld, 1985). These rates are likely to have increased over the last two decades as survival rates have improved for breast and other cancers that metastasize to the brain. Monitoring metastatic tumors is important in terms of health care planning and in assessment of therapy.

SOCIAL CLASS

It has been noted for 20 years that incidence rates for brain tumors are higher in the upper social classes (Barker, Weller and Garfield, 1976; Demers, Vaughan and Schommer, 1991). In Los Angeles County population-based data, this pattern was only apparent in males with glioma (Preston-Martin, Henderson and Peters, 1982), and further description by tumor subtype is needed.

Meningiomas are, again, an exception, with the highest incidence rates occurring in the lowest social classes (Preston-Martin, Henderson and Yu, 1983).

RELIGION

In Los Angeles County, Jews of both sexes have an excess of all types of brain tumors, an association that is strongest for meningiomas and nerve sheath tumors and that is consistent with an earlier report from New York City (Newill, 1961; Preston-Martin, 1989). A statistically significant excess of brain cancer in Mormon compared with non-Mormon men and women has been reported in Utah. Utah Mormons generally have less cancer than do non-Mormons, which has primarily been attributed to differences in lifestyle (Lyon *et al.*, 1976).

URBAN/RURAL

The observation that brain tumor rates are higher in rural than urban communities requires confirmation in population-based studies (Barker, Weller and Garfield, 1976). In the United States, the highest rates for primary intracranial tumors come from the relatively rural state of Minnesota, but these rates also reflect the inclusion of cases diagnosed at autopsy (Codd and Kurland, 1985). Clarifying urban/rural patterns may provide insight to those etiologic studies that suggest an increased rate in farmers.

REGIONAL VARIATION

Data to address the question of international variation for all primary malignant and benign brain tumor rates come from isolated reports of primary intracranial tumors. Little regional or temporal variation is apparent in these reports, with the exception of recent data from Italy (Table 1.4). Unfortunately, the site codes included in brain tumor estimates are not consistent across regions, which affects the interpretation of overall and histologic specific data.

International variation in brain cancer mortality rates, which has been about twofold, is far less than for other cancers (Kurtzke, 1969; Codd and Kurland, 1985; Bahemuka, Massey and Schoenberg, 1988). A four- to sixfold variation in incidence rates for malignant tumors across countries is seen using IARC data from the mid-1980s. Estimates are limited to adults aged 35–64. Excluding the older and younger populations, given the known diagnostic and reporting variations in these groups, was

Table 1.4 Incidence rates of primary intracranial tumors by region and time[a]

Region	Time period	Number	Rate/10^5	Comment
Rochester, Minn.	1935–77	145	9.2	Excludes cases diagnosed at autopsy
Rochester, Minn.	1950–77	123	10.0	Excludes cases diagnosed at autopsy
Connecticut	1955–64	1731	6.6	
Iceland	1954–63	132	8.3	
Carlisle, England	1955–61	33	6.4	
Israel	1960–64	741	7.8	Excludes pituitary tumors
Faroe Islands	1962–75	52	10.2	Includes cases diagnosed *in vivo*
Southern England	1965–74	894	6.4	Includes brain and spinal cord but excludes pituitary tumors
Finland	1978–82	209	11.2	
Los Angeles County	1972–85	8612	8.9 (M)[b] 8.1 (F)[b]	Brain, cranial nerves and cranial meninges only
Victoria, Australia	1982–90	3575	8.8 (M) 8.1 (F)	Brain, cranial nerves and cranial meninges only
Valle d'Aosta, Italy	1986–91	285	28.3	
Ten U.S. states	1990–93	13814	11.8	Ariz., Colo., Conn., Del., Idaho, Me., Minn., Mont., N.Car., Utah
Kumamoto Prefecture, Japan	1989–94	1117	9.5	Excludes angioma[c]

[a] Table adapted from Codd and Kurland (1985).
[b] (M), male; (F) female.
[c] Tumors selected using WHO classification.

Table 1.5 International variation: incidence of malignant brain/nervous system tumors (age 35–64 years) for selected high- and low-rate regions[a,b]

Registry	Males	Females
High-rate regions		
Sweden	16.9	16.9
Denmark	16.5	15.9
Norway	15.2	15.5
Israel: all Jews	14.3	15.3
U.K.: South Thames	13.4	10.1
Poland: Warsaw	12.5	8.1
U.S.: Bay area whites	11.8	7.5
Low-rate regions		
Slovenia	6.6	4.6
China: Tianjin	6.4	6.4
U.S.: Puerto Rico	6.4	3.3
Belarus	5.9	3.7
Hong Kong	5.1	4.5
Japan: Osaka	3.4	2.4
India: Bombay	3.3	2.4

[a] Selected regions were those reporting more than 100 male cases.
[b] Table compiled from IARC data for 1983–87 (Parkin *et al.*, 1992).

done to improve the comparability of these rates (Table 1.5) (Parkin *et al.*, 1992).

A few studies based on assessing rates by country of origin have been conducted. These studies have the advantage of comparable definitions and reporting procedures. Brain tumor rates have been reported to be higher among Europeans and Israelis and lower among Africans and Asians living in Israel (Cohen and Modan, 1968). Eastern Europeans have been reported to have higher brain tumor rates than other Los Angeles County residents (Preston-Martin, 1989). Women born in Eastern Europe and the Middle East have been reported to have higher incidence rates of meningioma, while women born in southern Europe had higher rates of glioma (Preston-Martin, 1989).

The study of brain tumor clusters has been uninformative with respect to providing clues to the etiology of these tumors. While reports of community clusters have appeared in the literature, most have failed to implicate any suspected risk factors (Preston-Martin and Mack, 1996).

MIGRANT STUDIES

Migrant studies have traditionally been useful in pointing to environmental versus inherited causes of cancer, and migrant data are now emerging that support the view of an environmental etiology for brain tumors. One early study from Minnesota demonstrated a two- to threefold excess of primary brain tumors in foreign-born compared with native-born populations (Choi, Schuman and Gullen, 1970a). A Canadian study showed an excess risk of brain tumor deaths in those born in Western Europe that was more pronounced in males (Neutel, Quinn and Brancker, 1989).

A mortality study noted that sub-Saharan migrants in France had a deficit of brain and CNS cancers compared with the French-born population. This deficit was statistically significant for males born in West Africa compared with males born in France [odds ratio (OR) 0.5, 95% confidence interval (CI) 0.1–1.0] (Bouchardy, Wanner and Parkin, 1995). Similarly, the mortality rates among immigrants born in West Africa or the Caribbean were half those of the same ethnic groups born in England and Wales (Grulich *et al.*, 1992). These data are consistent with the lower rates observed among blacks compared with whites (Table 1.3).

DISEASE OUTCOME

The overall survival rate of patients with brain tumors is poor, with a 27% 5-year relative survival estimate for all those with malignant brain tumors in the United States (Reis *et al.*, 1994) (Table 1.6). This survival rate is predominantly a reflection of the short survival of glioblastoma patients, who make up the largest proportion of the malignant tumor groups. Only a few population-based studies have examined survival data by histology internationally (Helseth and Mørk, 1989; Preston-Martin *et al.*, 1993; Shugg *et al.*, 1994) or within the United States (Mahaley *et al.*, 1989; Polednak and Flannery, 1995). Population-based studies have the advantage of reflecting changes in treatment and patterns of care and may be used to evaluate whether or not results experienced in clinical trials have been achieved on a larger scale. Population-based survival rates have improved for medulloblastoma, ependymoma, astrocytoma and oligodendroglioma over the last two decades, reflecting improvements in diagnosis and treatment made during this time period. Survival estimates for malignant tumors from clinical studies, in contrast to population-based studies, do not seem to vary by sex (Preston-Martin *et al.*, 1993; Shugg *et al.*, 1994), a discrepancy which suggests that access to care should be further explored as a contributing factor.

Table 1.6 shows 2- and 5-year relative survival rates for patients with malignant brain tumors by

Table 1.6 The 2- and 5-year relative survival rates for patients with malignant primary brain tumors by age and histology[a]

Histology grouping	Number of cases	Survival (years)	Age at diagnosis (years) <21	21–24	45–64	65+
Glioblastoma	9738	2	31.2	31.1	7.3	2.2
		5	21.6	13.3	1.9	–[b]
Astrocytoma, NOS[c]	6102	2	80.4	74.6	27.2	7.9
		5	74.8	52.0	15.6	4.6
Pilocytic astrocytoma	446	2	93.8	86.4	76.6	–[b]
		5	88.9	86.4	–[b]	
Diffuse astrocytoma	491	2	85.1	83.8	42.2	15.2
		5	79.1	56.2	26.6	–[b]
Anaplastic astrocytoma	1378	2	63.3	71.1	31.6	5.7
		5	50.6	47.1	15.5	–[b]
Oligodendroglioma	873	2	84.4	88.0	68.5	46.0
		5	78.4	76.1	44.4	22.6
Anaplastic oligodendroglioma	74	2	–[b]	74.3	55.3	–[b]
		5		–[b]	–[b]	–[b]
Ependymoma/anaplastic ependymoma	720	2	65.3	87.9	77.3	63.9
		5	46.4	81.1	60.7	63.9
Glioma, malignant, NOS[c]	1825	2	47.1	64.6	29.5	8.5
		5	40.9	49.5	20.0	3.9
Mixed glioma	447	2	79.0	85.5	61.6	42.4
		5	70.6	68.9	36.6	–[b]
Embryonal/primitive/medulloblastoma	860	2	67.4	72.8	67.9	–[b]
		5	49.8	54.9	52.7	–[b]
Neuroepithelial	202	2	78.5	66.7	30.0	–[b]
		5	69.0	52.3	22.0	–[b]
Malignant neuronal/glial, neuronal and mixed	125	2	64.2	67.3	–[b]	–[b]
		5	47.6	57.4		

[a] Table compiled from SEER data for 1973–93.
[b] Estimates were not reported when numbers of cases were less than 10.
[c] NOS, not otherwise specified.

age at diagnosis, as estimated from Surveillance, Epidemiology and End Results Program (SEER) data. Age at diagnosis is a strong determinant of prognosis.

Table 1.7 shows survival rates for patients with two tumors for which data are not readily available in cancer registries: meningiomas and nerve sheath tumors. These rates are based on data from the National Cancer Database, a large hospital-based reporting system in the United States. The 5-year survival rates for nerve sheath tumors are similar to those seen for pilocytic astrocytomas, while the rates for meningiomas are lower than those reported in an Australian study (Preston-Martin *et al.*, 1993).

As the survival rate of patients with primary brain tumors improves, the occurrence of second primary tumors and the posttreatment quality of life become important factors in evaluating treatment success. Data from Connecticut for pediatric tumors diagnosed between 1935 and 1974 were used to estimate the relative risk (RR) of developing a second primary in patients with a first brain tumor compared with the general population. The RR was estimated at 9.1 (95% CI 4.0–17.3); risk was higher in children with a family history of cancer (Farwell and Flannery, 1984). A Toronto series of medulloblastoma patients observed second primaries develop in 10% of the patients over a

Table 1.7 The 2- and 5-year observed survival rates for patients with selected primary brain tumors by age and histology[a]

Histology	Survival (years)	Age at diagnosis (years)				
		<21	21–44	45–64	65+	All
Meningioma	2	–[b]	0.94	0.87	0.72	0.81
	5	–[b]	0.87	0.79	0.56	0.69
Neurilemoma	2	–[b]	0.92	0.93	0.82	0.90
	5	–[b]	0.89	0.88	0.69	0.83

[a] Table compiled from data from the National Cancer Database for 1985–88 and 1990–92.
[b] Number of deaths were less than 20.

20-year period (Jenkin, 1996). In addition to treatment and familial factors, an irritative effect of one tumor influencing the development of a contiguous tumor in the brain has been suggested (Deen and Laws, 1981).

While there is little information on the long-term status of adults with brain tumors, some studies have been completed with children. Neuropsychologic and neuroendocrine damage have been recognized as a result of the treatment for these tumors (Packer *et al.*, 1987, 1989). Radiotherapy and the age at this treatment are known to affect the IQ levels of young patients (Mulhern *et al.*, 1992). Characteristics of the tumor, treatment and family environment have been related to decreased social competence scores and increased behavioral problems among children (Mulhern *et al.*, 1993). An instrument to assess quality of life, which has specifically been developed for use with brain tumor patients, is now available (Weitzner *et al.*, 1995; Weitzner, Meyers and Byrne, 1996) and will improve the assessment of sequelae.

Analytic epidemiology

Numerous epidemiology studies have been conducted on a wide range of putative agents to identify risk factors for brain tumors. The identification of risk factors may be useful in understanding the underlying biologic process of disease and, if modifiable, in preventing disease. Many analytic studies have grouped all brain tumors or brain cancers together, a practice that reduces the probability of being able to identify risk factors which may be histologically specific, although they may identify risk factors common to an array of tumor types. Potential agents or classes of agents are reviewed with a focus on the histologically specific information available from this body of evidence.

OVERVIEW

Analytic epidemiology studies are designed to test hypothesized exposure and disease relationships. They broadly fall into two categories, observational and experimental, with the most common observational studies being cohort or case-control study designs. Experimental studies, which could test the potential to prevent brain tumors, await further identification of preventable risk factors.

Cohort studies are usually the preferred approach to testing etiologic hypotheses in humans. They involve identifying a large group of individuals with an exposure of interest in common, selecting an appropriate unexposed group for comparison and documenting the development of disease. Their most important advantages: allowing the direct estimation of incidence rates in the study groups, allowing the investigators to ensure that exposure precedes disease and allowing observation of the time period after exposure in which an excess of disease may occur. Studies conducted retrospectively identify a cohort with a common past exposure and observe the development of disease up to the present, while studies conducted prospectively require establishment of a cohort with a common current exposure and following them to observe the development of disease in the future. In general, more retrospective cohort studies have been conducted because they are more feasible and provide a timely result; but study power, data quality and the subsequent results are constrained by the availability of an appropriate cohort and the availability of relevant data.

Case-control studies involve the selection of defined cases and nondiseased controls. Ideally, case-control studies identify all cases and a representative sampling of nondiseased individuals within a defined population. This ideal may be achieved in special circumstances: when a cohort has already been established or when population data are available. The major advantage of case-control studies is that they are more feasible to conduct than cohort studies; this is especially true for a rare disease such as brain tumors. Another important advantage is that various exposures can be evaluated in a single study. Their major disadvantages lie in the difficulty of identifying an unbiased control group and in clarifying the relevant timing and level of exposure. Population-based case-control studies are preferred as selection biases associated with case ascertainment are minimized.

Special precautions need to be taken in designing epidemiologic studies to address hypotheses specific to brain tumors. A major limitation of cohort studies is the expense associated with obtaining information on a large number of individuals over long time intervals in order to observe an adequate number of cases. Similarly, accruing a large homogeneous series of brain tumors for case-control studies, given the complex diagnostic and classification issues and the relatively rare nature of specific tumor types, is challenging. The poor prognosis associated with some tumor types also limits the feasibility of obtaining accurate information directly from patients.

Epidemiologic studies attempt to measure the magnitude of disease associated with the exposure of interest. An RR is estimated in cohort studies and an OR in case-control studies. An OR in case-control studies of rare diseases, for practical purposes, can be interpreted as an estimate of the RR. A value of 1 (OR or RR) indicates that the rate of disease is similar in the study groups; a value less than 1 suggests that the exposure of interest is a protective factor (may reduce disease) and a value greater than 1 suggests that the exposure of interest is a risk factor (may increase disease). An RR of 2 simply means that the rate of disease among the exposed is two times higher than the rate of disease among the nonexposed. Two and threefold relative effects tend to be observable using epidemiologic methods, while smaller effects are difficult to establish because of the potential for measurement error and biases.

The interpretation of observational studies must be approached with care. Statistics help to rule out chance associations and allow investigators to reject the null hypothesis (RR of 1.0). The CIs provide a statistical estimate of the range in which the true RR is likely to appear. 'Likely' is conventionally defined as 95%. Narrow CIs may reflect large sample sizes while wide unstable CIs may reflect small sample sizes. A range which does not include 1 is statistically significant. Bias and confounding errors which may distort estimates can never be eliminated, but can be minimized in the design and analysis of studies. Examples of biases are the propensity for patients to be more careful to recall accurate information than healthy controls (recall bias) and for health-conscious individuals to be more likely to participate in a study than health-abusing individuals (selection bias). Confounding may be present when some factor other than the exposure of interest is related to both exposure and disease. If this factor is not considered in the analysis, it may impact an association incorrectly attributed to the exposure of interest. When an association is observed and cannot be explained by chance, bias or confounding, then the question of causality arises. When no association is observed, methodologic issues that may mask an effect, such as inaccurate measurement of exposure or disease, inadequate sample size or time intervals, must also be considered (Hernberg, 1981).

Criteria for causality, as used in epidemiology, have evolved out of classic work on smoking and lung cancer (Cornfield *et al.*, 1959; Hill, 1965) and have recently been revisited (Rothman, 1986; Gordis, 1996). One necessary criterion is to establish that the putative causal factor preceded the occurrence of disease, for without this temporal sequence, an association cannot be causal. A temporal relationship is easier to establish in prospective cohort studies than in retrospective cohort or case-control studies. Other considerations include issues of biologic plausibility, consistency, the strength of association, the presence of a dose response and cessation effects. Biologic plausibility refers to the coherence of study results with the current body of scientific knowledge and, when present, lends support to an association being causal. However, there are examples in which the epidemiologic data are so strong that a factor is considered causal without having an established biologic basis. Consistency requires that study results agree with other data. A single study is rarely definitive, and findings replicated in several populations are less likely to be an artifact of some unknown bias. The strength of association is measured by the RR or OR, and moderate-to-large effects, those greater than 2.0, are less likely to be explained by confounding than small effects. Smaller effects may be causal, but substantial evidence that uses rigorous methodology is necessary before making this conclusion. A dose response is present when increases in exposure are related to increases in disease; but while this gradient may strengthen the support for causality, the lack of a dose response may simply reflect a threshold effect. Additionally, if an exposure is removed and the rate of disease declines, support for that exposure having caused the disease is strengthened. While these guidelines may assist in the interpretation of data, they are not rules, and the process of inference is a subjective one.

The public health importance of a causal risk factor is related to whether or not the risk factor is modifiable and is influenced by the prevalence of the risk factor in the population. Attributable risk estimates measure the amount of disease that is due to a risk factor. An uncommon factor with a large RR may actually cause fewer cases of disease than a common risk factor with a modest RR.

RADIATION

Three forms of radiation have been implicated with respect to the development of brain tumors: ionizing radiation and two wavelengths of nonionizing radiation – electromagnetic radiation associated with the use of 50–60 Hz electric power and radiofrequency (RF) exposures. Because the physical and biologic properties of these exposures varies, the human evidence for each type is reviewed separately.

Ionizing radiation

Ionizing radiation is an established risk factor for brain tumors. Human data are available that establish this risk from a variety of exposure settings: radiotherapy treatments for numerous medical conditions including cancers and brain tumors, atomic bomb exposures, diagnostic dental and medical x-rays, prenatal exposures for x-ray pelvimetry of pregnant women and job exposure for nuclear workers.

The risk to the brain with high doses of ionizing radiation is well established (Modan *et al.*, 1974). A cohort study of over 10 000 children with tinea capitis treated with x-ray for a mean neural tissue dose of 1.5 Gy demonstrated an overall increased RR of 8.4 (95% CI 4.8–14.8) for all brain and nervous system tumors. Large RRs were observed for predominantly benign tumors [nerve sheath tumors (RR 33.1, 95% CI 9.4–116.5) and meningiomas (RR 9.5, 95% CI 3.5–25.7)], while moderate RRs were observed for the malignant gliomas (RR 2.6, 95% CI 0.8–8.6). A strong dose response relationship was observed for doses in the range of 1.0–6.0 Gy (Ron *et al.*, 1988). A cohort of over 2500 individuals who received x-ray treatment in infancy for presumed thymic enlargement and were followed from 5 to 45 years of age also showed an elevated RR for benign nervous system tumors (RR 6.0, 95% CI 2.0–18.5), which was not apparent for malignant tumors (RR 0.3, 95% CI 0.02–2.9) (Hildreth *et al.*, 1985). Another cohort of over 4000 children irradiated for enlarged tonsils and adenoids also demonstrated an increased risk of developing subsequent benign brain tumors, which began to emerge in the treatment region within 10 years of exposure (Shore-Freedman *et al.*, 1983). Data from over 79 000 atomic bomb survivors who received a mean dose of 0.255 Sv (J/kg) and were followed to 1987 provide no evidence of a brain tumor effect, but do suggest a dose response effect for persons exposed before age 20 for other nervous system tumors (excess RR 1 Sv 2.9, 95% CI −0.05–11.3). These data also suggest a decreasing risk with increasing time since exposure and a decreasing risk with increased attained age (Thompson *et al.*, 1994). Data on approximately 200 children receiving nasopharynx radium implants with a range of exposures (44–78 Gy) to the brain suggests an excess of tumors, but the number of cases is small (Sandler, Comstock and Matanoski, 1982). In a cohort of children treated with radiation for thyroid conditions, an excess of benign brain tumors, including acoustic schwannomas, has been observed (Schneider *et al.*, 1985). A case-control study has also reported an elevated risk for meningiomas (OR 7.0) associated with radiation treatment to the head for benign conditions in childhood (Preston-Martin, Henderson and Yu, 1983).

Less well established are brain tumor risks associated with lower dose exposures to ionizing radiation, such as diagnostic x-rays. Dental x-rays have been the most frequently studied because they are the most common diagnostic x-ray in the United States, with a frequency estimated at 440 exams/1000 individuals in 1980 (NCRP, 1989). Three U.S. studies have shown an increasing risk of meningioma with the increasing frequency of dental exams, an effect that is stronger when exposure occurs at younger ages and in early years when doses were relatively high, and when restricted to tumors arising at or below the tentorium where the exposure is most direct (Preston-Martin *et al.*, 1980; Preston-Martin, Henderson and Yu, 1983; Preston-Martin, Mack and Henderson, 1989). A study based in Australia also reported a possible increase in meningiomas in males exposed to dental x-rays (Ryan *et al.*, 1992a). These results are consistent with higher dose studies which suggest that the meninges may be more radiosensitive than other parts of the brain and that exposures early in life may lead to tumors decades later. Studies of other brain tumor types are less persuasive. One study of glioma patients suggested an increased RR with increasing frequency of exams, which was stronger in those exposed over age 25 (Preston-Martin, Mack and Henderson, 1989). One very small study demonstrated a large increased risk for glioblastoma with any dental exam exposure (Neuberger *et al.*, 1991). This study was based on spouse interviews that may be subject to recall bias and did not consider timing of exposure relative to the current diagnosis. Other studies show elevated but unstable ORs (CIs that include 1.0) in adult (Burch *et al.*, 1987) and pediatric glioma patients (Howe *et al.*, 1989; Cordier *et al.*, 1994). Prior to the introduction of fast speed film in 1956, exposures from dental radiography were orders of magnitude higher than they are today (Preston-Martin *et al.*, 1988; Preston-Martin and White, 1990). Between 1970 and 1980, the number and rate of dental exams increased by approximately 50%, while the mean exposure at skin entrance measured using dental bitewing posterior films has declined from 695 mR in 1973 to 334 mR in 1981. Estimates of radiation exposure from dental films suggest overall exposures may be decreasing slightly (NCRP, 1989).

A modest increase in CNS tumor risk with *in utero* exposure to diagnostic x-rays, when mothers had x-ray pelvimetry late in pregnancy, was first reported in 1958 (Stewart and Kneale, 1968; Bithell and Stewart, 1975) and replicated in the early 1960s (MacMahon, 1962). A case-control study from Shanghai has recently reported elevated ORs for prenatal (OR 1.3, 95% CI 0.2–9.0) and postnatal (OR 1.5, 95% CI 0.8–3.0) x-ray exposures (Shu *et al.*, 1994); however, these are not statistically significant associations. These results are supported by studies in twins (Mole, 1974; Harvey *et al.*, 1985; Rodvall *et al.*, 1990), the most recent of which reported a modestly elevated RR (RR 1.5, 95% CI 0.5–4.2) that appeared not to be confounded by mother's age, obstetric complications or other factors. Studies of prenatal x-rays in twins have the advantage that the indication for pelvimetry is likely related to the twin status of the pregnancy, although unidentified confounders affecting the selection of mothers for pelvimetry cannot be ruled out (MacMahon, 1985).

Paternal exposures to ionizing radiation, as measured by industry of employment at birth, were associated with childhood brain tumors in one study (Nasca *et al.*, 1988), but not in another (Shu *et al.*, 1994). Tumors of the CNS have been reported to occur more often among children whose fathers were in the Air Force, raising speculation about a possible association with ionizing radiation exposures incurred while flying (Hicks *et al.*, 1984; Band *et al.*, 1990).

Increased risks of brain cancer among cohorts of nuclear workers have been seen in some studies (Hadjimichael *et al.*, 1983; Wilkinson *et al.*, 1987; Checkoway *et al.*, 1988), but not in others (Tolley *et al.*, 1983; Reyes *et al.*, 1984; Carpenter *et al.*, 1987a, 1987b, 1994; Gilbert *et al.* 1989; Wiggs, Cox-Devore and Voelz, 1991). A dose response has not been observed and associations with other exposures, including chemicals, did not explain these results (Checkoway *et al.*, 1985, 1988). One case-control study of astrocytoma patients has estimated a non-statistically significant increase in risk among those who handled radioactive material (OR 3.5) (Olin *et al.* 1987). As such, evidence for an association at the lower doses experienced in the workplace is equivocal, and other workplace exposures and/or biases have not been ruled out as an explanation for the elevated rates.

Nonionizing radiation

Electromagnetic fields

An increased risk of leukemia and brain tumors in people exposed to electric wiring configurations suggestive of high current flow was first reported in children in 1979 (Wertheimer and Leeper, 1979) and in adults in 1982 (Wertheimer and Leeper, 1982). Other studies demonstrate that electrical workers have a higher risk of cancer, including that of the brain and nervous system, which is possibly related to occupational electromagnetic field (EMF) exposure (Savitz, 1993). Studies of preconception exposure of fathers to occupations associated with EMF are inconclusive (Johnson and Spitz, 1989; Wilkins and Sinks, 1990).

A recent review concluded that the consistency of results regarding EMF exposures from occupational studies was such that they are unlikely to be due to chance, but whether they are due to some other workplace exposure correlated with EMF is unknown (Savitz, 1993). Additional occupational studies have now reported an association of nonionizing radiation with brain cancer (Mack, Preston-Martin and Peters, 1991; Tornqvist *et al.*, 1991; Floderus *et al.*, 1993; Sahl, Kelsh and Greenland, 1993; Theriault *et al.*, 1994; Savitz and Loomis, 1995; Grayson, 1996; Guénel *et al.*, 1996), while others have not (Armstrong *et al.*, 1994; Tynes, Jynge and Vistnes, 1994; Beall *et al.*, 1996). One case-control study suggests that risk from occupations with EMF exposures, as measured by complete occupational histories, may vary by histology. An elevated OR of 1.7 (94% CI 0.7–4.4) for all gliomas and a reduced OR of 0.3 (94% CI 0.03–3.2) for meningiomas was reported, although these estimates are not statistically significant. In contrast, a large elevated OR of 10.3 (95% CI 1.3–80.8) was observed for astrocytomas, with a statistically significant upward trend in risk observed with increasing length of employment (Mack, Preston-Martin and Peters, 1991).

Studies have now attempted to improve exposure measurements and address issues of confounding (Savitz, Pearce and Poole, 1989, 1993). A large and statistically significant risk estimate for astrocytoma (OR 12.3, 95% CI 1.1–144, $n = 5$) was associated with cumulative magnetic field exposures above the 90th percentile in a large case-control study. Measurements of current exposures were applied to working histories to estimate a cumulative exposure. This result was dismissed by the authors because of the small number of cases and the fact that smaller estimates were obtained when exact statistical tests were used. Estimates were unchanged when other chemical carcinogens were considered, and elevated risks were not suggested for glioblastoma, other and unknown brain cancers (Theriault *et al.*, 1994). A second study obtained cancer mortality data on a cohort of approximately 139 000 electric utility workers, and individual work histories were combined with magnetic field measurements to estimate a magnetic field cumulative index. An elevated risk for all brain cancer deaths was apparent. This risk was most strongly demonstrated with magnetic field indices and was most evident for those working in the electric utility industry for between 2 and 10 years, and a dose–response gradient was observed. An RR of 2.6 (95% CI 1.4–4.9) was estimated for the highest exposure group (>0.7 μ-year). Other potential carcinogenic workplace exposures, polychlorinated biphenyls and solvents, did not explain these results (Savitz and Loomis, 1995). A third case-control study was carried out among a cohort of 170 000 French electric utility workers. Exposures to electric fields were assessed using 5-day measurements from a subset of workers and these data were used to estimate exposures by job categories on all workers. Benign and malignant brain tumors were included and cases diagnosed after retirement were excluded. An RR of 3.0 (95% CI 1.0–8.8) was reported for all brain tumors when comparing those in the upper 90th percentile of exposure levels with those in the less than 50th percentile. This estimate was adjusted for socioeconomic status and other occupational exposures (benzene, chlorinated solvents, petroleum solvents, ionizing radiations, coal tars and herbicides). A dose–response effect was not apparent in these data and the risk could not be linked to a specific tumor type. However, the strongest association was apparent for exposures 5–10 years prior to diagnosis. These studies do implicate an association between brain tumor development and working in the electric utility industry, and suggest a latency period which is shorter than that usually expected for solid tumors. While intriguing, inconsistencies across studies and limitations in exposure measurements prevent the conclusion that the development of brain tumors is due to EMF exposure.

A recent review of residential EMF exposure studies considered this body of evidence to be equivocal with respect to brain tumors (Sagan, 1992). Since then, several cohort and case-control studies and one ecological study focusing on residential exposures have not shown an increased risk of brain cancer in children or adults (Myers *et al.*, 1990; Olsen, Nielsen and Schulgen, 1993; Schreiber *et al.*, 1993; Versakalo *et al.*, 1993; Feychting and Ahlbom, 1994; Kraut, Tate and Tran, 1994; Gurney *et al.*, 1996b; Preston-Martin *et al.*, 1996a; Li, Thériault and Lin, 1997; Tynes and Haldorsen, 1997). Using direct 24-hour exposure measurements, recent case-control studies of childhood brain tumors have shown no evidence of an increased risk of brain tumors with increasing exposure to EMFs (Preston-Martin *et al.*, 1996s; Tynes and Haldorsen, 1997). In-home measurements, such as those used in these studies, have been shown to be a good predictor of current residential and total magnetic field exposures in children (Friedman *et al.*, 1996). Studies addressing the use of specific electrical appliances also provide no consistent evidence of an increased risk of brain cancer (Preston-Martin *et al.*, 1996b; Gurney *et al.*, 1996b), an association that had been suggested earlier in a much smaller study (Savitz, John and Kleckner, 1990). These recent studies, which are methodologically more rigorous than previous studies, seem to rule out a large causation effect between EMF and brain cancer in children experiencing current residential exposure levels.

The results of early positive studies of EMF were viewed with skepticism, partly because, unlike ionizing radiation, no plausible mechanism of cancer induction was apparent. A number of biologic effects following EMF exposures have since been put forth as potential indicators of biologic damage (Stevens, 1993).

Radiofrequency radiation

Studies of the effect of RF exposure in humans have included microwave exposures, the use of radar equipment (occupational and hand-held), and direct occupational exposures such as RF heaters, sealers and plastic welders, medical exposures, amateur radio operator exposures and telecommunications worker exposures. While some studies suggest a possible effect of RF on all cancers, specific other cancers and/or brain cancer, the data are equivocal. The question of whether or not RF exposures associated with cellular telephone usage are implicated in the development of brain tumors has been raised in the legal arena. The rapid increase in the use of cellular telephones combined with their direct exposure to selected regions of the brain suggests that epidemiologic studies will be needed, and some studies are now in progress (SAG, 1994).

The biologic rationale for RF exposure affecting tumor development has not been established, although one study has suggested an increase of primary malignancies in chronic exposure of rats (Chou *et al.*, 1992), and studies of tumor progression are ongoing (Salford *et al.*, 1993). Data are too limited to implicate any biologic effects of RF exposure for the human CNS (Nilsson *et al.*, 1989). Exposure to higher frequency RF fields is known to increase heat and blood flow, and pressure changes may be expected to affect the blood–brain barrier (SAG, 1994).

Summary of ionizing and nonionizing radiation

Many lines of evidence point to ionizing radiation as being a cause of human brain tumors. The temporal sequence of exposure has been clearly established in cohort studies, although the latency period has not been well defined. The biologic plausibility for this is strong, based on animal and human studies for numerous types of malignancy (NRC, 1980). Studies that had adequate sample sizes and that carefully ascertained brain tumors are consistent in demonstrating elevated RRs after direct high-dose exposures: estimates that are quite large for meningiomas and nerve sheath tumors and more modest for malignant gliomas. A dose response has not been demonstrated specific to brain tumors, possibly due to sample size limitations, although dose responses have been demonstrated in studies of other cancers. As such, ionizing radiation is considered to be a cause of brain tumors, with meningiomas and nerve sheath tumors appearing to be the most radiosensitive.

While effects at the higher dose levels are becoming clear, effects at lower doses are equivocal. Future studies of diagnostic x-ray exposure would be informative with respect to cumulative exposures in the moderate dose range, but careful documentation of timing and frequency of exposures, validation of exposures, and estimates of total cumulative doses to specific regions of the brain are essential to furthering our understanding of risk. However, the lack of data in medical charts regarding doses or the radiation parameters of specific exams limits the feasibility of addressing these concerns. Rigorous studies of nonionizing radiation exposure in children provide no indication of an increased risk of brain cancer at levels experienced in the home environment. The excess brain tumor risk among adult utility workers remains provocative, but unexplained. Human data on the tumorigenic effects of RF exposures are lacking, and the biologic plausibility for such an effect is limited.

INHERITED AND GENETIC FACTORS

Several observations suggest a role for heredity in the development of CNS neoplasia: an increase in the rate of tumors in families of patients, the association of brain tumors with other hereditary diseases, variation in brain tumor occurrence according to blood type and genetic alterations in individuals with brain tumors. These observations may be due to an inherited susceptibility, but also may reflect a shared exposure to environmental risk factors or a chance occurrence. Inherited predisposition is estimated to account for approximately 5% of childhood CNS tumors (Bondy *et al.*, 1991).

Studies of families include estimates of the rate of disease among families, siblings and identical twins. The RRs for cancer at any site range from 1.0 to 1.8 in first- and second-degree relatives of brain cancer patients and from 1.0 to 8.9 for brain cancers in first- and second-degree relatives (Bondy *et al.*, 1994). Data suggest, but are inconclusive, that a family history of breast, lung or colon cancer may predispose to the development of brain tumors (Bondy *et al.*, 1994). Brain tumors are also the third most frequent tumor identified in the Li-Fraumeni cancer family syndrome (Li *et al.*, 1988). A study that used segregation analysis to explore cancer in the families of childhood brain tumor patients rejected the hypothesis that this pattern was due to chance (Bondy *et al.*, 1991). Few studies conducted to date are subtype specific and it seems likely that the inherited component will vary according to the type of brain tumor.

A number of inherited diseases have been associated with the occurrence of specific brain tumors, and while these conditions account for a very small portion of all brain tumors, the identification of associated genes may also help explain some portion of sporadic tumors. In families with neurofibromatosis (NF) type 1, one of the most common single-gene disorders, CNS tumors, particularly astrocytomas and optic gliomas, are known to occur approximately four times more frequently than expected (Sorensen, Mulvihill and Nielsen, 1986). Neurofibromatosis type 2, a much rarer disease entity than NF type 1, involves multiple tumors of the cranial and nerve roots, including bilateral acoustic schwannomas, meningiomas, gliomas and spinal neurofibromas (Rubio *et al.*, 1994). Turcot documented the occurrence of glioblastomas, astrocytomas and medulloblastomas in patients with inherited adenomatous polyps (Turcot, Despres and St. Pierre, 1959). Two germline defects have now been defined in association with Turcot's syndrome, and this discovery may influence the prognosis of patients with glioblastomas (Merlo, Rochlitz and Scott, 1996). Subependymal giant-cell astrocytoma has been reported to occur in 6% of patients with tuberous sclerosis complex, an autosomal dominant disease (Shepherd *et al.*, 1991). Cerebral and spinal hemangioblastomas occur in approximately 72% of patients with von Hippel-Lindau disease (Maher *et al.*, 1990). An estimated 2% of all patients with nevoid basal-cell carcinoma, or Gorlin's syndrome, develop medulloblastoma (Gorlin, 1987; Evans *et al.*, 1991). Patients with Wilms' tumor have also presented with medulloblastoma (Rainov *et al.*, 1995). Choroid plexus papilloma has been reported in association with Sturge-Weber disease. These inherited conditions and their associated genes are described in detail elsewhere.

Studies of blood groups suggest that a higher proportion of individuals with astrocytomas or gliomas have blood group A (Sowbhagya *et al.*, 1991) and fewer have blood group O compared with individuals in the general population (Buckwalter, Turner and Gamber, 1959; Yates and Pearce, 1960; Selverstone and Cooper, 1961; Strang, Tovi and Lopez, 1966; Sowbhagya *et al.*, 1991), although differences are not consistently reported in all populations studied (Garcia, Okazaki and Aronson, 1963; Carter, Hitchcock and Sato, 1964; Schlehofer *et al.*, 1992). One study has suggested a higher proportion of blood group O and a lower proportion of blood group A in individuals with pituitary adenomas compared with a control group (Mayr, 1956). The AB blood group antigens have been hypothesized to play a role in the modulation of cell membrane functions (Engelmann and Schumacher, 1993), and, if this role includes affecting transport through the blood–brain barrier, it may provide a potential mechanism for affecting brain tumor growth. A smaller proportion of U.S. blacks compared with U.S. whites have blood group A (Garcia, Okazaki and Aronson, 1963), an observation which is consistent with the lower incidence rate of most astrocytomas and other glioma subtypes in blacks compared with whites.

Molecular studies have identified numerous genetic markers for brain tumors, as outlined elsewhere in this book. Some markers are specific to selected tumors or tumor groups (e.g., chromosome 10 in astrocytic tumors), while others are involved in several cancer sites (e.g., *TP53*). A series of molecular events that activate oncogenes or inactivate tumor suppressor genes at various stages of the neoplastic process is being identified (Inskip, Linet and Heineman, 1995). This pattern of events has best been described for astrocytomas and may vary for each histologic type of tumor (Kleihues, Aguzzi and Ohgaki, 1995; Ohgaki *et al.* 1995). Data are now emerging which suggest that more than one type of glioblastoma may exist (Watanabe *et al.*, 1996). A statistically significant association of *GSTM1* (glutathione-*S*-transferase μ) deletions in women with early-onset glioma has been reported, suggesting that some gene–environment interactions may be important in the development of these tumors (Wiencke *et al.*, 1985).

Incorporating gene measurements and other molecular markers into epidemiologic studies should reduce the heterogeneity of tumor groups, assist in clarifying the inherited component of each tumor type, improve the ability to detect preventable environmental risk factors, and further our understanding of tumor progression.

N-NITROSO COMPOUNDS

Many *N*-nitroso compounds (NOCs) are potent carcinogens. While experimental data demonstrate that NOCs induce CNS tumors, only the nitrosamides induce tumors, and different NOCs have an affinity to develop tumors at different sites. The rate of tumors and the period of time it takes tumors to emerge vary with the route of administration. For example, intragastric administration of *N*-methyl-*N*-nitrosourea results in a longer latent period and overall fewer tumors than intravenous or intraperitoneal administration (Magee, 1972).

Transplacental administration of ethylnitrosourea (ENU) causes nervous system tumors in the offspring of pregnant rats. The fetus appears to be particularly sensitive to these compounds and rates vary depending on the timing of administration. Only 1/50 of the adult mg/kg dose of ENU is needed when exposure is transplacental. Exposure to ENU leads to the formation of O^6-ethylguanine, a mutagen removed more slowly from brain DNA than from DNA of other tissues (Rajewsky *et al.*, 1976). The inability of the brain to remove this mutagen quickly, coupled with the high rate of DNA replication in the fetal brain, may explain why fetal animals are more sensitive than adults and why the brain is more sensitive than other tissues (Rajewsky *et al.*, 1976); however, other investigators argue that this DNA alkylation may not be the key event in tumor development, although it may be a necessary one (Lijinsky, 1992). Other nitrosamides have also been shown to damage DNA by production of an O^6-alkylguanine–DNA adduct (Craddock, 1983). It has also been suggested that these alkylated bases cause base mispairing and point mutations that lead to uncontrollable expression of oncogenes and growth factor receptors, followed by permanently heightened cell proliferation (Bilzer, Reifenberger and Wechsler, 1989).

Human exposure to NOCs is estimated to derive equally from exogenously and endogenously formed compounds (NRC, 1981). The major sources of nitrosamide exposures have not been widely measured, presumably because of their instability, but the major sources of population exposure to nitrosamines are known: tobacco smoke, cosmetics, automobile interiors and cured meats (NRC, 1981). Some limited occupational exposures may also occur, particularly in the rubber industry. Measurable levels of NOCs are present in rubber baby-pacifiers and in rubber baby-bottle nipples and the liquids passed through them. A variety of drugs contain nitrosatable amides and amines, including some analgesics, antihistamines, diuretics, oral hypoglycemics, antibiotics, antialcoholics, tranquilizers and narcotics (Inskip, Linet and Heineman, 1995). *N*-nitrodiethanolamine, a compound that is carcinogenic at low levels in animals, occurs as a contaminant in cosmetics, soaps, shampoos and hand lotions, at levels that may be of concern in humans. Because some NOCs are carcinogenic in animals, efforts have been made to reduce the levels in consumer products and in industrial environments.

Endogenous formation of nitrosamines and nitrosamides takes place in the stomach when nitrite and amides or amines are present from the diet or from ingested drugs. A less important source of nitrite is reduction (e.g., by saliva) from nitrate that comes from vegetables in the diet. Vitamins C and E, among other compounds, are known inhibitors of this process, and caffeine potentiates the NOC effect. The level of NOCs in the body is influenced by the timing, presence and type of NOC precursors (i.e., nitrite, amides), presence of bacteria or other nitrosation catalysts, gastric pH and other physiologic factors. The complexity of this endogenous process makes measurement of total NOC exposure for epidemiologic studies very crude.

Limited support for the hypothesis that NOC exposure causes brain tumors in humans comes from a study that found an increased risk of brain tumors in children having maternal contact with substances that contain NOCs or NOC precursors, including burning incense, sidestream cigarette smoke, face make-up, diuretics, antihistamines and cured meats (Preston-Martin *et al.*, 1982). A protective effect of ascorbic acid foods was noted in this study, an effect that is consistent with the animal models (Preston-Martin *et al.*, 1982). Limited and inconclusive support for this hypothesis has subsequently emerged from studies that measure intake of foods high in nitrate or nitrite (e.g., high-nitrate vegetables such as spinach and celery, and meats cured with nitrite) and estimate overall intake from all food items (Boeing *et al.*, 1993; Bunin *et al.*, 1993; Giles *et al.*, 1994). A strong dose-related increase in risk is observed when nitrite from cured meats is considered alone (Preston-Martin *et al.*, 1996c). An elevated RR with smoked meats was also apparent in a case-control study of astrocytoma (Ahlbom *et al.*, 1986a), but this association was present with population and not hospital controls, which becomes difficult to interpret. Site-specific studies suggest elevated RRs in adult patients with high intakes of various NOC-forming food items; these occur with astrocytoma (Ahlbom *et al.*, 1986a) and with gliomas (Giles *et al.*, 1994), but not with meningioma (Mills *et al.*, 1989; Boeing *et al.*, 1993). Under the hypothesis that NOC exposures increase brain tumor risk, one would also expect to see a reduced risk associated with NOC-inhibiting foods and/or nutrients (e.g., fruits, vitamins C and E). Studies of maternal diet and PNETs and other brain tumors in children, and studies of adult patients, support this expectation to some extent (Burch *et al.*, 1987; Schlehofer *et al.*, 1992; Bunin *et al.*, 1993; Giles *et al.*, 1994; Preston-Martin *et al.*, 1996c).

The lack of human evidence for a carcinogenic role associated with NOC exposure may be an artifact of the complexity of measuring total (exogenous and endogenous) exposures (Choi, 1985). Because human exposures are modest and tend to mimic the intragastric exposures of animals, which are associated with a lower carcinogenic risk, one can predict that it will be extremely difficult to measure any risk associated with human exposures. While evidence from human studies does not suggest a large effect, further work in children should have some priority, as this is a group which may be particularly sensitive to these exposures, for whom the exposure period of primary interest (gestation) is clear, and for whom incidence rates are currently increasing.

DIET

Relatively few studies of brain tumors have focused on dietary components other than those related to NOC formation. Use of vitamin supplements has been found to reduce brain tumor risk in adults (Burch *et al.*, 1987; Preston-Martin, Mack and Henderson, 1989); in children, risk is reduced by their personal vitamin use (McCredie, Maisonneuve and Boyle, 1994b) and their mothers' use during pregnancy (Bunin *et al.*, 1993; Preston-Martin *et al.*, 1996c). The consumption of fruit or fruit juice has been linked to reduced risk of meningiomas in males (Preston-Martin *et al.*, 1983) and childhood tumors (Howe *et al.*, 1989). In contrast, a vegetarian lifestyle in childhood was a risk factor for meningioma in one study (Mills *et al.*, 1989), while other studies find no association (Ryan *et al.*, 1992b; Boeing *et al.*, 1993). A study of maternal diets of children with PNETs found that dietary factors varied according to tumor type. Protective trends were observed for vegetables, fruits, vitamins A, C and nitrate and folate (Bunin *et al.*, 1993).

An association between high serum cholesterol levels, which may have both a genetic and a dietary component, and primary brain tumors in adults has been noted and appears to be stronger for meningiomas (Abramson and Kark, 1985; Neugut, Fink and Radin, 1989; Davey-Smith *et al.*, 1992; Gatchev *et al.*, 1994), although this is not consistently reported (Knekt, Reunanen and Teppo, 1991;

Davey-Smith *et al.*, 1992). It is possible that cholesterol levels reflect dietary fat intake and may play a role in brain tumor development given their fundamental role in sex hormone biosynthesis (Inskip, Linet and Heineman, 1995). One study reports a positive association with β-lipoprotein level and the development of primary brain tumors in younger women, but not in older women; this finding is consistent with the hypothesis that menopausal status may affect risk (Gatchev *et al.*, 1994). Another study has also found an increased risk of brain tumors with use of vegetable fats for deep frying (Boeing *et al.*, 1993).

One study has suggested an association between obesity and the occurrence of meningioma (Bellur, Chandra and Anderson, 1983). This was not confirmed in a subsequent report, but associations with height were reported for several categories of tumors (Helseth and Tretli, 1989).

These results are consistent with the protective effects of antioxidants and trace elements reported at other cancer sites. These data indicate that diet may play a role independent of NOC formation and suggest that a broad spectrum of dietary components with biologic potential in the CNS should be explored. Studies of brain tumor patients that include more comprehensive dietary histories are indicated.

TOBACCO AND ALCOHOL

Limited and inconclusive data are available on smoking and alcohol exposure with respect to brain tumors. In a small case-control study, maternal smoking during pregnancy was reported to increase the risk of childhood brain tumors fivefold (Gold *et al.*, 1979). Similarly, women exposed to passive smoking during pregnancy have an increased risk of brain tumors (1.5) among their children (Preston-Martin *et al.*, 1982). Equivocal results have since been obtained in studies of direct maternal exposure to tobacco products, observing modest but not statistically significant findings among their children (Preston-Martin *et al.*, 1982; McKinney *et al.*, 1985; Stjernfeldt *et al.*, 1986; Howe *et al.*, 1989; John, Savitz and Sandler, 1991; Gold *et al.*, 1993; Filippini *et al.*, 1994; Norman, Holly and Preston-Martin, 1996; Norman *et al.*, 1996).

Among adults, the data on smoking exposures are also inconsistent. An early study that suggested a protective effect among smokers (Choi, Schuman and Gullen, 1970b) may have been biased in this direction by the use of smoking status at the time of interview rather than prior to diagnosis (Preston-Martin and Mack, 1996). An elevated risk with a statistically significant dose–response relationship has been reported with use of tobacco products specific to glioma patients (Burch *et al.*, 1987). No association has been reported with smoking and meningiomas (Preston-Martin *et al.*, 1980, 1983; Preston-Martin, Mack and Henderson, 1989). Adult women exposed to passive smoking have an increased risk of death from brain tumors; a rate that increased as the husbands' smoking increased (Hirayama, 1984). In contrast to direct exposures, one case-control study found an increased risk for meningioma in persons exposed to a smoking spouse (Ryan *et al.*, 1992b).

No type of alcoholic beverage, nor all types combined, was associated consistently with risk across studies (Choi, Schuman and Gullen, 1970b; Preston-Martin *et al.*, 1982, 1983; Burch *et al.*, 1987; Preston-Martin, Mack and Henderson, 1989; Kuijten *et al.*, 1990). Beer, which does have higher concentrations of nitrosamines than other alcoholic beverages, was reported to increase brain tumors in children when their mothers had consumed it during pregnancy according to one study (Howe *et al.*, 1989).

OCCUPATIONAL STUDIES

The initiation of brain tumors has been demonstrated in animals for several industrial chemicals (Maekawa and Mitsumori, 1990; see also Chapter 6 herein). Occupational studies have generally not focused on human exposures to known animal neurocarcinogens. Rather, elevated risks noted in groups of workers have been used to prompt searches for unknown carcinogens, and elevated risks for brain tumors have appeared in cohorts with no known exposure to animal neurocarcinogens. Because of the inherent methodologic difficulties and biases in these studies, the results have been largely inconclusive.

Occupational studies are frequently conducted in cohorts with workplace exposures in common. The inherent difficulty of identifying a comparable unexposed group often prevents the direct estimation of an RR. A measure of association, called the standardized mortality ratio (SMR), is then used as an estimate of the RR. This estimate compares the observed number of cases among an exposed group with the expected number of cases. This is sometimes called the standardized incidence ratio (SIR), when incidence rather than mortality is the outcome of interest. The expected number of cases is calculated using population rates of disease, and reflects the number of cases that would be expected to occur in the defined cohort if they experienced the same rate of disease as in the population. By convention, SMRs are multiplied by a factor of 100; ideally, an SMR of 100 is equivalent to an RR of 1.0.

In estimating expected values, care must then be taken to use a comparably defined (considering primary versus metastatic, site, behavior and histology of disease) rate of disease, which, as outlined previously, may be problematic for brain tumors. For example, if 10 brain tumors are observed in a cohort with an expected value of 5, the SMR would be 200. If this value of 5 is underestimated by 50%, as suggested earlier, then the appropriate SMR would be 10/(5*1.5) or 130, and the study SMR would overestimate this true value. Studies that are restricted to malignant tumors may be less likely to have this ascertainment error, but may still suffer from detection bias. Specifically, a cohort of working adults with health care coverage may be more likely to have used imaging diagnostics, making the identification of brain tumors in the exposed group more complete than that recorded in population rates; again, potentially overestimating the true association. This bias seems more likely in data involving case identification in the 1970s and early 1980s and will diminish as these diagnostic procedures become standard care.

Vinyl chloride

Interest in the relationship between vinyl chloride (VC) exposure and brain cancer has been strong because of the established causal relationship between VC exposure and liver cancer and because of reports that VC exposure induces brain tumors in rats. The basic scientific evidence for VC acting as an inducer of primary brain tumors in animals or humans has been called into question (see Chapter 6 herein). Several human studies have reported a modest excess risk of brain cancer in cohorts of VC-exposed workers, while others have not. Most of these negative studies have had insufficient statistical power to detect an elevated risk of brain cancer and should be considered noninformative rather than providing evidence of no association (Beaumont and Breslow, 1981). Data from a combined analysis of well-defined cohorts with extended follow-up suggest a modest elevation in death rates, but the role of chance could not be ruled out (Doll, 1988). A large U.S. cohort of VC workers reported a statistically significant elevated SMR (Cooper, 1981); this report has not held up with additional follow-up and a refined definition of exposure (Wu *et al.*, 1989). A second U.S. cohort reported an elevated but borderline statistically significant SMR in VC workers (Wong *et al.*, 1991), but workers exposed in more recent years accounted for the increased risk. If VC exposure were to explain this increase, one would expect that the higher dose exposures from the earlier years would account for the increase (Wong and Whorton, 1993), not the recent years. In addition, the liver cancer pattern in the same cohort followed the expected pattern, which also argues against a VC effect for brain cancer. A cohort study of over 12 000 VC workers from 1955 to 1986, from four countries and 19 factories, was conducted by the IARC and showed no increased incidence of brain cancer overall or by job title, level of exposure or cumulative exposure. However, a statistically significant excess of brain cancer deaths was reported among those workers with over 30 years of exposure (SMR 407, 95% CI 111–1041) (Simonato *et al.*, 1991). Other recent cohorts have either not had an adequate sample size or enough time between exposure and disease to add to this discussion (Smulevich, Fedotova and Filatova, 1988; Hagmar *et al.*, 1990; Laplanche *et al.*, 1992; Lundberg *et al.*, 1993). Two case-control studies of malignant brain tumors have also not observed an association with VC occupational exposures (Heinonen *et al.*, 1973; Burch *et al.*, 1987). One study of residents living near VC production facilities, presumably with lower levels of exposure than workers, has reported an increased rate of deaths from CNS cancer and an increased rate of congenital anomalies; both results are based on sparse data (Infante, 1976).

The epidemiologic data are not adequate to establish an association between VC exposure and brain cancer, and other factors that may explain an effect have not been ruled out in studies that have suggested an association. For example, the elevated SMR for brain cancer deaths in the IARC study may reflect underreporting of brain cancers on death certificates rather than an excess risk. Alternatively, the deaths may have been from metastatic tumors rather than primary malignancies. This uncertainty in the human data, combined with the re-evaluation of the earlier reports of animal neurocarcinogenicity of VC, argue against a causal relationship between these two factors.

Petrochemical industry

Numerous studies in the petroleum industry have suggested an increased risk of brain tumors in workers (Wong and Raabe, 1989; Demers, Vaughan and Schommer, 1991; Teta, Ott and Schnatter, 1991) or in residents living near a petroleum plant (Olin *et al.*, 1987), but this effect is not seen consistently (Wong and Raabe, 1989; Christie *et al.*, 1991; Marsh, Enterline and McCraw, 1991). A meta-analysis, including studies conducted through 1987, provided a summary estimated RR of 1.0 (Wong and Raabe, 1989). Detailed analyses of potential exposures and workplace factors have not been informative (Austin and Schnatter, 1983; Teta, Ott and Schnatter, 1991), and it seems unlikely that petrochemical workers are commonly exposed to animal neurocarcinogens such as acrylonitrile (Thomas and Waxweiler, 1986). It appears unlikely that there is an elevated risk of brain cancers in workers exposed to polycyclic aromatic hydrocarbons.

Rubber industry

Early studies in Ohio reported an excess rate of brain cancer mortality, which was subsequently attributed to workers in the rubber industry (Mancuso, 1963; Mancuso, Ciocco and El-Attar, 1968). Follow-up studies reported an approximately twofold excess rate of brain cancer among workers in the tire building department (McMichael, Spirtas and Kupper 1974; Monson and Nakano, 1976; Monson and Fine, 1978). With the exception of two recent reports (Solionova and Smulevich, 1993; Heineman *et al.*, 1995), studies of other large cohorts of rubber workers have not found an excess of brain cancer (Thomas and Waxweiler, 1986; Sorahan *et al.*, 1989), and no specific neurocarcinogen has been identified (Moss, 1985). A Moscow study reported a fivefold excess for brain cancer incidence in workers exposed to numerous chemicals (carbon black, benzopyrene and *N*-nitrosamines), but this observation is based on only three cases. A study among women in Shanghai also noted an increased rate for brain cancers (SIR 5.0, 95% CI 1.6–11.6) among rubber and products manufacturing workers, although this observation is based on only five cases. It would be interesting to know if *N*-nitrosamines were present in the Ohio and Shanghai plants, as they were in the Moscow plants.

Aircraft pilots

In separate cohorts of aircraft pilots, an excess of brain cancer has been reported (Band *et al.*, 1990; Salisbury *et al.*, 1991; Irvine and Davies, 1992), and the hypothesis that working at high altitude might increase the risk of brain tumors has emerged. Cohort studies of workers in aircraft manufacture or maintenance facilities have not demonstrated an increased risk for brain tumors (Park *et al.*, 1990; Spirtas *et al.*, 1991), but one case-control study has suggested this as a risk factor (Preston-Martin *et al.*, 1982).

Firefighters

Four studies of firefighters are consistent with a two- to fourfold excess risk of death from brain cancer (Vena and Fiedler, 1987; Grimes, Hirsch and Borgeson, 1991; Aronson, Tomlinson and Smith, 1994; Tornling, Gustavsson and Hogstedt, 1994). There is no known consistent exposure to an animal neurocarcinogen in this group of workers (Tornling, Gustavsson and Hogstedt, 1994).

Farmers

An elevated risk of brain cancer in farmers has been recognized, although specific risk factors in this environment have not been identified (Blair *et al.*, 1985; Reif, Pearce and Fraser, 1989; Brownson *et al.*, 1990; Blair, Dosemeci and Heineman, 1993; Figa-Talamanca *et al.*, 1993; Littorin *et al.*, 1993; Heineman *et al.*, 1995), and this risk does not appear in all studies (Thomas and Waxweiler, 1986; Giusti, Boyle and Zack, 1987; Corrao *et al.*, 1989; Stark *et al.*, 1990; Morrison *et al.*, 1992; Ronco, Costa and Lynge, 1992; Dean, 1994). Agents of most interest have been pesticides and viruses (Blair *et al.*, 1985), and an excess among white males in the central United States has been confirmed in regional studies (Mallin, Rubin and Joo, 1989; Brownson *et al.*, 1990).

A few studies have been specific to pesticide exposures. A Swedish study found a statistically significant increase in the risk of brain tumors in young and middle-aged horticulturists (SMR 3.2, 95% CI 1.6–5.7) and an increase of meningiomas in gardeners (SMR 6.0, 95% CI 1.2–17.5) (Littorin *et al.*, 1993). Italian studies have reported an increase in risk in farmers exposed to fungicides and copper sulfate (RR 2.0, $P = 0.006$) (Musicco *et al.*, 1988) and an increased risk in licensed pesticide users (SMR 270, 95% CI 109–557) (Figa-Talamanca *et al.*, 1993). Among Chinese farming women with probable exposure to high levels of pesticides, an elevated rate of brain cancer has been observed (SIR 3.6, 95% CI 1.2–8.5) (Heineman *et al.*, 1995). One small residential study has reported an elevated risk in children exposed to specific groups of pesticides (Davis *et al.*, 1993); this has not been confirmed.

In a large case-control study of brain cancers in New Zealand, livestock workers appeared to have the highest risk (OR 2.6, 95% CI 1.4–4.8) within the agricultural, forestry workers and fishing occupations (Reif, Pearce and Fraser, 1989), and a later study found this risk to be highest among dairy farmers, sheep handlers and other livestock workers (Preston-Martin *et al.*, 1993). Consistent with this are earlier studies that showed an elevated SMR among small-animal veterinarians (Blair and Hayes, 1982), a case-control study that reported a large elevated risk in workers associated with the production of meat and fish products (RR 9.7, 95%

CI 2.6–36.8) (Magnani *et al.*, 1987) and a small case-control study which showed that cases were more likely than controls to have had contact with horses or pet birds (Wrensch, 1983).

Given these moderate-to-large RR estimates, which are statistically significant in several studies, further work is needed to characterize types of pesticide exposures, possible animal virus exposures and the types of tumors potentially sensitive to these exposures.

Health professionals

An unexplained increase in the risk of brain tumors has been reported among occupations that use preservatives for biologic tissue: physicians (Mallin, Rubin and Joo, 1989), pathologists (Harrington and Oakes, 1984; Logue, Barrick and Jessup, 1986; Hall, Harrington and Aw, 1991), anatomists (Stroup, Blair and Erikson, 1986), embalmers (Walrath and Fraumeni, 1983, 1984), nurses (Katz, 1983), dentists and dental nurses (Ahlbom *et al.*, 1986b) and veterinarians (Blair and Hayes, 1980, 1982). The follow-up of a cohort of British pathologists recently observed an SMR of 218 (95% CI 80–475) for brain cancer deaths and suggests that an unusually large proportion of these were among hematologists, who comprised 16% of the cohort (Hall, Harrington and Aw, 1991). Formaldehyde exposures have been the primary agent suspected in these studies, although exposure to x-rays also needs to be considered.

Other workers

In addition to health professionals, numerous other occupational groups have been reported to have an excess of brain cancer. These observations are based on cohort studies from the early 1950s to the mid- and late 1970s, which had no internal comparison groups and focused on professional workers who presumably had minimal exposures to chemical agents. Exposure-specific studies have not emerged to support these observations, which may reflect the higher rates of brain tumors in higher socioeconomic groups who may be more likely, because of better access to medical care, to be diagnosed with brain cancer than the general population (Thomas and Waxweiler, 1986).

A study of gliomas among woodworkers showed that frequent exposure to organochlorine wood preservatives and to organic solvents occurred more often among cases than controls (Cordier *et al.*, 1988). Higher concentrations of organochlorines in patients with cancer (including glioblastoma) compared to patients with other diseases have been reported (Unger and Olsen, 1980).

Other occupational exposures

A second generation of occupational studies that are carefully focused on specific chemical exposures has been emerging in the last few years, with mixed results. A study of chloralkali workers exposed to inorganic mercury, and for whom biologic monitoring of exposure was available, showed no increase for all brain cancer (Barregard, Sallsten and Jarvholm, 1990). A cohort and nested case-control study of exposure to glycerol polyglycidyl ether among synthetic fiber workers showed no increase of brain cancer deaths among workers with more than 5 years employment, although the time interval of follow-up was limited (Lanes *et al.*, 1994). A cohort study of exposure to polychlorinated biphenyls among electric capacitor manufacturing workers estimated elevated, but unstable, rates of death from malignant CNS tumors (Sinks *et al.*, 1992). Brain cancer cases were identified using the underlying or contributing cause of death as listed on death certificates, with no additional verification. As such, metastatic and nonneoplastic brain lesions may have been included, making this estimate questionable.

A case-control study of malignant astrocytoma deaths and exposures to chlorinated aliphatic hydrocarbons showed that risk increased with duration of exposure to all organic solvents, and risk increased with duration of exposure and with increasing probability of exposure to methylene chloride. Controls were other randomly selected deaths. Direct exposure measures were not available, but a job exposure matrix was developed with the aid of industrial hygienists and was related to individual occupational histories. For methylene chloride, an OR of 2.4 (95% CI 0.9–6.4) was reported among the highest exposure group and an OR of 6.1 (1.1–43.8) was reported in workers with over 20 years employment (Heineman *et al.*, 1994).

Elevated risks, but not statistically significant results, were reported for epichlorohydrine exposures among chemical workers in a very small case-control study conducted within a cohort of workers at a dye and resin manufacturing facility (Barbone *et al.*, 1994). This is a chemical labeled as a possible carcinogen. Both an association with total cumulative exposure and a trend of increasing risk with longer duration of exposures were noted. Work in the anthraquinone dye area was strongly implicated, but was not independent of the epichlorohydrine exposure. Cases included astrocytomas, glioblastomas, meningiomas and other benign CNS tumors, although exposure to epichlorohydrine was most frequent in the meningioma cases. Control for smoking, radiation, trauma, epilepsy, antineoplastic drugs and other employment did not explain these results; however, many other chemicals were used in this environment.

While not focused on specific exposures, a population-based assessment of occupational risk and meningiomas in Sweden may stimulate exposure assessment in selected occupations at high risk of brain tumors. Large elevated RRs of 5–6 among glass, porcelain and ceramic workers and among men in headwear fabrication and book publishing were reported (McLaughlin *et al.*, 1987). These and other moderate associations require further study.

Parental occupations

Concern for transplacental tumor induction in humans is supported by work which shows that the rat fetal system is approximately 50 times more sensitive to the action of neurocarcinogens than the adult system (Maekawa and Mitsumori, 1990), and the pattern of brain tumors occurring in offspring of exposed rats is dependent on the timing of exposure. Occupational exposures of parents with children diagnosed with brain tumors have been reviewed elsewhere, and data were considered suggestive of excess leukemia and brain cancer rates for paternal work in ionizing radiation, petroleum, chemical, electrical and paper industries (Savitz and Chen, 1990). Accurate exposure classification of parents from preconception and conception to diagnosis is extremely difficult, but is important in understanding how an agent is transmitted to the fetus and in identifying what specific agent may be affecting offspring (Gold, Diener and Szklo, 1982). It seems unlikely that prospective cohort studies on this question will be feasible and the retrospective assessment of exposures in cohort or case-control studies will require extensive interviews and confirmation.

Summary

The data on occupational exposures and brain cancer are equivocal. The story of petrochemical exposures and brain cancer (that of elevated risks reported in early studies, followed by subsequent negative findings) should caution against conducting occupational studies without specific hypotheses regarding specific exposures. In addition, many of the negative studies do not rule out a moderate risk, largely because of the small numbers of brain cancer cases expected, the imprecise exposure measures, the noncomparable disease rates that may be used and the inability to control for bias and confounding. Rigorous case-control studies are needed to address the many possible associations that have emerged in the occupational literature over the last 20 years. Large cohort studies of farming families exposed to substances that are animal neurocarcinogenic may be justifiable since multiple agents and outcomes, including reproductive factors, could be addressed.

In the 1980s, the age-specific incidence pattern for brain cancers, which peaked between the ages of 45 and 65, was used as support for potential occupational risks (Thomas and Waxweiler, 1986). Today, that pattern has shifted to the older age groups (Fig. 1.1), and only two tumor types peak in early-to-middle adulthood: the oligodendrogliomas and mixed gliomas (Fig. 1.2). This is consistent with the hypothesis that mitotically active cells of the subependymal plate are the most susceptible target cells for neuro-oncogenic chemicals (Maekawa and Mitsumori, 1990). As such, oligodendrogliomas, mixed gliomas, astrocytomas and ependymomas may be the logical tumor types to prioritize when studying chemical exposures.

INFECTIONS

There are numerous reports in the literature of the isolation of viruses or virus-like particles from human cerebral tumors or tumor cell lines, but whether this finding has etiologic significance is uncertain (Bigner, 1978; Corallini *et al.*, 1987).

Clinical studies have clearly shown the presence of simian virus 40 (SV40) and related viruses in human brain tumors (Dorries, Loeber and Meixensberger, 1987; Negrini *et al.*, 1990; Bergsagel *et al.*, 1992; Martini *et al.*, 1995), and intracerebral inoculation of SV40 has induced malignant ependymomas and choroid plexus tumors in newborn hamsters. This virus is in the same family as the papilloma virus, which has been shown to cause epithelial cancers in humans. Other polyoma viruses that are closely related to SV40, specifically BK and JC viruses, were thought to have the capability of invading the brain, although a recent study questions this conclusion as a highly sensitive test was unable to detect BK or JC virus in patients with glioblastomas (Arthur *et al.*, 1994). Other nonpolyoma viruses, including adenoviruses, arboviruses, cytomegaloviruses, herpes viruses and retroviruses, have also been shown to infect the CNS and to induce brain tumors in animals. Few of these viruses have been investigated in epidemiologic studies of brain tumors, although they should be considered as potential carcinogens.

Questions about poliomyelitis vaccines used between 1955 and 1962 in the United States were raised because of contamination with SV40 (Geissler, 1990). While an initial study did not indicate a dramatic rise in childhood cancer during these years (Fraumeni, Ederer and Miller, 1963), subsequent studies have suggested a role for this class of viruses in CNS tumor formation, particularly for exposures during pregnancy (Heinonen *et al.*, 1973) and for medulloblastomas (Farwell *et al.*, 1979).

While the oncogenic potential of *Toxoplasma gondii* infection has not been clearly established, two case-control studies conducted 25 years apart in two countries have demonstrated a fairly strong association between the presence of *T. gondii* and brain tumors (Schuman, Choi and Gullen, 1967; Ryan *et al.*, 1993). This association was most apparent for astrocytoma cases in the earlier study (Schuman, Choi and Gullen, 1967) and for meningioma cases in the later study (Ryan *et al.*, 1993).

A few studies have reported an increased risk of childhood brain tumors in individuals whose mothers had infections during pregnancy (Adelstein and Donovan, 1972; Fedrick and Alberman, 1972; Bithell, Draper and Gorbach, 1973; Linet *et al.*, 1996), while other studies have not (Heinonen *et al.*, 1973; Gold *et al.*, 1979; Birch *et al.* 1990). Specific maternal infections implicated are chickenpox (Adelstein and Donovan, 1972; Bithell, Draper and Gorbach, 1973), influenza (Fedrick and Alberman, 1972), rubella and mumps (Adelstein and Donovan, 1972). A large study recently reported an association with neonatal infections and pediatric brain tumors (RR 2.4, 95% CI 1.5–4.0), a result that did not appear to be subtype specific (Linet *et al.*, 1996).

One study reported an association between previous tuberculosis infection and cerebral glioma (Ward, Mattison and Finn, 1973). This excess has not been observed in subsequent studies (MacPherson, 1976; Davis *et al.*, 1989).

Reports of family clusters and of high-grade astrocytomas in spouses suggest some focus on these tumors (Lossignol *et al.*, 1990; Osman *et al.*, 1992) with respect to an infectious etiology. The potential perinatal transmission of SV40 or related viruses suggests a focus on ependymomas and choroid plexus tumors in children (Bergsagel *et al.*, 1992). Other epidemiologic observations lend some support to a potential etiologic role of infections: exposure to zoonotic agents is a possible explanation for the reported increase in brain tumors in farmers (Preston-Martin *et al.*, 1993) and in children exposed to pets (Gold *et al.*, 1979).

In China, counties with high schistosomiasis death rates were observed to have high brain tumor mortality rates (Merz and Schwartzbaum, 1994). These authors suggest that this is a plausible association, as infections increase endogenous production of NOCs, which are known animal neurocarcinogens.

Overall, there is relatively little evidence supporting a role for infectious agents in human brain tumors, in spite of the clinical evidence of viruses in human tissue and experimental evidence that some viruses have an affinity for the CNS system. While methodologically difficult, this seems a promising area of further study.

TRAUMA

The potential for an association between physical trauma and the later development of brain tumors is supported by several observations: numerous case reports (Cushing, 1922; Reinhardt, 1928; Cushing and Eisenhardt, 1938; Walsh, Gye and Connelley, 1969; Hung, Chang and Yao, 1972; Whatmore and Hitchcock, 1973), case-control studies of meningiomas and glioblastomas (Preston-Martin *et al.*, 1980, 1983; Hochberg, Toniolo and Cole, 1984; Preston-Martin, Mack and Henderson, 1989), experimental evidence which suggests that trauma may act as a cocarcinogen (Morantz and Shain, 1978), and indirectly by the high rates of brain injuries noted in farmers, carpenters and building construction workers—occupational groups with unexplained excesses of brain tumors (Heyer and Franklin, 1994). However, this association has not been consistently reported (Annegers, Kurland and Hauser, 1979; Ahlbom *et al.*, 1986a; Burch *et al.*, 1987; Carpenter *et al.*, 1987a; Preston-Martin *et al.*, 1995), and issues of bias and confounding have not been ruled out.

The evidence associating head trauma and brain tumors is strongest for meningiomas. Three case-control studies found an excess of meningiomas: in women with histories of head trauma treated medically; in men who boxed as a sport; and in men with histories of serious head injuries (Preston-Martin *et al.*, 1980, 1983; Preston-Martin, Mack and Henderson, 1989). A strong dose response was observed with injuries occurring over 2 years prior to diagnosis in one study (Preston-Martin, Mack and Henderson, 1989). However, a recent study restricted to spinal meningiomas in women was negative with respect to trauma (Preston-Martin *et al.*, 1995). Benign tumors such as meningiomas are slow growing, so injuries in the distant past may be of most interest, but may also be the most difficult on which to obtain accurate data (Chang and Horoupian, 1994).

Pediatric gliomas have been associated with birth trauma or prior hospitalization for head injuries, but the attributable risk appears small (Choi, Schuman and Gullen, 1970b; Preston-Martin *et al.*, 1982). Some studies have noted small excesses of risk for cerebral tumors among firstborn children, which may be attributable to perinatal trauma (MacMahon, 1962; Gold *et al.*, 1979; Gurney *et al.*, 1996c). Characteristics of neonatal distress (e.g.,

Apgar score, asphyxia) or treatment for such have recently been associated with increased risk of pediatric brain tumors (OR 1.6, 95% CI 0.9–2.6) (Linet *et al.*, 1996). Other studies found either no association with birth order or a reduced risk among firstborn (Preston-Martin *et al.*, 1982; Howe *et al.*, 1989; Kuijten *et al.*, 1990; Schlehofer *et al.*, 1992; Bunin *et al.*, 1993; McCredie, Maisonneuve and Boyle, 1994b).

Acoustic trauma has been related to the development of acoustic schwannomas in the only epidemiologic study of this tumor to date. This study noted that during the period 10 or more years prior to the year of diagnosis of the case, more cases than controls had a job involving exposure to extremely loud noise (OR 2.2, 95% CI 1.1–4.7) and demonstrated a dose–response relationship. These findings may support the more general hypothesis that mechanical trauma may contribute to tumorigenesis (Preston-Martin *et al.*, 1989).

Separating out events interrelated with trauma becomes important as injuries are diagnosed by the use of x-rays, and ionizing radiation exposures from x-rays may increase the risk of brain tumors. Exposure to x-rays may also be more common in individuals who have repeated seizures and who are more likely to fall—such as in patients with epilepsy or with undiagnosed brain tumors (Hochberg, Toniolo and Cole, 1984; Inskip, Linet and Heineman, 1995). Differential recall of injuries, which may be a reflection of the severity of the injury or better recall on the part of cases compared with controls, may also introduce bias. In one analysis, no association was apparent when restricted to injuries for which people sought medical attention, although an association was apparent when all injuries were included (Burch *et al.*, 1987). As such, future studies need to attempt to confirm reports of injuries, to standardize the definition of trauma severity and to address issues of timing with respect to events intertwined with trauma and brain tumors.

HORMONAL FACTORS

There is some evidence to suggest a role for reproductive and hormonal factors in the development of meningioma and possibly acoustic schwannomas and pituitary adenomas. In addition to the fact that meningioma is a female-preponderant tumor, elevated risks have been observed among women with breast cancer, a disease for which hormonal involvement is widely accepted (Schoenberg, Christine and Whisnant, 1975). Steroid hormones readily cross the blood–brain barrier, and progesterones are thought to affect the growth of some tumors, specifically meningiomas, gliomas and vascular tumors (Roelvink *et al.*, 1987; Carroll *et al.*, 1993).

Few epidemiologic studies have addressed a hormonal hypothesis. Brain cancer risk was negatively associated with parity in two studies (Plesko *et al.*, 1985; Cantor, Lynch and Johnson, 1993), but not in others (Ryan *et al.*, 1992b; Schlehofer, Blettner and Wahrendorf, 1992). Parity has been associated with a reduced risk of pituitary adenomas, an effect that was stronger in younger than older women (Coogan, Baron and Lambe, 1995). Specific to meningiomas, a reduced risk associated with natural or surgical menopause and the use of postmenopausal hormone replacement therapy has also been observed (Schlehofer *et al.*, 1992). These results are intriguing and suggest that future studies consider both endogenous (age at menarche, age at menopause, number of pregnancies and weight) and exogenous (oral contraceptive use, surgical menopause, hormone replacement therapy and steroid hormone receptor status) hormonal factors.

In one study of childhood brain tumors oral contraceptive use prior to conception was associated with an increased risk of all brain tumors and was strongest for ependymoma (OR 8.8, 95% CI 2.1–37.5) (Linet *et al.*, 1996). This study suggests an indirect effect of exogenous hormone use as well.

The female preponderance of meningiomas has been well established in clinical and population studies (Preston-Martin *et al.*, 1989, 1993; Kuratsu and Ushio, 1996; Longstreth *et al.*, 1993) (Table 1.1). While a female preponderance of acoustic schwannomas (Chang and Horoupian, 1994) has been reported in clinical studies, this has not been confirmed in population studies (Preston-Martin *et al.*, 1989). However, schwannomas have been shown to have a peak incidence rate in the 20- to 29-year age group among Japanese females (Kuratsu and Ushio, 1996). A female preponderance of pituitary adenomas has been suggested in two clinical studies (Robinson, Beral and Ashley, 1979; Radhakrishnan *et al.*, 1995) and more recently in a Japanese population study (Kuratsu and Ushio, 1996). The age-specific pattern of rates in women in the Japanese study had two peaks: one in the childbearing years between ages 20 and 29, the other between ages 60 and 69 (Kuratsu and Ushio, 1996). Gender differences for these two tumors—schwannomas and pituitary adenomas—require further explanation. Discrepancies between population and clinical studies suggest that either some referral or health care bias may be overestimating female cases in clinical studies or that females are systematically underreported in population-based incidence studies. This underscores the importance of having accurate incidence data on which to base hypotheses.

MEDICAL FACTORS

Numerous medical conditions or treatments for medical conditions have been suggested as risk factors for brain tumors; however, few of these have been related to tumor type, and other explanations for a general association with brain tumors have not been adequately ruled out.

A large increased risk of primary brain tumors in patients with seizure disorders has been suggested in several studies (Gold *et al.*, 1979; White, McLean and Howland, 1979; Shirts *et al.*, 1986), but not in others (Heinonen *et al.*, 1973; Annegers, Kurland and Hauser, 1979; Clemmesen and Hjalgrim-Jensen, 1981). As most tumors were diagnosed within 5 years of the seizure diagnosis and a decrease in the RR has been observed over time, it has been suggested that the seizure itself is related to early tumor growth, not the medications used for the seizures or physical trauma associated with the presence of disease (Shirts *et al.*, 1986). In a large cohort of patients hospitalized for epilepsy (who received prolonged exposures to phenobarbital, phenytoin and other barbiturates), an increased RR was found for CNS cancers (RR 5.7, 95% CI 4.7–6.8); this decreased significantly over time (Olsen *et al.*, 1989). Seizures are the first manifestation of brain tumors in 11–50% of children and adults with such tumors. In children, seizures increase with age and are more frequent in patients with supratentorial tumors than with infratentorial tumors (Gilles *et al.*, 1992). A case-control study of barbiturate exposure *in utero* demonstrated that as duration of use increased, the OR associated with childhood brain tumors increased. However, these results disappeared after adjusting for epilepsy (Goldhaber *et al.*, 1990).

Other associations in children exposed to barbiturates early in life have been reported. In one study, six case mothers compared with no control mothers had used this drug during pregnancy (Gold *et al.*, 1978). A larger study found an association with intrauterine exposure to barbiturates administered to the mother for general anesthesia, and to children exposed to antiepileptics but not other barbiturates (Preston-Martin, Henderson and Peters, 1982). Maternal exposure to narcotics has been associated with high-grade astrocytomas in children (OR 2.3, 95% CI 1.1–4.7), and maternal exposure to a specific anesthetic, penthrane, has also been related to high-grade astrocytomas (OR 3.5, 95% CI 1.5–8.5) and medulloblastomas (OR 2.3, 95% CI 1.1–5.1) in offspring (Linet *et al.*, 1996). No association with barbiturates has been seen in other studies (Howe *et al.*, 1989; Kuijten *et al.*, 1990; McCredie, Maisonneuve and Boyle, 1994a).

Clinical studies have suggested that kidney transplant patients are at higher risk of developing cerebral lymphomas in addition to other cancers. A recent study reported one such death in a transplant population of approximately 2500 individuals over a 20-year period. Conservatively, this is a rate of approximately 2/100 000, which is six times higher than the rate of 0.3/100 000 reported in Table 1.1 (Hoover and Fraumeni, 1973; Schwechheimer and Hashemian, 1995). Studies have not considered the other risk factors of the recipient or those of the donor, although transmission of glioblastoma multiforme to two kidney transplant patients has been reported (Ruiz *et al.*, 1993).

A decreased frequency of primary brain tumors and metastatic brain tumors among the diabetic population has been reported. An autopsy study indicated that this decrease is limited to gliomas (Aronson and Aronson, 1965). This observation was not replicated in a cohort mortality study (Kessler, 1970), possibly due to limited brain tumor reporting on death certificates.

An increased rate of brain tumors, in addition to endocrine tumors, breast and colon cancers, has been observed in a cohort of patients with primary hyperthyroidism (RR 2.6, 95% CI 1.4–4.6) (Palmer *et al.*, 1988). The occurrence of hyperthyroidism and other endocrine neoplasia is well recognized in the multiple endocrine neoplasia syndrome. Whether this observation reflects a shared genetic component, some risk factor in common to all these tumors or a hormonal influence is unknown.

An increased risk of primary brain tumors has been reported in younger women in a cohort of patients with multiple sclerosis (Moller *et al.*, 1991). Whether this is an artifact of diagnostic complexities, some viral factor in common between the diseases or chance is unknown (Hunter, Ballinger and Rubin, 1987). History of multiple sclerosis was not associated with brain tumor risk in a more recent study (Schlehofer *et al.*, 1992).

In a large population of children with cancer, an excess of cases with cystic fibrosis (SIR 2.97, 95% CI 0.8–7.6) has been reported in one study (Robertson and Hawkins, 1995).

Asthma, eczema and other allergic diseases have been negatively associated with gliomas (Ryan *et al.*, 1992b; Schlehofer *et al.*, 1992) although one study reports a decreased susceptibility to allergies among adults with glioblastoma (Hochberg, Toniolo and Cole, 1990). Investigators have hypothesized that impaired immunity increases susceptibility, although no increase has been reported among groups with suppressed immunity or human immunodeficiency virus (HIV) infection (Kinlen, 1982; Blattner and Hoover, 1985; Biggar *et al.*, 1987; Rabkin and Yellin, 1994).

While these associations between medical factors and brain tumors are interesting, the lack of consistency across studies is remarkable, with wide variations in the magnitude and stability of estimated risks. Combining this with the difficulty in separating out the effects of underlying disease from those of the treatment, this evidence is difficult to interpret as anything more than separate clues that should be addressed systematically and rigorously. A unifying theory is needed about how each underlying disease or group of conditions potentially impacts the CNS. If prevalent medical conditions with some suspect biologic process in common were to hold up as a risk factor for brain tumors, this would be consistent with the descriptive data that suggest some globally prevalent component in the etiology of these tumors.

Summary

Many epidemiologic studies have been completed, exploring the potential for numerous noninherited causes of brain tumors. These studies have provided many provocative statistical associations and some intriguingly large RR estimates; but, frequently, limitations in methodology have prevented chance, bias and other confounding factors from being ruled out as explanations for these observations. Studies of ionizing radiation are the one exception, with the combination of biologic and epidemiologic evidence resulting in a consensus that this is an exposure which, at high levels, causes brain tumors in humans. There is also general agreement that some inherited and genetic factors influence the development of brain tumors. However, risk from these factors needs further characterization and the magnitude of disease that can be attributed to these factors is likely to be quite small, leaving room for work in other areas of study that do show promise. Studies also need to better characterize the potential risk associated with trauma and to sort out the possible role of bias and interaction. Studies specifically focused on cohorts exposed to known neurocarcinogens may be informative, and population-based case-control studies that identify high-risk occupational groups may assist in the identification of new neurocarcinogens. If the early suggestions for diet, medical factors, infections and hormones are replicated and clarified, ways to prevent brain tumors may emerge.

In spite of current data limitations, a few features of these tumors stand out to provide direction for further epidemiologic work. First, the distinct patterns of age-specific incidence and survival rates by histology suggest that different etiologic factors operate for different tumor types, and histologically specific studies are needed to identify risk factors. This has been demonstrated in the ionizing radiation literature where RRs from similar exposures vary greatly depending on tumor type. Second, as data on brain tumors become available with more accuracy, variations in rates according to demographic factors are emerging that may be etiologically important and need to be incorporated into hypotheses. For example, the female preponderance of meningioma may suggest that hormonal factors play a role in etiology; and regional variation suggests a role for cultural behaviors, such as diet. Third, the increasing rate of brain tumors, particularly in the younger age groups, suggests that changes in unknown etiologic factors may be taking place over time, and these need to be identified.

The next decade will increase our understanding of the molecular events that underlie the biology of these tumors. Combining this knowledge into hypotheses that can be tested with rigorous epidemiologic methods should clarify many of the suggested associations presented in this review, reveal new ones, and sort out those which have etiologic significance.

References

Abramson, Z.H. and Kark, J.D. (1985) Serum cholesterol and primary brain tumours: a case-control study. *British Journal of Cancer* **52**, 93–8.

Adelstein, A.M. and Donovan, J.W. (1972) Malignant disease in children whose mothers had chickenpox, mumps or rubella in pregnancy. *British Medical Journal* **4**, 629–31.

Ahlbom, A. and Rodvall, Y. (1989) Brain tumor trends. *Lancet* **2**, 1272.

Ahlbom, A., Navier, I.L., Norell, S., Olin, R. and Spannare, B. (1986a) Nonoccupational risk indicators for astrocytomas in adults. *American Journal of Epidemiology* **124**, 334–7.

Ahlbom, A., Norell, S., Rodvall, Y. and Nylander, M. (1986b) Dentists, dental nurses, and brain tumors. *British Medical Journal* **292**, 662.

Annegers, J.F. and Paleologos, N. (1994) Intracranial neoplasia. In Gorelick, P.B. and Alter, M. (eds), *Handbook of neuroepidemiology*. New York: Marcel Dekker, 295–313.

Annegers, J.F., Kurland, L.T. and Hauser, W.A. (1979) Brain tumors in children exposed to barbiturates. *Journal of the National Cancer Institute* **63**, 3–4.

Annegers, J.F., Schoenberg, B.S., Okazaki, H. and Kurland, L.T. (1981) Epidemiologic study of primary intracranial neoplasms. *Archives of Neurology* **38**, 217–19.

Armstrong, B., Theriault, G., Guenel, P., Deadman, J., Goldberg, M. and Heroux, P. (1994) Association between exposure to pulsed electromagnetic fields and cancer in electric utility workers in Quebec, Canada, and France. *American Journal of Epidemiology* **140**, 805–20.

Aronson, K.J., Tomlinson, G.A. and Smith, L. (1994) Mortality among fire fighters in metropolitan Toronto. *American Journal of Industrial Medicine* **26**, 89–101.

Aronson, S.M. and Aronson, B.E. (1965) Central nervous system in diabetes mellitus. *Archives of Neurology* **12**, 390–8.

Arthur, R.R., Grossman, S.A., Ronnett, B.M., Bigner, S.H., Vogelstein, B. and Shah, K.V. (1994) Lack of association of human polyomaviruses with human brain tumors. *Journal of Neuro-Oncology* **20**, 55–8.

Austin, S.G. and Schnatter, A.R. (1983) A case-control study of chemical exposures and brain tumors in petrochemical workers. *Journal of Occupational Medicine* **25**, 313–20.

Bahemuka, M., Massey, E.W. and Schoenberg, B.S. (1988) International mortality from primary nervous system neoplasms: distribution and trends. *International Journal of Epidemiology* **17**, 33–8.

Band, P.R., Spinelli, J.J., Ng, V.T.Y., Moody, J. and Gallagher, R.P. (1990) Mortality and cancer incidence in a cohort of commercial airline pilots. *Aviation Space and Environmental Medicine* **61**, 299–302.

Barbone, F., Delzell, E., Austin, H. and Cole, P. (1994) Exposure to epichlorohydrin and central nervous system neoplasms at a resin and dye manufacturing plant. *Archives of Environmental Health* **49**, 355–8.

Barker, D.J., Weller, R.O. and Garfield, J.S. (1976) Epidemiology of primary tumors of the brain and spinal cord: a regional survey in Southern England. *Journal of Neurology, Neurosurgery, and Psychiatry* **39**, 290–6.

Barregard, L., Sallsten, G. and Jarvholm, B. (1990) Mortality and cancer incidence in chloralkali workers exposed to inorganic mercury. *British Journal of Industrial Medicine* **47**, 99–104.

Beall, C., Delzell, E., Cole, R. and Brill, I. (1996) Brain tumors among electronic industry workers. *Epidemiology* **7**, 125–30.

Beaumont, J.J. and Breslow, N.E. (1981) Power considerations in epidemiologic studies of vinyl chloride workers. *American Journal of Epidemiology* **114**, 725–34.

Bellur, S.N., Chandra, V. and Anderson, R.J. (1983) Association of meningiomas with obesity. *Annals of Neurology* **13**, 346–7.

Ben-Shlomo, Y. and Smith, G.D. (1989) Brain tumor trends. *Lancet* **2**, 1272–3.

Bergsagel, D.J., Finegold, M.J., Butel, J.S., Kupsky, W.J. and Garcea, R.L. (1992) DNA sequences similar to those of simian virus 40 in ependymomas and choroid plexus tumors of childhood. *New England Journal of Medicine* **326**, 988–93.

Biggar, R.J., Horm, J., Goedert, J.J. and Melbye, M. (1987) Cancer in a group at risk of acquired immunodeficiency syndrome (AIDS) through 1984. *American Journal of Epidemiology* **126**, 578–86.

Bigner, D.D. (1978) Role of viruses in the causation of neural neoplasia. In Laerum, O.D., Bigner, D.D. and Rajewsky, M.F. (eds), *Biology of brain tumors*. UICC Technical Report Series, Vol. 30, Report 5. Geneva: International Union Against Cancer, 85–111.

Bilzer, T., Reifenberger, G. and Wechsler, W. (1989) Chemical induction of brain tumors in rats by nitrosoureas: molecular biology and neuropathology. *Neurotoxicology and Teratology* **11**, 551–6.

Birch, J.M., Hartley, A.L., Teare, M.D., Blair, V., McKinney, P.A., Mann, J.R., Stiller, C.A., Draper, G.J., Johnston, H.E., Cartwright, R.A. and Waterhouse, J.A.H. (1990) The inter-regional epidemiological study of childhood cancer (IRESCC): case-control study of children with central nervous system tumours. *British Journal of Neurosurgery* **4**, 17–25.

Bithell, J.F. and Stewart, A.M. (1975) Pre-natal irradiation and childhood malignancy: a review of British data from the Oxford survey. *British Journal of Cancer* **31**, 271–87.

Bithell, J.F., Draper, G.J. and Gorbach, P.D. (1973) Association between malignant disease in children and maternal virus infections. *British Medical Journal* **1**, 706–8.

Blair, A. and Hayes, H.M. Jr (1980) Cancer and other causes of death among U.S. veterinarians, 1966–1977. *International Journal of Cancer* **25**, 181–5.

——(1982) Mortality patterns among U.S. veterinarians, 1947–1977: an expanded study. *International Journal of Epidemiology* **11**, 391–7.

Blair, A., Dosemeci, M. and Heineman, E.F. (1993) Cancer and other causes of death among male and female farmers from twenty-three states. *American Journal of Industrial Medicine* **23**, 729–42.

Blair, A., Malker, H., Cantor, K.P., Burmeister, L. and Wiklund, K. (1985) Cancer among farmers. *Scandinavian Journal of Work, Environment and Health* **11**, 397–407.

Blattner, W.A. and Hoover, R.N. (1985) Cancer in the immunosuppressed host. In Devita, V.T., Hellman, S. and Rosenberg, S.A. (eds), *Cancer principles and practice of oncology*. Philadelphia: Lippincott, 1989–2006.

Boeing, H., Schlehofer, B., Blettner, M. and Wahrendoorf, J. (1993) Dietary carcinogens and the risk for glioma and meningioma in Germany. *International Journal of Cancer* **53**, 561–5.

Bondy, M.L., Lustbader, E.D., Buffler, P.A., Schull, W.J., Hardy, R.J. and Strong, L.C. (1991) Genetic epidemiology of childhood brain tumors. *Genetic Epidemiology* **8**, 253–67.

Bondy, M.L., Wiencke, J., Wrensch, M. and Kyritsis, A.P. (1994) Genetics of primary brain tumors: a review. *Journal of Neuro-Oncology* **18**, 69–81.

Bouchardy, C., Wanner, P. and Parkin, D.M. (1995) Cancer mortality among sub-Saharan African migrants in France. *Cancer Causes and Control* **6**, 539–44.

Boyle, P., Maisonneuve, P., Saracci, R. and Muir, C.S. (1990) Is the increased incidence of primary malignant brain tumors in the elderly real? *Journal of the National Cancer Institute* **82**, 1594–6.

Brownson, R.C., Reif, J.S., Chang, J.C. and Davis, J.R. (1990) An analysis of occupational risks for brain cancer. *American Journal of Public Health* **80**, 169–72.

Buckwalter, J.A., Turner, J.H. and Gamber, H.H. (1959) Psychoses, intracranial neoplasms and genetics. *Archives of Neurology and Psychiatry* **81**, 480–5.

Bunin, G.R., Kuijten, R.R., Buckley, J.D., Rorke, L.B. and Meadows, A.T. (1993) Relation between maternal diet and subsequent primitive neuroectodermal brain tumors in young children. *New England Journal of Medicine* **329**, 536–41.

Burch, J.D., Craib, K.J.P., Choi, B.C.K., Miller, A.B., Risch, H.A. and Howe, G.R. (1987) An exploratory case-control study of brain tumors in adults. *Journal of the National Cancer Institute* **78**, 601–9.

Burger, P.C. (1995) Revising the World Health Organization (WHO) blue book—histological typing of tumors of the central nervous system. *Journal of Neuro-Oncology* **24**, 3–7.

Cantor, K.P., Lynch, C.F. and Johnson, D. (1993) Reproductive factors and risk of brain, colon, and other malignancies in Iowa (United States). *Cancer Causes and Control* **4**, 505–11.

Carpenter, A.V., Flanders, W.D., Frome, E.L., Cole, P. and Fry, S.A. (1987a) Brain cancer and nonoccupational risk factors: a case-control study among workers at two nuclear facilities. *American Journal of Public Health* **77**, 1180–2.

Carpenter, A.V., Flanders, W.D., Frome, E.L., Crawford-Brown, D.J. and Fry, S.A. (1987b) CNS cancers and radiation exposure: a case-control study among workers at two nuclear facilities. *Journal of Occupational Medicine* **29**, 601–4.

Carpenter, L., Higgins, C., Douglas, D., Fraser, P., Beral, V. and Smith, P. (1994) Combined analysis of mortality in three United Kingdom nuclear industry workforces, 1946–1988. *Radiation Research* **138**, 224–38.

Carroll, R.S., Glowacka, D., Dashner, K. and Black, P.M. (1993) Progesterone receptor expression in meningiomas. *Cancer Research* **53**, 1312–16.

Carter, R.L., Hitchcock, E.R. and Sato, F. (1964) Malignant glioma and ABO blood group. (Letter) *British Medical Journal* **I**, 122.

CBTRUS (1996) *First annual report 1995*. Central Brain Tumor Registry of the United States.

——(1997) *1996 Annual Report*. Central Brain Tumor Registry of the United States.

Chang, Y. and Horoupian, D.S. (1994) Pathology of benign brain tumors. In Morantz, R.A. and Walsh, J.W. (ed), *Brain tumors: a comprehensive text*. New York: Marcel Dekker, 19–44.

Checkoway, H., Mathew, R.M., Shy, C.M., Watson, J.E. Jr, Tankersley, W.G., Wolf, S.H., Smith, S.H. and Fry, S.A. (1985) Radiation work experience and cause specific mortality among workers at an energy research laboratory. *British Journal of Industrial Medicine* **42**, 525–33.

Checkoway, H., Pearce, N., Crawford-Brown, D.J. and Cragle, D.L. (1988) Radiation doses and cause-specific mortality among workers at a nuclear materials fabrication plant. *American Journal of Epidemiology* **127**, 255–66.

Choi, B.K. (1985) *N*-Nitroso compounds and human cancer. *American Journal of Epidemiology* **121**, 737–43.

Choi, N.W., Schuman, L.M. and Gullen, W.H. (1970a) Epidemiology of primary central nervous system neoplasms. I. Mortality from primary central nervous system neoplasms in Minnesota. *American Journal of Epidemiology* **91**, 238–59.

——(1970b) Epidemiology of primary central nervous system neoplasms. II. Case-control study. *American Journal of Epidemiology* **91**, 467–85.

Chou, C.-K., Guy, A.W., Kunz, L.L., Johnson, R.B., Crowley, J.J. and Krupp, J.H., (1992) Long-term, low-level microwave irradiation of rats. *Bioelectromagnetics* **13**(6), 469–96.

Christie, D., Robinson, K., Gordon, I. and Bisby, J. (1991) A prospective study in the Australian petroleum industry. I. Mortality. *British Journal of Industrial Medicine* **48**, 507–10.

Clemmesen, J. and Hjalgrim-Jensen, S. (1981) Does phenobarbital cause intracranial tumors? A follow-up through 35 years. *Ecotoxicology and Environmental Safety* **5**, 255–60.

Codd, M.B. and Kurland, L.T. (1985) Descriptive epidemiology of primary intracranial neoplasms. *Progress in Experimental Tumor Research* **29**, 1–11.

Cohen, A. and Modan, B. (1968) Some epidemiologic aspects of neoplastic diseases in Israeli immigrant population. III. Brain tumors. *Cancer* **22**, 1323–8.

Cole, P. and Sateren, W. (1995) The evolving picture of cancer in America. *Journal of the National Cancer Institute* **87**, 159–60.

Coleman, M.P., Esteve, J., Damiecki, P., Arslan, A. and Renard, H. (1993) *Trends in cancer incidence and mortality*. IARC Scientific Publication 121. Lyon: International Agency for Research on Cancer.

Coogan, P.F., Baron, J.A. and Lambe, M. (1995) Parity and pituitary adenoma risk. *Journal of the National Cancer Institute* **87**, 1410–11.

Coons, S.W. and Johnson, P.C. (1991) Histopathology of astrocytomas: grading, patterns of spread, and correlation with modern imaging modalities. *Seminars in Radiation Oncology* **1**, 2–9.

Cooper, W.C. (1981) Epidemiologic study of vinyl chloride workers: mortality through December 31, 1972. *Environmental Health Perspective* **41**, 101–6.

Corallini, A., Pagnani, M., Viadana, P., Silini, E., Mottes, M., Melanesi, G., Gerna, G., Vettor, R., Trapella, G., Silvani, V., Gaist, G. and Barbanti-Brodano, G. (1987) Association of BK virus with human brain tumors and tumors of pancreatic islets. *International Journal of Cancer* **39**, 60–7.

Cordier, S., Poisson, M., Gerin, M., Varin, J., Conso, F. and Hemon, D. (1988) Gliomas and exposure to wood preservatives. *British Journal of Industrial Medicine* **45**, 705–9.

Cordier, S., Iglesias, M.J., Le Goaster, M.M., Guyot, M.M., Mandereau, L. and Hemon, D. (1994) Incidence and risk factors for childhood brain tumors in the Ile de France. *International Journal of Cancer* **59**, 776–82.

Cornfield, J., Haenszel, W., Hammond, E.C., Lilienfeld, A.M., Shimkin, M. and Wynder, E.L. (1959) Smoking and lung cancer: recent evidence and a discussion of some questions. *Journal of the National Cancer Institute* **22**, 173–203.

Corrao, G., Calleri, M., Carle, F., Russo, R., Bosia, S. and Piccioni, P. (1989) Cancer risk in a cohort of licensed pesticide users. *Scandinavian Journal of Work, Environment and Health* **15**, 203–9.

Cote, T.R., Manns, A., Hardy, C.R., Yellin, F.J., Hartge, P. and AIDS/Cancer Study Group (1996) Epidemiology of brain lymphoma among people with or without acquired immunodeficiency syndrome. *Journal of the National Cancer Institute* **88**, 675–9.

Craddock, V.M. (1983) Nitrosamines and human cancer: proof of an association? *Nature* **306**, 638.

Cushing, H. (1922) The meningiomas (dural endotheliomas). Their source and favored seats of origin. *Brain* **45**, 282–316.

Cushing, H. and Eisenhardt, L. (1938) *Meningiomas, their classification, regional behavior, life history and surgical end results*. Springfield, Ill.: Thomas.

D'Alessandro, G., Giovanni, M.D., Iannizzi, L., Guidetti, E. and Bottacchi, E. (1995) Epidemiology of primary intracranial tumors in the Valle d'Aosta (Italy) during the 6-year period 1986–1991. *Neuroepidemiology* **14**, 139–46.

Daumas-Duport, C., Scheithauer, B.W., O'Fallon, J. and Kelly, P. (1988) Grading of astrocytomas. A simple and reproducible method. *Cancer* **62**, 2152–65.

Davey-Smith, G., Neaton, J.D., Ben-Shlomo, Y., Shipley, M. and Wentworth, D. (1992) Serum cholesterol and primary malignant brain tumors: a prospective study. *American Journal of Epidemiology* **135**, 259–65.

Davis, D.L. and Schwartz, J. (1988) Trends in cancer mortality: U.S. white males and females, 1968–83. *Lancet*, **1**, 633–6.

Davis, D.L., Ahlbom, A., Hoel, D. and Percy, C. (1991) Is brain cancer mortality increasing in industrial countries? *American Journal of Industrial Medicine* **19**, 421–31.

Davis, F., Boice, J.D., Hrubec, Z. and Monson, R.R. (1989) Cancer mortality in a radiation exposed cohort of Massachusetts tuberculosis patients. *Cancer Research* **49**, 6130–6.

Davis, F.G., Malinski, N., Haenszel, W., Chang, J., Flannery, J., Gershman, S., Dibble, R. and Bigner, D.D. (1996) Primary brain tumor incidence rates in four United States regions, 1985–1989: a pilot study. *Neuroepidemiology* **15**, 103–12.

Davis, J.R., Brownson, R.C., Garcia, R., Bentz, B.J. and Turner, A. (1993) Family pesticide use and childhood brain cancer. *Archives of Environmental Contamination and Toxicology* **24**, 87–92.

Dean, G. (1994) Deaths from primary brain cancers, lymphatic and hematopoietic cancers in agricultural workers in the Republic of Ireland. *Journal of Epidemiology and Community Health* **48**, 364–8.

Deen, H.G. Jr and Laws, E.R. Jr (1981) Multiple primary brain tumors of different cell types. *Neurosurgery* **8**, 20–5.

Demers, P.A., Vaughan, T.L. and Schommer, R.R. (1991) Occupation, socioeconomic status, and brain tumor mortality: a death certificate-based case-control study. *Journal of Occupational Medicine* **33**, 1001–6.

Desmeules, M., Mikkelsen, T. and Mao, Y. (1992) Increasing incidence of primary malignant brain tumors: influence of diagnostic methods. *Journal of the National Cancer Institute* **84**, 442–5.

Devesa, S.S. and Silverman, D.T. (1978) Cancer incidence and mortality trends in the United States: 1935–74. *Journal of the National Cancer Institute* **60**, 545–71.

Devesa, S.S., Blot, W.J., Stone, B.J., Miller, B.A., Tarone, R.E. and Fraumeni, J.F. Jr (1995) Recent cancer trends in the United States. *Journal of the National Cancer Institute* **87**, 175–82.

Dobkin, B.H. (1985) Stroke associated with glioblastoma. *Bulletin of Clinical Neurosciences* **50**, 111–18.

Doll, R. (1988) Effects of exposure to vinyl chloride: an assessment of the evidence. *Scandinavian Journal of Work, Environment and Health* **14**, 61–78.

——(1991) Progress against cancer: an epidemiologic assessment. *American Journal of Epidemiology* **134**, 675–88.

Dorries, K., Loeber, G. and Meixensberger, J. (1987) Association of polyomaviruses JC, SV40, and BK with human brain tumors. *Virology* **160**, 268–70.

Eby, N., Grufferman, S., Flannelly, C.M., Schold, S.C. Jr, Vogel, F.V. and Burger, P.C. (1988) Increasing incidence of primary brain lymphoma in the U.S. *Cancer* **62**, 2461–5.

Elandt-Johnson, R.C. (1975) Definition of rates: some remarks on their use and misuse. *American Journal of Epidemiology* **102**, 267–71.

Engelmann, B. and Schumacher, U. (1993) The emerging role of ABH blood group antigens as modulators of cell membrane functions. *Comprehensive Biochemistry and Physiology*. **105A**, 197–203.

Ericsson, J.L., Karnstrom, L. and Mattsson, B. (1978) Childhood cancer in Sweden 1958–1974. I. Incidence and mortality. *Acta Paediatrica Scandinavica* **67**, 425–32.

Evans, D.G.R., Farndon, P.A., Burnell, L.D., Gattamaneni, H.R. and Birch, J.M. (1991) The incidence of Gorlin syndrome in 173 consecutive cases of medulloblastoma. *British Journal of Cancer* **64**, 959–61.

Farwell, J.R. and Flannery, J.T. (1984) Second primaries in children with central nervous system tumors. *Journal of Neuro-Oncology* **2**, 371–5.

Farwell, J.R., Dohrmann, G.J., Marrett, L.D. and Meigs, J.W. (1979) Effect of SV40 virus-contaminated polio vaccine on the incidence and type of CNS neoplasms in children: a population-based study. *Transactions of the American Neurological Association* **104**, 261–4.

Fedrick, J. and Alberman, E.D. (1972) Reported influenza in pregnancy and subsequent cancer in the child. *British Medical Journal* **2**, 485–8.

Feychting, M. and Ahlbom, A. (1994) Magnetic fields, leukemia, and central nervous system tumors in Swedish adults residing near high-voltage power lines. *Epidemiology* **5**, 501–9.

Figa-Talamanca, I., Mearelli, I., Valente, P. and Bascherini, S. (1993) Cancer mortality in a cohort of rural licensed pesticide users in the province of Rome. *International Journal of Epidemiology* **22**, 579–83.

Filippini, G., Farinotti, M., Lovicu, G., Maisonneuve, P. and Boyle, P. (1994) Mothers' active and passive smoking during pregnancy and risk of brain tumours in children. *International Journal of Cancer* **57**, 769–74.

Flannery, J.T., Boice, J.D. Jr, Devesa, S.S., Kleinerman, R.A., Curtis, R.E. and Fraumeni, J.F. Jr (1985) Cancer registration in Connecticut and the study of multiple primary cancers, 1935–82. *National Cancer Institute Monograph* **68**, 13–24.

Floderus, B., Persson, T., Stenlund, C., Wennberg, A., Ost, A. and Knave, B. (1993) Occupational exposure to electromagnetic fields in relation to leukemia and brain tumors: a case-control study in Sweden. *Cancer Causes and Control* **4**, 465–76.

Fraumeni, J.F. Jr, Ederer, F. and Miller, R.W. (1963) An evaluation of the carcinogenicity of Simian Virus 40 in man. *Journal of the American Medical Association* **185**, 713–18.

Frelick, R., Huang, P. and Topham, A. (1992) Brain and central nervous system tumors Delaware, 1980 to 1989. *Delaware Medical Journal* **64**, 571–3.

Friedman, D.R., Hatch, E.E., Tarone, R., Kaune, W.T., Kleinerman, R.A., Wacholder, S., Boice, J.D. Jr and Linet, M.S. (1996) Childhood exposure to magnetic fields: residential area measurements compared to personal dosimetry. *Epidemiology* **7**, 151–5.

Garcia, J.H., Okazaki, H. and Aronson, S.M. (1963) Blood-group frequencies and astrocytomata. *Journal of Neurosurgery* **20**, 397–9.

Garfinkel, L. and Sarokhan, B. (1982) Trends in brain cancer tumor mortality and morbidity in the United States. *Annals of the New York Academy of Sciences* **381**, 1–5.

Gatchev, O., Rastam, L., Lindberg, G., Gullberg, B., Tornberg, S. and Eklund, G.A. (1994) Tumours of the central nervous system and concentration of total serum cholesterol and beta-lipoprotein in men and women. *British Journal of Cancer* **70**, 668–71.

Geissler, E. (1990) SV40 and human brain tumors. *Progress in Medical Virology* **37**, 211–22.

Gilbert, E.S., Fry, S.A., Wiggs, L.D., Voelz, G.L., Cragle, D.L. and Petersen, G.R. (1989) Analyses of combined mortality data on workers at the Hanford site, Oak Ridge National Laboratory, and Rocky Flats Nuclear Weapons Plant. *Radiation Research* **120**, 19–35.

Giles, G.G., McNeil, J.J., Donnan, G., Webley, C., Staples, M.P., Ireland, P.D., Hurley, S.F. and Salzberg, M. (1994) Dietary factors and the risk of glioma in adults: results of a case-control study in Melbourne, Australia. *International Journal of Cancer* **59**, 357–62.

Gilles, F.H., Sobel, E., Leviton, A., Hedley-Whyte, E.T., Tavare, C.J., Adelman, L.S. and Sobel, R.A. (1992) Epidemiology of seizures in children with brain tumors. *Journal of Neuro-Oncology* **12**, 53–68.

Giusti, R., Boyle, C. and Zack, M. (1987) Brain cancer in South Georgia farmers. *American Journal of Epidemiology* **126**, 743.

Gold, E., Diener, M. and Szklo, M. (1982) Parental occupations and cancer in children. *Journal of Occupational Medicine* **24**(8), 578–84.

Gold, E., Gordis, L., Tonascia, J. and Szklo, M. (1978) Increased risk of brain tumors in children exposed to barbiturates. *Journal of the National Cancer Institute* **61**, 1031–4.

——(1979) Risk factors for brain tumors in children. *American Journal of Epidemiology* **109**, 309–19.

Gold, E., Leviton, A., Lopez, R., Gilles, F.H., Hedley-Whyte, E.T., Kolonel, L.N., Lyon, J.L., Swanson, G.M., Weiss, N.S., West, D., Aschenbrener, C. and Austin, D.F. (1993) Parental smoking and risk of childhood brain tumors. *American Journal of Epidemiology* **137**, 620–8.

Goldhaber, M.K., Selby, J.V., Hiatt, R.A. and Quesenberry, C.P. (1990) Exposure to barbiturates in utero and during childhood and risk of intracranial and spinal cord tumors. *Cancer Research* **50**, 4600–3.

Gordis, L. (1996) *Epidemiology*. Philadelphia: W.B. Saunders.

Gorlin, R.J. (1987) Nevoid basal cell carcinoma syndrome. *Medicine* **66**, 98–113.

Grayson, J.K. (1996) Radiation exposure, socioeconomic status, and brain tumor risk in the U.S. Air Force: a nested case-control study. *American Journal of Epidemiology* **143**, 480–6.

Greig, N.H., Ries, L.G., Yancik, R. and Rapoport, S.I. (1990) Increasing annual incidence of primary malignant brain tumors in the elderly. *Journal of the National Cancer Institute* **82**, 1621–4.

Grimes, G., Hirsch, D. and Borgeson, D. (1991) Risk of death among Honolulu fire fighters. *Hawaii Medical Journal* **50**, 82–5.

Grulich, A.E., Swerdlow, A.J., Head, J. and Marmot, M.G. (1992) Cancer mortality in African and Caribbean migrants to England and Wales. *British Journal of Cancer* **66**, 905–11.

Guénel, P., Nicolau, J., Imbernon, E., Chevalier, A. and Goldberg, M. (1996) Exposure to 50-Hz electric field and incidence of leukemia, brain tumors, and other cancers among French electric utility workers. *American Journal of Epidemiology* **144**, 1107–21.

Gurney, J.G., Davis, S., Severson, R.K., Fang, J.Y., Ross, J.A. and Robison, L.L. (1996a) Trends in cancer incidence among children in the U.S. *Cancer* **78**, 532–41.

Gurney, J.G., Mueller, B.A., Davis, S., Schwartz, S.M., Stevens, R.G. and Kopecky, K.J. (1996b) Childhood brain tumor occurrence in relation to residential power line configurations, electric heating sources, and electric appliance use. *American Journal of Epidemiology* **143**, 120–8.

Gurney, J.G., Preston-Martin, S., McDaniel, A.M., Mueller, B.A. and Holly, E.A. (1996c) Head injury as a risk factor for brain tumors in children: results from a multicenter case-control study. *Epidemiology* **7**, 485–9.

Hadjimichael, O.C., Ostfeld, A.M., D'Atri, D.A. and Brubaker, R.E. (1983) Mortality and cancer incidence experience of employees in a nuclear fuels fabrication plant. *Journal of Occupational Medicine* **25**, 48–61.

Hagmar, L., Akesson, B., Nielsen, J., Andersson, C., Linden, K., Attewell, R. and Moller, T. (1990) Mortality and cancer morbidity in workers exposed to low levels of vinyl chloride monomer at a polyvinyl chloride processing plant. *American Journal of Industrial Medicine* **17**, 553–65.

Hall, A., Harrington, J.M. and Aw, T. (1991) Mortality study of British pathologists. *American Journal of Industrial Medicine* **20**, 83–9.

Harrington, J.M. and Oakes, D. (1984) Mortality study of British pathologists 1974–80. *British Journal of Industrial Medicine* **41**, 188–91.

Harvey, E.B., Boice, J.D., Honeyman, M. and Flannery, J.T. (1985) Prenatal x-ray exposure and childhood cancer in twins. *New England Journal of Medicine* **312**, 541–5.

Heineman, E.F., Cocco, P., Gomez, M.R., Dosemeci, M., Stewart, P.A., Hayes, R.B., Zahm, S.H., Thomas, T.L. and Blair, A. (1994) Occupational exposure to chlorinated aliphatic hydrocarbons and risk of astrocytic brain cancer. *American Journal of Industrial Medicine* **26**, 155–69.

Heineman, E.F., Gao, Y., Dosemeci, M. and McLaughlin, J. (1995) Occupational risk factors for brain tumors among women in Shanghai, China. *Journal of Occupational and Environmental Medicine* **37**(3), 288–93.

Heinonen, O.P., Shapiro, S., Monson, R.R., Hartz, S.C., Rosenberg, L. and Slone, D. (1973) Immunization during pregnancy against poliomyelitis and influenza in relation to childhood malignancy. *International Journal of Epidemiology* **2**, 229–35.

Helseth, A. (1993) Increasing incidence of primary central nervous system tumors in the elderly: real increase or improved detection? *Journal of the National Cancer Institute* **85**, 1871–2.

——(1995) The incidence of primary central nervous system neoplasms before and after computerized tomography availability. *Journal of Neurosurgery* **83**, 999–1003.

Helseth, A. and Mørk, S.J. (1989) Neoplasms of the central nervous system in Norway. III. Epidemiological characteristics of intracranial gliomas according to histology. *APMIS* **97**, 547–55.

Helseth, A. and Tretli, S. (1989) Pre-morbid height and weight as risk factors for development of central nervous system neoplasms. *Neuroepidemiology* **8**, 277–82.

Helseth, A., Langmark, F. and Mørk, S.J. (1988) Neoplasms of the central nervous system in Norway II. Descriptive epidemiology of intracranial neoplasms 1955–1984. *APMIS* **96**, 1066–74.

Hernberg, S. (1981) Negative results in cohort studies – how to recognize fallacies. *Scandinavian Journal of Work, Environment and Health* **4**, 121–6.

Heshmat, M.Y., Kovi, J., Simpson, C., Kennedy, J. and Fan, K.J. (1976) Neoplasms of the central nervous system. *Cancer* **38**, 2135–42.

Heyer, N.J. and Franklin, G.M. (1994) Work-related traumatic brain injury in Washington State, 1988 through 1990. *American Journal of Public Health* **84**, 1106–9.

Hicks, N., Zack, M., Caldwell, G.G., Fernbach, D.J. and Falletta, J.M. (1984) Childhood cancer and occupational radiation exposure in parents. *Cancer* **53**, 1637–43.

Hildreth, N.G., Shore, R.E., Hempelmann, L.H. and Rosenstein, M. (1985) Risk of extrathyroid tumors following radiation treatment in infancy for thymic enlargement. *Radiation Research* **102**, 378–91.

Hill, A.B. (1965) The environment and disease: association or causation? *Proceedings of the Royal Society of Medicine* **58**, 295–300.

Hirayama, T. (1984) Cancer mortality in nonsmoking women with smoking husbands based on a large-scale cohort study in Japan. *Preventive Medicine* **13**, 680–90.

Hochberg, F., Toniolo, P. and Cole, P. (1984) Head trauma and seizures as risk factors of glioblastoma. *Neurology* **34**, 1511–14.

——(1990) Nonoccupational risk indicators of glioblastoma in adults. *Journal of Neuro-Oncology* **8**, 55–60.

Hoover, R. and Fraumeni, J.F. Jr (1973) Risk of cancer in renal-transplant recipients. *Lancet* **2**, 55–7.

Howe, G.R., Burch, J.D., Chiarelli, A.M., Risch, H.A. and Choi, B.C.K. (1989) An exploratory case-control study of brain tumors in children. *Cancer Research* **49**, 4349–52.

Howe, H.L., Lihner, M. and Derrick, L. (eds) (1996) *Cancer incidence in North America 1998–1992*. Sacramento, Calif.: North American Association of Central Cancer Registries.

Hung, C., Chang, W. and Yao, Y. (1972) Post-traumatic intracranial meningioma. *Journal of the Formosan Medical Association* **71**, 214–19.

Hunter, S.B., Ballinger, W.E. Jr and Rubin, J.J. (1987) Multiple sclerosis mimicking primary brain tumor. *Archives of Pathology and Laboratory Medicine* **111**, 464–8.

Infante, P.F (1976) Oncogenic and mutagenic risk in communities with polyvinyl chloride production facilities. *Annals of the New York Academy of Sciences* **271**, 49–57.

Inskip, P.D., Linet, M.S. and Heineman, E.F. (1995) Etiology of brain tumors in adults. *Epidemiologic Reviews* **17**, 382–414.

Irvine, D. and Davies, D.M. (1992) The mortality of British Airways pilots, 1966–1989: a proportional mortality study. *Aviation Space and Environmental Medicine* **63**, 276–9.

Jenkin, D. (1996) The radiation treatment of medulloblastoma. *Journal of Neuro-Oncology* **29**, 45–54.

John, E.M., Savitz, D.A. and Sandler, D.P. (1991) Prenatal exposure to parents' smoking and childhood cancer. *American Journal of Epidemiology* **133**, 123–32.

Johnson, C.C. and Spitz, M.R. (1989) Childhood nervous system tumours: an assessment of risk associated with paternal occupations involving use, repair or manufacture of electrical and electronic equipment. *International Journal of Epidemiology* **18**, 756–62.

Kallio, M. (1993) The incidence, survival, and prognostic factors of patients with intracranial glioma and meningioma in Finland from 1953–1987. Academic Dissertation, University of Helskinki, Finland.

Katz, R.M. (1983) Causes of death among registered nurses. *Journal of Occupational Medicine* **25**, 760–2.

Kessler, I.K. (1970) Cancer mortality among diabetics. *Journal of the National Cancer Institute* **44**, 673–86.

Kinlen, L.J. (1982) Immunosuppressive therapy and cancer. *Cancer Surveys* **1**, 565–83.

Kleihues, P., Aguzzi, A. and Ohgaki, H. (1995) Genetic and environmental factors in the etiology of human brain tumors. *Toxicology Letters* **82**, 601–5.

Kleihues, P., Burger, P.C. and Scheithauer, B.W. (1993) The new WHO classification of brain tumours. *Brain Pathology* **3**, 255–68.

Knekt, P., Reunanen, A. and Teppo, L. (1991) Serum cholesterol concentration and risk of primary brain tumours. *British Medical Journal* **302**, 90.

Kraut, A., Tate, R. and Tran, N. (1994) Residential electric consumption and childhood cancer in Canada (1971–1986). *Archives of Environmental Health* **49**, 156–9.

Kuijten, R.R., Bunin, G.R., Nass, C.C. and Meadows, A.T.(1990) Gestational and familial risk factors for childhood astrocytoma: results of a case-control study. *Cancer Research* **50**, 2608–12.

Kuratsu, J. and Ushio, Y. (1996) Epidemiological study of primary intracranial tumors: a regional survey in Kumamoto prefecture in the southern part of Japan. *Journal of Neurosurgery* **84**, 946–50.

Kurland, L.T., Schoenberg, B.S., Annegers, J.F., Okazaki, H. and Molgaad, C.A. (1982) The incidence of primary intracranial neoplasms in Rochester, Minnesota 1935–1977. *Annals of New York Academy of Sciences* **381**, 6–16.

Kurtzke, J.F. (1969) Geographic pathology of brain tumors. I. Distribution of deaths from primary tumors. *Acta Neurologica Scandinavica* **45**, 540–55.

Lanes, S.F., Rothman, K.J., Soden, K.J., Amsel, J. and Dreyer, N.A. (1994) Mortality among synthetic fiber workers exposed to glycerol polyglycidyl ether. *American Journal of Industrial Medicine* **25**, 689–96.

Laplanche, A., Clavel-Chapelon, F., Contassot, J., Lanouzier, C. and The French VCM Group (1992) Exposure to vinyl chloride monomer: results of a cohort study after a seven year follow up. *British Journal of Industrial Medicine* **49**, 134–7.

Levi, F., La Vecchia, C. and Te, V. (1990) Descriptive epidemiology of malignant brain tumors in the Swiss canton of Vaud. *Neuroepidemiology* **9**, 135–42.

Li, C.-Y., Thériault, G. and Lin, R.S. (1997) Residential exposure to 60-hertz magnetic fields and adult cancers in Taiwan. *Epidemiology* **8**, 25–30.

Li, F.P., Fraumeni, J.F. Jr, Mulvihill, J.J., Blattner, W.A., Dreyfus, M.G., Tucker, M.A. and Miller, R.W. (1988) A cancer family syndrome in twenty-four kindreds. *Cancer Research* **48**, 5358–62.

Lijinsky, W. (1992) *Chemistry and biology of N-nitroso compounds*. Cambridge: Cambridge University Press.

Linet, M.S., Gridley, G., Cnattingius, S., Nicholson, H.S., Martinsson, U., Glimelius, B., Adami, H. and Zack, M. (1996) Maternal and perinatal risk factors for childhood brain tumors (Sweden). *Cancer Causes and Control* **7**, 437–448.

Littorin, M., Attewell, R., Skerfving, S., Horstmann, V. and Moller, T. (1993) Mortality and tumour morbidity among Swedish market gardeners and orchardists. *International Archives of Occupational Environmental Health* **65**, 163–9.

Logue, J.N., Barrick, M.K. and Jessup, G.L. (1986) Mortality of radiologists and pathologists in the radiation registry of physicians. *Journal of Occupational Medicine* **28**(2), 91–9.

Longstreth, W.T. Jr, Dennis, L.K., McGuire, V.M., Drangsholt, M.T. and Koepsell, T.D. (1993) Epidemiology of intracranial meningioma. *Cancer* **72**, 639–48.

Lossignol, D., Grossman, S.A., Sheidler, V.R., Griffin, C.A. and Piantadosi, S. (1990) Familial clustering of malignant astrocytomas. *Journal of Neuro-Oncology* **9**, 139–45.

Lundberg, I., Gustavsson, A., Holmberg, B., Molina, G. and Westerholm, P. (1993) Mortality and cancer incidence among PVC-processing workers in Sweden. *American Journal of Industrial Medicine* **23**, 313–19.

Lutz, J.M. and Coleman, M.P. (1994) Trends in primary cerebral lymphoma. *British Journal of Cancer* **70**, 716–18.

Lyon, J.L., Klauber, M.R., Gardner, J.W. and Smart, C.R. (1976) Cancer incidence in Mormons and non-Mormons in Utah, 1966–1970. *New England Journal of Medicine* **294**, 129–33.

Mack, W., Preston-Martin, S. and Peters, J.M. (1991) Astrocytoma risk related to job exposure to electric and magnetic fields. *Bioelectromagnetics* **12**, 57–66.

MacMahon, B. (1962) Prenatal x-ray exposure and childhood cancer. *Journal of the National Cancer Institute* **28**, 1173–91.

——(1985) Prenatal x-ray exposure and twins. *New England Journal of Medicine* **312**, 576–7.

MacPherson, P. (1976) Association between previous tuberculous infection and glioma. *British Medical Journal* **2**, 1112.

Maekawa, A. and Mitsumori, K. (1990) Spontaneous occurrence and chemical induction of neurogenic tumors in rats– influence of host factors and specificity of chemical structure. *Clinical Reviews in Toxicology* **20**, 287–310.

Magee, P.N. (1972) Possibilities of hazard from nitrosamines in industry. *Annals of Occupational Hygiene* **15**, 19–23.

Magnani, C., Coggon, D., Osmond, C. and Acheson, E.D. (1987) Occupation and five cancers: a case-control study using death certificates. *British Journal of Industrial Medicine* **44**, 769–76.

Mahaley, M.S. Jr, Mettlin, C., Natarajan, N., Laws, E.R. Jr and Peace, B. (1989) National survey of patterns of care of brain-tumor patients. *Journal of Neurosurgery* **71**, 826–36.

Maher, E.R., Yates, J.R.W., Harries, R., Benjamin, C., Harris, R., Moore, A.T. and Ferguson-Smith, M.A. (1990) Clinical features and natural history of von Hippel-Lindau disease. *Quarterly Journal of Medicine* **77**, 1151–63.

Mallin, K., Rubin, M. and Joo, E. (1989) Occupational cancer mortality in Illinois white and black males, 1979–1984, for seven cancer sites. *American Journal of Industrial Medicine* **15**, 699–717.

Mancuso, T.F. (1963) Tumors of the central nervous system: industrial considerations. *Acta Union Internationale Contre le Cancer* **19**, 488.

Mancuso, T.F., Ciocco, A. and El-Attar, A.A. (1968) An epidemiological approach to the rubber industry: a study based on departmental experience. *Journal of Occupational Medicine* **10**, 213–32.

Mao, Y., Desmeules, M., Semenciw, R.M., Hill, G., Gaudette, L. and Wigle, D.T. (1991) Increasing brain cancer rates in Canada. *Canadian Medical Association Journal* **145**, 1583–91.

Marsh, G.M., Enterline, P.E. and McCraw, D. (1991) Mortality patterns among petroleum refinery and chemical plant workers. *American Journal of Industrial Medicine* **19**, 29–42.

Martini, F., De Mattei, M., Iaccheri, L., Lazzarin, L., Barbanti-Brodano, G., Tognon, M. and Gerosa, M. (1995) Human brain tumors and simian virus 40. *Journal of the National Cancer Institute* **87**, 1331.

Mayr, E. (1956) Suspected correlation between blood-group frequency and pituitary adenomas. *Science* **124**, 932–4.

McCredie, M., Maisonneuve, P. and Boyle, P. (1994a) Antenatal risk factors for malignant brain tumours in New South Wales children. *International Journal of Cancer* **56**, 6-10.

——(1994b) Perinatal and early postnatal risk factors for malignant brain tumours in New South Wales children. *International Journal of Cancer* **56**, 11–15.

McKinney, P.A., Cartwright, R.A., Stiller, C.A., Hopton, P.A., Mann, J.R., Birch, J.M., Hartley, A.L., Waterhouse, J.A.H. and Johnston, H.E. (1985) Inter-regional epidemiological study of childhood cancer (IRESCC): childhood cancer and the consumption of Debendox and related drugs in pregnancy. *British Journal of Cancer* **52**, 923–9.

McKinney, P.A., Ironside, J.W., Harkness, E.F., Arango, J.C., Doyle, D. and Black, R.J. (1994) Registration quality and descriptive epidemiology of childhood brain tumours in Scotland 1975–90. *British Journal of Cancer* **70**(5), 973–9.

McLaughlin, J.K., Malker, H.S.R., Blot, W.J., Malker, B.K., Stone, B.J., Weiner, J.A., Ericsson, J.L.E. and Fraumeni, J.F. Jr (1987) Occupational risks for intracranial gliomas in Sweden. *Journal of the National Cancer Institute* **78**, 253–7.

McMichael, A.J., Spirtas, R. and Kupper, L.L. (1974) An epidemiologic study of mortality within a cohort of rubber workers, 1964–72. *Journal of Occupational Medicine* **16**, 458–64.

Merlo, A., Rochlitz, C. and Scott, R. (1996) Survival of patients with Turcot's syndrome and glioblastoma. *New England Journal of Medicine* **334**(11), 736–7.

Merz, D. and Schwartzbaum, J. (1994) The role of infection in the etiology of brain tumors. *American Journal of Epidemiology* (Suppl.) **139**, 11845.

Mills, P.K., Preston-Martin, S., Annegers, J.F., Beeson, W.L., Phillips, R.L. and Fraser, G.E. (1989) Risk factors for tumors of the brain and cranial meninges in Seventh-Day Adventists. *Neuroepidemiology* **8**, 266–75.

Modan, B., Baidatz, D., Mart, H., Steinitz, R. and Levin, S.G. (1974) Radiation-induced head and neck tumours. *Lancet* **1**, 277–9.

Modan, B., Wagener, D.K., Feldman, J.J., Rosenberg, H.M. and Feinleib, M. (1992) Increased mortality from brain tumors: a combined outcome of diagnostic technology and change of attitude toward the elderly. *American Journal of Epidemiology* **135**, 1349–57.

Mole, R.H. (1974) Antenatal irradiation and childhood cancer: causation or coincidence? *British Journal of Cancer* **30**, 199–208.

Moller, H., Kneller, R.W., Boice, J.D. Jr and Olsen, J.H. (1991) Cancer incidence following hospitalization for multiple sclerosis in Denmark. *Acta Neurologica Scandinavica* **84**, 214–20.

Monson, R.R and Fine, L.J. (1978) Cancer mortality and morbidity among rubber workers. *Journal of the National Cancer Institute* **61**, 1047–53.

Monson, R.R. and Nakano, K.K. (1976) Mortality among rubber workers. I. White male union employees in Akron, Ohio. *American Journal of Epidemiology* **103**, 284–96.

Morantz, R.A. and Shain, W. (1978) Trauma and brain tumors: an experimental study. *Neurosurgery* **3**, 181–6.

Morrison, H.I., Semenciw, R.M., Morison, D., Magwood, S. and Mao, Y. (1992) Brain cancer and farming in western Canada. *Neuroepidemiology* **11**, 267–76.

Moss, A.R. (1985) Occupational exposure and brain tumors. *Journal of Toxicology and Environmental Health* **16**, 703–11.

Mosso, M.L., Colombo, R., Giordano, L., Pastore, G., Terracini, B. and Magnani, C. (1992) Childhood cancer registry of the province of Torino, Italy. *Cancer* **69**, 1300–6.

Mulhern, R.K., Hancock, J., Fairclough, D. and Kun, L. (1992) Neuropsychological status of children treated for brain tumors: a critical review and integrative analysis. *Medical and Pediatric Oncology* **20**, 181–91.

Mulhern, R.K., Carpenteri, S., Shema, S., Stone, P. and Fairclough, D. (1993) Factors associated with social and behavioral problems among children recently diagnosed with brain tumor. *Journal of Pediatric Psychology* **18**, 339–50.

Musicco, M., Sant, M., Molinari, S., Filippini, G., Gatta, G. and Berrino, F. (1988) A case-control study of brain gliomas and occupational exposure to chemical carcinogens: the risk to farmers. *American Journal of Epidemiology* **128**, 778–85.

Myers, A., Clayden, A.D., Cartwright, R.A. and Cartwright, S.C. (1990) Childhood cancer and overhead powerlines: a case-control study. *British Journal of Cancer* **62**, 1008–14.

Nasca, P.C., Baptiste, M.S., MacCubbin, P.A., Metzger, B.B., Carlton, K., Greenwald, P., Armbrustmacher, V.W., Earle, K.M. and Waldman, J. (1988) An epidemiologic case-control study of central nervous system tumors in children and parental occupational exposures. *American Journal of Epidemiology* **128**, 1256–65.

NCRP (National Council on Radiation Protection and Measurements) (1989) *Exposure of the U.S. population from diagnostic medical radiation*. NCRP Report 100. Bethesda, Md: National Council on Radiation Protection and Measurements.

Negrini, M., Rimessi, P., Mantovani, C., Sabbioni, S., Corallini, A., Gerosa, M.A. and Barbanti-Brodano, G. (1990) Characterization of BK virus variants rescued from human tumours and lamour cell lines. *Journal of General Virology* **71**, 2731–6.

Neuberger, J.S., Brownson, R.C., Morantz, R.A. and Chin, T.D.Y. (1991) Association of brain cancer with dental x-rays and occupation in Missouri. *Cancer, Detection and Prevention* **15**, 31–4.

Neugut, A.I., Fink, D.J. and Radin, D. (1989) Serum cholesterol and primary brain tumours: a case-control study. *International Journal of Epidemiology* **18**, 798–801.

Neutel, C.I., Quinn, A. and Brancker, A. (1989) Brain tumour mortality in immigrants. *International Journal of Epidemiology* **18**, 60–6.

Newill, V.A. (1961) Distribution of cancer mortality among ethnic subgroups of the white population of New York City, 1953–58. *Journal of the National Cancer Institute* **26**, 405–17.

Nilsson, R., Hamnerius, Y., Mild, K.H., Hansson, H.A., Hjelmqvist, E., Olanders, S. and Persson, L.I. (1989) Microwave effects on the central nervous system – a study of radar mechanics. *Health Physics* **56**, 777–9.

Norman, M.A., Holly, E.A. and Preston-Martin, S. (1996) Childhood brain tumors and exposure to tobacco smoke. *Cancer, Epidemiology, Biomarkers and Prevention* **5**, 85–91.

Norman, M.A., Holly, E.A., Ahn, D.K., Preston-Martin, S., Mueller, B.A. and Bracci, P.M. (1996) Prenatal exposure to tobacco smoke and childhood brain tumors: results from the U.S. West Coast Childhood Brain Tumor Study. *Cancer Epidemiology, Biomarkers and Prevention* **5**, 127–33.

NRC (National Research Council) U.S. Committee on the Biological Effects of Ionizing Radiations (1980) *The effects on populations of exposure to low levels of ionizing radiation: 1980.* Washington, D.C.: National Academy Press.

NRC (National Research Council) (1981) *The health effects of nitrate, nitrite, and N-nitroso compounds*, Part 1. Washington D.C.: National Academy Press.

Ohgaki, H., Schauble, B., zur Hausen, A., von Ammon, K. and Kleihues, P. (1995) Genetic alteration associated with the evolution and progression of astrocytic brain tumours. *Virchows Archiv* **427**, 113–18.

Olin, R.G., Ahlbom, A., Lindberg-Navier, I., Norell, S.E. and Spannare, B. (1987) Occupational factors associated with astrocytomas: a case-control study. *American Journal of Industrial Medicine* **11**, 615–25.

Olsen, J.H., Nielsen, A. and Schulgen, G. (1993) Residence near high voltage facilities and risk of cancer in children. *British Medical Journal* **307**, 891–5.

Olsen, J.H., Boice, J.D. Jr, Jensen, J.P.A. and Fraumeni, J.F. Jr (1989) Cancer among epileptic patients exposed to anticonvulsant drugs. *Journal of the National Cancer Institute* **81**, 803–8.

Osman, M., Grossman, S.A., Guffin, C., Hrulan, R. and Shuldler, V.R. (1992) Primary brain tumors in spouses and relatives. A report from the National Familial Brain Tumor Registry. (Abstract) *Proceedings of the American Society of Clinical Oncology* **11**, 149.

Packer, R.J., Meadows, A.T., Rorke, L.B., Goldwein, J.L. and D'Angio, G. (1987) Long term sequelae of cancer treatment on the central nervous system in childhood. *Medical and Pediatric Oncology* **15**, 241–53.

Packer, R.J., Sutton, L.N., Atkins, T.E., Radcliffe, J., Bunin, G.R., D'Angio, G., Siegel, K.R. and Schut, L. (1989) A prospective study of cognitive function in children receiving whole-brain radiotherapy and chemotherapy: 2-year results. *Journal of Neurosurgery* **70**, 707–13.

Palmer, M., Adami, H., Krusemo, U.B. and Ljunghall, S. (1988) Increased risk of malignant diseases after surgery for primary hyperparathyroidism: a nationwide cohort study. *American Journal of Epidemiology* **127**, 1031–40.

Park, R.M., Silverstein, M.A., Green, M.A. and Mirer, F.E. (1990) Brain cancer mortality at a manufacturer of aerospace electromechanical systems. *American Journal of Industrial Medicine* **17**, 537–52.

Parkin, D.M., Muir, C.S., Whelan, S.L., Gao, Y.T., Ferlay, J. and Powel, J. (eds) (1992) *Cancer incidence in five continents*, Vol. VI. IARC Scientific Publication 120. Lyon: International Agency for Research on Cancer.

Percy, C. (1985) VI. Alterations of cancer statistical data by the 8th and 9th revisions of the international classification of diseases. *Current Problems in Cancer* **9**, 61–77.

Plesko, I., Preston-Martin, S., Day, N.E., Tzonou, A., Dimitrova, E. and Somogyi, J. (1985) Parity and cancer risk in Slovakia. *International Journal of Cancer* **36**, 529–33.

Polednak, A.P. (1991) Time trends in incidence of brain and central nervous system cancers in Connecticut. *Journal of the National Cancer Institute* **83**, 1679–81.

——(1994) Increased mortality from brain tumors: a combined outcome of diagnostic technology and change of attitude toward the elderly. *American Journal of Epidemiology* **140**, 1138–43.

Polednak, A.P. and Flannery, T. (1995) Brain, other central nervous system, and eye cancer. *Cancer Supplement* **75**, 330–7.

Preston-Martin, S. (1989) Descriptive epidemiology of primary tumors of the brain, cranial nerves and cranial meninges in Los Angeles county. *Neuroepidemiology* **8**, 283–95.

Preston-Martin, S. and Mack, W. (1996) Neoplasms of the nervous system. In Schottenfeld, D. and Fraumeni, J. (eds), *Cancer epidemiology and prevention*. Second edition. Oxford: Oxford University Press, 1231–81.

Preston-Martin, S. and White, S.C. (1990) Brain and salivary gland tumors related to prior dental radiography: implications for current practice. *Journal of the American Dental Association* **120**, 151–8.

Preston-Martin, S., Henderson, B.E. and Peters, J.M. (1982) Descriptive epidemiology of central nervous system neoplasms in Los Angeles County, Los Angeles, California. *Annals of the New York Academy of Sciences* **381**, 202–8.

Preston-Martin, S., Henderson, B.E. and Yu, M.C. (1983) Epidemiology of intracranial meningiomas: Los Angeles County, California. *Neuroepidemiology* **2**, 164–78.

Preston-Martin, S., Mack, W. and Henderson, B.E. (1989) Risk factors for gliomas and meningiomas in males in Los Angeles county. *Cancer Research* **49**, 6137–43.

Preston-Martin, S., Paganini-Hill, A., Henderson, B.E., Pike, M.C. and Wood, C. (1980) Case-control study of intracranial meningiomas in women in Los Angeles county, California. *Journal of the National Cancer Institute* **65**, 67–73.

Preston-Martin, S., Yu, M.C., Benton, B. and Henderson, B.E. (1982) *N*-Nitroso compounds and childhood brain tumors: a case-control study. *Cancer Research* **42**, 5240–5.

Preston-Martin, S., Yu, M.C., Henderson, B.E. and Roberts, C. (1983) Risk factors for meningiomas in men in Los Angeles County. *Journal of the National Cancer Institute* **70**, 863–6.

Preston-Martin, S., Thomas, D.C., White, S.C. and Cohen, D. (1988) Prior exposure to medical and dental x-rays related to tumors of the parotid gland. *Journal of the National Cancer Institute* **80**, 943–9.

Preston-Martin, S., Thomas, D.C., Wright, W.E. and Henderson, B.E. (1989) Noise trauma in the aetiology of acoustic neuromas in men in Los Angeles county, 1978–1985. *British Journal of Cancer* **59**, 783–6.

Preston-Martin, S., Staples, M., Farrugia, H. and Giles, G. (1993) Primary tumors of the brain, cranial nerves and cranial meninges in Victoria, Australia, 1982–1990: patterns of incidence and survival. *Neuroepidemiology* **12**, 270–9.

Preston-Martin, S., Monroe, K., Lee, P.J., Bernstein, L., Kelsey, J., Henderson, S., Forrester, D. and Henderson, B. (1995) Spinal meningiomas in women in Los Angeles County: investigation of an etiological hypothesis. *Cancer Epidemiology, Biomarkers and Prevention* **4**, 333–9.

Preston-Martin, S., Navidi, W., Thomas, D., Lee, P., Bowman, J. and Pogoda, J. (1996a) Los Angeles study of residential magnetic fields and childhood brain tumors. *American Journal of Epidemiology* **143**, 105–19.

Preston-Martin, S., Gurney, J.G., Pogoda, J.M., Holly, E.A. and Mueller, B.A. (1996b) Brain tumor risk in children in relation to use of electric blankets and water bed heaters: results from the United States West Coast Childhood Brain Tumor Study. *American Journal of Epidemiology* **143**, 1116–22.

Preston-Martin, S., Pogoda, J.M., Mueller, B.A., Holly, E.A., Lijinsky, W. and Davis, R.L. (1996c) Maternal consumption of cured meats and vitamins in relation to pediatric brain tumors. *Cancer Epidemiology, Biomarkers and Prevention* **5**, 599–605.

Rabkin, C.S. and Yellin, F. (1994) Cancer incidence in a population with a high prevalence of infection with human immunodeficiency virus type 1. *Journal of the National Cancer Institute* **86**, 1711–16.

Radhakrishnan, K., Mokri, B., Parisi, J.E., O'Fallon, W.M., Sunku, J. and Kurland, L.T. (1995) The trends in incidence of primary brain tumors in the population of Rochester, Minnesota. *Annals of Neurology* **37**, 67–73.

Rainov, N.G., Lubbe, J., Renshaw, J., Pritchard-Jones, K., Luthy, A.R. and Aguzzi, A. (1995) Association of Wilms' tumor with primary brain tumor in siblings. *Journal of Neuropathology and Experimental Neurology* **54**, 214–23.

Rajewsky, M.F., Goth, R., Laerum, O.D., Biessmann, H. and Hülser, D.F (1976) Molecular and cellular mechanisms in nervous system-specific carcinogenesis by *N*-ethyl-*N*-nitrosourea. In Magee, P.N., Takayama, S., Sugimura, T. and Matsushima, T. (eds), *Fundamentals in cancer prevention*. Baltimore: University Park Press, 313–34.

Reif, J.S., Pearce, N. and Fraser, J. (1989) Occupational risks for brain cancer: a New Zealand cancer registry-based study. *Journal of Occupational Medicine* **31**, 863–7.

Reinhardt, G. (1928) Trauma-Fremdkorper-Hirngeschwulst. *Munich Med Worchenschr* **75**, 399–401.

Reis, L.A.G., Miller, B.A., Hankey, B.F., Kosary, C.L., Harras, A. and Edwards, B.K. (eds) (1994) *SEER cancer statistics review, 1973–1991*. NIH Publication No. 94-2789. Bethesda, Md: National Institutes of Health.

Reyes, M., Wilkinson, G.S., Tietjen, G., Voelz, G.L., Acquavella, J.F. and Bistline, R. (1984) Brain tumors at a nuclear facility. *Journal of Occupational Medicine* **26**, 721–4.

Robertson, C.M. and Hawkins, M.M. (1995) Childhood cancer and cystic fibrosis. *Journal of the National Cancer Institute* **87**, 1486–7.

Robinson, N., Beral, V. and Ashley, J.S. (1979) Incidence of pituitary adenoma in women. *Lancet* **2**, 630.

Rodvall, Y., Pershagen, G., Hrubec, Z., Ahlbom, A., Pedersen, N.L. and Boice, J.D. (1990) Prenatal x-ray exposure and childhood cancer in Swedish twins. *International Journal of Cancer* **46**, 362–5.

Roelvink, N.C.A., Kamphorst, W., van Alphen, H.A.M. and Rao, B.R. (1987) Pregnancy-related primary brain and spinal tumors. *Archives of Neurology* **44**, 209–15.

Ron, E., Modan, B., Boice, J.D. Jr, Alfandary, E., Stovall, M., Chetrit, A. and Katz, L. (1988) Tumors of the brain and nervous system after radiotherapy in childhood. *New England Journal of Medicine* **319**, 1033–9.

Ronco, G., Costa, G. and Lynge, E. (1992) Cancer risk among Danish and Italian farmers. *British Journal of Industrial Medicine* **49**, 220–5.

Rothman, K.J. (1986) *Modern epidemiology*. Boston, Mass.: Little, Brown and Company.

Rubio, M.P., Correa, K.M., Ramesh, V., MacCollin, M.M., Jacoby, L.B., von Deimling, A., Gusella, J.F. and Louis, D.N. (1994) Analysis of the neurofibromatosis 2 gene in human ependymomas and astrocytomas. *Cancer Research* **54**, 45–7.

Ruiz, J.C., Cotorruelo, J.G., Tudela, V., Ullate, P.G., Van-Bernal, F., de Francisco, A.L.M., Zukimendi, J.A., Prieto, M., Conga, E. and Arias, M. (1993) Transmission of glioblastoma multiforme to two kidney transplant recipients from the same donor in the absence of ventricular shunt. *Transplantion* **55**, 682–3.

Ryan, P., Lee, M.W., North, B. and McMichael, A.J. (1992a) Amalgam fillings, diagnostic dental x-rays and tumours of the brain and meninges. *European Journal of Cancer, Part B. Oral Oncology* **28B**, 91–5.

——(1992b) Risk factors for tumors of the brain and meninges: results from the Adelaide adult brain tumor study. *International Journal of Cancer* **51**, 20–7.

Ryan, P., Hurley, S.F., Johnson, A.M., Salzberg, M., Lee, M.W., North, B., McNeil, J.J. and McMichael, A.J. (1993) Tumours of the brain and presence of antibodies to toxoplasma gondii. *International Journal of Epidemiology* **22**, 412–19.

SAG (Scientific Advisory Group) (1994) *Potential public health risks from wireless technology: research agenda for the development of data for science-based decision making*. Washington, D.C.: Scientific Advisory Group on Cellular Telephone Research.

Sagan, L.A. (1992) Epidemiological and laboratory studies of power frequency electric and magnetic fields. *Journal of the American Medical Association* **268**, 625–9.

Sahl, J.D., Kelsh, M.A. and Greenland, S. (1993) Cohort and nested case-control studies of hematopoietic cancers and brain cancer among electric utility workers. *Epidemiology* **4**, 104–14.

Salford, L.G., Brun, A., Persson, B.R.R. and Eberhardt, J. (1993) Experimental studies of brain tumor development during exposure to continuous and pulsed 915 mHz radiofrequency radiation. *Bioelectrochemistry and Bioenergetics* **30**, 313–18.

Salisbury, D.A., Band, P.R., Threlfall, W.J. and Gallagher, R.P. (1991) Mortality among British Columbia pilots. *Aviation Space and Environmental Medicine* **62**, 351–2.

Sandler, D.P., Comstock, G.W. and Matanoski, G.M. (1982) Neoplasms following childhood radium irradiation of the nasopharynx. *Journal of the National Cancer Institute* **68**, 3–8.

Sant, M., Crosignani, P., Bordo, B.M., Nicola, G.N., Bianchi, M. and Berrino, F. (1988) Incidence and survival of brain tumors: a population-based study. *Tumori* **74**, 243–52.

Savitz, D.A. (1993) Overview of epidemiologic research on electric and magnetic fields and cancer. *American Industrial Hygiene Association Journal* **54**, 197–204.

Savitz, D.A. and Chen, J. (1990) Parental occupation and childhood cancer: review of epidemiologic studies. *Environmental Health Perspectives* **88**, 325–37.

Savitz, D.A. and Loomis, D.P. (1995) Magnetic field exposure in relation to leukemia and brain cancer mortality among electric utility workers. *American Journal of Epidemiology* **141**, 123–34.

Savitz, D.A., John, E.M. and Kleckner, R.C. (1990) Magnetic field exposure from electric appliances and childhood cancer. *American Journal of Epidemiology* **131**, 763–73.

Savitz, D.A., Pearce, N.E. and Poole, C. (1989) Methodological issues in the epidemiology of electromagnetic fields and cancer. *Epidemiologic Reviews* **11**, 59–78.

——(1993) Update on methodological issues in the epidemiology of electromagnetic fields and cancer. *Epidemiology Reviews* **15**, 558–66.

Schlehofer, B., Blettner, M. and Wahrendorf, J. (1992) Association between brain tumors and menopausal status. *Journal of the National Cancer Institute* **84**, 1346–9.

Schlehofer, B., Blettner, M., Becker, N., Martinsohn, C. and Wahrendorf, J. (1992) Medical risk factors and the development of brain tumors. *Cancer* **69**, 2541–7.

Schneider, A.B., Shore-Freedman, E., Ryo, U.Y., Beckerman, C., Faves, M. and Pensky, S. (1985) Radiation-induced tumors of the head and neck following childhood irradiation – prospective studies. *Medicine* **64**, 1–15.

Schoenberg, B.S., Christine, B.W. and Whisnant, J.P. (1975) Nervous system neoplasms and primary malignancies of other sites: the unique association between meningiomas and breast cancer. *Neurology* **25**, 705–12.

——(1976) The descriptive epidemiology of primary intracranial neoplasms: the Connecticut experience. *American Journal of Epidemiology* **104**, 499–510.

Schreiber, G.H., Swaen, G.M.H., Meijers, J.M.M., Slangen, J.J.M. and Sturmans, F. (1993) Cancer mortality and residence near electricity transmission equipment: a retrospective cohort study. *International Journal of Epidemiology* **22**, 9–15.

Schuman, L.M., Choi, N.W. and Gullen, W.H. (1967) Relationship of central nervous system neoplasms to toxoplasma gondii infection. *American Journal of Public Health* **57**, 848–56.

Schwechheimer, K. and Hashemian, A. (1995) Neuropathologic findings after organ transplantation. An autopsy study. *General Diagnosis and Pathology* **1**, 35–9.

Selverstone, B. and Cooper, D.R. (1961) Astrocytomas and ABO blood groups. *Journal of Neurosurgery* **18**, 602–4.

Shepherd, C.W., Gomez, M.R., Lie, J.T. and Crowson, C.S. (1991) Causes of death in patients with tuberous sclerosis. *Mayo Clinic Proceedings* **66**, 792–6.

Shirts, S.B., Annegers, J.F., Hauser, W.A. and Kurland, L.T. (1986) Cancer incidence in a cohort of patients with seizure disorders. *Journal of the National Cancer Institute* **77**, 83–7.

Shore-Freedman, E., Abrahams, C., Recant, W. and Schneider, A.B. (1983) Neurilemomas and salivary gland tumors of the head and neck following childhood irradiation. *Cancer* **51**, 2159–63.

Shu, X.O., Jin, F., Linet, M.S., Zheng, W., Clemens, J., Mills, J. and Gao, Y.T. (1994) Diagnostic X-ray and ultrasound exposure and risk of childhood cancer. *British Journal of Cancer* **70**, 531–6.

Shugg, D., Allen, B.J., Blizzard, L., Dwyer, T. and Roder, D. (1994) Brain cancer incidence, mortality and case survival: observations from two Australian cancer registries. *International Journal of Cancer* **59**, 765–70.

Simonato, L., L'Abbe, K.A., Andersen, A., Belli, S., Comba, P., Engholm, G., Ferro, G., Hagmar, L., Langard, S., Lundberg, I., Pirastu, R., Thomas, P., Winkelman, R. and Saracci, R. (1991) A collaborative study of cancer incidence and mortality among vinyl chloride workers. *Scandinavian Journal of Work, Environment and Health* **17**, 159–69.

Sinks, T., Steele, G., Smith, A.B., Watkins, K. and Shults, R.A. (1992) Mortality among workers exposed to polychlorinated biphenyls. *American Journal of Epidemiology* **136**, 389–98.

Smulevich, V.B., Fedotova, I.V. and Filatova, V.S. (1988) Increasing evidence of the rise of cancer in workers exposed to vinylchloride. *British Journal of Industrial Medicine* **45**, 93–7.

Solionova, L.G. and Smulevich, V.B. (1993) Mortality and cancer incidence in a cohort of rubber workers in Moscow. *Scandinavian Journal of Work, Environment and Health* **19**, 96–101.

Sorahan, T., Parkes, H.G., Veys, C.A., Waterhouse, J.A.H., Straughan, J.K. and Nutt, A., (1989) Mortality in the British rubber industry 1946–85. *British Journal of Industrial Medicine* **46**, 1–11.

Sorensen, S.A, Mulvihill, J.J. and Nielsen, A. (1986) Long-term follow-up of von Recklinghausen neurofibromatosis survival and malignant neoplasms. *New England Journal of Medicine* **314**, 1010–15.

Sowbhagya, P., Kolluri, V.R.S., Krishna, D.K.S., Das, B.S. and Narayana Reddy, G.N. (1991) Intracranial tumours and blood groups. *European Journal of Cancer* **27**, 221–2.

Spirtas, R., Stewart, P.A., Lee, J.S., Marano, D.E., Forbes, C.D., Grauman, D.J., Pettigrew, H.M., Blair, A., Hoover, R.N. and Cohen, J.L. (1991) Retrospective cohort mortality study of workers at an aircraft maintenance facility. I. Epidemiological results. *British Journal of Industrial Medicine* **48**, 515–30.

Stark, A.D., Chang, H., Fitzgerald, E.F., Riccardi, K. and Stone, R.R. (1990) A retrospective cohort study of cancer incidence among New York State Farm Bureau Members. *Archives of Environmental Health* **45**, 155–62.

Stevens, R.G. (1993) Biologically based epidemiological studies of electric power and cancer. *Environmental Health Perspectives* **101**, 93–100.

Stewart, A. and Kneale, G.W. (1968) Changes in the cancer risk associated with obstetric radiography. *Lancet* **1**, 104–7.

Stiller, C.A. and Nectoux, J. (1994) International incidence of childhood brain and spinal tumours. *International Journal of Epidemiology* **23**, 458–64.

Strang, R.R., Tovi, D. and Lopez, J. (1966) Astrocytomas and the ABO blood groups. *Journal of Medical Genetics* **3**, 274–5.

Stjernfeldt, M., Berglund, K., Lindsten, J. and Ludvigsson, J. (1986) Maternal smoking during pregnancy and risk of childhood cancer. *Lancet* **1**, 1350–2.

Stroup, N.E., Blair, A. and Erikson, G.E. (1986) Brain cancer and other causes of death in anatomists. *Journal of the National Cancer Institute* **77**, 1217–24.

Teppo, L., Salonen, T. and Hakulinen, T. (1975) Incidence of childhood cancer in Finland. *Journal of the National Cancer Institute* **55**, 1065–7.

Teta, M.J., Ott, M.G. and Schnatter, A.R. (1991) An update of mortality due to brain neoplasms and other causes among employees of a petrochemical facility. *Journal of Occupational Medicine* **33**, 45–51.

Theriault, G., Goldberg, M., Miller, A.B., Armstrong, B., Guenel, P., Deadman, J., Imbernon, E., To, T., Chevalier, A., Cyr, D. and Wall, C. (1994) Cancer risks associated with occupational exposure to magnetic fields among electric utility workers in Ontario and Quebec, Canada, and France: 1970–1989. *American Journal of Epidemiology* **139** 550–72.

Thomas, T.L. and Waxweiler, R.J. (1986) Brain tumors and occupational risk factors. *Scandinavian Journal of Work, Environment and Health* **12**, 1–15.

Thompson, D.E., Mabuchi, K., Ron, E., Soda, M., Tokunaga, M., Ochikubo, S., Sugimoto, S., Ikeda, T., Terasaki, M., Izumi, S. and Preston, D.L. (1994) Cancer incidence in atomic bomb survivors. Part II. Solid tumors, 1958–1987. *Radiation Research* **137**, S17–S67.

Thorne, R.N., Pearson, A.D.J., Nicoll, J.A.R., Coakham, H.B., Oakhill, A., Mott, M.G. and Foreman, N.K. (1994) Decline in incidence of medulloblastoma in children. *Cancer* **74**, 3240–4.

Tolley, H.D., Marks, S., Buchanan, J.A. and Gilbert, E.S. (1983) A further update of the analysis of mortality of workers in a nuclear facility. *Radiation Research* **95**, 211–13.

Tornling, G., Gustavsson, P. and Hogstedt, C. (1994) Mortality and cancer incidence in Stockholm fire fighters. *American Journal of Industrial Medicine* **25**, 219–28.

Tornqvist, S., Knave, B., Ahlbom, A. and Persson, T. (1991) Incidence of leukaemia and brain tumours in some electrical occupations. *British Journal of Industrial Medicine* **48**, 597–603.

Turcot, J., Despres, J.P. and St. Pierre, F. (1959) Malignant tumors of central nervous system associated with familial polyposis of the colon: report of two cases. *Diseases of the Colon and Rectum* **2**, 465–8.

Tynes, T. and Haldorsen, T. (1997) Electromagnetic fields and cancer in children residing near Norwegian high-voltage power lines. *American Journal of Epidemiology* **145**, 219–26.

Tynes, T., Jynge, H. and Vistnes, A.I. (1994) Leukemia and brain tumors in Norwegian railway workers, a nested case-control study. *American Journal of Epidemiology* **139**, 645–53.

Unger, M. and Olsen, J. (1980) Organochlorine compounds in the adipose tissue of deceased people with and without cancer. *Environmental Research* **23**, 257–63.

Velema, J.P. and Percy, C.L. (1987) Age curves of central nervous system tumor incidence in adults: variation of shape by histologic type. *Journal of the National Cancer Institute* **79**, 623–9.

Vena, J.E. and Fiedler, R.C. (1987) Mortality of a municipal-worker cohort. IV. Fire fighters. *American Journal of Industrial Medicine* **11**, 671–84.

Verkasalo, P.K., Pukkala, E., Hongisto, M.Y., Valjius, J.E., Jarvinen, P.J., Heikkila, K.V. and Koskenvuo, M. (1993) Risk of cancer in Finnish children living close to power lines. *British Medical Journal* **307**, 895–9.

Vick, N.A. (1994) Commentary. In Gorelick, P.B. and Alter, M. (eds), *Handbook of neuroepidemiology*. New York: Marcel Dekker, 313–15.

Walker, A.E., Robins, M. and Weinfeld, F.D. (1985) Epidemiology of brain tumors: the national survey of intracranial neoplasms. *Neurology* **35**, 219–26.

Walrath, J. and Fraumeni, J.F. Jr (1983) Mortality patterns among embalmers. *International Journal of Cancer* **31**, 407–11.

——(1984) Cancer and other causes of death among embalmers. *Cancer Research* **44**, 4638–41.

Walsh, J., Gye, R. and Connelley, T.J. (1969) Meningioma: a late complication of head injury. *Medical Journal of Australia* **1**, 906–8.

Ward, D.W., Mattison, M.L. and Finn, R. (1973) Association between previous tuberculous infections and cerebal glioma. *British Medical Journal* **1**, 83–4.

Watanabe, K., Sato, K., Yonekawa, Y., Kleihues, P. and Ohgaki, H. (1996) Overexpression of the EGF receptor and *p53* mutations are mutually exclusive in the evolution of primary and secondary glioblastomas. *Brain Pathology* **6**, 217–23.

Weitzner, M.A., Meyers, C.A. and Byrne, K.S. (1996) Psychosocial functioning and quality of life in patients with primary brain tumors. *Journal of Neurosurgery* **84**, 29–34.

Weitzner, M.A., Meyers, C.A., Gelke, C.K., Byrne, K.S., Cella, D.F. and Levin, V.A. (1995) The functional assessment of cancer therapy (FACT) scale. *Cancer* **75**, 1151–61.

Werner, M.H., Phuphanich, S. and Lyman, G.H. (1995) The increasing incidence of malignant gliomas and primary central nervous system lymphoma in the elderly. *Cancer* **76**, 1634–42.

Wertheimer, N. and Leeper, E. (1979) Electrical wiring configurations and childhood cancer. *American Journal of Epidemiology* **109**, 273–84.

——(1982) Adult cancer related to electrical wires near the home. *International Journal of Epidemiology* **11**, 345–55.

Whatmore, W.J. and Hitchcock, E.R. (1973) Meningioma following trauma. *British Journal of Surgery* **60**, 496–8.

White, S.J., McLean, A.E.M. and Howland, C. (1979) Anticonvulsant drugs and cancer. A cohort study in patients with severe epilepsy. *Lancet* **2**, 458–61.

World Health Organization (WHO) (1976) *International classification of diseases for oncology*. First edition. Geneva: World Health Organization.

——(1990) *International classification of diseases for oncology*. Second edition. Geneva: World Health Organization.

Wiencke, J.K., Wrensch, M., Miike, R. and Kelsy, K.T. (1985) Early onset brain cancer in women associated with glutathione s-transferase mu gene deletion: a population based study. (Abstract) *Proceedings of the American Association for Cancer Research* **36**, 118.

Wiggs, L.D., Cox-DeVore, C.A. and Voelz, G.L. (1991) Mortality among a cohort of workers monitored for ^{210}Po exposure 1944–72. *Health Physics* **61**, 71–6.

Wilkins, J.R. and Sinks, T. (1990) Parental occupational and intracranial neoplasms of childhood: results of a case-control interview study. *American Journal of Epidemiology* **132**(2), 275–92.

Wilkinson, G.S., Tietjen, G.L., Wiggs, L.D., Galke, W.A., Acquavella, J.F., Reyes, M., Voelz, G.L. and Waxweiler, R.J. (1987) Mortality among plutonium and other radiation workers at a plutonium weapons facility. *American Journal of Epidemiology* **125**, 231–50.

Wong, O. and Raabe, G.K. (1989) Critical review of cancer epidemiology in petroleum industry employees, with a quantitative meta-analysis by cancer site. *American Journal of Industrial Medicine* **15**, 283–310.

Wong, O. and Whorton, M.D. (1993) Diagnostic bias in occupational epidemiologic studies: an example based on the vinyl chloride literature. *American Journal of Industrial Medicine* **24**, 251–6.

Wong, O., Whorton, M.D., Foliart, D.E. and Ragland, D. (1991) An industry-wide epidemiologic study of vinyl chloride workers, 1942–1982. *American Journal of Industrial Medicine* **20**, 317–34.

Wrensch, M.R. (1983) Epidemiology of malignant brain tumors with emphasis on occupational, residential, and familial factors. *Dissertation Abstracts International* **44**, 2390-B.

Wu, W., Steenland, K., Brown, D., Wells, V., Jones, J., Schulte, P. and Halperin, W. (1989) Cohort and case-control analyses of workers exposed to vinyl chloride: an update. *Journal of Occupational Medicine* **31**, 518–23.

Yates, P.O. and Pearce, K.M. (1960) Recent change in blood-group distribution of astrocytomas. *Lancet* **1**, 194–5.

Zulch, K.J. (1979) *Histological typing of tumors of the central nervous system*. Geneva: World Health Organization.

CHAPTER 2

Mechanisms of altered growth control

Cytogenetics, oncogenes and suppressor genes

SANDRA H. BIGNER, SURINDER K. BATRA AND B.K. AHMED RASHEED

Introduction

Tumors of the nervous system are among the neoplasms that were studied earliest by cytogenetics. In the prebanding era, Zang and Singer (1967) described loss of a G-group chromosome as a nonrandom finding in meningiomas. Some of the first reports of double-minute chromosomes (Dmins) included examples of neuroblastomas and medulloblastomas containing these structures (Cox, Yuncken and Spriggs, 1965; Lubs and Salmon, 1965; Cox, 1968; Levan, Manolov and Clifford, 1968).

The first large series of adult brain tumor karyotypes was reported by Mark in 1971. He observed that near-diploid stemlines predominated in these tumors, with smaller proportions of cases having stemlines in the near-triploid and near-tetraploid regions. He also noted the presence of Dmins in 13/50 cases.

With the development of chromosome banding techniques in the early 1970s, the missing G-group chromosome in meningiomas was identified as chromosome 22 (Mark, Levan and Mitelman, 1972; Zankl and Zang, 1972). The first descriptions of banded glioma karyotypes were from studies of permanent cultured cell lines (Mark, 1974a, 1974b; Mark, Pontén and Westermark, 1974; Mark *et al.*, 1977). In contrast to findings in the direct chromosome preparations in the prebanding era, these studies yielded mainly near-triploid and near-tetraploid stemlines with numerous numerical and structural deviations. Gains and losses of specific chromosomes were difficult to determine in these reports, due to the high chromosome counts, but increased copies of chromosomes 7 and 19 and decreased copies of chromosomes 4, 10, 12 and 22 were noted. The chromosomes most frequently involved in structural deviations were 1, 7, 8, 12, 13, 14 and 15.

In the early 1980s, reports by Al Saadi and Latimer (1980, 1983) and Bigner *et al.* (1984) described gains of chromosome 7 and losses of chromosome 10 in the majority of near-diploid tumors. The chromosomes involved most frequently in structural deviations were 1, 6, 9 and 13, and Dmins were seen in 50% of cases. Later studies by Bigner *et al.* (1986, 1988b) confirmed these numerical deviations and showed that the most common structural abnormalities involved 9p and, to a lesser extent, 19q. Since these early publications, more than 300 glioma karyotypes have been reported (detailed in the next section). Although additional changes, such as loss of chromosome 22 and structural abnormalities of 19q and 13q, have been noted in subgroups of cases, the abnormalities of chromosomes 7, 9 and 10 and the presence of Dmins have remained the most prevalent features.

Studies of medulloblastoma have revealed the most consistent finding to be the presence of isochromosome 17q, resulting in loss of 17p in approximately 1/3 cases (Bigner *et al.*, 1988c; Griffin *et al.*, 1988). The Dmins are seen in 5–10% of cases (Bigner *et al.*, 1988c). Other notable observations include loss of chromosome 22 in a subset of ependymomas and rhabdoid tumors.

With the dawning of the molecular era in the mid-1980s, many of these karyotypic observations were explained. The majority of glioblastomas multiforme (GBMs) with Dmins contain amplification of the epidermal growth factor receptor (*EGFR*) gene (Bigner *et al.*, 1987), while a few cases bearing these structures have amplified *MYCN, GLI,* murine double-minute 2 (*MDM2*), platelet-derived growth factor receptor (*PDGFR*), *CDK4*, or *CCND1* genes. Medulloblastomas with Dmins, in contrast, have amplification of the *MYC* or *MYCN* genes (Rouah *et al.*, 1989; Bigner *et al.*, 1990a). Loss of 9p is associated with homozygous deletion and loss of expression of the *CDKN2A* and *CDKN2B* genes located in this chromosomal region. The neurofibromatosis (NF) type 2 (*NF2*) gene has been localized to 22q. With cloning and characterization of this gene, it has been found to be mutated or inactivated in most meningiomas and schwannomas bearing loss of this chromosomal region.

But some of the karyotypic observations remain unexplained. While loss of 17p has been documented by loss of heterozygosity (LOH) studies in a subset of medulloblastomas, the *TP53* gene, which is located in this region, is mutated in only a few of these tumors. These observations suggest that a novel, as yet undescribed, suppressor gene on 17p is important in these tumors (Steck *et al.*, 1997). The region of chromosome 10 that is lost in gliomas has been narrowly localized to 10q25–6, and the *PTEN* gene (Li *et al.*, 1997), located near this region, is mutated in a subset of these tumors. Whether or not *PTEN* is the only relevant chromosome 10 tumor suppressor gene in gliomas has not yet been determined. Furthermore, the molecular explanation for gain of chromosome 7 remains obscure.

Molecular studies, particularly LOH analysis, have also revealed new findings not suspected by cytogenetic studies. For example, approximately 1/3 of GBMs have loss of 17p, which is frequently associated with *TP53* gene mutations in these tumors, although abnormalities of 17p are not particularly striking in glioma karyotypes.

In this chapter, the karyotypic deviations of central nervous system (CNS) tumors will be reviewed along with the molecular alterations of these tumors. We will focus on the enormous strides that have brought us closer to an understanding of the molecular events responsible for the genesis and evolution of these tumors, but we will also acknowledge the vast gaps in our present knowledge.

Gliomas

CYTOGENETIC ANALYSIS

The earliest reports of glioma karyotypes included only small numbers of cases. These observations on unbanded spreads included high-grade astrocytomas with near-diploid stems, although near-tetraploid sidelines were sometimes seen (Lubs and Salmon, 1965; Bicknell, 1967; Wilson, Kaufmann and Barker, 1970), and the first description of Dmins in a GBM was made by Hansteen in 1967. The first large series of GBM karyotypes was published in 1971 by Mark. He observed that approximately 75% of these tumors had pseudodiploid, diploid or near-diploid stemlines and that near-tetraploid tumors were more than twice as common as near-triploid tumors. Structural deviations were seen in approximately 75% of cases, and the C and D groups contained the most abnormalities. Four of the 50 gliomas studied contained Dmins in their stemlines, and an additional nine cases had these structures in sporadic cells.

The first reports of banded glioma karyotypes were performed on permanent, cultured cell lines (Mark, 1974a, 1974b; Mark, Pontén and Westermark, 1974; Mark *et al.*, 1977). In contrast to direct preparations, 4/7 lines in these initial studies had stemlines in the near-triploid region, with two lines having diploid/near-diploid stemlines and one line having a hypotetraploid stemline. Taken together, these lines had a proportional increase in chromosomes 7 and 19, and decreases of chromosomes 4 and 22 and, most likely, also of chromosomes 10 and 12. The chromosomal regions with the highest incidence of structural changes were the near-centromeric region of chromosome 1, the centromeric/near-centromeric regions of chromosomes 7 and 8, the middle regions of the long arms of chromosomes 12, 13 and 14, and the centromeric region of chromosome 15.

In 1980, Yamada *et al.* described loss of a chromosome 22 in two resected high-grade astrocytomas and a translocation involving a chromosome 22 in an oligodendroglioma. That same year, an abstract published by Al Saadi and Latimer (1980) included descriptions of loss of a chromosome 22 in one glioma, and a second glioma with 48,XX,+7,+8. One glioma was 46,XX, one was hypertriploid and the remaining seven cases had 45,X0 or 47,XX or XY,+7 populations. In 1983, Rey *et al.* also described loss of a chromosome 22 in a high-grade glioma. Al Saadi and Latimer, in 1983, noted abnormalities of chromosomes 7, 22 and the Y in a series of GBMs as part of an abstract publication. In 1984, Bigner *et al.* described nonrandom findings in a series of GBMs. They demonstrated that 5/6 GBMs with abnormal, near-diploid stemlines had gain of one or more chromosome 7 and loss of a chromosome 10. Six of the total 12 tumors showed Dmins. Other deviations included loss of a chromosome 22 and structural abnormalities of chromosomes 1, 6, 9 and 13. In 1986, in a series of 15 additional glioma karyotypes, Bigner *et al.* demonstrated that aside from Dmins, 9p alterations were the most common structural deviations. During the past decade, more than 300 karyotypes of high-grade adult gliomas have been published. Gains of chromosome 7, occurring in up to 80% of near-diploid tumors; losses of all or part of chromosome 10, occurring in up to 60% of near-diploid tumors; the presence of Dmins, occurring in 15–50% of tumors; and structural abnormalities of 9p, occurring in about 33% of cases, have remained the most prevalent findings (Rey *et al.*, 1987b; Bigner *et al.*, 1988b; Jenkins *et al.*, 1989; Thiel *et al.*, 1992; Debiec-Rychter *et al.*, 1995; Hecht *et al.*, 1995) (Fig. 2.1).

Subsets of GBMs and small numbers of low-grade astrocytomas and oligodendrogliomas have shown stemlines or sidelines of 45,X0 or 47,XX or XY,+7. Initially, the significance of these observations was controversial, with opinions divided as to whether these abnormalities were occurring in neoplastic cells or whether these populations were normal brain cells exhibiting these changes in short-term culture. The demonstration that cultures of normal brain from patients without tumors may show 45,X0 or trisomy 7 has fairly conclusively proven that cells with these changes alone are not necessarily neoplastic (Heim *et al.*, 1989; Lindström *et al.*, 1991; Moertel *et al.*, 1993). Furthermore, fluorescence *in situ* hybridization (FISH) analysis has shown retention of sex chromosomes in specimens of normal and gliotic brain tissue that showed sex chromosome loss by karyotype (Dalrymple *et al.*, 1994).

Low-grade gliomas

Reports of glioma karyotypes in the prebanding era contain few accounts of low-grade tumors. Mark (1971) describes one oligodendroglioma with a hypodiploid stemline, and Lubs and Salmon (1965) include one oligodendroglioma with a tetraploid stemline. Using banding, Rey *et al.* (1987c) showed in their series that all four low-grade adult astrocytomas had normal stemline karyotypes, although one case had a sideline with monosomy 22 and two cases had sidelines with gains of chromosome 7, loss of chromosome 10 and additional abnormalities. Griffin *et al.* (1992) report five adult low-grade astrocytomas, three of which had normal or 45,X0 stemlines and two of which had abnormal stemlines with structural changes. Among 21 low-grade astrocytomas described by Thiel *et al.* (1992), 17 cases had normal karyotypes, or stemlines or sidelines with isolated sex chromosome loss or trisomy 7. The remaining four cases included three tumors with sidelines, each lacking a single autosome, and one tumor with a pseudodiploid stemline containing multiple deletions and unbalanced translocations.

Banding studies of oligodendrogliomas revealed normal cells with sidelines containing isolated sex chromosome losses in 5/10 cases studies by Rey *et al.* (1987c). Four of the five remaining cases had near-diploid sides and one had a hypertriploid sideline. Chromosome 7 was involved in numerical and/or structural deviations in three of these cases with near-diploid sidelines, and one tumor also had deletions of chromosomes 9 and 10. Among 15 successful karyotypic preparations from oligodendrogliomas, 11 cases had normal stemlines, often with associated nonclonal changes, and/or isolated sex chromosome loss (Ransom *et al.*, 1992a). The remaining four cases had structural abnormalities involving chromosomes 7 and 10 in one case and chromosome 9 in another case. Six mixed oligoastrocytomas also described by these investigators (Ransom *et al.*, 1992b) showed similar findings of normal or 45,X0 populations, sometimes with variant cells, in five cases, and one case with structural abnormalities involving the Y and other unidentified chromosomes. Griffin *et al.* (1992) described 10 oligodendroglioma karyotypes, including one atypical oligodendroglioma, one mixed oligoastrocytoma and one anaplastic oligodendroglioma. All 10 cases had normal stemlines. Three cases had 45,X0 sidelines and one case had a 45,XY,–22 sideline. Thiel *et al.* (1992) reported 12 oligodendroglioma karyotypes. Their findings were

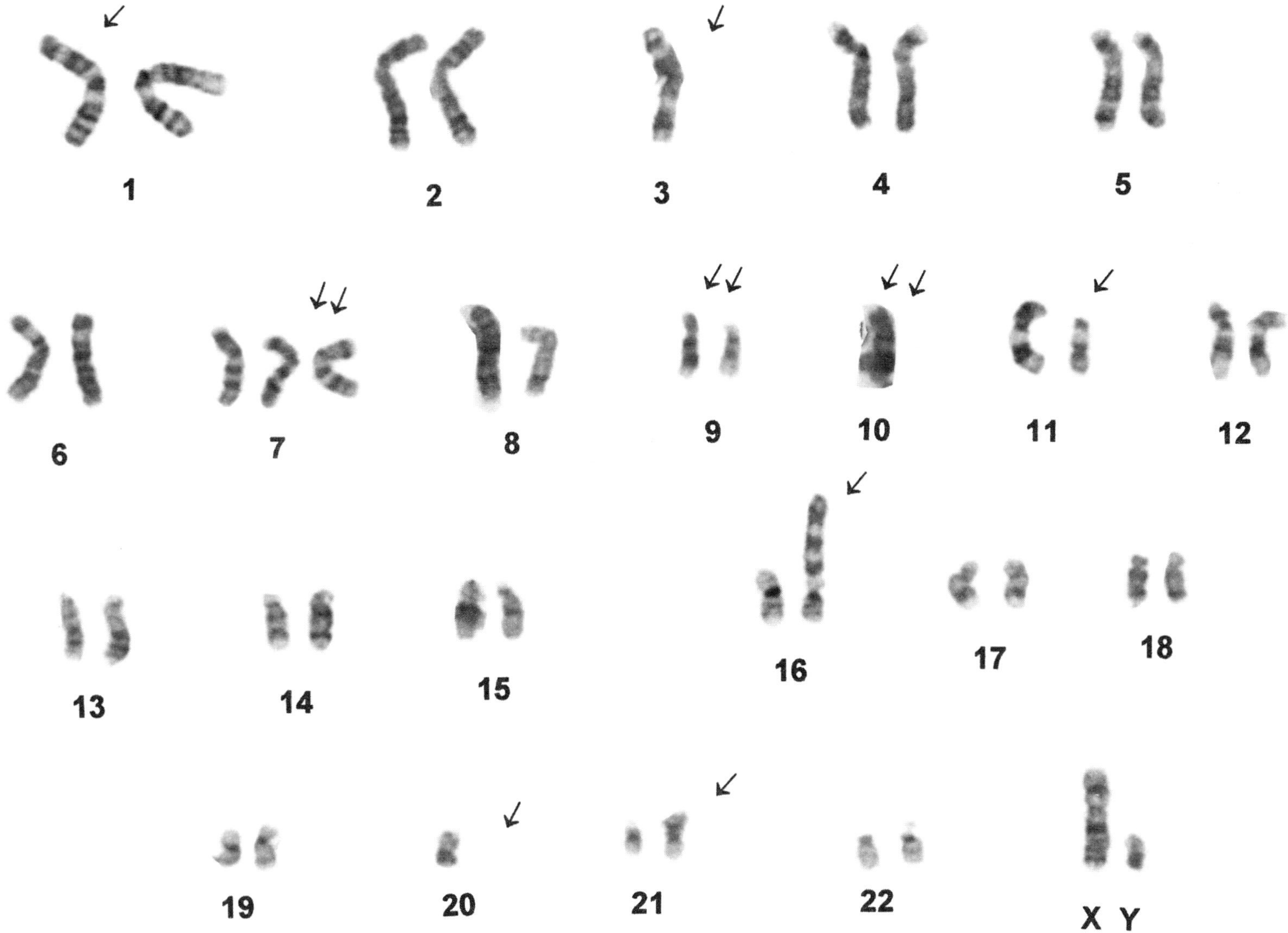

Fig 2.1 Karyotype, with Giemsa-trypsin banding of glioblastoma D-904 MG. The most prevalent features of glioblastoma are present: gain of chromosome 7 (double arrows), loss of chromosome 10 (double arrows), structural abnormalities of both copies of 9p (double arrows), as well as additional numerical and structural alterations (single arrows).

similar to those in the series reported by others (Rey *et al.*, 1987c; Griffin *et al.*, 1992; Ransom *et al.*, 1992a, 1992b) in that most cases had normal stemlines, often with 45,X0 sidelines. Four of the 12 cases had loss or deletion of a chromosome 22, and five cases contained sidelines with simple chromosomal gains and losses.

Childhood gliomas

In the prebanding era there are few reports of childhood glioma karyotypes. Bicknell (1967) describes a recurrent ependymoma in a 16-year-old boy with a stemline in the triploid–tetraploid range, with numerical and structural abnormalities, including small fragments. In his series of childhood brain tumor karyotypes, Mark (1970) includes a pseudodiploid ependymoma with markers and an ependymoma with a sharp mode of 83 and structural abnormalities from a 15-year-old girl and a 4-year-old boy, respectively. He also reports an optic nerve glioma with an apparently normal karyotype.

As in the adult, banding studies revealed that the majority of low-grade astrocytomas in children have normal stemlines, with occasional cases containing variant cells. Interestingly, one cerebellar astrocytoma from a 12-year-old girl showed extensive telomeric association, and a pilocytic astrocytoma from a 10-year-old girl showed telomeric association as well as additional numerical and structural abnormalities (Bigner *et al.*, 1996). Telomeric association with ring formation has been reported by Sawyer *et al.* in a case of recurrent pleomorphic xanthoastrocytoma (1992) and in another of cerebellar astrocytoma (1993).

For high-grade astrocytic tumors [anaplastic astrocytomas (AAs) and GBMs], occasional examples of gains of chromosome 7 have been reported in near-diploid tumors, but this alteration does not appear with the high (approximately 80%) frequency that it does in adult gliomas. However, the series of childhood tumors reported by Vagner-Capodano *et al.* (1992), Neumann *et al.* (1993) and Bigner *et al.* (1996) include a total of nine astrocytic tumors with hyperdiploid (greater than 50 chromosomes) stemlines; eight of these nine cases contain gains of one or two copies of chromosome 7. A significant inconsistency among these reports, however, is that Neumann *et al.* (1993) found this pattern in a subset of low-grade pilocytic astrocytomas while Vagner-Capodano *et al.* (1992) and Bigner *et al.* (1996) describe these findings in high-grade tumors. In addition, Bigner *et al.* (1996) include four cases of astrocytic tumors with deletions of portions of 7q that have not been seen in other series. Monosomy 10 was seen in 2/4 near-diploid gliomas described by Bigner *et al.* (1996), and loss of chromosome 10 or portions of 10q have been reported in occasional cases in other series (Chadduck, Boop and Sawyer, 1991–92; Vagner-Capodano *et al.*, 1992; Neumann *et al.*, 1993). The true incidence of chromosome 10 loss is difficult to define in childhood gliomas because of polyploidy in many of the cases.

The chromosomes most frequently reported to have structural abnormalities are 9 and 17. Neumann *et al.* (1993) describe loss of 9p through deletion and unbalanced translocations in two cases of AA. Karnes *et al.* (1992) report an unbalanced translocation involving 9p in an AA and Fujii, Hongo and Hayashi (1994) describe monosomy 9 in an optic nerve glioma and a GBM. Bigner *et al.* (1996) report loss of 9p in four childhood gliomas through unbalanced translocations and i(9q). Loss of 17p through unbalanced translocation or i(17q) was seen in five gliomas by Bigner *et al.* (1996) and i(17q) was observed in an AA by Griffin *et al.* (1988). In contrast to adult high-grade gliomas and medulloblastomas, Dmins are uncommon in childhood gliomas and have been reported in only a few cases (Fujii, Hongo and Hayashi, 1994; Agamanolis and Malone, 1995; Bigner *et al.*, 1996).

Ependymomas differ from other low-grade gliomas in that abnormal stemlines are encountered in a substantial proportion of cases, exceeding 50% in some series (Vagner-Capodano *et al.*, 1992; Neumann *et al.*, 1993). The stemlines are most frequently in the near-diploid range, but there is considerable variation among cases, with some tumors exhibiting only numerical deviations, while others contain complex numerical and structural changes. The most common abnormality is loss or structural alteration of chromosome 22, which is seen as an isolated finding in some cases and as part of a more complex picture in others. Although some observers have noted this abnormality in a high proportion of their cases (Weremowicz *et al.*, 1992; Rogatto *et al.*, 1993; Wernicke *et al.*, 1995), the overall incidence of chromosome 22 involvement in childhood ependymomas by karyotype is approximately 10–20% in cases with abnormal stemlines (Bown *et al.*, 1988; Stratton *et al.*, 1989; Chadduck, Boop and Sawyer, 1991–92; Vagner-Capodano *et al.*, 1992; Weremowicz *et al.*, 1992; Neumann *et al.*, 1993; Rogatto *et al.*, 1993, Sawyer *et al.*, 1994; Agamanolis and Malone, 1995; Wernicke *et al.*, 1995; Bigner *et al.*, 1996).

ALLELOTYPING STUDIES

Adult gliomas

In the earliest allelotyping study reported by James *et al.* (1988), 37 tumor samples were analyzed with at least one probe from each chromosome, and nonrandom loss of loci from chromosomes 10 (>90%), 13 (14%), 17 (22%) and 22 (19%) were found. The chromosome 10 loss was restricted to GBM. Other chromosomal losses were found in at least one tumor of each malignancy grade. Allelotyping using at least one marker for each nonacrocentric arm (26 GBMs and 15 AAs), Fults *et al.* (1990) demonstrated LOH for 10p, 10q and 17p loci in about 35% of tumors, and LOH for 5q, 7p, 11p, 14q and 15q loci in about 20% of tumors. The median fractional allelic loss (FAL) for GBM patients (0.224) was twice that of AA patients (0.108), indicating a correlation between number of chromosomal abnormalities and malignancy grade. Ransom *et al.* (1992b), in a series containing 45 astrocytomas (39 grade 4, four grade 3 and two grade 2) and seven mixed oligoastrocytomas, observed frequent LOH for 10p (52%), 10q (62%) and 17p (47%) loci. Nonrandom loss (>18%) of loci was seen in 5p, 6p, 7q, 9p, 13q, 14q and 19p. The median FAL ratio for astrocytomas was 0.17 and much less for mixed oligoastrocytomas. Karlbom *et al.* (1993) noted frequent loss of loci on chromosome 9 (55%), 10 (87%), 13 (18%) and 17 (31%) among high-grade gliomas (29 GBMs and 4 AAs). Analysis of 37 tumors of oligodendroglial origin (21 oligodendrogliomas and 16 mixed oligoastrocytomas) revealed LOH for 19q (81%), 1p (67%), 9p (19%), 10q (19%) and 17p (19%) (J. Reifenberger *et al.*, 1994).

Childhood gliomas

Among tumors of young adults and children, LOH for chromosome 22 loci was seen in 3/4 ependymomas. None of the tested loci showed LOH in three pilocytic astrocytomas included in this study (James *et al.*, 1990). Similar analysis carried out on 17 tumors of children and young adults (eight oligodendrogliomas, six ependymomas and three pilocytic astrocytomas) found LOH for 19q loci in four oligodendrogliomas. Cytogenetics showed that four ependymomas exhibited abnormalities of chromosome 22 and there was no consistent abnormality among pilocytic astrocytomas (Ransom *et al.*, 1992a). Extensive allelotyping of nine high-grade childhood tumors using microsatellite markers revealed LOH for 2p in three cases, 9p in two cases, 9q in two cases, 10q in three cases and 16q in three cases. Three of 13 ependymomas showed allelic loss of 22q. Among the 12 pilocytic astrocytomas, the only abnormalities detected were a deletion in 17q and another in 9q (Blaeker *et al.*, 1996).

COMPARATIVE GENOMIC HYBRIDIZATION

Comparative genomic hybridization (CGH) of nine high-grade adult tumors (seven GBMs and two AAs) displayed gain of chromosome 7 (in eight cases), loss of 9p (five cases), loss of chromosome 10 (eight cases), loss of chromosome 17 (three cases), gain of chromosome 19 (five cases), gain of chromosome 20 (three cases) and loss of 22q (five cases). Amplification at the *EGFR* locus (7p12) was seen in four cases. Six new amplification sites mapped to 1q32, 4q12, 7q21.1, 7q21.2, 12p and 22q12 were also seen (Schröck *et al.*, 1994). Among 10 low-grade astrocytomas, gain of 7q occurred in five cases; gain of 12p, loss at 1p, 4q, X and amplification of 8q occurred in two cases each (Schröck *et al.*, 1996). In another study using DNA from four tumors and five xenografts, amplification sites on 7p12 (five cases), 1q32 (two cases), 4q12, 5p15, 7q31 and 8q24 (one case each) were found (Muleris *et al.*, 1994). Gains of chromosome 7 and losses of chromosomes 10, 18, 13, 11, 9, 14, 4, 6, 1 and X (in order of frequency) were found in CGH analysis of 10 glioma cell lines (Mohapatra, Kim and Feuerstein, 1995). There were no consistent abnormalities found in five pediatric low-grade astrocytomas (Schröck *et al.*, 1996).

SUMMARY OF FINDINGS BY KARYOTYPE, ALLELOTYPE AND COMPARATIVE GENOMIC HYBRIDIZATION

When taken together, the results of karyotyping, allelotyping and CGH of adult GBMs demonstrate that gains of chromosome 7 and losses of all or part of chromosome 10 occur in at least 80% of cases. Subsets of between 1/3 and 1/2 of cases contain losses of 9p, 13, 17p and 22q, and possess Dmins (Table 2.1). More than 50% of childhood AAs and GBMs have abnormal stemlines. Although subsets have gains of chromosome 7, and losses of 9p, 10q and 17p, these abnormalities do not occur with the high frequency that they do in adult tumors. The most common abnormalities in LOH studies of oligodendroglial tumors are losses of 19q and 1p, occurring in 81% and 67% of tumors, respectively, while the most frequent abnormality in ependymomas is loss of 22q, occurring in more than 75% of cases in some series. The known suppressor genes *CDKN2, RB1* and *TP53* are located on 9p, 13q and 17p, respectively; and, in a number of LOH cases, mutations in the remaining allele of *TP53*, and to a

Table 2.1 Chromosomal and genetic alterations in glioblastoma

Chromosomal deviation	Genetic alteration	Approximate incidence (%)
+7	Unknown	80
–9p	*CDKN2A* deletion	30–40
–10	Unknown	60–90
–17p	*TP53* mutation	33
Dmins	*EGFR* gene amplification (often with rearrangement)	30–50

lesser extent in *RB* and *CDKN2* genes, have been demonstrated, confirming that they are the target of allele loss. The *NF2* gene is located on 22q, but its role as a suppressor gene in astrocytomas and ependymomas has not been established. For other frequent LOH regions, studies have mainly focused on defining critical deletion regions, but the target genes remain unknown.

Cytogenetic and allelotypic studies of low-grade adult astrocytomas have revealed few deviations, while CGH has demonstrated the provocative finding of gain of 7q in 50% of tumors studied. Aside from some cases of 17p loss and *TP53* gene mutation as discussed in the following sections, few abnormalities have been described in low-grade childhood gliomas.

ALTERATIONS OF GENES INVOLVED IN CELL CYCLE CONTROL

In mammalian cells, the cyclin D–CDK4 complexes phosphorylate RB1 protein and abolish its negative control over G1 exit and entry into the S phase. The protein p16 encoded by the tumor suppressor gene *CDKN2A* exerts negative control over cell proliferation by binding to CDK4 and preventing the cyclin D–CDK4 phosphorylation of RB1 protein. Recent studies suggest that alteration of one of the components of the regulatory mechanism composed of CDKN2, CDK4 and RB1 is common among subgroups of gliomas.

Deletions in 9p

Structural abnormalities with loss of 9p are one of the most common specific findings seen in gliomas. Molecular characterization of these deletions was first carried out using markers for the α and β interferon genes. When genomic DNA from 19 cell lines established from malignant glioma were probed with the *IFNA* and *IFNB* genes, Miyakoshi *et al.* (1990) found complete loss of both the *IFNA* and *IFNB* genes in five cell lines and loss of *IFNA* sequences in three other cell lines. Both *IFNA* and *IFNB* genes have been mapped to 9p22. In tumor biopsies, James *et al.* (1991) found LOH for *IFNB1* in 10/15 informative cases. Deletion of *IFNA* gene sequences were observed in all the tumors lacking *IFNB*, and in two additional tumors positive for *IFNB*. All of the tumors that lost interferon genes were high-grade tumors (AAs and GBMs). Olopade *et al.* (1992) reported hemizygous or homozygous deletion of interferon genes in 13/37 tumor samples that included 23 high-grade tumors. The homozygous deletions in interferon gene clusters pointed to the possibility of either the interferon genes, or genes in close proximity to them, being the target tumor suppressor genes on 9p. Similar deletions were also reported in various tumors, including melanomas, acute lymphoblastic leukemias, and lung and bladder cancers.

CDKN2A

Inactivation of the *CDKN2A* gene (mapped to 9p21) by homozygous deletion is observed in various types of tumors, including gliomas (Kamb *et al.*, 1994). In a study using xenografts, exon 1 of *CDKN2A* was homozygously deleted in 26/38 GBMs, but not in 14 medulloblastomas and five ependymomas. The gene was also deleted in four corresponding primary tumors tested. No mutations in *CDKN2A* were found in the 12 remaining xenografts without deletion. Similarly, 27/38 xenografts contained deletions of *CDKN2B*, with no mutations in the remaining 11 xenografts (Jen *et al.*, 1994). Data collected in several laboratories indicate an overall incidence of homozygous deletions of 33% (98/300) in GBMs and 24% in AAs (19/79); and hemizygous deletion or LOH for 9p loci in 24% of GBMs and 18% of AAs. Among the 23 low-grade astrocytomas analyzed, none exhibited homozygous deletion, although five showed LOH. Altogether, there were only three cases of mutations, all in GBMs (Giani and Finocchiaro, 1994; He *et al.*, 1994a; Schmidt *et al.*, 1994; Ueki *et al.*, 1994, 1996; Li *et al.*, 1995a; Moulton *et al.*, 1995; Nishikawa *et al.*, 1995; Sonoda, Yoshimoto and Sekiya, 1995; Walker *et al.*, 1995b). By sequencing clones from polymerase chain reaction (PCR) product, Kyritsis *et al.* (1996b) have reported a higher incidence of mutation (5/35), but in only a fraction of tumor cells (1.3–22%). The high frequency of homozygous deletions on chromosome 9, and the inclusion of *CDKN2A* and *CDKN2B* gene sequences in the deleted region in most cases, indicated that *CDKN2A* and *CDKN2B* are the target suppressor genes. Unlike the *TP53* gene, the *CDKN2A* gene is inactivated in gliomas mostly by homozygous deletions. However, alternative mechanisms, such as transcriptional silencing by hypermethylation of CpG islands, may be responsible for reduced expression in some gliomas with intact *CDKN2A* and *CDKN2B* genes (Herman *et al.*, 1995). It has been demonstrated that the introduction of *CDKN2A* gene into glioma cell lines results in marked growth suppression in cells lacking the endogenous gene, but had little effect on wild-type cells (Arap *et al.*, 1995, Tenan, Benedetti and Finocchiaro, 1995). Attempts to find *CDKN2A* deletions in nonastrocytic tumors have been unsuccessful (Jen *et al.*, 1994, Walker *et al.*, 1995a).

CDK4 *amplification*

It was first noted in human sarcomas that *CDK4* gene located on 12q13 was amplified as part of the amplification unit that also includes *MDM2* and *GLI* genes (Khatib *et al.*, 1993). In an analysis of 234 primary tumors comprising all grades of gliomas, G. Reifenberger *et al.* (1994) found amplification of *CDK4* and *SAS* (sarcoma amplified sequence) in 18 cases of high-grade tumors. Amplification was always associated with overexpression and, in some high-grade gliomas and PNETs, increased transcript without gene amplification was detected. Also, *MDM2* was coamplified in 11 tumors, and *GLI* in six cases. Based on the finding that *CDK4* was amplified in 2/10 cell lines that had intact *CDKN2* gene, He *et al.* (1994a) proposed that *CDKN2* inactivation and *CDK4* amplification are alternate mechanisms. Among 14 GBM tumors with intact *CDKN2*, Schmidt *et al.* (1994) found amplification of *CDK4* in seven tumors compared with 2/32 GBMs with *CDKN2* loss. The *CDK4* gene was also amplified in 3/11 AA cases without *CDKN2* alteration. Nishikawa *et al.* (1995) noted amplification of *CDK4* in 3/5 high-grade tumors that exhibited increased expression of *CDKN2A*.

Retinoblastoma gene: loss of heterozygosity in 13q

The *RB1* locus is mapped to chromosome 13q14. The observation of structural abnormalities of chromosome 13 in a subset of gliomas raised the possibility of *RB1* gene alterations in gliomas. By restriction fragment length polymorphism (RFLP) analysis using chromosome 13 probes, loss of 13q loci was found in 5/37 GBMs (James *et al.*, 1988), 2/32 tumors (one GBM and one AA) (Fults *et al.*, 1990), 10/45 tumors (Ransom *et al.*, 1992b), 0/40 tumors (Frankel *et al.*, 1992), 6/37 tumors (Karlbom *et al.*, 1993) and 4/9 tumors (Venter *et al.*, 1991). Loss of heterozygosity for a repeat within the *RB1* locus was seen in 0/12 astrocytomas, 2/10 grade III astrocytomas and 14/44 GBMs. Among the LOH cases, single-strand conformation polymorphism (SSCP), followed by sequencing, revealed mutations in two cases, and immunohistochemistry showed altered expression in four cases, three of which were LOH tumors (Henson *et al.*, 1994). He, Olson and James (1995), in an analysis of 45 gliomas by Western blot, found lack of p16 in 15 cases (10 homozygous deletion, three hemizygous), increased *CDK41* in six cases, and lack of RB1 protein in 10 cases. The lack of *RB1* expression was more common among tumors that had a normal complement of *CDKN2A* and *CDK4*. In only three cases, lack of *RB1* coexisted with lack of *CDKN2A* or *CDK4* overexpression. Similarly, of the 42 GBM tumors studied in another series, 26 had *CDKN2* alterations; 14 tumors had LOH at the *RB1* locus, including three cases with point mutations; and except for four cases, these two abnormalities were mutually exclusive (Ueki *et al.*, 1996).

Loss of heterozygosity in 17p

The overall frequency of 17p LOH is about 29% in GBMs (81/276), 41% in AAs (42/103) and 31% (13/42) in astrocytomas (El-Azouzi *et al.*, 1989; Fults *et al.*, 1989, 1992a; James *et al.*, 1989; Venter and Thomas, 1991; Frankel *et al.*, 1992; von Deimling *et al.*, 1992a; Lang *et al.*, 1994a; Leenstra *et al.*, 1994; Rasheed *et al.*, 1994; Tenan *et al.*, 1994; Hermanson *et al.*, 1996). The nearly equal frequency of 17p loss seen in both high- and low-grade tumors suggested the presence of a suppressor gene on 17p associated with early steps of tumorigenesis common to both astrocytomas and GBMs.

TP53 *mutations*

It is now established that *TP53* is the target tumor suppressor gene in a number of tumor types with LOH for 17p. Point mutations in the coding region of the remaining allele of *TP53* have been discovered, confirming the functional inactivation of both copies of *TP53* in these tumors. In the initial study where *TP53* mutations were described in a various types of cancer, five GBM tumors were analyzed and point mutations were identified in four tumors (Nigro *et al.*, 1989). The mutations were clustered in the same hot spots as were seen in colon, breast and lung carcinomas. The incidence of *TP53* mutations confirmed by sequence data in various reports is about 25% (73/295) in GBMs, 34% (49/144) in AAs and 30% (33/111) in astrocytomas (Chung *et al.*, 1991; Mashiyama *et al.*, 1991; Frankel *et al.*, 1992; Fults *et al.*, 1992a; von Deimling *et al.*, 1992a; Louis *et al.*, 1993; Kraus *et al.*, 1994; Lang *et al.*, 1994b; Rasheed *et al.*, 1994; Tenan *et al.*, 1994; Alderson *et al.*, 1995; Chen *et al.*, 1995; Hermanson *et al.*, 1996; Kyritsis *et al.*, 1996a). Most of the *TP53* studies concentrated on conserved exons 5–8. However, some of the studies that included the entire coding sequences (exons 2–11) have uncovered only a handful of mutations outside of exons 5–8 (Chung *et al.*, 1991; Mashiyama *et al.*, 1991; Frankel *et al.*, 1992; Fults *et al.*, 1992a; Lang *et al.*, 1994b). As in colon cancer, codons 175, 248 and 273 are frequently mutated in brain tumors; however, the codon most frequently mutated in brain is codon 273, whereas in colon it is codon 175 (Bogler *et al.*, 1995). The incidence of *TP53* mutations is lower in nonastrocytic tumors than in astrocytomas. The few examples of mutations include 2/17 oligodendrogliomas, 0/15 ependymomas (Ohgaki *et al.*, 1991); 1/8 oligodendrogliomas, 0/10 ependymomas (Rasheed *et al.*, 1994); 0/9 oligodendrogliomas and mixed oligoastrocytomas (J. Reifenberger *et al.*, 1994); 0/17 ependymomas (Bijlsma *et al.*, 1995) and 1/7 oligodendrogliomas (Hermanson *et al.*, 1996). Mutations of *TP53* are also rare among pediatric patients: 1/7 pilocytic astrocytomas (Lang *et al.*, 1994b); 1/6 high-grade, 0/28 astrocytomas (Rasheed *et al.*, 1994); 0/14 high-grade, 0/17 pilocytic astrocytomas (Litofsky, Hinton and Raffel, 1994); 1/8 AA, 1/20 pilocytic astrocytomas (Willert *et al.*, 1995); 0/8 pilocytic astrocytomas, 0/2 astrocytomas, 0/6 high-grade (Chen *et al.*, 1995); and 0/17 pilocytic astrocytomas (Hermanson *et al.*, 1996). However, there is one report of high incidence of *TP53* mutations (8/13) among pontine gliomas of juvenile onset (Zhang *et al.*, 1993). Most of the *TP53* mutations, both sporadic and germline, identified in astrocytomas are G:C→A:T transitions located at CpG sites, and resemble the pattern of mutations found in colon cancer, sarcomas and lymphomas. Such mutations are believed to result from spontaneous deamination of 5-methyl cytosine common at CpG sites, rather than being caused by environmental carcinogens. The type of *TP53* mutations found in non-small-cell lung cancer and liver cancer are different, and are considered to be associated with tobacco-related carcinogens and aflatoxin B1 (Kleihues, Aguzzi and Ohgaki, 1995).

p53 accumulation

The p53 protein is not detectable immunologically in normal tissue because of its short half-life. Many p53 missense mutants have a longer half-life and are detectable by immunological techniques. Overall incidence of immunostaining using antibodies against the p53 protein is about 34% (63/185) in GBMs, 52% (49/94) in AAs and 37% (30/81) in astrocytomas. However, there is no strict correlation between LOH on 17p and p53 mutations identified by immunostaining or by PCR/SSCP sequencing. Mutation in the remaining allele has not been found in about 30–40% of tumors with 17p loss, and not all cases with *TP53* mutations are immunopositive (Frankel *et al.*, 1992; Fults *et al.*, 1992a; Louis, 1994; Rasheed *et al.*, 1994, Kyritsis *et al.*, 1996a). Accumulation of p53 protein in the absence of mutation has been detected in adult tumors (Rubio *et al.*, 1993) as well as pediatric tumors (Lang *et al.*, 1994b). These findings have led some investigators to suggest the existence of another suppressor gene on 17p (Frankel *et al.*, 1992; Fults *et al.*, 1992a; Saxena *et al.*, 1992).

MDM2 *amplification*

Another mechanism implicated in the abnormal functioning of the *TP53* gene, mainly seen in soft tissue sarcomas, is the amplification of the *MDM2* gene located at 12q13. The *MDM2* gene product forms a complex with p53 protein and can inhibit p53-mediated transactivation (Momand *et al.*, 1992). It is suggested that amplification and overexpression of *MDM2* may provide an alternative mechanism of *TP53* inactivation distinct from *p53* mutations. In the largest series of tumors tested, *MDM2* was amplified in 6/75 GBMs and 3/27 AAs. Amplification was associated with mRNA overexpression. Two of the tumors exhibited amplification of *EGFR*. No amplification was seen in 22 astrocytomas, 18 oligodendrogliomas and eight ependymomas (Reifenberger *et al.*, 1993). Other studies have found only rare cases of *MDM2* amplification: in 0/40 (Saxena *et al.*, 1992), 0/10 (Rubio *et al.*, 1993), 1/120 (Rasheed *et al.*, 1994) and 0/65 (Lang *et al.*, 1994b) primary tumors and 2/30 GBM-derived cell lines (He *et al.*, 1994b). These results suggest that *MDM2*-mediated *TP53* alteration is uncommon among gliomas.

BCL2 *expression*

Wild-type p53 is part of the cellular machinery responsible for arresting proliferation or inducing apoptosis in response to DNA damage. The p53-mediated apoptosis is inhibited by the oncogene

BCL2. Alderson *et al.* (1995) found *BCL2* expression in 7/7 gliomas with wild-type p53 and in only 1/7 tumors with mutant p53. Weller *et al.* (1995) reported a higher number of *BCL2* immunoreactive cells in grade III/IV tumors than in I/II tumors. However, another study detected expression of *BCL2* in all the 63 high- and low-grade tumors analyzed. There was no correlation between expression and malignancy grade. The p53 status in these tumors is unknown (Krishna, Smith and Recht, 1995). Tachibana *et al.* (1995) found a correlation between expression of *APT1*, an apoptosis-signal receptor gene, and malignancy grade. By reverse transcriptase (RT)-PCR, mRNA coding for *APT1* was found in 1/4 pilocytic astrocytomas, 1/9 astrocytomas, 6/12 AAs and 9/9 GBMs (Tachibana *et al.*, 1995). A novel gene, *BRAG1* (brain-related apoptosis gene), related to *BCL2,* has been cloned from a human glioma cell line. The gene is expressed predominantly in brain tissue, and aberrant-size transcript is found in gliomas (Das *et al.*, 1996)

TP53 *germline mutations*

Germline *TP53* mutations are a predisposing factor in Li-Fraumeni syndrome, in which affected family members are at increased risk of developing many types of tumors, including gliomas (Malkin *et al.*, 1990; Srivastava *et al.*, 1990). Kyritsis *et al.* (1994) found an overall rate of 12% germline mutations among 51 glioma patients. Included in this group were 19 patients with multifocal glioma, additional primary tumor or family history of cancer. The mutation rate was 43% if two factors were present, and increased to 67% if all three factors were present. Germline mutations were not seen in patients with unifocal glioma without a family history of cancer or another primary tumor. On the contrary, van Meyel *et al.* (1994) did not find inherited *TP53* mutations among 26 members of 16 families with a history of glioma. Li *et al.* (1995b) found germline mutations in 1/80 among unselected, and 3/15 among selected, familial cancer patients. Chen *et al.* (1995) described germline mutations in two patients who developed GBM before the age of 31. Chung *et al.* (1991) reported a case of germline mutation in an NF type 1 patient with a GBM tumor. Metzger *et al.* (1991) reported a germline *TP53* mutation in a patient with malignant ependymoma. Lübbe *et al.* (1995) identified a germline mutation of the *TP53* gene in a family with four brain tumors in two generations. Taken together, the data suggest that germline *TP53* mutations may have a role in some cases, but it is not the primary predisposing factor among most familial cases of glioma. Turcot's syndrome patients are characterized by the simultaneous occurrence of primary brain tumors and multiple colon adenomas. In a study of two Turcot's syndrome patients, germline *TP53* mutations were not found, although both patients carried somatic mutations in the tumor tissue (one GBM and one astrocytoma). The results suggested that inherited *TP53* mutations may play a role in progression but are not responsible for initiation of tumors in Turcot's syndrome patients (Kikuchi *et al.*, 1993).

OTHER TUMOR SUPPRESSOR GENES

Reduced expression of the *DCC* (deleted in colon cancer, located on 18q) gene was reported in 15/22 glioma samples, including 7/8 GBMs (Scheck and Coons, 1993). Western blotting revealed lack of *DCC* expression in 15/28 GBMs, and RNase protection assays showed lack of transcripts in 12/28 tumors. In another study, no mutations in the *DCC* gene were detected, but in a few cases with LOH for 18q; *DCC* abnormalities resulted from aberrant splicing of transcripts (Ekstrand *et al.*, 1995). Attempts to identify mutations in another colon cancer-related gene, *APC*, were negative in 42 brain tumor samples (8 GBMs, 22 astrocytomas, 2 oligodendrogliomas and 10 GBM cell lines). Only 1/11 informative tumors had LOH at the *APC* locus (Mori *et al.*, 1994). Microsatellite instability, usually seen in tumors with mutant DNA mismatch repair gene, is rare among gliomas in most studies, although one report described this abnormality in 5/10 GBMs and 1/6 astrocytomas (Dams *et al.*, 1995). The *NF2* gene located on 22q was considered a candidate suppressor gene in glioma tumorigenesis because of higher incidence of ependymomas and astrocytomas among NF type 2 patients and the frequent deletions of 22q loci in ependymomas and, to a lesser extent, in gliomas. Three independent studies have failed to uncover somatic *NF2* mutations among gliomas, including those that showed 22q LOH (Rubio *et al.*, 1994a; Hoang-Xuan *et al.*, 1995; Ng *et al.*, 1995), although there was one case of germline mutation in an astrocytoma (Hoang-Xuan *et al.*, 1995) and a somatic mutation in 1/8 ependymomas (Rubio *et al.*, 1994a). Similarly, *NF1* somatic mutations are uncommon among gliomas: 1/10 (Li *et al.*, 1992), 0/18 (Tenan *et al.*, 1993), 0/26 familial glioma cases (van Meyel *et al.*, 1994) and 0/51 childhood brain tumors (Scheurlen and Senf, 1995).

ALLELIC DELETIONS

Loss of heterozygosity in 1p

Loss of heterozygosity for 1p along with LOH for 19q are frequently found in oligodendrogliomas.

Bello *et al.* (1994b) reported LOH for loci on 1p in 6/6 oligodendrogliomas, 5/6 anaplastic oligodendrogliomas and 2/3 mixed oligoastrocytomas. Among other types of glioma, only 2/11 GBMs exhibited 1p LOH, suggesting that 1p LOH is characteristic of tumors of oligodendroglial origin. J. Reifenberger *et al.* (1994) observed 1p loss in 7/8 oligodendrogliomas, 7/13 anaplastic oligodendrogliomas, 1/8 oligoastrocytomas and 2/8 anaplastic oligoastrocytomas, and in all cases it was accompanied by LOH on 19q. Similarly, microsatellite markers revealed 1p loss in 3/9 oligodendrogliomas, 3/6 anaplastic oligodendrogliomas and 12/25 mixed oligoastrocytomas. Among astrocytomas, 6/79 GBMs and 5/26 AAs exhibited 1p loss. There was no LOH at 1p in 19 astrocytomas and 26 pilocytic astrocytomas (Kraus *et al.*, 1995). In a study of a variety of tumors of the nervous system, LOH at 1p was seen in 12/58 gliomas and 17/18 tumors of oligodendroglial origin (Bello *et al.*, 1995). By using FISH, Hashimoto *et al.* (1995) found deletion of a 1p locus in 9/9 oligodendrogliomas, 3/4 mixed oligoastrocytomas, 2/8 astrocytomas, 0/2 AAs and 1/4 GBMs.

Loss of heterozygosity in 2p

Loss of 2p loci was detected in 4/4 informative high-grade pediatric gliomas and 1/9 ependymomas. Unlike LOH on other chromosomes, which includes large deletions, the LOH on 2p is highly localized. The deletion region is mapped to 2p21–p23 (Blaeker *et al.*, 1996).

Loss of chromosome 10 loci

The most frequent molecular abnormality seen in GBM tumors is LOH at chromosome 10 loci (Fig. 2.2). The incidence calculated from published reports is 68% (275/402) in GBMs, 20% (17/86) in AAs and 0% (0/45) in astrocytomas (James *et al.*, 1988; Fujimoto *et al.*, 1989; Watanabe *et al.*, 1990; Venter *et al.*, 1991; Fults *et al.*, 1992a; Ransom *et al.*, 1992b; Rasheed *et al.*, 1992, 1995; Fults and Pedone, 1993; Karlbom *et al.*, 1993; von Deimling *et al.*, 1993; Lang *et al.*, 1994a; Leenstra *et al.*, 1994). The high frequency of chromosome 10 allele loss clearly indicates that critical gene(s) associated with glial tumor initiation/progression are located on chromosome 10. In the majority of cases, allelic loss on chromosome 10 includes loss of a complete copy or large regions of chromosome 10. The limited number of tumors with partial deletions of the chromosome has made mapping of the critical region of loss difficult.

From the allelic loss pattern of 11 tumors with partial loss, we reported a minimal deletion region

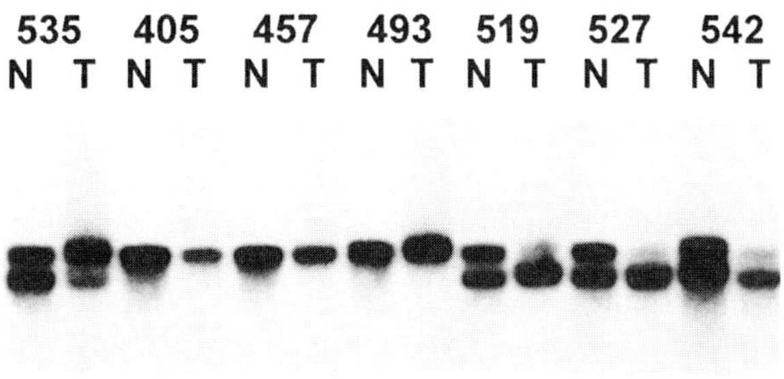

Fig 2.2 Loss of heterozygosity for probes on chromosome 10 in glioblastoma samples as demonstrated by Southern blot. A Southern blot of *Eco*RI-digested DNA (5 μg) from blood (N) and tumor (T) was hybridized to a 10q marker CRI-L368. The alleles were 20 and 17 kb in size. Tumors 535, 519, 527 and 542 show LOH, whereas tumors 405, 457 and 493 are uninformative relative to this marker.

in 10q24–q26 (Rasheed *et al.*, 1992). Ransom *et al.* (1992b) have suggested two deletion intervals: one on the long arm (10q22–q26), and another on the short arm or near the centromere. The data from Karlbom *et al.* (1993) pointed to three separate minimal deletion locations on chromosome 10. One telomeric region is on 10p, and both telomeric and centromeric loci are on the long arm. The availability of more precisely mapped RFLP markers and the highly informative microsatellite markers have helped to refine the critical regions on chromosome 10. Based on the LOH data from six tumors with partial deletion of chromosome 10, Fults and Pedone (1993) indicated an overlapping deletion region in 10q25.1-qter. This region corresponds to 33.4 centimorgans (cM) near the telomere on 10q. Using microsatellite markers, we have defined a deletion region of approximately 5 cM mapped to 10q25.1. This interval was deleted in all but 2/17 tumors that showed partial deletion (Rasheed *et al.*, 1995). In tumors preselected for heterozygosity at a centromeric locus, Kimmelman, Ross and Liang (1996) reported a high rate (69%) of LOH for distal 10p alleles. The allelic loss was seen in both high- and low-grade tumors and included two deletion regions: one at 10p15 and another at a more centromeric locus.

The presence of tumor suppressor genes on chromosome 10 is also supported by chromosome transfer studies. Partial reversion of tumor phenotype in a GBM cell line upon transfer of chromosome 10 has been reported (Pershouse *et al.*, 1993; Steck *et al.*, 1995). Microcell-mediated transfer of chromosome 10 into glioma cell line U-251 MG resulted in suppression of transformed and tumorigenic phenotypes of recipient cells. The hybrid cells containing most of the chromosome 10, as assessed by the gain of heterozygosity at tested loci, had reduced capacity to proliferate in soft agarose and were incapable of forming tumors upon injection into athymic nude mice. However, further characterization of hybrid cells containing portions of chromosome 10 appears to distinguish two functional loci on chromosome 10. The subclones that retained both the distal region of the long arm (10q24–q26) and portions of the short arm lost both their colony-forming and tumor-forming capacity. Subclones lacking most of the long arm of chromosome 10, with portions of 10p retained, grew in soft agarose, but were not able to form tumors in nude mice. In another study, transfection of *RSU1* (*ras* suppressor), mapped to 10p, into glioma cell line U-251 MG and production of the protein resulted in marked reduction of growth rate and inhibition of tumor formation in mice (Tsuda *et al.*, 1995). These observations lend support to the idea of two suppressor loci on chromosome 10. It is speculated that the loss of an entire copy of chromosome 10 in most GBMs is because of the presence of two suppressor loci on this chromosome.

The minimal deletion region in distal 10q defined in gliomas is also one of the common deletion regions in prostate cancer, renal cell carcinoma, malignant melanoma and endometrial cancer (Carter *et al.*, 1990; Morita *et al.*, 1991; Isshiki *et al.*, 1993; Peiffer *et al.*, 1995). This suggests that the tumor suppressor gene on 10q may also be relevant in the development of other types of human tumors. The *PAX2* gene that codes for a transcription factor is localized to 10q25 (Stapleton *et al.*, 1993). The *MXI1* gene encoding a negative regulator of the MYC family of oncoproteins is mapped to 10q24–q25. In 4/10 prostate tumors with 10q LOH, mutations in the remaining allele were identified, suggesting a suppressor gene role for *MXI1* in prostate cancer. Mutations were observed in only a small fraction of cells from each tumor (Eagle *et al.*, 1995). Gray *et al.* (1995) failed to detect *MXI1* mutations in 23 prostate tumors with 10q LOH, and specific loss of *MXI1* as opposed to loss of another 10q23–q25 region was seen in only 1/23 tumors. The deletion data in this series of prostate tumors is suggestive of a suppressor gene located in the 10q23–24 boundary. Recently, homozygous deletions in another newly identified gene, *DMBT1*, located in 10q25, are reported in approximately 20% of GBMs and 10% of medulloblastomas. So far, no mutations are detected in this gene, suggesting that a closely located gene rather than this one may be the real target of these deletions.

PTEN is a putative protein tyrosine phosphatase gene that is located on chromosome 10 at 10q23. This gene has been shown to be deleted or mutated in glioblastoma cell lines and xenografts and in 9/44 (20%) of glioblastoma biopsies, which raises the possibility that this gene may be the target for chromosome 10 loss in gliomas (Li *et al.*, 1997; Steck *et al.*, 1997). *PTEN* is also mutated in prostate and breast cancer cell lines and xenografts, which suggests that it may be an important tumor suppressor gene in a variety of human malignancies. The predicted protein sequence of *PTEN* has extensive homology to tensin, in addition to bearing a protein tyrosine phosphatase domain, suggesting a role both in cellular adhesion and motility and as an antagonist for protein tyrosine kinases.

Deletions in 11p

Fults *et al.* (1992b) found an LOH on chromosome 11 in 11/43 high-grade tumors. The minimal deletion interval was at 11p15, the location of the *HRAS* gene. However, *HRAS* PCR/SSCP assay results were negative, indicating that a gene other than *HRAS* may be the target of 11p deletions in human gliomas. Using microsatellite markers, Sonoda *et al.* (1995) found LOH at 11p in 8/26 high-grade gliomas but not in any of the 12 low-grade gliomas. Deletion mapping studies point to a 21 cM common deletion region in 11p15.5-pter as the likely location of a tumor suppressor gene.

Loss of 19q

Although abnormalities of chromosome 19 are not particularly striking in cytogenetic studies of gliomas, molecular studies have uncovered a high incidence of 19q LOH among oligodendrogliomas. Loss of heterozygosity for 19q loci was seen in 4/4 informative oligodendrogliomas, including one possible homozygous deletion for the marker D19S8 mapped to 19q13.2 (Ransom *et al.*, 1992a). In a survey of 122 tumors (54 grade 4 GBMs, nine grade 3 AAs, six grade 2 astrocytomas, 20 pilocytic astrocytomas, three grade 3 anaplastic oligodendrogliomas, five grade 2 oligodendrogliomas and 25 other tumors), LOH for 19q RFLP markers was found in 11/46 GBMs, 4/9 grade 3 AAs, 2/3 grade 3 anaplastic oligodendrogliomas, 2/5 grade 2 oligodendrogliomas and 10/15 mixed oligoastrocytomas. Low-grade astrocytomas, pilocytic astrocytomas and ependymomas did not show LOH (von Deimling *et al.*, 1992b). Analysis with microsatellite markers showed LOH in 16/76 GBMs, 12/27 AAs, 3/19 astrocytomas, 3/5 anaplastic oligodendrogliomas, 4/9 oligodendrogliomas and 13/19 mixed oligoastrocytomas. Among tumors that lost alleles on chromosome 19, LOH at all informative loci suggestive of complete loss of a copy was more common among oligodendrogliomas than astrocytomas. In 19 gliomas there was partial deletion of chromosome 19 and the common deletion interval was in 19q13.2–q13.4 (von Deimling *et al.*, 1994b). Similarly, Reifenberger *et al.* (1996a), in their series, detected LOH for 19q in 7/8 oligodendrogliomas and 10/13 anaplastic oligodendrogliomas. Among mixed gliomas, the allele loss was less common (5/16). In a related study, LOH on 19p with retention of 19q loci was more frequent among astrocytomas (17/23), and the converse was true among oligodendrogliomas and mixed oligoastrocytomas (12/14) (Ritland, Ganju and Jenkins, 1995). A comparative study of 19q LOH among astrocytomas (grade 2) and AAs (grade 3) revealed LOH in 2/18 astrocytomas and 12/26 AAs, and it has been suggested that the 19q locus may be involved in tumor progression (von Deimling *et al.*, 1994a). The 19q minimal deletion region has been mapped to a 425-kilobase (kb) region on 19q13.3 (Rubio *et al.*, 1994b; Yong *et al.*, 1995a).

Loss of 22q

Allelotyping studies have confirmed loss of 22q alleles in gliomas (James *et al.*, 1988; Fults *et al.*, 1990; Ransom *et al.*, 1992b). In 3/19 high-grade malignant gliomas, loss of 22q loci was detected both by cytogenetics and by RFLP markers. There was no LOH in six astrocytomas and six oligodendrogliomas (Rey *et al.*, 1992). In a larger series, 6/56 (four high-grade and two low-grade) tumors exhibited 22q LOH (Rey *et al.*, 1993). In another series, microsatellite markers revealed LOH for 22q loci in 12/42 GBMs, 4/13 anaplastic astrocytomas, 1/5 astrocytomas, 0/7 oligodendrogliomas and 0/3 mixed oligoastrocytomas (Hoang-Xuan *et al.*, 1995). Bijlsma *et al.* (1995) have reported LOH at 22q loci in 3/17 ependymomas studied.

ONCOGENES

About 50% of GBM tumors contain Dmins, and in the majority of tumors containing Dmins the *EGFR* gene is amplified. Other genes found to be amplified in small numbers of gliomas include *GLI, MDM2, CDK4, CCND1, PDGFRA, MYC, MYCN, MET, REN*, and marker D17S67.

EGFR *gene amplification, rearrangement and overexpression*

The *EGFR* gene was the first gene shown to be amplified in gliomas (Libermann *et al.*, 1985). Data from several laboratories confirm that the *EGFR* gene is amplified in one-third to one-half of GBMs, but only in isolated cases of AAs and rarely in other lower grade tumors. In all cases where amplification of the *EGFR* gene has occurred, high levels of *EGFR* mRNA or protein have been demonstrated (Wong *et al.*, 1987, 1992; Humphrey *et al.*, 1988, 1990; Malden *et al.*, 1988; Yamazaki *et al.*, 1988; Sugawa *et al.*, 1990; Ekstrand *et al.*, 1991, 1992, 1994; Tuzi *et al.*, 1991; Nishikawa *et al.*, 1994; Schwechheimer, Huang and Cavenee, 1995). Overexpression of *EGFR* is reported in a number of neoplasms, including those of lung, breast, esophagus and bladder (reviewed in Gullick, 1991), and J. Reifenberger *et al.* (1994) have described overexpression without amplification in a high proportion of oligodendroglial tumors.

The human *EGFR* gene is highly homologous to the viral oncogenes collectively termed v-*erb*B. The *EGFR* gene is 110 kb in size, has 26 exons and is localized to chromosome arm 7p11–p13. The mature receptor is a 170-kilodalton (kDa) transmembrane glycoprotein composed of three functional domains: an extracellular ligand binding domain, a transmembrane domain and an intracellular tyrosine kinase domain (reviewed in Yarden and Ullrich, 1988). Rearrangements of the *EGFR* gene in gliomas, seen as loss or altered size of bands in Southern blots, are often the result of extensive deletions in the coding sequence of the gene. In most cases, both the normal and a rearranged copy of the gene are amplified, which may suggest that rearrangement follows amplification of the normal copy.

Cumulative results indicate that the rearrangements produce a limited number of alterations at the transcript level, despite variable rearrangements at the genomic level. The class I mutants contain deletion in the extracellular domain, resulting in a mutant receptor similar to that of the v-*erb*B oncogene except for an eight-amino-acid internal extension (Wong *et al.*, 1992). The class II mutants undergo deletions in the extracellular domain of the *EGFR* gene, resulting in an in-frame deletion of 83 amino acids outside the ligand binding domain. Both the ligands, EGF and TGF-α, bind to the mutant EGFR with high affinity and enhance the intrinsic mutant EGFR kinase activity. This mutant is capable of transducing EGF-stimulated glioma cell proliferation and invasiveness in an *in vitro* spheroid model system (Humphrey *et al.*, 1991). This type of mutant is reported in two tumors (Wong *et al.*, 1992). The class III mutants bear deletion of exons 2–7 of the gene, resulting in an in-frame deletion of 801 base pairs of coding sequence and generation of a glycine residue at the fusion point. This variant receptor, designated EGFRvIII, is the most common type of mutant and has been reported in 17–62% of GBMs (Wong *et al.*, 1987; Bigner *et al.*, 1990b; Humphrey *et al.*, 1990; Sugawa *et al.*, 1990; Ekstrand *et al.*, 1991, 1992; Moscatello *et al.*, 1995; Wikstrand *et al.*, 1995) (Fig. 2.3). The tumor cell membrane fractions, containing the mutant 140-kDa receptor, show a significant elevation in tyrosine kinase activity without its ligand. The mutant is still capable of binding with its ligand,

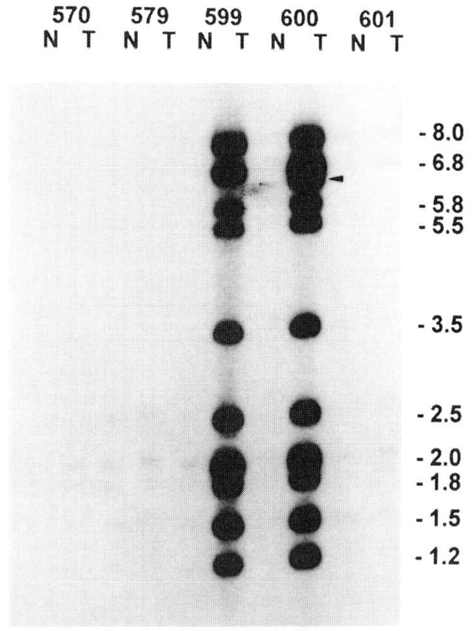

Fig 2.3 Amplification of the *EGFR* gene in glioblastoma samples. A Southern blot of *Eco*RI-digested DNA (5 μg) from blood (N) and tumor (T) was hybridized with the *EGFR* gene probe. In samples with a normal gene copy number, the hybridizing fragments appear as faint bands, and their sizes (in kb) are marked on the right. In tumor 599, the *EGFR* gene is amplified; in tumor 600, the gene is amplified and rearranged. The arrowhead indicates the variant band from the rearranged gene.

but at a significantly reduced affinity. The class IV–VII mutants carry deletions in the cytoplasmic domain, often coexisting with deletion in the extracellular domain. The intracellular deletions, in the limited number of cases studied to date, mostly result in frame shift and truncation of the receptor after the tyrosine kinase domain. All the mutants in the cytoplasmic domain lack amino acid residues between 991 and 1022 and lack Ca^{2+} influx and receptor internalization regions. The lack of regulatory regions in the mutant receptor affects the down regulation of the ligand-bound receptor and, in the absence of this attenuation mechanism, low concentration of ligands would result in uncontrolled proliferation and transformation (Ekstrand *et al.*, 1992).

A high incidence of EGFRvIII expression and the presence of a functional, potentially immunogenic segment in the extracellular portion of the mutant EGFR has provoked the investigation of EGFRvIII as an oncogene and eventual target for therapy. The EGFRvIII cDNA has been demonstrated to transform rodent immortalized fibroblast cells in culture and to develop tumors in nude mice independent of the pressure of EGF or TGF-α (Yamazaki *et al.*, 1988; Batra *et al.*, 1995a; Hills, Rowlinson-Busza and Gullick, 1995). In GBM cells expressing wild-type EGFR, tranfection of EGFRvIII cDNA led to increased tumorigenicity and a shorter latent period for tumor formation as compared with untransfected cells (Nishikawa *et al.*, 1994). This ligand-independent malignant transformation caused by EGFRvIII does not appear to be a consequence of activation of intrinsic kinase activity as judged by direct enzymatic autophosphorylation (Batra *et al.*, 1995a). Some elevation of constitutive phosphorylation actually has been reported (Ekstrand *et al.*, 1994; Nishikawa *et al.*, 1994, Hills, Rowlinson-Busza and Gullick, 1995), and the role of phosphorylation of substrates other than the EGFRvIII itself, such as messengers erb2, phosphatase C and others, remains to be addressed. Montgomery *et al.* (1995) observed that the EGFRvIII constitutively activates downstream ligand transduction via mitogen-activated protein kinase (MAPK).

GLI *gene*

The 12q13–q15 region is rearranged or amplified in a variety of human sarcomas, such as malignant fibrous histiocytoma, rhabdomyosarcoma, osteosarcoma and liposarcoma (Turc-Carel *et al.*, 1986; Mandahl *et al.*, 1987). The GLI gene was the first amplified gene identified from this region (Kinzler *et al.*, 1987). The GLI gene product has a predominantly nuclear localization and is presumed to function as a transcriptional regulator, although its specific targets and function remain unknown. Only isolated instances of GLI gene amplification in gliomas are reported: 6/234 all grades of tumors (G. Reifenberger *et al.*, 1994) and 1/46 GBMs (Rasheed *et al.*, 1994). Normal adult tissues, including brain, do not express detectable levels of mRNA for GLI. Studies to detect GLI gene expression in gliomas have been mostly negative (Salgaller, Pearl and Stephens, 1991; Watkins *et al.*, 1994; Xiao, Goldthwait and Mapstone, 1994).

PDGFRA *gene*

A few tumors exhibit amplification and rearrangement of the *PDGFRA* gene. Kumabe *et al.* (1992) reported amplification of a truncated version of the *PDGFRA* gene in 1/9 gliomas tested. The deletion resulted in the expression of a mutant receptor lacking a portion of the extracellular region. Subsequent studies have documented amplification of *PDGFRA* in 4/50 GBMs (Fleming *et al.*, 1992) and 1/46 GBMs (Rasheed *et al.*, 1994), and 0/37 oligodendroglial tumors (G. Reifenberger *et al.*, 1994). By PCR methods, Hermanson *et al.* (1996) detected gene amplification in 7/43 GBMs. By *in situ* hybridization, higher expression was detected in 13/39 GBMs, 2/7 AAs and 1/6 astrocytomas. Hermanson *et al.* also reported a correlation between overexpression of *PDGFRA* and LOH on 17p. In two independent CGH studies, the chromosomal location of the *PDGFRA* gene, region 4q11–q12, was amplified in 2/18 cases studied (Muleris *et al.*, 1994; Schröck *et al.*, 1994).

OTHER ONCOGENES

The *MET* oncogene, mapped to 7q31, encodes a transmembrane tyrosine kinase and is the receptor for hepatocyte growth factor. In gliomas, it was first reported to be amplified in T3095, a cell line derived from a GBM tumor (Wullich *et al.*, 1993). Fischer *et al.* (1995) reported *MET* amplification in 6/40 cases analyzed, five of which were high-grade tumors.

Birchmeier, Sharma and Wigler (1987) found an elevated level (up to 60-fold) of the *ROS1* oncogene mRNA in 8/12 glioma-derived cell lines, but not in cell lines derived from other tumors. Expression of the *ROS1* gene was observed in 3/11 malignant tumors, but not in more benign tumors or normal glial cells (Mapstone, McMichael and Goldthwait, 1990). Using RNase protection assay, Wu and Chikaraishi (1990) failed to detect overexpression of the *ROS1* gene in 25 primary astrocytomas of all histological grades. By dot-blot screening, Watkins *et al.* (1994) found elevated levels of *ROS1* transcript in 6/17 mostly high-grade gliomas.

Elevated levels of the *ABL1* gene located on 9q34 were first found in the glioma cell line HeRo (Blin *et al.*, 1987). Rearrangement of *ABL1*, with a sequence originating from chromosome 16, was shown in the GBM cell line A172 (Heisterkamp *et al.*, 1990). The cell line lacks germline alleles of *ABL1*. This is the only report of *ABL1* gene alteration in gliomas.

Point mutations of the *RAS* gene are very frequent in human neoplasia, but appear to be rare among human gliomas. Loss of heterozygosity for 11p, where *HRAS* is located, was seen in both high-grade gliomas (11/43) and medulloblastomas (3/11). However, *HRAS* PCR amplification/SSCP screening results were negative for mobility shift in this series of tumors (Fults *et al.*, 1992b). The *KRAS* gene was amplified in one case (Bigner *et al.*, 1988a). Increased expression of *NRAS* at the RNA level has been reported in malignant glioma cell lines and 5/5 patient biopsies (Gerosa *et al.*, 1989). Reduced levels of *HRAS* mRNA were reported in 13/18 primary tumors (Blumenstock *et al.*, 1991). The level of RAS protein expression, determined by immunohistochemistry, is correlated with the severity of 55 gliomas examined in one clinical study (Salgaller, Pearl and Stephens, 1991). Welter *et al.* (1990) reported amplification, rearrangement and overexpression of the *MYB* gene in 2/4 GBM cell lines. In another study, 17/20 glioma cell lines expressed mRNA for the *MYB* gene in roughly equal amounts (LaRocca *et al.*, 1989). Because the reported studies in gliomas were performed in cultured cells, the expression levels of *MYB* may not reflect those in the original tumors.

Members of the *MYC* gene family are infrequently amplified in glioma cell lines and primary biopsies. LaRocca *et al.* (1989) showed expression of MYC in 20/20 glioma cell lines. In another study with anti-*MYC* antibodies, cell lines derived from GBM as well as GBM tissue showed at least a four-fold increase in immunofluorescence compared with normal brain (Engelhard, Butler and Bauer, 1989). It is possible that the increased MYC protein in tumor tissue reflects the increased proliferative state of these cells. Isolated cases of amplification and rearrangement of *MYC* and *MYCN* have been reported. Amplification and rearrangement of *MYC* was seen in a cell line derived from a childhood GBM (Trent *et al.*, 1986), and amplification of *MYC* was seen in another cell line derived from adult GBM (Rasheed *et al.*, 1994). Amplification of *MYCN* was found in 2/63 (Wong *et al.*, 1987) and 0/120 (Rasheed *et al.*, 1994) tumors tested. These results suggest that the *MYC* family of genes have a minimal role in the development of gliomas.

OTHER ABNORMALITIES

Amplification of *REN*, located at 1q32, is reported in one anaplastic oligodendroglioma (J. Reifenberger *et al.*, 1994), *CCND1* gene in one GBM (He, Olson and James, 1995) and marker D17S67 in 3/30 GBMs (Bijlsma *et al.*, 1994a). Approximately 20–30% of glioma cell lines lack the O^6-methylguanine-DNA methyltransferase enzyme, which protects tumor cells from the cytotoxic effects of certain chemotherapeutic alkylating drugs (Day *et al.*, 1983). The gene for this enzyme is located on 10q, and studies have found lack of mRNA and protein but no deletion, rearrangement or amplification of this gene (Ostrowski *et al.*, 1991). The gene expression is regulated at the promoter level by methylation of CpG nucleotides. Many tumor cell lines, including malignant gliomas, are deficient in methylthioadenosine phosphorylase enzyme because of codeletion of the *MTAP* gene, located on 9p21, along with *CDKN2A* and the interferon gene cluster (Nobori *et al.*, 1991; Della Ragione *et al.*, 1995).

MOLECULAR MARKERS IN PROGNOSIS AND PROGRESSION OF GLIOMAS

Investigations of relationships between molecular and cytogenetic abnormalities and histologic and clinical parameters have disclosed several consistent observations. For example, although losses of the q arm of chromosome 19 and of chromosome 22 are seen in subsets of astrocytic tumors, there is a strong association between these deviations and oligodendroglial and ependymal differentiation, respectively. Among astrocytomas, *EGFR* gene amplification and loss of all or part of chromosome 10 are seen mainly in GBMs, occurring infrequently in lower grade tumors. By contrast, *TP53* mutations occur in all grades of astrocytomas; and there is a strong relationship with age of the patient in that young adults (ages 18–50 years) have a considerably higher incidence of this change than do older patients, and *TP53* mutations are uncommon in childhood astrocytomas (Leenstra *et al.*, 1994; Rasheed *et al.*, 1994; Tenan *et al.*, 1994). Furthermore, within GBMs, *TP53* mutations and *EGFR* gene amplification are largely mutually exclusive (von Deimling *et al.*, 1993). These observations have led to the concept of two pathways for GBM: *de novo* tumors, which occur in older patients and often have gene amplification, and the progressive pathway, occurring in young adults, possessing *TP53* mutations and progressing from lower grade tumors (Lang *et al.*, 1994a; Ohgaki *et al.*, 1995; Louis, 1996; Reifenberger *et al.*, 1996b; Watanabe *et al.*, 1996).

Another interesting observation concerns the relationship between abnormalities of the various genes involved in proliferation. Deletions of the *CDKN2A* gene, amplification of *CDK4* or *CCND1* and loss of expression of the retinoblastoma gene *RB1* appear to be mutually exclusive, with most gliomas bearing only one of these changes (He, Olson and James, 1995; Ueki *et al.*, 1996).

Attempts have been made to relate molecular parameters to prognosis. Most studies have shown that although molecular alterations may be associated with clinical parameters, such as age, and histologic parameters, such as grade, which have a bearing on prognosis, the molecular markers described to date do not have independent prognostic significance (Bigner *et al.*, 1988a; Chozick *et al.*, 1994; Kraus *et al.*, 1994; Rasheed *et al.*, 1994; Danks *et al.*, 1995). However, in the series reported by Leenstra *et al.* (1994), patients who had 17p LOH survived longer compared with patients who had 10 LOH and *EGFR* amplification; and studies by Hurtt *et al.* (1992) and Diedrich *et al.* (1995) have found shorter survival times associated with *EGFR* gene amplification. Schlegel *et al.* (1994) found that, following therapy, tumors regrew in a shorter time (9 weeks) in GBM patients with *EGFR* amplification compared with patients without amplification (32 weeks).

In summary, most typical adult GBMs occurring in the older adult contain an aberration of one of the cell-cycle-related genes, such as deletion of *CDKN2A*, or loss of all or part of chromosome 10, and often have amplification of the *EGFR* gene. Astrocytomas in the younger patient, in contrast, start as low-grade tumors, often containing *TP53* gene mutations, and progress to higher grade lesions with acquisition of cell-cycle gene abnormalities and loss of all or part of chromosome 10.

Medulloblastomas

CYTOGENETIC ANALYSIS

Initial reports on karyotypic analysis of medulloblastomas demonstrated that most have near-diploid stemlines, with only occasional near-tetraploid stemlines (Cox, 1968; Mark, 1970); a few cases contain Dmins (Cox, Yuncken and Spriggs, 1965; Lubs and Salmon, 1965). More precise banded karyotypic analysis reveals that the chromosome most commonly involved in structural abnormalities is chromosome 1, although there is no consistency with regard to breakpoints or type of rearrangement (Bigner *et al.*, 1988c; Griffin *et al.*, 1988; Fujii, Hongo and Hayashi, 1994). Abnormalities of chromosome 17 resulting in loss of all or part of the p arm occur in approximately 1/3 of the tumors (Bigner *et al.*, 1988c; Griffin *et al.*, 1988; Biegel *et al.*, 1989; Chadduck, Boop and Sawyer, 1991–92; Karnes *et al.*, 1992; Vagner-Capodano *et al.*, 1992; Neumann *et al.*, 1993; Fujii, Hongo and Hayashi, 1994; Agamanolis and Malone, 1995). These changes include isochromosome 17q [i(17q)] and unbalanced translocations (Figs 2.4 and 2.5). The next most frequent abnormality is monosomy 22, occurring in 25–40% of cases. Biegel *et al.* (1990) noted frequent monosomy 22 in rhabdoid tumors of the CNS, which, according to some observers, represents a variant of medulloblastoma when they occurr in the cerebellum. Rorke, Packer and Biegel (1995) consider these

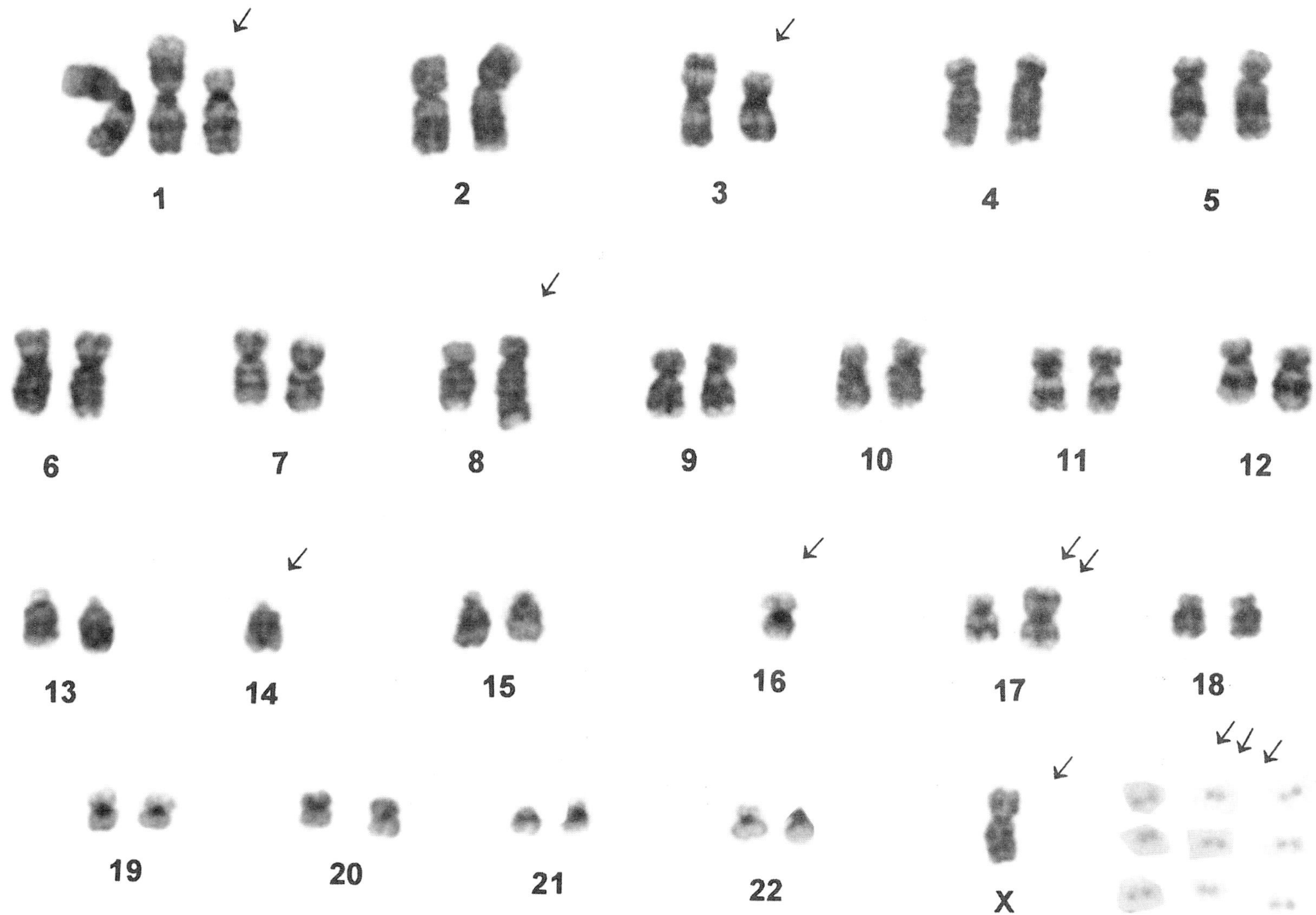

Fig 2.4 Karyotype, with Giemsa-trypsin banding, of cultured medulloblastoma D487 Med showing i(17q) (double arrows) and Dmins (triple arrows). Additional numerical and structural alterations are indicated by single arrows.

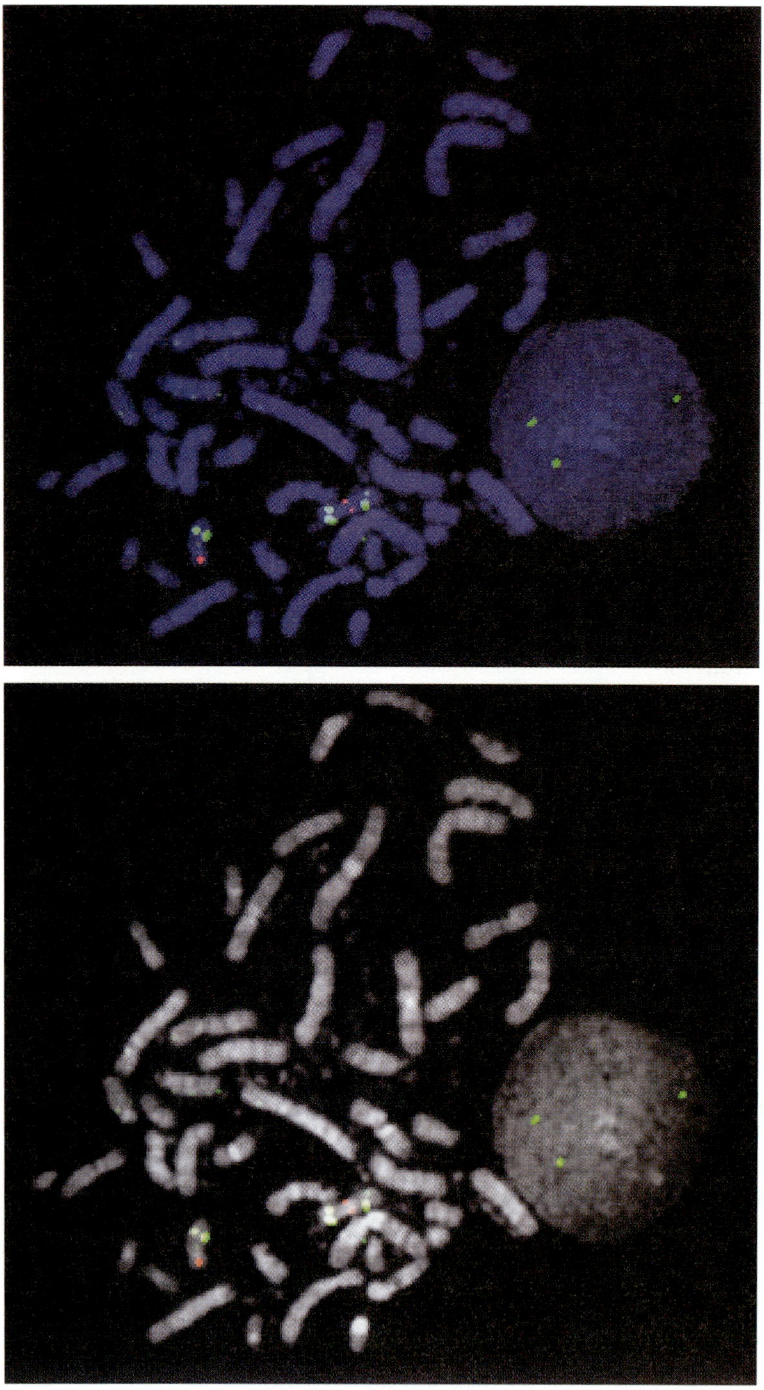

Fig 2.5 Fluorescence *in situ* hybridization using probes that localize to proximal 17p (DI7S122) and 17q (*MPO*) in medulloblastoma cell line D425 Med stained with Dapi. The normal chromosome 17 shows one red signal corresponding to the proximal 17p probe and one double-green signal corresponding to the 17q probe. The i(17q) shows the red signal for the 17p probe near the centromere and two double-green signals indicating two copies of 17q as expected. With the filter set in the lower panel, the banding pattern of the chromosomes and Dmins can be seen.

neoplasms to represent a unique class of CNS tumor. They have named these lesions atypical teratoid/rhabdoid tumors and stress their poor prognosis and their association with monosomy 22. Although some of the small-cell childhood tumors with monosomy 22 may belong to this class of tumor, we believe that there is a subgroup of medulloblastomas bearing monosomy 22, either alone or along with other abnormalities (Bigner *et al.*, 1996).

Other less frequent cytogenetic changes in medulloblastomas are deletions of 6q, 9q, 10q, 11 and 16q (Bigner *et al.*, 1988c; Griffin *et al.*, 1988; Chadduck, Boop and Sawyer, 1991–92; Thomas and Raffel, 1991; Vagner-Capodano *et al.*, 1992). However, these changes are not consistently found in various cytogenetic series, an observation that may be due, in part, to the small number of cases represented in most studies.

ALLELOTYPING STUDIES

The first allelotypic study on 11 medulloblastomas utilized one probe for each of the chromosomal arms (James *et al.*, 1990). This investigation confirmed loss of 17p as the most frequent abnormality, seen in 5/11 informative cases. The next most frequent loss was from chromosome 11, followed by losses of chromosomes 10 and 22. A single case with loss of chromosome 16 was reported in this series. Blaeker *et al.* (1996) recently used 200 microsatellite markers, evenly distributed over the 22 autosomes, to analyze a series of childhood brain tumors, including seven medulloblastomas. This study confirmed frequent loss of 17p (four cases), 10q (five cases), 11p (three cases), 11q (three cases) and 16q (three cases), and also identified new regions of deletion on 2p (four cases) and 8p (three cases).

LOSS OF HETEROZYGOSITY FOR 17P AND MUTATIONS OF THE TP53 GENE

Most LOH studies of medulloblastomas have focused on only a few chromosomal regions. In one such study of 23 tumors, LOH for 17p was found in six cases (Thomas and Raffel, 1991). In another study, a higher incidence of 45% (5/11) for loss of 17p was found (Cogen *et al.*, 1990). Using both cytogenetic and molecular genetic approaches on the same tumor specimens, Biegel *et al.* (1992) found loss of allelic loci for 17p in 50% of tumors (7/14). Albrecht *et al.* (1994) also detected LOH on chromosome 17p in 7/19 medulloblastoma specimens. Using both microsatellite and minisatellite analyses, Batra *et al.* (1995b) observed an LOH for 17p in 8/28 (29%) medulloblastomas (Fig. 2.6). Unlike many other pediatric tumors where the maternal allele is preferentially deleted or disrupted, there was no evidence for preferential loss of one parental allele over the other for chromosome 17p in medulloblastomas (Scheurlen, Krauss and Kuhl, 1995).

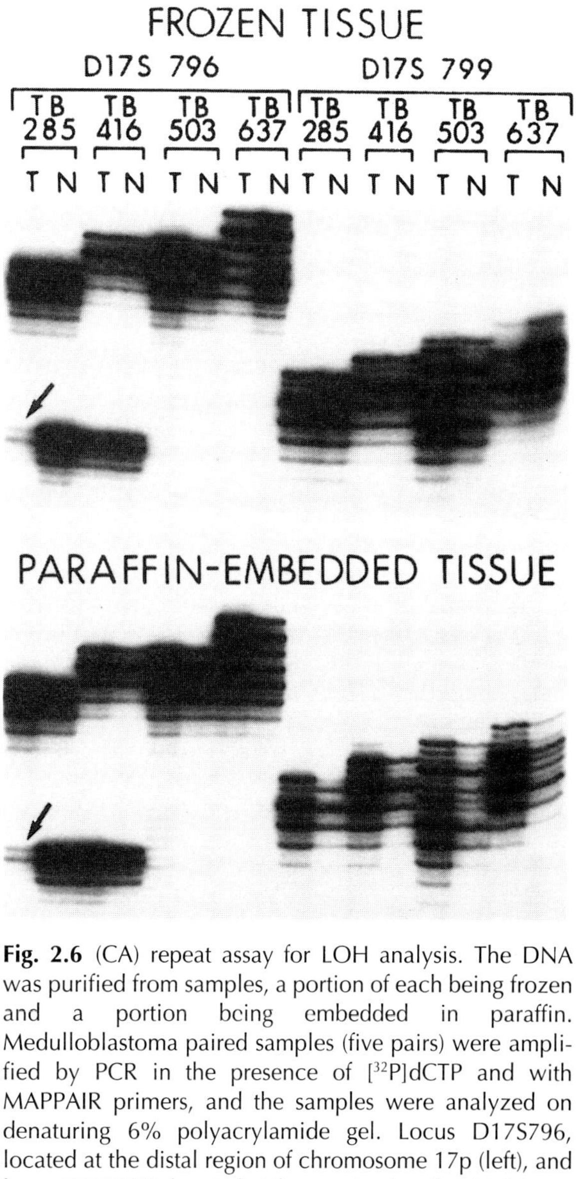

Fig. 2.6 (CA) repeat assay for LOH analysis. The DNA was purified from samples, a portion of each being frozen and a portion being embedded in paraffin. Medulloblastoma paired samples (five pairs) were amplified by PCR in the presence of [^{32}P]dCTP and with MAPPAIR primers, and the samples were analyzed on denaturing 6% polyacrylamide gel. Locus D17S796, located at the distal region of chromosome 17p (left), and locus D17S799, located at the proximal region (right), are presented. The pattern obtained from frozen tissue (upper panel) can be compared with the similar pattern obtained from the paraffin-embedded tissues (lower panel). The PCR products are designated from tumor (T) and normal blood (N). Arrows indicate LOH in specimen TB285 (shown in lane 1).

The most commonly deleted region on chromosome 17 is 17p13.1–13.3, which harbors the tumor suppressor gene *TP53*. This association raises the possibility that its mutant allele may play a role in the malignant transformation. Nevertheless, a low incidence of *TP53* mutations in medulloblastomas has been reported by several groups: 2/19 cases (Ohgaki *et al.*, 1991), 0/12 cases (Saylors *et al.*, 1989), 0/14 cases (Biegel *et al.*, 1992), 2/20 cases (Cogen *et al.*, 1992), 2/22 cases (Badiali *et al.*, 1993), 1/14 cases (Raffel *et al.*, 1993), 1/9 cases (Adesina, Nalbantoglu and Cavenee, 1994) and 2/46 cases (Batra *et al.*, 1995b). The lissencephaly gene 1 (*MDCR*) is also located on chromosome 17p, in the region 17p13.3 most commonly deleted in medulloblastomas. The *MDCR* gene is altered in the Mieler-Dieker lissencephaly, as well as in isolated lissencephaly. Based on the chromosomal localization of *MDCR*, which is distal to *TP53*, Koch *et al.* (1996) examined medulloblastomas for alterations of the *MDCR* gene. Loss of heterozygosity for this region was detected in 13/24 (54%) tumors, whereas none of the tumors showed a somatic mutation in the *MDCR* coding region.

The demonstration of *TP53* mutations in rare cases suggests that it might contribute to the pathogenesis of a small subset of medulloblastomas. In support of this idea, transfer of the wild-type *TP53* gene into a human medulloblastoma cell line, Daoy, containing a mutant copy of *TP53*, induced cell-cycle arrest of the majority of the transduced cells (Rosenfeld *et al.*, 1995). However, most observers believe that it is unlikely that the *TP53* gene is the target of 17p loss in the majority of medulloblastomas.

In addition to intragenic mutations in *TP53*, other proteins involved in the regulation of its function can be targeted and produce the same physiological consequences as direct *TP53* alterations. The human homolog of the *MDM2* gene has been shown to be a potential regulator of p53 activity and is amplified in sarcomas where *TP53* mutations are uncommon (Oliner *et al.*, 1992). Overexpression of MDM2 protein can abolish p53-mediated transactivation (Momand *et al.*, 1992). Cytogenetic analysis of medulloblastomas has shown the presence of Dmins in a subset of cases (Biegel *et al.*, 1989; Bigner *et al.*, 1990a). However, none of the tumors with or without *TP53* mutations showed amplification of the *MDM2* gene, suggesting that amplification of *MDM2* is not an alternative molecular mechanism by which medulloblastoma escapes p53-regulated growth control (Adesina, Nalbantoglu and Cavenee, 1994; Batra *et al.*, 1995b).

The frequent deletion of 17p regions (30–50%) and infrequent *TP53* inactivations (5–10%) in medulloblastomas may be explained in several ways: (1) the *TP53* gene may be inactivated by another unusual mechanism compared with other tumors; or (2) the *TP53* gene is not the target for allelic loss in the majority of medulloblastomas with 17p loss, and a second tumor suppressor gene may be located on the short arm of chromosome 17. In support of the latter explanation, deletion mapping has indicated another telomeric locus distal to *TP53* (Biegel *et al.*, 1992; Cogen *et al.*, 1992). Using pulsed-field gel electrophoresis, McDonald *et al.* (1994) identified an *ABR* gene locus in this region, which is deleted in 88% of informative medulloblastomas.

LOSS OF HETEROZYGOSITY FOR OTHER CHROMOSOMAL REGIONS

Loss of heterozygosity for 11p and 11q was seen in allelotypic studies by James *et al.* (1990) and Blaeker *et al.* (1996). Fults *et al.* (1992b) described LOH of 11p, with the region of common overlap being 11p15.4-pter in 3/11 medulloblastomas. This observation was not confirmed in an LOH study of medulloblastomas from 16 patients by Albrecht *et al.* (1994).

Interestingly, a loss of chromosomal segment 2p21–p23 was also observed in 3/4 informative cases of medulloblastomas (Blaeker *et al.*, 1996). Although cytogenetic studies have failed to identify this area in medulloblastomas, it could be due to the smaller size of the lost region.

As in childhood high-grade gliomas, a partial loss of chromosome 10 was observed in a subset of medulloblastomas (James *et al.*, 1990; Blaeker *et al.*, 1996), which is in contrast to adult high-grade gliomas where the entire chromosome 10 is lost in the majority of cases. Loss of heterozygosity of chromosomal arms 6q, 9q, 10q, 16q and 22q has also been reported in a few cases (James *et al.*, 1990; Thomas and Raffel, 1991; Schofield *et al.*, 1995; Blaeker *et al.*, 1996).

TUMOR SUPPRESSOR GENES

In recent studies, another tumor suppressor gene, adenomatous polyposis coli (*APC*), has been implicated in the pathogenesis of medulloblastomas. The *APC* gene originally showed mutations in germline DNA of patients with familial adenomatous polyposis and sporadic colorectal adenomas and carcinomas (Groden *et al.*, 1991; Nishisho *et al.*, 1991). In Turcot's syndrome, which is characterized clinically by symptoms of both primary brain tumors and adenomatous polyposis coli, Hamilton *et al.* (1995) demonstrated a frequent occurrence [10/12 families (83%)] of germline mutations for *APC* in families classified as having polyposis. Interestingly, the authors reported that the predominant brain tumor in the families who had mutations in the *APC* gene was medulloblastoma (79%), and that both copies of the *APC* gene were inactivated in the medulloblastomas of the patients studied. The patients with familial adenomatous polyposis were 92 times higher at risk than the general population for developing medulloblastomas. It is possible that in patients carrying germline mutations in the *APC* gene, inactivation of the second copy of the gene may lead to the pathogenesis of medulloblastoma. In another study, Mori *et al.* (1994) reported germline mutations in the *APC* gene of Turcot's syndrome patients (3/3) and somatic mutations in the other normal copy of the *APC* gene of all three colorectal adenomas, but could not demonstrate somatic mutations in the *APC* gene of corresponding medulloblastomas of these Turcot's syndrome patients (2/3). These results could have been either due to the technical difficulty of identifying alterations in the large gene without DNA sequencing, or merely coincidental due to the small number of tumors. It is common for LOH to occur at the chromosomal locus where an inactivated tumor suppressor gene is located. However, Yong *et al.* (1995b) observed no LOH at the locus of the *APC* gene on chromosome 5q in 27 sporadic medulloblastomas. Also, no mutations of the *APC* gene were found in 41 sporadic medulloblastomas (Mori *et al.*, 1994). These studies indicate that the role of the *APC* gene in medulloblastomas from patients with Turcot's syndrome is unique and that somatic mutations of the *APC* gene are rare in sporadic medulloblastomas. Recently, mutations in the *PTCH* gene, located on 9q22, have been demonstrated in medulloblastomas that occurred in nevoid basal cell carcinoma syndrome (NBCCS) patients and in medulloblastomas (approximately 15%) that were sporadic.

ONCOGENE AMPLIFICATION

The Dmins, which are cytogenetic evidence for gene amplification, are seen in occasional medulloblastoma karyotypes, but are present in the majority of medulloblastoma cell lines and xenografts. Although *MYC* amplification is infrequent in primary biopsies as determined by Southern blot analysis: 2/7 cases (Bigner *et al.*, 1990a), 1/10 cases (Raffel, Gilles and Weinberg, 1990), 0/20 cases (Wasson *et al.*, 1990), 0/27 cases (Badiali *et al.*, 1991) and 3/43 cases (Batra *et al.*, 1995b), the majority of medulloblastoma cell lines and xenografts have amplification, sometimes with rearrangement, and overexpression of the *MYC* gene (Friedman *et al.*, 1988; Bigner *et al.*, 1990a; Wasson *et al.*, 1990; Batra *et al.*, 1994; Pietsch *et al.*, 1994). The discrepancy between the incidence of *MYC* amplification in biopsies and in culture or xenograft suggests that this property may be necessary for medulloblastoma cells to establish in culture and to be propagated as xenografts. Since it is predominantly biopsies taken at the time of diagnosis that have been examined, the incidence of *MYC* amplification in recurrent or progressed medulloblastomas is not known with any degree of accuracy. Interestingly, an analysis of medulloblastoma biopsies using CGH showed high copy number of regions on 2p24 and 8q24, suggesting amplification of *MYCN* and *MYC* genes, respectively, in 4/18 (22%) cases (Schütz *et al.*, 1996).

Amplification of *MYCN* occurs in about one-third of neuroblastomas and is established as an indicator of poor prognosis (Brodeur *et al.*, 1984). Although medulloblastoma has a strong histologic resemblance to neuroblastoma, *MYCN* amplification is limited in medulloblastomas: 0/9 cases (Garson *et al.*, 1989), 1/20 cases (Wasson *et al.*, 1990), 0/27 cases (Badiali *et al.*, 1991) and 0/43 cases (Batra *et al.*, 1995b). Rouah *et al.* (1989) reported two cases of primitive neuroectodermal tumors that showed *MYCN* amplification and exhibited neuroblastic differentiation. In another study, an increased expression of the *MYCN* gene was observed in 6/11 medulloblastoma samples as determined by immunocytochemistry using an antiserum raised against a synthetic peptide of a sequence unique to the *MYCN* gene product (Garson *et al.*, 1989). Of the 12 medulloblastoma samples collected over a 2-year period, a trend towards longer disease-free survival was observed in patients having low levels of *MYCN* in their tumors (Garson *et al.*, 1989).

Other oncogenes studied in medulloblastomas include *EGFR, GLI, ERBB2, HRAS, KRAS, NRAS, PDGFB* and *SRC*. Amplification of *EGFR* has been reported in 1/20 tumors (Wasson *et al.*, 1990) and 0/43 tumors (Batra *et al.*, 1995b). It seems that oncogene amplification is infrequent in medulloblastomas, and it represents the principal mechanism of oncogene activation only in a small subset of medulloblastomas. Precise information on the incidence of oncogene mutations in medulloblastomas is limited. Iolascon *et al.* (1991) found mutation of the *NRAS* gene at codon 61 in 3/32 (9%) medulloblastomas. Moscatello *et al.* (1995) reported a high incidence 86% (6/7) of *EGFRvIII* expression in medulloblastomas. Further studies are necessary to confirm the high incidence of *RAS* activation or *EGFRvIII* expression in medulloblastomas.

MOLECULAR MARKERS OF PROGNOSIS IN MEDULLOBLASTOMAS

Loss of 17p loci has been correlated with poor response to treatment in a limited number of medulloblastoma cases (Cogen, 1991; Cogen *et al.*, 1992).

Table 2.2 Chromosomal and genetic alterations in nonastrocytic brain tumors

Tumor type	Chromosomal deviation	Genetic alteration	Approximate incidence (%)
Oligodendroglioma	–19q	Unknown	90–100
	–1p	Unknown	50–100
Ependymoma	–22	Unknown	10–20
Medulloblastoma	–17p	Unknown	33
	Dmins	*MYC* or *MYCN* gene amplification	5–18
Meningioma	–22	*NF2* gene mutation	60
Schwannoma	–22	*NF2* gene mutation	60

In a recent study, Batra *et al.* (1995b) observed that LOH for 17p (8/28 cases) was associated with a shortened survival period ($P = 0.045$ by the logrank test). These results suggest that LOH of chromosome 17p is indicative of a significantly worse prognosis among patients with these tumors. Rorke, Packer and Biegel (1995) have noted that atypical teratoid/rhabdoid tumors have a high incidence of monosomy 22 and are associated with a poor prognosis. Although the relationship between these tumors and medulloblastomas is unclear, it is possible that medulloblastomas with loss of chromosome 22 may also belong to a poor prognostic group.

Another possible indicator of prognosis in medulloblastomas is gene amplification. Although too few cases have been identified to determine whether patients whose tumors contain amplified genes do more poorly than patients whose tumors lack this feature, there are anecdotal cases linking amplified *MYC* genes and shortened survival of the patient (Badiali *et al.*, 1991; Tomlinson *et al.*, 1994; Batra *et al.*, 1995b) (Table 2.2).

Meningiomas and schwannomas

CHROMOSOME 22

In 1967, Zang and Singer observed that 8/8 meningiomas studied by them had consistent loss of one G-group chromosome. In 1972, Zankl and Zang and also Mark, Levan and Mitelman used fluorescent banding techniques to determine that the missing chromosome was 22. Overall, approximately 60% of meningiomas showed loss of all or part of chromosome 22 (Mark, 1977; Zankl and Zang, 1980), although in a review of meningioma karyotypes, published in 1982 by Zang, it was noted that chromosome 22 was involved in over 95% of cases with abnormal stemlines or sidelines (Fig. 2.7)

The first clues concerning the molecular basis for this cytogenetic observation came in 1987, when LOH for regions of 22q was demonstrated in 43% (Seizinger *et al.*, 1987a) and 55% (Dumanski *et al.*, 1987) of informative meningiomas. These observations were of particular interest since LOH for 22q was also shown in 44% of informative acoustic neuromas (Seizinger, Martuza and Gusella, 1986). These findings, taken together with linkage studies implicating chromosome 22 in NF type 2, lead to the hypothesis that the same defective gene on chromosome 22 that is responsible for NF type 2 might also be responsible for sporadic meningiomas and schwannomas (Rouleau *et al.*, 1987; Seizinger *et al.*, 1987b; Wertelecki *et al.*, 1988). Deletion mapping studies of chromosome 22 in meningiomas in the early 1990s supported the idea that the critical region of deletion overlapped with the *NF2* locus, as defined by linkage studies, in the majority of cases (Dumanski *et al.*, 1990; Cogen *et al.*, 1991).

For schwannomas, cytogenetic studies revealed loss of all or part of chromosome 22 in the stemlines or sidelines of 60% (Rey *et al.*, 1987a) or 100% (Stenman *et al.*, 1991) of cases with abnormal stemlines.

In 1993, Rouleau *et al.* and Trofatter *et al.* isolated and characterized a novel gene that encodes a 595-amino-acid protein, called 'merlin' or 'schwannomin', related to the moesin–ezrin–radixin family, which links cytoskeletal components with proteins in the cell membrane. Alterations of this gene in the germlines of several NF type 2 families and in sporadic meningiomas and schwannomas supported the concept that this gene is responsible for NF type 2 and also supported its role in the development of these sporadic tumors. Mutations of the *NF2* gene have been demonstrated in up to 60% of meningiomas, 50–60% of schwannomas and in virtually all tumors in NF type 2 patients (Bijlsma *et al.*, 1994b; Deprez *et al.*, 1994; Irving *et al.*, 1994; Jacoby *et al.*, 1994; Ruttledge *et*

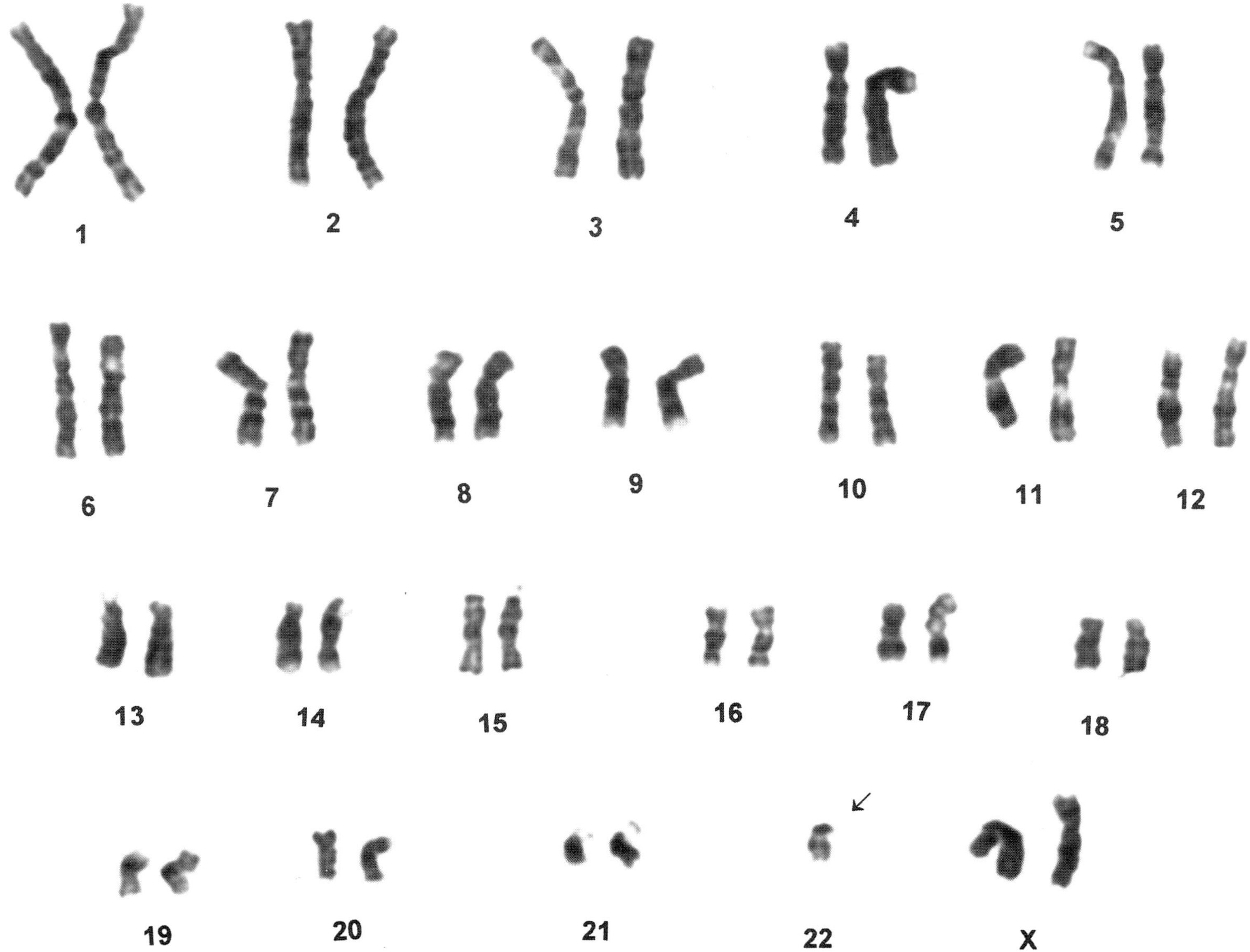

Fig. 2.7 Karyotype, with Giemsa-trypsin banding, of a meningioma,. The only abnormality in this tumor is loss of one copy of chromosome 22 (arrow).

al., 1994a, 1994b). In most cases, the mutations would result in truncation, splicing abnormalities or an altered reading frame of the predicted protein.

Interestingly, Wellenreuther *et al.* (1995) found a relationship between incidence of *NF2* gene mutation and histologic type of meningioma. They demonstrated mutations in 70% of fibroblastic meningiomas and 83% of transitional meningiomas, but in only 25% of meningothelial meningiomas. Mutations of the *NF2* gene have not been seen in intracranial hemangiopericytomas, supporting the concept that this tumor type is histogenetically separate from meningioma (Joseph *et al.*, 1995).

CHROMOSOMAL ABNORMALITIES IN PROGRESSION OF MENINGIOMAS

Although the majority of meningiomas with abnormal karyotypes display loss of all or part of chromosome 22 only, a smaller subset of cases shows additional abnormalities. Loss of chromosomes 1 and 14 and the sex chromosomes are the most consistently reported findings, followed by losses of chromosomes 6, 10, 18 and 19 and gains of chromosome 20 (Al Saadi *et al.*, 1987; Casalone *et al.*, 1987; Maltby, Ironside and Battersby, 1988; Griffin *et al.*, 1994; Deprez *et al.*, 1995). In most cases, the entire chromosome is lost, while some cases show deletions of particular regions. Balanced and unbalanced translocations are uncommon in this tumor type. Although more complex karyotypes are sometimes seen in otherwise typical meningiomas, cases with atypical or malignant histologic features have a higher incidence of karyotypic deviations in addition to monosomy 22. Several observers have noted that, while there is a female predominance in meningiomas, cases from males have a higher incidence of complex karyotypes (Maltby, Ironside and Battersby, 1988; Deprez *et al.*, 1995), and complex karyotypes are more likely to occur in older individuals (Al Saadi *et al.*, 1987). Al Saadi *et al.* (1987) found that complex karyotypes occur mainly in the fibroblastic type of meningioma, and Griffin *et al.* (1994) found 100% of fibroblastic meningiomas to have monosomy 22, either alone or with other abnormalities. Maltby, Ironside and Battersby (1987), however, noted a relationship between structural abnormalities and the meningotheliomatous pattern.

Studies of recurrent meningiomas have shown that, although some recurrent tumors have benign histology and normal or monosomy 22 karyotypes, grade II and grade III tumors, often with complex karyotypes, account for more than half of the recurrent cases (López-Ginés *et al.*, 1995).

Loss of regions of chromosomes 1, 10 and 14, particularly in atypical and malignant meningiomas, has been confirmed by LOH studies and FISH (Bello *et al.*, 1994a; Lindblom *et al.*, 1994; Schneider *et al.*, 1995). Rempel *et al.* (1993) found LOH for loci on chromosome 22 in 5/15 grade I meningiomas, 2/2 grade II tumors, and 5/10 grade III tumors, while LOH for regions on 10q was detected in 0/20 grade I tumors, 1/2 grade II tumors and 4/13 grade III tumors. Simon *et al.* (1995) found loss of 1p in 11% of grade I tumors, 40% of grade II tumors and 70% of grade III tumors; loss of 14q in 0% of grade I tumors, 47% of grade II tumors and 55% of grade III tumors, and loss of 10q in 12% of grade I tumors, 27% of grade II tumors and 40% of grade III tumors. Thus, these studies confirm the cytogenetic observations that the most frequent abnormalities in the small subset of cases with alterations in addition to chromosome 22 loss are losses from chromosomes 1, 10 and 14. In addition, there is an association between histologic grade and incidence of chromosomal loss, in that grade 2 and grade 3 tumors are more likely to show these additional chromosomal changes than are grade I tumors.

References

Adesina, A.M., Nalbantoglu, J. and Cavenee, W.K. (1994) *p53* Gene mutation and *mdm2* gene amplification are uncommon in medulloblastoma. *Cancer Research* **54**, 5649–51.

Agamanolis, D.P. and Malone, J.M. (1995) Chromosomal abnormalities in 47 pediatric brain tumors. *Cancer Genetics and Cytogenetics* **81**, 125–34.

Albrecht, S., von Deimling, A., Pietsch, T., Giangaspero, F., Brandner, S. Kleihues, P. and Wiestler, O.D. (1994) Microsatellite analysis of loss of heterozygosity on chromosomes 9q, 11p, and 17p in medulloblastoma. *Neuropathology and Applied Neurobiology* **20**, 74–81.

Alderson, L.M., Castleberg, R.L., Harsh, G.R., Louis, D.N. and Henson, J.W. (1995) Human gliomas with wild-type p53 express *bcl-2*. *Cancer Research* **55**, 999–1001.

Al Saadi, A. and Latimer, F. (1980) Nonrandom chromosomal abnormalities in human brain tumors. (Abstract) *American Journal of Human Genetics* **32**, 61A.

——(1983) Cytogenetic and clinical correlations in neoplasms of the human nervous system. (Abstract) *Proceedings of the American Association for Cancer Research* **24**, 10.

Al Saadi, A., Latimer, F., Madercic, M. and Robbins, T. (1987) Cytogenetic studies of human brain tumors and their clinical significance. II. Meningioma. *Cancer Genetics and Cytogenetics* **26**, 127–41.

Arap, W., Nishikawa, R., Furnari, F.B., Cavenee, W.K. and Huang, H.J. (1995) Replacement of the *p16/CDKN2* gene suppresses human glioma cell growth. *Cancer Research* **55**, 1351–4.

Badiali, M., Pession, A., Basso, G., Andreini, L., Rigobello, L., Galassi, E. and Giangaspero, F. (1991) N-*myc* and c-*myc* oncogenes amplification in medulloblastomas. Evidence of particularly aggressive behavior of a tumor with *c-myc* amplification. *Tumori* **77**, 118–21.

Badiali, M., Iolascon, A., Loda, M., Scheithauer, B.W., Basso, G., Trentini, G.P. and Giangaspero, F. (1993) p53 Gene mutations in medulloblastoma. Immunohistochemistry, gel shift analysis, and sequencing. *Diagnostic Molecular Pathology* **2**, 23–8.

Batra, S.K., Rasheed, B.K.A., Bigner, S.H. and Bigner, D.D. (1994) Oncogenes and anti-oncogenes in human central nervous system tumors. *Laboratory Investigation* **71**, 621–37.

Batra, S.K., Castelino-Prabhu, S., Wikstrand, C.J., Zhu, X., Humphrey, P.A., Friedman, H.S. and Bigner, D.D. (1995a) Epidermal growth factor ligand-independent, unregulated, cell-transforming potential of a naturally occurring human mutant *EGFRvIII* gene. *Cell Growth and Differentiation* **6**, 1251–9.

Batra, S.K., McLendon, R.E., Koo, J.S., Castelino-Prabhu, S., Fuchs, H.E., Krischer, J.P., Friedman, H.S., Bigner, D.D. and Bigner, S.H. (1995b) Prognostic implications of chromosome 17q deletions in human medulloblastomas. *Journal of Neuro-Onocology* **24**, 39–45.

Bello, M.J., de Campos, J.M., Kusak, M.E., Vaquero, J., Sarasa, J.L., Pestana, A. and Rey, J.A. (1994a) Allelic loss at 1p is associated with tumor progression of meningiomas. *Genes, Chromosomes and Cancer* **9**, 296–8.

Bello, M.J., Vaquero, J., de Campos, J.M., Kusak, M.E., Sarasa, J.L., Saez-Castresana, J., Pestana, A. and Rey, J.A. (1994b). Molecular analysis of chromosome 1 abnormalities in human gliomas reveals frequent loss of 1p in oligodendroglial tumors. *International Journal of Cancer* **57**, 172–5.

Bello, M.J., Leone, P.E., Nebreda, P., de Campos, J.M., Kusak, M.E., Vaquero, J., Sarasa, J.L., Garcia-Miguel, P., Queizan, A., Hernandez-Moneo, J.L., Pestana, A. and Rey, J.A. (1995) Allelic status of chromosome 1 in neoplasms of the nervous system. *Cancer Genetics and Cytogenetics* **83**, 160–4.

Bicknell, J.M. (1967). Chromosome studies of human brain tumors. *Neurology* **17**, 485–90.

Biegel, J.A., Rorke, L.B., Packer, R.J., Sutton, L.N., Schut, L., Bonner, K. and Emanuel, B.S. (1989) Isochromosome 17q in primitive neuroectodermal tumors of the central nervous system. *Genes, Chromosomes and Cancer* **1**, 139–47.

Biegel, J.A., Rorke, L.B., Packer, R.J. and Emanuel, B.S. (1990) Monosomy 22 in rhabdoid or atypical tumors of the brain. *Journal of Neurosurgery* **73**, 710–14.

Biegel, J.A., Burk, C.D., Barr, F.G. and Emanuel, B.S. (1992) Evidence for a 17p tumor related locus distinct from *p53* in pediatric primitive neuroectodermal tumors. *Cancer Research* **52**, 3391–5.

Bigner, S.H., Mark, J., Mahaley, M.S. Jr and Bigner, D.D. (1984) Patterns of early, gross chromosomal changes in malignant human gliomas. *Hereditas* **101**, 103–13.

Bigner, S.H., Mark, J., Bullard, D.E., Mahaley, M.S. Jr, and Bigner, D.D. (1986) Chromosomal evolution in malignant human gliomas starts with specific and usually numerical deviations. *Cancer Genetics and Cytogenetics* **22**, 121–35.

Bigner, S.H., Wong, A.J., Mark, J., Muhlbaier, L.H., Kinzler, K.W., Vogelstein, B. and Bigner, D.D. (1987) Relationship between gene amplification and chromosomal deviations in malignant human gliomas. *Cancer Genetics and Cytogenetics* **29**, 165–70.

Bigner, S.H., Burger, P.C., Wong, A.J., Werner, M.H., Hamilton, S.R., Muhlbaier, L.H., Vogelstein, B. and Bigner, D.D. (1988a). Gene amplification in malignant gliomas: clinical and histopathologic aspects. *Journal of Neuropathology and Experimental Neurology* **47**, 191–205.

Bigner, S.H., Mark, J., Burger, P.C., Mahaley, M.S. Jr, Bullard, D.E., Muhlbaier, L.H. and Bigner, D.D. (1988b) Specific chromosomal abnormalities in malignant human gliomas. *Cancer Research* **48**, 405–11.

Bigner, S.H., Mark, J., Friedman, H.S., Biegel, J.A. and Bigner, D.D. (1988c) Structural chromosomal abnormalities in human medulloblastomas. *Cancer Genetics and Cytogenetics* **30**, 91–101.

Bigner, S.H., Friedman, H.S., Vogelstein, B., Oakes, W.J. and Bigner, D.D. (1990a) Amplification of the *c-myc* gene in human medulloblastoma cell lines and xenografts. *Cancer Research* **50**, 2347–50.

Bigner, S.H., Humphrey, P.A., Wong, A.J., Vogelstein, B., Mark, J., Friedman, H.S. and Bigner, D.D. (1990b) Characterization of the epidermal growth factor receptor in human glioma cell lines and xenografts. *Cancer Research* **50**, 8017–22.

Bigner, S.H., McLendon, R.M., Fuchs, H., McKeever, P.E. and Friedman, H.S. (1997) Chromosomal characteristics of childhood brain tumors. *Cancer Genetics and Cytogenetics*, in press.

Bijlsma, E.K., Leenstra, S., Westerveld, A., Bosch, D.A. and Hulsebos, T.J.M. (1994a) Amplification of the anonymous marker D17S67 in malignant astrocytomas. *Genes, Chromosomes and Cancer* **9**, 148–52.

Bijlsma, E.K., Mérel, P., Bosch, D.A., Westerveld, A., Delattre, O., Thomas, G. and Hulsebos, T.J.M. (1994b) Analysis of mutations in the *SCH* gene in schwannomas. *Genes, Chromosomes and Cancer* **11**, 7–14.

Bijlsma, E.K., Voesten, A.M.J., Bijleveld, E.H., Troost, D., Westerveld, A., Mérel, P., Thomas, G. and Huslebos, T.J.M. (1995) Molecular analysis of genetic changes in ependymomas. *Genes, Chromosomes and Cancer* **13**, 272–7.

Birchmeier, C., Sharma, S. and Wigler, M. (1987) Expression and rearrangement of the *ROS1* gene in human glioblastoma cells. *Proceedings of the National Academy of Sciences U.S.A.* **84**, 9270–4.

Blaeker, H., Rasheed, B.K.A., McLendon, R.E., Friedman, H., Batra, S.K., Fuchs, H.E. and Bigner, S.H. (1996). Microsatellite analysis of childhood brain tumors. *Genes, Chromosomes and Cancer* **15**, 54–63.

Blin, N., Muller-Brechlin, R., Carstens, C., Meese, E. and Zang, K.D. (1987) Enhanced expression of four cellular oncogenes in a human glioblastoma cell line. *Cancer Genetics and Cytogenetics* **25**, 285–92.

Blumenstock, M., Prosenc, N., Patt, S., Pfanne, K., Drum, F. and Cervos-Navarro, J. (1991) In contrast to *EGFr* gene overexpression, H-*ras* gene expression decreases in human gliomas. *Anticancer Research* **11**, 1353–7.

Bogler, O., Huang, H.J.S., Kleihues, P. and Cavenee, W.K. (1995) The *p53* gene and its role in human brain tumors. *Glia* **15**, 308–27.

Bown, N.P., Pearson, A.D.J., Davison, E.V., Gardner-Medwin, D., Crawford, P. and Perry, R. (1988) Multiple chromosome rearrangements in a childhood ependymoma. *Cancer Genetics and Cytogenetics* **36**, 25–30.

Brodeur, G.M., Seeger, R.C., Schwab, M., Varmus, H.E. and Bishop, J.M. (1984) Amplification of N-*myc* in untreated human neuroblastomas correlates with advanced disease stage. *Science* **224**, 1121–4.

Carter, B.S., Ewing, C.M., Ward, W.S., Treiger, B.F., Aalders, T.W., Schalken, J.A., Epstein, J.I. and Isaacs, W.B. (1990) Allelic loss of chromosomes 16q and 10q in human prostate cancer. *Proceedings of the National Academy of Sciences U.S.A.* **87**, 8751–5.

Casalone, R., Granata, P., Simi, P., Tarantino, E., Butti, G., Buonaguidi, R., Faggionato, F., Knerich, R. and Solero, L. (1987) Recessive cancer genes in meningiomas? An analysis of 31 cases. *Cancer Genetics and Cytogenetics* **27**, 145–59.

Chadduck, W.M., Boop, F.A. and Sawyer, J.R. (1991–92) Cytogenetic studies of pediatric brain and spinal cord tumors. *Pediatric Neurosurgery* **17**, 57–65.

Chen, P., Iavarone, A., Fick, J., Edwards, M., Prados, M. and Israel, M.A. (1995) Constitutional *p53* mutations associated with brain tumors in young adults. *Cancer Genetics and Cytogenetics* **82**, 106–15.

Chozick, B.S., Pezzullo, J.C., Epstein, M.H. and Finch, P.W. (1994) Prognostic implications of *p53* overexpression in supratentorial astrocytic tumors. *Neurosurgery* **35**, 837–8.

Chung, R., Whaley, J., Kley, N., Anderson, K., Louis, D., Menon, A., Hettlich, C., Freiman, R., Hedley-Whyte, E.T., Martuza, R., Jenkins, R., Yandell, D. and Seizinger, B.R. (1991) *TP53* gene mutations and 17p deletions in human astrocytomas. *Genes, Chromosomes and Cancer* **3**, 323–31.

Cogen, P.H. (1991) Prognostic significance of molecular genetic markers in childhood brain tumors. *Pediatric Neurosurgery* **92**, 245–50.

Cogen, P.H., Daneshvar, L., Metzger, A.K. and Edwards, M.S.B. (1990) Deletion mapping of the medulloblastoma locus on chromosome 17p. *Genomics* **8**, 279–85.

Cogen, P.H., Daneshvar, L., Bowcock, A.M., Metzger, A.K. and Cavalli-Sforza, L.L. (1991) Loss of heterozygosity for chromosome 22 DNA sequences in human meningioma. *Cancer Genetics and Cytogenetics* **53**, 271–7.

Cogen, P.H., Daneshvar, L., Metzger, A.K., Duyk, G., Edwards, M.S.B. and Sheffield, V.C. (1992) Involvement of multiple chromosome 17p loci in medulloblastoma tumorigenesis. *American Journal of Human Genetics* **50**, 584–9.

Cox, D. (1968) Chromosomal studies in 12 solid tumours from children. *British Journal of Cancer* **22**, 402–14.

Cox, D., Yuncken, C. and Spriggs, A.I. (1965) Minute chromatin bodies in malignant tumours of childhood. *Lancet* **2**, 55–8.

Dalrymple, S.J., Herath, J.F., Borell, T.J., Moertel, C.A. and Jenkins, R.B. (1994) Correlation of cytogenetic and fluorescence *in situ* hybridization (FISH) studies in normal and gliotic brain. *Journal of Neuropathology and Experimental Neurology* **53**, 448–56.

Dams, E., Van de Kelft, E.J., Martin, J.-J., Verlooy, J. and Willems, P.J. (1995) Instability of microsatellites in human gliomas. *Cancer Research* **55**, 1547–9.

Danks, R.A., Chopra, G., Gonzales, M.F., Orian, J.M. and Kaye, A.H. (1995) Aberrant *p53* expression does not correlate with the prognosis in anaplastic astrocytoma. *Neurosurgery* **37**, 246–54.

Das, R., Reddy, E.P., Chatterjee, D. and Andrews, D.W. (1996) Identification of a novel *Bcl-2* related gene, *BRAG-1*, in human glioma. *Oncogene* **12**, 947–51.

Day, R.S., Scudiero, D.A., Mattern, M.R. and Yarosh D.B. (1983) Repair of O^6-methylguanine by normal and transformed cells. (Abstract) *Proceedings of the American Association for Cancer Research* **24**, 335–7.

Debiec-Rychter, M., Alwasiak, J., Liberski, P.P., Nedoszytko, B., Babinska, M., Mrózek, K., Imielinski, B., Borowska-Lehman, J. and Limon, J. (1995) Accumulation of chromosomal changes in human glioma progression. A cytogenetic study of 50 cases. *Cancer Genetics and Cytogenetics* **85**, 61–7.

Della Ragione, F., Russo, G., Oliva, A., Mastropietro, S., Mancini, A., Borrelli, A., Casero, R.A., Iolascon, A. and Zappia, V. (1995) 5'-Deoxy-5'-methylthioadenosine phosphorylase and $p16^{INK4}$ deficiency in multiple tumor cell lines. *Oncogene* **10**, 827–33.

Deprez, R.H.L., Bianchi, A.B., Groen, N.A., Seizinger, B.R., Hagemeijer, A., van Drunen, E., Bootsma, D., Koper, J.W., Avezaat, C.J.J., Kley, N. and Zwarthoff, E.C. (1994) Frequent *NF2* gene transcript mutations in sporadic meningiomas and vestibular schwannomas. *American Journal of Human Genetics* **54**, 1022–9.

Deprez, R.H.L., Reigman, P.H., van Drunen, E., Warringa, U.L., Groen, N.A., Stefanko, S.Z., Koper, J.W., Avezaat, C.J.J., Mulder, P.G.H., Zwarthoff, E.C. and Hagemeuer, A. (1995) Cytogenetic, molecular genetic and pathological analyses in 126 meningiomas. *Journal of Neuropathology and Experimental Neurology* **54**, 224–35.

Diedrich, U., Lucius, J., Baron, E., Behnke, J., Pabst, B. and Zoll, B. (1995) Distribution of epidermal growth factor receptor gene amplification in brain tumours and correlation to prognosis. *Journal of Neurology* **242**, 683–8.

Dumanski, J.P., Carlbom, E., Collins, V.P. and Nordenskjöld, M. (1987) Deletion mapping of a locus on human chromosome 22 involved in the oncogenesis of meningioma. *Proceedings of the National Academy of Sciences U.S.A.* **84**, 9275–9.

Dumanski, J.P., Rouleau, G.A., Nordenskjöld, M. and Collin, V.P. (1990) Molecular genetic analysis of chromosome 22 in 81 cases of meningioma. *Cancer Research* **50**, 5863–7.

Eagle, L.R., Yin, X., Brothman, A.R., Williams, B.J., Atkin, N.B. and Prochownik, E.V. (1995) Mutation of the *MXI1* gene in prostate cancer. *Nature Genetics* **9**, 249–55.

Ekstrand, A.J., James, C.D., Cavenee, W.K., Seliger, B., Pettersson, R.F. and Collins, V.P. (1991) Genes for epidermal growth factor receptor, transforming growth factor alpha, and epidermal growth factor and their expression in human gliomas *in vivo*. *Cancer Research* **51**, 2164–72.

Ekstrand, A.J., Sugawa, N., James, C.D. and Collins, V.P. (1992) Amplified and rearranged epidermal growth factor receptor genes in human glioblastomas reveal deletions of sequences encoding portions of the N- and/or C-terminal tails. *Proceedings of the National Academy of Sciences U.S.A.* **89**, 4309–13.

Ekstrand, A.J., Longo, N., Hamid, M.L., Olson, J.J., Liu, L., Collins, V.P. and James, C.D. (1994) Functional characterization of an EGF receptor with a truncated extracellular domain expressed in glioblastomas with *EGFR* gene amplification. *Oncogene* **9**, 2313–20.

Ekstrand, B.C., Mansfield, T.A., Bigner, S.H. and Fearon, E.R. (1995) DCC expression is altered by multiple mechanisms in brain tumors. *Oncogene* **11**, 2393–402.

El-Azouzi, M., Chung, R.Y., Farmer, G.E., Martuza, R.L., Black, P.M., Rouleau, G.A., Hettlich, C., Hedley-Whyte, E.T., Zervas, N.T., Panagopoulos, K., Nakamura, Y., Gusella, J.F. and Sizinger, B.R. (1989) Loss of distinct regions on the short arm of chromosome 17 associated with tumorigenesis of human astrocytomas. *Proceedings of the National Academy of Sciences U.S.A.* **86**, 7186–90.

Engelhard, H.H. III, Butler, A.B. IV and Bauer, K.D. (1989) Quantification of the c-*myc* oncoprotein in human glioblastoma cells and tumor tissue. *Journal of Neurosurgery* **71**, 224–32.

Fischer, U., Müller, H.W., Sattler, H.P., Feiden, K., Zang, K.D. and Meese, E. (1995) Amplification of the *MET* gene in glioma. *Genes, Chromosomes and Cancer* **12**, 63–5.

Fleming, T.P., Saxena, A., Clark, W.C., Robertson, J.T., Oldfield, E.H., Aaronson, S.A. and Ali, I.U. (1992) Amplification and/or overexpression of platelet-derived growth factor receptors and epidermal growth factor receptor in human glial tumors. *Cancer Research* **52**, 4550–3.

Frankel, R.H., Bayona, W., Koslow, M. and Newcomb, E.W. (1992) *p53* Mutations in human malignant gliomas: comparison of loss of heterozygosity with mutation frequency. *Cancer Research* **52**, 1427–33.

Friedman, H.S., Burger, P.C., Bigner, S.H., Trojanowski, J.Q., Brodeur, G.M., He, X., Wikstrand, C.J., Kurtzberg, J., Berens, M.E., Halperin, E.C. and Bigner, D.D. (1988) Phenotypic and genotypic analysis of a human medulloblastoma cell line and transplantable xenograft (D341 Med) demonstrating amplification of c-myc. *American Journal of Pathology* **130**, 472–84.

Fujii, Y., Hongo, T. and Hayashi, Y. (1994) Chromosome analysis of brain tumors in childhood. *Genes, Chromosomes and Cancer* **11**, 205–15.

Fujimoto, M., Fults, D.W., Thomas, G.A., Nakamura, Y., Heilbrun, M.P., White, R., Story, J.L., Naylor, S.L., Kagan-Hallet, K.S. and Sheridan, P.J. (1989) Loss of heterozygosity on chromosome 10 in human glioblastoma multiforme. *Genomics* **4**, 210–14.

Fults, D. and Pedone, C. (1993) Deletion mapping of the long arm of chromosome 10 in glioblastoma multiforme. *Genes, Chromosomes and Cancer* **7**, 173–7.

Fults, D., Tippets, R.H., Thomas, G.A., Nakamura, Y. and White, R. (1989). Loss of heterozygosity for loci on chromosome 17p in human malignant astrocytoma. *Cancer Research* **49**, 6572–7.

Fults, D., Pedone, C.A., Thomas, G.A. and White, R. (1990) Allelotype of human malignant astrocytoma. *Cancer Research* **50**, 5784–9.

Fults, D., Brockmeyer, D., Tullous, M.W., Pedone C.A. and Cawthon, R.M. (1992a) *p53* Mutation and loss of heterozygosity on chromosomes 17 and 10 during human astrocytoma progression. *Cancer Research* **52**, 674–9.

Fults, D., Petronio J., Noblett, B.D. and Pedone C.A. (1992b) Chromosome 11p15 deletions in human malignant astrocytomas and primitive neuroectodermal tumors. *Genomics* **14**, 799–801.

Garson, J.A., Pemberton, L.F., Sheppard, P.W., Varndell, I.M., Coakham, H.B. and Kemshead, J.T. (1989) N-*myc* gene expression and oncoprotein characterization in medulloblastoma. *British Journal of Cancer* **59**, 889–94.

Gerosa, M.A., Talarico, D., Fognani, C., Raimondi, E., Colombatti, M., Tridente, G., De Carli, L. and Della Valle, G. (1989) Overexpression of N-*ras* oncogene and epidermal growth factor receptor gene in human glioblastomas. *Journal of the National Cancer Institute* **81**, 63–7.

Giani, C. and Finocchiaro, G. (1994) Mutation rate of the *CDKN2* gene in malignant gliomas. *Cancer Research* **54**, 6338–9.

Gray, I.C., Phillips, S.M.A., Lee, S.J., Neoptolemos, J.P., Weissenbach, J. and Spurr, N.K. (1995) Loss of the chromosomal region 10q23-25 in prostate cancer. *Cancer Research* **55**, 4800–3.

Griffin, C.A., Hawkins, A.L., Packer, R.J., Rorke, L.B. and Emanuel, B.S. (1988) Chromosome abnormalities in pediatric brain tumors. *Cancer Research* **48**, 175–80.

Griffin, C.A., Long, P.P., Carson, B.S. and Brem, H. (1992) Chromosome abnormalities in low-grade central nervous system tumors. *Cancer Genetics and Cytogenetics* **60**, 67–73.

Griffin, C.A., Hruban, R.H., Long, P.P., Miller, N., Volz, P., Carson, B. and Brem, H. (1994) Chromosome abnormalities in meningeal neoplasms: do they correlate with histology? *Cancer Genetics and Cytogenetics* **78**, 46–52.

Groden, J., Thliveris, A., Samowitz, W., Carlson, M., Gelbert, L., Albertsen, H., Joslyn, G., Stevens, J., Spirio, L., Robertson, M., Sargeant, L., Krapcho, K., Wolff, E., Burt, R., Hughes, J.P., Warrington, J., McPherson, J., Wasmuth, J., Le Paslier, D., Abderrahim, H., Cohen, D., Leppert, M. and White, R. (1991) Identification and characterization of the familial adenomatous polyposis coli gene. *Cell* **66**, 589–600.

Gullick, W.J. (1991) Prevalence of aberrant expression of the epidermal growth factor receptor in human cancers. *British Medical Bulletin* **47**, 87–98.

Hamilton, S.R., Liu, B., Parsons, R.E., Papadopoulos, N., Jen, J., Powell, S.M., Krush., A.J., Berk, T., Cohen, Z., Tetu, B., Burger, P.C., Wood., P.A., Taqi, F., Booker, S.V., Petersend, G.M., Offerhaus, G.J.A., Tersmette, A.C., Giardiello, F.M., Vogelstein, B. and Kinzler, K.W. (1995) The molecular basis of Turcot's syndrome. *New England Journal of Medicine* **332**, 839–47.

Hansteen, I.L. (1967) Chromosome studies in glial tumours. *European Journal of Cancer* **3**, 183–91.

Hashimoto, N., Ichikawa, D., Arakawa, Y., Date, K., Ueda, S., Nakagawa, Y., Horii, A., Nakamura, Y., Abe, T. and Inazawa, J. (1995) Frequent deletions of material from chromosome arm 1p in oligodendroglial tumors revealed by double-target fluorescence *in situ* hybridization and microsatellite analysis. *Genes, Chromosomes and Cancer* **14**, 295–300.

He, J., Olson, J.J. and James, C.D. (1995) Lack of $p16^{INK4}$ or retinoblastoma protein (pRb), or amplification-associated overexpression of *cdk4* is observed in distinct subsets of malignant glial tumors and cell lines. *Cancer Research* **55**, 4833–6.

He, J., Allen, J.R., Collins, V.P., Allalunis-Turner, M.J., Godbout, R., Day, R.S. III and James, C.D. (1994a) *CDK4* amplification is an alternative mechanism to *p16* gene homozygous deletion in glioma cell lines. *Cancer Research* **54**, 5804–7.

He, J., Reifenberger, G., Liu, L., Collins, V.P. and James C.D. (1994b) Analysis of glioma cell lines for amplification and overexpression of *MDM2*. *Genes, Chromosomes and Cancer* **11**, 91–6.

Hecht, B.K., Turc-Carel, C., Chatel, M., Grellier, P., Gioanni, J., Attias, R., Gaudray, P. and Hecht, F. (1995) Cytogenetics of malignant gliomas. 1. The autosomes with reference to rearrangements. *Cancer Genetics and Cytogenetics* **84**, 1–8.

Heim, S., Mandahl N., Jin, Y., Strömblad, S., Lindstrom, E., Salford, L.G. and Mitelman, F. (1989) Trisomy 7 and sex chromosome loss in human brain tissue. *Cytogenetics and Cell Genetics* **52**, 136–8.

Heisterkamp, N., Morris, C., Sender, L., Knoppel, E., Uribe, L., Cui, M.Y. and Groffen, J. (1990) Rearrangement of the human *ABL* oncogene in a glioblastoma. *Cancer Research* **50**, 3429–34.

Henson, J.W., Schnitker, B.L., Correa, K.M., von Deimling, A., Fasshender, F., Xu, H.J., Benedict, W.F., Yandell, D.W. and Louis, D.N. (1994) The retinoblastoma gene is involved in malignant progression of astrocytomas. *Annals of Neurology* **36**, 714–21.

Herman, J.G., Merlo, A., Mao, L., Lapidus, R.G., Issa, J.-P.J., Davidson, N.E., Sidransky, D. and Baylin, S.B. (1995) Inactivation of the *CDKN2/p16/MTS1* gene is frequently associated with aberrant DNA methylation in all common human cancers. *Cancer Research* **55**, 4525–30.

Hermanson, M., Funa, K., Koopmann, J., Maintz, D., Waha, A., Westermark, B., Heldin, C.H., Wiestler, O.D., Louis, D.N., von Deimling, A. and Nister, M. (1996) Association of loss of heterozygosity on chromosome 17p with high platelet-derived growth factor alpha receptor expression in human malignant gliomas. *Cancer Research* **56**, 164–71.

Hills, D., Rowlinson-Busza, G. and Gullick, W.J. (1995) Specific targeting of a mutant, activated EGF receptor found in glioblastoma using a monoclonal antibody. *International Journal of Cancer* **63**, 537–43.

Hoang-Xuan, K., Merel, P., Vega, F., Hugot, J.-P., Cornu, P., Delattre, J.Y., Poisson, M., Thomas, G. and Delattre, O. (1995) Analysis of the *NF2* tumor-suppressor gene and of chromosome 22 deletions in gliomas. *International Journal of Cancer* **60**, 478–81.

Hurtt, M.R., Moossy, J., Donovan-Peluso, M. and Locker, J. (1992) Amplification of epidermal growth factor receptor gene in gliomas: histopathology and prognosis. *Journal of Neuropathology and Experimental Neurology* **51**, 84–90.

Humphrey, P.A., Wong, A.J., Vogelstein, B., Friedman, H.S., Werner, M.H., Bigner, D.D. and Bigner, S.H. (1988) Amplification and expression of the epidermal growth factor receptor gene in human glioma xenografts. *Cancer Research* **48**, 2231–8.

Humphrey, P.A., Wong, A.J., Vogelstein, B., Zalutsky, M.R., Fuller, G.N., Archer, G.E., Friedman, H.S., Kwatra, M.M., Bigner, S.H. and Bigner, D.D. (1990) Anti-synthetic peptide antibody reacting at the fusion junction of deletion-mutant epidermal growth factor receptors in human glioblastoma. *Proceedings of the National Academy of Sciences U.S.A.* **87**, 4207–11.

Humphrey, P.A., Gangarosa, L.M., Wong, A.J., Archer, G.E., Lund-Johansen, M., Bjerkvig, R., Laerum, O.D., Friedman, H.S. and Bigner, D.D. (1991) Deletion-mutant epidermal growth factor receptor in human gliomas: effects of type II mutation on receptor function. *Biochemical and Biophysical Research Communication* **178**, 1413–20.

Iolascon, A., Lania, A., Badiali, M., Pession, A., Saglio, G., Giangaspero, F., del Giudice, E.M., Perrotta, S. and Cutillo, S. (1991) Analysis of N-*ras* gene mutations in medulloblastomas by polymerase chain reaction and oligonucleotide probes in formalin-fixed, paraffin-embedded tissues. *Medical and Pediatric Oncology* **19**, 240–5.

Irving, R.M., Moffat, D.A., Hardy, D.G., Barton, D.E., Xuereb, J.H. and Maher, E.R. (1994) Somatic *NF2* gene mutations in familial and non-familial vestibular schwannoma. *Human Molecular Genetics* **3**, 347–50.

Isshiki, K., Elder, D.E., Guerry, D. and Linnenbach, A.J. (1993) Chromosome 10 allelic loss in malignant melanoma. *Genes, Chromosomes and Cancer* **8**, 178–84.

Jacoby, L.B., MacCollin, M., Louis, D.N., Mohney, T., Rubio, M.P., Pulaski, K., Trofatter, J.A., Kley, N., Seizinger, B., Ramesh, V. and Gusella, J.F. (1994) Exon scanning for mutations of the *NF2* gene in schwannomas. *Human Molecular Genetics* **3**, 413–19.

James, C.D., Carlbom, E., Dumanski, J.P., Hansen, M., Nordenskjöld, M., Collins, V.P. and Cavenee, W.K. (1988) Clonal genomic alterations in glioma malignancy stages. *Cancer Research* **48**, 5546–51.

James, C.D., Carlbom, E., Nordenskjöld, M., Collins, V.P. and Cavenee, W.K. (1989) Mitotic recombination of chromosome 17 in astrocytomas. *Proceedings of the National Academy of Sciences U.S.A.* **86**, 2858–62.

James, C.D., He, J., Carlbom, E., Mikkelsen, T., Ridderheim, P.A., Cavenee, W.K. and Collins, V.P. (1990) Loss of genetic information in central nervous system tumors common to children and young adults. *Genes, Chromosomes and Cancer* **2**, 94–102.

James, C.D., He, J., Carlbom, E., Nordenskjöld, M., Cavenee, W.K. and Collins, V.P. (1991) Chromosome 9 deletion mapping reveals interferon alpha and interferon beta-1 gene deletions in human glial tumors. *Cancer Research* **51**, 1684–8.

Jen, J., Harper, J.W., Bigner, S.H., Bigner, D.D., Papadopoulos, N., Markowitz, S., Wilson, J.K.V., Kinzler, K.W. and Vogelstein, B. (1994) Deletion of *p16* and *p15* genes in brain tumors. *Cancer Research* **54**, 6353–8.

Jenkins, R.B., Kimmel, D.W., Moertel, C.A., Schultz, C.G., Schiethauer, B.W., Kelly, P.J. and Dewald, G.W. (1989) A cytogenetic study of 53 human gliomas. *Cancer Genetics and Cytogenetics* **39**, 253–79.

Joseph, J.T., Lisle, D.K., Jacoby, L.B., Paulus, W., Barone, R., Cohen, M.L., Roggendorf, W.H., Bruner, J.M., Gusella, J.F. and Louis, D.N. (1995) *NF2* gene analysis distinguishes hemangiopericytoma from meningioma. *American Journal of Pathology* **147**, 1450–5.

Kamb, A., Gruis, N.A., Weaver-Feldhaus, J., Liu, Q., Harshman, K., Tavtigian, S.V., Stockert, E., Day, R.S. III, Johnson, B.E. and Skolnick, M.H. (1994) A cell cycle regulator potentially involved in genesis of many tumor types. *Science* **264**, 436–40.

Karlbom, A.E., James, C.D., Boethius, J., Cavenee, W.K., Collins, V.P., Nordenskjöld, M. and Larsson, C. (1993) Loss of heterozygosity in malignant gliomas involves at least three distinct regions on chromosome 10. *Human Genetics* **92**, 169–74.

Karnes, P.S., Tran, T.N., Cui, M.Y., Raffel, C., Gilles, F.H., Barranger, J.A. and Ying, K.L. (1992) Cytogenetic analysis of 39 pediatric central nervous system tumors. *Cancer Genetics and Cytogenetics* **59**, 12–19.

Khatib, Z.A., Matsushime, H., Valentine, M., Shapiro, D.N., Sherr, C.J. and Look, A.T. (1993) Coamplification of *CDK4* gene with *MDM2* and *GLI* in human sarcoma. *Cancer Research* **53**, 5535–41.

Kikuchi, T., Rempel, S.A., Rutz, H.-P., de Tribolet, N., Mulligan, L., Cavenee, W.K., Jothy, S., Leduy, L. and Van Meir, E.G. (1993) Turcot's syndrome of glioma and polyposis occurs in the absence of germ line mutations of exons 5 to 9 of the *p53* gene. *Cancer Research* **53**, 957–61.

Kimmelman, A.C., Ross, D.A. and Liang, B.C. (1996) Loss of heterozygosity of chromosome 10p in human gliomas. *Genomics* **34**, 250–4.

Kinzler, K.W., Bigner, S.H., Bigner, D.D., Trent, J.M., Law, M.L., O'Brien, S.J., Wong, A.J. and Vogelstein, B. (1987). Identification of an amplified, highly expressed gene in a human glioma. *Science* **236**, 70–3.

Kleihues, P., Aguzzi, A. and Ohgaki, H. (1995) Genetic and environmental factors in the etiology of human brain tumors. *Toxicology Letters* **82/83**, 601–5.

Koch, A., Tonn, J., Kraus, J.A., Sörensen, N., Albrecht, S., Wiestler, O.D. and Pietsch, T. (1996) Molecular analysis of the lissencephaly gene 1 (*LIS-1*) in medulloblastomas. *Neuropathology and Applied Neurobiology* **22**, 233–42.

Kraus, J.A., Bolln, C., Wolf, H.K., Neumann, J., Kindermann, D., Fimmers, R., Forster, F., Baumann, A. and Schlegel, U. (1994) *TP53* alterations and clinical outcome in low grade astrocytomas. *Genes, Chromosomes and Cancer* **10**, 143–9.

Kraus, J.A., Koopmann, J., Kaskel, P., Maintz, D., Brandner, S., Schramm, J., Louis, D.N., Wiestler, O.D. and von Deimling, A. (1995) Shared allelic losses on chromosomes 1p and 19q suggest a common origin of oligodendroglioma and oligoastrocytoma. *Journal of Neuropathology and Experimental Neurology* **54**, 91–5.

Krishna, M., Smith, T.W. and Recht, L.D. (1995) Expression of *bcl-2* in reactive and neoplastic astrocytes: lack of correlation with presence or degree of malignancy. *Journal of Neurosurgery* **83**, 1017–22.

Kumabe, T., Sohma, Y., Kayama, T., Yoshimoto, T. and Yamamoto, T. (1992) Amplification of alpha-platelet-derived growth factor receptor gene lacking an exon coding for a portion of the extracellular region in a primary brain tumor of glial origin. *Oncogene* **7**, 627–33.

Kyritsis, A.P., Bondy, M.L., Xiao, M., Berman, E.L., Cunningham, J.E., Lee, P.S., Levin, V.A. and Saya, H. (1994) Germline *p53* gene mutations in subsets of glioma patients. *Journal of the National Cancer Institute* **86**, 344–9.

Kyritsis, A.P., Xu, R.S., Bondy, M.L., Levin, V.A. and Bruner, J.M. (1996a). Correlation of p53 immunoreactivity and sequencing in patients with glioma. *Molecular Carcinogenesis* **15**, 1–4.

Kyritsis, A.P., Zhang, B., Zhang, W., Xiao, M., Takeshima, H., Bondy, M.L., Cunningham, J.E., Levin, V.A. and Bruner, J. (1996b). Mutations of the *p16* gene in gliomas. *Oncogene* **12**, 63–7.

Lang, F.F., Miller, D.C., Koslow, M. and Newcomb, E.W. (1994a) Pathways leading to glioblastoma multiforme: a molecular analysis of genetic alterations in 65 astrocytic tumors. *Journal of Neurosurgery* **81**, 427–36.

Lang, F.F., Miller, D.C., Pisharody, S., Koslow, M. and Newcomb, E.W. (1994b) High frequency of p53 protein accumulation without *p53* gene mutation in human juvenile pilocytic, low grade and anaplastic astrocytomas. *Oncogene* **9**, 949–54.

LaRocca, R.V., Rosenblum, M., Westermark, B. and Israel, M.A. (1989) Patterns of proto-oncogene expression in human glioma cell lines. *Journal of Neuroscience Research* **24**, 97–106.

Leenstra, S., Bijlsma, E.K., Troost, D., Oosting, J., Westerveld, A., Bosch, D.A. and Huslebos, T.J.M. (1994) Allele loss on chromosomes 10 and 17p and epidermal growth factor receptor amplification in human malignant astrocytoma related to prognosis. *British Journal of Cancer* **70**, 684–9.

Levan, A., Manolov, G. and Clifford, P. (1968) Chromosomes of a human neuroblastoma: a new case with accessory minute chromosomes. *Journal of the National Cancer Institute* **41**, 1377–87.

Li, J., Yen, C., Liaw, D., Podsypanina, K., Bose, S., Wang, S.I., Puc, J., Miliaresis, C., Rodgers, L., McCombie, R., Bigner, S.H., Giovanella, B.C., Ittman, M., Tycko, B., Hibshoosh, H., Wigler, M.H. and Parsons, R. (1997) *PTEN,* a putative protein tyrosine phosphatase gene mutated in human brain, breast, and prostrate cancer. *Science* **275**, 1943–7.

Li, Y., Bollag, G., Clark, R., Stevens, J., Conroy, L., Fults, D., Ward, K., Friedman, E., Samowitz, W., Robertson,

M., Bradley, P., McCormick, F., White, F., White, R. and Cawthon, R. (1992) Somatic mutations in the neurofibromatosis 1 gene in human tumors. *Cell* **69**, 275–81.

Li, Y.J., Hoang-Xuan, K., Delattre, J.Y., Poisson, M., Thomas, G. and Hamelin, R. (1995a) Frequent loss of heterozygosity on chromosome 9, and low incidence of mutations of cyclin-dependent kinase inhibitors *p15 (MTS2)* and *p16 (MTS1)* genes in gliomas. *Oncogene* **11**, 597–600.

Li Y.J., Sanson, M., Hoang-Xuan, K., Delattre, J.-Y., Poisson, M., Thomas, G. and Hamelin, R. (1995b) Incidence of germline *p53* mutations in patients with gliomas. *International Journal of Cancer* **64**, 383–7.

Libermann, T.A., Nusbaum, H.R., Razon, N., Kris, R., Lax, I., Soreq, H., Whittle, N., Waterfield, M.D., Ullrich, A. and Schlessinger, J. (1985) Amplification, enhanced expression and possible rearrangement of EGF receptor gene in primary human brain tumours of glial origin. *Nature* **313**, 144–7.

Lindblom, A., Ruttledge, M., Collins, V.P., Nordenskjöld, M. and Dumanski, J.P. (1994) Chromosomal deletions in anaplastic meningiomas suggest multiple regions outside chromosome 22 as important in tumor progression. *International Journal of Cancer* **56**, 354–7.

Lindström, E., Salford, L.G., Heim, S., Mandahl, N., Stromblad, S., Brun, A. and Mitelman, F. (1991) Trisomy 7 and sex chromosome loss need not be representative of tumor parenchyma cells in malignant glioma. *Genes, Chromosomes and Cancer* **3**, 474–9.

Litofsky, N.S., Hinton, D. and Raffel, C. (1994) The lack of a role for *p53* in astrocytomas in pediatric patients. *Neurosurgery* **34**, 967–73.

López-Ginés, C., Cerda-Nicolas, M., Barcia-Salorio, J.L. and Llombart-Bosch, A. (1995) Cytogenetical findings of recurrent meningiomas. A study of 10 tumors. *Cancer Genetics and Cytogenetics* **85**, 113–17.

Louis, D.N. (1994) The *p53* gene and protein in human brain tumors. *Journal of Neuropathology and Experimental Neurology* **53**, 11–21.

——(1996) Clinicopatho-genetic subsets of glioblastoma multiforme: from both sides now. *Brain Pathology* **6**, 217–24.

Louis, D.N., Rubio, M.P., Correa, K.M., Gusella, J.F. and von Deimling, A. (1993) Molecular genetics of pediatric brain stem gliomas. Application of PCR techniques to small and archival brain tumor specimens. *Journal of Neuropathology and Experimental Neurology* **52**, 507–15.

Lübbe, J., von Ammon, K., Watanabe, K., Hegi, M.E. and Kleihues, P. (1995) Familial brain tumour syndrome associated with a *p53* germline deletion of codon 236. *Brain Pathology* **5**, 15–23.

Lubs, H.A. and Salmon, J.H. (1965) The chromosomal complement of human solid tumors. II. Karyotypes of glial tumors. *Journal of Neurosurgery* **22**, 160–8.

Malden, L.T., Novak, U., Kaye, A.H. and Burgess, A.W. (1988) Selective amplification of the cytoplasmic domain of the epidermal growth factor receptor gene in glioblastoma multiforme. *Cancer Research* **48**, 2711–14.

Malkin, D., Li, F.P., Strong, L.C., Fraumeni, J.F. Jr, Nelson, C.E., Kim, D.H., Kassel, J., Gryka, M.A., Bischoff, F.Z., Tainsky, M.A. and Friend, S.H. (1990) Germ line *p53* mutations in a familial syndrome of breast cancer, sarcomas, and other neoplasms. *Science* **250**, 1233–8.

Maltby, E.L., Ironside, J.W. and Battersby, R.D.E. (1988) Cytogenetic studies in 50 meningiomas. *Cancer Genetics and Cytogenetics* **31**, 199–210.

Mandahl, N., Heim, S., Johansson, B., Bennet, K., Mertens, F., Olsson, G., Rooser, B., Rydholm, A., Willen, H. and Mitelman, F. (1987) Lipomas have characteristic structural chromosomal rearrangements of 12q13–q14. *International Journal of Cancer* **39**, 685–8.

Mapstone, T., McMichael, M. and Goldthwait, D. (1990) Expression of platelet-derived growth factors, transforming growth factors and the *ros* gene in a variety of primary human brain tumors. *Neurosurgery* **28**, 216–22.

Mark, J. (1970) Chromosomal characteristics of neurogenic tumors in children. *Acta Cytologica* **14**, 510–18.

——(1971) Chromosomal characteristics of neurogenic tumours in adults. *Hereditus* **68**, 61–100.

——(1974a) G-band analyses of an established cell line of a human malignant glioma. *Humangenetik* **22**, 323–6.

——(1974b) Origin of the marker chromosomes in an established hypotriploid glioma cell line studied with G-band technique. *Acta Neuropathologica* **29**, 223–8.

——(1977) Chromosomal abnormalities and their specificity in human neoplasm. An assessment of recent observations by banding techniques. *Advances in Cancer Research* **24**, 165–222.

Mark, J., Levan, G. and Mitelman, F. (1972) Identification by fluorescence of the G chromosome lost in human meningiomas. *Hereditas* **71**, 163–8.

Mark, J., Pontén, J. and Westermark, B. (1974) Cytogenetical studies with G-band technique of established cell lines of human malignant gliomas. *Hereditas* **78**, 304–7.

Mark, J., Westermark, B., Pontén, J. and Hugosson, R. (1977) Banding patterns in human glioma cell lines. *Hereditas* **87**, 243–60.

Mashiyama, S., Murakami, Y., Yoshimoto, T., Sekiya, T. and Hayashi, K. (1991) Detection of *p53* gene mutations in human brain tumors by single-strand conformation polymorphism analysis of polymerase chain reaction products. *Oncogene* **6**, 1313–18.

McDonald, J.D., Daneshvar, L., Willert, J.R., Matsumura, K., Waldman, F. and Cogen, P.H. (1994) Physical mapping of chromosome 17p13.3 in the region of a putative tumor suppressor gene important in medulloblastoma. *Genomics* **23**, 229–32.

Metzger, A.K., Sheffield, V.C., Duyk, G., Daneshvar, L., Edwards, M.S.B. and Cogen, P.H. (1991) Identification of a germ line mutation in the *p53* gene in a patient with an intracranial ependymoma. *Proceedings of the National Academy of Sciences U.S.A.* **88**, 7825–9.

Miyakoshi, J., Dobler, K.D., Allalunis-Turner, J., McKean, J.D., Petruk, K., Allen, P.B.R., Aronyk, K.N., Weir, B., Huyser-Wierenga, D., Fulton, D., Urtsun, R.C. and Day, R.S. III (1990) Absence of *IFNA* and *IFNB* genes from human malignant glioma cell lines and lack of correlation with cellular sensitivity to interferons. *Cancer Research* **50**, 278–83.

Moertel, C.A., Dahl, R.J., Stalboerger, P.G., Kimmel, D.W., Scheithauer, B.W. and Jenkins, R.B. (1993) Gliosis specimens contain clonal cytogenetic abnormalities. *Cancer Genetics and Cytogenetics* **67**, 21–7.

Mohapatra, G., Kim, D.H. and Feuerstein, B.G. (1995) Detection of multiple gains and losses of genetic material in ten glioma cell lines by comparative genomic hybridization. *Genes, Chromosomes and Cancer* **13**, 86–93.

Mollenhauer, J., Wiemann, S., Scheurlen, W., Korn, B., Hayashi, Y., Wilgenbus, K.K., von Deimling, A. and Poustka, A. (1997) DMBT1, a new member of the SRCR superfamily on chromosome 10q25.3–26.1 is deleted in malignant brain tumours. *Nature Genetics* **17**, 32–9.

Momand, J., Zambetti, G.P., Olson, D.C., George, D. and Levine, A.J. (1992) The *mdm*-2 oncogene product forms a complex with the p53 protein and inhibits p53-mediated transactivation. *Cell* **69**, 1237–45.

Montgomery, R.B., Moscatello, D.K., Wong, A.J., Cooper, J.A. and Stahl, W.L. (1995) Differential modulation of mitogen-activated protein (MAP) kinase/extracellular signal-related kinase and MPA kinase activities by a mutant epidermal growth factor receptor. *Journal of Biological Chemistry* **270**, 30562–6.

Mori, T., Nagase, H., Horii, A., Miyoshi, Y., Shimano, T., Nakatsuru, S., Aoki, T., Arakawa, H., Yanagisawa, A., Ushio, Y., Takano, S., Ogawa, M., Nakamura, M., Shibuya, M., Nishikawa, R., Matsutani, M., Hayashi, Y., Takahashi, H., Ikuta, F., Nishihira, T., Mori, S. and Nakamura, Y. (1994) Germ-line and somatic mutations of the *APC* gene in patients with Turcot syndrome and analysis of *APC* mutations in brain tumors. *Genes, Chromosomes and Cancer* **9**, 168–72.

Morita, R., Saito, S., Ishikawa, J., Ogawa, O., Yoshida, O., Yamakawa, K. and Nakamura, Y. (1991) Common regions of deletion on chromosomes 5q, 6q, and 10q in renal cell carcinoma. *Cancer Research* **51**, 5817–20.

Moscatello, D.K., Holgado-Madruga, M., Godwin, A.K., Ramirez, G., Gunn, G., Zoltick, P.W., Biegel, J.A., Hayes, R.L. and Wong, A.J. (1995) Frequent expression of a mutant epidermal growth factor receptor in multiple human tumors. *Cancer Research* **55**, 5536–9.

Moulton, T., Samara, G., Chung, W.Y., Yuan, L., Desai, R., Sisti, M., Bruce, J. and Tycko, B. (1995) *MTS1/p16/CDKN2* lesions in primary glioblastoma multiforme. *American Journal of Pathology* **146**, 613–19.

Muleris, M., Almeida, A., Dutrillaux, A.M., Pruchon, E., Vega, F., Delattre, J.Y., Poisson, M., Malfoy, B. and Dutrillaux, B. (1994) Oncogene amplification in human gliomas: a molecular cytogenetic analysis. *Oncogene* **9**, 2717–22.

Neumann, E., Kalousek, D.K., Norman, M.G., Steinbok, P., Cochrane, D.D. and Goddard, K. (1993) Cytogenetic analysis of 109 pediatric central nervous system tumors. *Cancer Genetics and Cytogenetics* **71**, 40–9.

Ng, H., Lau, K., Tse, J.Y.M., Lo, K.W., Wong, J.H.C., Poon, W.S. and Huang, D.P. (1995) Combined molecular genetic studies of chromosome 22q and the neurofibromatosis type 2 gene in central nervous system tumors. *Neurosurgery* **37**, 764–73.

Nigro, J.M., Baker, S.J., Presisinger, A.C., Jessup, J.M., Hostetter, R., Cleary, K., Bigner, S.H., Davidson, N., Baylin, S., Devilee, P., Glover, T., Collins, F.S., Weston, A., Modali, R., Harris, C.C. and Vogelstein, B. (1989) Mutations in the *p53* gene occur in diverse human tumour types. *Nature* **342**, 705–8.

Nishikawa, R., Ji, X.-G., Harmon, R.C., Lazar, C.S., Gill, G.N., Cavenee, W.K. and Huang, H.J.S. (1994) A mutant epidermal growth factor receptor common in human glioma confers enhanced tumorigenicity. *Proceedings of the National Academy of Sciences U.S.A.* **91**, 7727–31.

Nishikawa, R., Furnari, F.B., Lin, H., Arap, W., Berger, M.S., Cavenee, W.K. and Huang, H.J.S. (1995) Loss of $P16^{INK4}$ expression is frequent in high grade gliomas. *Cancer Research* **55**, 1941–5.

Nishisho, I., Nakamura, Y., Miyoshi, Y., Miki, Y., Ando, H., Horri, A., Koyama, K., Utsunomiya, J., Baba, S., Hedge, P., Markham, A., Krush, A.J., Petersen, G., Hamilton, S.R., Nilbert, M.C., Levy, D.B., Bryan, T.M., Preisinger, A.C., Smith, K.J., Su, K.-L., Kinzler, K.W. and Vogelstein, B. (1991) Mutations of the chromosome 5q21 genes in FAP and colorectal cancer patients. *Science* **253**, 665–9.

Nobori, T., Karras, J.G., Ragione, F.D., Waltz, T.A., Chen, P.P. and Carson, D.A. (1991) Absence of methyladenosine phosphorylase in human gliomas. *Cancer Research* **51**, 3193–7.

Ohgaki, H., Eibl, R.H., Wiestler, O.D., Yasargil, M.G., Newcomb, E.W. and Kleihues, P. (1991) *p53* Mutations in nonastrocytic human brain tumors. *Cancer Research* **51**, 6202–5.

Ohgaki, H., Schäuble, B., zur Hausen, A., von Ammon, K. and Kleihues, P. (1995) Genetic alterations associated with the evolution and progression of astrocytic brain tumours. *Virchows Archiv* **427**, 113–18.

Oliner, J.D., Kinzler, K.W., Meltzer, P.S., George, D.L. and Vogelstein, B. (1992) Amplification of a gene encoding p53-associated protein in human sarcomas. *Nature* **358**, 80–3.

Olopade, O.I., Jenkins, R.B., Ransom, D.T., Malik, K., Pomykala, H., Nobori, T., Cowan, J.M., Rowley, J.D. and Diaz, M.O. (1992) Molecular analysis of deletions of the short arm of chromosome 9 in human gliomas. *Cancer Research* **52**, 2523–9.

Ostrowski, L.E., von Wronski, M.A., Bigner, S.H., Rasheed, A., Schold, S.C. Jr, Brent, T.P., Mitra, S. and Bigner, D.D. (1991) Expression of O^6-methylguanine-DNA methyltransferase in malignant human glioma cell lines. *Carcinogenesis* **12**, 1739–44.

Peiffer, S.L., Herzog, T.J., Tribune, D.J., Mutch, D.G., Gerssell, D.J. and Goodfellow, P.J. (1995) Allelic loss of sequences from the long arm of chromosome 10 and replication errors in endometrial cancers. *Cancer Research* **55**, 1922–6.

Pershouse, M.A., Stubblefield, E., Hadi, A., Killary, A.M., Yung, W.K.A. and Steck, P.A. (1993) Analysis of the functional role of chromosome 10 in human glioblastomas. *Cancer Research* **53**, 5043–50.

Pietsch, T., Scharman, T., Fonatsch, C.F., Schmidt, D., Ockler, R., Freihoff, D., Albrecht, S., Wiestler, O.D., Zeltzer, P. and Riehm, H. (1994) Characterization of five new cell lines derived from human primitive neuroectodermal tumors of the central nervous system. *Cancer Research* **54**, 3278–87.

Raffel, C., Gilles, F.E. and Weinberg, K.I. (1990) Reduction to homozygosity and gene amplification in central nervous system primitive neuroectodermal tumors of childhood. *Cancer Research* **50**, 587–91.

Reffel, C., Jenkins, R.B., Frederick, L., Hebrink, D., Aldrete, B., Fults, D.W. and James, C.D. (1997) Sporadic medulloblastomas contain PTCH mutations. *Cancer Research* **57**, 842–5.

Raffel, C., Thomas, G.A., Tishler, D.M., Lassof, S. and Allen, J.C. (1993) Absence of *p53* mutations in childhood central nervous system primitive neuroectodermal tumors. *Neurosurgery* **33**, 301–6.

Ransom, D.T., Ritland, S.R., Kimmel, D.W., Moertel, C.A., Dahl, R.J., Scheithauer, B.W., Kelly, P.J. and Jenkins, R.B. (1992a) Cytogenetic and loss of heterozygosity studies in ependymomas, pilocytic astrocytomas, and oligodendrogliomas. *Genes, Chromosomes and Cancer* **5**, 348–56.

Ransom, D.T., Ritland, S.R., Moertel, C.A., Dahl, R.J., O'Fallon, J.R., Scheithauer, B.W., Kimmel, D.W., Kelly, P.J., Olopade, O.I., Diaz, M.O. and Jenkins, R.B. (1992b) Correlation of cytogenetic analysis and loss of heterozygosity studies in human diffuse astrocytomas and mixed oligo-astrocytomas. *Genes, Chromosomes and Cancer* **5**, 357–74.

Rasheed, B.K.A., Fuller, G.N., Friedman, A.H., Bigner, D.D. and Bigner, S.H. (1992) Loss of heterozygosity for 10q loci in human gliomas. *Genes, Chromosomes and Cancer* **5**, 75–82.

Rasheed, B.K.A., McLendon, R.E., Herndon, J.E., Friedman, H.S., Friedman, A.H., Bigner, D.D. and Bigner, S.H. (1994) Alterations of the *TP53* gene in human gliomas. *Cancer Research* **54**, 1324–30.

Rasheed, B.K.A., McLendon, R.E., Friedman, H.S., Friedman, A.H., Fuchs, H.E., Bigner, D.D. and Bigner, S.H. (1995) Chromosome 10 deletion mapping in human gliomas: a common deletion region in 10q25. *Oncogene* **10**, 2243–6.

Reifenberger, G., Liu, L., Ichimura, K., Schmidt, E.E. and Collins, V.P. (1993) Amplification and overexpression of the *MDM2* gene in a subset of human malignant gliomas without *p53* mutations. *Cancer Research* **53**, 2736–9.

Reifenberger, G., Reifenberger, J., Ichimura, K., Meltzer, P.S. and Collins, V.P. (1994) Amplification of multiple genes from chromosomal region 12q13–14 in human malignant gliomas: preliminary mapping of the amplicons shows preferential involvement of *CDK4, SAS*, and *MDM2*. *Cancer Research* **54**, 4299–303.

Reifenberger, J., Reifenberger, G., Liu, L., James, C.D., Wechsler, W. and Collins, V.P. (1994) Molecular genetic analysis of oligodendroglial tumors shows preferential allelic deletions on 19q and 1p. *American Journal of Pathology* **145**, 1175–90.

Reifenberger, J., Reifenberger, G., Ichimura, K., Schmidt, E.E., Wechsler, W. and Collins, V.P. (1996a) Epidermal growth factor receptor expression in oligodendroglial tumors. *American Journal of Pathology* **149**, 29–35.

Reifenberger, J., Ring, G.U., Gies, U., Cobbers, J.M.J.L., Oberstrass, J., An, H.-X., Niederacher, D., Wechsler, W. and Reifenberger, G. (1996b) Analysis of *p53* mutation and epidermal growth factor receptor amplification in recurrent gliomas with malignant progression. *Journal of Neuropathology and Experimental Neurology* **55**, 822–31.

Rempel, S.A., Schwechheimer, K., Davis, R.L., Cavenee, W.K. and Rosenblum, M.L. (1993) Loss of heterozygosity for loci on chromosome 10 is associated with morphologically malignant meningioma progression. *Cancer Research* **53**, 2386–92.

Rey, J.A., Bello, M.J., de Campos, J.M., Benitez, J., Ayuso, M.C. and Valcàrcel, E. (1983) Chromosome studies in two human brain tumors. *Cancer Genetics and Cytogenetics* **10**, 159–65.

Rey, J.A., Bello, M.J., de Campos, J.M., Kusak, M.E. and Moreno, S. (1987a) Cytogenetic analysis in human neurinomas. *Cancer Genetics and Cytogenetics* **28**, 187–8.

Rey, J.A., Bello, M.J., de Campos, J.M., Kusak, M.E., Ramos, C. and Benitez, J. (1987b) Chromosomal patterns in human malignant astrocytomas. *Cancer Genetics and Cytogenetics* **29**, 201–21.

Rey, J.A., Bello, M.J., de Campos, J.M., Kusak, M.E. and Moreno, S. (1987c) Chromosomal composition of a series of 22 human low grade gliomas. *Cancer Genetics and Cytogenetics* **29**, 223–37.

Rey, J.A., Bello, M.J., Jimenez-Lara, A.M., Vaquero, J., Kusak, M.E., de Campos, J.M., Sarasa, J. and Pestana A. (1992) Loss of heterozygosity for distal markers on 22q in human gliomas. *International Journal of Cancer* **51**, 703–6.

Rey, J.A., Bello, M.J., de Campos, J.M., Vaquero, J., Kusak, M.E., Sarasa, J.L., Pestana, A. (1993) Abnormalities of chromosome 22 in human brain tumors determined by combined cytogenetic and molecular genetic approaches. *Cancer Genetics and Cytogenetics* **66**, 1–10.

Ritland, S.R., Ganju, V. and Jenkins, R.B. (1995) Region-specific loss of heterozygosity on chromosome 19 is related to the morphologic type of human glioma. *Genes, Chromosomes and Cancer* **12**, 277–82.

Rogatto, S.R., Casartelli, C., Rainho, C.A. and Barbieri-Neto, J. (1993) Chromosomes in the genesis and progression of ependymomas. *Cancer Genetics and Cytogenetics* **69**, 146–52.

Rorke, L.B., Packer, R. and Biegel, J. (1995) Central nervous system typical teratoid/rhabdoid tumors of infancy and childhood. *Journal of Neuro-Oncology* **24**, 21–8.

Rosenfeld, M.R., Meneses, P., Dalmau, J., Drobnjak, M., Cordon-Cardon, C. and Kaplitt, M.G. (1995) Gene transfer of wild type *p53* results in restoration of tumor suppressor function in a medulloblastoma cell line. *Neurology* **45**, 1533–9.

Rouah, E., Wilson, D.R., Armstrong, D.L. and Darlington, G.J. (1989) N-*myc* amplification and neuronal differentiation in human primitive neuroectodermal tumors of the central nervous system. *Cancer Research* **49**, 1797–801.

Rouleau, G.A., Wertelecki, W., Haines, J.L., Hobbs, W.J., Trofatter, J.A., Seizinger, B.R., Martuza, R.L., Superneau, D.W., Conneally, P.M. and Gusella, J.F. (1987) Genetic linkage of bilateral acoustic neurofibromatosis to a DNA marker on chromosome 22. *Nature* **329**, 246–8.

Rouleau, G.A., Merel, P., Lutchman, M., Sanson, M., Zucman, J., Marineau, C., Hoang-Xuan, K., Demczuk, S., Desmaze, C., Plougastel, B., Pulst, S.M., Lenoir, G., Bijlsma, E., Fashold, R., Dumanski, J., deJong, P., Parry, D., Eldrige, R., Aurias, A., Delattre, O. and Thomas, G. (1993) Alteration in a new gene encoding a putative membrane-organizing protein causes neurofibromatosis type 2. *Nature* **363**, 515–21.

Rubio, M.P., von Deimling, A., Yandell, D.W., Wiestler, O.D., Gusella, J.F. and Louis, D.N. (1993) Accumulation of wild type p53 protein in human astrocytomas. *Cancer Research* **53**, 3465–7.

Rubio, M.P., Correa, K.M., Ramesh, V., MacCollin, M.M., Jacoby, L.B., von Deimling, A., Gusella, J.F. and Louis, D.N. (1994a) Analysis of the neurofibromatosis 2 gene in human ependymomas and astrocytomas. *Cancer Research* **54**, 45–7.

Rubio, M.P., Correa, K.M., Ueki, K., Mohrenweiser, H.W., Gusella, J.F., von Deimling, A. and Louis, D.N. (1994b) The putative glioma tumor suppressor gene on chromosome 19q maps between *APOC2* and *HRC*. *Cancer Research* **54**, 4760–3.

Ruttledge, M.H., Sarrazin, J., Rangaratnam, S., Phelan, C.M., Twist, E., Merel, P., Delattre, O., Thomas, G., Nordenskjöld, M., Collins, V.P., Dumanski, J.P. and Rouleau, G.A. (1994a) Evidence of the complete inactivation of the *NF2* gene in the majority of sporadic meningiomas. *Nature Genetics* **6**, 180–4.

Ruttledge, M.H., Xie, Y.-G., Han, F.-Y., Peyrard, M., Collins, V.P., Nordenskjöld, M. and Dumanski, J.P. (1994b) Deletions on chromosome 22 in sporadic meningioma. *Genes, Chromosomes and Cancer* **10**, 122–30.

Salgaller, M., Pearl, D. and Stephens, R. (1991) *In situ* hybridization with single-stranded RNA probes to demonstrate infrequently elevated *gli* mRNA and no increased *ras* mRNA levels in meningiomas and astrocytomas. *Cancer Letters* **57**, 243–53.

Sawyer, J.R., Thomas, E.L., Roloson, G.J., Chadduck, W.M. and Boop, F.A. (1992) Telomeric associations evolving to ring chromosomes in a recurrent pleomorphic xanthoastrocytoma. *Cancer Genetics and Cytogenetics* **60**, 152–7.

Sawyer, J.R., Sammartino, G., Husain, M., Lewis, J.M., Anderson, B. and Boop, F.A. (1993) Ring chromosome 12 resulting from nonrandom telomeric associations with the short arm of chromosome 15 in a cerebellar astrocytoma. *Genes, Chromosomes and Cancer* **8**, 69–73.

Sawyer, J.R., Sammartino, G., Husain, M., Boop, F.A. and Chadduck, W.M. (1994) Chromosome aberrations in four ependymomas. *Cancer Genetics and Cytogenetics* **74**, 132–8.

Saxena, A., Clark, W.C., Robertson, J.T., Ikejiri, B., Oldfield, E.H. and Ali, I.U. (1992) Evidence for the involvement of a potential second tumor suppressor gene on chromosome 17 distinct from *p53* in malignant astrocytomas. *Cancer Research* **52**, 6716–21.

Saylors, R.L., Sidransky, D., Friedman, H.S., Bigner, S.H., Bigner, D.D., Vogelstein, B. and Brodeur, G.M. (1989) Infrequent *p53* gene mutations in medulloblastomas. *Cancer Research* **51**, 4721–3.

Scheck, A.C. and Coons, S.W. (1993) Expression of the tumor suppressor gene *DCC* in human gliomas. *Cancer Research* **53**, 5605–9.

Scheurlen, W.G. and Senf, L. (1995) Analysis of the GAP-related domain of the neurofibromatosis type 1 (*NF1*) gene in childhood brain tumors. *International Journal of Cancer* **64**, 234–8.

Scheurlen, W.G., Krauss, J. and Kuhl, J. (1995) No preferential loss of one parental allele of chromosome 17p13.3 in childhood medulloblastoma. *International Journal of Cancer* **63**, 372–4.

Schlegel, J., Merdes, A., Stumm, G., Albert, F.K., Forsting, M., Hynes, N. and Kiessling, M. (1994) Amplification of the epidermal-growth-factor-receptor gene correlates with different growth behaviour in human glioblastoma. *International Journal of Cancer* **56**, 72–7.

Schmidt, E.E., Ichimura, K., Reifenberger, G. and Collins, V.P. (1994) *CDKN2 (p16/MTS1)* gene deletion or *CDK4* amplification occurs in the majority of glioblastomas. *Cancer Research* **54**, 6321–4.

Schneider, B.F., Shashi, V., von Kap-herr, C. and Golden, W.L. (1995) Loss of chromosomes 22 and 14 in the malignant progression of meningiomas. A comparative study of fluorescence *in situ* hybridization (FISH) and standard cytogenetic analysis. *Cancer Genetics and Cytogenetics* **85**, 101–4.

Schofield, D., West, D.C., Anthony, D.C., Marshal, R. and Sklar, J. (1995) Correlation of loss of heterozygosity at chromosome 9q with histological subtype in medulloblastomas. *American Journal of Pathology* **146**, 472–80.

Schröck, E., Thiel, G., Lozanova, T., du Manoir, S., Meffert, M.-C., Jauch, A., Speicher, M.R., Nurnberg, P., Vogel, S., Janisch, W., Donis-Keller, H., Ried, T., Witkowski, R. and Cremer, T. (1994) Comparative genomic hybridization of human malignant gliomas reveals multiple amplification sites and nonrandom chromosomal gains and losses. *American Journal of Pathology* **144**, 1203–18.

Schröck, E., Blume, C., Meffert, M.-C., du Manoir, S., Bersch, W., Kiessling, M., Lozanowa, T., Thiel, G., Witkowski, R. and Cremer, T. (1996) Recurrent gain of chromosome arm 7q in low grade astrocytic tumors studied by comparative genomic hybridization. *Genes, Chromosomes and Cancer* **15**, 199–205.

Schütz, B.R., Scheurlen, W., Krauss, J., du Manoir, S., Joos, S., Bentz, M. and Lichter, P. (1996) Mapping of chromosomal gains and losses in primitive neuroectodermal tumors by comparative genomic hybridization. *Genes, Chromosomes and Cancer* **16**, 196–203.

Schwechheimer, K., Huang, S. and Cavenee, W.K. (1995) EGFR gene amplification—rearrangement in human glioblastomas. *International Journal of Cancer* **62**, 145–8.

Seizinger, B.R., Martuza, R.L. and Gusella, J.F. (1986) Loss of genes on chromosome 22 in tumorigenesis of human acoustic neuroma. *Nature* **322**, 644–7.

Seizinger, B.R., de la Monte, S., Atkins, L., Gusella, J.F. and Martuza, R.L. (1987a) Molecular genetic approach to human meningioma: loss of genes on chromosome 22. *Proceedings of the National Academy of Sciences U.S.A.* **84**, 5419–23.

Seizinger, B.R., Rouleau, G., Ozelius, L.J., Lane, A.H., St. George-Hyslop, P., Huson, S., Gusella, J.F. and

Martuza, R.L. (1987b) Common pathogenetic mechanism for three tumor types in bilateral acoustic neurofibromatosis. *Science* **236**, 317–19.

Simon, M., von Deimling, A., Larson, J.J., Wellenreuther, R., Kaskel, P., Waha, A., Warnick, R.E., Tew, J.M. Jr and Menon, A.G. (1995) Allelic losses on chromosomes 14, 10, and 1 in atypical and malignant meningiomas: a genetic model of meningioma progression. *Cancer Research* **55**, 4696–701.

Sonoda, Y., Yoshimoto, T. and Sekiya, T. (1995) Homozygous deletion of the *MTS1/p16* and *MTS2/p15* genes and amplification of the *CDK4* gene in glioma. *Oncogene* **11**, 2145–9.

Sonoda, Y., Iizuka, M., Yasuda, J., Makino, R., Ono, T., Kayama, T., Yoshimoto, T. and Sekiya, T. (1995) Loss of heterozygosity at 11p15 in malignant glioma. *Cancer Research* **55**, 2166–8.

Srivastava, S., Zou, Z.Q., Pirollo, K., Blattner, W. and Chang, E.H. (1990) Germ-line transmission of a mutated *p53* gene in a cancer-prone family with Li-Fraumeni syndrome. *Nature* **348**, 747–9.

Steck, P.A., Ligon, A.H., Cheong, P., Yung, W.K.A. and Pershouse, M.A. (1995) Two tumor suppressor loci on chromosome 10 involved in human glioblastomas. *Genes, Chromosomes and Cancer* **12**, 255–61.

Steck, P.A., Pershouse, M.A., Jasser, S.A., Yung, W.K.A., Lin, H., Ligon, A.H., Langford, L.A., Baumgard, M.L., Hattier, T., Davis, T., Frye, C., Hu, R., Swedlund, B., Teng, D.H.F. and Tavtigian, S.V. (1997) Identification of a candicate tumour suppressor gene, *MMAC1*, at chromosome 10q23.3 that is mutated in multiple advanced cancers. *Nature Genetics* **15**, 356–62.

Stenman, G., Kindblom, L.-G., Johansson, M. and Angervall, L. (1991) Clonal chromosome abnormalities and *in vitro* growth characteristics of classical and cellular schwannomas. *Cancer Genetics and Cytogenetics* **57**, 121–31.

Stapleton, P., Weith, A., Urbanek, P., Kozmik, Z. and Busslinger, M. (1993). Chromosomal localization of seven *PAX* genes and cloning of a novel family member, *PAX-9. Nature Genetics* **3**, 292–8.

Stratton, M.R., Darling, J., Lantos, P.L., Cooper, C.S. and Reeves, B.R. (1989) Cytogenetic abnormalities in human ependymomas. *International Journal of Cancer* **44**, 579–81.

Sugawa, N., Ekstrand, A.J., James, C.D. and Collins, V.P. (1990) Identical splicing of aberrant epidermal growth factor receptor transcripts from amplified rearranged genes in human glioblastomas. *Proceedings of the National Academy of Sciences U.S.A.* **87**, 8602–6.

Tachibana, O., Nakazawa, H., Lampe, J., Watanabe, K., Kleihues, P. and Ohgaki, H. (1995) Expression of *Fas/APO-1* during the progression of astrocytomas. *Cancer Research* **55**, 5528–30.

Tenan, M., Benedetti, S. and Finocchiaro, G. (1995) Deletion and transfection analysis of the *p15/MTS2* gene in malignant gliomas. *Biochemical and Biophysical Research Communications* **217**, 195–202.

Tenan, M., Colombo, B.M., Cajola, L., Pollo, B., Broggi, G. and Finocchiaro, G. (1993) Low frequency of *NF1* gene mutations in malignant gliomas. (Abstract) *European Journal of Cancer* **29A**, 1217–18.

Tenan, M., Colombo, B.M., Pollo, B., Cajola, L., Broggi, G. and Finocchiaro, G. (1994) *p53* Mutations and microsatellite analysis of loss of heterozygosity in malignant gliomas. *Cancer Genetics and Cytogenetics* **74**, 139–43.

Thiel, G., Losanowa, T., Kintzel, D., Nisch, G., Martin, H., Vorpahl, K. and Witkowski, R. (1992) Karyotypes in 90 human gliomas. *Cancer Genetics and Cytogenetics* **58**, 109–20.

Thomas, G.A. and Raffel, C. (1991) Loss of heterozygosity on 6q, 16q and 17p in human central nervous system primitive neuroectodermal tumors. *Cancer Research* **51**, 639–43.

Tomlinson, F.H., Jenkins, R.B., Scheithauer, B.W., Keelan, P.A., Ritland, S., Parisi, J.E., Cunningham, J. and Olsen, K.D. (1994) Aggressive medulloblastoma with high-level N-*myc* amplification. *Mayo Clinic Proceedings* **69**, 359–65.

Trent, J., Meltzer, P., Rosenblum, M., Harsh, G., Kinzler, K., Mashal, R., Feinberg, A. and Vogelstein, B. (1986) Evidence for rearrangement, amplification, and expression of c-*myc* in a human glioblastoma. *Proceedings of the National Academy of Sciences U.S.A.* **83**, 470–3.

Trofatter, J.A., MacCollin, M.M., Rutter, J.L., Murrell, J.R., Duyao, M.P., Parry, D.M., Eldridge, R., Kley, N., Menon, A.G., Pulaski, K., Haase, V.H., Ambrose, C.M., Munroe, D., Bove, C., Haines, J.L., Martuza, R.L., MacDonald, M.E., Seizinger, B.R., Short, M.P., Buckler, A.J. and Gusella, J.F. (1993) A novel moesin-, ezrin-, radixin-like gene is a candidate for the neurofibromatosis 2 tumor suppressor. *Cell* **72**, 791–800.

Tsuda, T., Marinetti, M.R., Masuelli, L. and Cutler, M.L. (1995) The *Ras* suppressor *RSU-1* localizes to 10p13 and its expression in the U251 glioblastoma cell line correlates with a decrease in growth rate and tumorigenic potential. *Oncogene* **11**, 397–403.

Turc-Carel, C., Limon, J., Cin, P.D., Rao, U., Karakousis, C. and Sandberg, A.A. (1986) Cytogenetic studies of adipose tissue tumors. II. Recurrent reciprocal translocation t(12;16)(q13;p11) in myxoid liposarcomas. *Cancer Genetics and Cytogenetics* **23**, 291–9.

Tuzi, N.L., Venter, D.J., Kumar, S., Staddon, S.L., Lemoine, N.R. and Gullick, W.J. (1991) Expression of growth factor receptors in human brain tumours. *British Journal of Cancer* **63**, 227–33.

Ueki, K., Rubio, M.P., Ramesh, V., Correa, K.M., Rutter, J.L., von Deimling, A., Buckler, A.J., Gusella, J.F. and Louis, D.N. (1994) *MTS1/CDKN2* gene mutations are rare in primary human astrocytomas with allelic loss of chromosome 9p. *Human Molecular Genetics* **3**, 1841–5.

Ueki, K., Ono, Y., Henson, J.W., Efird, J.T., von Deimling, A. and Louis, D.N. (1996) *CDKN2/p16* or *RB* alterations occur in the majority of glioblastomas and are inversely correlated. *Cancer Research* **56**, 150–3.

Vagner-Capodano, A.M., Gentet, J.C., Gambarelli, D., Pellissier, J.F., Gouzien, M., Lena, G., Genitori, L., Choux, M. and Raybaud, C. (1992) Cytogenetic studies in 45 pediatric brain tumors. *Pediatric Hematology and Oncology* **9**, 223–35.

van Meyel, D.J., Ramsay, D.A., Chambers, A.F., Macdonald, D.R. and Cairncross, J.G. (1994) Absence of hereditary mutations in exons 5 through 9 of the *p53* gene and exon 24 of the neurofibrin gene in families with glioma. *Annals of Neurology* **35**, 120–2.

Venter, D.J. and Thomas, D.G.T. (1991) Multiple sequential molecular abnormalities in the evolution of human gliomas. *British Journal of Cancer* **63**, 753–7.

Venter, D.J., Bevan, K.L., Ludwig, R.L., Riley, T.E.W., Jat, P.S., Thomas, D.G.T. and Noble, M.D. (1991) Retinoblastoma gene deletions in human glioblastomas. *Oncogene* **6**, 445–8.

von Deimling, A., Eibl., R.H., Ohgaki, H., Louis, D.N., von Ammon, K., Petersen, I., Kleihues, P., Chung, R.Y., Wiestler, O.D. and Seizinger, B.R. (1992a) *p53* Mutations are associated with 17p allelic loss in grade II and grade III astrocytoma. *Cancer Research* **52**, 2987–90.

von Deimling, A., Louis, D.N., von Ammon, K., Petersen, I., Wiestler, O.D. and Seizinger, B.R. (1992b) Evidence for a tumor suppressor gene on chromosome 19q associated with human astrocytomas, oligodendrogliomas, and mixed gliomas. *Cancer Research* **52**, 4277–9.

von Deimling, A., von Ammon, K., Schoenfeld, D., Wiestler, O.D., Seizinger, B.R. and Louis, D.N. (1993) Subsets of glioblastoma multiforme defined by molecular genetic analysis. *Brain Pathology* **3**, 19–26.

von Deimling, A., Bender, B., Jahnke, R., Waha, A., Kraus, J., Albrecht, S., Wellenreuther, R., Fasbbender, F., Nagel, J., Menon, A.G., Louis, D.N., Lenartz, D., Schramm, J. and Wiestler, O.D. (1994a) Loci associated with malignant progression in astrocytomas: a candidate on chromosome 19q. *Cancer Research* **54**, 1397–401.

von Deimling, A., Nagel, J., Bender, B., Lenartz, D., Schramm, J., Louis, D.N. and Wiestler, O.D. (1994b) Deletion mapping of chromosome 19 in human gliomas. *International Journal of Cancer* **57**, 676–80.

Walker, D.G., Duan, W., Kaye, A.H. and Lavin, M.F. (1995a) Homozygous deletions of the *MTS1* gene are rare in non-astrocytic brain tumors. *Biochemical and Biophysical Research Communications* **211**, 404–9.

Walker, D.G., Duan, W., Popovic, E.A., Kaye, A.H., Tomlinson, F.H. and Lavin, M. (1995b) Homozygous deletions of the multiple tumor suppressor gene 1 in the progression of human astrocytomas. *Cancer Research* **55**, 20–3.

Wasson, J.C., Saylors, R.L. III, Zeltzer, P., Friedman, H.S., Bigner, S.H., Burger, P.C., Bigner, D.D., Look, A.T., Douglass, E.C. and Brodeur, G.M. (1990) Oncogene amplification in pediatric brain tumors. *Cancer Research* **50**, 2987–90.

Watanabe, K., Nagai, M., Wakai, S., Arai, T. and Kawashima, K. (1990) Loss of constitutional heterozygosity in chromosome 10 in human glioblastoma. *Acta Neuropathologica* **80**, 251–4.

Watanabe, K., Tachibana, O., Sato, K., Yonekawa, Y., Kleihues, P. and Ohgaki, H. (1996) Overexpression of the EGF receptor and *p53* mutations are mutually exclusive in the evolution of primary and secondary glioblastomas. *Brain Pathology* **6**, 217–24.

Watkins, D., Dion, F., Poisson, M., Delattre, J.Y. and Rouleau, G.A. (1994) Analysis of oncogene expression in primary human gliomas: evidence for increased expression of the *ros* oncogene. *Cancer Genetics and Cytogenetics* **72**, 130–6.

Wellenreuther, R., Kraus, J.A., Lenartz, D., Menon, A.G., Schramm, J., Louis, D.N., Ramesh, V., Gusella, J.F., Wiestler, O.D. and von Deimling, A. (1995) Analysis of the neurofibromatosis 2 gene reveals molecular variants of meningioma. *American Journal of Pathology* **146**, 827–32.

Weller, M., Malipiero, U., Aguzzi, A., Reed, J.C. and Fontana, A. (1995) Protooncogene *bcl-2* gene transfer abrogates *Fas/APO-1* antibody-mediated apoptosis of human malignant glioma cells and confers resistance to chemotherapeutic drugs and therapeutic irradiation. *Journal of Clinical Investigation* **95**, 2633–43.

Welter, C., Henn, W., Theisinger, B., Fischer, H., Zang, K.D. and Blin, N. (1990) The cellular *myb* oncogene is amplified, rearranged and activated in human glioblastoma cell lines. *Cancer Letters* **52**, 57–62.

Weremowicz, S., Kupsky, W.J., Morton, C.C. and Fletcher, J.A. (1992) Cytogenetic evidence for a chromosome 22 tumor suppressor gene in ependymoma. *Cancer Genetics and Cytogenetics* **61**, 193–6.

Wernicke, C., Thiel, G., Lozanova, T., Vogel, S., Kintzel, D., Jänisch, W., Lehmann, K. and Witkowski, R. (1995) Involvement of chromosome 22 in ependymomas. *Cancer Genetics and Cytogenetics* **79**, 173–6.

Wertelecki, W., Rouleau, G.A., Superneau, D.W., Forehand, L.W., Williams, J.P., Haines, J.L. and Gusella, J.F. (1988) Neurofibromatosis 2: clinical and DNA linkage studies of a large kindred. *New England Journal of Medicine* **319**, 278–83.

Wikstrand, C.J., Hale, L.P., Batra, S.K., Hill, M.L., Humphrey, P.A., Kurpad, S.N., McLendon, R.E., Moscatello, D., Pegram, C.N., Reist, C.J., Traweek, S.T., Wong, A.J., Zalutsky, M.R. and Bigner, D.D. (1995) Monoclonal antibodies against EGFRvIII are tumor specific and react with breast and lung carcinomas and malignant gliomas. *Cancer Research* **55**, 3140–8.

Willert, J.R., Daneshvar, L., Sheffield, V.C. and Cogen, P.H. (1995) Deletion of chromosome arm 17p DNA sequences in pediatric high-grade and juvenile pilocytic astrocytomas. *Genes, Chromosomes and Cancer* **12**, 165–72.

Wilson, C.B., Kaufmann, L. and Barker, M. (1970) Chromosome analysis of glioblastoma multiforme. *Neurology* **20**, 821–7.

Wong, A.J., Bigner, S.H., Bigner, D.D., Kinzler, K.W., Hamilton, S.R. and Vogelstein, B. (1987) Increased expression of the epidermal growth factor receptor gene in malignant gliomas is invariably associated with gene amplification. *Proceedings of the National Academy of Sciences U.S.A.* **84**, 6899–903.

Wong, A.J., Rupert, J.M., Bigner, S.H., Grzeschik, C.H., Humphrey, P.A., Bigner, D.D. and Vogelstein, B. (1992) Structural alterations of the epidermal growth factor receptor gene in human gliomas. *Proceedings of the National Academy of Sciences U.S.A.* **89**, 2965–9.

Wu, J.K. and Chikaraishi, D.M. (1990) Differential expression of *ros* oncogene in primary human astrocytomas and astrocytoma cell lines. *Cancer Research* **50**, 3032–5.

Wullich, B., Müller, H.W., Fischer, U., Zang, K.D. and Meese, E. (1993) Amplified *MET* gene linked to double minutes in human glioblastoma. *European Journal of Cancer* **29A**, 1991–5.

Xiao, H., Goldthwait, D.A. and Mapstone, T. (1994) A search for *gli* expression in tumors of the central nervous system. *Pediatric Neurosurgery* **20**, 178–82.

Yamada, K., Kondo, T., Yoshika, M. and Oami, H. (1980) Cytogenetic studies in twenty human brain tumors: association of No. 22 chromosome abnormalities with tumors of the brain. *Cancer Genetics and Cytogenetics* **2**, 293–307.

Yamazaki, H., Fukui, Y., Ueyama, Y., Tamaoki, N., Kawamoto, T., Taniguchi, S. and Shibuya, M. (1988) Amplification of the structurally and functionally altered epidermal growth factor receptor gene (*c-erbB*) in human brain tumors. *Molecular and Cellular Biology* **8**, 1816–20.

Yarden, Y. and Ullrich, A. (1988) Growth factor receptor tyrosine kinases. *Annual Review of Biochemistry* **57**, 443–78.

Yong, W.H., Chou, D., Ueki, K., Harsh, G.R. IV, von Deimling, A., Gusella, J.F., Mohrenweiser, H.W. and Louis, D.N. (1995a) Chromosome 19q deletions in human gliomas overlap telomeric to D19S219 and may target a 425 kb region centromeric to D19S112. *Journal of Neuropathology and Experimental Neurology* **54**, 622–6.

Yong, W.H., Raffel, C., von Deimling, A. and Louis, D.N. (1995b) The *APC* gene in Turcot's syndrome. *New England Journal of Medicine* **333**, 524.

Zang, K.D. (1982) Cytological and cytogenetical studies on human meningioma. *Cancer Genetics and Cytogenetics* **6**, 249–74.

Zang, K.D. and Singer, H. (1967) Chromosomal constitution of meningiomas. *Nature* **216**, 84–5.

Zankl, H. and Zang, K.D. (1972) Cytological and cytogenetical studies on brain tumors. IV. Identification of the missing G chromosome in human meningiomas as No. 22 by fluorescence technique. *Humangenetik* **14**, 167–9.

——(1980) Correlations between clinical and cytogenetical data in 180 meningiomas. *Cancer Genetics and Cytogenetics* **1**, 351–6.

Zhang, S., Feng, X., Koga, H., Ichikawa, T., Abe, S. and Kumanishi, T. (1993) *p53* Gene mutations in pontine gliomas of juvenile onset. *Biochemical and Biophysical Research Communications* **196**, 851–7.

CHAPTER 3

Mechanisms of altered growth control

Growth factors

MONICA NISTÉR AND BENGT WESTERMARK

Growth factors and their receptors

Growth factors are polypeptides that are active at nanomolar concentrations and mediate their effects via binding to cell surface receptors with a high degree of specificity. Most growth factor receptors are protein tyrosine kinases (PTKs) (van der Geer, Hunter and Lindberg, 1994). The PTK receptors were first subclassified, based on their structure, into four major groups of transmembrane receptors (Ullrich and Schlessinger, 1990); the classification now extends to ten major groups with additional nonclassified species (Fantl, Johnson and Williams, 1993; Heldin, 1996, and references therein) (Table 3.1). The PTK receptors function as ligand-induced allosteric enzymes and are composed of an extracellular ligand-binding domain, a single hydrophobic transmembrane stretch and a cytoplasmic tyrosine kinase domain. The transmembrane receptor conveys the growth factor signal to the cytoplasm, and the enzyme

Table 3.1 Growth factor receptors of the protein tyrosine kinase and serine/threonine kinase families and their corresponding ligands

Receptor family	Receptor characteristics	Ligand characteristics
Protein tyrosine kinase receptors		
Epidermal growth factor receptor family	Two cysteine-rich domains; long C-terminal tail where phosphorylation sites are clustered.	Monomeric ligands with conserved EGF-like domains characterized by six cysteine residues and synthesized as transmembrane precursors. EGF, TGF-α and AREG are members of the EGF-like structural superfamily of growth factors; HGL belongs to the mosaic family.
Insulin receptor family	Disulfide-linked preformed heterotetramer of two α (extracellular) and two β (transmembrane and intracellular) polypeptide chains, one cysteine-rich domain and two fibronectin type III domains in each α-chain; receptor associates with the intracellular transducer IRS1 (insulin receptor substrate 1).	Insulin, IGF-1 and IGF-2 are homologous, originally single-chained molecules containing 2–3 disulfide bridges. Insulin-like structural superfamily.
Platelet-derived growth factor receptor family	Five immunoglobulin-like domains; split tyrosine kinase domain with a long insert.	Dimeric molecules with similarity to VEGF. PDGF and CSF-1 are disulfide-linked dimers; SCF is noncovalently linked. PDGF is a member of the cystine knot structural superfamily.
Fibroblast growth factor receptor family	Two to three immunoglobulin-like domains, extracellular acidic stretch; split tyrosine kinase domain with a short insert. Several splice variants of the receptors.	Heparin and heparan sulfate stabilize dimeric binding. FGFs are members of the β-trefoil structural superfamily.
Neurotrophin receptor family	Two immunoglobulin-like domains, leucin-rich motif; short tyrosine kinase domain.	NGF is a homodimeric molecule and a member of the cystine knot structural superfamily; NGF binds with high affinity to TrkA and also to a member of the TNF-α receptor superfamily, which serves as a low-affinity receptor.
Hepatocyte growth factor receptor family	Large extracellular domain that undergoes proteolytic cleavage near the N-terminal end whereafter the two resulting subunits are held together as a disulfide-linked dimer.	HGF is a dimeric disulfide-linked molecule derived from one single polypeptide chain. HGF has four kringle domains and one domain with homology to the serine proteases.

Table 3.1 Continued

Receptor family	Receptor characteristics	Ligand characteristics
Vascular endothelial growth factor receptor family	Seven immunoglobulin-like domains, split tyrosine kinase domain. Receptors expressed only on endothelial cells.	Dimeric disulfide-linked molecules with similarity to PDGF.
Eph-like receptor family	N-terminal immunoglobulin-like domain, one cysteine-rich domain and two fibronectin type III repeats. Receptors predominantly expressed in the CNS.	Transmembrane or membrane-anchored ligands with juxtacrine action.
Tie receptor family	Three EGF-like domains, three fibronectin type III domains and two immunoglobulin-like domains. Receptors expressed on endothelial cells.	Ligands partly unknown. Angiopoietin-1 is a ligand for Tie-2.
Serine/threonine kinase receptors		
Transforming growth factor-β receptor family	Many variant receptor molecules of, in principle, two types, i.e., TGF-β type I and TGF-β type II receptors. TGF-β type I receptors are characterized by a glycine–serine rich intracellular juxtamembrane domain. Both receptors are needed for signaling and mediate the effect by sequential binding and phosphorylation in hetero-oligomeric complexes most likely of two type I and two type II receptors.	TGF-β superfamily—dimeric molecules synthesized as large precursors. TGF-β belongs to the cystine knot structural superfamily. Additional TGF-β receptors are the type III proteoglycan receptor and endoglin.

The PTK receptors are glycosylated transmembrane proteins. The subclassification of these receptors is based on the structure of their extracellular (amino terminal) domain, such as the presence of cysteine-rich fibronectin type III and immunoglobulin-like domains and the intracellular (carboxy terminal) domain (length and arrangement of the tyrosine kinase domain). It is also based on the mono- or oligomeric composition of the receptor molecule. Information was obtained from Ullrich and Schlessinger (1990), Fantl, Johnson and Williams (1993), van der Geer, Hunter and Lindberg (1994), Heldin (1996), McDonald and Hendrickson (1993), and references therein.

EGF, epidermal growth factor; TGF, transforming growth factor; AREG, amphiregulin; HGL, heregulin; IGF, insulin-like growth factor; IRS, insulin receptor substrate; VEGF, vascular endothelial growth factor; PDGF, platelet-derived growth factor; CSF, colony-stimulating factor; SCF, stem-cell factor; FGF, fibroblast growth factor; NGF, nerve growth factor; TNF, tumor necrosis factor; HGF, hepatocyte growth factor; CNS, central nervous system.

activity of the intrinsic kinase domain is absolutely essential for signal transduction.

The growth factor ligands specific for a given PTK receptor class are structurally partly related, partly unrelated (Table 3.1) (McDonald and Hendrickson, 1993). Binding of the growth factor leads to dimerization of receptor molecules into homo- or heterodimers (Heldin, 1995), transphosphorylation of the receptors and activation of their intrinsic receptor tyrosine kinases. Several tyrosine residues in the intracellular domains of the receptors become phosphorylated and form docking sites for intracellular substrates, some of which also become phosphorylated. These docking molecules contain Src homology 2 (SH2) or phosphotyrosine binding (PTB) domains that confer binding specificity by recognizing phosphotyrosine residues in specific amino acid environments. Receptor dimerization is thus crucial for activation and is brought about by association of two homologous receptor molecules [e.g., the platelet-derived growth factor receptors (PDGFRs)], juxtaposition of the two intracellular PTK domains of an originally tetrameric receptor [e.g., the insulin receptor (InsulinR) family] or recruitment of other intracellular tyrosine kinases that associate with the receptor molecule (e.g., members of the cytokine receptor family). The PTK receptors exert their mitogenic effects most probably via the Ras, Raf and mitogen-activated protein kinase (MAPK) signal transduction pathway. The growth factor receptor kinase activity is normally transient due to down regulation, internalization and dephosphorylation of the ligand-activated receptor molecules (Hunter, 1995). Furthermore, cellular sorting mechanisms determine whether the internalized receptors are recycled to the cell surface or degraded.

The receptors of the transforming growth factor (TGF)-β superfamily of growth factors are serine/threonine protein kinases (ten Dijke, Miyazono and Heldin, 1996). The intracellular downstream effects of TGF-β are not known to the same extent as are those of tyrosine kinase receptors, but they involve Smad (i.e., Sma + Mad) proteins, which are encoded by vertebrate homologs of developmental genes in *Cænorhabditis elegans* and *Drosophila (Sma and Mad)*. These intracellular proteins become phosphorylated, dimerize and translocate to the nucleus upon TGF-β stimulation (Derynck and Zhang, 1996). Other types of receptors (e.g., certain neuropeptide and hormone receptors) belong to the seven-transmembrane-spanning receptor family and are G-protein coupled (Strader *et al.*, 1994); some of them function through activation of adenylate cyclase.

Receptors for interferons, interleukins, and colony-stimulating factors (CSF-Rs) except for CSF-1R, belong to the cytokine receptor family (Kishimoto, Taga and Akira, 1994). These receptors lack catalytic domains, but recruit and activate intracytoplasmic PTKs and transduce signals via the signal transducers and activators of transcription (Jak-STAT) pathway. In this family, there are a plethora of receptors and substrates that signal via partly overlapping pathways. Shared substrates enable cross-talk between signals of the family of cytokine receptors and the family of PTK receptors, a mechanism that constitutes one of several whereby cytokines can modulate growth factor signals. The receptors for tumor necrosis factor (TNF)-α and TNF-β constitute a group of their own, also without an intracellular kinase domain. In this case, binding of a trimeric ligand induces trimeric receptor complexes (Smith, Farrah and Goodwin, 1994).

Growth factors are soluble molecules or they are bound to extracellular matrix (ECM). Members of the fibroblast growth factor (FGF) family are, for example, characterized by their high specific binding to heparin; *in vivo* they are bound to heparan sulfate-containing ECM components. Growth factors act locally, and their mode of activation may be juxtacrine (cell-bound ligand activates receptor on adjacent cells by direct cell–cell contact), autocrine (ligand activates receptor, both of which are produced by the same cell) or paracrine (secreted ligand activates receptors on nearby cells) as opposed to classic hormonal activation where the ligand derives from a distant organ and is presented to the target tissue via the bloodstream.

Binding of a growth factor to its cognate receptor elicits an array of cellular responses, including those directly involved in the regulation of the cell cycle, such as induction of certain immediate early genes, cyclins, and cyclin-dependent kinases (CDKs) and their inhibitors (CDKIs). Thus, the transduced growth factor signal is integrated into the system of positive and negative regulators of G1/S phase transition and checkpoint controls, and thereby drives the cell through G1 into S phase.

The normal function of growth factors is to regulate cell proliferation, differentiation, apoptosis and cell motility. Thus, growth factors are indispensable during embryonic development and in regenerative processes. They are also important mediators of these functions in oncogenesis. Several of the PTK receptors, as well as certain growth factors [e.g., of the platelet-derived growth factor (PDGF) and FGF families] have been identified as proto-oncogene products. Thus, they may potentially cause transformation and induce tumors when activated through retroviral transduction or insertion, gene amplification, recombination or point mutation (Aaronson, 1991). A number of genes encoding intracellular transducer molecules, the normal function of which is to transmit the growth factor signal, can, when aberrantly activated, also act as oncogenes (described in Chapter 2 of this book). Moreover, tumor cells synthesize many different types of growth factors [Table 3.2(a)] that may elicit various cellular responses through autocrine as well as paracrine routes. Finally, tumor cells express growth factor receptors [Table 3.2(b)], that may be activated by mitogens released not only by the tumor cells themselves, but also by resident or invading normal cells.

In summary, growth factor function in tumor cells can be aberrantly triggered or subverted by several mechanisms (cf. Fig. 3.1):

- improper expression of ligand with respect to time, tissue localization and cell specificity, leading to abnormal paracrine stimulation
- co-expression of ligand and receptor in the same cell at the cell surface or in an intracellular compartment, leading to autocrine receptor activation

Table 3.2(a) Growth factors of relevance for brain tumors, with special reference to their expression in gliomas

Ligand		Reference
Ligands for the EGFR family		
TGF-α	Transforming growth factor α	Nistér *et al.*, 1988; Schlegel *et al.*, 1990; Yung *et al.*, 1990; Ekstrand *et al.*, 1991
EGF	Epidermal growth factor	Ekstrand *et al.*, 1991
HGL	Heregulin/Neu differentiation factor/glial growth factor	
AREG/SDGF	Amphiregulin/schwannoma-derived growth factor	Mishima *et al.*, 1996
Ligands for the insulinR family		
Insulin		
IGF-1 and -2	Insulin-like growth factor 1 and 2	Grunberger *et al.*, 1986; Sandberg *et al.*, 1988; Antoniades *et al.*, 1992; Sandberg-Nordqvist *et al.*, 1993; Trojan *et al.*, 1993; D'Ambrosio *et al.*, 1996
Ligands for the PDGFR family		
PDGF-B	Platelet-derived growth factor B-chain; Sis	Eva *et al.*, 1982; Pantazis *et al.*, 1985; Maxwell *et al.*, 1990b; Mauro *et al.*, 1991; Strawn *et al.*, 1994; Vassbotn *et al.*, 1994
PDGF-A	Platelet-derived growth factor A-chain	Nistér, Heldin and Westermark 1986; Nistér *et al.*, 1987; Nistér *et al.*, 1988; Hermanson *et al.*, 1992; Shamah, Stiles and Guha, 1993; Potapova, Fakhrai and Mercola, 1996
SCF	Stem-cell factor	Stanulla *et al.*, 1995
CSF-1	Colony-stimulating factor 1	Alterman and Stanley, 1994
Ligands for the FGFR family		
FGF-1/aFGF	Fibroblast growth factor 1/acidic FGF	Libermann *et al.*, 1987; Stefanik *et al.*, 1991; Myers *et al.*, 1995
FGF-2/bFGF	Fibroblast growth factor 2/basic FGF	Morrison *et al.*, 1990, 1994; Takahashi *et al.*, 1990, 1991, 1992; Zagzag *et al.*, 1990; Morrison, 1991; Alvarez *et al.*, 1992; Murphy, Sato and Knee, 1992; Ueba *et al.*, 1994; Stan *et al.*, 1995
FGF-9	Fibroblast growth factor 9	Miyamoto *et al.*, 1993
Ligands for the neurotrophin receptor family		
NGF	Nerve growth factor	Hamel *et al.*, 1993
BDNF	Brain-derived neurotrophic factor	
NT-3	Neurotrophin 3	
NT-4	Neurotrophin 4	
Ligands for the hepatocyte growth factor receptor family		
HGF	Hepatocyte growth factor; scatter factor (SF)	Moriyama *et al.*, 1995, 1996; Rosen *et al.*, 1996
Ligands for the vascular endothelial growth factor receptor family		
VEGF/VPF	Vascular endothelial growth factor/vascular permeability factor	Criscuolo, Merrill and Oldfield, 1988; Plate *et al.*, 1992b, 1994; Berkman *et al.*, 1993; Weindel *et al.*, 1994; Hatva *et al.*, 1995; Samoto *et al.*, 1995; Stein *et al.*, 1995; Cheng *et al.*, 1996; Saleh, Stacker and Wilks, 1996; Takano *et al.*, 1996
PlGF	Placental growth factor	Weindel *et al.*, 1994; DiSalvo *et al.*, 1995

Table 3.2(a) Continued

Ligand		Reference
Ligands for the Tie receptor family		
	Partly unknown	
	Angiopoietin-1	
Ligands for other protein tyrosine kinase receptors		
Ros ligand	Unknown	
Transforming growth factor-β family		
TGF-βs	Transforming growth factor-βs	de Martin *et al.*, 1987; Kuppner *et al.*, 1988; Bodmer *et al.*, 1989; Constam *et al.*, 1992; Olofsson *et al.*, 1992; Tucker and Gillespie, 1994; Saitoh *et al.*, 1995; Weller and Fontana, 1995; Yamada *et al.*, 1995; Fakhrai *et al.*, 1996; Jachimczak *et al.*, 1996
BMPs	Bone morphogenetic proteins	Yamada *et al.*, 1996

Human tumor tissues and cell lines, as well as rodent cell lines, were used in the investigations referenced. Some of the articles describe experimental *in vivo* and *in vitro* systems for inhibition of glioma cell growth.

Table 3.2(b) Growth factor receptors relevant to brain tumors, with special reference to gliomas

Receptor		Reference
Epidermal growth factor receptor family		
EGFR/ErbB	Epidermal growth factor receptor	Westermark, Magnusson and Heldin, 1982; Libermann *et al.*, 1985; Malden *et al.*, 1988; Sugawa *et al.*, 1990; Ekstrand *et al.*, 1991, 1992, 1994; Wong *et al.*, 1992; Nishikawa *et al.*, 1994
ErbB2/HER-2/Neu	Human epidermal growth factor receptor 2	LaRocca *et al.*, 1989; Torp *et al.*, 1993; Schwechheimer *et al.*, 1994; Haapasalo *et al.*, 1996
ErbB3/HER-3	Human epidermal growth factor receptor 3	
ErbB4/HER-4	Human epidermal growth factor receptor 4	
Insulin receptor family		
InsulinR	Insulin receptor	Gammeltoft *et al.*, 1988
IGF-1R	Insulin-like growth factor receptor 1	Glick *et al.*, 1989; Merrill and Edwards, 1990; Antoniades *et al.*, 1992; Baserga, 1995; Resnicoff *et al.*, 1995
Platelet-derived growth factor receptor family		
PDGFR-β	Platelet-derived growth factor β-receptor	Hermansson *et al.*, 1988; Nistér *et al.*, 1991; Plate *et al.*, 1992a; Strawn *et al.*, 1994; Vassbotn *et al.*, 1994

Table 3.2(b) Continued

Receptor		Reference
PDGFR-α	Platelet-derived growth factor α-receptor	Nistér *et al.*, 1991; Fleming *et al.*, 1992; Hermanson *et al.*, 1992, 1996; Kumabe *et al.*, 1992; Shamah, Stiles and Guha, 1993; Guha *et al.*, 1995
SCFR/Kit	Stem-cell factor receptor	Berdel *et al.*, 1992; Stanulla *et al.*, 1995
CSF-1R/Fms	Colony-stimulating factor 1 receptor	
Flk-2/Flt-3		
Fibroblast growth factor receptor family		
FGFR-1/Flg	Fibroblast growth factor receptor 1	Morrison *et al.*, 1990; Morrison *et al.*, 1994; Ueba *et al.*, 1994
FGFR-2/Bek/KGFR	Fibroblast growth factor 2	
FGFR-3	Fibroblast growth factor 3	
FGFR-4	Fibroblast growth factor 4	
Neurotrophin receptor family		
TrkA/NGFR	Nerve growth factor receptor	Hutton, DeVellis and Perez-Polo, 1992
TrkB/BDNR/NT-4R	Brain-derived neurotrophic receptor/neurotrophin 4 receptor	
TrkC/NT3R	Neurotrophin 3 receptor	
Hepatocyte growth factor receptor family		
HGFR/Met	Hepatocyte growth factor receptor	Muleris *et al.*, 1994; Wullich *et al.*, 1994; Fischer *et al.*, 1995; Matsumoto, Kagoshima and Nakamura, 1995; Moriyama *et al.*, 1995, 1996
Vascular endothelial growth factor receptor family		
VEGFR-1/Flt-1	Vascular endothelial growth factor receptor 1	
VEGFR-2/KDR/Flk-1	Vascular endothelial growth factor receptor 2/kinase insert domain-containing receptor	Millauer *et al.*, 1994; Plate *et al.*, 1994; Hatva *et al.*, 1995
Flt-4		
Tie receptor family		
Tie-1		Hatva *et al.*, 1995
Tie-2/Tek		
Other protein tyrosine kinase receptors		
Ros		Birchmeier, Sharma and Wigler, 1987; Sharma *et al.*, 1989; Birchmeier *et al.*, 1990; Wu and Chikaraishi, 1990; Watkins *et al.*, 1994
Receptors for the transforming growth factor-β family of growth factors		
Receptors for TGF-βs	TGF-β type I and type II receptors	Helseth *et al.*, 1988; Jennings *et al.*, 1991
Receptors for BMPs	BMP type II receptor, activin type II and IIB receptors, BMP type IA and IB receptors and activin type I receptor	Perides *et al.*, 1994; Yamada *et al.*, 1996

Human tumor tissues and cell lines, as well as rodent cell lines, were used in the investigations referenced. Some of the articles describe experimental *in vivo* and *in vitro* systems for inhibition of glioma cell growth.

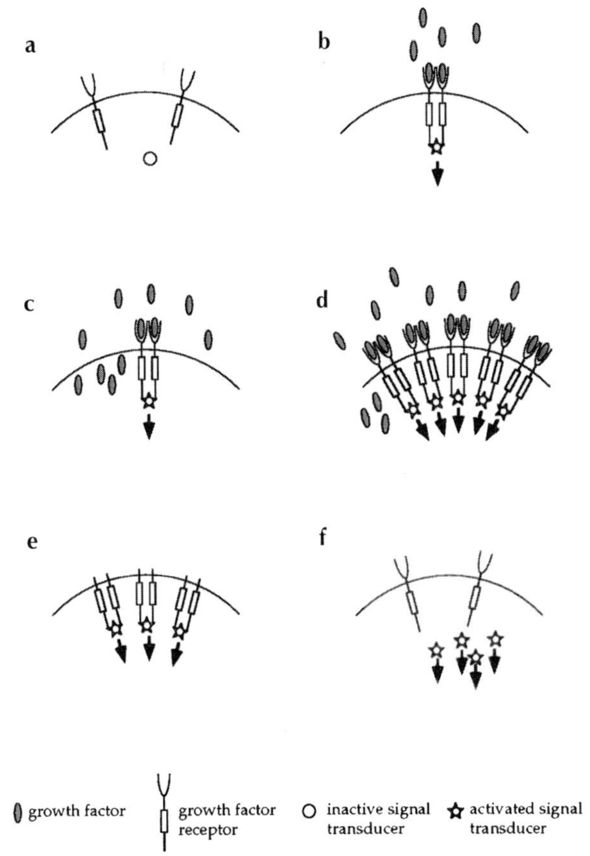

Fig. 3.1 Mechanisms of aberrant activation of growth factor function in tumorigenesis. (a) Resting cells with unoccupied, monomeric growth factor receptors and inactive signal transducer; (b) paracrine activation whereby binding of a growth factor leads to receptor dimerization, activation of the signal transducer and mitogenic stimulation; (c) autocrine receptor activation; (d) overexpression of cell-surface growth factor receptors, caused by receptor gene amplification, overexpression of a normal copy gene or deficient receptor down regulation; (e) constitutive signaling of a rearranged growth factor receptor; and (f) constitutive signaling of a mutated and activated signal transducer.

- increased receptor activation due to overexpression of a normal gene
- amplification of the growth factor receptor gene
- mutational activation of receptor
- mutational activation of transducer molecule
- uncoupling of inhibitory feedback mechanisms for receptor down regulation

The normal function of certain growth factors, such as members of the TGF-β family, is inhibition of cell proliferation. The loss of function of these growth factors may therefore also contribute to the oncogenic process. Loss of an inhibitory growth factor signal can, in principle, be effected by the following:

- loss of receptor expression
- inactivation of receptor due to mutation
- inactivation of downstream mediators and/or abnormal activation of stimulatory pathways

In the context of neuro-oncogenesis, the biologic effects of aberrant growth factor receptor activation may be described in terms of deregulation of cell proliferation, cell differentiation and cell death; other effects are an increase in cell motility, the modulation of cell adhesion and the recruitment of a nonneoplastic, supportive, mainly vascular stroma. Thus, soluble and matrix-bound growth factors constitute part of a functional network of cellular interactions within brain tumors. The tumors of the central nervous system (CNS) are typically not demarcated from the surrounding normal brain tissue, but are intermingled with normal astrocytic and neuronal cells and infiltrated by vessels. Blood cells capable of secreting cytokines are recruited into the tumor area. Neuronal cells contain an array of neuropeptides that may have functional effects on both neuronally and glially derived tumor cells. Similarly, reactive glial cells may release various types of growth factors and cytokines. Thus, both neoplastic cells and nonneoplastic cells may provide important sources of growth factors.

In this chapter, we focus on receptor-mediated events in neuro-oncogenesis. We will provide evidence that growth factors and growth factor receptors are important players in tumor growth and invasion and that information on their structure and mechanism of action may be of great potential value in the design of novel treatment modalities. Details are provided in the tables, one of which includes information on the loci for selected growth factor and growth factor receptor genes (Table 3.3).

Human cell lines are valuable tools for studying the cell biology of brain tumors and for addressing specific questions concerning the functions of growth factors, oncogenes and tumor suppressor genes. An introduction to this field is therefore provided. An overall understanding of the mechanisms of perturbed growth control in human tumors requires that the reader be familiar with the process of tumor angiogenesis and the heterogeneity of tumor cells. These subjects are of utmost importance to such an understanding and are, therefore, also covered in this chapter.

Table 3.3 Chromosomal location of growth factor and receptor genes relevant to CNS oncogenesis and their chromosomal location

Gene name	Gene abbreviation	Locus
Tyrosine kinase with immunoglobulin and epidermal growth factor homology domains-1	*TIE1*	1p34–p33
Transforming growth factor-β receptor type III	*TGFBR3*	1p33–p32
Colony-stimulating factor-1	*CSF1* (*MCSF*)	1p21–p13
Nerve growth factor-β subunit	*NGFB* (*NGF*)	1p13.1
Neurotrophic tyrosine kinase receptor 1	*NTRK1* (*TRKA*)	1q21–q22
Transforming growth factor-β2	*TGFB2*	1q41
Transforming growth factor-α	*TGFA*	2p13
Human epidermal growth factor receptor 4	*ERBB4* (*HER4*)	2q33.3–q34
Transforming growth factor-β receptor type II	*TGFBR2*	3p22
Fibroblast growth factor receptor-3	*FGFR3*	4p16.3
Kinase insert domain receptor (vascular endothelial growth factor receptor 2)	*KDR* (*FLK1*; *VEGFR2*)	4q12
Platelet-derived growth factor receptor-α	*PDGFRA* (*PDGFR2*)	4q12
Mast/stem-cell growth factor receptor (oncogene *kit*)	*KIT*	4q12
Amphiregulin; schwannoma-derived growth factor	*AREG; SDGF*	4q13–q21
Fibroblast growth factor-5	*FGF5*	4q21
Fibroblast growth factor-2 (basic fibroblast growth factor)	*FGF2* (*FGFB*)	4q25–q27
Fibroblast growth factor-1 (acidic fibroblast growth factor)	*FGF1* (*FGFA*)	5q31
Platelet-derived growth factor receptor-β	*PDGFRB* (*PDGFR1*)	5q31–q32
Colony-stimulating factor-1 receptor (oncogene *fms*)	*CSF1R* (*FMS*)	5q33.2–q33.3
Fms-like tyrosine kinase-4	*FLT4*	5q34–q35
Fibroblast growth factor receptor-4	*FGFR4*	5q35.1–qter
Bone morphogenetic protein-5	*BMP5*	6
Bone morphogenetic protein-6	*BMP6*	6
Vascular endothelial growth factor	*VEGF* (*VEGFA*)	6p12
Oncogene *ros*	*ROS1*	6q22
Insulin-like growth factor-2 receptor (mannose 6-phosphate receptor)	*IGF2R*	6q26
Platelet-derived growth factor A chain	*PDGFA*	7p22
Epidermal growth factor receptor	*EGFR* (*HER*; *ERBB1*)	7p12.3–p12.1
Hepatocyte growth factor (scatter factor)	*HGF*	7q21.1
Hepatocyte growth factor receptor (oncogene *met*)	*MET* (*HGFR*)	7q31
Heregulin; Neu differentiation factor	*HGL; NDF*	8p22–p11
Fibroblast growth factor receptor-1 (Fms-like tyrosine kinase-2; flt 2 *fms*-like gene)	*FGFR1* (*FLG*)	8p11.2–p11.1
Tek endothelial tyrosine kinase	*TEK* (*TIE2*)	9p21
Neurotrophic tyrosine kinase receptor 2	*NTRK2* (*TRKB*)	9q22.1
Transforming growth factor-β receptor type I	*TGFBR1*	9q33–q34
Endoglin	*ENG*	9q34.1
Fibroblast growth factor-8	*FGF8*	10q25–26
Fibroblast growth factor receptor-2 (keratinocyte growth factor receptor)	*FGFR2* (*BEK*; *KGFR*)	10q26

Table 3.3 Continued

Gene name	Gene abbreviation	Locus
Insulin	*INS*	11p15.5
Insulin-like growth factor-2 (somatomedin A)	*IGF2*	11p15.5
Brain-derived neurotrophic factor	*BDNF*	11p13
Fibroblast growth factor-3 (oncogene *int*-2)	*FGF3* (*INT2*)	11q13
Fibroblast growth factor-4 (Kaposi's sarcoma oncogene; heparin secretory transforming protein-1)	*FGF4* (*KFGF; HSTF1*)	11q13
Fibroblast growth factor-6 (oncogene *hst*-2)	*FGF6* (*HST2*)	12p13
Neurotrophin-3 (neurotrophic factor-3)	*NTF3* (*NT3*)	12p13
Human epidermal growth factor receptor 3	*ERBB3* (*HER3*)	12q13
Stem-cell factor (mast-cell growth factor; steel factor)	*MGF* (*SCF*)	12q22
Insulin-like growth factor-1 (somatomedin C)	*IGF1*	12q22–q24.1
Fibroblast growth factor-9	*FGF9*	13q11–q12
Fms-like tyrosine kinase-1 (vascular endothelial growth factor receptor 1)	*FLT1* (*VEGFR1*)	13q12
Fms-like tyrosine kinase-3 (stem-cell tyrosine kinase-1)	*FLT3* (*STK1*)	13q12
Bone morphogenetic protein-4	*BMP4* (*BMP2B1*)	14q22–q23
Transforming growth factor-β3	*TGFB3*	14q24
Placental growth factor (vascular endothelial growth factor-related protein)	*PGF* (*PLGF*)	14q24–q31
Fibroblast growth factor-7 (keratinocyte growth factor)	*FGF7* (*KGF*)	15q13–q22
Neurotrophic tyrosine kinase receptor 3 (neurotrophin-3 receptor)	*NTRK3* (*TRKC*)	15q24–q25
Insulin-like growth factor-1 receptor	*IGF1R*	15q25–q26
Human epidermal growth factor receptor 2 (oncogene *neu*)	*ERBB2* (*HER2; NEU*)	17q12–q21
Insulin receptor	*INSR*	19p13.2
Transforming growth factor-β1	*TGFB1*	19q13.1–q13.3
Nerve growth factor-γ subunit	*NGFG*	19q13.3
Bone morphogenetic protein-7 (osteogenic protein-1)	*BMP7* (*OP1*)	20
Bone morphogenetic protein-2	*BMP2* (*BMP2A*)	20p12
Platelet-derived growth factor B chain (oncogene *sis*)	*PDGFB* (*SIS*)	22q12.3–q13.1

Information about chromosomal location of genes was obtained from the OMIM database (OMIM™, 1995). Further detailed information can be found therein. Most of the members of the FGF family of growth factors have been included, although the major importance of some of them and their action as oncogenes might be in tumors outside rather than within the CNS. The information given for the TGF-β family is incomplete, due to the fact that the whole spectrum of expression of these factors is not yet known and also the fact that the identification of these factors and receptors is still ongoing. For a description of the chromosome localization of genes for interferons, interleukins and tumor necrosis factors and their ligands we refer the reader to Van Meir (1995).

The growth factor and growth factor receptor genes are, to some extent, located in clusters in the genome. For example, there is one homologous cluster of PTK receptor genes on the long arm of chromosome 4 and one on the long arm of chromosome 5 that have evolved through gene duplication. The growth factor receptor genes so far known to be amplified in glioma are *PDGFRA* (4q12), *EGFR* (7p12) and *MET* (7q31) (Muleris *et al.*, 1994; Collins, 1995).

Growth factors and growth factor receptors in gliomas

PATTERNS OF EXPRESSION

Various PTK receptors and their ligands are expressed in glioma. They are often coexpressed, indicating that autocrine stimulation is a common mechanism by which the growth factor receptor signal is activated in glioma cells. Many reports have focused on receptor and ligand partners from the following families: epidermal growth factor receptor (EGFR), PDGFR, fibroblast growth factor receptor (FGFR) and insulin-like growth factor receptor (IGFR). Table 3.2 summarizes these findings. Most of these factors have a proven mitogenic effect on normal cells of the CNS and on tumor cells. Although stimulation of cell proliferation may be their major function in oncogenesis, it should be remembered that growth factors are multifunctional signaling molecules, and their effects on cell differentiation, motility, survival and angiogenesis may be equally important. Table 3.2 also provides information on members of the TGF-β family of growth factors and receptors.

GROWTH FACTORS THAT PROMOTE CELL PROLIFERATION

Epidermal growth factor receptor family

The major ligands of this group, EGF and TGF-α (Lee, 1996), are synthesized as large transmembrane precursor molecules from which a soluble [approximately 6 kilodalton (kDa)] mature protein, as well as larger, incompletely processed forms, are split off by proteolytic cleavage. In addition, the membrane-anchored form of TGF-α serves as a growth factor that may stimulate adjacent cells through juxtacrine receptor activation (Wong *et al.*, 1989). The addition of EGF to EGFR-expressing cells leads to increased cell proliferation (Carpenter and Cohen, 1976; Westermark, 1976), while co-expression of either EGF or TGF-α and EGFR in immortalized rodent cells in culture leads to cell transformation via autocrine receptor activation (Di Fiore *et al.*, 1987a, 1987b). The *in vivo* transforming potential of TGF-α in EGFR-expressing epithelial cells has been proven in transgenic mice (Jhappan *et al.*, 1990).

A body of evidence has accumulated in which abnormal EGFR activation is shown to be operative in human glioma development. Thus, EGFR mRNA and protein are overexpressed in a majority of malignant gliomas; in many of these cases, but not in all (Chaffanet *et al.*, 1992; Schlegel *et al.*, 1994b), overexpression is caused by *EGFR* gene amplification (Libermann *et al.*, 1985; Agosti *et al.*, 1992; Collins, 1993, and references therein; Schlegel *et al.*, 1994a; Hoi *et al.*, 1995; Schwechheimer, Huang and Cavenee, 1995). The EGF and/or TGF-α are usually co-expressed with the receptor in glioma cell lines (Nistér *et al.*, 1988) and tissue (Ekstrand *et al.*, 1991), and thereby the stage is set for autocrine activation of the EGFR.

Amplification of the *EGFR* gene in glioma is often accompanied by structural alterations of the amplified gene, which can be regarded as a sign of further genetic progression. These alterations appear with a striking similarity from case to case, and the most common type is a deletion of exons 2 through 7. This rearranged gene codes for a receptor protein (EGFRvIII) lacking 267 amino acids in the amino terminal, EGF-binding extracellular domain (Malden *et al.*, 1988; Yamazaki *et al.*, 1988; Humphrey *et al.*, 1990; Sugawa *et al.*, 1990; Yamazaki *et al.*, 1990; Wong *et al.*, 1992). The functional consequence of this deletion is twofold: the ligand binding capacity is lost (Ekstrand *et al.*, 1994; Batra *et al.*, 1995) and the receptor tyrosine kinase is spontaneously activated. This is associated with an increased proliferation rate in the absence of ligand as shown by studies of transduced Chinese hamster ovary (CHO) cells (Yamazaki *et al.*, 1990; Ekstrand *et al.*, 1994; Batra *et al.*, 1995). Experimental transfection of murine fibroblasts (Yamazaki *et al.*, 1990; Batra *et al.*, 1995), CHO cells (Ekstrand *et al.*, 1994) or human U-87 MG glioma cells (Nishikawa *et al.*, 1994) with the variant receptor cDNA suggests that EGFRvIII may be an oncoprotein because it mediates soft agar focus formation and an increased tumorigenic capacity in nude mice (Nishikawa *et al.*, 1994; Batra *et al.*, 1995).

Specific high-affinity monoclonal antibodies (MAbs) to the EGFRvIII receptor have been characterized and are rapidly internalized within 5 minutes of binding to the cell surface receptor in EGFRvIII-expressing cells (Reist *et al.*, 1995; Wikstrand *et al.*, 1995; this book, Chapter 8). Although Ekstrand *et al.* (1994) reported that the EGFRvIII protein expressed in CHO transfectants appeared to be abnormally processed and sequestered intracellularly, Wikstrand *et al.* (1997) showed by quantitative cell-surface immunofluorescence and confocal microscopy of variably fixed cells that the EGFRvIII protein expressed by transfected murine fibroblasts, by transfected U-87 MG human glioma cells and by cells isolated from 10/20 human glioma biopsies all demonstrate the same transmembrane localization of the variant molecule that has been described as typical of wild-type EGFR (Suarez-Quian and Byers, 1993). In summary, this aberrant-activated variant EGFR molecule most likely exerts its effect at the cell surface.

Interestingly, the truncated form of the *EGFR* gene in glioma bears a striking similarity to the retroviral oncogene *v-erbB*, the product of which lacks most of the extracellular portion (Downward *et al.*, 1984) and also has ligand-independent transforming and oncogenic potential. Another, less consistent EGFR variant in glioma has a short deletion in the carboxy terminal end (Ekstrand *et al.*, 1992). The functional effect of this type of alteration is most probably sustained receptor activation due to defective receptor down regulation; a similar experimentally introduced mutation inhibits internalization of the EGFR (Wells *et al.*, 1990).

The EGFR family of growth factor receptors—class I according to Ullrich and Schlessinger (1990)—now comprises four members that can be combined into heterodimeric complexes upon ligand binding (Carraway and Cantley, 1994). The second family member to be identified was HER-2/Neu, and it was isolated as an oncogene from a chemically induced tumor in the rat peripheral nervous system. Expression of Neu has been described as being present in glioma, but the frequency of expression in this type of tumor seems to be relatively low compared with meningioma (Torp *et al.*, 1993 and references therein; Schwechheimer *et al.*, 1994; Haapasalo *et al.*, 1996). Interestingly, a single point mutation and amino acid change in the transmembrane region of Neu leads to spontaneous activation and oligomerization and has a transforming effect as described in other cell types (Bargmann, Hung and Weinberg, 1986; Yarden and Ullrich, 1988; Weiner *et al.*, 1989).

Only recently has a ligand for HER-2/Neu been identified (Holmes *et al.*, 1992). Heregulin, also named Neu differentiation factor and glial growth factor, is known to be a Schwann cell mitogen (Falls *et al.*, 1993; Marchionni *et al.*, 1993) and is expressed in the nervous system during development (Orr-Urtreger *et al.*, 1993). Heregulin is also a ligand for the other two members in this group of receptors, and the binding of heregulin leads to heterodimer formation between HER-2 and HER-3 or HER-4. Likewise, the binding of EGF leads to heterodimer formation between EGFR and HER-2 in cells where both receptor proteins are expressed. These complex binding patterns, and the fact that HER-3 has a low intrinsic kinase activity, lead to a substantial diversity of transduced signals, depending on which setup of receptor molecules a cell expresses. Amphiregulin/schwannoma-derived growth factor is another growth factor in this group, distinct from heregulin. It was purified from a sciatic nerve tumor (Shoyab *et al.*, 1989; Kimura, Fischer and Schubert, 1990).

Platelet-derived growth factor receptor family

The PDGF is a dimeric molecule composed of two homologous polypeptide chains, A and B, in different combinations (Heldin, 1992). The growth factor effect is mediated by two homologous receptor molecules, the α- and the β-receptors, which are the prototypes of class III PTK receptors (Ullrich and Schlessinger, 1990). PDGF-A binds only to the α-receptor, while PDGF-B binds to both α- and β-receptors (Claesson-Welsh, 1994), a fact that contributes to the cell type-specific effects of each of the two PDGF chains. The two PDGF chains, as well as the two receptors, are encoded by separate genes (Table 3.3). As with EGF and TGF-α, PDGF has a transforming effect when expressed in receptor-bearing rodent cells (Leal *et al.*, 1985; Beckman *et al.*, 1988).

Thorough examination of the expression of these genes in human glioma cell lines and tissues has revealed an intricate pattern. Many glioma cell lines express PDGF ligand and receptor (Nistér *et al.*, 1991), suggesting autocrine stimulation of glioma cell growth. The PDGFR-α is expressed at a high level on the tumor cells in all grades of astrocytic tumors, whereas the PDGF-A, and to some degree PDGF-B, are overexpressed in glioblastomas but not in astrocytomas (Hermanson *et al.*, 1992; Guha *et al.*, 1995). Co-expression of PDGFR-α and the PDGF-A can thus be regarded as a progressional phenomenon in glioma. Another autocrine PDGF loop may help drive the vascular proliferations in glioblastoma, since the PDGF-B and the β-receptor are co-expressed in those structures (Hermansson *et al.*, 1988; Hermansson *et al.*, 1992).

In a minority of cases, overexpression of PDGFR-α is associated with amplification of the *PDGFRA* gene (Fleming *et al.*, 1992; Muleris *et al.*, 1994), and, in a single case, an interstitial deletion of 81 amino acids in the extracellular part of the receptor has been described (Kumabe *et al.*, 1992). In most cases, however, mechanisms other than gene amplification are the cause of overexpression. Interestingly, there is a significant correlation in glioma tumors between increased levels of expression of PDGFR-α mRNA and loss of heterozygosity on chromosome 17p, where the *TP53* gene is a gene of interest. Whether this reflects a direct or indirect involvement of the p53 protein in the regulation of *PDGFRA* gene expression, or whether PDGFR-α stimulation and loss of p53 function have complementary effects in glioma development, is not known.

Amplification of the *PDGFRA* and *EGFR* genes in glioma is mutually exclusive (Fleming *et al*., 1992; Hermanson *et al*., 1996), and there is a significant correlation between *EGFR* gene amplification and loss of genetic material on chromosome 10 (von Deimling *et al*., 1993). This has been taken to indicate the existence of two biologically different groups of gliomas originating from different precursor cells, one driven by PDGF, the other by EGF. Consistent with this notion, Noble *et al*. (1995) described a glioblastoma with striking similarity to the oligodendrocyte type 2 astrocyte (O-2A) progenitor cells, which are characterized by their expression of PDGFR-α (Hart *et al*., 1989). PDGF-A is a mitogen and an inhibitor of differentiation for these precursor cells (Raff *et al*., 1988; Richardson *et al*., 1988). On the other hand, PDGFR-β is expressed on vascular structures and neuronal cells in the developing brain (Smits *et al*., 1991). In the adult CNS, large amounts of PDGF are present in neurons (Sasahara *et al*., 1991; Yeh *et al*., 1991).

Other members of the PDGFR family are Kit and the colony-stimulating factor-1 receptor (CSF-1R), i.e., receptors for stem-cell factor (SCF) and for macrophage stimulatory factor (MCSF or CSF-1), respectively. The *KIT* and the *CSF1R* genes are the human homologs of the oncogenes of Hardy-Zuckerman 4 feline sarcoma virus (Besmer *et al*., 1986) and McDonough feline sarcoma virus (Donner *et al*., 1982), respectively. The *KIT* gene is located close to the *PDGFRA* gene on chromosome 4 (Vandenbark *et al*., 1992), while the *CSF1R* gene is located close to the *PDGFRB* gene on chromosome 5 in a head-to-tail arrangement (Roberts *et al*., 1988). The Kit protein is of importance for hematopoietic and melanoblastic cells during development, and both ligand and receptor are expressed in the CNS during embryonic development (Matsui, Zsebo and Hogan, 1990; Keshet *et al*., 1991). Co-expression of Kit and SCF in glioma cells is suggestive of autocrine stimulation (Berdel *et al*., 1992; Stanulla *et al*., 1995). Whether SCF is mitogenic to glioma cells or has other major functional effects has been discussed. There is evidence that CSF-1 is necessary for the normal development of microglia (Blevins and Fedoroff, 1995). CSF-1 can also be produced by glioma cells and may, in concert with other cytokines, contribute to the recruitment of macrophages into the tumor area (Alterman and Stanley, 1994; Van Meir, 1995).

Insulin receptor family

The effect of the insulin family of growth factors is mediated mainly via InsulinR and IGF-1R (White and Kahn, 1994), which both belong to the class II PTK receptors (Ullrich and Schlessinger, 1990). In this group, each mature receptor molecule is a tetramer wherein all parts are encoded by a single gene. In contrast, IGF-2R is a completely different type of cell-surface receptor lacking catalytic activity and identical to the mannose 6-receptor (Morgan *et al*., 1987). Binding to IGF-2R leads rather to degradation of the ligand than to a mitogenic response.

Binding sites for insulin and insulin-like growth factors (IGFs) are abundant in the fetal and adult brain. Several reports describe the expression of IGF-1 and IGF-2 also on human glioma cell lines and tissues, suggesting that an autocrine stimulation prevails in the malignant tumor. Genomic alterations in the corresponding genes have, to our knowledge, not been reported in glioma, but the importance especially of IGF-1R signaling for maintaining the tumorigenic phenotype of glioma cells is illustrated by many reports using antisense IGF-1, and more recently a dominant negative IGF-1 receptor construct to inhibit tumor cell growth and/or to induce apoptosis (Trojan *et al*., 1993; Baserga, 1995, and references therein; D'Ambrosio *et al*., 1996). Particularly intriguing is the finding that inhibition of tumor cell-produced IGF-1 not only leads to the inhibition of local tumor growth, but also protects the experimental animal from establishing tumors at distant locations and at later time points (Trojan *et al*., 1993). This phenomenon has been suggested to occur via IGF-1-dependent escape from the host immune system. From the therapeutic point of view, it is also interesting to note that transformation via several other growth factor receptor pathways seems to depend ultimately on an intact IGF-1R (Baserga, 1995, and references therein).

Fibroblast-derived growth factor receptor family

The family of FGFs (Mason, 1994; Spivak-Kroizman *et al*., 1994) now comprises nine members: FGF-1 [aFGF, endothelial cell growth factor (ECGF), heparin-binding growth factor 1 (HBGF1)], FGF-2 (bFGF), FGF-3 (Int2), FGF-4 (Hst, K-FGF), FGF-5, FGF-6 (Hst2), FGF-7 (KGF), FGF-8 and FGF-9 (glial activating factor). Several members exert important functions in the CNS (Eckenstein, 1994). The normal expression of FGF-2 in neurons and the involvement of this factor in neuronal survival is well established. Expression of FGF-2 also occurs in reactive astrocytes, and it is a mitogen for oligodendrocyte type-2 astrocyte precursors (Bögler *et al*., 1990). Other members of this group have been identified due to their involvement in mouse mammary carcinogenesis (FGF-3) (Nussc *et al.*, 1991), in human stomach carcinoma and Kaposi's sarcoma (FGF-4) and in keratinocyte growth (FGF-7). Recently, four factors homologous to the family of FGFs, fibroblast growth factor homologous factors 1–4 (FHF1–4), were identified and their expression was localized to the CNS (Smallwood *et al.*, 1996).

The FGFRs (Fantl, Peters and Williams, 1996) constitute class IV of the PTK receptors (Ullrich and Schlessinger, 1990). Four receptors have been identified in this group, and each of the FGF ligands specifically bind to a certain setup of receptors. The specificity of binding is also influenced by the existence of several splice variants of receptors. The FGF-2 protein is known to bind to FGFR-1 and FGFR-2 with high affinity.

The FGF-2 protein has been described as one major autocrine stimulator of glioma cell growth. It is co-expressed with FGFRs, mainly FGFR-1, on glioma cells *in vitro* (Morrison *et al.*, 1990) and in glioma tissue (Takahashi *et al.*, 1990; Morrison *et al.*, 1994). Moreover, the degree of FGF-2 expression correlation with the degree of vascularity and of malignancy (Zagzag *et al.*, 1990; Takahashi *et al.*, 1992). Finally, blocking of FGF-2 autocrine loops in glioma cells has led to the inhibition of tumor cell growth. This was accomplished by the addition of antibodies to FGF-2 expressing glioma cells *in vitro* and *in vivo* (Takahashi *et al.*, 1991; Stan *et al.*, 1995) and by the addition of antisense oligonucleotides (Morrison, 1991; Murphy, Sato and Knee, 1992).

Glioma cells also express FGF-1 (Libermann *et al.*, 1987; Myers *et al.*, 1995). The FGF-9 protein has been purified and molecularly cloned from a glioma cell line (Miyamoto *et al.*, 1993). The FGF-1, FGF-2 and FGF-9 molecules all lack a signal peptide and, subsequently, many investigators have addressed the question of how these factors can be secreted and act as growth factors.

GROWTH FACTORS IN GLIOMA CELL MOTILITY

The intrinsic motility of tumor cells is crucial for their invasive property, and the ability to increase cell motility is therefore an important function of growth factors in the oncogenesis of CNS cells. The motility of cultured human glioma cells varies widely (Chicoine and Silbergeld, 1995) and can be increased by the addition of several growth factors such as EGF and TGF-α (Westermark, Magnusson and Heldin, 1982; Pedersen *et al.*, 1994; Chicoine, Madsen and Silbergeld, 1995). Thus, the activation of EGFR in gliomas might result in both increased cell proliferation and cell motility. These two types of effects are seemingly transduced by separate pathways (Chen, Gupta and Wells, 1994).

Several other factors involved in cell motility are secreted from glioma cells. Among these factors is the hepatocyte growth factor (HGF) (Rubin, Bottaro and Aaronson, 1993), also named scatter factor (SF) (Gherardi *et al.*, 1989; Nakamura *et al.*, 1989). The HGF mediates its effect via a PTK receptor, the hepatocyte growth factor receptor (HGFR), which is the homolog of the *c-met* oncogene product (Park *et al.*, 1987; Bottaro *et al.*, 1991; Cooper, 1992). The HGF has a generalized function as a motility factor. It is essential during embryonic development, operates during liver regeneration, and induces the migration and scattering of epithelial cells (Gherardi *et al.*, 1989). Both HGF and HGFR are expressed in the CNS, which implies a normal function also in this tissue (Di Renzo *et al.*, 1993; Jung *et al.*, 1994).

Addition of HGF to glioma cells in culture leads to scattering, i.e., outward cell movements in all directions, and thereby to dissolution of cell colonies. This occurs in the absence of obvious cell proliferation (Matsumoto, Kagoshima and Nakamura, 1995). The activation of the HGFR in glioma may be executed by autocrine stimulation since ligand and receptor can be expressed in the same cells (Moriyama *et al.*, 1995, 1996). Further support for the involvement of HGFR activation in glioma development is gained from the finding that the *HGFR* gene is amplified in a subset of gliomas. The amplified gene was shown to be localized to double-minute chromosomes (Dmins) (Wullich *et al.*, 1994; Fischer *et al.*, 1995).

GROWTH FACTORS WITH MAINLY INHIBITORY FUNCTIONS

Transforming growth factor-β

The TGF-β family of growth factors comprises TGF-βs, bone morphogenetic proteins (BMPs), activins, inhibins and Müllerian inhibiting substance (Kingsley, 1994; Derynck and Zhang, 1996; Massagué, 1996). As the names imply, these factors serve important functions during embryonic development. The molecules are synthesized as large precursor proteins, latent TGF-βs where the active ligand is proteolytically cleaved from the carboxy terminal end. Each factor in this family binds to a set of receptor molecules from the two major classes of receptors, type I and type II receptors, and binding most likely leads to the formation of a heterotetrameric receptor complex (Wrana *et al.*, 1994). According to the current model for receptor activation, TGF-β1 first binds to the type II receptor, whereupon the type I receptor is recruited into the complex and gets phosphorylated in its glycine–serine rich juxtamembrane domain. The signaling pathway thereby becomes activated. The TGF-β modulates cell proliferation and differentiation, largely by inducing the activities of CDKIs. The TGF-β stimulates the production of ECM and, in glioma, it may also influence the host immune response.

Members of the TGF-β family of growth factors and of the TGF-β receptor family are expressed in glioma cell lines and tissues (Kuppner *et al.*, 1988; Bodmer *et al.*, 1989; Olofsson *et al.*, 1992; Yamada *et al.*, 1995), and glioma cells may potentially activate the precursor form of TGF-β (Huber, Fontana and Bodmer, 1991). While the normal function of this family of growth factors is to inhibit cell proliferation, TGF-β was found to stimulate the growth of some glioma cells (Helseth *et al.*, 1988; Jennings *et al.*, 1991). As yet unidentified alterations in TGF-β receptors and/or in signal transduction components may occur in gliomas, as has been described in other types of tumors (Markowitz *et al.*, 1995; Azuma *et al.*, 1996; Eppert *et al.*, 1996). It is possible that tumor cells may loose the growth inhibitory response but retain other favorable types of responses, such as modulation of ECM and the induction of angiogenesis. In this way, TGF-β might contribute to glioma cell progression. Consistent with this notion, the administration of TGF-β antisense constructs to glioma cells had a growth inhibitory effect (Fakhrai *et al.*, 1996). Receptors for BMPs have also been identified in glioma tissue, and glioma cells are responsive to BMPs (Perides *et al.*, 1994; Yamada *et al.*, 1996).

GROWTH FACTORS IN TUMOR ANGIOGENESIS

Angiogenesis is the process whereby constituent endothelial cells are activated and recruited to develop into new vessels by sprouting (Folkman, 1971, 1990). This process is promoted by growth factors and involves activation of enzymes that degrade the vascular basement membrane and surrounding ECM, as well as directed movement of the endothelial cells, endothelial cell proliferation and differentiation into tubular structures. It is assumed that the *in vivo* growth of a solid tumor occurs in two phases. Being primarily avascular, it changes into a vascular phase as the size of the tumor increases. Folkman indicated that a tumor is unable to grow over a few millimeters in size in the absence of a vascular support. The polypeptide factors that take part in this process during tumor formation are most likely to be found among the factors that mediate normal vascularization during embryonic development (Plate, Breier and Risau, 1994; Breier *et al.*, 1992).

Malignant glioma is one of the most vascularized human tumors and it has been used as a model system in the search for angiogenic mechanisms (Plate, Breier and Risau, 1994; Plate and Risau, 1995). In an *in vivo* experiment where the size of implanted mouse glioma cell spheroids was monitored by the nuclear magnetic resonance (NMR) imaging technique, vascularization was found to accompany successful tumor growth (Abramovitch, Meir and Neeman, 1995). Angiogenic mechanisms *in vivo* can also be studied in models where endothelial cells are implanted in experimental tumors (Lal *et al.*, 1994).

Over the years, several glioma cell-produced angiogenic polypeptides have been identified (Folkman and Klagsburn, 1987; Zagzag, 1995). The angiogenic effects of FGF-1 and FGF-2 and of TGF-α and TGF-β are well known. Also, PDGF-B has an angiogenic effect *in vivo* (Risau *et al.*, 1992; Forsberg *et al.*, 1993). The effects of FGFs have been most studied in this respect, and more recently it was shown that the ECM heparan sulfate proteoglycan perlecan, which promotes FGFR binding, greatly potentiates the angiogenic effect of FGF-2 (Aviezer *et al.*, 1994).

The identification and characterization of vascular endothelial growth factor (VEGF) as an endothelial cell-specific mitogen (Ferrara *et al.*, 1992; Neufeld *et al.*, 1994) has, however, been a major contribution to the understanding of the angiogenic process (Mustonen and Alitalo, 1995; Plate and Risau, 1995). The VEGF is a dimeric protein that binds to two different vascular endothelial growth factor receptors (VEGFRs), VEGFR-1 and VEGFR-2, which belong to a separate group of PTK receptors. Among them, the VEGFR-2/KDR/Flk-1 seems to be responsible for transducing most of the VEGF-induced effects. This receptor is abundant on vascular sprouts of embryonic brain, while VEGFR-1/Flt-1 and Flt-4 are expressed at relatively later stages of angiogenesis (Millauer *et al.*, 1993). The functions of VEGF are, for example, endothelial cell proliferation, differentiation and induction of plasminogen activator. Types of cells other than endothelial cells do not express VEGFRs and are thus unable to respond to this factor.

Glioma cells produce VEGF, high-grade gliomas, in particular, and also cells adjacent to necrotic areas (Plate *et al.*, 1992b; Shweiki *et al.*, 1992). Simultaneously, VEGF receptors, mainly VEGFR-1 and VEGFR-2 but not Flt-4, are up regulated on endothelial cells in gliomas (Plate *et al.*, 1994; Hatva *et al.*, 1995), consistent with a model of paracrine stimulation of endothelial cells by tumor cell-produced VEGF. The vessels that form in glioma are leaky, which contributes to the peritumoral edema. The VEGF, also named vascular permeability factor (VPF), has the potential also to promote this effect. The microvascular proliferations of malignant gliomas, however, also have a substantial component of nonendothelial mesenchyme-like elements with pericyte or smooth muscle characteristics (McComb *et al.*, 1982; Haddad *et al.*, 1992). Due to the restricted distribution of VEGF receptors on endothelial cells, the stimulatory effect on these nonendothelial mesenchymal elements must be promoted by some of the other factors that have a 'direct or indirect' angiogenic effect *in vivo*.

Microvascular proliferations are characteristic of anaplastic astrocytoma and glioblastoma multiforme and provide the basis for malignancy grading of astrocytic tumors. Angiogenesis, therefore, seems to be closely associated with tumor progression, and efforts have been made to understand the mechanisms by which VEGF is induced during glioma progression. Hypoxic conditions (Shweiki *et al.*, 1992; Stein *et al.*, 1995), mutated tumor suppressor genes (Kieser *et al.*, 1994) and tumor cell-produced growth factors (Goldman *et al.*, 1993) can potentially induce VEGF. Expression of the VEGF family of growth factors is, however, not confined to malignant tumor cells, but is found also in meningioma and hemangioblastoma (Berkman *et al.*, 1993; Weindel *et al.*, 1994; Samoto *et al.*, 1995; Wizigmann-Vos *et al.*, 1995).

The Tie-1 and Tie-2/Tek group of PTK receptors (Sato *et al.*, 1993) are also specifically expressed on endothelial cells of the brain. They are required for normal endothelial function (Dumont *et al.*, 1994), but their ligands and specific functions are still partly unknown. Angiopoietin-1 was recently identified as a ligand for Tie-2 (Davis *et al.*, 1996). The expression of Tie on glioma vessels has been described (Hatva *et al.*, 1995).

OTHER FACTORS

Other members of the PTK receptor superfamily are also expressed in glioma, like the neurotrophin receptors and their ligands (Kaplan *et al.*, 1991; Barbacid, 1995). The neurotrophin receptor signals are of major importance in the differentiation and survival of neuronal cell types. Likewise, these receptors might be major players in tumors of neuronal derivation (Segal *et al.*, 1994).

Ros, a yet unclassified tyrosine kinase receptor (Heldin, 1996), is differentially expressed in glioma cell lines (Birchmeier, Sharma and Wigler, 1987) and seemingly rearranged in U-118 MG (Sharma *et al.*, 1989). The role for Ros in glioma development, however, remains unproven.

Some additional members of the PTK receptor superfamily that are expressed in the CNS have been included in Table 3.1. The Eph family (Davis *et al.*, 1994; Friedman and O'Leary, 1996; Holland *et al.*, 1996) is an especially interesting group of receptors with membrane-bound ligands. These receptors have the unique capacity of signaling in two directions. They can thereby mediate mutual signaling between adjacent cells and have been suggested to direct the formation of axonal networks in the CNS. Whether these or other as yet unidentified tyrosine kinase receptors are additional players in the development of CNS tumors remains to be seen.

As described above and in the legend to Table 3.3, certain PTK receptor genes have been identified as amplified in human glioblastoma. Such findings are compelling evidence for the involvement of these genes in glioma development. Results from studies using comparative genomic hybridization (CGH) illustrate the location of other potentially amplified genomic regions (Muleris *et al.*, 1994; Schröck *et al.*, 1994). Whether some of these regions correspond to growth factor or growth factor receptor genes is, of course, an open question, but future research to identify the genes of interest, and analogously to identify growth inhibitory genes in areas of genomic deletions, will provide further information about the mechanisms of disturbed growth control in CNS tumors.

Growth factors and growth factor receptors in other types of brain tumors

It can be taken as a general paradigm that tumor cells are stimulated by the same type of growth factors as are their normal counterparts during CNS development. Growth factors and growth factor receptors are most probably as important in other types of brain tumors as in glioma and some examples are given below. High expression of EGFR been described in oligodendroglioma (Reifenberger *et al.*, 1996), and oligodendrogliomas express PDGFR-α (Hermanson, M., Funa, K. and Nistér, M., unpublished observation). Likewise, meningiomas have binding sites for EGF (Weisman, Raguet and Kelly, 1987; Schlegel *et al.*, 1993) and express the Neu oncoprotein product at a high frequency (Torp *et al.*, 1993; Schwechheimer *et al.*, 1994); they have binding sites for insulin and IGF-1 and express the corresponding ligands (Glick *et al.*, 1989; Lichtor, Kurpakus and Gurney, 1991; Antoniades *et al.*, 1992). PDGF-B and the β-receptors are co-expressed in meningioma (Wang *et al.*, 1990; Maxwell *et al.*, 1990a; Figarella-Branger *et al.*, 1994), and intron deletions in the *PDGFB* gene have been described (Bolger *et al.*, 1985; Smidt, Kirsch and Ratner, 1990).

Similarly, medulloblastomas/PNETs express PDGF receptors (Smits *et al.*, 1996) and, in comparison with other types of tumors, PDGF-B is expressed at a high level in medulloblastoma (Nakamura *et al.*, 1993). This is consistent with their neuronal derivation since PDGF is known to be expressed at high levels in neurons. Moreover, PNETs synthesize neurotrophin receptors and their ligands, which may act as inducers of differentiation. High levels of TrkC expression are associated with a favourable outcome in patients with PNETs (Segal *et al.*, 1994; Washiyama *et al.*, 1996).

Experimental evidence for the involvement of growth factors in brain tumor development

TRANSFORMING EFFECT OF RETROVIRALLY TRANSDUCED PDGF-B

Simian sarcoma virus

The acutely transforming retrovirus simian sarcoma virus (SSV) has transduced the cellular gene encoding PDGF-B (Doolittle *et al.*, 1983; Waterfield *et al.*, 1983). The retroviral *onc* gene (v-*sis*) is integrated within the *env* gene as a 5' and 3' truncated gene segment that contains all protein coding sequences except for the segment that codes for the hydrophobic leader sequence (Devare *et al.*, 1983). However, translation of the *sis* mRNA is initiated within the 5' flanking region of the *env* gene that codes for a stretch of hydrophobic amino acid residues that function as a leader peptide.

Cultured cells transformed with either v-*sis* or c-*sis*/PDGF-B, have been used as model systems for studies of autocrine stimulation and transformation. Whether encoded by the v-*sis* or c-*sis*/PDGF-B, the protein products seem to be identically synthesized, processed and externalized, and there is no indication that the viral gene product has any structural or functional characteristics different from those of the normal PDGF B-chain (Westermark and Heldin, 1991, and references therein). However, there is ample evidence that in the *sis*-transformed cell, the growth factor and the receptor are associated in a proximal intracellular compartment, probably both in the endoplasmic reticulum and in the Golgi complex. Although ligand-activated, tyrosine-phosphorylated PDGF receptors are present in an intracellular compartment (Keating and Williams, 1988; Bejcek, Li and Deuel, 1989), there is compelling evidence that the mitogenic signal is generated at the cell surface (Hannink and Donoghue, 1988; Valgeirsdóttir *et al.*, 1994). Consequently, agents that block extracellular ligand binding, such as suramin or PDGF antibodies, inhibit autocrine receptor activation and revert the transformed phenotype (Johnsson *et al.*, 1985; Betsholtz *et al.*, 1986). Similarly, autocrine activation of the EGF receptor, in cells that synthesize EGF or TGF-α along with the EGF receptor, seems to take place at the cell surface (Di Marco *et al.*, 1989). It should be emphasized that these findings do not preclude that the intracellular, receptor-associated tyrosine kinase lacks functional activities. Studies of *sis*/PDGF-B-transformed NIH 3T3 cells have shown that the intracellular PDGF receptor is associated with some of the signaling substrates, and these may elicit responses that remain to be identified.

Gliomas induced by simian sarcoma virus

Injection of SSV together with its helper virus into the brain of newborn marmosets gave rise to brain tumors (Deinhardt, 1980) with a strong resemblance to human gliomas (Fig. 3.2). This striking similarity, together with the fact that PDGF and PDGF receptors are expressed in human tumors, implies a role for PDGF also in human glioma development. The presence of both astrocytoma-like/glioblastoma and oligodendroglioma-like areas in the same individual tumor is consistent with the notion that the target cell of a PDGF-driven glioma is a common oligodendrocyte–astrocyte precursor.

EXPERIMENTS USING ANTIBODIES, DOMINANT NEGATIVE AND ANTISENSE CONSTRUCTS TO INHIBIT GLIOMA CELL GROWTH

Several growth factors and their specific growth factor receptors are co-expressed on glioma cells. The functional significance of such an autocrine growth factor stimulation has, in several cases, been unequivocally proven. Thus, addition of anti-FGF-2 antibodies (Takahashi *et al.*, 1991) and antisense RNA (Morrison, 1991) to FGF-2-expressing cells,

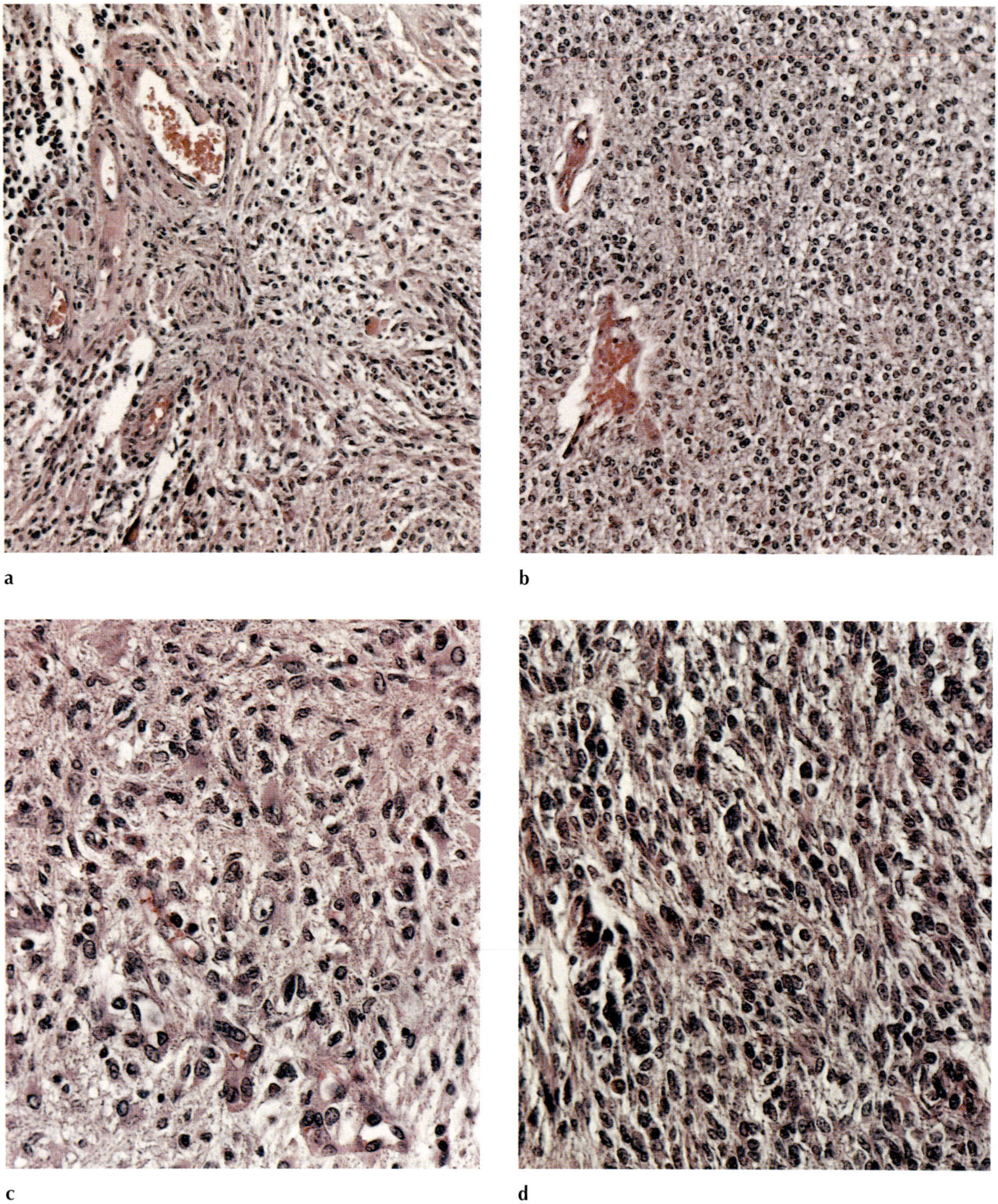

Fig. 3.2 Simian sarcoma virus-induced gliomas in the brains of newborn marmosets. The SSV-induced brain tumors were described by Deinhardt (1980). The experimentally induced tumors show a mixed histologic picture with a striking similarity to human gliomas. (a) A glioblastoma-like area with vascular proliferations and heterogeneous tumor cells. ×100 (b) An oligodendroglioma-like area characterized by clear cells with rounded nuclei and by thin-walled vessels. ×100 (c) A closer view showing astrocytic tumor cells and vascular proliferations. ×175 (d) A cell-dense anaplastic area. In addition, the tumors had a rich supply of vessels, several hemorrhagic areas and a few areas of necrosis. H & E ×175 (Formalin-fixed and paraffin-embedded material from these tumors was generously provided by Dr D.D. Bigner.)

inhibits their growth. Moreover, anti-PDGF-BB antibodies inhibit the growth of PDGF-B-expressing glioma cells (Vassbotn *et al.*, 1994), as do antisense IGF-1 mRNA in IGF-1-expressing cells (Trojan *et al.*, 1993). Finally, dominant negative PDGF (Shamah, Stiles and Guha, 1993) and PDGF receptor (Strawn *et al.*, 1994) constructs negatively affect growth of glioma cells *in vitro* and *in vivo*. The fact that antibodies against VEGF (Kim *et al.*, 1993), as well as a dominant negative mutant of VEGFR-2/Flk-1 (Millauer *et al.*, 1994), can inhibit glioma cell growth *in vivo* highlights the crucial importance of angiogenesis for tumor growth *in vivo*.

Therapeutic implications

As described above, a substantial amount of evidence has emerged that growth factor receptor-mediated events are instrumental in the development of human brain tumors. Knowledge of the structure of growth factors and growth factor receptors and of the biochemical mechanisms of growth factor action may help to design specific inhibitors of growth factor action. The PTK inhibitors (tyrphostins) (Levitzki and Gazit, 1995) may be especially potent in this respect since most of the perturbed growth regulatory pathways in the malignant tumor ultimately involve PTKs. Interestingly, the rearranged, amino terminal-deleted, EGF receptor found in glioma seems to confer higher sensitivity to tyrphostins, which may increase their value in glioma treatment (Han *et al.*, 1996). Other potentially clinically useful inhibitors of growth factor action are antibodies, peptides and other compounds that interfere with ligand binding, inhibit receptor oligomerization or interfere with the interaction between phosphorylated receptor and intracellular substrates. The finding that receptor activation mostly occurs at the cell surface increases the likelihood that the therapeutic compounds will reach the site of action.

Growth factors and growth factor receptors are often expressed at a higher level in glioma cells than in the adjacent normal tissue, which is why it is possible to preferentially target tumor cells as compared with normal cells. Especially potent targeting can, however, be obtained if the compounds can be directed towards tumor-specific molecules. For instance, a specific antibody was developed towards the fusion junction in the external domain of the rearranged EGFR (Humphrey *et al.*, 1990); since this antibody is targeted with high specificity to cells expressing the mutated receptor (Hills, Rowlinson-Busza and Gullick, 1995), it may become clinically useful. Radioactive nuclides linked to EGF receptor antibodies (Miyamoto *et al.*, 1996), or to the ligand itself (Andersson *et al.*, 1991), can be mediators of cytotoxicity.

The fact that tumor growth *in vivo* is dependent on a vascular support has led to several experimental ways of modifying tumor angiogenesis (Folkman, 1995). Tumor cell-produced inhibitors of angiogenesis, like angiogenin, may be prototypes for future therapeutic agents.

Glioma cells also express several types of cytokine receptors and even secrete their own cytokines; the latter are most likely to modulate the tumorigenic phenotype. The fact that interferon genes are frequently deleted in gliomas indicates that these factors might have some important regulatory function. Glioma cells also have receptors for TNFs, which are potential mediators of apoptosis and cytotoxicity. These types of factors are the subjects for immunotherapeutic strategies discussed elsewhere in this book.

Glioma cells carry binding sites for neuropeptides, e.g., sites for bombesin/gastrin-releasing peptide (GRP) (Moody *et al.*, 1989), vasoactive intestinal peptide (VIP) (Nielsen *et al.*, 1990), substance P (Hennig *et al.*, 1995; Luo, Sharif and Sharif, 1996) and somatostatin (Reubi *et al.*, 1987). These receptors are members of the G protein-coupled, seven-transmembrane-domain receptor family and activators of adenylate cyclase. Agonists and antagonists of neuropeptides and neuropeptide receptors (Buscail *et al.*, 1994) may potentially be included in future therapeutic strategies for modulating glioma cell growth. Pinski *et al.* (1994) reported that analogs of somatostatin and antagonists of bombesin/GRP inhibited the growth of human glioma cells in the nude mouse brain.

Culture systems: established tumor cell lines

MONOLAYER CULTURES

Many established cell lines, i.e., tumor cells that can be passaged indefinitely *in vitro*, are available from human malignant brain tumors. The pioneering work in this field was by Manuelidis (1965, 1969) and by Pontén and Macintyre (1968), who managed to establish cell lines from glioblastoma tumors at a high frequency. Today, many laboratories have their own selection of established brain tumor cell lines (for review see Collins, 1983; Nistér and Westermark, 1994). Anaplastic astrocytomas, glioblastomas, oligodendrogliomas and PNETs/medulloblastomas are mainly represented.

Glioma cell lines

Glioblastoma multiforme is one of the human tumor types that most easily gives rise to established cell lines. In spite of this, the frequency of successful establishment from glioblastoma biopsies is only around 20%; the capacity to form established cell lines seems to be an inherent property of each individual tumor sample. Often, the cells that establish as cell lines are fibroblast-like spindle-shaped cells, while astrocyte-like glial fibrillary acidic protein (GFAP)-expressing (GFAP$^+$) tumor cells differentiate in culture (Lumsden, 1971; Westermark, Pontén and Hugosson, 1973).

Established glioma cell lines have been categorized according to cell morphology, with cells resembling either astrocytes or fibroblasts or epithelial cells (Bullard, Bigner and Bigner, 1981; Nistér *et al.*, 1988). The presence of GFAP or fibronectin (FN), or the lack thereof, correlates quite well with cell morphology, and these have been used as biologic markers for the previously mentioned cell types. Most permanent glioma cell lines are composed of fibroblast-like GFAP$^-$ cells; only a minority of cell lines express GFAP. The FN$^+$ cells resemble mesenchymal elements (Paetau *et al.*, 1980; Kennedy *et al.*, 1987; McKeever *et al.*, 1987). While there is no doubt that GFAP$^+$ cell lines are derived from glioma tumors, whether or not GFAP$^-$/FN$^+$ cell lines are representative of gliomas has been questioned. It might, however, be argued that the FN$^+$ cells must be of neoplastic origin since nonneoplastic normal human cells never give rise to established cell lines *in vitro*.

Shapiro, Yung and Shapiro (1981) showed that astrocyte-like and squamous-like cells of human gliomas were mostly near-diploid, while fibroblast-like cells were mostly hyperploid and fast growing. A recent finding from the culture of mouse astrocytes that lack a normal *TP53* gene is that of a shift in phenotype during *in vitro* culture, with down modulation of GFAP expression and appearance of FN that occurs in parallel with the development of an aneuploid cell population (Yahanda *et al.*, 1995). This can be interpreted as a progressional phenomenon and seemingly parallels similar events in cultured glioma cells. Additional evidence for a shift between the two phenotypes during tumor progression was provided by the finding that transformation of GFAP$^+$ astrocyte progenitor cells by SV40 T resulted in a GFAP$^-$/FN$^+$ phenotype (Geller and Dubois-Dalcq, 1988). Our interpretation is, therefore, that the large number of GFAP$^-$ aneuploid malignant glioma cell lines represent glioma cells that have undergone further progressional changes during *in vitro* culture (Fig. 3.3). This interpretation gains support from the finding of exactly the same specific chromosomal translocation in both GFAP$^+$/FN$^-$ and GFAP$^-$/FN$^+$ clones isolated from one and the same original biopsy (Nistér *et al.*, 1987). It was also found that GFAP$^-$ cell lines retained the same karyotypic abnormalities as were seen in the original tumor tissue from which they were derived (Bigner *et al.*, 1986).

In addition to GFAP, the expression of various types of intermediate filaments has been described in glioma, e.g., expression of neurofilament, keratin and nestin. Thus, from the biologic point of view, the glioblastoma can be regarded as a multipotent cell population that is continually proliferating and aberrantly differentiating along multiple lineages.

Oligodendroglioma cell lines

Some oligodendroglioma-derived cell lines have been established in culture, e.g., HOG (Post and Dawson, 1992), TC 620 (Merrill and Matsushima, 1988; Kashima *et al.*, 1993) and ONS-21 (Okamoto *et al.*, 1990). These cell lines are characterized by the expression of myelin basic protein (MBP) and galactocerebroside (GalC).

Cell lines from primitive neuroectodermal tumors/medulloblastomas

Primitive neuroectodermal tumors (PNETs)/ medulloblastomas are suggested to originate from immature bipotential neuroepithelial cells that differentiate into either neuronal or glial cells (Molenaar *et al.*, 1989; Kilpatrick, Richards and Bartlett, 1995). By careful adjustment of cell culture media and other *in vitro* conditions, quite a few PNET/medulloblastoma cell lines have been established *in vitro* (Friedman *et al.*, 1985; Trojanowski *et al.*, 1987; Friedman *et al.*, 1988; Wasson *et al.*, 1990; for a review Friedman *et al.*, 1991; He *et al.*, 1991; Fults *et al.*, 1992; Pietsch *et al.*, 1994). Many medulloblastoma cell lines grow in suspension and spontaneously form rounded spheroid-like structures, while others are adherent. Most lines express nestin, which is a characteristic of an immature neuroepithelial phenotype (Tohyama *et al.*, 1992), but also display neuroblastic characteristics by expressing the adhesion molecules N-CAM and L1 (Wikstrand, Friedman and Bigner, 1991).

TUMOR PROGRESSION IN CULTURE

During the establishment of tumor cells as cell lines, the environmental conditions and thereby the selective forces are completely changed as compared with the *in vivo* situation. The capacity

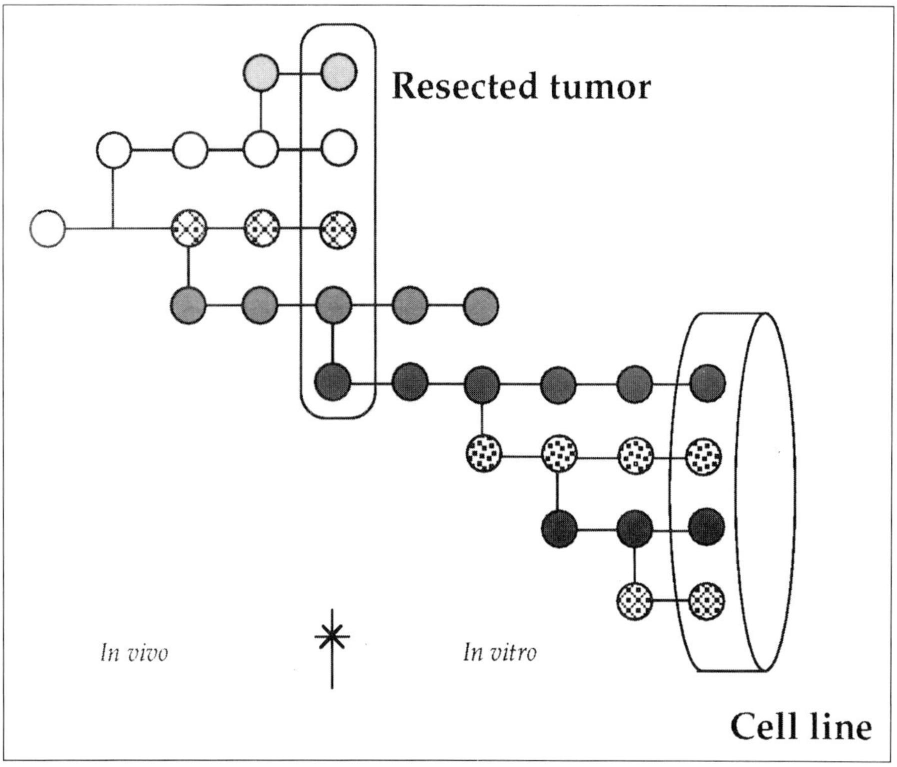

Fig. 3.3 A schematic representation of tumor progression *in vivo* and continued progression during the establishment and propagation of cell lines *in vitro*.

of tumor cells to recruit vessels, which is crucial for *in vivo* growth (Folkman, 1971), has, for example, no selective advantage *in vitro*. Continual proliferation *in vitro* requires that the cells have been or become immortalized, a selective force that might be stronger *in vitro* than *in vivo*. In this context, it is interesting to note that several medulloblastoma cell lines have an amplified *MYC* gene, which is seldom seen in original tumor tissues (Bigner *et al.*, 1990), and deletion of the *CDKN2A* gene, coding for the p16 CDKI, is more frequent in established glioma cell lines than in tumor samples (Kamb *et al.*, 1994; He, Olsson and James, 1995). Double-minute chromosomes, often harboring the amplified *EGFR* gene, while present in about 50% of human glioblastoma multiforme, are generally absent from established glioma cell lines. This finding suggests that the tumor cells are less dependent on the EGF receptor kinase activity *in vitro* than *in vivo*. Analogously, further tumor progression and selection of clones suited for *in vitro* growth, such as those expressing fibronectin, may occur in culture (Fig. 3.3). Established cell lines are, therefore, only partially representative of the original tumor.

Although experiments on glioma cells in culture must be interpreted with caution, this does not invalidate them as tools for the understanding of the molecular biology of glioma. For instance, they may constitute a valuable source for the studies of specific biologic functions of defined gene products. They are good candidates for studies of the biologic and biochemical function of specific gene products involved in brain tumor development. As an example, the introduction and expression of a normal p53 (Mercer *et al.*, 1990) or p16 (Arap *et al.*, 1995; Fueyo *et al.*, 1996) coding sequence in cells lacking a normal gene product results in growth arrest or senescence (Uhrbom *et al.*, 1997), proving the *in vivo* function of these gene products. Future testing of the mechanisms of action and the target specificity of therapeutic compounds will also have to be performed in cell lines (Han *et al.*, 1996).

SPHEROID CULTURES

Human glioma cell lines can be grown as suspensions of free-floating spheroids. This method makes large-scale culturing possible and is advantageous because it mimics the human tumor more closely than do monolayer cultures. Thus, the cells are grown in a three-dimensional structure with hypoxic regions and a central necrotic area. Spheroids are used for testing the penetrance and effect of radioactive ligands or antibodies in the development of treatment strategies (Carlsson, 1992; Pettersson, Carlsson and Grusell, 1992; Lindström and Carlsson, 1993). They are also useful tools in the studies of glioma cell invasion and for the application and testing of specific inhibitors to this process (de Ridder *et al.*, 1987; Lund-Johansen *et al.*, 1990).

Glioma cell heterogeneity

Brain tumors, like most malignant tumors, are genotypically and phenotypically heterogeneous. The heterogeneity presents as a variation between individual cells, as regional heterogeneity and as an intertumoral heterogeneity. Among the astrocytic brain tumors, astrocytoma grade I has the least and glioblastoma multiforme the highest degree of heterogeneity. From the practical point of view, heterogeneity leads to an obvious sampling difficulty, such that biopsies from glioblastomas frequently fail to contain diagnostically relevant information. As partly elucidated by studies on cell lines, heterogeneity is presented as variation in the expression of ECM proteins, intermediate filaments, growth factors, growth factor receptors (Nistér, Heldin and Westermark, 1986) and other cell surface proteins, as well as in the expression of intracellular tyrosine kinases and other proto-oncogene products. From the biologic point of view, this provides a basis for multiple paracrine interactions between tumor cells.

Areas of morphologically low-grade malignancy appear within high-grade gliomas, indicating that high-grade tumors, at least in certain cases, evolve from initially low-grade tumors as a progressional phenomenon. Nowell (1976) proposed that the mechanisms leading to tumor progression are sequential mutations, selection and clonal expansion of the fittest clone. Through careful dissection of one single case of low-grade oligoastrocytoma, Coons, Johnson and Shapiro (1995) described an intricate pattern of local karyotype heterogeneity. Against a background of near-diploid cells, characterized by numeric gains and losses of single chromosomes, microscopic foci of aneuploid cells characterized by chromosomal deletions and unique marker chromosomes were found. These foci were randomly distributed within the tumor, and their location was not necessarily evident from the histopathology. The existence of such microfoci of aneuploid cells in low-grade tumors sets the stage for clonal selection and further progression into high-grade tumors.

The understanding of mechanisms that protect a cell against mutagenic events has increased tremendously over the last decade. Protection against genomic instability leading to gene amplification, chromosomal deletions, translocations and inadequate chromosomal segregation is tightly coupled to cell cycle checkpoint control. So far, the involvement of the *TP53* tumor suppressor gene in this process seems well established. Mutations of the *TP53* gene have been recognized as an early event in many malignant gliomas of the astrocyte lineage since they occur at a similar frequency in astrocytomas and in glioblastomas. Furthermore, the results of Sidransky *et al.* (1992) suggest that *TP53* mutations facilitate tumor progression from foci of mutated cells in astrocytomas.

The use of homologous recombination techniques for gene disruption in mice has provided experimental systems for the study of tumor suppressor gene function. Astrocytes derived from *TP53* knockout mice (Yahanda *et al.*, 1995) become aneuploid when cultured *in vitro* and acquire angiogenic and invasive properties when transplanted to the subcutaneous tissue of nude mice. The tumorigenic phenotype is also associated with increased growth factor expression.

However, the loss of p53 function cannot be the sole explanation why genomic instability and heterogeneity occur in malignant glioma. The *TP53* gene mutations/deletions occur only in a subset of human malignant gliomas. Another subset of glioblastomas is, for example, characterized by amplification of the *EGFR* gene and loss of heterozygosity on chromosome 10 (von Deimling *et al.*, 1993). Other genes, the products of which are involved in different aspects of cell cycle control and cell division, will most likely be found to have a major importance in this context. Genes that encode key factors in the regulation of pRb phosphorylation, e.g., CDKIs and pRb itself, are possible candidates.

Acknowledgment Our own work cited in this text was supported by grants from the Swedish Cancer Society and the Children's Cancer Foundation.

References

Aaronson, S.A. (1991) Growth factors and cancer. *Science* **254**, 1146–53.

Abramovitch, R., Meir, G. and Neeman, M. (1995) Neovascularization induced growth of implanted C6 glioma multicellular spheroids: magnetic resonance microimaging. *Cancer Research* **55**, 1956–62.

Agosti, R.M., Leuthold, M., Gullick, W.J., Yasargil, M.G. and Wiestler, O.D. (1992) Expression of the epidermal growth factor receptor in astrocytic tumours is specifically associated with glioblastoma multiforme. *Virchows Archiv A, Pathological Anatomy and Histopathology* **420**, 321–5.

Alterman, R.L. and Stanley, E.R. (1994) Colony stimulating factor-1 expression in human glioma. *Molecular and Chemical Neuropathology* **21**, 177–88.

Alvarez, J.A., Baird, A., Tatum, A., Daucher, J., Chorsky, R., Gonzalez, A.M. and Stopa, E.G. (1992) Localization of basic fibroblast growth factor and vascular endothelial growth factor in human glial neoplasms. *Modern Pathology* **5**, 303–7.

Andersson, A., Holmberg, A., Carlsson, J., Pontén, J. and Westermark, B. (1991) Binding of epidermal growth factor-dextran conjugates to cultured glioma cells. *International Journal of Cancer* **47**, 439–44.

Antoniades, H.N., Galanopoulos, T., Neville-Golden, J. and Maxwell, M. (1992) Expression of insulin-like growth factors 1 and 2 and their receptor mRNAs in primary human astrocytomas and meningiomas; *in vivo* studies using *in situ* hybridization and immunocytochemistry. *International Journal of Cancer* **50**, 215–22.

Arap, W., Nishikawa, R., Furnari, F.B., Cavenee, W.K. and Huang, H.J. (1995) Replacement of the *p16/CDKN2* gene suppresses human glioma cell growth. *Cancer Research* **55**, 1351–4.

Aviezer, D., Hecht, D., Safran, M., Eisinger, M., David, G. and Yayon, A. (1994) Perlecan, basal lamina proteoglycan, promotes basic fibroblast growth factor-receptor binding, mitogenesis, and angiogenesis. *Cell* **79**, 1005–13.

Azuma, M., Yuki, T., Tamatani, T., Motegi, K., Yoshida, H. and Sato, M. (1996) Lack of expression of transforming growth factor β type II receptor associated with malignant progression in human salivary gland cell clones. *International Journal of Cancer* **66**, 802–5.

Barbacid, M. (1995) Neurotrophic factors and their receptors. *Current Opinion in Cell Biology* **7**, 148–55.

Bargmann, C.I., Hung, M.-C. and Weinberg, R.A. (1986) The *neu* oncogene encodes an epidermal growth factor receptor-related protein. *Nature* **319**, 226–30.

Baserga, R. (1995) The insulin-like growth factor 1 receptor: a key to tumor growth? *Cancer Research* **55**, 249–52.

Batra, S.K., Castelino-Prabhu, S., Wikstrand, C.J., Zhu, X., Humphrey, P.A., Friedman, H.S. and Bigner, D.D. (1995) Epidermal growth factor receptor ligand-independent, unregulated, cell-transforming potential of a naturally occurring human mutant *EGFRvIII* gene. *Cell Growth and Differentiation* **6**, 1251–9.

Beckmann, M.P., Betsholtz, C., Heldin, C.-H., Westermark, B., Di Marco, E., Di Fiore, P.P., Robbins, K.C. and Aaronson, S.A. (1988) Comparison of biological properties and transforming potential of human PDGF-A and PDGF-B chains. *Science* **241**, 1346–9.

Bejcek, B.E., Li, D.Y. and Deuel, T.F. (1989) Transformation by v-*sis* occurs by an internal autoactivation mechanism. *Science* **245**, 1496–9.

Berdel, W.E., de Vos, S., Maurer, J., Oberberg, D., von Marschall, Z., Schroeder, J.K., Li, J., Ludwig, W.-D., Kreuser, E.D., Thiel, E. and Herrmann, F. (1992) Recombinant human stem cell factor stimulates growth of a human glioblastoma cell line expressing *c-kit* protooncogene. *Cancer Research* **52**, 3498–502.

Berkman, R.A., Merrill, M.J., Reinhold, W.C., Monacci, W.T., Saxena, A., Clark, W.C., Robertson, J.T., Ali, I.U. and Oldfield, E.H. (1993) Expression of the vascular permeability factor/vascular endothelial growth factor gene in central nervous system neoplasms. *Journal of Clinical Investigation* **91**, 153–9.

Besmer, P., Murphy, J.E., George, P.C., Qiu, F.H., Bergold, P.J., Lederman, L., Snyder, H.W.Jr, Brodeur, D., Zuckerman, E.E. and Hardy, W.D. (1986) A new acute transforming feline retrovirus and relationship of its oncogene v-*kit* with the protein kinase gene family. *Nature* **320**, 415–21.

Betsholtz, C., Johnsson, A., Heldin, C.-H. and Westermark, B. (1986) Efficient reversion of simian sarcoma virus-transformation and inhibition of growth factor-induced mitogenesis by suramin. *Proceedings of the National Academy of Sciences U.S.A* **83**, 6440–4.

Bigner, S.H., Friedman, H.S., Biegel, J.A., Wikstrand, C.J., Mark, J., Gebhardt, R., Eng, L.F. and Bigner, D.D. (1986) Specific chromosomal abnormalities characterize four established cell lines derived from malignant human gliomas. *Acta Neuropathologica* **72**, 86–97.

Bigner, S.H., Friedman, H.S., Vogelstein, B., Oakes, W.J. and Bigner, D.D. (1990) Amplification of the c-*myc* gene in human medulloblastoma cell lines and xenografts. *Cancer Research* **50**, 2347–50.

Birchmeier, C., Sharma, S. and Wigler, M. (1987) Expression and rearrangement of the *ROS1* gene in human glioblastoma cells. *Proceedings of the National Academy of Sciences U.S.A.* **84**, 9270–4.

Birchmeier, C., O'Neill, K., Riggs, M. and Wigler, M. (1990) Characterization of ROS1 cDNA from a human glioblastoma cell line. *Proceedings of the National Academy of Sciences U.S.A.* **87**, 4799–803.

Blevins, G. and Fedoroff, S. (1995) Microglia in colony-stimulating factor 1-deficient op/op mice. *Journal of Neuroscience Research* **40**, 535–44.

Bodmer, S., Strommer, K., Frei, K., Siepl, C., de Tribolet, N., Heid, I. and Fontana, A. (1989) Immunosuppression and transforming growth factor-β in glioblastoma. Preferential production of transforming growth factor-β2. *Journal of Immunology* **143**, 3222–9.

Bögler, O., Wren, D., Barnett, S.C., Land, H. and Noble, M. (1990) Cooperation between two growth factors promotes extended self-renewal and inhibits differentiation of oligodendrocyte-type-2 astrocyte (O-2A) progenitor cells. *Proceedings of the National Academy of Sciences U.S.A.* **87**, 6368–72.

Bolger, G.B., Stamberg, J., Kirsch, I.R., Hollis, G.F., Schwarz, D.F. and Thomas, G.H (1985) Chromosomal translocation t(14;22) and oncogene (c-*sis*) variant in a pedigree with familial meningioma. *New England Journal of Medicine* **312**, 564–7.

Bottaro, D.P., Rubin, J.S., Faletto, D.L., Chan, A.M.-L., Kmiecik, T.E., Vande Woude, G.F. and Aaronson, S.A. (1991) Identification of the hepatocyte growth factor receptor as the c-*met* proto-oncogene product. *Science* **251**, 802–4.

Breier, G., Albrecht, U., Sterrer, S. and Risau, W. (1992) Expression of vascular endothelial growth factor during embryonic angiogenesis and endothelial cell differentiation. *Development* **114**, 521–32.

Bullard, D.E., Bigner, S.H. and Bigner, D.D. (1981) The morphologic response of cell lines derived from human gliomas to dibutyryl adenosine 3':5' cyclic monophosphate. *Journal of Neuropathology and Experimental Neurology* **40**, 230–46.

Buscail, L., Delesque, N., Esteve, J.-P., Saint-Laurent, N., Prats, H., Clerc, P., Robberecht, P., Bell, G.I., Liebow, C., Schally, A.V., Vaysse, N. and Susini, C. (1994) Stimulation of tyrosine phosphatase and inhibition of cell proliferation by somatostatin analogues: mediation by human somatostatin receptor subtypes SSTR1 and SSTR2. *Proceedings of the National Academy of Sciences U.S.A.* **91**, 2315–19.

Carlsson, J. (1992) Tumor spheroids in studies of immunotherapy. In Bjerkvig, R. (ed.), *Spheroid culture in cancer research*. Boca Raton, Fla.: CRC Press, 277–306.

Carpenter, G. and Cohen, S. (1976) Human epidermal growth factor and the proliferation of human fibroblasts. *Journal of Cellular Physiology* **88**, 227–37.

Carraway, K.L. III and Cantley, L.C. (1994) A neu acquaintance for erbB3 and erbB4: a role for receptor heterodimerization in growth signalling. *Cell* **78**, 5–8.

Chaffanet, M., Chauvin, C., Laine, M., Berger, F., Chedin, M., Rost, N., Nissou, M.F. and Benabid, A.L. (1992) EGF receptor amplification and expression in human brain tumours. *European Journal of Cancer* **28**, 11–17.

Chen, P., Gupta, K. and Wells, A. (1994) Cell movement elicited by epidermal growth factor receptor requires kinase and autophosphorylation but is separable from mitogenesis. *Journal of Cell Biology* **124**, 547–55.

Cheng, S.Y., Huang, H.J., Nagane, M., Ji, X.D., Wang, D., Shih, C.C., Arap, W., Huang, C.M. and Cavenee, W.K. (1996) Suppression of glioblastoma angiogenicity and tumorigenicity by inhibition of endogeneous expression of vascular endothelial growth factor. *Proceedings of the National Academy of Sciences U.S.A.* **93**, 8502–7.

Chicoine, M.R. and Silbergeld, D.L. (1995) The *in vitro* motility of human gliomas increases with increasing grade of malignancy. *Cancer* **75**, 2904–9.

Chicoine, M.R., Madsen, C.L. and Silbergeld, D.L. (1995) Modification of human glioma locomotion *in vitro* by cytokines EGF, bFGF, PDGFBB, NGF, and TNF-α. *Neurosurgery* **36**, 1165–71.

Claesson-Welsh, L. (1994) Platelet-derived growth factor receptor signals. *Journal of Biological Chemistry* **269**, 32023–6.

Collins, V.P. (1983) Cultured human glial and glioma cells. *International Review of Experimental Pathology* **24**, 135–202.

——(1993) Amplified genes in human gliomas. *Seminars in Cancer Biology* **4**, 27–32.

——(1995) Gene amplification in human gliomas. *Glia* **15**, 289–96.

Constam, D.B., Philipp, J., Malipiero, U.V., ten Dijke, P., Schachner, M. and Fontana, A. (1992) Differential expression of transforming growth factor-β1, -β2, and -β3 by glioblastoma cells, astrocytes, and microglia. *Journal of Immunology* **148**, 1404–10.

Coons, S.W., Johnson, P.C. and Shapiro, J.R. (1995) Cytogenetic and flow cytometry DNA analysis of regional heterogeneity in a low grade human glioma. *Cancer Research* **55**, 1569–77.

Cooper, C.S. (1992) The *met* oncogene: from detection by transfection to transmembrane receptor for hepatocyte growth factor. *Oncogene* **7**, 3–7.

Criscuolo, G.R., Merrill, M.J. and Oldfield, E.H. (1988) Further characterization of malignant glioma-derived vascular permeability factor. *Journal of Neurosurgery* **69**, 254–62.

D'Ambrosio, C., Ferber, A., Resnicoff, M. and Baserga, R. (1996) A soluble insulin-like growth factor 1 receptor that induces apoptosis of tumor cells *in vivo* and inhibits tumorigenesis. *Cancer Research* **56**, 4013–20.

Davis, S., Aldrich, T.H., Jones, P.F., Ácheson, A., Compton, D.L., Jain V., Ryan, T.E., Bruno, J., Radziejewski, G., Maisonpierre, P.C. and Yancopoulos, G.D. (1996) Isolation of angiopoietin-1, a ligand for the TIE2 receptor, by secretion-trap expression cloning. *Cell* **87**, 1161–9.

Davis, S., Gale, N.W., Aldrich, T.H., Maisonpierre, P.C., Lhotak, V., Pawson, T., Goldfarb, M. and Yancopoulos, G.D. (1994) Ligands for EPH-related receptor tyrosine kinases that require membrane attachment or clustering for activity. *Science* **266**, 816–19.

Deinhardt, F. (1980) Biology of primate retroviruses. In Klein, G. (ed.), *Viral oncology*. New York: Raven Press, 357–98.

de Martin, R., Haendler, B., Hofer-Warbinek, R., Gaugitsch, H., Wrann, M., Schlüsener, H., Seifert, J.M., Bodmer, S., Fontana, A. and Hofer, E. (1987) Complementary DNA for human glioblastoma-derived T cell suppressor factor, a novel member of the transforming growth factor-β gene family. *EMBO Journal* **6**, 3673–7.

de Ridder, L.I., Laerum, O.D., Mørk, S.J. and Bigner, D.D. (1987) Invasiveness of human glioma cell lines *in vitro*: relation to tumorigenicity in athymic mice. *Acta Neuropathologica* **72**, 207–13.

Derynck, R. and Zhang, Y. (1996) Intracellular signalling: the Mad way to do it. *Current Biology* **6**, 1226–9.

Devare, S.G., Reddy, E.P., Law, J.D., Robbins, K.C. and Aaronson, S.A. (1983) Nucleotide sequence of the simian sarcoma virus genome: demonstration that its acquired cellular sequences encode the transforming gene product $p28^{sis}$. *Proceedings of the National Academy of Sciences U.S.A.* **80**, 731–5.

Di Fiore, P.P., Pierce, J.H., Fleming, T.P., Hazan, R., Ullrich, A., King, C.R., Schlessinger, J. and Aaronson, S.A. (1987a) Overexpression of the human EGF receptor confers an EGF-dependent transformed phenotype to NIH 3T3 cells. *Cell* **51**, 1063–70.

Di Fiore, P.P., Pierce, J.H., Kraus, M.H., Segatto, O., King, C.R. and Aaronson, S.A. (1987b) *erb*B-2 is a potent oncogene when overexpressed in NIH/3T3 cells. *Science* **237**, 178–82.

Di Marco, E., Pierce, J.H., Fleming, T.P., Kraus, M.H., Molloy, C.J., Aaronson, S.A. and Di Fiore, P.P. (1989) Autocrine interaction between TGF α and the EGF-receptor: quantitative requirements for induction of the malignant phenotype. *Oncogene* **4**, 831–8.

Di Renzo, M.F., Bertolotto, A., Olivero, M., Putzolu, P., Crepaldi, T., Schiffer, D., Pagni, C.A. and Comoglio, P.M. (1993) Selective expression of the Met/HGF receptor in human central nervous system microglia. *Oncogene* **8**, 219–22.

DiSalvo, J., Bayne, M.L., Conn, G., Kwok, P.W., Trivedi, P.G., Soderman, D.D., Palisi, T.M., Sullivan, K.A. and Thomas, K.A. (1995) Purification and characterization of a naturally occurring vascular endothelial growth factor•placenta growth factor heterodimer. *Journal of Biological Chemistry* **270**, 7717–23.

Donner, L., Fedele, L.A., Garon, C.F., Anderson, S.J. and Sherr, C.J. (1982) McDonough feline sarcoma virus: characterization of the molecularly cloned provirus and its feline oncogene (v-*fms*). *Journal of Virology* **41**, 489–500.

Doolittle, R.F., Hunkapiller, M.W., Hood, L.E., Devare, S.G., Robbins, K.C., Aaronson, S.A. and Antoniades, H.N. (1983) Simian sarcoma virus *onc* gene, v-*sis*, is derived from the gene (or genes) encoding a platelet-derived growth factor. *Science* **221**, 275–7.

Downward, J., Yarden, Y., Mayes, E., Scrace, G., Totty, N., Stockwell, P., Ullrich, A., Schlessinger, J. and Waterfield, M.D. (1984) Close similarity of epidermal growth factor receptor and v-*erb*-B oncogene protein sequences. *Nature* **307**, 521–7.

Dumont, D.J., Gradwohl, G.J., Fong, G.-H., Puri, M.C., Gertsenstein, M., Auerbach, A. and Breitman, M.L. (1994) Dominant negative and targeted null mutations in the endothelial receptor tyrosine kinase, *tek*, reveal a critical role in vasculogenesis of the embryo. *Genes and Development* **8**, 1897–909.

Eckenstein, F.P. (1994) Fibroblast growth factors in the nervous system. *Journal of Neurobiology* **25**, 1467–80.

Ekstrand, A.J., James, C.D., Cavenee, W.K., Seliger, B., Pettersson R.F. and Collins, V.P. (1991) Genes for epidermal growth factor receptor, transforming growth factor α, and epidermal growth factor and their expression in human gliomas *in vivo*. *Cancer Research* **51**, 2164–72.

Ekstrand, A.J., Sugawa, N., James, C.D. and Collins, V.P. (1992) Amplified and rearranged epidermal growth factor receptor genes in human glioblastomas reveal deletions of sequences encoding portions of the N- and/or C-terminal tails. *Proceedings of the National Academy of Sciences U.S.A.* **89**, 4309–13.

Ekstrand, A.J., Longo, N., Hamid, M.L., Olson, J.J., Liu, L., Collins, V.P. and James, C.D. (1994) Functional characterization of an EGF receptor with a truncated extracellular domain expressed in glioblastomas with *EGFR* gene amplification. *Oncogene* **9**, 2313–20.

Eppert, K., Scherer, S.W., Ozcelik, H., Pirone, R., Hoodless, P., Kim, H., Tsui, L.-C., Bapat, B., Gallinger, S., Andrulis, I.L., Thomsen, G.H., Wrana, J.L. and Attisano, L. (1996) *MADR2* maps to 18q21 and encodes a TGFβ-regulated MAD-related protein that is functionally mutated in colorectal carcinoma. *Cell* **86**, 543–52.

Eva, A., Robbins, K.C., Andersen, P.R., Srinivasan, A., Tronick, S.R., Reddy, E.P., Ellmore, N.W., Galen, A.T., Lautenberger, J.A., Papas, T.S., Westin, E.H., Wong-Staal, F., Gallo, R.C. and Aaronson, S.A. (1982) Cellular genes analogous to retroviral *onc* genes are transcribed in human tumor cells. *Nature* **295**, 116–19.

Fakhrai, H., Dorigo, O., Shawler, D.L., Lin, H., Mercola, D., Black, K.L., Royston, I. and Sobol, R.E. (1996) Eradication of established intracranial rat gliomas by transforming growth factor β antisense gene therapy. *Proceedings of the National Academy of Sciences U.S.A.* **93**, 2909–14.

Falls, D.L., Rosen, K.M., Corfas, G., Lane, W.S. and Fischbach, G.D. (1993) ARIA, a protein that stimulates acetylcholine receptor synthesis, is a member of the Neu ligand family. *Cell* **72**, 801–15.

Fantl, W.J., Johnson, D.E. and Williams, L.T. (1993) Signalling by receptor tyrosine kinases. *Annual Review of Biochemistry* **62**, 453–81.

Fantl, W.J., Peters, K.G. and Williams, L.T. (1996) PDGF and FGF receptors in health and disease. In Leroith, D. and Bondy, C. (eds), *Growth factors in health and disease*, Vol. 1A. Greenwich, Conn.: JAI Press, 179–228.

Ferrara, N., Houck, K., Jakeman, L. and Leung, D.W. (1992) Molecular and biological properties of the vascular endothelial growth factor family of proteins. *Endocrine Reviews* **13**, 18–32.

Figarella-Branger, D., Vagner-Capodano, A.M., Bouillot, P., Graziani, N., Gambarelli, D., Devictor, B., Zattara-Cannoni, H., Bianco, N., Grisoli, F. and Pellissier, J.F. (1994) Platelet-derived growth factor (PDGF) and receptor (PDGFR) expression in human meningiomas: correlations with clinicopathological features and cytogenetic analysis. *Neuropathology and Applied Neurobiology* **20**, 439–47.

Fischer, U., Müller, H.-W., Sattler, H.-P., Feiden, K., Zang, K.D. and Meese, E. (1995) Amplification of the *MET* gene in glioma. *Genes, Chromosomes and Cancer* **12**, 63–5.

Fleming, T.P., Saxena, A., Clark, W.C., Robertson, J.T., Oldfield, E.H., Aaronson, S.A. and Ali, I.U. (1992) Amplification and/or overexpression of platelet-derived growth factor receptors and epidermal growth factor receptor in human glial tumors. *Cancer Research* **52**, 4550–3.

Folkman, J. (1971) Tumor angiogenesis: therapeutic implications. *New England Journal of Medicine* **285**, 1182–6.

——(1990) What is the evidence that tumors are angiogenesis dependent? *Journal of the National Cancer Institute* **82**, 4–6.

——(1995) Angiogenesis in cancer, vascular, rheumatoid and other diseases. *Nature Medicine* **1**, 27–31.

Folkman, J. and Klagsburn, M. (1987) Angiogenic factors. *Science* **235**, 442–7.

Forsberg, K., Valyi-Nagy, I., Heldin, C.-H., Herlyn, M. and Westermark, B. (1993) Platelet-derived growth factor (PDGF) in oncogenesis: development of a vascular connective tissue stroma in xenotransplanted human melanoma producing PDGF-BB. *Proceedings of the National Academy of Sciences U.S.A.* **90**, 393–7.

Friedman, G.C. and O'Leary, D.D. (1996) Eph receptor tyrosine kinases and their ligands in neural development. *Current Opinion in Neurobiology* **6**, 127–33.

Friedman, H.S., Burger, P.C., Bigner, S.H., Trojanowski, J.Q., Wikstrand, C.J., Halperin, E.C. and Bigner, D.D. (1985) Establishment and characterization of the human medulloblastoma cell line and transplantable xenograft D283 Med. *Journal of Neuropathology and Experimental Neurology* **44**, 592–605.

Friedman, H.S., Burger, P.C., Bigner, S.H., Trojanowski, J.Q., Brodeur, G.M., He, X., Wikstrand, C.J., Kurtzberg, J., Berens, M.E., Halperin, E.C. and Bigner, D.D. (1988) Phenotypic and genotypic analysis of a human medulloblastoma cell line and transplantable xenograft (D341 Med) demonstrating amplification of c-*myc*. *American Journal of Pathology* **130**, 472–84.

Friedman, H.S., Oakes, W.J., Bigner, S.H., Wikstrand, C.J. and Bigner, D.D. (1991) Medulloblastoma: tumor biological and clinical perspectives. (Review) *Journal of Neuro-Oncology* **11**, 1–15.

Fueyo, J., Gomez-Manzano, C., Yung, W.K., Clayman, G.L., Liu, T.J., Bruner, J., Levin, V.A. and Kyritsis, A.P. (1996) Adenovirus-mediated *p16/CDKN2* gene transfer induces growth arrest and modifies the transformed phenotype of glioma cells. *Oncogene* **12**, 103–10.

Fults, D., Pedone, C.A., Morse, H.G., Rose, J.W. and McKay, R.D.G. (1992) Establishment and characterization of a human primitive neuroectodermal tumor cell line from the cerebral hemisphere. *Journal of Neuropathology and Experimental Neurology* **51**, 272–80.

Gammeltoft, S., Ballotti, R., Kowalski, A., Westermark, B. and Van Obberghen, E. (1988) Expression of two types of receptor for insulin-like growth factors in human malignant glioma. *Cancer Research* **48**, 1233–7.

Geller, H.M. and Dubois-Dalcq, M. (1988) Antigenic and functional characterization of a rat central nervous system-derived cell line immortalized by a retroviral vector. *Journal of Cell Biology* **107**, 1977–86.

Gherardi, E., Gray, J., Stoker, M., Perryman, M. and Furlong, R. (1989) Purification of scatter factor, a fibroblast-derived basic protein that modulates epithelial interactions and movement. *Proceedings of the National Academy of Sciences U.S.A.* **86**, 5844–8.

Glick, R.P., Gettleman, R., Patel, K., Lakshman, R. and Tsibris, J.C.M. (1989) Insulin and insulin-like growth factor 1 in brain tumors: binding and *in vitro* effects. *Neurosurgery* **24**, 791–7.

Goldman, C.K., Kim, J., Wong, W.-L., King, V., Brock, T. and Gillespie, G.Y. (1993) Epidermal growth factor stimulates vascular endothelial growth factor production by human malignant glioma cells: a model of glioblastoma multiforme pathophysiology. *Molecular and Cellular Biology* **4**, 121–33.

Grunberger, G., Lowe, W.L. Jr, McElduff, A. and Glick, R.P. (1986) Insulin receptor of human cerebral gliomas. Structure and function. *Journal of Clinical Investigation* **77**, 997–1005.

Guha, A., Dashner, K., Black, P.M., Wagner, J.A. and Stiles, C.D. (1995) Expression of PDGF and PDGF receptors in human astrocytoma operation specimens supports the existence of an autocrine loop. *International Journal of Cancer* **60**, 168–73.

Haapasalo, H., Hyytinen, E., Sallinen, P., Helin, H., Kallioniemi, O.P. and Isola, J. (1996) c-*erb*B-2 in astrocytomas: infrequent overexpression by immunohistochemistry and absence of gene amplification by fluorescence *in situ* hybridization. *British Journal of Cancer* **73**, 620–3.

Haddad, S.F., Moore, S.A., Schelper, R.L. and Goeken, J.A. (1992) Vascular smooth muscle hyperplasia underlies the formation of glomeruloid vascular structures of glioblastoma multiforme. *Journal of Neuropathology and Experimental Neurology* **51**, 488–92.

Hamel, W., Westphal, M., Szönyi, É., Escandón, E. and Nikolics, K. (1993) Neurotrophin gene expression by cell lines derived from human gliomas. *Journal of Neuroscience Research* **34**, 147–57.

Han, Y., Caday, C.G., Nanda, A., Cavenee, W.K. and Huang, H.-J.S. (1996) Tyrphostin AG 1478 preferentially inhibits human glioma cells expressing truncated rather than wild-type epidermal growth factor receptors. *Cancer Research* **56**, 3859–61.

Hannink, M. and Donoghue, D.J. (1988) Autocrine stimulation by the v-*sis* gene product requires a ligand-receptor interaction at the cell surface. *Journal of Cell Biology* **107**, 287–98.

Hart, I.K., Richardson, W.D., Heldin, C.-H., Westermark, B. and Raff, M.C. (1989) PDGF receptors on cells of the oligodendrocyte-type-2 astrocyte (O-2A) cell lineage. *Development* **105**, 595–603.

Hatva, E., Kaipainen, A., Mentula, P., Jääskeläinen, J., Paetau, A., Haltia, M. and Alitalo, K. (1995) Expression of endothelial cell-specific receptor tyrosine kinases and growth factors in human brain tumors. *American Journal of Pathology* **146**, 368–78.

He, J., Olsson, J.J. and James, C.D. (1995) Lack of $p16^{INK4}$ or retinoblastoma protein (pRb), or amplification-associated overexpression of cdk4 is observed in distinct subsets of malignant glial tumors and cell lines. *Cancer Research* **55**, 4833–6.

He, X., Wikstrand, C.J., Friedman, H.S., Bigner, S.H., Pleasure, S., Trojanowski, J.Q. and Bigner, D.D. (1991) Differentiation characteristics of newly established medulloblastoma cell lines (D384 Med, D425 Med and D458 Med) and their transplantable xenografts. *Laboratory Investigation* **64**, 833–43.

Heldin, C.-H. (1992) Structural and functional studies on platelet-derived growth factor. *EMBO Journal* **11**, 4251–9.

——(1995) Dimerization of cell surface receptors in signal transduction. *Cell* **80**, 213–23.

——(1996) Protein tyrosine kinase receptors. *Cancer Surveys* **27**, 7–24.

Helseth, E., Unsgaard, G., Dalen, A. and Vik, R. (1988) The effect of type β transforming growth factor on proliferation of clonogenic cells from human gliomas. *Acta Neurochirurgica* **43**, 118–20.

Hennig, I.M., Laissue, J.A., Horisberger, U. and Reubi, J.C. (1995) Substance-P receptors in human primary neoplasms: tumoral and vascular localization. *International Journal of Cancer* **61**, 786–92.

Hermanson, M., Funa, K., Hartman, M., Claesson-Welsh, L., Heldin, C.-H., Westermark, B. and Nistér, M.

(1992) Platelet-derived growth factor (PDGF) and its receptors in human glioma tissue. Expression of mRNA and protein suggests the presence of autocrine and paracrine loops. *Cancer Research* **52**, 3213–19.

Hermanson, M., Funa, K., Koopmann, J., Maintz, D., Waha, A., Westermark, B., Heldin, C.-H., Wiestler, O.D., Louis, D.N., von Deimling, A. and Nistér, M. (1996) Association of high platelet-derived growth factor (PDGF) α-receptor expression with loss of heterozygosity (LOH) on chromosome 17p in human malignant gliomas. *Cancer Research* **56**, 164–71.

Hermansson, M., Nistér, M., Betsholtz, C., Heldin, C.-H., Westermark, B. and Funa, K. (1988) Endothelial cell hyperplasia in human glioblastoma: coexpression of mRNA for platelet-derived growth factor (PDGF) B chain and PDGF receptor suggests autocrine growth stimulation. *Proceedings of the National Academy of Sciences U.S.A.* **85**, 7748–52.

Hills, D., Rowlinson-Busza, G. and Gullick, W.J. (1995) Specific targeting of a mutant, activated EGF receptor found in glioblastoma using a monoclonal antibody. *International Journal of Cancer* **63**, 537–43.

Hoi, S.U., Espiritu, O.D., Kelley, P.Y., Klauber, M.R. and Hatton, J.D. (1995) The role of the epidermal growth factor receptor in human gliomas: I. The control of cell growth. *Journal of Neurosurgery* **82**, 841–6.

Holland, S.J., Gale, N.W., Mbamalu, G., Yancopoulos, G.D., Henkemeyer, M. and Pawson, T. (1996) Bidirectional signalling through the EPH-family receptor Nuk and its transmembrane ligands. *Nature* **383**, 722–5.

Holmes, W.E., Sliwkowski, M.X., Akita, R.W., Henzel, W.J., Lee, J., Park, J.W., Yansura, D., Abadi, N., Raab, H., Lewis, G.D., Shepard, H.M., Kuang, W.-J., Wood, W.I., Goeddel, D.V. and Vandlen, R.L. (1992) Identification of heregulin, a specific activator of $p185^{erbB2}$. *Science* **256**, 1205–10.

Huber, D., Fontana, A. and Bodmer, S. (1991) Activation of human platelet-derived latent transforming growth factor-β1 by human glioblastoma cells. Comparison with proteolytic and glycosidic enzymes. *Biochemical Journal* **277**, 165–73.

Humphrey, P.A., Wong, A.J., Vogelstein, B., Zalutsky, M.R., Fuller, G.N., Archer, G.E., Friedman, H.S., Kwatra, M.M., Bigner, S.H. and Bigner, D.D. (1990) Anti-synthetic peptide antibody reacting at the fusion junction of deletion-mutant epidermal growth factor receptors in human glioblastoma. *Proceedings of the National Academy of Sciences U.S.A.* **87**, 4207–11.

Hunter, T. (1995) Protein kinases and phosphatases: the yin and yang of protein phosphorylation and signaling. *Cell* **80**, 225–36.

Hutton, L.A., DeVellis, J. and Perez-Polo, J.R. (1992) Expression of $p75^{NGFR}$ TrkA, and TrkB mRNA in rat C6 glioma and type 1 astrocyte cultures. *Journal of Neuroscience Research* **32**, 375–83.

Jachimczak, P., Hessdörfer, B., Fabel-Schulte, K., Wismeth, C., Brysch, W., Schlingensiepen, K.H., Bauer, A., Blesch, A. and Bogdahn, U. (1996) Transforming growth factor-β-mediated autocrine growth regulation of gliomas as detected with phosphorothioate antisense oligonucleotides. *International Journal of Cancer* **65**, 332–7.

Jennings, M.T., Maciunas, R.J., Carver, R., Bascom, C.C., Juneau, P., Misulis, K. and Moses, H.L. (1991) $TGF\beta_1$ and $TGF\beta_2$ are potential growth regulators for low-grade and malignant gliomas *in vitro*: evidence in support of an autocrine hypothesis. *International Journal of Cancer* **49**, 129–39.

Jhappan, C., Stahle, C., Harkins, R.N., Fausto, N., Smith, G.H. and Merlino, G.T. (1990) TGF-α overexpression in transgenic mice induces liver neoplasia and abnormal development of the mammary gland and pancreas. *Cell* **61**, 1137–46.

Johnsson, A., Betsholtz, C., Heldin, C.-H. and Westermark, B. (1985) Antibodies against platelet-derived growth factor inhibit acute transformation by simian sarcoma virus. *Nature* **317**, 438–40.

Jung, W., Castren, E., Odenthal, M., Vande Woude, G.F., Ishii, T., Dienes, H.P., Lindholm, D. and Schirmacher, P. (1994) Expression and functional interaction of hepatocyte growth factor-scatter factor and its receptor c-*met* in mammalian brain. *Journal of Cell Biology* **126**, 485–94.

Kamb, A., Gruis, N.A., Weaver-Feldhaus, J., Liu, Q., Harshman, K., Tavtigian, S.V., Stockert, E., Day, R.S. III, Johnson, B.E. and Skolnick, M.H. (1994) A cell cycle regulator potentially involved in genesis of many tumor types. *Science* **264**, 436–40.

Kaplan, D.R., Hempstead, B.L., Martin-Zanca, D., Chao, M.V. and Parada, L.F. (1991) The *trk* proto-oncogene product: a signal transducing receptor for nerve growth factor. *Science* **252**, 554–8.

Kashima, T., Tiu, S.N., Merrill, J.E., Vinters, H.V., Dawson, G. and Campagnoni, A.T. (1993) Expression of oligodendrocyte-associated genes in cell lines derived from human gliomas and neuroblastomas. *Cancer Research* **53**, 170–5.

Keating, M.T. and Williams, L.T. (1988) Autocrine stimulation of intracellular PDGF receptors in v-*sis* transformed cells. *Science* **239**, 914–16.

Kennedy, P.G.E., Watkins, B.A., Thomas, D.G.T. and Noble, M.D. (1987) Antigenic expression by cells derived from human gliomas does not correlate with morphological classification. *Neuropathology and Applied Neurobiology* **13**, 327–47.

Keshet, E., Lyman, S.D., Williams, D.E., Anderson, D.M., Jenkins, N.A., Copeland, N.G. and Parada, L.F. (1991) Embryonic RNA expression patterns of the *c-kit* receptor and its cognate ligand suggest multiple functional roles in mouse development. *EMBO Journal* **10**, 2425–35.

Kieser, A., Weich, H.A., Brandner, G., Marmé, D. and Kölch, W. (1994) Mutant p53 potentiates protein kinase C induction of vascular endothelial growth factor expression. *Oncogene* **9**, 963–9.

Kilpatrick, T.J., Richards, L.J. and Bartlett, P.F. (1995) The regulation of neural precursor cells within the mammalian brain. *Molecular and Cellular Neurosciences* **6**, 2–15.

Kim, K.J., Li, B., Winer, J., Armanini, M., Gillett, N., Phillips, H.S. and Ferrara, N. (1993) Inhibition of vascular endothelial growth factor-induced angiogenesis suppresses tumour growth *in vivo*. *Nature* **362**, 841–4.

Kimura, H., Fischer, W.H. and Schubert, D. (1990) Structure, expression and function of a schwannoma derived growth factor. *Nature* **348**, 257–60.

Kingsley, D.M. (1994) The TGF-β superfamily: new members, new receptors, and new genetic tests of function in different organisms. *Genes and Development* **8**, 133–46.

Kishimoto, T., Taga, T. and Akira, S. (1994) Cytokine signal transduction. *Cell* **76**, 253–62.

Kumabe, T., Sohma, Y., Kayama, T., Yoshimoto, T. and Yamamoto, T. (1992) Amplification of the platelet-derived growth factor receptor gene lacking an exon coding for a portion of the extracellular region in a primary brain tumor of glial origin. *Oncogene* **7**, 627–33.

Kuppner, M.C., Hamou, M.-F., Bodmer, S., Fontana, A. and de Tribolet, N. (1988) The glioblastoma-derived T-cell suppressor factor/transforming growth factor β_2 inhibits the generation of lymphokine-activated killer (LAK) cells. *International Journal of Cancer* **42**, 562–7.

Lal, B., Indurti, R.R., Couraud, P.O., Goldstein, G.W. and Laterra, J. (1994) Endothelial cell implantation and survival within experimental gliomas. *Proceedings of the National Academy of Sciences U.S.A.* **91**, 9695–9.

LaRocca, R.V., Rosenblum, M., Westermark, B. and Israel, M.A. (1989) Patterns of proto-oncogene expression in human glioma cell lines. *Journal of Neuroscience Research* **24**, 97–106.

Leal, F., Williams, L.T., Robbins, K.C. and Aaronson, S.A. (1985) Evidence that the v-*sis* gene product transforms by interaction with the receptor for platelet-derived growth factor. *Science* **230**, 327–30.

Lee, D.C. (1996) TGF-α: a member of the EGF receptor ligand family. In Leroith, D. and Bondy, C. (eds), *Growth factors and cytokines in health and disease*, Vol. 1B. Greenwich, Conn.: JAI Press, 277–318.

Levitzki, A. and Gazit, A. (1995) Tyrosine kinase inhibition: an approach to drug development. *Science* **267**, 1782–8.

Libermann, T.A., Nusbaum, H.R., Razon, N., Kris, R., Lax, I., Soreq, H., Whittle, N., Waterfield, M.D., Ullrich, A. and Schlessinger, J. (1985) Amplification, enhanced expression and possible rearrangement of EGF receptor gene in primary human brain tumors of glial origin. *Nature* **313**, 144–7.

Libermann, T.A., Friesel, R., Jaye, M., Lyall, R.M., Westermark, B., Drohan, W., Schmidt, A., Maciag, T. and Schlessinger, J. (1987) An angiogenic growth factor is expressed in human glioma cells. *EMBO Journal* **6**, 1627–32.

Lichtor, T., Kurpakus, M.A. and Gurney, M.E. (1991) Differential expression of insulin-like growth factor-2 in human meningiomas. *Neurosurgery* **29**, 405–10.

Lindström, A. and Carlsson, J. (1993) Penetration and binding of epidermal growth factor-dextran conjugates in spheroids of human glioma origin. *Cancer Biotherapy* **8**, 145–58.

Lumsden, C.E. (1971) The study by tissue culture of tumors of the nervous system. In Russell, D.S. and Rubinstein, L.J. (eds), *Pathology of tumours of the nervous system*. Third edition. London: Edward Arnold, 334–420.

Lund-Johansen, M., Bjerkvig, R., Humphrey, P.A., Bigner, S.H., Bigner, D.D. and Laerum, O.-D. (1990) Effect of epidermal growth factor on glioma cell growth, migration, and invasion *in vitro*. *Cancer Research* **50**, 6039–44.

Luo, W., Sharif, T.R. and Sharif, M. (1996) Substance P-induced mitogenesis in human astrocytoma cells correlates with activation of the mitogen-activated protein kinase signaling pathway. *Cancer Research* **56**, 4983–91.

Malden, L.T., Novak, U., Kaye, A.H. and Burgess, A.W. (1988) Selective amplification of the cytoplasmic domain of the epidermal growth factor receptor gene in glioblastoma multiforme. *Cancer Research* **48**, 2711–14.

Manuelidis, E.E. (1965) Long-term lines of tissue cultures of intracranial tumors. *Journal of Neurosurgery* **22**, 368–73.

——(1969) Experiments with tissue culture and heterologous transplantation of tumors. In Scheinberg, L.C. (ed.), *Research in the experimental and clinical aspects of brain tumors*. Annals of the New York Academy of Sciences, Vol. 159, Part 1, Art. 2. New York: New York Academy of Sciences, 409–31.

Marchionni, M.A., Goodearl, A.D., Chen, M.S., Bermingham-McDonogh, O., Kirk, C., Hendricks, M., Danehy, F., Misumi, D., Sudhalter, J., Kobayashi, K., Wroblewski, D., Lynch, C., Baldassare, M., Hiles, I., Davis, J.B., Hsuan, J.J., Totty, N.F., Otsu, M., McBurney, R.N., Waterfield, M.D., Stroobant, P. and Gwynne, D. (1993) Glial growth factors are alternatively spliced erbB2 ligands expressed in the nervous system. *Nature* **362**, 312–18.

Markowitz, S., Wang, J., Myeroff, L., Parsons, R., Sun, L., Lutterbaugh, J., Fan, R.S., Zborowska, E., Kinzler, K.W., Vogelstein, B., Brattain, M. and Willson, K.V. (1995) Inactivation of the type II TGF-β receptor in colon cancer cells with microsatellite instability. *Science* **268**, 1336–8.

Mason, I.J. (1994) The ins and outs of fibroblast growth factors. *Cell* **78**, 547–52.

Massagué, J. (1996) TGF-β signaling: receptors, transducers, and Mad proteins. *Cell* **85**, 945–50.

Matsui, Y., Zsebo, K.M. and Hogan, B.L.M. (1990) Embryonic expression of a haematopoietic growth factor encoded by the *Sl* locus and the ligand for c-kit. *Nature* **347**, 667–9.

Matsumoto, K., Kagoshima, M. and Nakamura, T. (1995) Hepatocyte growth factor as a potent survival factor for rat pheochromocytoma PC12 cells. *Experimental Cell Research* **220**, 71–8.

Mauro, A., Bulfone, A., Turco, E. and Schiffer, D. (1991) Coexpression of platelet-derived growth factor (PDGF) B chain and PDGF B-type receptor in human gliomas. *Child's Nervous System* **7**, 432–6.

Maxwell, M., Galanopoulos, T., Hedley-Whyte, E.T., Black, P.M. and Antoniades, H.N. (1990a) Human meningiomas co-express platelet-derived growth factor (PDGF) and PDGF-receptor genes and their protein products. *International Journal of Cancer* **46**, 16–21.

Maxwell, M., Naber, S.P., Wolfe, H.J., Galanopoulos, T., Hedley-Whyte, E.T., Black, P. McL. and Antoniades,

H.N. (1990b) Coexpression of platelet-derived growth factor (PDGF) and PDGF-receptor genes by primary human astrocytomas may contribute to their development and maintenance. *Journal of Clinical Investigation* **86**, 131–40.

McComb, R.D., Jones, T.R., Pizzo, S.V. and Bigner, D.D. (1982) Immunohistochemical detection of factor VIII/von Willebrand factor in hyperplastic endothelial cells in glioblastoma multiforme and mixed gliomasarcoma. *Journal of Neuropathology and Experimental Neurology* **41**, 479–89.

McDonald, N.Q. and Hendrickson, W.A. (1993) A structural superfamily of growth factors containing a cystine knot motif. *Cell* **73**, 421–4.

McKeever, P.E., Smith, B.H., Taren, J.A., Wahl, R.L., Kornblith, P.L. and Chronwall, B.M. (1987) Products of cells cultured from gliomas. VI. Immunofluorescent, morphometric, and ultrastructural characterization of two different cell types growing from explants of human gliomas. *American Journal of Pathology* **127**, 358–72.

Mercer, W.E., Shields, M.T., Amin, M., Sauve, G.J., Appella, E., Romano, J.W. and Ullrich, S.J. (1990) Negative growth regulation in a glioblastoma tumor cell line that conditionally expresses human wild-type p53. *Proceedings of the National Academy of Sciences U.S.A.* **87**, 6166–70.

Merrill, J.E. and Matsushima, K. (1988) Production of and response to interleukin 1 by cloned human oligodendroglioma cell lines. *Journal of Biological Regulators and Homeostatic Agents* **2**, 77–86.

Merrill, M.J. and Edwards, N.A. (1990) Insulin-like growth factor-1 receptors in human glial tumors. *Journal of Clinical Endocrinology and Metabolism* **71**, 199–209.

Millauer, B., Wizigmann-Voos, S., Schnurch, H., Martinez, R., Moller, N.P.H., Risau, W. and Ullrich, A. (1993) High affinity VEGF binding and developmental expression suggest Flk-1 as a major regulator of vasculogenesis and angiogenesis. *Cell* **72**, 835–46.

Millauer, B., Shawver, L.K., Plate, K.H., Risau, W. and Ullrich, A. (1994) Glioblastoma growth inhibited *in vivo* by a dominant-negative Flk-1 mutant. *Nature* **367**, 576–9.

Mishima, K., Asai, A., Sugiyama, A., Miyagi, Y., Kitanaka, C., Kagaya, S., Kirino, T. and Kuchino, Y. (1996) Increased expression of schwannoma-derived growth factor (SDGF) mRNA in rat tumor cells: involvement of SDGF in the growth promotion of rat gliomas. *International Journal of Cancer* **66**, 352–7.

Miyamoto, C.T., Brady, L.W., Rackover, M.A., Emrich, J., Class, R., Bender, H., Micaily, B. and Steplewski, Z. (1996) The use of epidermal growth factor receptor-425 monoclonal antibodies radiolabeled with iodine-125 in the adjuvant treatment of patients with high grade gliomas of the brain. *Recent Results in Cancer Research* **141**, 183–92.

Miyamoto, M., Naruo, K.-I, Seko, C., Matsumoto, S., Kondo, T. and Kurokawa, T. (1993) Molecular cloning of a novel cytokine cDNA encoding the ninth member of the fibroblast growth factor family, which has a unique secretion property. *Molecular and Cellular Biology* **13**, 4251–9.

Molenaar, W.M., Jansson, D.S., Gould, V.E., Rorke, L.B., Franke, W.W., Lee, V.M.-Y., Packer, R.J. and Trojanowski, J.Q. (1989) Molecular markers of primitive neuroectodermal tumors and other pediatric central nervous system tumors. Monoclonal antibodies to neuronal and glial antigens distinguish subsets of primitive neuroectodermal tumors. *Laboratory Investigation* **61**, 635–43.

Moody, T.W., Mahmoud, S., Staley, J., Naldini, L., Cirillo, D., South, V., Felder, S. and Kris, R. (1989) Human glioblastoma cell lines have neuropeptide receptors for bombesin/gastrin-releasing peptide. *Journal of Molecular Neuroscience* **1**, 235–42.

Morgan, D.O., Edman, J.C., Standring, D.N., Fried, V.A., Smith, M.C., Roth, R.A. and Rutter, W.J. (1987) Insulin-like growth factor 2 receptor as a multifunctional binding protein. *Nature* **329**, 301–7.

Moriyama, T., Kataoka, H., Tsubouchi, H. and Koono, M. (1995) Concomitant expression of hepatocyte growth factor (HGF), HGF activator and c-met genes in human glioma cells *in vitro*. *FEBS Letters* **372**, 78–82.

Moriyama, T., Kataoka, H., Seguchi, K., Tsubouchi, H. and Koono, M. (1996) Effects of hepatocyte growth factor (HGF) on human glioma cells *in vitro*: HGF acts as a motility factor in glioma cells. *International Journal of Cancer* **66**, 678–85.

Morrison, R.S. (1991) Suppression of basic fibroblast growth factor expression by antisense oligodeoxynucleotides inhibits the growth of transformed human astrocytes. *Journal of Biological Chemistry* **266**, 728–34.

Morrison, R.S., Gross, J.L., Herblin, W.F., Reilly, T.M., LaSala, P.A., Alterman, R.L., Moskal, J.R., Kornblith, P.L. and Dexter, D.L. (1990) Basic fibroblast growth factor-like activity and receptors are expressed in a human glioma cell line. *Cancer Research* **50**, 2524–9.

Morrison, R.S., Yamaguchi, F., Bruner, J.M., Tang, M., McKeehan, W. and Berger, M.S. (1994) Fibroblast growth factor receptor gene expression and immunoreactivity are elevated in human glioblastoma multiforme. *Cancer Research* **54**, 2794–9.

Muleris, M., Almeida, A., Dutrillaux, A.M., Pruchon, E., Vega, F., Delattre, J.Y., Poisson, M., Malfoy, B. and Dutrillaux, B. (1994) Oncogene amplification in human gliomas: a molecular cytogenetic analysis. *Oncogene* **9**, 2717–22.

Murphy, P.R., Sato, Y. and Knee, R.S. (1992) Phosphorothioate antisense oligonucleotides against basic fibroblast growth factor inhibit anchorage-dependent and anchorage-independent growth of a malignant glioblastoma cell line. *Molecular Endocrinology* **6**, 877–84.

Mustonen, T. and Alitalo, K. (1995) Endothelial receptor tyrosine kinases involved in angiogenesis. *Journal of Cell Biology* **129**, 895–8.

Myers, R.L., Chedid, M., Tronick, S.R. and Chiu, I.-M. (1995) Different fibroblast growth factor 1 (FGF-1) transcripts in neural tissues, glioblastomas and kidney carcinoma cell lines. *Oncogene* **11**, 785–9.

Nakamura, T., Nishizawa, T., Hagiya, M., Seki, T., Shimonishi, M., Sugimura, A., Tashiro, K. and Shimizu, S. (1989) Molecular cloning and expression of human hepatocyte growth factor. *Nature* **342**, 440–3.

Nakamura, T., Takeshita, I., Inamura, T., Tashima, T. and Fukui, M. (1993) Expression of the B-chain of platelet-derived growth factor and proliferative activity of human brain tumors. *Neurologia Medico-Chirurgica* **33**, 205–11.

Neufeld, G., Tessler, S., Gitay-Goren, H., Cohen, T. and Levi, B.-Z. (1994) Vascular endothelial growth factor and its receptors. *Progress in Growth Factor Research* **5**, 89–97.

Nielsen, F.C., Gammeltoft, S., Westermark, B. and Fahrenkrug, J. (1990) High affinity receptors for vasoactive intestinal peptide on a human glioma cell line. *Peptides* **11**, 1225–31.

Nishikawa, R., Ji, X.D., Harmon, R.C., Lazar, C.S., Gill, G.N., Cavenee, W.K. and Huang, H.J. (1994) A mutant epidermal growth factor receptor common in human glioma confers enhanced tumorigenicity. *Proceedings of the National Academy of Sciences U.S.A.* **91**, 7727–31.

Nistér, M. and Westermark, B. (1994) Human glioma cell lines. In Hay, R.J., Park, J.G. and Gazdar, A. (eds), *Atlas of human tumor cell lines*. San Diego: Academic Press, 17–42.

Nistér, M., Heldin, C.-H. and Westermark, B. (1986) Clonal variation in the production of a platelet-derived growth factor-like protein and expression of corresponding receptors in a human malignant glioma. *Cancer Research* **46**, 332–40.

Nistér, M., Wedell, B., Betsholtz, C., Bywater, M., Pettersson, M., Westermark, B. and Mark, J. (1987) Evidence for progressional changes in the human malignant glioma cell line U-343 MGa: analysis of karyotype and expression of genes encoding the subunit chains of platelet-derived growth factor. *Cancer Research* **47**, 4953–60.

Nistér, M., Libermann, T.A., Betsholtz, C., Pettersson, M., Claesson-Welsh, L., Heldin, C.-H., Schlessinger, J. and Westermark, B. (1988) Expression of messenger RNAs for platelet-derived growth factor and transforming growth factor α and their receptors in human malignant glioma cell lines. *Cancer Research* **48**, 3910–18.

Nistér, M., Claesson-Welsh, L., Eriksson, A., Heldin, C.-H. and Westermark, B. (1991) Differential expression of platelet-derived growth factor receptors in human malignant glioma cell lines. *Journal of Biological Chemistry* **266**, 16755–63.

Noble, M., Gutowski, N., Bevan, K., Engel, U., Linskey, M., Urenjak, J., Bhakoo, K. and Williams, S. (1995) From rodent glial precursor cell to human glial neoplasia in the oligodendrocyte-type-2 astrocyte lineage. *GLIA* **15**, 222–30.

Nowell, P.C. (1976) The clonal evolution of tumor cell populations. *Science* **194**, 23–8.

Nusse, R., Brown, A., Papkoff, J., Scambler, P., Shackleford, G., McMahon, A., Moon, R. and Varmus, H. (1991) A new nomenclature for *int-1* and related genes: the *Wnt* gene family. *Cell* **64**, 231–2.

Okamoto, Y., Minamoto, S., Shimizu, K., Mogami, H. and Taniguchi, T. (1990) Interleukin 2 receptor β chain expressed in an oligodendroglioma line binds interleukin 2 and delivers growth signal. *Proceedings of the National Academy of Sciences U.S.A.* **87**, 6584–8.

Olofsson, A., Miyazono, K., Kanzaki, T., Colosetti, P., Engström, U. and Heldin, C.-H. (1992) Transforming growth factor-β1, -β2, and -β3 secreted by a human glioblastoma cell line. Identification of small and different forms of large latent complexes. *Journal of Biological Chemistry* **267**, 19482–8.

OMIM™ *online Mendelian inheritance in man database.* (1995) Database online. Baltimore, Md.: Johns Hopkins University. Updated daily (cited 2/28/97). OMIM data type: gene map. Available from Internet: <http://www3.ncbi.nlm.nih.gov/omim/>.

Orr-Urtreger, A., Trakhtenbrot, L., Ben-Levy, R., Wen, D., Rechavi, G., Lonai, P. and Yarden, Y. (1993) Neural expression and chromosomal mapping of Neu differentiation factor to 8p12-p21. *Proceedings of the National Academy of Sciences U.S.A.* **90**, 1867–71.

Paetau, A., Mellström, K., Vaheri, A. and Haltia, M. (1980) Distribution of a major connective tissue protein, fibronectin, in normal and neoplastic human nervous tissue. *Acta Neuropathologica* **51**, 47–51.

Pantazis, P., Pelicci, P.G., Dalla-Favera, R. and Antoniades, H.N. (1985) Synthesis and secretion of proteins resembling platelet-derived growth factor by human glioblastoma and fibrosarcoma cells in culture. *Proceedings of the National Academy of Sciences U.S.A.* **82**, 2404–8.

Park, M., Dean, M., Kaul, K., Braun, M.J., Gonda, M.A. and Vande Woude, G. (1987) Sequence of *MET* protooncogene cDNA has features characteristic of the tyrosine kinase family of growth-factor receptors. *Proceedings of the National Academy of Sciences U.S.A.* **84**, 6379–83.

Pedersen, P.H., Ness, G.O., Engebraaten, O., Bjerkvig, R., Lillehaug, J.R. and Laerum, O.D. (1994) Heterogeneous response to the growth factors [EGF, PDGF(BB), TGF-α, bFGF, IL-2] on glioma spheroid growth, migration and invasion. *International Journal of Cancer* **56**, 255–61.

Perides, G., Safran, R.M., Downing, L.A. and Charness, M.E. (1994) Regulation of neural cell adhesion molecule and L1 by the transforming growth factor-β superfamily. Selective effects of the bone morphogenetic proteins. *Journal of Biological Chemistry* **269**, 765–70.

Pettersson, O.-A., Carlsson, J. and Grusell, E. (1992) Accumulation of ^{10}B in the central degenerative areas of human glioma and colon carcinoma spheroids after sulfhydryl boron hydride administration. *Cancer Research* **52**, 1587–91.

Pietsch, T., Scharmann, T., Fonatsch, C., Schmidt, D., Ockler, R., Freihoff, D., Albrecht, S., Wiestler, O.D., Zeltzer, P. and Riehm, H. (1994) Characterization of five new cell lines derived from human primitive neuroectodermal tumors of the central nervous system. *Cancer Research* **54**, 3278–87.

Pinski, J., Schally, A.V., Halmos, G., Szepeshazi, K. and Groot, K. (1994) Somatostatin analogues and bombesin/gastrin-releasing peptide antagonist RC-3095 inhibit the growth of human glioblastomas *in vitro* and *in vivo*. *Cancer Research* **54**, 5895–901.

Plate, K.H. and Risau, W. (1995) Angiogenesis in malignant gliomas. *GLIA* **15**, 339–47.

Plate, K.H., Breier, G. and Risau, W. (1994) Molecular mechanisms of developmental and tumor angiogenesis. *Brain Pathology* **4**, 207–18.

Plate, K.H., Breier, G., Farrell, C.L. and Risau, W. (1992a) Platelet-derived growth factor receptor-β is induced during tumor development and upregulated during tumor progression in endothelial cells in human gliomas. *Laboratory Investigation* **67**, 529–34.

Plate, K.H., Breier, G., Weich, H.A. and Risau, W. (1992b) Vascular endothelial growth factor is a potential tumour angiogenesis factor in human gliomas *in vivo*. *Nature* **359**, 845–8.

Plate, K.H., Breier, G., Weich, H.A., Mennel, H.D. and Risau, W. (1994) Vascular endothelial growth factor and glioma angiogenesis: coordinate induction of VEGF receptors, distribution of VEGF protein and possible *in vivo* regulatory mechanisms. *International Journal of Cancer* **59**, 520–9.

Pontén, J. and Macintyre, E.H. (1968) Long term culture of normal and neoplastic human glia. *Acta Pathologica et Microbiologica Scandinavica* **74**, 465–86.

Post, G.R. and Dawson, G. (1992) Regulation of carbachol- and histamine-induced inositol phospholipid hydrolysis in a human oligodendroglioma. *GLIA* **5**, 122–30.

Potapova, O., Fakhrai, H. and Mercola, D. (1996) Growth factor PDGF-B/v-*sis* confers a tumorigenic phenotype to human tumor cells bearing PDGF receptors but not to cells devoid of receptors: evidence for an autocrine, but not a paracrine, mechanism. *International Journal of Cancer* **66**, 669–77.

Raff, M.C., Lillien, L.E., Richardson, W.D., Burne, J.F. and Noble, M.D. (1988) Platelet-derived growth factor from astrocytes drives the clock that times oligodendrocyte development in culture. *Nature* **333**, 562–5.

Reifenberger, J., Reifenberger, G., Ichimura, K., Schmidt, E.E., Wechsler, W. and Collins, V.P. (1996) Epidermal growth factor receptor expression in oligodendroglial tumors. *American Journal of Pathology* **149**, 29–35.

Reist, C.J., Archer, G.E., Kurpad, S.N., Wikstrand, C.J., Vaidyanathan, G., Willingham, M.C., Moscatello, D.K., Wong, A.J., Bigner, D.D. and Zalutsky, M.R. (1995) Tumor-specific anti-epidermal growth factor receptor variant III monoclonal antibodies: use of the tyramine-cellobiose radioiodination method enhances cellular retention and uptake in tumor xenografts. *Cancer Research* **55**, 4375–82.

Resnicoff, M., Abraham, D., Yutanawiboonchai, W., Rotman, H.L., Kajstura, J., Rubin, R., Zoltick, P. and Baserga, R. (1995) The insulin-like growth factor 1 receptor protects tumor cells from apoptosis *in vivo*. *Cancer Research* **55**, 2463–9.

Reubi, J.C., Lang, W., Maurer, R., Koper, J.W. and Lamberts, S.W.J. (1987) Distribution and biochemical characterization of somatostatin receptors in tumors of the human central nervous system. *Cancer Research* **47**, 5758–64.

Richardson, W.D., Pringle, N., Mosley, M.J., Westermark, B. and Dubois-Dalcq, M. (1988) A role for platelet-derived growth factor in normal gliogenesis in the central nervous system. *Cell* **53**, 309–19.

Risau, W., Drexler, H., Mironov, V., Smits, A., Siegbahn, A., Funa, K. and Heldin, C.-H. (1992) Platelet-derived growth factor is angiogenic *in vivo*. *Growth Factors* **7**, 261–6.

Roberts, W.M., Look, A.T., Roussel, M.F. and Sherr, C.J. (1988) Tandem linkage of human CSF-1 receptor (c-*fms*) and PDGF receptor genes. *Cell* **55**, 655–61.

Rosen, E.M., Laterra, J., Joseph, A., Jin, L., Fuchs, A., Way, D., Witte, M., Weinand, M. and Goldberg, I.D. (1996) Scatter factor expression and regulation in human glial tumors. *International Journal of Cancer* **67**, 248–55.

Rubin, J.S., Bottaro, D.P. and Aaronson, S.A. (1993) Hepatocyte growth factor/scatter factor and its receptor, the c-*met* proto-oncogene product. *Biochimica et Biophysica Acta* **1155**, 357–71.

Saitoh, Y., Kuratsu, J.-I., Takeshima, H., Yamamoto, S. and Ushio, Y. (1995) Expression of osteopontin in human glioma: its correlation with the malignancy. *Laboratory Investigation* **72**, 55–63.

Saleh, M., Stacker, S.A. and Wilks, A.F. (1996) Inhibition of growth of C6 glioma cells *in vivo* by expression of antisense vascular endothelial growth factor sequence. *Cancer Research* **56**, 393–401.

Samoto, K., Ikezaki, K., Ono, M., Shono, T., Kohno, K., Kuwano, M. and Fukui, M. (1995) Expression of vascular endothelial growth factor and its possible relation with neovascularization in human brain tumors. *Cancer Research* **55**, 1189–93.

Sandberg, A.-C., Engberg, C., Lake, M., von Holst, H. and Sara, V.R. (1988) The expression of insulin-like growth factor 1 and insulin-like growth factor 2 genes in the human fetal and adult brain and in glioma. *Neuroscience Letters* **93**, 114–19.

Sandberg-Nordqvist, A.-C., Ståhlbom, P.-A., Reinecke, M., Collins, V.P., von Holst, H. and Sara, V. (1993) Characterization of insulin-like growth factor 1 in human primary brain tumors. *Cancer Research* **53**, 2475–8.

Sasahara, M., Fries, J.W.U., Raines, E.W., Gown, A.M., Westrum, L.E., Frosch, M.P., Bonthron, D.T., Ross, R. and Collins, T. (1991) PDGF B-chain in neurons of the central nervous system, posterior pituitary, and in a transgenic model. *Cell* **64**, 217–27.

Sato, T.N., Qin, Y., Kozak, C.A. and Audus, K.L. (1993) *tie-1* and *tie-2* define another class of putative receptor tyrosine kinase genes expressed in early embryonic vascular system. *Proceedings of the National Academy of Sciences U.S.A.* **90**, 9355–8.

Schlegel, J., Ullrich, B., Stumm, G., Gass, P., Harwerth, I.-M., Hynes, N.E. and Kiessling, M. (1993) Expression of the c-*erb*B-2-encoded oncoprotein and progesterone receptor in human meningiomas. *Acta Neuropathologica* **86**, 473–9.

Schlegel, J., Merdes, A., Stumm, G., Albert, F.K., Forsting, M., Hynes, N.E. and Kiessling, M. (1994a) Amplification of the epidermal-growth-factor-receptor gene correlates with different growth behaviour in human glioblastoma. *International Journal of Cancer* **56**, 72–7.

Schlegel, J., Stumm, G., Brandle, K., Merdes, A., Mechtersheimer, G., Hynes, N.E. and Kiessling, M.

(1994b) Amplification and differential expression of members of the *erb*B-gene family in human glioblastoma. *Journal of Neuro-Oncology* **22**, 201–7.

Schlegel, U., Moots, P.L., Rosenblum, M.K., Thaler, H.T. and Furneaux, H.M. (1990) Expression of transforming growth factor α in human gliomas. *Oncogene* **5**, 1839–42.

Schröck, E., Thiel, G., Lozanova, T., du Monoir, S., Meffert, M.-C., Jauch, A., Speicher, M.R., Nürnberg, P., Vogel, S., Jänisch, W., Donis-Keller, H., Ried, T., Witkowski, R. and Cremer, T. (1994) Comparative genomic hybridisation of human malignant gliomas reveals multiple amplification sites and nonrandom chromosomal gains and losses. *American Journal of Pathology* **144**, 1203–18.

Schwechheimer, K., Huang, S. and Cavenee, W.K. (1995) EGFR gene amplification—rearrangement in human glioblastomas. *International Journal of Cancer* **62**, 145–8.

Schwechheimer, K., Läufle, R.M., Schmahl, W., Knödlseder, M., Fischer, H. and Höfler, H. (1994) Expression of Neu/c-erbB-2 in human brain tumors. *Human Pathology* **25**, 772–80.

Segal, R.A., Goumnerova, L.C., Kwon, Y.K., Stiles, C.D. and Pomeroy, S.L. (1994) Expression of the neurotrophin receptor TrkC is linked to a favourable outcome in medulloblastoma. *Proceedings of the National Academy of Sciences U.S.A.* **91**, 12867–71.

Shamah, S.M., Stiles, C.D. and Guha, A. (1993) Dominant-negative mutants of platelet-derived growth factor revert the transformed phenotype of human astrocytoma cells. *Molecular and Cellular Biology* **13**, 7203–12.

Shapiro, J.R., Yung, W.-K.A. and Shapiro, W.R. (1981) Isolation, karyotype and clonal growth of heterogeneous subpopulations of human malignant gliomas. *Cancer Research* **41**, 2349–59.

Sharma, S., Birchmeier, C., Nikawa, J., O'Neill, K., Rodgers, L. and Wigler, M. (1989) Characterization of the *ros*1-gene products expressed in human glioblastoma cell lines. *Oncogene Research* **5**, 91–100.

Shoyab, M., Plowman, G.D., McDonald, V.L., Bradley, J.G. and Todaro, G.J. (1989) Structure and function of human amphiregulin: a member of the epidermal growth factor family. *Science* **243**, 1074–6.

Shweiki, D., Itin, A., Soffer, D. and Keshet, E. (1992) Vascular endothelial growth factor induced by hypoxia may mediate hypoxia-initiated angiogenesis. *Nature* **359**, 843–5.

Sidransky, D., Mikkelsen, T., Schwechheimer, K., Rosenblum, M.L., Cavanee, W. and Vogelstein, B. (1992) Clonal expansion of p53 mutant cells is associated with brain tumour progression. *Nature* **355**, 846–7.

Smallwood, P.M., Munoz-Sanjuan, I., Tong, P., Macke, J.P., Hendry, S.H.C., Gilbert, D.J., Copeland, N.G., Jenkins, N.A. and Nathans, J. (1996) Fibroblast growth factor (FGF) homologous factors: new members of the FGF family implicated in nervous system development. *Proceedings of the National Academy of Sciences U.S.A.* **93**, 9850–7.

Smidt, M., Kirsch, I. and Ratner, L. (1990) Deletion of *Alu* sequences in the fifth c-*sis* intron in individuals with meningiomas. *Journal of Clinical Investigation* **86**, 1151–7.

Smith, C.A., Farrah, T. and Goodwin, R.G. (1994) The TNF receptor superfamily of cellular and viral proteins: activation, costimulation, and death. *Cell* **76**, 959–62.

Smits, A., Kato, M., Westermark, B., Nistér, M., Heldin, C.-H. and Funa, K. (1991) Neurotrophic activity of platelet-derived growth factor (PDGF): rat neuronal cells possess functional PDGF β-type receptors and respond to PDGF. *Proceedings of the National Academy of Sciences U.S.A.* **88**, 8159–63.

Smits, A., van Grieken, D., Hartman, M., Lendahl, U., Funa, K. and Nistér, M. (1996) Coexpression of platelet-derived growth factor α and β receptors on medulloblastomas and other primitive neuroectodermal tumors is consistent with an immature stem cell and neuronal derivation. *Laboratory Investigation* **74**, 188–98.

Spivak-Kroizman, T., Lemmon, M.A., Dikic, I., Ladbury, J.E., Pinchasi, D., Huang, J., Jaye, M. Crumley, G., Schlessinger, J. and Lax, I. (1994) Heparin-induced oligomerization of FGF molecules is responsible for FGF receptor dimerization, activation, and cell proliferation. *Cell* **79**, 1015–24.

Stan, A.C., Nemati, M.N., Pietsch, T., Walter, G.F. and Dietz, H. (1995) *In vivo* inhibition of angiogenesis and growth of the human U-87 malignant glial tumor by treatment with an antibody against basic fibroblast growth factor. *Journal of Neurosurgery* **82**, 1044–52.

Stanulla, M., Welte, K., Hadam, M.R. and Pietsch, T. (1995) Coexpression of stem cell factor and its receptor c-Kit in human malignant glioma cell lines. *Acta Neuropathologica* **89**, 158–65.

Stefanik, D.F., Rizkalla, L.R., Soi, A., Goldblatt, S.A. and Rizkalla, W.M. (1991) Acidic and basic fibroblast growth factors are present in glioblastoma multiforme. *Cancer Research* **51**, 5760–5.

Stein, I., Neeman, M., Shweiki, D., Itin, A. and Keshet, E. (1995) Stabilization of vascular endothelial growth factor mRNA by hypoxia and hypoglycemia and coregulation with other ischemia-induced genes. *Molecular and Cellular Biology* **15**, 5363–8.

Strader, C.D., Fong, T.M., Tota, M.R., Underwood, D and Dixon, R.A. (1994) Structure and function of G protein-coupled receptors. *Annual Review of Biochemistry* **63**, 101–32.

Strawn, L.M., Mann, E., Elliger, S.S., Chu, L.M., Germain, L.L., Niederfellner, G., Ullrich, A. and Shawver, L.K. (1994) Inhibition of glioma cell growth by a truncated platelet-derived growth factor β-receptor. *Journal of Biological Chemistry* **269**, 21215–22.

Suarez-Quian, C.A. and Byers, S.W. (1993) Redistribution of epidermal growth factor receptor as a function of cell density, cell-cell adhesion and calcium in human (A431) cells. *Tissue and Cell* **25**, 1–17.

Sugawa, N., Ekstrand, A.J., James, C.D. and Collins, V.P. (1990) Identical splicing of aberrant epidermal growth factor receptor transcripts from amplified rearranged genes in human glioblastomas. *Proceedings of the National Academy of Sciences U.S.A.* **87**, 8602–6.

Takahashi, J.A., Mori, H., Fukumoto, M., Igarashi, K., Jaye, M., Oda, Y., Kikuchi, H. and Hatanaka, M. (1990) Gene expression of fibroblast growth factors in human gliomas and meningiomas: demonstration of cellular source of basic fibroblast growth factor mRNA and peptide in tumor tissues. *Proceedings of the National Academy of Sciences U.S.A.* **87**, 5710–14.

Takahashi, J.A., Fukumoto, M., Kozai, Y., Ito, N., Oda, Y., Kikuchi, H. and Hatanaka, M. (1991) Inhibition of cell growth and tumorigenesis of human glioblastoma cells by a neutralizing antibody against human basic fibroblast growth factor. *FEBS Letters* **288**, 65–71.

Takahashi, J.A., Fukumoto, M., Igarashi, K., Oda, Y., Kikuchi, H. and Hatanaka, M. (1992) Correlation of basic fibroblast growth factor expression levels with the degree of malignancy and vascularity in human gliomas. *Journal of Neurosurgery* **76**, 792–8.

Takano, S., Yoshii, Y., Kondo, S., Suzuki, H., Maruno, T., Shirai, S. and Nose, T. (1996) Concentration of vascular endothelial growth factor in the serum and tumor tissue of brain tumor patients. *Cancer Research* **56**, 2185–90.

ten Dijke, P., Miyazono, K. and Heldin, C.-H, (1996) Signaling via hetero-oligomeric complexes of type I and type II serine/threonine kinase receptors. *Current Opinion in Cell Biology* **8**, 139–45.

Tohyama, T., Lee, V.M.-Y., Rorke, L.B., Marvin, M., McKay, R.D.G. and Trojanowski, J.Q. (1992) Nestin expression in embryonic human neuroepithelium and in human neuroepithelial tumor cells. *Laboratory Investigation* **66**, 303–13.

Torp, S.H., Helseth, E., Unsgaard, G. and Dalen, A. (1993) C-erbB-2/HER-2 protein in human intracranial tumours. *European Journal of Cancer* **29A**, 1604–6.

Trojan, J., Johnson, T.R., Rudin, S.D., Ilan, J., Tykocinski, M.L. and Ilan, J. (1993) Treatment and prevention of rat glioblastoma by immunogenic C6 cells expressing antisense insulin-like growth factor 1 RNA. *Science* **259**, 94–7.

Trojanowski, J.Q., Friedman, H.S., Burger, P.C. and Bigner, D.D. (1987) A rapidly dividing human medulloblastoma cell line (D283 MED) expresses all three neurofilament subunits. *American Journal of Pathology* **126**, 358–63.

Tucker, M.A. and Gillespie, G.Y. (1994) Production of a bioactive high molecular weight transforming growth factor β-like molecule by human malignant glioma cell lines. *Growth Factors* **11**, 153–62.

Ueba, T., Takahashi, J.A., Fukumoto, M., Ohta, M., Ito, N., Oda, Y., Kikuchi, H. and Hatanaka, M. (1994) Expression of fibroblast growth factor receptor-1 in human glioma and meningioma tissues. *Neurosurgery* **34**, 221–5.

Uhrbom, L., Nistér, M. and Westermark, B. (1997) Induction of senescence in human malignant glioma cells by $p16^{INKYA}$. *Oncogene* **15**, 505–14.

Ullrich, A. and Schlessinger, J. (1990) Signal transduction by receptors with tyrosine kinase activity. *Cell* **61**, 203–12.

Valgeirsdóttir, S., Eriksson, A., Nistér, M., Heldin, C.-H., Westermark, B. and Claesson-Welsh, L. (1994) Compartmentalization of autocrine signal transduction pathways in *sis*-transformed NIH 3T3 cells. *Journal of Biological Chemistry* **270**, 10161–70.

Vandenbark, G.R., deCastro, C.M., Taylor, H., Dew-Knight, S. and Kaufman, R.E. (1992) Cloning and structural analysis of the human c-*kit* gene. *Oncogene* **7**, 1259–66.

van der Geer, P., Hunter, T. and Lindberg, R.A. (1994) Receptor protein-tyrosine kinases and their signal transduction pathways. *Annual Review of Cell Biology* **10**, 251–337.

Van Meir, E.G. (1995) Cytokines and tumors of the central nervous system. *GLIA* **15**, 264–88.

Vassbotn, F.S., Östman, A., Langeland, N., Holmsen, H., Westermark, B., Heldin, C.-H. and Nistér, M. (1994) Activated platelet-derived growth factor autocrine pathway drives the transformed phenotype of a human glioblastoma cell line. *Journal of Cellular Physiology* **158**, 381–9.

von Deimling, A., von Ammon, K., Schoenfeld, D., Wiestler, O.D., Seizinger, B.R. and Louis, D.N. (1993) Subsets of glioblastoma multiforme defined by molecular genetic analysis. *Brain Pathology* **3**, 19–26.

Wang, J.-L., Nistér, M., Hermansson, M., Westermark, B. and Pontén, J. (1990) Expression of PDGF β-receptors in human meningioma cells. *International Journal of Cancer* **46**, 772–8.

Washiyama, K., Muragaki, Y., Rorke, L.B., Lee, V.M., Feinstein, S.C., Radeke, M.J., Blumberg, D., Kaplan, D.R. and Trojanowski, J.Q. (1996) Neurotrophin and neurotrophin receptor proteins in medulloblastomas and other primitive neuroectodermal tumors of the pediatric central nervous system. *American Journal of Pathology* **148**, 929–40.

Wasson, J.C., Saylors, R.L. III, Zeltzer, P., Friedman, H.S., Bigner, S.H., Burger, P.C., Bigner, D.D., Look, A.T., Douglass, E.C. and Brodeur, G.M. (1990) Oncogene amplification in pediatric brain tumors. *Cancer Research* **50**, 2987–90.

Waterfield, M.D., Scrace, G.T., Whittle, N., Stroobant, P., Johnsson, A., Wasteson, Å., Westermark, B., Heldin, C.-H., Huang, J.S. and Deuel, T.F. (1983) Platelet-derived growth factor is structurally related to the putative transforming protein $p28^{sis}$ of simian sarcoma virus. *Nature* **304**, 35–9.

Watkins, D., Dion, F., Poisson, M., Delattre, J.Y. and Rouleau, G.A. (1994) Analysis of oncogene expression in primary human gliomas: evidence for increased expression of the *ros* oncogene. *Cancer Genetics and Cytogenetics* **72**, 130–6.

Weindel, K., Moringlane, J.R., Marmé, D. and Weich, H.A. (1994) Detection and quantification of vascular endothelial growth factor/vascular permeability factor in brain tumor tissue and cyst fluid: the key to angiogenesis? *Neurosurgery* **35**, 439–49.

Weiner, D.B., Liu, J., Cohen, J.A., Williams, W.V. and Greene, M.I. (1989) A point mutation in the *neu* oncogene mimics ligand induction of receptor aggregation. *Nature* **339**, 230–1.

Weisman, A.S., Raguet, S.S. and Kelly, P.A. (1987) Characterization of the epidermal growth factor receptor in human meningioma. *Cancer Research* **47**, 2172–6.

Weller, M. and Fontana, A. (1995) The failure of current immunotherapy for malignant glioma. Tumor-derived TGF-β, T-cell apoptosis, and the immune privilege of the brain. *Brain Research. Brain Research Reviews* **21**, 128–51.

Wells, A., Welsh, J.B., Lazar, C.S., Wiley, H.S., Gill, G.N. and Rosenfeld, M.G. (1990) Ligand-induced transformation by a noninternalizing epidermal growth factor receptor. *Science* **247**, 962–4.

Westermark, B. (1976) Density dependent proliferation of human glia cells stimulated by epidermal growth factor. *Biochemical and Biophysical Research Communications* **69**, 304–10.

Westermark, B. and Heldin, C.-H. (1991) Platelet-derived growth factor in autocrine transformation. *Cancer Research* **51**, 5087–92.

Westermark, B., Magnusson, A. and Heldin, C.-H. (1982) Effect of epidermal growth factor on membrane motility and cell locomotion in cultures of human clonal glioma cells. *Journal of Neuroscience Research* **8**, 491–507.

Westermark B., Pontén, J. and Hugosson, R. (1973) Determinants for the establishment of permanent tissue culture lines from human gliomas. *Acta Pathologica et Microbiologica Scandinavica Section A* **81**, 791–805.

White, M.F. and Kahn, C.R. (1994) The insulin signaling system. *Journal of Biological Chemistry* **269**, 1–4.

Wikstrand, C.J., Friedman, H.S. and Bigner, D.D. (1991) Medulloblastoma cell-substrate interaction *in vitro*. *Invasion Metastasis* **11**, 310–24.

Wikstrand, C.J., Hale, L.P., Batra, S.K., Hill, M.L., Humphrey, P.A., Kurpad, S.N., McLendon, R.E., Moscatello, D., Pegram, C.N., Reist, C.J., Traweek, S.T., Wong, A.J., Zalutsky, M.R. and Bigner, D.D. (1995) Monoclonal antibodies against EGFRvIII are tumor specific and react with breast and lung carcinomas and malignant gliomas. *Cancer Research* **55**, 3140–8.

Wikstrand, C.J., McLendon, R.E., Friedman, A.H. and Bigner, D.D. (1997) Cell surface localization and density of the tumor-associated variant of the epidermal growth factor receptor EGFRvIII. *Cancer Research* **57**, 4130–40.

Wizigmann-Voos, S., Breier, G., Risau, W. and Plate, K.H. (1995) Up-regulation of vascular endothelial growth factor and its receptors in von Hippel-Lindau disease-associated and in sporadic hemangioblastomas. *Cancer Research* **55**, 1358–64.

Wong, A.J., Ruppert, J.M., Bigner, S.H., Grzeschik, C.H., Humphrey, P.A., Bigner, D.S. and Vogelstein, B. (1992) Structural alterations of the epidermal growth factor receptor gene in human gliomas. *Proceedings of the National Academy of Sciences U.S.A.* **89**, 2965–9.

Wong, S.T., Winchell, L.F., McCune, B.K., Earp, H.S., Teixidó, J., Massagué, J., Herman, B. and Lee, D.C. (1989) The TGF-α precursor expressed on the cell surface binds to the EGF receptor on adjacent cells, leading to signal transduction. *Cell* **56**, 495–506.

Wrana, J.L., Attisano, L., Wieser, R., Ventura, F. and Massagué, J. (1994) Mechanism of activation of the TGF-β receptor. *Nature* **370**, 341–7.

Wu, J.K. and Chikaraishi, D.M. (1990) Differential expression of *ros* oncogene in primary human astrocytomas and astrocytoma cell lines. *Cancer Research* **50**, 3032–5.

Wullich, B., Sattler, H.-P., Fischer, U. and Meese, E. (1994) Two independent amplification events on chromosome 7 in glioma: amplification of the epidermal growth factor receptor gene and amplification of the oncogene *MET*. *Anticancer Research* **14**, 577–9.

Yahanda, A.M., Bruner, J.M., Donehower, L.A. and Morrison, R.S. (1995) Astrocytes derived from p53-deficient mice provide a multistep *in vitro* model for development of malignant gliomas. *Molecular and Cellular Biology* **15**, 4249–59.

Yamada, N., Kato, M., Yamashita, H., Nistér, M., Miyazono, K., Heldin, C.-H. and Funa, K. (1995) Enhanced expression of transforming growth factor-β and its type I and type II receptors in human glioblastoma. *International Journal of Cancer* **62**, 386–92.

Yamada, N., Kato, M., ten Dijke, P., Yamashita, H., Sampath, T.K., Heldin, C.-H., Miyazono, K. and Funa, K. (1996) Bone morphogenetic protein type 1B receptor is progressively expressed in malignant glioma tumors. *British Journal of Cancer* **73**, 624–9.

Yamazaki, H., Fukui, Y., Ueyama, Y., Tamaoki, N., Kawamoto, T., Taniguchi, S. and Shibuya, M. (1988) Amplification of the structurally and functionally altered epidermal growth factor receptor gene (*c-erb*B) in human brain tumors. *Molecular and Cellular Biology* **8**, 1816–20.

Yamazaki, H., Ohba, Y., Tamaoki, N. and Shibuya, M. (1990) A deletion mutation within the ligand binding domain is responsible for activation of epidermal growth factor receptor gene in human brain tumors. *Japanese Journal of Cancer Research* **81**, 773–9.

Yarden, Y. and Ullrich, A. (1988) Growth factor receptor tyrosine kinases. *Annual Review of Biochemistry* **57**, 443–78.

Yeh, H.-J., Ruit, K.G., Wang, Y.-X., Parks, W.C., Snider, W.D. and Deuel, T.F. (1991) PDGF A-chain gene is expressed by mammalian neurons during development and in maturity. *Cell* **64**, 209–16.

Yung, W.K.A., Zhang, X., Steck, P.A. and Hung, M.-C. (1990) Differential amplifications of the TGF-α gene in human gliomas. *Cancer Communications* **2**, 201–5.

Zagzag, D. (1995) Angiogenic growth factors in neural embryogenesis and neoplasia. (Review) *American Journal of Pathology* **146**, 293–309.

Zagzag, D., Miller, D.C., Sato, Y., Rifkin, D.B. and Burstein, D.E. (1990) Immunohistochemical localization of basic fibroblast growth factor in astrocytomas. *Cancer Research* **50**, 7393–8.

CHAPTER 4

Mechanisms of altered growth control

Invasion and metastasis

OLE DIDRIK LAERUM AND SVERRE J. MØRK

Introduction

Although primary brain tumors characteristically are confined to the skull and only rarely metastasize, they have a poor prognosis. In contrast to cancers elsewhere in the body, primary central nervous system (CNS) neoplasms are rarely circumscribed 'tumors'. The malignant cells are dispersed among normal cells and structures of the brain from the earliest stages of neoplastic disease. Thus, a brain tumor must be comprehended as a tissue composed of neoplastic cells, normal macro- and microglia, neurons, myelin and extracellular matrix (ECM), vasculature and immunocompetent cells. These tumors are ill defined in relation to the surrounding brain tissue. In addition to invading tumor cells, the border zone consists of axons and nerve cell bodies, more or less reactive astrocytes, oligodendrocytes, myelin, microglia and blood vessels with pericytes and a varying number of mononuclear cells. Morphologically, it may be impossible to discriminate reactive from neoplastic glial cells and, thereby, it may be problematic to establish eventual radicality of a surgical procedure. The extensive invasive nature of neuroepithelial tumors makes curative surgery a viable option for only a few patients. Even wide surgical excisions of primary brain tumors are sooner or later followed by local recurrence. This may be due to invasion of cells outside the borders of surgery. The invasive behavior of primary neoplasms of the nervous system is, therefore, of great clinical and biologic importance.

The growth patterns of brain tumors were highlighted in the 1930s when the Belgian pathologist Hans-Joachim Scherer presented thorough studies of gliomas in relation to the brain as a whole (Scherer, 1935, 1938, 1940). He made careful analyses of the interaction between primary brain tumors and the adjacent brain tissue, and showed on whole-mount sections of human brains that tumor cells grow along fiber tracts of the white matter, along the subpial interface, in the subependymal area, and that they can invade the perivascular space of Virchow-Robin. In particular, Scherer emphasized that cell shape and tissue pattern mirrored the microenvironment of the tumor cells. The migratory properties of the brain tumor cells were particularly important for the appearance of the tumor.

Following is a survey of the histologic and biologic features of brain tumor invasion. Cell properties related to invasion are described and compared with their normal counterparts. This comparison is important since invasion, in principle, is closely related to basically normal cell properties. To analyze the complex cellular interactions in brain tumors, investigators have widely employed *in vitro* and animal experiments. In recent years, investigators, using several newly developed *in vitro* and animal models, have produced extensive research on interactions between brain tumor cells and non-neoplastic tissues (for review, see Bjerkvig, 1991).

General features of invasive and metastasizing tumor cells

Classically, invasion can be described as a condition where malignant cells gradually replace normal tissue. There is destruction of the normal cells, and the process is progressive in time. In primary brain tumors, however, destruction of the normal tissue is not always evident.

Migrating tumor cells are dependent on a functioning cytoskeleton and specific cell-surface receptors associated with the locomotory system. Although cell proliferation is important for tumor progression, it is, as such, not a necessary condition for cell invasion. Neovascularization is not necessary since invasion can occur by single cells entering the neighboring vascularized tissue.

Generally, the formation of metastases depends on invasion into normal tissue, by which the cells reach other sites either as direct intercellular spread along existing structures, or by blood or lymphatic circulation. In the brain, the characteristic patterns of invasion and the biologic cell properties of invading cells are somewhat different from the situation in other organs (Laerum *et al.*, 1984; Mareel and Calman, 1984).

Normal neural cell properties related to invasiveness

Although the spreading of malignant neuroepithelial cells among different structures in the brain may seem rather unique, it should be remembered that normal brain cells are capable of a similar migratory activity (Jessen and Richardson, 1996). In addition to knowledge about the nervous system during embryonic and fetal life, there are now several experimental systems where such migration can be shown directly. For example, when prelabeled cortical astrocytes from 14-day-old rat fetuses are homografted into the cerebral cortex, a rapid migration takes place over a period of 30–60 days. The transplanted astrocytes are found along the entire circumference of the brain. They enter the spaces of Virchow-Robin and migrate along parenchymal blood vessels and also within the subependymal zone adjacent to the ventricles. The nerve fiber bundles are important for directing this migration (Goldberg and Bernstein, 1988; Bernstein and Goldberg, 1989). It has also been shown that immature neurons from the subependymal zone can migrate over long distances and differentiate into mature neurons at various locations when transplanted into adult mice (Lois and Alvarez-Buylla, 1994).

Interestingly, the patterns of migration of fetal rat cells and human glioma cells are indistinguishable, and both cell types migrate over long distances when transplanted into the adult rat brain (Pedersen *et al.*, 1993). However, there is one important difference between normal neural cells and their malignant counterparts–a difference that can be shown directly in organ cultures *in vitro*. When spheroids from human gliomas are cultured together with fetal rat brain tissue *in vitro*, the malignant cells will rapidly invade and replace most of the nervous tissue. When two fetal rat brain aggregates are put together, the fetal tissues will intermingle and not destroy each other. In contrast, mature rat brain cells show a tendency to adhere, but otherwise keep apart as separate structures, when confronted as cell aggregates. In addition, their migratory capacity, upon transplantation to the brain, is relatively low (Marienhagen *et al.*, 1994). Thus, the migratory properties of malignant glioma cells seem to resemble fetal more than adult neural cells.

Some of the destructive properties of glioma cells are associated with proteolytic enzymes. It should be noted that such enzymes are important for development, regeneration and repair in the nervous system. The molecules that constitute the ECM of the brain are assembled in a highly organized manner and contribute to the local structural integrity (Jones, 1996). Proteinases that degrade and modulate the ECM are important for maintaining this integrity. They include matrix metalloproteinases and plasminogen activators. Several specific inhibitors of such proteinases are important for brain development and neural outgrowth, as well as in diseases of the nervous system (for review, see Romanic and Madri, 1994).

The process of invasion in the nervous system involves a series of complex interactions between tumor cells, normal cells and their ECM, as well as interactions between physiologic regulatory circuits and their eventual disturbed version in malignant cells and tissues. Various cytokines and growth factors act as signals within the brain, and are involved in neuronal degeneration and repair of both the peripheral and the central nervous systems. In particular, cytokines are important mediators of the inflammatory process (for review, see Hopkins and Rothwell, 1995; Rothwell and Hopkins, 1995). Interestingly, the identification of proto-oncogenes coding for growth factor receptors and their ligands in malignant cells has led to the discovery of their normal function in the nervous system (Marchionni *et al.*, 1993). Theoretically, normally occurring growth factors and cytokines might enhance invasive behavior of tumor cells that carry an increased density of their receptors.

Patterns of invasion by malignant brain tumors

Morphologic studies on the infiltration and spread of human brain tumors have been done mainly on autopsy material. Therefore, most of the existing data are based on knowledge from the end stage of tumor progression. This is rapidly changing in light of modern imaging techniques, where even small tumors may be studied three-dimensionally. From experimental studies on carcinogen-induced brain tumors in rats, it has been shown that, from the stage of microtumors, malignant gliomas are already mixed with nonneoplastic cells and have an unclear demarcation from the surrounding brain tissue (Lantos and Pilkington, 1979). Destructive invasion seems to be a late phenomenon in experimental carcinogenesis of the nervous system (de Ridder and Laerum, 1981). In line with this, a selective clinicopathologic study on small human gliomas (< 2 cm in diameter) concluded that most of them were histologically benign, localized and removable. However, some of the cases appeared, histologically, as high-grade gliomas from the start (Tamura, Ohye and Nakazato, 1993).

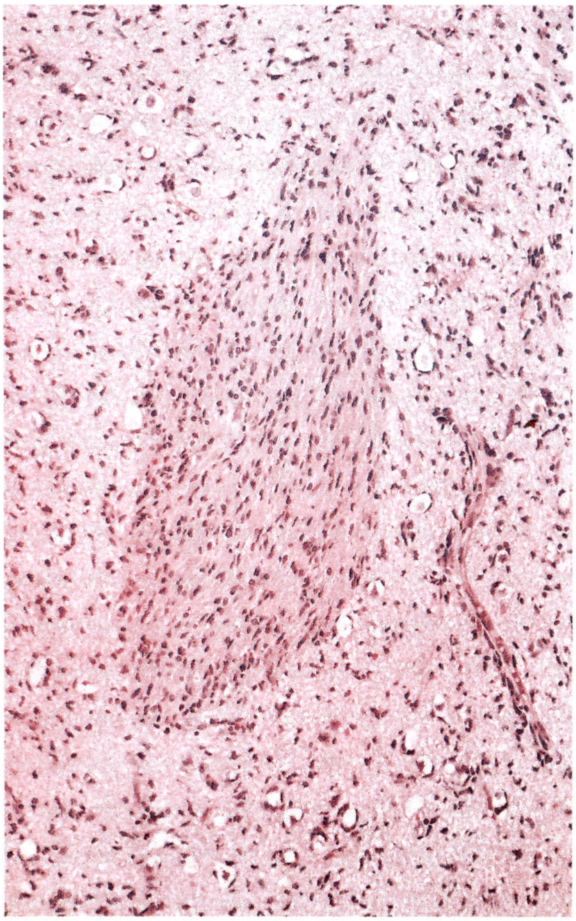

Fig. 4.1 Diffuse growth of neoplastic glia in stereotactic biopsy material from central portion of the brain (corpus striatum). Note the orientation of tumor cells along a blood vessel (right), aligned with fiber systems in white matter (center) and around neurons (round 'empty' spaces). Hematoxylin and eosin (H&E), × 140

The growth patterns of gliomas are determined by the anatomic relations of the infiltrated areas. To distinguish them from the structure in the primary tumor itself, Scherer used the term 'secondary structures' for the organization of tumor cells according to pre-existing neural tissue elements (Scherer, 1935, 1938, 1940). Examples are organization of tumor cells around nerve cells and vessels; along interfaces in the brain, such as where gray and white substances meet; and along the parenchymal and ventricular linings. Tumor cells infiltrating fiber tracts in the brain, brainstem or spinal medulla will, therefore, tend to be elongated by orientation of their long axes parallel to the nerve fibers (Fig. 4.1). Impaired circulation, hemorrhage and necrosis may lead to mesenchymal reaction and alterations of the

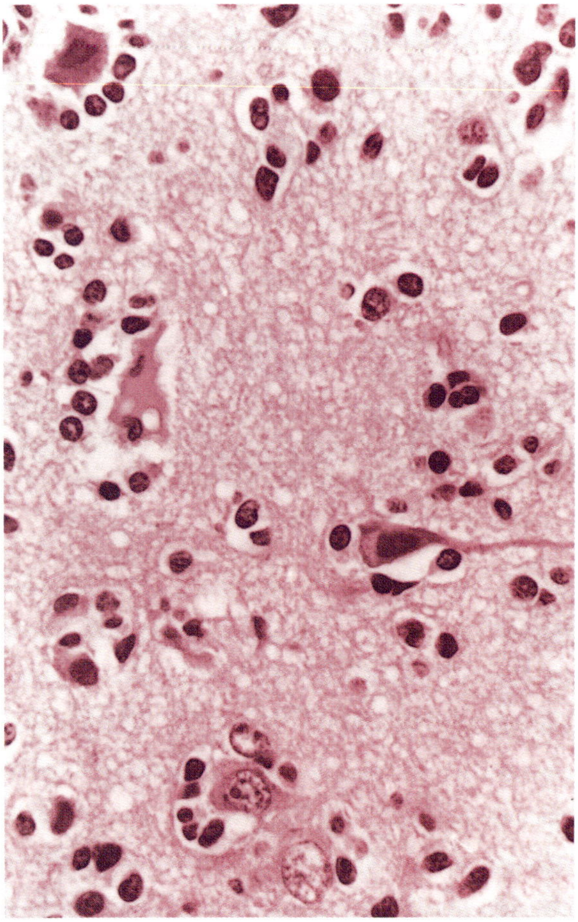

Fig. 4.2 Glioma cells crowding around normal (bottom) and pathological neurons (right, top left). H&E, × 560

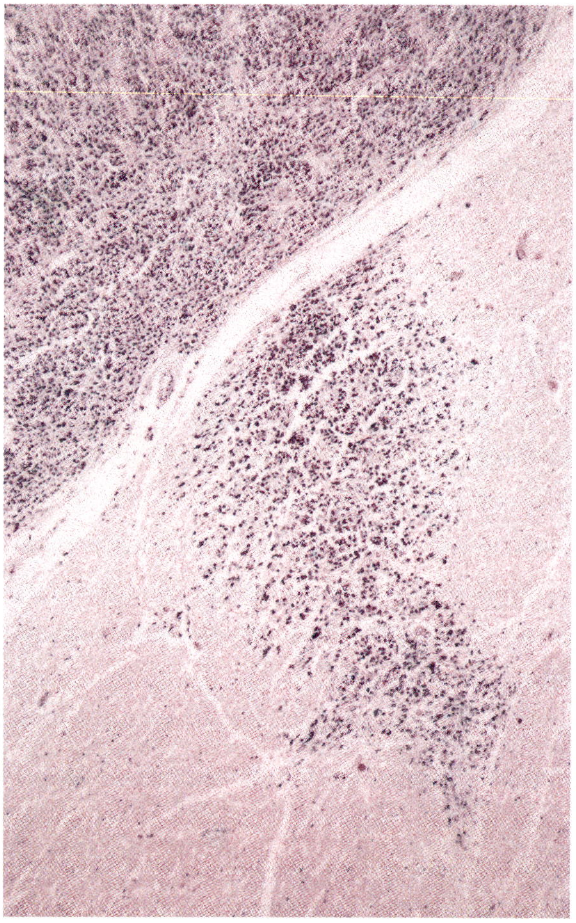

Fig. 4.3 An anaplastic ependymoma of the cerebellum with massive leptomeningeal spread and focal diffuse re-entry into the pons. H&E, × 70

tissues infiltrated by tumor cells: changes that were denoted 'tertiary structures' and that may also result from invasion of the dura. These structures may occur late in the progression of a tumor, imprinting the tissues with a pattern considerably different from that of their 'primary structure', and alluding to the type of glioma irrespective of its location, i.e., ependymal canals and rosettes in ependymomas, pseudopalisading of nuclei adjacent to necrosis in glioblastomas or characteristic rosettes in medulloblastomas.

When glioma cells penetrate the neural parenchyma, both glial and neural cells may become surrounded by tumor cells and gradually be destroyed (Fig. 4.2). Pre-existing nerve fibers and healthy-looking neurons can, however, often be identified, even deeply within the solid tumor. Large parts of the pre-existing nervous parenchyma can remain morphologically intact among tumor tissue. Therefore, neural tissue may show resistance to the cytolytic effect mediated by malignant cells.

In the invasion zone, complex tissue reactions occur, such as edema and anoxic changes due to local pressure, as well as necrosis and apoptosis. Characteristically, reactive astrocytes with abundant cytoplasm and short cell processes are seen, both in the tumor periphery and peritumorally. Such reactive astrocytes are easy to see by hematoxylin and eosin staining, but immunostaining for glial fibrillary acidic protein (GFAP) makes their elaborate branches stand out. Mitotic activity may also be seen in the reacting astrocytes, sometimes making their discrimination from the malignant cells difficult (Schiffer, 1993). A central position for microglia in normal and pathologic conditions has emerged during recent years (Graeber, 1994). In response to changes in the microenvironment (e.g., invasion), microglia produce proteinases, cytokines, reactive

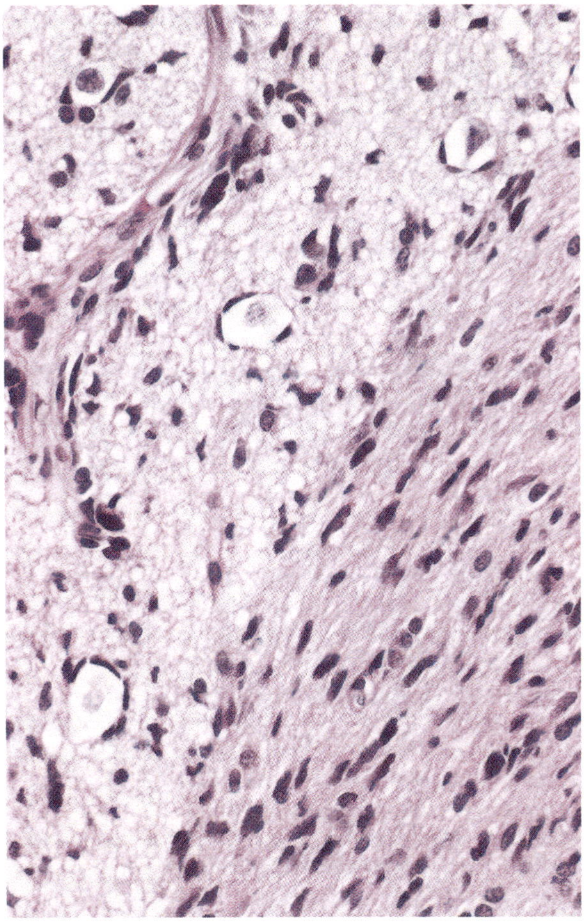

Fig. 4.4 Diffuse invasive growth of neoplastic glial cells without tissue destruction in gliomatosis cerebri. The stereotactic biopsy was from the basal ganglia. H&E, × 450

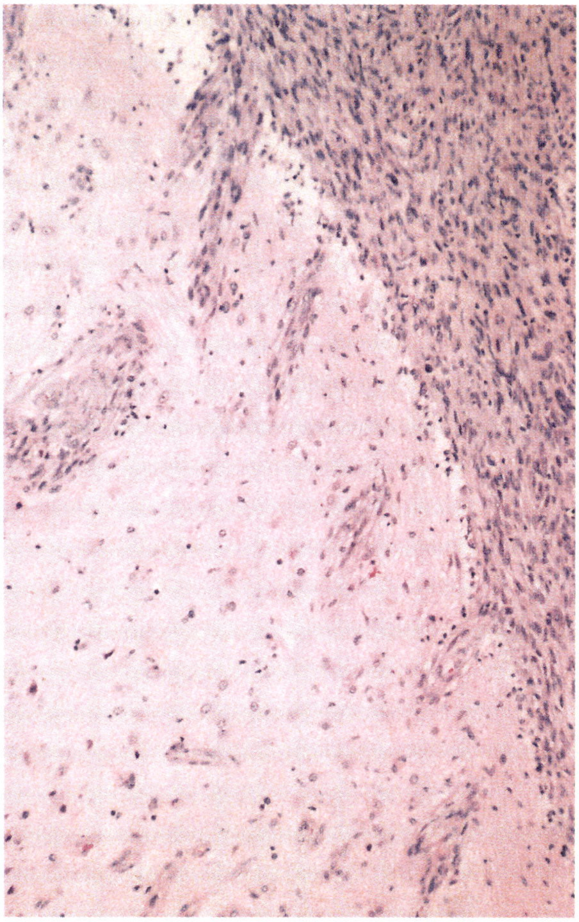

Fig. 4.5 An anaplastic meningioma invading the cerebral cortex through the Virchow-Robin space. Note the diffuse astrogliosis and the well-demarcated tumor 'fingers'. H&E, ×140

oxygen intermediates and reactive nitrogen intermediates (Banati *et al.*, 1993).

Glioma cells tend to invade the superficial pia mater, but seldom proceed to the outer border of the perivascular spaces. Invasion of the Virchow-Robin space is common. Blood vessels within this space are intact, and penetration into the lumen of the blood vessels, including capillaries, is not usual. The adjacent leptomeninges can be infiltrated, but, as will be discussed later, a barrier to further spread seems to exist. From the leptomeninges, tumor cells may also re-enter the brain tissue and form secondary tumors (Fig. 4.3). When neoplastic infiltration occurs in the pia mater, invasion of the cortex of the opposite convulsion may also occur.

As a rare event, both glioblastomas and anaplastic astrocytomas may invade the adjacent dura mater and even cranial bone tissue (Pompili *et al.*, 1993). This may occur spontaneously during tumor progression, but is most often seen after surgical intervention. Invasion through the ventricular walls with local ependymal spread may lead to development of metastases by way of the cerebrospinal fluid (CSF) (Tamura, Ohye and Nakazato, 1993).

Diffuse infiltrative growth, which is characteristic of most cerebral astrocytomas, is exemplified in extreme in the condition gliomatosis cerebri, where diffuse infiltration (Fig. 4.4) is seen over large parts of the brain without a localized tumor (Dunn and Kernohan, 1957).

Invasive growth by anaplastic meningiomas mainly occurs locally (Fig. 4.5) and seldom gives remote metastases. However, neoplastic meningitis from anaplastic meningioma has been described (Vinchon *et al.*, 1995).

Morphology of invasion by the different tumor types

Following is a brief description of the characteristic macroscopic and histologic patterns of invasion by common types of primary brain tumors. An outline of the invasive properties is presented in Table 4.1.

ASTROCYTOMAS

Diffuse cerebral astrocytomas of the white matter are most common in the cerebral hemispheres of adults. They do not appear as a solid tumor, but rather as a diffuse proliferation of neoplastic astrocytes. The lesions are firmer than the normal brain substance, they show some cystic changes and they are not well demarcated from the surrounding brain. Microscopic analysis usually shows invasion by astrocytes that are slightly larger and have more irregular nuclei and higher cell density than the normal brain parenchyma. Characteristically, spread of neoplastic cells is seen over a wide area. In some sectors, the border zone between tumor and brain tissue may be relatively sharp, due to a more intense infiltration of tumor cells. Clusters of astrocytoma cells may be found around nerve cells, under the ependymal lining of the ventricles, in the perivascular space of the brain parenchyma and under the pia mater. When the tumor invades fiber tracts of the corpus callosum, pons or spinal cord, the tumor cells are often elongated with a bipolar or piloid shape.

Pilocytic astrocytoma has a varied but characteristic appearance, with piloid cells and elongated eosinophilic extracellular structures (Rosenthal fibers). Glial cells of varying shape with hyperchromatic, often bizarre, nuclei; some clear, oligodendroglia-like cells; cystic spaces; varying amounts of blood vessels; microvascular proliferations (relatively common); and decalcified foci make up the composite tumor tissue of a pilocytic astrocytoma. These tumors have a tendency to invade the subarachnoid space (Fig. 4.6), but dissemination through the CSF is a very rare event. Thus, astrocytoma invasion into the leptomeninges is not an unfavorable prognostic sign *per se*. Nonneoplastic gliotic elements separate the lesion from normal, or slightly disorganized, cerebellar tissue, and this probably explains the very good prognosis after surgery in these cases.

Astrocytomas of the diffuse type (fibrillary, protoplasmic and gemistocytic) almost invariably reappear after surgical removal.

GLIOBLASTOMAS

Comprising more than one half of all gliomas (Helseth and Mørk, 1989), glioblastomas are most frequently found in the white matter of the cerebral hemispheres. Although they may seem grossly well circumscribed, microscopy shows the border with normal brain tissue to be indistinct. In histologic sections, the tumors often have areas of necrosis surrounded by a rim of tumor with a high density of cells (pseudopalisading). Outside this, a peripheral zone of infiltrating tumor cells is seen, often with distinct microvascular proliferation. Invasion of the Virchow-Robin space (Fig. 4.7) may lead to subsequent infiltration to the leptomeninges, although they may also be directly invaded. When meningeal infiltration occurs, a characteristic fasciculated pattern of connective tissue proliferation can be seen, both in the meninges and in the perivascular and Virchow-Robin spaces. Seeding through the cerebrospinal pathways is not uncommon. This occurs after glioblastoma cells have invaded the ventricular walls of the brain or after tumor has infiltrated the subarachnoid space. Rapid

Table 4.1 Invasive behavior of some primary central nervous system tumors

	Structures involved					
Type of CNS tumor	Gray matter	White matter	Perineuronal area	Subpial area	Subarachnoid space	CSF
Astrocytoma	++	+++	+	+	+	–
Oligodendroglioma	++	+++	++	++	++	–
Ependymoma	+	+++	–	–	+	+
Glioblastoma	++	+++	+	++	++	+
Medulloblastoma	+++	+++	–	+++	+++	++

–, usually not present; +, may be present; ++, often present; +++, usually present.

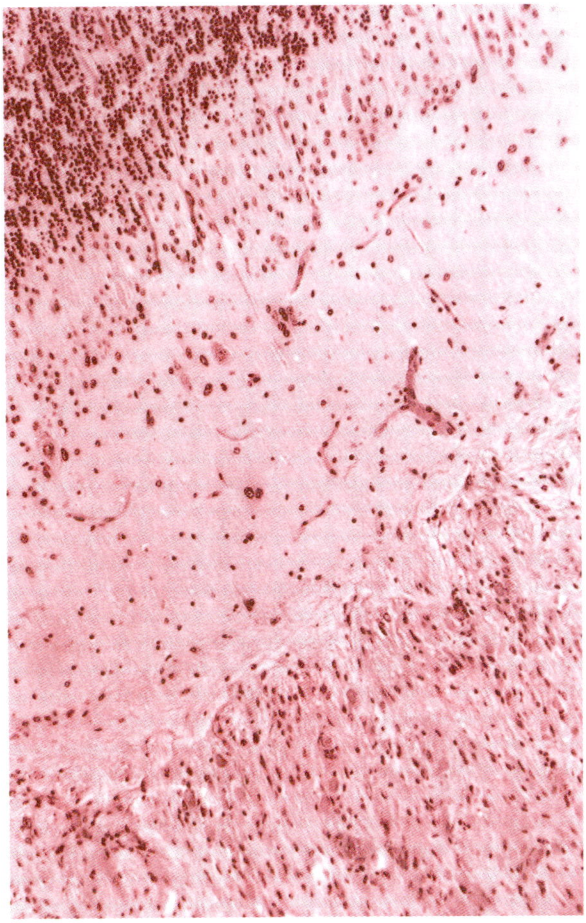

Fig. 4.6 Piloid astrocytes and Rosenthal fibers in a pilocytic astrocytoma (bottom). Reactive gliosis is present in the molecular and Purkinje cell layer. The granular cell layer is seen in the upper left corner. H&E, × 140

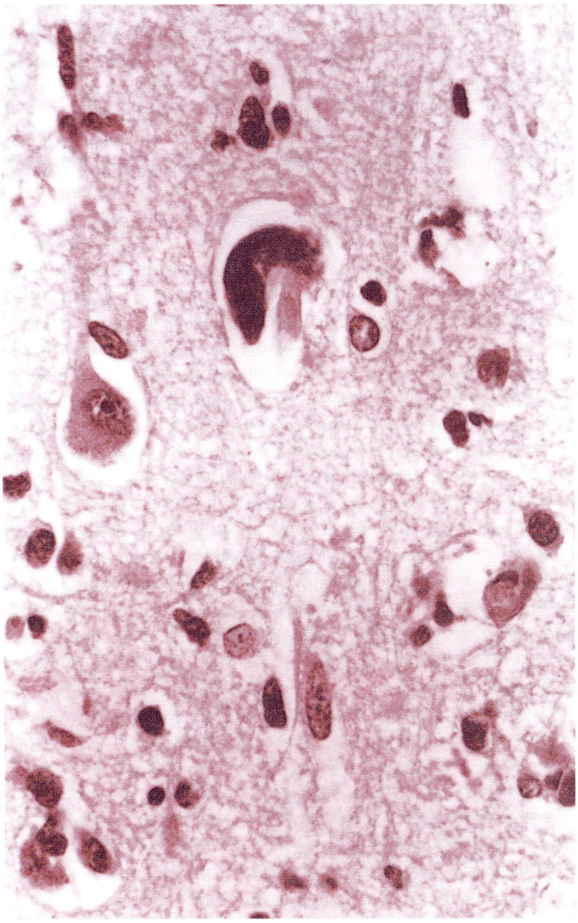

Fig. 4.7 Bizarre tumor cell nucleus in the Virchow-Robin space at the periphery of an anaplastic glioma. H&E, × 560

subarachnoid dissemination in some glioblastomas of the spinal cord may give symptoms resembling meningitis. Extracranial spread usually appears after craniotomy or after shunting procedures.

The progression of gliomas with well-differentiated astrocytic elements to lower differentiated (anaplastic) forms has been elucidated by whole-brain mapping of glioblastomas *post mortem* (Burger and Kleihues, 1989). In some cases, multifocal glioblastomas appeared to be emerging on a background of well-differentiated neoplastic astrocytes. The hypercellular foci showed increased mitotic rate, a higher percentage of cycling cells and increased capacity to invade throughout the CNS. An intimate mixture of well- and poorly differentiated tumor cells could be found. The investigators also studied the topographic anatomy and correlated this to images from computer tomography in cases of untreated glioblastoma multiforme (Burger *et al.*, 1988). Tumor cells often infiltrated far outside the area of the localized tumor and extended irregularly and asymmetrically as 'fingers' of neoplastic tissue. These formations emphasized the spread of glioma cells along fiber pathways. Often, microscopically detectable neoplasm extended outside the area of tumor and the edema zone, the regions identifiable by computer tomographic examination. These studies confirm the highly invasive character of gliomas and emphasize the care that must be taken in evaluating small biopsies in the diagnosis and grading of astrocytic neoplasms.

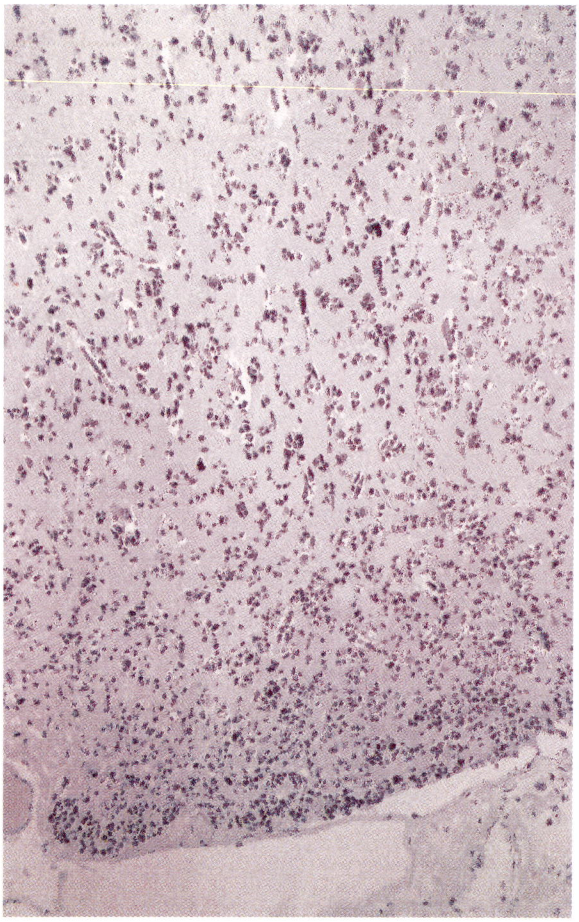

Fig. 4.8 An oligodendroglioma invading the cortex, with degeneration of neurons (partly calcified) and subpial condensation of tumor cells (lower left). H&E, × 140

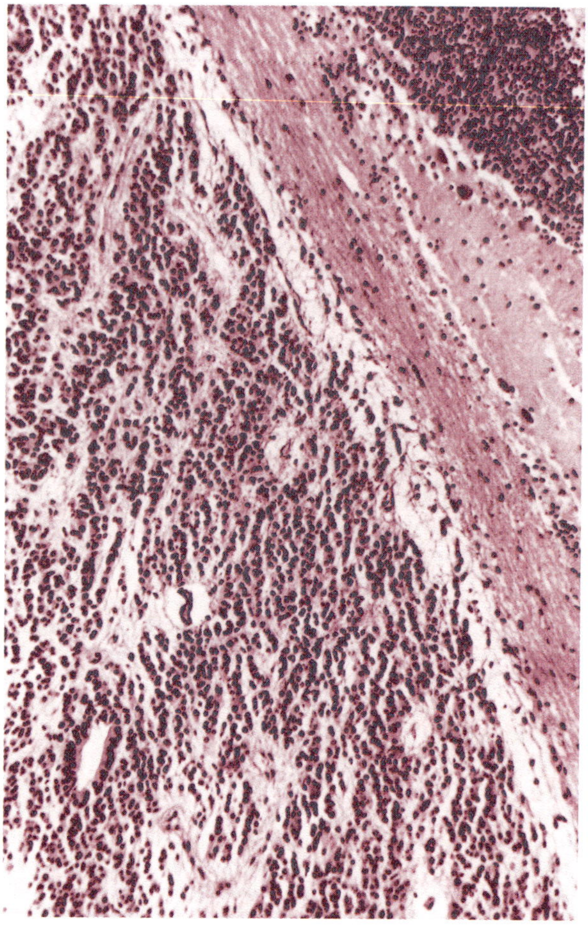

Fig. 4.9 An infratentorial ependymoma with sharp interface to the cerebellum. H&E, × 140

OLIGODENDROGLIOMAS

Oligodendrogliomas are diffusely infiltrating tumors, usually solid and without gross cysts. Some oligodendrogliomas are grossly well defined, and this seems to be an advantage for surgery. Postoperative survival has been reported to be significantly longer in patients whose oligodendrogliomas, at operation, were noted to be well demarcated (Mørk *et al.*, 1985).

The round, uniform cells of oligodendrogliomas characteristically have a more or less empty-looking cytoplasm with a 'central' round to oval nucleus. Often, however, the neoplastic oligodendrocytes are not classical in their appearance. They tend to disguise themselves as glia, and only the pattern of cell distribution gives a signal of the cell of origin. Oligodendrogliomas tend to grow within both the white and gray matter; they may be compact and often contain calcifications. In the cortex, characteristic clusters of neoplastic oligodendrocytes accumulate around neurons, and they tend to crowd subpially (Fig. 4.8). Infiltration of tumor cells and growth through the cortex into the leptomeninges does not seem to signal a more aggressive behavior (Mørk *et al.*, 1986).

EPENDYMOMAS

These tumors tend to grow solid (Fig. 4.9) in relation to the fourth ventricle, with a relatively sharp, narrow tumor–brain interface, although they are focally invasive (Fig. 4.10). Seeding to the CSF is rare. Attachment to the ventricular ependyma is not necessarily present in cerebral ependymomas,

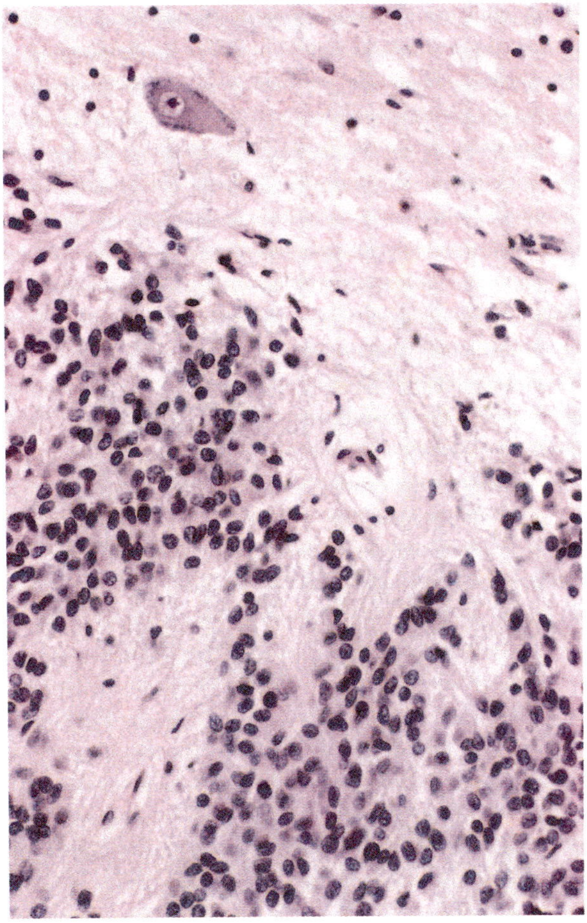

Fig. 4.10 An infratentorial ependymoma with infiltrating single cells near a large neuron. H&E, × 450

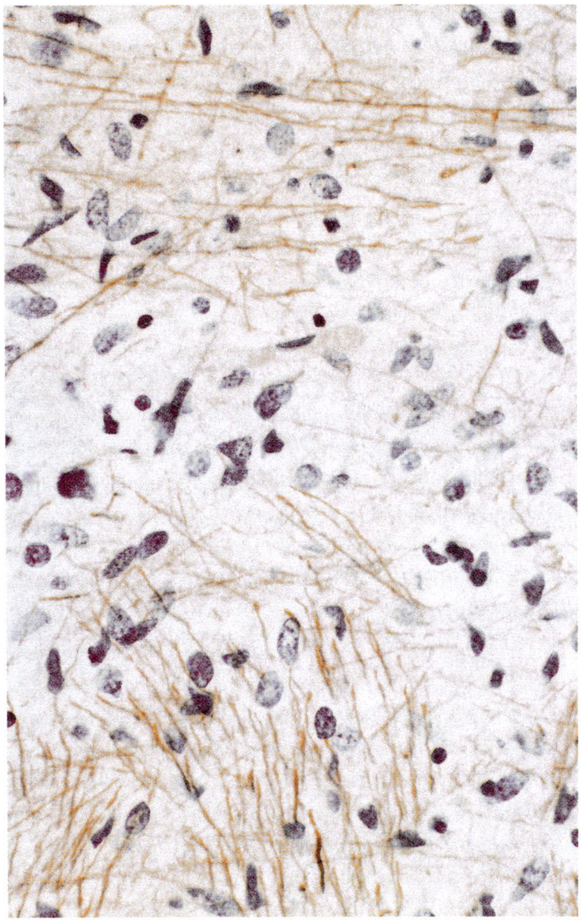

Fig. 4.11 Diffuse infiltrative growth of a neoplastic glia seemingly independently oriented in relation to nerve fibers (axons). The stereotactic biopsy was from a case of gliomatosis cerebri and was immunostained for neurofilament. × 450

and they are not as demarcated as their infratentorial counterparts (Mørk and Løken, 1977).

GLIOMATOSIS CEREBRI

This extremely diffuse infiltration of neoplastic glial cells involves one or both cerebral hemispheres, with preservation of neuronal elements (Fig. 4.4). The prominent, elongated tumor cells may be accompanied by more rounded and stellate cells as well. A spindle-shape morphology may be secondary to the infiltration of fiber tracts. In some diffuse lesions, the shape is independent of the polarity of the fiber tracts (Fig. 4.11). Whether this gliomatosis represents diffuse neoplastic transformation with multicentric origin of transformed glia cells or direct spread from one or more localized neoplastic foci is, at present, not known.

MEDULLOBLASTOMAS

These tumors may originate in the cerebellum and predominantly affect midline structures, the vermis cerebelli and the fourth ventricle. They may more or less fill the latter and often affect the ventricular floor. Invasion of the cerebellar peduncles is often seen. Laterally situated medulloblastomas may be lobulated, firm and circumscribed, presenting on the surface of the cerebellar hemisphere.

At the microscopic level, the border between tumor tissue and normal structures is indefinite due to diffuse tumor cell infiltration. Local infiltration of the molecular and granular layers, white matter centrally, and cerebellar folia are common, as is invasion into the leptomeninges. This may lead to an intense proliferation of fibroblasts (desmoplastic reaction). Metastatic spread within the subarachnoid space is common.

Metastasizing tumors of the nervous system

While cerebral metastases from malignant tumors elsewhere in the body are quite common, usually reported in the magnitude of around 10% of all metastasizing tumors, the opposite is very rare. A collection of case reports of extraneural metastases of brain tumors indicates that the incidence is lower than 0.5%, including cases where surgical intervention and shunting procedures may have facilitated metastasis (Liwnicz and Rubinstein, 1979).

However, invasion of primary neuroepithelial neoplasms into the ventricular spaces and seeding through the CSF are not uncommon (Onda *et al.*, 1990; Grabb, Albright and Pang, 1992; Umezu *et al.*, 1992). In a large study of case material from 1986, Choucair *et al.* estimated the frequency of cerebrospinal metastasis at 5–9% of the patients. In general, metastasis to remote areas of the leptomeninges, to ependyma or to spinal cord, either by seeding or as nodular growth, may be seen. In particular, medulloblastomas tend to show spinal metastases, although glioblastomas and anaplastic astrocytomas may spread along the same pathway (Pezeshkpour, Henry and Armbrustmacher, 1984). The cellular character of these metastases generally resembles the parent growth, although some of the architectural features, e.g., the rosettes of medulloblastomas, may be lost.

Once the malignant cells have obtained access to the CSF, they may be rapidly transported. Although tumor cell migration is an important feature of malignancy, the rapid production of the fluid, amounting to 500 mL per day (Rowland, Fink and Rubin, 1991), and the circulation may make passive transport an important contributing mechanism for cell spread (Pedersen *et al.*, 1993).

In their large case material with review of the literature on brain tumor metastasis, Liwnicz and Rubinstein (1979) found that previous craniotomy procedures and artificial openings through different shunting operations, as well as topographic distribution of the tumor and the glioma types, were important predisposing factors. The most critical step in the progression of malignant gliomas leading to metastasis appears to be the ability to permeate blood vessels. Figure 4.12 shows the distribution of extraneural metastases according to the type of glioma, based on a compilation of known cases up to 1979 (Liwnicz and Rubinstein,

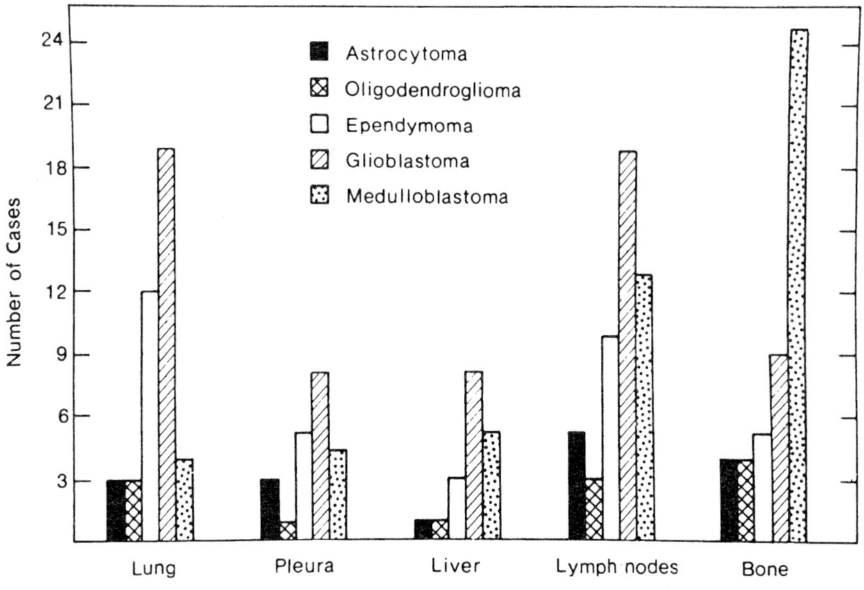

Fig. 4.12 Distribution of extraneural metastases according to type of brain tumor in 116 cases, as reviewed by Liwnicz and Rubinstein (1979). (From Liwnicz and Rubinstein, 1979)

1979). There seem to exist defined structural and biologic barriers to the exit of glioma cells from the nervous system until the malignant progression eventually goes beyond a certain level (Pansera and Pansera, 1992; Pedersen *et al.*, 1994b). To what extent the progression—the number of tumor doublings—must occur before the barrier is breached, as hypothesized by Alvord (1976), is presently unknown.

Different case reports demonstrate a highly heterogeneous, invasive and metastatic behavior of brain tumors. Thus, a primary astrocytoma can present as diffuse primary leptomeningeal gliomatosis (Davila *et al.*, 1993). Histologically benign intracranial astrocytomas may still disseminate within the neuraxis (Pollack *et al.*, 1994). After shunting procedures, malignant glioma cells can be transported over longer distances, as is apparent from the description of several cases of seeding to peritoneum (Declercq *et al.*, 1992; Newton, Rosenblum and Walker, 1992). Multiple bone metastases from malignant gliomas have been described, as has lymph node metastasis (Kleinman, Hochberg and Richardson, 1981; Morild, Mørk and Nyland, 1982; Morild, Bang and Mørk, 1984; Malca, Roche and Pellet, 1993; Pireyre *et al.*, 1993; Sheikh and Kanaan, 1994).

At one extreme, metastases from intracranial tumors may occur after a long latency time. For oligodendrogliomas, metastases have been reported as seeding to the CSF up to 17 years after the primary operation (Natelson, Dyer and Harp, 1992). At the other extreme, extracranial metastases from a primitive neuroectodermal tumor with astrocytic differentiation have been described in a 28-day-old infant (Yu *et al.*, 1990). Malignant extra-CNS tumors may even metastasize to intracranial primaries (Chambers *et al.*, 1980; Mørk and Rubinstein, 1988; Franke, Altmannsberger and Schachenmayr, 1990).

In the 1960s, several attempts were made to perform subcutaneous implantation of malignant gliomas to patients as part of an immunization procedure. Retransplanted glioma cells grew slowly and formed subcutaneous nodules, but these were sharply demarcated and did not metastasize (Bloom *et al.*, 1960; Battista *et al.*, 1961; Grace *et al.*, 1961). This further indicates that connective tissue components may act as a barrier to glioma cell invasion and metastasis at the time when these activities are clinically detectable and are locally progressive in the brain. Therefore, in the metastatic process, primary intracranial neoplasms seem to behave differently than do malignant primaries elsewhere in the body (Mareel, Van Roy and Bracke, 1993; Kerbel, Hart and Frost, 1995).

Models for the study of brain tumor invasion in vivo *and* in vitro

In recent years, several different models for the study of brain tumor invasiveness have been designed, both *in vitro* and *in vivo*. A brief survey of these methods will be given here, together with an evaluation of their potential for elucidating mechanisms related to invasiveness. Basically, the methods imply that invasion and migration are studied in relation to a target tissue, either *in vivo* or in organ culture *in vitro* (Fig. 4.13). Another approach is to use an artificial substrate whereby more controlled conditions can be achieved, but at the expense of the complexity under which cells invade normal tissues during the malignant process.

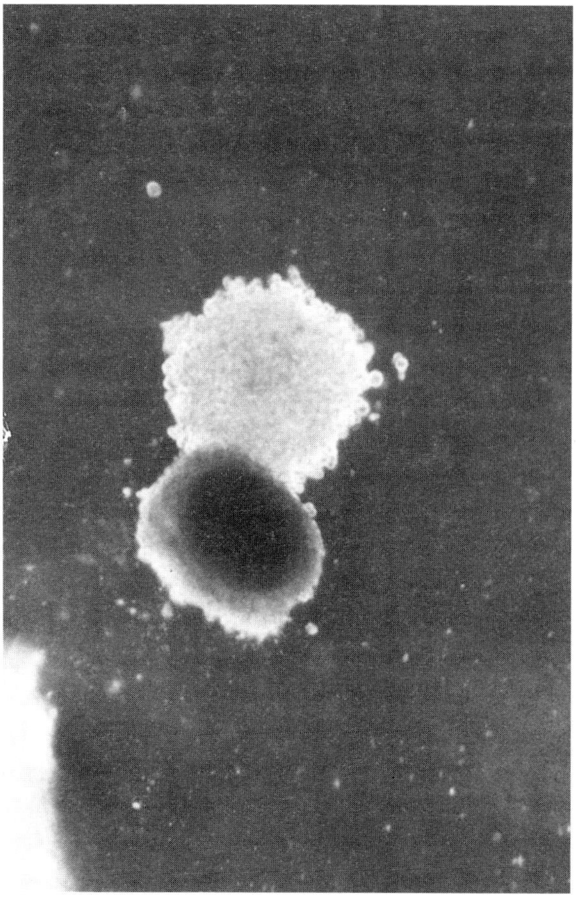

Fig. 4.13 Initial phase of coculture between glioma spheroid (top) and precultured fetal rat brain aggregate (bottom). (Phase contrast; courtesy of Dr R. Bjerkvig)

IN VIVO *MODELS*

Although transplantation of malignant tumors to the brain is not a new approach, several transplantation models have, in recent years, more specifically addressed the question of invasion and further spread of glioma cells in the nervous system. Comparative studies have shown that brain tumor invasion can be observed in a variety of animals, including fishes, reptiles, snails and other animals that could serve as models for studies on invasiveness (Kaiser, 1993).

After microinjection of C6 glioma cells into rat brain, tumor cell processes could be observed attached to the perivascular basement membrane and in close connection to the astroglia. The tumor cells invaded along the pre-existing blood vessels and showed classic brain parenchymal infiltration (Nagano *et al.*, 1993). When the same cell line was prelabeled with a plant lectin, the cells could be identified as growing in the brain after transplantation (Bernstein *et al.*, 1990; Goldberg, Laws and Bernstein, 1991). Within a period of days to weeks, the malignant cells had migrated and spread over large areas of the brain, showing that these cells actively migrated as individual cells in addition to invading as a solid mass. Similar migration was seen when fresh cells from human grade 3 astrocytomas were xenografted into rat cerebral cortex. The astrocytoma cells entered the spaces of Virchow-Robin and migrated along parenchymal blood vessels and between the ependymal and subependymal layers of the third and lateral ventricles. Also, in this case, the corpus callosum was a major migration route for the astrocytoma cells (Bernstein, Goldberg and Laws, 1989). In elegant studies, Marienhagen and coworkers compared the migration of fetal rat brain cells and human glioma cells after xenotransplantation to rat brains (Marienhagen *et al.*, 1994). Beforehand, the cells were vitally stained with a fluorochrome (DiO) with which migrating cells could be traced by their fluorescence. The CSF circulation seems to be of great importance for the rapid transport of malignant cells, although active migration and invasion are equally important contributing factors.

Further refinements were made by Lampson, Lampson and Dunne (1993) and Pedersen *et al.* (1995). These were based on the finding that transfer of the *lacZ* gene to human malignant cells by use of a virus vector could be used for tracing invading cells (Brünner *et al.*, 1992). The *lacZ* gene codes for a bacterial β-galactosidase for which the enzyme activity can be detected by staining with a chromogenic substrate, giving a dark blue reaction product. Since the identification of single invading cells in the nervous system has been extremely difficult by conventional histologic methods, such labeling techniques are powerful tools for the direct observation of single-cell invasion.

It should be noted that other tumor cells, some related to those just discussed, have been studied as models for invasiveness in the brain, including melanoma cells (Hatton, Lechtman and U, 1992; Hatton *et al.*, 1992; McGrady, McCormick and Toner, 1993). *In vivo* transplantation of glioma cells to syngeneic BD IX rats has been standardized as a model for therapy of both growth and invasion (Mella *et al.*, 1990).

In conclusion, new methods employing invasive and migrating malignant cells in the nervous system have considerably increased the potential for direct *in vivo* studies of mechanisms related to invasiveness.

IN VITRO *MODELS*

The migratory capacity of rat and human malignant astrocytoma cells can be directly studied on permissive substrates (Bernstein *et al.*, 1991; Bernstein, Goldberg and Laws, 1993). In these studies, hydrated gel wafers composed of artificial basement membrane or collagen I were used as substrates. Similar studies have been made with different types of ECMs and cell adhesion molecules adsorbed to substrate (Friedlander *et al.*, 1996). By this procedure, the specific substrates permissive for different malignant cells can be identified. Migration, as such, can be studied by outgrowth of tumor spheroids attached to a plastic surface and quantitated over time (see Lund-Johansen, Bjerkvig and Rucklidge, 1991).

Matrix-containing gel has also been used for direct invasion studies, e.g., of hamster brain tumor cells, showing that the invasion was dependent on the number of cells seeded, as well as on the stage of malignant progression (Boghaert, Simpson and Zimmer, 1992).

A limitation with the use of plastic surfaces, coated substrate or reconstituted basal membrane is that such methods make a microenvironment very different from the *in vivo* situation. On the other hand, malignant cells will usually not invade normal cells growing on a surface. One is therefore dependent on three-dimensional culture systems. Since 1981, several such approaches have been described. Using an organ culture of 9-day-old chick heart fragments in gyratory shakers (Mareel, Kint and Meyvisch, 1979), de Ridder and Laerum (1981) showed that malignant neurogenic cells from rat brains invaded the heart tissue in a progressive manner. Later, they were able to show that the histologic pattern and the type of invasion were similar to the growth pattern in the brain (Mørk, de Ridder and Laerum, 1982). Electron microscopy revealed that the glioma cells were penetrating between the heart cells (Mørk, Laerum and de Ridder, 1983). When human tumor lines were tested, their ability for invasiveness corresponded to their tumorigenicity in athymic mice (de Ridder *et al.*, 1987). Since then, it has been shown that the invasive propensity of spheroids from malignant human brain tumors *in vitro* reflects their clinical behavior *in vivo* (de Ridder and Calliauw, 1990, 1992a). The same system can also be used for studying invasiveness of anaplastic meningiomas *in vitro* (de Ridder and Calliauw, 1992b).

These studies led us to search for a natural substrate for brain tumor invasion by using coculture between normal brain and tumor tissue. Two different types of organotypic cultures were found to be suitable as target tissue when the brains from rat fetuses at the 18th day of gestation were used. By either explantation of solid tissue fragments from the hemispheres (Steinsvåg, Laerum and Bjerkvig, 1985) or reaggregation of cultures with reconstituted brain tissue (Bjerkvig, Laerum and Mella, 1986), malignant glioma cells would invade progressively under standardized conditions. For large-scale experiments, the reaggregating cultures were found to be most suitable as target tissue, since a higher yield was achieved and the cultures could be maintained stable over a longer time. These methods made it possible to study directly, outside the body, the sequential interactions between glioma cells and normal brain tissue (Steinsvåg, 1985; Bjerkvig, Laerum and Mella, 1986). Later, it was demonstrated that multicellular tumor spheroids from both human cell lines and primary human gliomas showed gradual invasion, destruction and replacement of the normal brain tissue. Generally, glioma cell lines induce more normal cell destruction in such cocultures than do spheroids from solid tumors (Bjerkvig *et al.*, 1990; Engebraaten, Bjerkvig and Berens, 1991). Other groups have similarly studied long-term cultures of organotypic glioma spheroids (Kaaijk *et al.*, 1995) and short-term cocultures between gliomas and human cortex and dura as supporting matrices (Ibayashi *et al.*, 1990). Compared with invasion into Gelfoam sponges as a growth matrix, human brain tissue as the target seems to modify the behavior of the malignant cells. An important improvement has been the use of confocal laser scanning microscopy (CLSM) (Murray, 1992) for studying cocultures between human gliomas and rat brain tissues after the cultures have been stained differentially by red and green fluorochromes (Fig. 4.14)

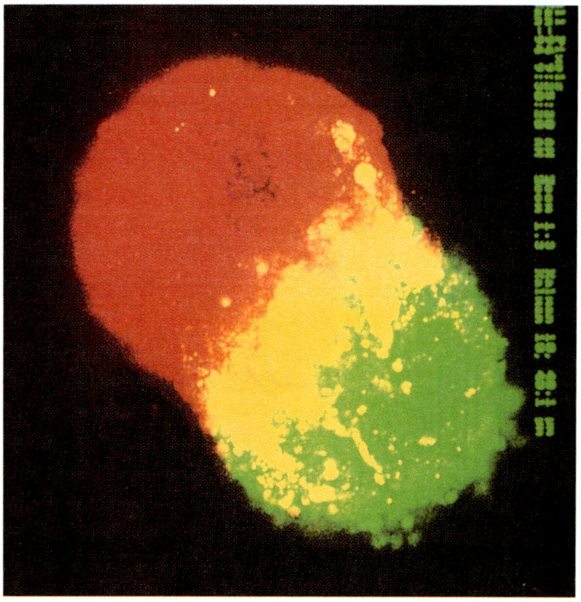

Fig. 4.14 An image of vitally stained coculture between rat brain aggregate (green) and human glioma spheroid (red) after 48 hours. The zone of invasion appears yellow. (Courtesy of Dr S.J.T. Nygaard)

(Nygaard *et al.*, 1995). With this approach the same cultures can be followed from day to day, making sequential studies easier and reducing the necessary number of parallel samples. Confocal microscopy, in general, seems to offer important progress in such studies on tumors of the nervous system.

The clinical potential of such coculture methods is illustrated by the case described by Wester *et al.* (1994), where a patient showed unusually long survival with a glioblastoma (over 7 years). In coculture with brain tissue, this tumor was rapidly growing and also invasive, but a high degree of spontaneous cell loss (apoptosis) could be visualized directly, resulting in reduction of spheroid growth and reduced malignant potential.

Mechanisms of invasion

Biologic properties of malignant brain tumor cells related to invasion will be surveyed here, together with a description of mechanisms underlying invasion. Since this is largely based on experimental studies, their direct relevance for the clinical situation is not always clear. The heterogeneity of brain neoplasms also makes such studies difficult. Much of the data are based on *in vitro* studies where a comparison to the *in vivo* situation may be difficult. With these reservations, some key features will be described.

GENETIC MARKERS

As dealt with in Chapter 2 of this book, several genetic alterations have been identified as possible determinants of biologic malignancy in brain tumor cells. Some of these may also be related to invasion, in addition to loss of growth control (Diedrich, 1992; Ohgaki *et al.*, 1995). Thus, amplification of the epidermal growth factor receptor (*EGFR*) gene may cause the malignant cells to respond more strongly to EGF than do normal cells (Torp *et al.*, 1991; von Deimling *et al.*, 1992; Van Meir *et al.*, 1994). Genetic alterations may lead to a more 'fetal' pattern in the malignant cell properties related to progression and altered differentiation (Leenstra *et al.*, 1992 ; Kashima *et al.*, 1993), and loss of tumor suppressor genes may represent other important biologic determinants (Scheck and Coons, 1993; Rubio *et al.*, 1994). It has been shown that transfection of normal and transformed glial cells, from hamster cerebral cortex, with activated c-H-*ras*-1 gene leads to the acquisition of a diffusely invasive phenotype (Fetherston *et al.*, 1989). Similarly, alterations in SV40 virus DNA integration patterns are associated with acquisition of an invasive phenotype in hamster brain tumors (Duigou *et al.*, 1990). On the other hand, overexpression of oncogene products can also cause tumor progression *without* brain tumor invasion in the rat (Schwartz, Morris and Sarid, 1991).

MIGRATION

The ability to migrate in connection with invasion is an important property of malignant cells, although the migration, as such, may not be abnormal. Recent *in vitro* studies indicate that the underlying substrate is of great importance as a determinant for glioma migration. Rat glioma cells were able to digest collagen type I and migrate into hydrated collagen gels (Goldberg *et al.*, 1992). However, human glioma cells capable of growing into matrix-containing gel showed poor growth on short-term culture of human cortex (Ibayashi *et al.*, 1990). Human astrocytoma cells migrating on substrates coated with ECM proteins frequently showed correlation between high adhesion and rapid migration *in vitro* (Giese et al., 1994). Laminin was frequently the most permissive for adhesion and migration. It has also been shown that human astrocytoma cells may migrate on a variety of substrates with ECM molecules, in contrast to cells from primitive neuroectodermal tumors that only migrate well on laminin, fibronectin or type IV collagen (Friedlander *et al.*, 1996). Human medulloblastoma cells showed poor ability to attach to surfaces coated with ECM components corresponding to those expressed by leptomeningeal tissue (Wikstrand, Friedman and Bigner, 1992). *In vivo*, complex interactions between cell adhesion molecules, glycosaminoglycans, gangliosides and different growth and motility factors, as well as matrix metalloproteinases, may play important and interdependent roles in the migration of neoplastic cells (Bertolotto *et al.*, 1982; Delpech *et al.*, 1993; Pilkington, 1994; Jaworski *et al.*, 1996). Thus, both adhesion and migration seem to be dependent on a complex interaction between the cell surface and ECM.

CYTOSKELETON

It is well established that invasive and migratory capacity is dependent on cytoskeletal components in the malignant cells (Mareel and Calman, 1984). Glial fibrillary acidic protein may be of importance for both astrocytoma morphology and adhesion, as well as for invasive potential, as shown by transfection with cDNA (Rutka and Smith, 1993; Rutka *et al.*, 1994). The content of GFAP in malignant cells may be actively regulated by hormones, cytokines and growth factors, indicating that it should not be considered as a fixed cell property (Laping *et al.*, 1994).

It has already been mentioned that glioma cells may express phenotypic properties of fetal cells. In this connection, it is interesting that an overexpression of the class VI intermediate filament nestin has been observed in malignant gliomas, as it has been in immature neural cells (Dahlstrand, Collins and Lendahl, 1992).

ADHESION MOLECULES AND EXTRACELLULAR MATRIX PROTEINS

Adhesion molecules play important roles for cellular interactions in normal brain tissue. Several of them also seem to be involved in the process of invasion. Thus, CD44 expression has been found on the surface of human gliomas, and this seems to play an active role in cell invasion *in vitro*, probably through interactions with ECM proteins (Merzak, Koocheckpour and Pilkington, 1994). Transfection of glioma cells with the neural cell adhesion molecule (NCAM) in rat gliomas reduced the metastatic capability after transplantation *in vivo* (Edvardsen *et al.*, 1993). In addition, its growth pattern in the brain was altered, causing more solid growth on the brain surface and less single-cell infiltration (Edvardsen *et al.*, 1994). This could indicate that increased NCAM expression reduced the malignant potential. Otherwise, expression of *N*-cadherin and α-catenin in astrocytomas and glioblastomas does not seem to restrict the invasive potential (Shinoura *et al.*, 1995).

In the same family of NCAMs, human and rat glioma cells express short types of L1 on the cell surface. In soluble form, these adhesion molecules stimulate adhesion and migration and may thus be related to invasiveness (Izumoto *et al.*, 1996).

Integrins are heterodimeric adhesion molecules that mediate cell-to-cell and cellular–extracellular interactions in the CNS, particularly during neural development (Jones, 1996). Altered integrin patterns have been described in both astrocytoma and neuroblastoma cells. In addition, invasiveness may be related to abnormally expressed integrins (Gladson and Cheresh, 1991).

It is generally known that tumor invasion may be regulated by ECM interaction (Ruoslahti, 1992). This also applies to cell motility (Schor, 1994). Interestingly, Rutka *et al.* (1987) reported that normal leptomeningeal ECM protein may inhibit growth and induce differentiation in malignant human glioma cells, while Wikstrand, Friedman and Bigner (1992) found that glioma cells did not attach and spread on components of the leptomeningeal ECM *in vitro*. Similar findings have been made by Pedersen *et al.* (1995). In coculture, human glioma cells readily invaded rat brain tissue, while they were not capable of invading spheroids from human leptomeningeal spheroids. In line with this, Reith, Bjerkvig and Rucklidge (1994) recently found that laminin coating of glioma spheroids reduced invasive capability *in vitro*. Hence, the ECM in the brain seems to be a critical factor in the inability of tumor cells to spread outside the brain. In contrast, metastases to the brain from carcinomas readily invade leptomeningeal tissue *in vitro* (Pedersen *et al.*, 1995).

This brings us back to the question of spread by glioma cells into and within the Virchow-Robin and subarachnoid spaces, which was addressed earlier. In the vicinity of blood vessels traversing the leptomeninges, there seems to be a complex continuation between the pial and arachnoid spaces. Tumor cells may be able to move freely once they have gained access there (Pedersen *et al.*, 1994b). This could explain the not uncommon finding of tumor cells present within the leptomeninges in all glioma grades (Rubinstein, 1972). The presence of fenestrations in the leptomeningeal cell lining of arterial walls (Zhang, Inman and Weller, 1990) may also allow tumor cell migration. Therefore, malignant cells within the leptomeninges are, as such, not a proof of aggressive invasion. In contrast, the leptomeninges may, according to experimental evidence, constitute a real barrier to invasion of glioma cells; and this may, at least in part, contribute to the scarcity of extracranial metastases (Pedersen *et al.*, 1994b).

Detailed studies have also been made of the collagen subtypes, including types I–IV, in human gliomas, since collagen may be related to the tumor's capacity for invasion (Paulus, Roggendorf and Schuppan, 1988; Han, Daniel and Pappas, 1995). These subtypes have also been tested as substrates for glioma invasion *in vitro* where, in contrast to merosin and tenascin, collagen, fibronectin and vitronectin were less supportive for migration (Giese *et al.*, 1995). Stromal expression of the transcription factor c-Ets1 facilitated invading neoplastic cells, while noninvasive lesions were consistently negative (Wernert *et al.*, 1994). Thus, the permissiveness of the stroma may also depend on cellular factors different from the collagen type.

ENZYMES

Generally, lysosomal enzymes are important not only for degradation of phagocytosed material, but also for the turnover of ECM components. Thus, proteases are key factors in the dynamic processes related to turnover of ECM. In line with this, the process of penetration into, and destruction of, normal neighboring cells by malignant brain tumors seems to be strongly dependent on secretion of different proteolytic enzymes. This includes urokinase-type plasminogen activator (Lund-Johansen *et al.*, 1991; Reith and Rucklidge, 1992; Mohanam *et al.*, 1994), membrane metalloendoprotease and cathepsin B as important factors (Amberger *et al.*, 1994; Rempel *et al.*, 1994). The plasminogen activator receptor on the cell also seems to be a critical factor, since the invasive phenotype can be modulated by receptor antibodies (Mohanam *et al.*, 1993). The same applies to tissue inhibitors of metalloproteinases as negative regulators of glioblastoma invasion *in vivo* (Mohanam *et al.*, 1995). Theoretically, both enzyme secretion and membrane-bound enzymes may be responsible for the splitting of normal cell junctions in the vicinity of glioma cells (Fig. 4.15) (Mørk, Laerum and de Ridder, 1983).

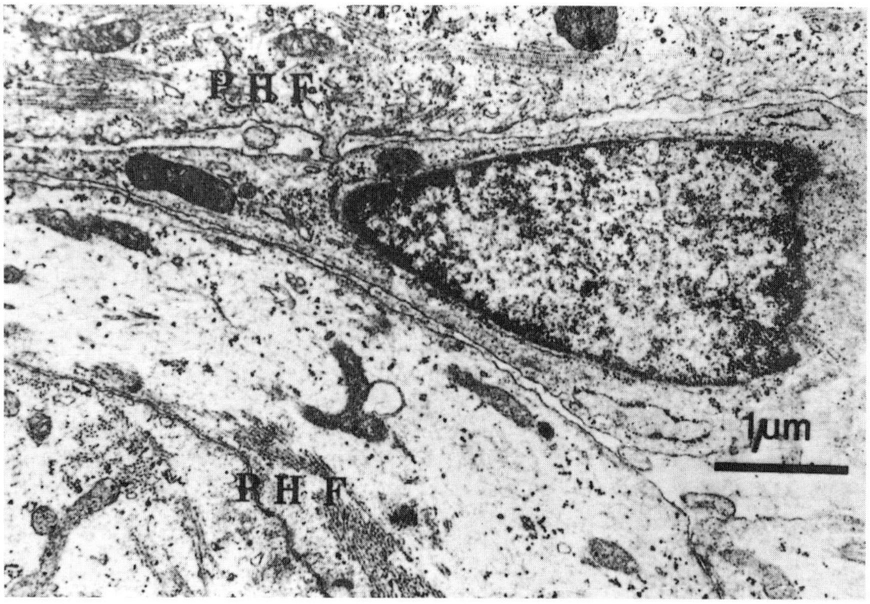

Fig. 4.15 A rat glioma cell invading between two heart muscle cells. The cells were present in a coculture between a glioma spheroid and chick heart fragment. Note that the glioma cell seems to split the normal cell junctions by an interposing cytoplasmic extension. PHF, precultured heart fragment. (From Mørk, Laerum and de Ridder, 1983)

CYTOKINES AND GROWTH FACTORS

It is generally known that, among factors controlling cell motility, both cytokines and ECM components may participate (Schor, 1994; Chicoine, Madsen and Silbergeld, 1995). In line with this, several different growth factors have been found to modify invasive behavior of brain tumor cells *in vitro*. Thus, it has been found that not only EGF, but also fibroblast growth factor (FGF) and platelet-derived growth factor (PDGF) may increase the invasiveness of human glioma cells into rat brain tissue *in vitro* (Lund-Johansen *et al.*, 1992; Engebraaten *et al.*, 1993; Pedersen *et al.*, 1994a). Possibly, this potentiation of invasiveness may be related to an overexpression of growth factor receptors observed in human gliomas (Fleming *et al.*, 1992; Bernstein *et al.*, 1993; Khazaie, Schirrmacher and Lichtner, 1993; Morrison *et al.*, 1994). Therefore, acceleration of invasion should be considered as an important growth factor effect, in addition to stimulation of cell proliferation and migration of malignant cells (Lund-Johansen *et al.*, 1990, 1992; Pollack *et al.*, 1991, 1994).

In line with this, cells transfected with the basic *FGF* gene are invasive *in vitro* and *in situ* in the brain (Gately *et al.*, 1995). Other cytokines, such as tumor necrosis factor-α (TNF-α) and interleukin-6 (IL-6), are weakly expressed in malignant gliomas and most prominent in infiltrating macrophages (Schneider *et al.*, 1992). The TNF-α is inhibitory and stimulatory to invasion (Iwasaki *et al.*, 1993; Merzak *et al.*, 1994). As an example of dual effects of growth factors, it has recently been found that hepatocyte growth factor stimulates both motility and proteolytic enzyme excretion in human gliomas *in vitro* (Moriyama *et al.*, 1996).

Since soluble growth factors secreted from gliomas may also stimulate proliferation of normal astrocytes, it is possible that the gliosis seen at the invasion zone *in situ* is induced by the tumor cells, thus modifying the invasion pattern and tissue reaction (Couldwell *et al.*, 1992).

When *in vitro* studies are performed, the type of culture can influence autocrine production of growth factors. It has been shown that three-dimensional growth in glioma cell lines as multicellular spheroids, as compared with monolayers, increases specific mRNA for different growth factors (Ness *et al.*, 1994). Thus, studies on monolayer cultures of glioma cells may not be representative for growth factor excretion in invasive tumor tissue.

OTHER CELL FUNCTIONS

Since various ligands, such as growth factors, may influence invasiveness, the question arises as to whether a similar action can be achieved by interfering with various components in the signal transduction processes. In line with this, stimulation of metabolic pathways under the control of protein kinase C (PKC) can accelerate glioma growth, migration and invasion *in vitro* (Tysnes and Laerum, 1993). A high PKC level seems to be related to high proliferative activity in gliomas *in vitro* as an indicator of enhanced signal transduction activity (Couldwell, Antel and Yong, 1992). On the other hand, Janik *et al.* (1992) found that the lack of PKC in rat glioma cells facilitated migration *in vitro*. This indicates that inducing PKC down regulation can also create a permissive event for vigorous migration.

It has also been shown that an increase in the intracellular calcium concentration inhibits both growth and invasion by glioma cells *in vitro* (Nygaard, Laerum and Tysnes, 1994). Dibutyryl cyclic adenosine monophosphate (dBcAMP) stimulation, on the other hand, did not appear to interfere with hamster brain tumor invasion *in vitro* (Boghaert *et al.*, 1991).

The interaction between glioma cells and their vascular supply seems to be rather complex with regard to invasiveness. Gliomas induce tumor angiogenesis through up regulation of the vascular endothelial growth factor (Plate *et al.*, 1993). Cultured human astrocytoma cells also induce transformational changes in normal endothelial cells, indicating that autocrine and paracrine mechanisms may affect the circulatory system in the tumors as well (Silbergeld, Ali-Osman and Winn, 1991). On the other hand, glioma cells are usually not capable of invading blood vessels (Bernstein and Woodard, 1995). As discussed above, this may be due to the inability of tumor cells to degrade ECM components in the vessel walls in the same way as in the meninges. This could be another important factor limiting metastatic formations by gliomas.

Anti-invasive brain tumor therapy: potentials and current developments

Since invasiveness, as already mentioned, is, in principle, overexpression and abnormal expression of basically normal cell functions, and since limited invasion may be exerted by normal fetal and embryonal cells, the possibility of stopping malignant invasion is not obvious. Thus, modern cancer chemotherapy is able to stop and kill proliferating malignant cells, but often has little or no effect on invasion (Mareel and Calman, 1984). A good example of this is the recent finding that antifolate drugs were not able to stop glioma invasion into brain tissue *in vitro*, although toxic effects on the malignant cells were obvious (Terzis *et al.*, 1993).

As mentioned above, brain tumor invasion *in vitro* can be retarded by addition of various molecules including laminin or inhibitory cytokines such as TNF-α and tumor growth factor–β (TGF-β) (Reith, Bjerkvig and Rucklidge, 1994). However, such modes of therapy may be difficult to employ in the brain.

Blocking of EGFRs on the tumor cell surface by use of monoclonal antibodies can also retard invasion, as shown by Lund-Johansen *et al.* (1992). In this study, however, it was not possible to stop invasion completely. In this connection, it is interesting that a recently described polypeptide, tumor invasion-inhibiting factor 2, was a potent inhibitor of cytokine-induced stimulation of tumor cell motility and, in addition, suppressed invasion and dissemination of a variety of different tumor cells (Isoai *et al.*, 1994). To what extent this factor acts through intervention with different growth factor regulatory loops is, at present, not known.

The inhibition of different proteolytic enzymes can be used to retard invasion both *in vitro* and *in vivo*. An angiotensin-converting enzyme inhibitor (captopril) has recently been found to inhibit glioma cell invasion into matrix-containing gel *in vitro* (Nakagawa *et al.*, 1995). It has also been shown that transfection of malignant cells with an inhibitor of metalloproteinases suppresses local tissue invasion, and down regulation of this metalloproteinase activity has a striking effect on local invasion and hematogenous metastases of fibrosarcomas (DeClerck *et al.*, 1992).

Although now in its infancy, anti-invasive therapy through chemical substances that act on the cytoskeleton, the cell membrane or other components of the malignant cells has been tried in culture (Storme *et al.*, 1987). Interestingly, an alkyl-lysophospholipid known to accumulate on the cell surface induced a dose-dependent inhibition of human glioma invasion into fetal rat brain tissue (Engebraaten, Bjerkvig and Berens, 1991).

In conclusion, intervention with invasive cells via biologic mechanisms is a great challenge. Nevertheless, specific anti-invasive therapy, including gene therapy, at this time needs further exploration.

Conclusions, unresolved issues and future prospects

- Invasiveness appears to be the most critical malignant cell property determining the fatal outcome in patients with malignant gliomas.
- Invasiveness may be due to a combination of different cell properties, including migratory ability combined with attachment and penetration through a substratum, *secretion* of different proteolytic enzymes that dissolve the ECM, and destruction combined with infiltration through the neighboring tissue.
- Malignant neoplasms of the CNS have a high invasive potential and, in most cases, only grow locally and kill by their invasiveness within the brain. Metastasis outside the nervous system is rare, and, when it occurs, is often mediated through surgical intervention and/or shunting procedures.
- That most malignant brain neoplasms do not metastasize seems to be due to their inability to invade through the leptomeninges and vascular vessel walls. Laminin may exert one of the barriers that many gliomas are unable to dissolve and penetrate. With tumor progression, these barriers may be overcome.
- Invading malignant glioma cells have a preference for existing structures in the brain, where fiber tracts are important routes of migration.
- At present, several different models for the specific study of brain tumor invasion are available, both *in vitro* and *in vivo*, including standardized systems for studying human brain tumor cells. In recent years, such models have contributed considerably to the understanding of underlying biologic factors and processes of importance for the invasive course. These include various growth factors, adhesion molecules, components of the ECM and different types of enzymes secreted by the tumor cells.
- At present, specific anti-invasive therapy seems to be a promising experimental approach, although clinically applicable therapy modalities are not yet available.

References

Alvord, E.C. Jr (1976) Why do gliomas not metastasize? *Archives of Neurology* **33**, 73–5.

Amberger, V.R., Paganetti, P.A., Seulberger, H., Eldering, J.A. and Schwab, M.E. (1994) Characterization of a membrane-bound metalloendoprotease of rat C6 glioblastoma cells. *Cancer Research* **54**, 4017–25.

Banati, R.B., Gehrmann, J., Schubert, P. and Kreutzberg, G.W. (1993) Cytotoxicity of microglia. *Glia* **7**, 111–18.

Battista, A.F., Bloom, W., Loffman, M. and Feigin, I. (1961) Autotransplantation of anaplastic astrocytoma into the subcutaneous tissue of man. *Neurology* **11**, 977–81.

Bernstein, J.J. and Goldberg, W.J. (1989) Rapid migration of grafted cortical astrocytes from suspension grafts placed in host thoracic spinal cord. *Brain Research* **491**, 205–11.

Bernstein, J.J. and Woodard, C.A. (1995) Glioblastoma cells do not intravasate into blood vessels. *Neurosurgery* **36**, 124–32.

Bernstein, J.J., Goldberg, W.J. and Laws, E.R. Jr (1989) Human malignant astrocytoma xenografts migrate in rat brain: a model for central nervous system cancer research. *Journal of Neuroscience Research* **22**, 134–43.

——(1993) Migration of fresh human malignant astrocytoma cells into hydrated gel wafers *in vitro*. *Journal of Neuro-Oncology* **18**, 151–61.

Bernstein, J.J., Goldberg, W.J., Laws, E.R. Jr, Conger, D., Morreale, V. and Wood, L.R. (1990) C6 glioma cell invasion and migration of rat brain after neural homografting: ultrastructure. *Neurosurgery* **26**, 622–8.

Bernstein, J.J., Laws, E.R. Jr, Levine, K.V., Wood, L.R., Tadvalkar, G. and Goldberg, W.J. (1991) C6 glioma-astrocytoma cell and fetal astrocyte migration into artificial basement membrane: a permissive substrate for neural tumors but not fetal astrocytes. *Neurosurgery* **28**, 652–8.

Bernstein, J.J., Anagnostopoulos, A.V., Hattwick, E.A. and Laws, E.R. Jr (1993) Human-specific *c-neu* proto-oncogene protein overexpression in human malignant astrocytomas before and after xenografting. *Journal of Neurosurgery* **78**, 240–51.

Bertolotto, A., Giordana, M.T., Magrassi, M.L., Mauro, A. and Schiffer, D. (1982) Glycosaminoglycans (GAGs) in human cerebral tumors. Part 1. Biochemical findings. *Acta Neuropathologica* **58**, 115–19.

Bjerkvig, R. (ed.) (1991) *Spheroid culture in cancer research*. Boca Raton, Fla.: CRC Press.

Bjerkvig, R., Laerum, O.D. and Mella, O. (1986) Glioma cell interactions with fetal rat brain aggregates *in vitro* and with brain tissue *in vivo*. *Cancer Research* **46**, 4071–9.

Bjerkvig, R., Tønnesen, A., Laerum, O.D. and Backlund, E.O. (1990) Multicellular tumor spheroids from human gliomas maintained in organ culture. *Journal of Neurosurgery* **72**, 463–75.

Bloom, W.H., Carstairs, K.C., Crompton, M.R. and McKissock, W. (1960) Autologous glioma transplantation. *Lancet* **2**, 77–8.

Boghaert, E.R., Simpson, J.F. and Zimmer, S.G. (1992) Invasion *in vitro* of malignant hamster brain tumor cells is influenced by the number of cells and the mode of malignant progression. *Invasion and Metastasis* **12**, 12–23.

Boghaert, E.R., Simpson, J., Jacob, R.J., Lacey, T., Walsh, J.W. and Zimmer, S.G. (1991) The effect of dibutyryl camp (dBcAMP) on morphological differentiation, growth and invasion *in vitro* of a hamster brain-tumor cell line: a comparative study of dBcAMP effects in 2- and 3-dimensional cultures. *International Journal of Cancer* **47**, 610–18.

Brünner, N., Thompson, E.W., Spang-Thomsen, M., Rygaard, J., Danø, K. and Zwiebel, J.A. (1992) *lacZ* Transduced human breast cancer xenografts as an *in vivo* model for the study of invasion and metastasis. *European Journal of Cancer* **28A**, 1989–95.

Burger, P.C. and Kleihues, P. (1989) Cytologic composition of the untreated glioblastoma with implications for the evaluation of needle biopsies. *Cancer* **63**, 2014–23.

Burger, P.C., Heinz, E.R., Shibata, T. and Kleihues, P. (1988) Topographic anatomy and CT correlations in the untreated glioblastoma multiforme. *Journal of Neurosurgery* **68**, 698–704.

Chambers, P.W., Davis, R.L., Blanding, J.D. and Buck, F.S. (1980) Metastases to primary ultracranial meningiomas and neurilemomas. *Archives of Pathology and Laboratory Medicine* **104**, 350–4.

Chicoine, M.R., Madsen, C.L. and Silbergeld, D.L. (1995) Modification of human glioma locomotion *in vitro* by cytokines EGF, bFGF, PDGFbb, NGF, and TNF-α. *Neurosurgery* **36**, 1165–71.

Choucair, A.K., Levin, V.A., Gutin, P.H., Davis, R.L., Silver, P., Edwards, M.S.B. and Wilson, C.B. (1986) Development of multiple lesions during radiation therapy and chemotherapy in patients with gliomas. *Journal of Neurosurgery* **65**, 654–8.

Couldwell, W.T., Antel, J.P. and Yong, V.W. (1992) Protein kinase C activity correlates with the growth rate of malignant gliomas: Part II. Effects of glioma mitogens and modulators of protein kinase C. *Neurosurgery* **31**, 717–24.

Couldwell, W.T., Fraser, G., De Vellis, G., Antel, J.P., Villemure, J.-G. and Yong, V.W. (1992) Malignant glioma-derived soluble factors regulate proliferation of normal adult human astrocytes. *Journal of Neuropathology and Experimental Neurology* **51**, 506–13.

Dahlstrand, J., Collins, V.P. and Lendahl, U. (1992) Expression of the class VI intermediate filament nestin in human central nervous system tumors. *Cancer Research* **52**, 5334–41.

Davila, G., Duyckaerts, C., Lazareth, J.P., Poisson, M. and Delattre, J.Y. (1993) Diffuse primary leptomeningeal gliomatosis. *Journal of Neuro-Oncology* **15**, 45–9.

DeClerck, Y.A., Perez, N., Shimada, H., Boone, T.C., Langley, K.E. and Taylor, S.M. (1992) Inhibition of invasion and metastasis in cells transfected with an inhibitor of metalloproteinases. *Cancer Research* **52**, 701–8.

Declercq, H., De Man, R., Vanderperre, H., De Praetere, P. and Wilms, G. (1992) Peritoneal seeding of a cerebral malignant astrocytoma via a ventriculo-peritoneal shunt. *Journal Belge de Radiologie* **75**, 191–3.

Delpech, B., Maingonnat, C., Girard, N., Chauzy, C., Maunoury, R., Olivier, A., Tayot, J. and Creissard, P. (1993) Hyaluronan and hyaluronectin in the extracellular matrix of human brain tumour stroma. *European Journal of Cancer* **29A**, 1012–17.

de Ridder, L. and Calliauw, L. (1990) Invasion of human brain tumors *in vitro*: relationship to clinical evolution. *Journal of Neurosurgery* **72**, 589–93.

——(1992a) Invasiveness of primary and secondary brain tumors *in vitro* correlated with clinical results. *Neurosurgery* **31**, 1043–7.

de Ridder, L.I. and Calliauw, L.J. (1992b) Invasiveness in *in vitro* and clinical evaluation of meningiomas. *Surgical Neurology* **37**, 269–73.

de Ridder, L.I. and Laerum, O.D. (1981) Invasion of rat neurogenic cell lines in embryonic chick heart fragments *in vitro*. *Journal of the National Cancer Institute* **66**, 723–8.

de Ridder, L.I., Laerum, O.D., Mørk, S.J. and Bigner, D.D. (1987) Invasiveness of human glioma cell lines *in vitro*: relation to tumorigenicity in athymic mice. *Acta Neuropathologica* **72**, 207–13.

Diedrich, U. (1992) Der Einfluß von Onkogenen in neuroepithelialen Tumoren. *Fortschritte der Neurologie-Psychiatrie* **60**, 146–53.

Duigou, G.J., Walsh, J.W., Oeltgen, J. and Zimmer, S.G. (1990) Alterations in SV40 DNA integration patterns are associated with acquisition of the invasive phenotype in hamster brain tumors. *Anticancer Research* **10**, 1683–92.

Dunn, J. Jr and Kernohan, J.W. (1957) Gliomatosis cerebri. *Archives of Pathology and Laboratory Medicine* **64**, 82–91.

Edvardsen, K., Brunner, N., Spang-Thomsen, M., Walsh, F.S. and Bock, E. (1993) Migratory, invasive and metastatic capacity of NCAM transfected rat glioma cells. *International Journal of Developmental Neuroscience* **11**, 681–90.

Edvardsen, K., Pedersen, P.-H., Bjerkvig, R., Hermann, G.G., Zeuthen, J., Laerum, O.D., Walsh, F.S. and Bock, E. (1994) Transfection of glioma cells with the neural-cell adhesion molecule NCAM: effect on glioma-cell invasion and growth *in vivo*. *International Journal of Cancer* **58**, 116–22.

Engebraaten, O., Bjerkvig, R. and Berens, M.E. (1991) Effect of alkyl-lysophospholipid on glioblastoma cell invasion into fetal rat brain tissue *in vitro*. *Cancer Research* **51**, 1713–19.

Engebraaten, O., Bjerkvig, R., Pedersen, P.-H. and Laerum, O.D. (1993) Effects of EGF, bFGF, NGF and PDGF(bb) on cell proliferative, migratory and invasive capacities of human brain-tumour biopsies *in vitro*. *International Journal of Cancer* **53**, 209–14.

Fetherston, J.D., Cotton, J.P., Walsh, J.W. and Zimmer, S.G. (1989) Transfection of normal and transformed hamster cerebral cortex glial cells with activated c-H-*ras*-1 results in the acquisition of a diffusely invasive phenotype. *Oncogene Research* **5**, 25–30.

Fleming, T.P., Saxena, A., Clark, W.C., Robertson, J.T., Oldfield, E.H., Aaronson, S.A. and Ali, I.U. (1992) Amplification and/or overexpression of platelet-derived growth factor receptors and epidermal growth factor receptor in human glial tumors. *Cancer Research* **52**, 4550–3.

Franke, F.E., Altmannsberger, M. and Schachenmayr, W. (1990) Metastasis of renal carcinoma colliding with glioblastoma. Carcinoma to glioma: an event only rarely detected. *Acta Neuropathologica* **80**, 448–52.

Friedlander, D.R., Zagzag, D., Shiff, B., Cohen, H., Allen, J.C., Kelly, P.J. and Grumet, M. (1996) Migration of brain tumor cells on extracellular matrix proteins *in vitro* correlates with tumor type and grade and involves α_v and β_1 integrins. *Cancer Research* **56**, 1939–47.

Gately, S., Tsanaclis, A.M., Takano, S., Klagsbrun, M. and Brem, S. (1995) Cells transfected with the basic fibroblast growth factor gene fused to a signal sequence are invasive *in vitro* and *in situ* in the brain. *Neurosurgery* **36**, 780–8.

Giese, A., Rief, M.D., Loo, M.A. and Berens, M.E. (1994) Determinants of human astrocytoma migration. *Cancer Research* **54**, 3897–904.

Giese, A., Loo, M.A., Rief, M.D., Tran, N. and Berens, M.E. (1995) Substrates for astrocytoma invasion. *Neurosurgery* **37**, 294–302.

Gladson, C.L. and Cheresh, D.A. (1991) Glioblastoma expression of vitronectin and the $\alpha v\beta 3$ integrin. Adhesion mechanism for transformed glial cells. *Journal of Clinical Investigation* **88**, 1924–32.

Goldberg, W.J. and Bernstein, J.J. (1988) Fetal cortical astrocytes migrate from cortical homografts throughout the host brain and over the glia limitans. *Journal of Neuroscience Research* **20**, 38–45.

Goldberg, W.J., Laws, E.R. Jr and Bernstein, J.J. (1991) Individual C6 glioma cells migrate in adult rat brain after neural homografting. *International Journal of Developmental Neuroscience* **9**, 427–37.

Goldberg, W.J., Levine, K.V., Tadvalkar, G., Laws, E.R. Jr and Bernstein, J.J. (1992) Mechanisms of C6 glioma cell and fetal astrocyte migration into hydrated collagen I gels. *Brain Research* **581**, 81–90.

Grabb, P.A., Albright, A.L. and Pang, D. (1992) Dissemination of supratentorial malignant gliomas via the cerebrospinal fluid in children. *Neurosurgery* **30**, 64–71.

Grace, J.T. Jr, Perese, D.M., Metzgar, R.S., Sasabe, T. and Holdridge, B.S. (1961) Tumor autograft responses in patients with glioblastoma multiforme. *Journal of Neurosurgery* **18**, 159–67.

Graeber, M.B. (1994) Development of the microglia literature. *Neuropathology and Applied Neurobiology* **20**, 215–16.

Han, J., Daniel, J.C. and Pappas, G.D. (1995) Expression of type VI collagen during glioblastoma cell invasion in brain tissue cultures. *Cancer Letters* **88**, 127–32.

Hatton, J.D., Lechtman, A.N. and U, H.S. (1992) Formation of PC12 tumors after transplantation into rat brains: dependence of time course on host age. *Cancer Research* **52**, 1933–7.

Hatton, J.D., Jackson, B.C., Kelley, P.Y. and U, H.S. (1992) Migratory behavior of PC12 cells transplanted into neonatal rat brain. *Cancer Research* **52**, 1938–42.

Helseth, A. and Mørk, S.J. (1989) Neoplasms of the central nervous system in Norway. III. Epidemiological characteristics of intracranial gliomas according to histology. *APMIS (Copenhagen)* **97**, 547–55.

Hopkins, S.J. and Rothwell, N.J. (1995) Cytokines and the nervous system. I: Expression and recognition. *Trends in Neurosciences* **18**, 83–8.

Ibayashi, N., Herman, M.M., Boyd, J.C. and Rubinstein, L.J. (1990) Relationship of invasiveness to proliferating activity and to cytoskeletal protein production in human neuroepithelial tumors maintained in an organ culture system: use of human cortex and dura as supporting matrices. *Neurosurgery* **26**, 629–37.

Isoai, A., Goto-Tsukamoto, H., Yamori, T., Oh-hara, T., Tsuruo, T., Silletti, S., Raz, A., Watanabe, H., Akedo, H. and Kumagai, H. (1994) Inhibitory effects of tumor invasion-inhibiting factor 2 and its conjugate on disseminating tumor cells. *Cancer Research* **54**, 1264–70.

Iwasaki, K., Rogers, L.R., Barnett, G.H., Estes, M.L. and Barna, B.P. (1993) Effect of recombinant tumor necrosis factor-alpha on three-dimensional growth, morphology, and invasiveness of human glioblastoma cells *in vitro*. *Journal of Neurosurgery* **78**, 952–8.

Izumoto, S., Ohnishi, T., Arita, N., Hiraga, S., Taki, T. and Hayakawa, T. (1996) Gene expression of neural cell adhesion molecule L1 in malignant gliomas and biological significance of L1 in glioma invasion. *Cancer Research* **56**, 1440–4.

Janik, P., Szaniawska, B., Miloszewska, J., Pietruszewska, E. and Kowalczyk, D. (1992) The role of protein kinase c in migration of rat glioma cells from spheroid cultures. *Cancer Letters* **63**, 167–70.

Jaworski, D.M., Kelly, G.M., Piepmeier, J.M. and Hockfield, S. (1996) BEHAB (brain enriched hyaluronan binding) is expressed in surgical samples of glioma and in intracranial grafts of invasive glioma cell lines. *Cancer Research* **56**, 2293–8.

Jessen, K.R. and Richardson, W.R. (eds) (1996) *Glial cell development*. Oxford: Bios Scientific.

Jones, L.S. (1996) Integrins: possible functions in the adult CNS. *Trends in Neurosciences* **19**, 68–72.

Kaaijk, P., Troost, D., Das, P.K., Leenstra, S. and Bosch, D.A. (1995) Long-term culture of organotypic multicellular glioma spheroids: a good culture model for studying gliomas. *Neuropathology and Applied Neurobiology* **21**, 386–91.

Kaiser, H.E. (1993) Comparative aspects of neoplastic invasion of the brain. *Journal of Neuro-Oncology* **18**, 163–70.

Kashima, T., Tiu, S.N., Merrill, J.E., Vinters, H.V., Dawson, G. and Campagnoni, A.T. (1993) Expression of oligodendrocyte-associated genes in cell lines derived from human gliomas and neuroblastomas. *Cancer Research* **53**, 170–5.

Kerbel, R.S., Hart, I. and Frost, P. (eds) (1995) Special Issue: Tumor host interactions in the metastatic process. *Cancer and Metastasis Reviews* **14**(4).

Khazaie, K., Schirrmacher, V. and Lichtner, R.B. (1993) EGF receptor in neoplasia and metastasis. *Cancer and Metastasis Reviews* **12**, 255–74.

Kleinman, G.M., Hochberg, F.H. and Richardson, E.P. Jr (1981) Systemic metastases from medulloblastoma: report of two cases and review of the literature. *Cancer* **48**, 2296–309.

Laerum, O.D., Bjerkvig, R., Steinsvåg, S.K. and de Ridder, L. (1984) Invasiveness of primary brain tumors. *Cancer Metastasis Reviews* **3**, 223–36.

Lampson, L.A., Lampson, M.A. and Dunne, A.D. (1993) Exploiting the *lacZ* reporter gene for quantitative analysis of disseminated tumor growth within the brain: use of the *lacZ* gene product as a tumor antigen, for evaluation of antigenic modulation, and to facilitate image analysis of tumor growth in situ. *Cancer Research* **53**, 176–82.

Lantos, P.L. and Pilkington, G.J. (1979) The development of experimental brain tumours. A sequential light and electron microscopy study of the subependymal plate. 1. Early lesions (abnormal cell clusters). *Acta Neuropathology* **45**, 167–75.

Laping, N.J., Teter, B., Nichols, N.R., Rozovsky, I. and Finch, C.E. (1994) Glial fibrillary acidic protein: regulation by hormones, cytokines, and growth factors. *Brain Pathology* **1**, 259–75.

Leenstra, S., Troost, D., Westerveld, A., Bosch, D.A. and Hulsebos, T.J.M. (1992) Molecular characterization of areas with low grade tumor or satellitosis in human malignant astrocytomas. *Cancer Research* **52**, 1568–72.

Liwnicz, B.H. and Rubinstein, L.J. (1979) The pathway of extraneural spread in metastasizing gliomas. A report of three cases and critical review of the literature. *Human Pathology* **10**, 453–67.

Lois, C. and Alvarez-Buylla, A. (1994) Long-distance neuronal migration in the adult mammalian brain. *Science* **264**, 1145–8.

Lund-Johansen, M., Bjerkvig, R. and Rucklidge (1991) Tumor spheroids from monolayer cultures. In Bjerkvig, R. (ed.), *Spheroid culture in cancer research*. Boca Raton, Fla.: CRC Press, 3–18.

Lund-Johansen, M., Bjerkvig, R., Humphrey, P.A., Bigner, S.H., Bigner D.D. and Laerum, O.D. (1990) Effect of epidermal growth factor on glioma cell growth, migration, and invasion *in vitro*. *Cancer Research* **50**, 6039–44.

Lund-Johansen, M., Rucklidge, G.J., Milne, G. and Bjerkvig, R. (1991) A metalloproteinase, capable of destroying cultured brain tissue isolated from rat glioma cells. *Anticancer Research* **11**, 1001–6.

Lund-Johansen, M., Forsberg, K., Bjerkvig, R. and Laerum, O.D. (1992) Effects of growth factors on a human glioma cell line during invasion into rat brain aggregates in culture. *Acta Neuropathologica* **84**, 190–7.

Malca, S.A., Roche, P.H. and Pellet, W. (1993) Secondary localizations of cerebral glioblastoma. Pathogenic and anatomoclinical focus apropos of a case of multiple bone metastases disclosed by vertebral involvement. *Neuro-chirurgie* **39**, 315–21.

Marchionni, M.A., Goodearl, A.D.J., Chen, M.S., Bermingham-McDonogh, O., Kirk, C., Hendricks, M., Danehy, F., Misumi, D., Sudhalter, J., Kobayashi, K., Wroblewski, D., Lynch, C., Baldassare, M., Hiles, I., Davis, J.B., Hsuan, J.J., Totty, N.F., Otsu, M., McBurney, R.N., Waterfield, M.D., Stroobant, P. and Gwynne, D. (1993) Glial growth factors are alternatively spliced *erb*B2 ligands expressed in the nervous system. *Nature* **362**, 312–18.

Mareel, M.M. and Calman, K.C. (eds) (1984) *Invasion. Experimental and clinical implications*. Oxford: Oxford University Press.

Mareel, M., Kint, J. and Meyvisch, C. (1979) Methods of study of the invasion of malignant C3H-mouse fibroblasts into embryonic chick heart *in vitro*. *Virchows Archiv B, Cell Pathology including Molecular Pathology* **30**, 95–111.

Mareel, M.M., Van Roy, F.M. and Bracke, M.E. (1993) How and when do tumor cells metastasize? *Critical Reviews in Oncogenesis* **4**, 559–94.

Marienhagen, K., Pedersen, P.-H., Terzis, A.J.A., Laerum, O.D., Arnold, H. and Bjerkvig, R. (1994) Interactions between fetal rat brain cells and mature brain tissue *in vivo* and *in vitro*. *Neuropathology and Applied Neurobiology* **20**, 130–43.

McGrady, B.J., McCormick, D.F. and Toner, P.G. (1993) Ultrastructural aspects of tumour invasion in the central nervous system. *Journal of Pathology* **169**, 89–97.

Mella, O., Bjerkvig, R., Schem, B.C., Dahl, O. and Laerum, O.D. (1990) A cerebral glioma model for experimental therapy and *in vivo* invasion studies in syngeneic BD IX rats. *Journal of Neuro-Oncology* **9**, 93–104.

Merzak, A., Koocheckpour, S. and Pilkington, G.J. (1994) CD44 mediates human glioma cell adhesion and invasion *in vitro*. *Cancer Research* **54**, 3988–92.

Merzak, A., McCrea, S., Koocheckpour, S. and Pilkington, G.J. (1994) Control of human glioma cell growth, migration and invasion *in vitro* by transforming growth factor beta 1. *British Journal of Cancer* **70**, 199–203.

Mohanam, S., Sawaya, R.E., McCutcheon, I., Ali-Osman, F., Boyd, D. and Rao, J.S. (1993) Modulation of *in vitro* invasion of human glioblastoma cells by urokinase-type plasminogen activator receptor antibody. *Cancer Research* **53**, 4143–7.

Mohanam, S., Sawaya, R.E., Yamamoto, M., Bruner, J.M., Nicholson, G.L. and Rao, J.S. (1994) Proteolysis and invasiveness of brain tumors: role of urokinase-type plasminogen activator receptor. *Journal of Neuro-Oncology* **22**, 153–60.

Mohanam, S., Wang, S.W., Rayford, A., Yamamoto, M., Sawaya, R.E., Nakajima, M., Liotta, L.A., Nicolson, G.L., Stetler-Stevenson, W.G. and Rao, J.S. (1995) Expression of tissue inhibitors of metalloproteinases: negative regulators of human glioblastoma invasion *in vivo*. *Clinical and Experimental Metastasis* **13**, 57–62.

Morild, I., Bang, G. and Mørk, S. (1984) Hemangiopericytic meningioma with extracranial spread to multiple sites without intracranial recurrence. *Clinical Neuropathology* **3**, 128–30.

Morild, I., Mørk, S. and Nyland, H. (1982) Metastasizing neuroectodermal tumour. *Journal of Neurology* **227**, 151–5.

Moriyama, T., Kataoka, H., Seguchi, K., Tsubouchi, H. and Koono, M. (1996) Effects of hepatocyte growth factor (HGF) on human glioma cells *in vitro*: HGF acts as a motility factor in glioma cells. *International Journal of Cancer* **66**, 678–85.

Mørk, S.J. and Løken, A.C. (1977) Ependymoma. A follow-up study of 101 cases. *Cancer* **40**, 907–15.

Mørk, S.J. and Rubinstein, L.J. (1988) Metastatic carcinoma to glioma. A report of three cases with a critical review of the literature. *Journal of Neurology, Neurosurgery and Psychiatry* **51**, 256–9.

Mørk, S., de Ridder, L. and Laerum, O.D. (1982) Invasive pattern and phenotypic properties of malignant neurogenic rat cells *in vivo* and *in vitro*. *Anticancer Research* **2**, 1–9.

Mørk, S.J., Laerum, O.D. and de Ridder, L. (1983) Transmission electron microscopy of malignant neurogenic rat cells during invasion into embryonic chick heart fragments *in vitro*. *Anticancer Research* **3**, 373–83.

Mørk, S.J., Lindegaard, K.-F., Halvorsen, T.B., Lehmann, E.H., Solgaard, T., Hatlevoll, R., Harvei, S. and Ganz, J. (1985) Oligodendroglioma: incidence and biological behavior in a defined population. *Journal of Neurosurgery* **63**, 881–9.

Mørk, S.J., Halvorsen, T.B., Lindegaard, K.-F. and Eide, G.E. (1986) Oligodendroglioma. Histologic evaluation and prognosis. *Journal of Neuropathology and Experimental Neurology* **45**, 65–78.

Morrison, R.S., Yamaguchi, F., Bruner, J.M., Tang, M., McKeehan, W. and Berger, M.S. (1994) Fibroblast growth factor receptor gene expression and immunoreactivity are elevated in human glioblastoma multiforme. *Cancer Research* **54**, 2794–9.

Murray, J.M. (1992) Neuropathology in depth: the role of confocal microscopy. *Journal of Neuropathology and Experimental Neurology* **51**, 475–87.

Nagano, N., Sasaki, H., Aoyagi, M. and Hirakawa, K. (1993) Invasion of experimental rat brain tumor: early morphological changes following microinjection of C6 glioma cells. *Acta Neuropathologica* **86**, 117–25.

Nakagawa, T., Kubota, T., Kabuto, M. and Kodera, T. (1995) Captopril inhibits glioma cell invasion *in vitro*: involvement of matrix metalloproteinases. *Anticancer Research* **15**, 1985–9.

Natelson, S.E., Dyer, M.L. and Harp, D.L. (1992) Delayed CSF seeding of benign oligodendroglioma. *Southern Medical Journal* **85**, 1011–12.

Ness, G.O., Pedersen, P.-H., Bjerkvig, R., Laerum, O.D. and Lillehaug, J.R. (1994) Three-dimensional growth of glial cell lines affects growth factor and growth factor receptor mRNA levels. *Experimental Cell Research* **214**, 433–6.

Newton, H.B., Rosenblum, M.K. and Walker, R.W. (1992) Extraneural metastases of infratentorial glioblastoma multiforme to the peritoneal cavity. *Cancer* **69**, 2149–53.

Nygaard, S.J.T., Laerum, O.D. and Tysnes, O.-B. (1994) Heterogeneous effects of bradykinin and A23187 on glioma growth, migration and invasion. *International Journal of Oncology* **5**, 69–75.

Nygaard, S.J.T., Pedersen, P.-H., Mikkelsen, T., Terzis, A.J.A., Tysnes, O.-B. and Bjerkvig, R. (1995) Glioma cell invasion visualized by scanning confocal laser microscopy in an *in vitro* co-culture system. *Invasion and Metastasis* **15**, 179–88.

Ohgaki, H., Schäuble, B., zur Hausen, A., von Ammon, K. and Kleihues, P. (1995) Genetic alterations associated with the evolution and progression of astrocytic brain tumours. *Virchows Archiv* **427**, 113–18.

Onda, K., Tanaka, R., Takahashi, H., Takeda, N. and Ikuta, F. (1990) Symptomatic cerebrospinal fluid dissemination of cerebral glioblastoma. Computed tomographic findings in 11 cases. *Neuroradiology* **32**, 146–50.

Pansera, F. and Pansera, E. (1992) An explanation for the rarity of extraaxial metastases in brain tumors. *Medical Hypotheses* **39**, 88–9.

Paulus, W., Roggendorf, W. and Schuppan, D. (1988) Immunohistochemical investigation of collagen subtypes in human glioblastomas. *Virchows Archiv A. Pathological Anatomy and Histopathology* **413**, 325–32.

Pedersen, P.-H., Marienhagen, K., Mørk, S. and Bjerkvig, R. (1993) Migratory pattern of fetal rat brain cells and human glioma cells in the adult rat brain. *Cancer Research* **53**, 5158–65.

Pedersen, P.-H., Ness, G.O., Engebraaten, O., Bjerkvig, R., Lillehaug, J.R. and Laerum, O.D. (1994a) Heterogeneous response to the growth factors [EGF, PDGF (bb), TGF-α, bFGF, IL-2] on glioma spheroid growth, migration and invasion. *International Journal of Cancer* **56**, 255–61.

Pedersen, P.-H., Rucklidge, G.J., Mørk, S.J., Terzis, A.J., Engebraaten, O., Lund-Johansen, M., Backlund, E.O., Laerum, O.D. and Bjerkvig, R. (1994b) Leptomeningeal tissue: a barrier against brain tumor cell invasion. *Journal of the National Cancer Institute* **86**, 1593–9.

Pedersen, P.-H., Edvardsen, K., Garcia-Cabrera, I., Mahesparan, R., Thorsen, J., Mathisen, B., Rosenblum, M.L. and Bjerkvig, R. (1995) Migratory patterns of *lac-z* transfected human glioma cells in the rat brain. *International Journal of Cancer* **62**, 767–71.

Pezeshkpour, G.H., Henry, J.M. and Armbrustmacher, V.W. (1984) Spinal metastases. A rare mode of presentation of brain tumors. *Cancer* **54**, 353–6.

Pilkington, G.J. (1994) Tumour cell migration in the central nervous system. *Brain Pathology* **4**, 157–66.

Pireyre, C., Gaudin, P., Falt-Rolachon, I., Pasquier, B., Juvin, R. and Phelip, X. (1993) Osteo-medullary metastases from cerebral glioblastoma. *Revue du Rhumatisme et des Maladies Osteo-Articulaires* **60**, 827–30.

Plate, K.H., Breier, G., Millauer, B., Ullrich, A. and Risau, W. (1993) Up-regulation of vascular endothelial growth factor and its cognate receptors in a rat glioma model of tumor angiogenesis. *Cancer Research* **53**, 5822–7.

Pollack, I.F., Randall, M.S., Kristofik, M.P., Kelly, R.H., Selker, R.G. and Vertosick, F.T. (1991) Response of low-passage human malignant gliomas *in vitro* to stimulation and selective inhibition of growth factor-mediated pathways. *Journal of Neurosurgery* **75**, 284–93.

Pollack, I.F., Hurtt, M., Pang, D. and Albright, A.L. (1994) Dissemination of low grade intracranial astrocytomas in children. *Cancer* **73**, 2869–78.

Pompili, A., Calvosa, F., Caroli, F., Mastrostefano, R., Occhipinti, E., Raus, L. and Sciarretta, F. (1993) The transdural extention of gliomas. *Journal of Neuro-Oncology* **15**, 67–74.

Reith, A. and Rucklidge, G.J. (1992) Invasion of brain tissue by primary glioma: evidence for the involvement of urokinase-type plasminogen activator as an activator of type IV collagenase. *Biochemical and Biophysical Research Communications* **186**, 348–54.

Reith, A., Bjerkvig, R. and Rucklidge, G.J. (1994) Laminin: a potential inhibitor of rat glioma cell invasion *in vitro*. *Anticancer Research* **14**, 1071–6.

Rempel, S.A., Rosenblum, M.L., Mikkelsen, T., Yan, P.-S., Ellis, K.D., Golembieski, W.A., Sameni, M.,

Rozhin, J., Ziegler, G. and Sloane, B.F. (1994) Cathepsin B expression and localization in glioma progression and invasion. *Cancer Research* **54**, 6027–31.

Romanic, A.M. and Madri, J.A. (1994) Extracellular matrix-degrading proteinases in the nervous system. *Brain Pathology* **4**, 145–56.

Rothwell, N.J. and Hopkins, S.J. (1995) Cytokines and the nervous system II: actions and mechanisms of action. *Trends in Neurosciences* **18**, 130–6.

Rowland, L.P., Fink, M.E. and Rubin, L. (1991) Cerebrospinal fluid: blood–brain barrier, brain edema, and hydrocephalus. In Kandel, E.R., Schwartz, J.H. and Jessell, T.M. (eds), *Principles of neural science*. Third edition. New York: Elsevier, 1050–60.

Rubinstein, L.J. (1972) *Tumors of the central nervous system*. Atlas of tumor pathology, second series, fascicle 6. Washington, D.C.: Armed Forces Institute of Pathology.

Rubio, M.-P., Correa, K.M., Ueki, K., Mohrenweiser, H.W., Gusella, J.F., von Deimling, A. and Louis, D.N. (1994) The putative glioma tumor suppressor gene on chromosome 19q maps between *APOC2* and *HRC*. *Cancer Research* **54**, 4760–3.

Ruoslahti, E. (1992) Control of cell motility and tumour invasion by extracellular matrix interactions. *British Journal of Cancer* **66**, 239–42.

Rutka, J.T. and Smith, S.L. (1993) Transfection of human astrocytoma cells with glial fibrillary acidic protein complementary DNA: analysis of expression, proliferation, and tumorigenicity. *Cancer Research* **53**, 3624–31.

Rutka, J.T., Giblin, J.R., Apodaca, G., DeArmond, S.J., Stern, R. and Rosenblum, M.L. (1987) Inhibition of growth and induction of differentiation in a malignant human glioma cell line by normal leptomeningeal extracellular matrix proteins. *Cancer Research* **47**, 3515–22.

Rutka, J.T., Hubbard, S.L., Fukuyama, K., Matsuzawa, K., Dirks, P.B. and Becker, L.E. (1994) Effects of antisense glial fibrillary acidic protein complementary DNA on the growth, invasion, and adhesion of human astrocytoma cells. *Cancer Research* **54**, 3267–72.

Scheck, A.C. and Coons, S.W. (1993) Expression of the tumor suppressor gene DCC in human gliomas. *Cancer Research* **53**, 5605–9.

Scherer, H.-J. (1935) Gliomstudien. I. Problemstellung, Methodik. *Virchows Archiv* **294**, 790–861.

Scherer, H.J. (1938) Structural development in gliomas. *American Journal of Cancer* **34**, 333–51.

Scherer, H. (1940) A critical review; the pathology of cerebral gliomas. *Journal of Neurology, Neurosurgery and Psychiatry* **3**, 147–77.

Schiffer, D. (1993) *Brain tumors. Pathology and its biological correlates*. Berlin, New York: Springer-Verlag.

Schneider, J., Hofman, F.M., Apuzzo, M.L.J. and Hinton, D.R. (1992) Cytokines and immunoregulatory molecules in malignant glial neoplasms. *Journal of Neurosurgery* **77**, 265–73.

Schor, S.L. (1994) Cytokine control of cell motility: modulation and mediation by the extracellular matrix. *Progress in Growth Factor Research* **5**, 223–48.

Schwartz, M.S., Morris, J. and Sarid, J. (1991) Overexpression of oncogene products can cause tumor progression without parenchymal infiltration in the rat brain. *Cancer Research* **51**, 3595–601.

Sheikh, B. and Kanaan, I. (1994) Lymph node metastasis in medulloblastoma. *Pediatric Neurosurgery* **20**, 269–71.

Shinoura, N., Paradies, N.E., Warnick, R.E., Chen, H., Larson, J.J., Tew, J.J., Simon, M., Lynch, R.A., Kanai, Y., Hirohashi, S., Hemperly, J.J., Menon, A.G. and Brackenbury, R. (1995) Expression of N-cadherin and α-catenin in astrocytomas and glioblastomas. *British Journal of Cancer* **72**, 627–33.

Silbergeld, D.L., Ali-Osman, F. and Winn, H.R. (1991) Induction of transformational changes in normal endothelial cells by cultured human astrocytoma cells. *Journal of Neurosurgery* **75**, 604–12.

Steinsvåg, S.K. (1985) Interaction between glioma cells and normal brain tissue in organ culture studied by scanning electron microscopy. *Invasion and Metastasis* **5**, 255–69.

Steinsvåg, S.K., Laerum, O.D. and Bjerkvig, R. (1985) Interaction between rat glioma cells and normal rat brain tissue in organ culture. *Journal of the National Cancer Institute* **74**, 1095–104.

Storme, G.A., Bruyneel, E.A., Schallier, D.C.C., Bolscher, J.G.M., Berdel, W.E. and Mareel, M.M.K. (1987) Effect of lipid derivates on invasion *in vitro* and on surface glycoproteins of three rodent cell types. *Lipids* **22**, 847–50.

Tamura, M., Ohye, C. and Nakazato, Y. (1993) Pathological anatomy of autopsy brain with malignant glioma. *Neurologia Medico-Chirurgica* **33**, 77–80.

Terzis, A.J.A., Fiskerstrand, T., Refsum, H., Ueland, P.M., Arnold, H. and Bjerkvig, R. (1993) Proliferation, migration and invasion of human glioma cells exposed to antifolate drugs. *International Journal of Cancer* **54**, 112–18.

Torp, S.H., Helseth, E., Ryan, L., Stølan, S., Dalen, A. and Unsgaard, G. (1991) Amplification of the epidermal growth factor receptor gene in human gliomas. *Anticancer Research* **11**, 2095–8.

Tysnes, O.-B. and Laerum, O.D. (1993) Differential effects of 12-O-tetradecanoyl-13-phorbol acetate (TPA) on growth, migration and invasion of a human glioma cell line. *Anticancer Research* **13**, 1325–30.

Umezu, H., Seki, Y., Aiba, T. and Matsuya, S. (1992) Intracranial seeding following surgery for spinal cord astrocytoma – case report. *Neurologia Medico-Chirurgica* **32**, 281–4.

Van Meir, E.G., Kikuchi, T., Tada, M., Li, H., Diserens, A.-C., Wojcik, B.E., Huang, H.-J.S., Friedmann, T., de Tribolet, N. and Cavenee, W.K. (1994) Analysis of the p53 gene and its expression in human glioblastoma cells. *Cancer Research* **54**, 649–52.

Vinchon, M., Ruchoux, M.-M., Lejeune, J.-P., Assaker, R. and Christiaens, J.-L. (1995) Carcinomatous meningitis in a case of anaplastic meningioma. *Journal of Neuro-Oncology* **23**, 239–43.

von Deimling, A., Louis, D.N., von Ammon, K., Petersen, I., Hoell, T., Chung, R.Y., Martuza, R.L., Schoenfeld, D.A., Yasargil, M.G., Wiestler, O.D. and Seizinger, B.R. (1992) Association of epidermal growth factor receptor gene amplification with loss of chromosome 10 in human glioblastoma multiforme. *Journal of Neurosurgery* **77**, 295–301.

Wernert, N., Gilles, F., Fafeur, V., Bouali, F., Raes, M.-B., Pyke, C., Dupressoir, T., Seitz, G., Vandenbunder, B. and Stéhelin, D. (1994) Stromal expression of c-Ets1 transcription factor correlates with tumor invasion. *Cancer Research* **54**, 5683–8.

Wester, K., Bjerkvig, R., Cressey, L., Engebraaten, O. and Mørk, S. (1994) Organ culture of a glioblastoma from a patient with an unusually long survival. *Neurosurgery* **35**, 428–33.

Wikstrand, C.J., Friedman, H.S. and Bigner, D.D. (1992) Medulloblastoma cell-substratc interaction *in vitro*. *Invasion and Metastasis* **11**, 310–24.

Yu, I.T., Ho, D.M., Wong, T.T. and Liu, H.C. (1990) Congenital cerebral primitive neuroectodermal tumor with astrocytic differentiation and extracranial metastases. *Child's Nervous System* **6**, 179–82.

Zhang, E.T., Inman, C.B. and Weller, R.O. (1990) Interrelationships of the pia mater and the perivascular (Virchow-Robin) spaces in the human cerebrum. *Journal of Anatomy* **170**, 111–23.

CHAPTER 5

Neurocarcinogens and experimentally induced brain tumors

DNA damage and repair

VERNON E. WALKER, DALE M. WALKER AND JAMES A. SWENBERG

Introduction

The incidence and mortality rates for primary neoplasms of the central nervous system have been rising for several decades, but the only causal relationship established for human brain tumors is ionizing (therapeutic) radiation (Jones, 1986; Burch *et al.*, 1987; Davis *et al.*, 1991; Mueller and Gurney, 1992; Berleur and Cordier, 1995), as discussed in Chapter 6. Co-occurrences with hereditary genetic syndromes are discussed in Chapter 6. The age–incidence curve for primary brain tumors is bimodal, with peaks occurring in childhood and around the seventh decade of life (Rubinstein, 1972; Solleveld *et al.*, 1986; Polednak and Flannery, 1995). Because of the differing distributions of morphology and behavior of brain tumors of children and adults, it has been postulated that different risk factors and causes may be operating in childhood and adulthood (Burch *et al.*, 1987). This bimodal distribution in human brain tumors may be due, in part, to differences in genetics and exposure to agents that damage DNA and to age-related differences in DNA repair. DNA damage and progressive accumulation of mutations are thought to be critical events in both aging (Mazzarello *et al.*, 1992; Subba Rao and Loeb, 1992; Subba Rao, 1993) and tumorigenesis (Loeb, 1989; Fearon and Vogelstein, 1990). To date, however, no DNA-reactive carcinogen, other than the physical agent of ionizing (therapeutic) radiation, has been unequivocally identified as a causative agent in human brain cancer.

The results of research conducted over the last three decades have considerably advanced our understanding of the relationships between carcinogen exposure, DNA damage and the induction of neoplasia (Loeb, 1989; Swenberg *et al.*, 1990). Much of this research has evaluated and extended concepts originally formulated by Miller and Miller (1966, 1974); namely, that the induction of mutations and the initiation of cancer by chemical carcinogens is a consequence of damage produced by electrophilic attack of the compound or its metabolites at critical sites in DNA. Studies relating DNA damage and cancer in brain and other tissues clearly indicate that tumorigenesis is a multistep process that involves two or more genetic events and requires cell proliferation (Foulds, 1958; Kleihues and Rajewsky, 1984; Knudson, 1987; Fearon and Vogelstein, 1990; Watkins and Rouleau, 1992).

A simplified model that attempts to relate DNA damage to the genesis of mutations and cancer is presented in Fig. 5.1. This cascade of events begins with exposure to agents that may be exogenous or endogenous in origin. The actual amount of carcinogen that reacts with DNA, or the *molecular dose* to DNA, is extremely small relative to the total exposure. Some of the host factors that determine the molecular dose of a carcinogen include absorption, distribution, metabolic activation,

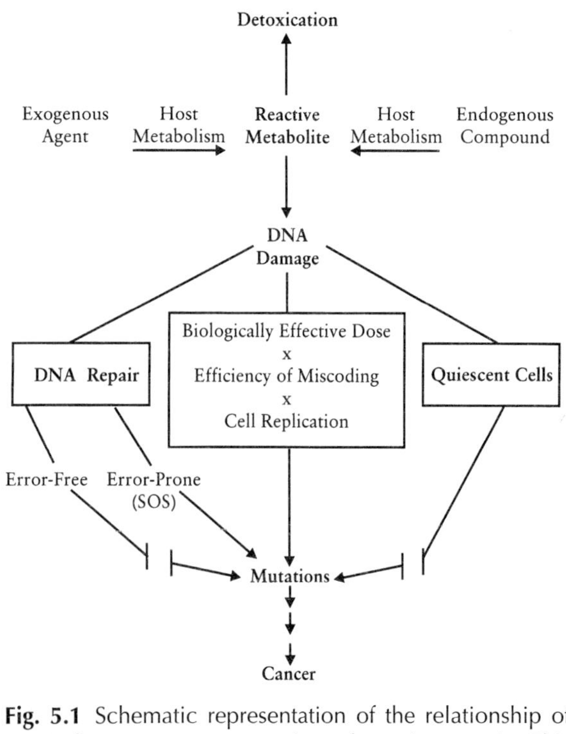

Fig. 5.1 Schematic representation of the relationship of DNA damage to mutagenesis and carcinogenesis. This scheme emphasizes the importance of cell proliferation for the conversion of unrepaired, premutagenic damage to mutation.

detoxification and DNA repair. Many of these processes can be saturated; for example, the enzymatic reactions associated with metabolic activation, detoxification and DNA repair exhibit dose-dependent saturable kinetics (Swenberg *et al.*, 1990). In this model, the amount of DNA damage that ultimately leads to mutation is considered to be the *biologically effective dose*, while cell proliferation is required for conversion of the unrepaired damage to mutation and for the clonal expansion of initiated cells (Swenberg *et al.*, 1987, 1990). Mutations do not result from error-free DNA repair or from unrepaired lesions that are copied without a change in DNA sequence during replication. Furthermore, mutations do not occur in cells that fail to undergo DNA replication (Loeb, 1989). The mutations that do occur, whether induced by exogenous or endogenous agents, may be located in genes of little consequence or in genes that are key to tumorigenesis (Loeb, 1989; Albertini, 1994). Most of the critical genes that are mutated in the development of human cancer have been broadly classified as either proto-oncogenes or tumor suppressor genes (Bishop, 1991; Marshall, 1991), and their activity can be altered by a range of genetic/mutational events, including point mutations, chromosomal rearrangements, insertions or deletions of genes and gene amplification (Akbasak and Sunar-Akbasak, 1992). Clonal expansion of initiated cells and the occurrence of additional genetic events in crucial genes are thought to be required for progression to malignancy (Swenberg *et al.*, 1987; Loeb, 1989). At present, the genetic events associated with initiation and progression of neoplasia in humans can probably be described best for colorectal carcinoma (Fearon and Vogelstein, 1990; Chung and Rustgi, 1995).

Because cell proliferation is necessary for initiation and progression of cancer, DNA damage and repair assume special significance in the long-lived cells of the nervous system. The majority of neurons lose their ability to divide around birth (Rakic, 1985), and even in glial cells only a small fraction of them are dividing in adult and aged animals (Korr, 1980). Thus, it has been hypothesized that the brain accumulates DNA damage with age, and may tolerate higher levels of DNA damage compared with tissues that have rapidly dividing cells (Mazzarello *et al.*, 1992; Subba Rao and Loeb, 1992; Subba Rao, 1993; Evans, Burbach and van Leeuwen, 1995).

It is the purpose of this chapter to review briefly the existing literature concerning DNA damage and repair in the brain, with respect to tumorigenesis. First, a concise overview of the variety of DNA damage induced by chemical and physical agents will be given, with the focus placed primarily upon data obtained from animal studies of experimental neurocarcinogens. Next, the mechanisms through which such DNA damage could be reversed or repaired are briefly reviewed, with references to DNA repair activities in mammalian brain at different ages. Finally, a closer look is taken at the relationships between DNA damage, DNA repair and drug resistance in brain tumors.

DNA damage in brain

Chemical and physical agents can react with DNA to cause a variety of structural and chemical lesions in the genome. The major kinds of DNA damage can be categorized as: (1) DNA adducts or modified bases, (2) abasic [apurinic/apyrimidinic (AP)] sites, (3) single- and double-strand breaks, (4) DNA intra- and interstrand cross-links and (5) cross-links between DNA and other cellular constituents (Friedberg, 1985, 1990, pp. 145–314; Sancar and Sancar, 1988; Sancar and Tang, 1993; Friedberg, Walker and Siede, 1995). These DNA modifications can result from both exogenous and endogenous exposures or events, and if not repaired they can lead to mutations in subsequent replication cycles (Subba Rao and Loeb, 1992).

Ionizing radiation was the first environmental agent shown to be mutagenic and is a recognized risk factor for cancers of many tissues, including the brain (Breimer, 1988; Berleur and Cordier, 1995). The deposition of energy from ionizing radiation results in the formation of excited and ionized molecules, particularly oxygen free radicals, which can randomly damage all cellular components and induce an array of DNA lesions, including modified bases, single- and double-strand breaks, and AP sites (Breimer, 1988; Friedberg, Walker, and Siede, 1995). The mechanisms of DNA damage and/or repair in ionizing radiation-induced mutation have been considered in several comprehensive reviews (Breimer, 1988; Goodhead, 1989; Frankenberg-Schwager, 1990; Price, 1993; Riley, 1994; Friedberg, Walker and Siede, 1995). However, the relative importance of individual lesions is difficult to establish and varies in different systems, due, in part, to the large number of ionizing radiation products induced in DNA (possibly more than 100), and thus the mutagenic and carcinogenic mechanisms of ionizing radiation are not as clearly understood as they are for ultraviolet irradiation and some alkylating agents (Breimer, 1988; Friedberg, Walker, and Siede, 1995).

DNA adducts from alkylating agents are the best studied of all DNA modifications, due mainly to the fact that they are formed following treatment with certain classical carcinogens, including neurocarcinogens such as the nitrosoureas and nitrosamines (Singer and Grunberger, 1983; Swenberg *et al.*, 1990; Marnett and Burcham, 1993; Dipple, 1995). However, covalently modified bases are also formed by oxidizing agents and ionizing radiation (Friedberg, 1990, pp. 145–314; Sancar and Tang, 1993; Friedberg, Walker and Siede, 1995). Singer and Grunberger (1983) have published an excellent review of the molecular mechanisms involved in the reaction of mutagens and carcinogens with DNA.

DNA adducts produced by many chemicals or their metabolites result from the reaction of electrophilic moieties with nucleophilic centers in DNA (Miller and Miller, 1966; Singer and Grunberger, 1983; Swenberg *et al.*, 1990; Friedberg, Walker and Siede, 1995). Simple alkylating agents react with DNA at 15 different sites (Singer and Grunberger, 1983; Swenberg *et al.*, 1990; Friedberg, Walker and Siede, 1995), with the relative reaction rates depending upon the nucleophilicity of the reaction site, the Swain-Scott substrate constants (*s* values) and steric factors (Ehrenberg and Hussain, 1981; Friedberg, Walker and Siede, 1995). Alkylating agents with high substrate constants, such as the rat neurocarcinogen ethylene oxide, generate 'soft' electrophiles that have a greater affinity for centers of high nucleophilicity, such as the N^7 position of guanine and the N^3 position of adenine; this alkylation involves bimolecular (S_N2) mechanisms and primarily produces adducts that give rise to AP sites in DNA (Golberg, 1986; Segerbäck, 1990). In contrast, chemicals with low substrate constants, such as the experimental neurocarcinogen ethylnitrosourea (ENU), generate 'hard' electrophiles that have reduced selectivity and react more efficiently at both oxygens and nitrogens in DNA by unimolecular (S_N1) mechanisms (Golberg, 1986; Lee *et al.*, 1992). Adducts generated at several oxygen sites, including O^6-guanine, O^2- and O^4-thymine, and O^2-cytidine, have the potential to cause base pair mismatch during DNA replication and are considered to be premutagenic DNA lesions (Singer and Essigmann, 1991; Bhanot *et al.*, 1992; Dosanjh *et al.*, 1993). Other classes of chemicals favor distinctly different sites for electrophilic attack. For instance, the N^2 position of guanine and the N^6 position of adenine are frequent sites of DNA adduct formation with one group of experimental neurocarcinogens, the polycyclic aromatic hydrocarbons.

Depending upon their structure, DNA adducts may (1) block or significantly slow DNA replication, leading to arrested cell division or chromosomal aberrations; (2) direct the mispairing of bases during replication, leading to mutations; or (3) undergo hydrolysis, leading to AP sites and increasing the probability of strand scission or misincorporation opposite the missing base (Marnett and Burcham, 1993). For example, DNA adducts of ethylene oxide appear to lead to a combination of these events, resulting in cell death or a mixture of point mutations, deletions, insertions and chromosomal rearrangements in replicating cells *in vitro* (Bastlová, *et al.*, 1993) and *in vivo* (Walker *et al.*, 1993). In contrast, *in vitro* or *in vivo* exposure to ENU produces predominantly premutagenic adducts that, if not repaired, lead to base substitutions in proliferating cells (Bronstein *et al.*, 1991; Skopek *et al.*, 1992; Walker *et al.*, 1996). The ability to relate chemical exposures and formation of specific DNA adducts to the structural basis of DNA repair and mutagenesis has been aided greatly by recent advances in oligonucleotide synthesis and the development of recombinant DNA technology (Basu and Essigmann, 1988; Singer and Essigmann, 1991), plus the development of mammalian *in vivo* mutation assays (Walker *et al.*, 1996).

DNA DAMAGE BY EXPERIMENTAL, ENVIRONMENTAL AND THERAPEUTIC AGENTS

Brain tumors have been induced experimentally by a wide variety of procedures, including irradiation; intracerebral injection of chemicals or oncogenic viruses; transplacental, parenteral or topical exposure to chemical carcinogens; and production of transgenic mice. Models for the induction of brain tumors in experimental animals have been examined in several comprehensive reviews (Zimmerman, 1973; Kleihues, Lantos and Magee, 1976; Bigner and Swenberg, 1977; Swenberg, 1982; Walker and Bigner, 1985a, 1985b, 1985c; Hanahan, 1986; Cuthbertson and Klintworth, 1988; Maekawa and Mitsumori, 1990; Peterson, Sheridan and Brown, 1994; Walker *et al.*, 1994), including Chapter 6 of this book. Chemical agents capable of inducing experimental brain tumors range from large polycyclic aromatic hydrocarbons to small alkylating agents.

The alkylating *N*-nitrosamides are a class of experimental carcinogens that cause nervous system tumors in various animals following systemic administration, and the results of rodent studies using nitrosamides have contributed greatly to our understanding of the relationships between chemical carcinogenesis and DNA adducts (Kleihues and Rajewsky, 1984; Swenberg *et al.*, 1985, 1990). Experiments on initiating events in neuro-oncogenesis demonstrated that the premutagenic DNA adduct, O^6-alkylguanine, persists in rat brain, but is repaired in several other tissues following exposure to ENU (Goth and Rajewsky, 1974; Den Engelse *et al.*, 1987) or methylnitrosourea (MNU) (Kleihues and Margison, 1974). The persistence of O^6-alkylguanine correlated well with the organotropism of nitrosourea carcinogenesis in rats and suggested that the O^6-guanine adduct was responsible for brain tumor induction. However, subsequent investigations showed that brains of mice exposed to ENU (Nakamura, Walker and Swenberg, 1993) and of mice and gerbils exposed to MNU (Bücheler and Kleihues, 1977; Kleihues, Bamborschke and Doerjer, 1980) had concentrations of O^6-alkylguanine similar to those in brains of exposed rats, but mice and gerbils developed few or no brain tumors. Furthermore, the rate of removal of O^6-methylguanine from cerebral DNA was similar in MNU-treated A/J and C3HeB/FeJ mice, although these strains differ significantly in their susceptibility to the neuro-oncogenic effects of MNU and related carcinogens (Kleihues and Rajewsky, 1984). Thus, the molecular basis for strain and species differences in susceptibility to brain tumor induction by alkylating agents remains unknown (Swenberg *et al.*, 1985), but the data indicate that the formation and persistence of O^6-alkylguanine, as well as other *O*-alkyl adducts in the case of ENU (Den Engelse *et al.*, 1987; Nakamura, Walker and Swenberg, 1993), may constitute necessary events that are not solely sufficient for the initiation of organ-specific carcinogenesis (Kleihues and Rajewsky, 1984). Swenberg *et al.* (1985) have proposed that a balance between the formation and repair of all DNA adducts leading to mutation and the extent of cell replication for each population of cells exposed to a chemical carcinogen determines the probability of neoplasia.

In contrast to numerous examinations of the events associated with the initiation of brain tumors, limited research has been conducted to investigate the role of promotion in experimental neuro-oncogenesis. Ethylnitrosourea has been used as the initiating agent in several initiation–promotion studies assessing the promoting potential of phenobarbital for neurogenic tumors induced in rodents. In mice, continuous administration of 0.05% phenobarbital in drinking water had no promoting effect on neurogenic tumors induced by neonatal exposure to 40 mg ENU/kg subcutaneously (Naito, Naito and Ito, 1982). Similar results were obtained in rats exposed first to ENU *in utero* (Walker and Swenberg, 1989) or as neonates (Naito, Aoyama and Ito, 1985), and then given phenobarbital in drinking water. In a more recent study, Tanigawa, Ondera, and Maekawa (1995) reported that barbital (in drinking water) had no neuro-oncogenic activity in rats after they were treated transplacentally with a different nitroso compound, butylnitrosourea. However, Kokunai, Tamaki and Matsumoto (1987) reported that

12-*O*-tetradecanoylphorbol-13-acetate promoted earlier occurrence of neurogenic tumors in SD-JCL rats treated transplacentally with ENU. Purves and Dayan (1992), who observed no brain tumor promotion in Sprague-Dawley rats exposed to ENU first and then hexachlorophane, considered Kokunai, Tamaki and Matsumoto's (1987) results concerning putative experimental brain tumor promotion with 12-*O*-tetradecanoylphorbol-13-acetate to be equivocal because of the short experimental time scale and the small number of animals used. More research is needed to establish the role of promotion in experimental neuro-oncogenesis.

Only a small number of the many other chemicals that have been tested for carcinogenicity in 2-year or lifetime bioassays in rodents have been found to be neuro-oncogenic. This group of compounds, which includes ethylene oxide, acrylonitrile, acrylamide, glycidol, propylene imine and propane sultone, were shown to cause glial tumors in chronically exposed rats (Ward and Rice, 1982; Haseman *et al.*, 1984; Snellings, Weil and Maronpot, 1984; Garman, Snellings and Maronpot, 1985; Bigner *et al.*, 1986; Johnson *et al.*, 1986; National Toxicology Program, 1990). Four of these rat brain carcinogens have an important chemical feature in common: ethylene oxide is an epoxide that reacts directly with DNA; and acrylonitrile, acrylamide and glycidol are metabolized to epoxide intermediates that alkylate DNA and form DNA adducts (Hogy and Guengerich, 1986; Segal, Solomon and Mukai, 1990; Walker *et al.*, 1990, 1992; Yates *et al.*, 1993; Bergmark *et al.*, 1994). The carcinogenicity of acrylonitrile and acrylamide has not been tested in mice, whereas ethylene oxide and glycidol induce tumors in several mouse tissues other than brain (National Toxicology Program, 1988, 1990). Furthermore, none of these four agents has been associated with a statistically significant increase in the incidence of brain tumors in epidemiologic studies of occupationally exposed people (Jones, 1986; Collins *et al.*, 1989; Mastrangelo, Serena and Marzia, 1993; Berleur and Cordier, 1995; Norman *et al.*, 1995).

Ethylene oxide is a major industrial chemical and gaseous sterilant that was recently reclassified by the International Agency for Research on Cancer (1994) from a group 2A carcinogen (probably carcinogenic to humans) to a group 1 carcinogen (carcinogenic to humans). This change was based largely upon the carcinogenicity of this chemical in rodents, the associations between exposure and mortality in ethylene oxide workers with lymphatic cancers, and the increased values for several biologic indicators of exposure in experimental animals and human populations. For several decades, ethylene oxide has served as a model compound for studying the relationships between chemical exposure and formation of adducts (in DNA and hemoglobin) and mutagenesis, and for evaluating the utility of adducts as biomarkers of exposure in the evolving field of molecular epidemiology (Walker *et al.*, 1990, 1993; Mayer *et al.*, 1991; Tates *et al.*, 1991; Schulte *et al.*, 1992; Walker and Skopek, 1993).

Extensive studies have been undertaken to identify and quantify adducts of ethylene oxide, to determine the source and significance of background levels of these adducts and to generate molecular dosimetry data for these adducts (Walker *et al.*, 1990, 1993). Reaction of ethylene oxide with DNA *in vitro* and *in vivo* leads mainly to the formation of N^7-(2-hydroxyethyl)guanine. After DNA is treated *in vitro* with ethylene oxide, greater than 98% of the alkylated DNA sites can be accounted for by N^7-(2-hydroxyethyl)guanine, N^3-(2-hydroxyethyl)adenine and several other DNA adducts that give rise to abasic sites (Segerbäck, 1990; Li, Segal and Solomon, 1992). Two of us (V.E.W. and J.A.S.) have conducted comprehensive molecular dosimetry studies investigating the relationships between exposure and DNA adduct formation and persistence during the course of repeated exposures of mice and rats to ethylene oxide (Walker *et al.*, 1990, 1992, 1993). N^7-(2-hydroxyethyl)guanine was found to accumulate to a similar extent in target (rat: brain and spleen; mouse: lung and spleen) and non-target (both species: kidney and testis) tissues of animals exposed to 100 ppm ethylene oxide by inhalation for up to 4 weeks, but concurrent exposures of rats and mice led to two- to threefold greater concentrations of this adduct in rat DNA of all tissues compared with mouse DNA (Walker *et al.*, 1992). Results of analyses for the premutagenic DNA adduct, O^6-(2-hydroxyethyl)guanine, demonstrated that similar concentrations of this adduct accumulated in brain, kidney, lung and spleen during multiple exposures of rats. However, the steady-state concentrations of O^6-(2-hydroxyethyl)guanine were 250- to 300-fold lower than the steady-state levels of N^7-(2-hydroxyethyl)guanine in the same tissues, indicating that these two adducts do not accumulate to the concentrations predicted by the *in vitro* ratios of the adducts (Segerbäck, 1990; Walker *et al.*, 1992). The lower than predicted levels of O^6-(2-hydroxyethyl)-guanine in brain and other tissues of ethylene oxide-exposed rats is probably due to differences in repair, *in vivo*, and stability of the adducts (see section on 'DNA repair proteins in brain'). Thus, these molecular dosimetry studies did not demonstrate any correlations between DNA adduct concentrations and tissue specificity for ethylene oxide-induced carcinogenesis in rats and mice.

Nevertheless, our research group recognized that an examination of the types of mutations induced by ethylene oxide should indicate which adduct(s) are causal for mutagenesis and, consequently, an *in vivo* model was developed to investigate the mutagenic specificity (location and types of mutations) of ethylene oxide and other DNA-reactive agents in experimental animals (Walker and Skopek, 1993).

Studies investigating the relationship between acrylonitrile exposure and the formation of adducts in hemoglobin have been conducted using rats exposed subchronically with treated drinking water (Osterman-Golkar *et al.*, 1994); however, little is known about the formation of acrylonitrile-induced DNA adducts *in vivo*. The chemistry of acrylonitrile has been compared with that of vinyl chloride, a known human carcinogen, but DNA adducts identical or similar to those formed by vinyl chloride do not appear to accumulate in acrylonitrile-exposed rats (Fedtke, Walker and Swenberg, 1989). On the contrary, recent *in vitro* experiments with cyanoethylene oxide, the putative carcinogenic metabolite of acrylonitrile, suggest that the epoxide intermediate ring may open and react with DNA to produce adducts analogous to those formed by ethylene oxide (Yates *et al.*, 1993). If this hypothesis is correct, the overlapping spectrum of tumors induced by acrylonitrile and ethylene oxide in the rat may be attributable, in part, to similar mutagenic and carcinogenic mechanisms (Melnick and Kohn, 1995).

Two of us (V.E.W. and D.M.W.) are presently conducting investigations to define the spectrum of mutations induced by acrylonitrile and ethylene oxide in the marker gene, hypoxanthine-guanine phosphoribosyltransferase (*HPRT1*), of exposed rats (and mice) (Walker and Skopek, 1993) and to identify the transforming genes and activating mutations occurring in acrylonitrile-induced brain tumors. The resulting data will be compared with the existing molecular genetic information concerning human brain tumors (Bigner *et al.*, 1990; Akbasak and Sunar-Akbasak, 1992; Watkins and Rouleau, 1992). These and additional studies are needed to advance our current understanding of the etiology of human brain tumors and of the potential role that environmental carcinogens may play in that etiology.

While naturally occurring ionizing radiation is a prevalent environmental source of damage to DNA, man-made therapeutic, diagnostic or occupational sources of ionizing radiation are of far greater importance (Friedberg, Walker and Siede, 1995). Nevertheless, only therapeutic irradiation is associated with a neurocarcinogenic effect in humans (Berleur and Cordier, 1995). This association has been shown for radiation therapy of acute lymphoblastic leukemia (moderate doses of 18–24 Gy) (Neglia *et al.*, 1991) and tinea capitis (low doses averaging 1.5 Gy) (Ron *et al.*, 1988) in children and for radiation therapy of pituitary adenoma (total doses limited to 50 Gy) (Tsang *et al.*, 1993) and skin hemangioma (doses of 5–10 Gy) (Fürst *et al.*, 1988) in adults. The health risks from diagnostic radiographs, ionizing radiation exposure in occupational settings and nonoccupational exposure to other types of radiation (e.g., magnetic fields, low-frequency electric fields) is less clear and highly debated (Berleur and Cordier, 1995).

Both ionizing radiation and several cancer chemotherapy drugs used in the treatment of human brain tumors have been found to induce neoplasia in a number of rat tissues, including the brain (Weisburger, 1977; Habs, Eisenbrand and Schmahl, 1979; Zeller *et al.*, 1989). This group of chemotherapeutic agents, which includes several chloroethylnitrosoureas (CENUs), has also been associated with secondary cancers in human patients (Cohen, Wiernik and Walker, 1976). The CENUs react with DNA through 2-hydroxyethylation and 2-chloroethylation to produce a spectrum of adducts analogous to that of ethylating agents, except that CENUs can cross-link bases on the same or opposite strands via subsequent reactions of monoalkylation products (Tong, Kirk and Ludlum, 1981; Gonzaga *et al.*, 1992). While cross-linking is probably the most important cytotoxic lesion associated with CENU therapy, the mutagenic and carcinogenic effects have been attributed to premutagenic adducts such as O^6-(2-hydroxyethyl)guanine and 3, N^4–ethanodeoxycytidine (Tong, Kirk and Ludlum, 1981; Bodell *et al.*, 1985). The roles of DNA interstrand cross-links and DNA repair in CENU chemotherapy of brain tumors will be reviewed later in this chapter.

Few data are available on the detection of DNA damage or specific types of DNA adducts in the brains or brain tumors of people exposed to low levels of agents suspected to be neurocarcinogens in humans or known to be neuro-oncogenic in animals. In one of the few studies in this area, Lee *et al.* (1993) reported the presence of DNA adducts of polycyclic aromatic hydrocarbons in human brain tumors. Low levels of large aromatic DNA adducts were detected in a variety of malignant brain tissues by ^{32}P postlabeling techniques. Matched normal brain tissues from the same individuals were not available for analysis, but aromatic DNA adducts were not detected in nontumorous brain tissues from epilepsy patients undergoing surgical intervention. The authors concluded that the aromatic adducts detected in brain tumors could result from environmental exposures to undetermined genotoxic agent(s) or from the aging process. It is noteworthy, however, that polycyclic aromatic hydrocarbon exposure has not been linked through epidemiologic studies to the occurrence of brain tumors in humans (Zülch, 1986, pp. 85–114).

DNA DAMAGE BY ENDOGENOUS EVENTS

Loeb (1989) has presented an excellent consideration of the possibility that certain normal endogenous cellular processes are inherently mutagenic and that this intrinsic mutagenesis is a significant factor in the etiology and pathogenesis of some human cancers. Also, recent advances in methodology permitting the detection, identification and quantitation of endogenous DNA adducts have contributed to a growing awareness of the potential importance of the DNA damage that amasses in multiple cellular genes during neoplastic transformation and aging. Based upon the accumulating evidence of endogenous DNA damage, Marnett and Burcham (1993) have made a comprehensive survey of several classes of spontaneous or background DNA adducts from a structural, analytical and biological perspective.

Since the brain is compartmentalized and somewhat protected from the outside environment, endogenous cellular processes that give rise to DNA damage may constitute a proportionately greater source of DNA damage than in other tissues. Potential endogenous sources of DNA damage can be classified into three groups (Loeb, 1989; Subba Rao and Loeb, 1992; Evans, Burbach and van Leeuwen, 1995; Friedberg, Walker and Siede, 1995). First, DNA is not entirely stable in aqueous solution and is subjected to spontaneous hydrolytic processes, including depurination, depyrimidination, deamination and cleavage of phosphodiester bonds. Depurination is the most frequent of these DNA damaging events (Lindahl and Nyberg, 1972). Although cells possess multiple pathways for the repair of apurinic sites, Loeb (1989) has suggested that many AP sites could filter through this DNA repair screen and that replication and misplacement of bases opposite these noncoding lesions may be a major source of spontaneous mutations. Second, DNA can be damaged by reactive species derived from normal cellular metabolism, producing DNA adducts. Such species include reactive alkyl groups (e.g., methyl, ethyl and hydroxyethyl groups), lipid peroxides and oxygen free radicals. Quantitatively, oxidized bases constitute the most important class of endogenous base modifications, with the total number of oxidized adducts formed daily rivaling the rate of spontaneous depurination of DNA (Loeb, 1989; Ames and Gold, 1991). Third, although neurons are nonreplicating cells, mutations may be introduced in DNA by infidelity of DNA polymerases during the repair of DNA damage (Fig. 5.1). This repair synthesis is thought to be catalyzed by DNA polymerase β (Fry and Loeb, 1986), the most error prone of mammalian DNA polymerases (Loeb and Kunkel, 1982).

Most studies concerning DNA damage in brain have focused on the relationship between single-strand breaks and age (Subba Rao and Loeb, 1992; Subba Rao, 1993). Several studies have indicated an accumulation of single-strand breaks in brain with age, while others have reported no change with age. Reasons for these discrepancies are not known.

A few reports are available on the occurrence of specific types of background DNA adducts in brain, including data on simple alkyl adducts, free-radical-induced adducts and a series of unidentified putative adducts called I-compounds. An increase in N^7-methylguanine, a major adduct formed *in vivo* by methylating agents, has been associated with age in the brains of untreated mice (Tan, Bencsath and Gaubatz, 1990). A comparison of adduct values in male mice at 11, 23 and 25 months of age suggested that N^7-methylguanine increased approximately twofold between young and old animals. The age-specific adduct levels observed should represent steady-state concentrations, since N^7-methylguanine is lost from DNA by a combination of spontaneous depurination and repair.

N^7-(2-hydroxyethyl)guanine has also been measured, presumably at steady-state concentrations, in brain and other tissues of untreated male rats and mice and is thought to result via the *in vivo* conversion of endogenously formed ethylene to ethylene oxide (Walker *et al.*, 1992; Wu *et al.*, 1996). Numerous studies have shown that ethylene from both endogenous and exogenous sources is metabolized to ethylene oxide *in vivo* in rats, mice and humans (Walker *et al.*, 1990). Other possible exogenous sources of background hydroxyethyl adducts in humans include several industrial and environmental pollutants, such as ethylene oxide, *N*-nitrosomorpholine, and *N*-nitrosodiethanolamine and its metabolites (Koepke *et al.*, 1988; Ludeke and Kleihues, 1988; Törnqvist, 1988). However, ethylene as a precursor of ethylene oxide is considered the main source of background hydroxyethylation. Exogenous sources of ethylene that are not occupational in nature include active and passive smoking and urban air pollution, mainly from motor exhausts (Törnqvist, 1988). In addition, studies in humans, rats and mice have shown that ethylene is produced endogenously by a variety of processes, including lipid peroxidation of unsaturated fats and metabolism by intestinal bacteria

(Törnqvist *et al.*, 1989; Walker *et al.*, 1990). Not surprisingly then, background levels of N^7-(2-hydroxyethyl)guanine have been found in liver (Wu *et al.*, 1996) and lymphocytes (Föst *et al.*, 1989) in humans and should be present in DNA of other human tissues, including brain.

A number of different free-radical-induced DNA adducts have been shown to occur in human tissues, including brain (Olinski *et al.*, 1992; Marnett and Burcham, 1993). In the most relevant study, Olinski *et al.* (1992) investigated endogenous levels of several typical hydroxyl radical-induced DNA adducts in chromatin of various human cancerous tissues and their cancer-free surrounding tissues. Five different types of surgically removed tissues (brain, colon, lung, ovary and stomach) were analyzed for five purine-derived and five pyrimidine-derived modified DNA bases, namely 8-hydroxyguanine, 8-hydroxyadenine, 2-hydroxyadenine, 2,6-diamino-4-hydroxy-5-formamidopyrimidine, 4,6-diamino-5-formamidopyrimidine, 5-hydroxycytosine, 5,6-dihydroxycytosine, 5-(hydroxymethyl) uracil, 5-hydroxyhydantoin and 5-hydroxy-5-methylhydantoin. In isolated chromatin samples, these adducts were identified and quantified by gas chromatography/mass spectrometry with selected-ion monitoring. In all tissue types examined, endogenous amounts of adducts were consistently higher in cancerous tissues than in their respective cancer-free tissues. In the case of brain cancer, the highest increases over control tissue levels of adducts were observed for 2-hydroxyadenine (≈fourfold), 8-hydroxyadenine (≈threefold) and 2,6-diamino-4-hydroxy-5-formamidopyrimidine (≈threefold). Reasons for the higher steady-state levels in cancerous tissues are unknown, but they may be due to the production of large amounts of H_2O_2, which is characteristic of human tumor cells (Szatrowski and Nathan, 1991). Subba Rao and Loeb (1992) have suggested that the exceptionally high rate of respiration in brain may predispose it to greater free-radical-induced DNA damage compared with other tissues; however, in the Olinski *et al.* (1992) study, the amount of each modified base was similar in all cancer-free tissues (of nonsmokers). A few of these oxidative lesions are known to be premutagenic, but the roles that individual types of oxidized bases play in carcinogenesis remain to be determined (Olinski *et al.*, 1992; Marnett and Burcham, 1993).

Development of the high-sensitivity version of ^{32}P postlabeling has enabled Randerath, Reddy and Disher (1986) to detect bulky, covalently modified nucleotides in DNA samples from humans and untreated animals. They have found multiple adduct spots that are detectable in DNA digests from several tissues, including brain (Randerath *et al.*, 1993). Randerath terms these putative adducts *I-compounds* (I-spots) because the evidence suggests that they arise indigenously. In analyses of rat brain DNA, two I-compounds were found to increase with animal age (1, 4 and 10 months). However, there was little variation in the intensity of the I-spots within each age group. Brain DNA from 20 humans ranging in age from neonatal to 100 years exhibited the same age-related increase in the same two I-spots. In humans, though, considerable individual variation of brain I-compound levels was observed, especially at ages greater than 60 years. This variation in human brains was presumed to reflect environmental, lifestyle or genetic factors. Interpretation of the significance of these findings awaits the additional work needed to determine the structural identities and the biological consequences of I-compounds.

DNA repair in brain

The variety of DNA damage caused by endogenous and exogenous factors is mirrored by an array of DNA repair systems that have evolved to remove the damage and to restore genomic integrity. Because of the relevance of DNA repair to cancer (Fig. 5.1), research concerning DNA repair mechanisms has ramifications for both the prevention and treatment of neoplasia (Orren and Sancar, 1987). A detailed discussion of known repair mechanisms is beyond the scope of this chapter; however, a brief overview of the DNA repair systems described thus far in mammals will be given as a prelude to a review of DNA repair activities in brain. For greater details of what is currently known about the interaction of repair enzymes with damaged DNA, the reader is referred to comprehensive reviews of DNA repair in general (Friedberg, 1985, 1990, pp. 145–314; Collins, Johnson and Boyle, 1987; Orren and Sancar, 1987; Sancar and Sancar, 1988; Kaufmann, 1989; Sancar and Tang, 1993; Friedberg, Walker and Siede, 1995) as well as to several papers considering the role of DNA repair in neurodegenerative diseases and the aging brain (Mazzarello *et al.*, 1992; Subba Rao and Loeb, 1992; Subba Rao, 1993; Evans, Burbach and van Leeuwen, 1995).

DNA repair mechanisms can be roughly grouped into the four categories listed in Table 5.1. The first category includes systems that simply reverse DNA damage via a single enzymatic step. Examples of this mode of repair include the monomerization of pyrimidine dimers by enzymatic photoreactivation, the removal of simple alkyl groups from O^6-alkylguanine and the rejoining of single-strand breaks. The second category of DNA repair mechanisms

Table 5.1 DNA repair systems

Mode of repair	Enzyme/proteins implicated
I. Reversal of damage	
Photoreactivation	DNA photolyase
Demethylation	MGMT
Ligation of single-strand breaks	DNA ligase
II. DNA excision repair	
Base excision repair	DNA glycosylases, AP endonucleases, DNA ploymerase and ligase
Nucleotide excision repair, including mismatch repair	Excision nuclease(s) (excinucleases), DNA polymerase and ligase
III. Recombinational repair	RecABC gene products in *Escherichia coli*, S_1 nuclease, single-strand binding protein, and other unknown factors
IV. Inducible SOS response	RecA and LexA gene products in *E. coli*, plus yet-to-be identified factors

Based upon information from Friedberg, 1985, 1990; Orren and Sancar, 1987; Mazzarello *et al.*, 1992; Subba Rao and Loeb, 1992; Friedberg, Walker and Siede, 1995.
MGMT, O^6-methylguanine-DNA methyltransferase; AP, apurinic/apyrimidinic.

includes excision repair, which relies upon redundant information in the DNA duplex or secondary signals within the helix to remove a damaged base (*base excision repair*), a mismatched base (*mismatch excision repair* or simply *mismatch repair*) or a damaged nucleotide (*nucleotide excision repair*) and to restore normal nucleotide sequence using the complementary strand as a template (Modrich, 1994; Sancar, 1994; Friedberg, Walker and Siede, 1995). Base excision repair has a more limited substrate range because some of the various DNA glycosylases that initiate the repair process are very specific for a particular type of base damage (Orren and Sancar, 1987). In contrast, nucleotide excision repair has a broader substrate range and plays a backup role for other repair systems (Sancar and Tang, 1993). The third type of repair system includes recombination repair, which is essentially a postreplication bypass mechanism that corrects replication gaps formed across damaged nucleotides by filling the gaps via recombination with the sister duplex (Kaufmann, 1989). The damaged bases/nucleotides are not eliminated by this process but can be removed later by other repair systems such as excision repair (Orren and Sancar, 1987). The final category includes an inducible repair mechanism called the 'SOS response', wherein more than 20 genes can be expressed consequent to DNA damage, either spontaneous or inducted. RecA and LexA proteins regulate the mechanism (Friedberg, Walker and Siede, 1995), which has been studied mainly in bacteria but which contains phenomena analagous to those in mammalian cells (Herrlich *et al.*, 1984).

From the knowledge currently available, DNA excision repair appears to be an important means by which many types of structural DNA damage are removed from brain and other mammalian tissues. In base excision repair, DNA lesions are removed by the action of specific DNA glycosylases that hydrolyze the glycosylic bond between the deoxyribose and the damaged base, resulting in an apurinic or apyrimidinic sugar (AP site). Subsequent steps of this repair process include incision of the sugar phosphate backbone of DNA by AP endonucleases, excision of the base-free sugar phosphate residue by an excision endonuclease and filling of the gap by DNA repair synthesis and ligation, thus restoring the correct DNA sequence. One example of base excision repair in brain is the removal of N^3-methyladenine, which is initiated by the action of 3-methyladenine (3MeA) DNA glycosylase. If unrepaired, N^3-methyladenine lesions are cytotoxic because they block DNA replication in prokaryotic (Karran, Hjelmgren and Lindahl, 1982) and eukaryotic cells (Engelward *et al.*, 1996).

Both prokaryotic and eukaryotic cells are capable of repairing mismatched base pairs that arise in DNA from replication errors, certain recombination events, deamination of 5-methylcytosine and occurrence of a base analog or a chemically modified base derivative opposite a normal base (Modrich, 1994; Friedberg, Walker and Siede, 1995). Depending upon the nature of the lesion, mispaired bases in DNA can be corrected by several mechanisms, including base excision repair, nucleotide excision repair or mismatch repair. Because many mismatches consist of normal Watson-Crick bases, mismatch repair systems rely upon secondary signals within the DNA helix to identify and correct mispaired bases (Modrich, 1994). The general phenomenon of mismatch repair is described in brief herein (see next section on 'DNA repair proteins in brain'), but for details of the mismatch repair systems, the reader is referred to several reviews (Modrich, 1994; Chung and Rustgi, 1995; Friedberg, Walker and Siede, 1995). It is noteworthy that studies of mismatch repair and cytotoxicity in human mutator cell lines exposed to simple alkylating agents indicate that the mismatch repair system recognizes lesions other than conventional mispairs, and the studies suggest that this pathway is involved in the death of those cells that suffer unacceptable levels of certain types of chemically induced DNA damage (Goldmacher, Cuzick and Thilly, 1986; Kat *et al.*, 1993; Modrich, 1994).

Nucleotide excision repair appears to be the major DNA repair mechanism in all species studied, from bacteria to humans (Sancar and Tang, 1993). This repair system is the sole mechanism for removing bulky adducts from DNA, including, for example, benzo[a]pyrene-guanine adducts caused by smoking and cisplatin-guanine adducts caused by chemotherapy (Sancar, 1994). However, bulky lesions are not the only substrate for nucleotide excision repair; this enzyme system repairs many other lesions that do not distort the DNA helix, including O^6-methylguanine and other methylated bases (Huang *et al.*, 1994). In nucleotide excision repair, an enzyme system recognizes and removes the DNA damage by incising, in a precise manner, on both sides of the lesion to generate an oligonucleotide carrying the damage (Matsunaga *et al.*, 1995). The excised oligonucleotide is released from the DNA duplex, and the resulting gap is filled in and ligated in steps similar to those of base excision repair (Subba Rao, 1993). In both prokaryotes and eukaryotes, nucleotide excision is carried out by a multisubunit ATP-dependent nuclease called excision nuclease or excinuclease to distinguish it from endonucleases and exonucleases that perform other functions in the cell (Sancar, 1994).

Much of the current knowledge concerning the enzymology of DNA repair is derived from prokaryotic systems, and information about homologous enzymes from mammalian cells is scant or just becoming available as human repair genes are cloned and characterized (Subba Rao, 1993; Sancar, 1994). As evidenced below, comparatively little is known about DNA repair mechanisms in cells of the mammalian nervous system. Nevertheless, it is believed that DNA repair systems in mammalian cells resemble those found in prokaryotes, except that the DNA repair pathways in the higher systems appear to be more complicated (Subba Rao and Loeb, 1992). For instance, the reaction mechanism of human excinuclease is far more complex, requiring the participation of 16 or 17 polypeptides, whereas (A)BC excinuclease activity in *Escherichia coli* requires three subunits (Sancar, 1994; Matsunaga *et al.*, 1995).

Part of the information available on DNA repair in brain has originated from studies investigating DNA repair activities as a function of age. Evidence suggests that, after birth, there is a decline in the DNA repair capacity of postmitotic or slowly dividing cells in brain, heart and liver; whereas induction of DNA repair activity seems to be linked to DNA replication (Mazzarello *et al.*, 1992). Nevertheless, it is logical to postulate that postmitotic cells such as neurons, with high transcriptional activity and with a high number of single-copy essential genes, would possess efficient DNA repair mechanisms to maintain fidelity of vital processes like transcription and translation throughout the life-span of the species (Subba Rao, 1993). In fact, results from several different laboratories indicate that DNA repair is not completely absent, but reduced, in the brains of adults as compared with newborns (Subba Rao and Loeb, 1992). For instance, Korr and Schultze (1989) found, by autoradiography, low but significant levels of *in vivo* DNA repair in various cell types of adult mouse brain. In agreement with this report, DNA polymerase β, which is generally considered to be a repair enzyme, was found in significant amounts in the brains of adult and aged mice (Subba Rao and Subba Rao, 1982), and there was no apparent difference in the fidelity of this enzyme among young, adult and old ages (Subba Rao, Martin and Loeb, 1985). In addition, the nonspecific alkaline DNase of rat brain, a putative 'housekeeping' DNA repair enzyme, exhibited high activity in adult and aged animals (Subba Rao and Subba Rao, 1982). Analogous findings regarding several other enzymes will be referred to in the following discussion of specific repair proteins in brain tissue. Results of studies evaluating the relative amounts of DNA repair potential in young versus aged adults are conflicting and inconclusive, and have been reviewed in detail elsewhere (Mazzarello *et al.*, 1992; Subba Rao and Loeb, 1992; Subba Rao, 1993). Overall, the experimental data indicate that adult brain could lack some DNA repair pathways

Table 5.2 DNA repair proteins in brain[a]

DNA repair system	Implicated protein	Mechanism of action	Reference(s)
I. Reversal of damage			
Photoreactivation	Photolyase of marsupial brain	Monomerizes pyrimidine dimers	Rupert, 1975
Demethylation	MGMT of human, mouse, rat and porcine brain and/or brain tumors	Transfer of simple methyl group from O^6-methylguanine to cys^{321} residue of MGMT	Washington *et al.*, 1989; Fong *et al.*, 1992; Silber *et al.*, 1993
Ligation of single-strand breaks	DNA ligase of neuronal glial cells of guinea pig and rat	Rejoining of DNA strands at single-strand break	Inoue, Ono and Kato, 1979; Inoue and Kato, 1980
II. DNA excision repair			
Base excision repair	Uracil DNA glycosylase of rat brain and human fetal brain	Releases uracil from DNA specifically	Krokan *et al.*, 1983; Weng and Sirover, 1993
	3MeA DNA glycosylase in mouse brain	Releases 3MeA, 7-methylguanine, and some other *N*-methylpurines	Washington *et al.*, 1988, 1989
	AP endonucleases in rat and mouse brain	Excision of abasic sites	Ivanov, Tretyak and Afonin, 1988; Ono *et al.*, 1995
	Exonuclease (DNAase BIII) from rat brain neuronal nuclei	Excises single-strand DNA of single-strand termini in a duplex DNA in 5'→3' direction	Ivanov, Gaziev and Tretyak, 1983
	DNA polymerase β of rat and mouse brain	Polymerization of deoxynucleoside triphosphate	Hübscher, Kuenzle and Spadari, 1979
	DNA ligase of neuronal and glial cells of guinea pig and rat	Sealing of repair patches	Inoue, Ono and Kato, 1979; Inoue and Kato, 1980
Nucleotide excision repair	Excinuclease factor, ERCC1 protein in human brain tumors	Component of protein complex that carries the nuclease active sites	Dabholkar *et al.*, 1995
	Excinuclease factor, ERCC2 protein in human brain tumors	Component of protein complex linking repair with transcription	Dabholkar *et al.*, 1995
	PCNA in rat brain	Facilitates catalytic turnover of excinuclease	Verri *et al.*, 1992
	DNA polymerase δ and ϵ in rat and mouse brain	Polymerization of deoxynucleoside triphosphates	Hübscher, Kuenzle and Spadari, 1979; Spadari, Focher and Hübscher, 1988
	DNA ligase of neuronal and glial cells of guinea pig and rat	Sealing of repair patches	Inoue, Ono and Kato, 1979; Inoue and Kato 1980

Based, in part, upon information from Friedberg, 1985, 1990; Orren and Sancar, 1987; SubbaRao, 1993; Friedberg, Walker and Siede, 1995.
MGMT, O^6-methylguanine-DNA methyltransferase; 3MeA, 3-methyladenine; AP, apurinic/apyrimidinic; PCNA, proliferating cell nuclear antigen.

normally present in other tissues, but the various cells of the adult and even the aged brain possess the necessary machinery to repair some forms of DNA damage (Mazzarello *et al.*, 1992; Subba Rao and Loeb, 1992).

Although the DNA repair systems in brain have yet to be well characterized, brain tissue contains a fairly impressive number of enzymes that are either proven or generally accepted to participate in DNA repair (Table 5.2) (Subba Rao and Loeb, 1992). Much of the information about these enzymes is based upon DNA repair studies in the brains of experimental animals, but it is believed that similar repair proteins will ultimately be demonstrated to occur in the nervous tissues of humans.

DNA REPAIR PROTEINS IN BRAIN

It is noteworthy that some of the enzymes required for semiconservative DNA synthesis are also associated with DNA repair in brain (Mazzarello *et al.*, 1992). In rat and/or mouse brain, for instance, several enzymes involved in the replication of nuclear DNA have been found at low levels in adult animals. These enzymes include DNA polymerases α, β, δ and ϵ; uracil DNA glycosylase and DNA ligase (Table 5.2) (Hübscher, Kuenzle and Spadari, 1979; Inoue, Ono and Kato, 1979; Inoue and Kato, 1980; Subba Rao and Subba Rao, 1982; Spadari, Focher and Hübscher, 1988; Focher *et al.*, 1990). Among these enzymes, DNA polymerase α, at least in proliferating cells, is considered to play some role in DNA repair (Friedberg, 1985), DNA polymerase β is thought to be responsible for DNA synthesis in base excision repair (Hübscher, Kuenzle and Spadari, 1979; Waser *et al.*, 1979), and DNA polymerases δ or ϵ are believed to be involved in nucleotide excision repair (Sancar, 1994).

Uracil DNA glycosylase has the main reparative role in the removal of uracil from DNA. Uracil occurs in DNA by misincorporation of this base instead of thymine, and by spontaneous deamination of cytosine (Friedberg, 1985). Uracil DNA glycosylase has been demonstrated in the fetal brains of humans and in the brains of rats ranging in age from 4 days before birth to 106 days after birth (Weng and Sirover, 1993). Rat brain, heart and lung had low uracil DNA glycosylase activity compared with liver, kidney and spleen. During development, uracil DNA glycosylase activity paralleled the regulation of DNA synthesis in all organs except liver. Furthermore, repair activity was highest around birth and then declined to relatively stable levels during postnatal growth.

DNA ligase, the key enzyme joining DNA fragments during DNA replication, sealing repair patches during excision repair and ligating single-strand breaks, has been found in neurons at levels that are about 11-fold higher than in glial cells (Inoue, Ono and Kato, 1979; Inoue and Kato, 1980). Its activity in rat brain was similar to the activities observed in kidney, liver and lung, but several times lower than that found in thymus. Developmental expression studies have demonstrated that DNA ligase activity remains constant in pooled noncerebellar nervous tissue, while it increases in cerebellar tissues through postnatal day 6, and then declines markedly (Nakaya *et al.*, 1977).

Among the repair enzymes found in both normal and tumorous brain tissue of humans and several other species, O^6-alkylguanine-DNA alkyltransferase [O^6-methylguanine-DNA methyltransferase (MGMT)] is the best studied because the enzyme removes the predominant premutagenic DNA adduct formed by the experimental nitroso compounds (Pegg, 1990), and its activity has been associated with resistance to chemotherapy in brain tumors. In mammals, MGMT is a 22-kDa protein that is involved in the repair of O^6-alkylguanine DNA adducts in brain and other tissues. Its known *in vitro* action is to accept small adducts of O^6-alkylguanine; the preferred substrate is O^6-methylguanine, but larger alkyl adducts are also removed at a rate inversely proportional to their size (Pegg, 1990). For instance, O^6-ethylguanine adducts are removed efficiently by MGMT, while O^6-(2-hydroxyethyl)guanine adducts are believed to be removed less efficiently by MGMT and by excision repair (Koepke *et al.*, 1988; Ludeke and Kleihues, 1988). Following removal from DNA, the adduct becomes irreversibly bound to the receptor site of MGMT (Edara, Goodtzova and Pegg, 1995); since these sites are not regenerated, the rate of removal of O^6-methylguanine and other O^6-alkylguanine adducts depends on the total number of MGMT molecules available and their rate of synthesis. The role of MGMT in normal brain tissue is considered to be the same as that demonstrated for other tissues: it has been shown to provide protection against both spontaneous mutagenesis (Aquilina *et al.*, 1992) and chemical mutagenesis (Maher *et al.*, 1990; Lukash *et al.*, 1991; Bronstein *et al.*, 1992). Because of the demonstrated action for this protein, MGMT has been hypothesized to play a role in tumor cell resistance to specific chemotherapeutic agents, and, more recently, to represent a potential risk factor for neoplasms of the brain and lung (Citron *et al.*, 1992; Silber *et al.*, 1993).

A number of enzymes associated with base excision repair have been found in mammalian brain, including 3MeA DNA glycosylase, AP endonucleases, exonucleases and other enzymes discussed above (see Table 5.2). Homologs of 3MeA DNA glycosylase have now been cloned from many eukaryotic organisms, and the characterization of their biochemical properties has revealed that these homologs can initiate repair of a surprising variety of damaged DNA bases, including numerous different N^3- and N^7-alkyl purines, O^2-alkyl pyrimidines, deaminated adenine, oxidized guanine (8-oxoguanine), oxidized derivatives of thymine, bases with cyclic etheno adducts (formed endogenously or by metabolites of the human carcinogen, vinyl chloride) and haloethylated and cross-linked bases (Engelward *et al.*, 1996; Hang *et al.*, 1996). However, no single homolog of 3MeA DNA glycosylase has been assayed for repair of all these DNA lesions. Thus, while all of the 3MeA DNA glycosylases are able to repair simple *N*-methylated purine bases, some may also play important roles in protecting cells against a variety of other cytotoxic and mutagenic DNA lesions (Engelward *et al.*, 1996).

Both 3MeA DNA glycosylase and MGMT have been measured in the brains of mice at various ages, and the activities of both repair proteins were found to be consistently lower in preweanling animals (9 days old) than in young adults (7–8 weeks old) (Washington *et al.*, 1988, 1989). However, MGMT levels in adults did not decrease with age, while 3MeA DNA glycosylase levels were significantly lowered with age (to 17 months old). Moreover, activities of both repair proteins were generally lower in brain than in other tissues.

Two examples of AP endonucleases have been demonstrated in the brains of rodents: an AP endodeoxyribonuclease was isolated from rat neocortex chromatin (Ivanov, Tretyak and Afonin, 1988), while developmental expression studies of an AP endonuclease, designated APE nuclease (Hapl, APEX or Ref-1 gene product), were conducted in mice. In addition, rat brain was found to contain a specific exonuclease, DNase BIII, that acted to excise the AP site incised by the AP endodeoxyribonuclease and to stimulate DNA synthesis with DNA polymerase β (Ivanov, Tretyak and Afonin, 1988). In mice, APEX nuclease expression was high in the proliferative zone of various brain regions during embryonic and postnatal growth, and then declined to basal levels in adulthood (Ono *et al.*, 1995). APEX nuclease is a mammalian multifunctional DNA repair enzyme having 5' endonuclease, DNA 3' repair diesterase, 3'–5' exonuclease and DNA 3'-phosphatase activities, and is considered the major AP endonuclease in human cells (Seki *et al.*, 1991, 1992; Robson *et al.*, 1992). Although APEX nuclease activity has yet to be assessed in human brain cells, the human *APE* (human AP endonuclease 1) gene has been cloned and characterized (Seki *et al.*, 1991, 1992; Robson *et al.*, 1992).

Several other endonucleases, not listed in Table 5.2, have been identified in brain; these proteins include an endonuclease of lamb brain (Healy *et al.*, 1963), and acid DNase (UV DNase) and alkaline DNase (AP DNase) of rat brain (Rajagopal and Subba Rao, 1992; Venugopal and Subba Rao, 1993). Their proposed catalytic actions have been considered elsewhere (Subba Rao, 1993), and one or more may be involved in excision repair (Venugopal and Subba Rao, 1993).

Although a few proteins involved in nucleotide excision repair (NER) have been found in brain or brain tumors (see Table 5.2), efforts to evaluate the expression of the multiple subunits of human excinuclease in specific tissues are just beginning (Dabholkar *et al.*, 1995). The mechanistic details of human excinuclease have become available only in the past 4–5 years, since the cloning of human repair genes (Sancar and Tang, 1993; Sancar, 1994; Matsunaga *et al.*, 1995). Actually, it was the landmark discovery of defective NER in patients with xeroderma pigmentosum (Cleaver, 1968) and the subsequent isolation of UV-sensitive mutants of rodent cell lines (Thompson *et al.*, 1981) that made cloning of human repair genes possible (Sancar, 1994). Consequently, the human NER genes are referred to by the *XP* (xeroderma pigmentosum) or *ERCC* (excision repair cross complementing) designations (Sancar, 1994).

In one of the few studies concerning NER in human brain tumors, Dabholkar *et al.* (1995) assessed the relationships between subtle abnormalities in DNA repair competency and the process of malignant transformation. To study this question, they assayed malignant and nonmalignant brain tissues, taken from the same individual patients, for mRNA expression levels of two human NER-associated genes, *ERCC1* and *ERCC2*. The first step of NER (DNA damage recognition and excision) involves at least two protein complexes. One of these complexes, which has ERCC2 protein as one component, has helicase activity and may link DNA repair with DNA transcription. The complex that performs incision of the DNA strand has ERCC1 protein as one component (Matsunaga *et al.*, 1995). In nonmalignant brain tissues, mRNA levels of ERCC1 and ERCC2 were tightly coordinated, particularly with respect to the full-length transcript of ERCC1, which is associated with efficient NER (Dabholkar *et al.*, 1995). In contrast, this coordination was completely lost in malignant brain tissues. These investigators suggest that the discordance of the full-length ERCC1 transcript with ERCC2 in malignant brain tissues may indicate the development of a disruption in NER machinery as cells transit from the nonmalignant to the malignant state (Dabholkar *et al.*, 1995). Furthermore, a subtle change of this type in the NER mechanism may be analogous to the abnormality in mismatch repair that is associated with the development of human nonpolyposis colon cancer (Parsons *et al.*, 1993). In support of studies of this nature, Sancar (1994) has pointed out that, as the precise roles of each protein in NER are elucidated, it will be especially important to determine whether defects in NER genes (both known and yet to be discovered) are involved in common human cancers, as has been shown for mismatch repair and some hereditary cancers, such as hereditary nonpolyposis colorectal cancer.

Leach *et al.* (1996) have begun to address basic questions about the expression of mismatch repair (MMR) proteins in normal and neoplastic human tissues, following the recent development of monoclonal antibodies to the prototype human MMR gene, *MSH2*. This prototype human MMR gene is a homolog of the bacterial *mutS* gene (Modrich, 1991, 1994). The MSH2 gene product binds to a second MutS homolog, GT-binding protein, and both together initiate the repair process by recognizing mismatched DNA pairs (Leach *et al.*, 1996). In prokaryotes, the MutL gene products interact with MutS proteins to recruit nucleases, polymerases and other proteins required for the repair. The *MSH2* gene and three human *MLH* homologs (*MLH1, PMS1* and *PMS2*) have been associated with hereditary nonpolyposis colorectal cancer when inherited in the mutant form (Modrich, 1994; Chung and Rustgi, 1995; Friedberg, Walker and Siede, 1995).

Immunohistochemistry studies with monoclonal antibodies against the carboxy-terminal end of the MSH2 gene product revealed that the protein was expressed in a variety of human tissues, including thyroid, heart, smooth muscle and the germinal centers of lymphoid follicles (Leach *et al.*, 1996). Staining was most prominent in the esophageal and intestinal epithelia, where expression was limited to the replicating compartment. The protein was also expressed in benign and malignant mismatch repair-proficient tumors of the colon, but no MSH2 immunoreactivity was observed in colorectal tumors of patients with germline *MSH2* mutation. These results have important implications for tumorigenic mechanisms, and lay a foundation for future investigations of the potential role of MMR deficiencies in the genesis of tumors of the brain and other tissues.

EXPRESSION OF DNA REPAIR GENES IN TRANSGENIC ANIMALS

The advent of transgenic animals expressing DNA repair genes provides new opportunities to evaluate the role of DNA alkylation and repair processes in both spontaneous and experimentally induced carcinogenesis. Accordingly, a number of laboratories have focused on the development of relevant transgenic mouse models, including mice carrying expression constructs for the *MGMT* gene (either the *MGMT* cDNA or the bacterial *ADA* gene) (Gerson *et al.*, 1994). Cells and tissue in which the *MGMT* gene is expressed are specifically protected from the DNA-damaging effects of *N*-nitroso compounds. For instance, mice expressing the human *MGMT* gene in thymus are more resistant to MNU-induced thymic lymphomas than nontransgenic mice (Dumenco *et al.*, 1993), providing clear evidence that removal of O^6-methylguanine adducts by MGMT gives protection from cancer in this tissue. Because DNA is methylated endogenously and many mouse strains have a relatively high incidence of spontaneous thymic lymphomas, a natural question to consider is whether expression of the *MGMT* transgene would reduce the background occurrence of this cancer in mice. The recent development of transgenic animals overexpressing the human *MGMT* gene in brain should permit the manipulation of repair enzyme levels and facilitate heretofore unfeasible studies of the relationships between DNA alkylation, repair and the induction of gliomas (Fan *et al.*, 1990; Walter *et al.*, 1993).

Relationship between DNA damage, DNA repair and chemotherapy of brain tumors

The activity of MGMT has been extensively studied in relation to the use of CENUs in the treatment of neoplasms of the brain. As noted above, CENUs are alkylating and cross-linking agents that are believed to exert their cytotoxic effects primarily through the formation of DNA interstrand cross-links, thereby preventing the strand separation required for DNA replication and mitosis (Tong, Kirk and Ludlum, 1982). Since MGMT has been demonstrated to have the capacity to repair one of the cytotoxic DNA lesions associated with CENU therapy, it has been postulated that measurement of MGMT activity in tumor cells could be used as an indicator of tumor cell susceptibility to this class of agents.

Chloroethylnitrosoureas are thought to produce their tumoricidal effects largely through a multistep mechanism in which formation of O^6-(2-chloroethyl)guanine is the initial alkylation event. This short-lived DNA adduct (*in vitro* half-life ≅ 18 minutes; Parker, Kirk and Ludlum, 1987) undergoes an intramolecular rearrangement to a cyclized intermediate, N^1,O^6-ethanoguanine, that reacts with cytosine in the complementary strand to produce a 1-(1-guanyl)-2-(3-cytosinyl)ethane interstrand cross-link (Tong, Kirk and Ludlum, 1982; Gonzaga *et al.*, 1992). *In vitro* studies have shown that MGMT prevents cross-link formation by opening the exocyclic ring of N^1,O^6-ethanoguanine and becoming covalently bound through an ethyl group to the N^1 position of guanine (Gonzaga *et al.*, 1992). The chloroethyl group is bound to a cysteine moiety within the MGMT active site, resulting in the generation of guanine and S-alkyl cysteine (Olsson and Lindahl, 1980; Pegg, 1990; Pegg and Byers, 1992) and preventing the formation of interstrand cross-links (Gonzaga *et al.*, 1992). That the same events occur *in vivo* remains to be demonstrated (Silber *et al.*, 1993).

O^6-METHYLGUANINE-DNA METHYLTRANSFERASE ACTIVITY IN NORMAL AND TUMOROUS BRAIN TISSUE

Activity of MGMT has been studied in multiple organ systems. Among human tissues, liver has the highest MGMT activity, brain has the lowest; colon and colon tumors also have low activity (Mineura *et al.*, 1993). MGMT is unique: it is expressed at highly variable levels between tissues and between individuals (Eberhagen, Bankmann and Kaina, 1995). In surgically removed brain tumor specimens, variations in protein activity between individuals have been found to range up to 100-fold (Citron *et al.*, 1991); in brain tumor cell lines, 200-fold variations have been found (Bobola *et al.*, 1995).

Because of the difficulty of obtaining normal brain tissue, a paucity of studies of MGMT activity in this tissue are available. Silber *et al.* (1993) performed one of the few studies to evaluate MGMT activity in tumorigenic and nontumorigenic brain tissue removed from the same patient. This study found that MGMT activity levels in normal brain ranged from 0.5 to 21.8 fmol/10^6 cells. Fifty-two per cent of the samples had MGMT activity levels of less than 0.5 fmol/10^6cells, consistent with the phenotypic classification of Mer$^-$. The activity range in the remaining samples varied by approximately 30-fold. In the tumorigenic tissues, 27% had no detectable MGMT activity, and the remaining samples had activities that varied by two orders of magnitude. No significant sex differences were observed, but MGMT activity in both normal and tumorigenic tissue was found to decrease with increasing age.

When tumorigenic tissue was compared with nontumorigenic tissue, a significant difference in MGMT activity was observed (Silber *et al.*, 1993). The activity of MGMT protein was found to be higher in tumor tissue than in normal adjacent brain tissue for 15/25 cases, lower in tumor than adjacent brain in 4/25 cases, and undetectable in both tumor and normal tissue for 6/25 cases. The hypothesis—that the increase in MGMT activity was due to the proliferative state of the tumor cells—would appear to be incorrect because no strong correlation between the fraction of cells in S phase and MGMT activity was found. Silber *et al.* (1993) have postulated that some changes associated with the expression of the tumorigenic phenotype may also affect MGMT expression. In support of this theory are the observations that expression of MGMT mRNA can be regulated by methylation of genomic 5' regulatory sequences, and expression can be affected by loss or rearrangement of sequences on chromosome 10, a change associated with glioblastoma (Silber *et al.*, 1993). The authors also note that the apparent high incidence of Mer$^-$ individuals (52%) in the study population suggests that this phenotype may constitute a potential risk factor for the development of brain tumors. They were able to test six brain biopsies from patients without evidence of neoplasia, and only one case was phenotypically Mer$^-$. Citron *et al.* (1992) found similar results in a study of lung tumors, and they suggest that low MGMT activity may constitute a predisposing factor for lung cancer.

Several investigators have evaluated both surgical specimens and cell lines derived from brain tumors; a diverse group of tumor types have been assayed, and some studies have also tested lesions metastatic to the brain. Mineura *et al.* (1991) found a significant difference between the MGMT activity of glial versus nonglial tumors. No significant difference in MGMT activity between types of nonglial tumors was noted. Glial tumors showed the widest variation in activity; 5/22 gliomas had low levels of MGMT activity compatible with the Mer$^-$ phenotype. Other investigators have also found that about 25% of gliomas have no detectable MGMT activity (Citron *et al.*, 1991; Silber *et al.*, 1993). No significant difference between the MGMT activity of high- and low-grade gliomas was found. In subsequent work, Mineura *et al.* (1993) found that MGMT activity of nonglial tumors and brain metastases was significantly higher than MGMT activity of glial tumors; but, in a similar study, Hotta *et al.* (1994) found a wide range of MGMT activity, with no significant difference between glioblastomas and anaplastic astrocytomas, or between primary and recurrent tumors. Mineura *et al.* (1993) suggest that the wide variation in protein activity may be related to the morphology of glial tumors, which includes viable portions, central necrosis and areas of peritumoral infiltration. This hypothesis may also account for variations between studies. Consistent with the above work is the additional hypothesis that the differences between tumor groups may reflect different genetic lesions that impinge upon MGMT expression, and which, in turn, may reflect differences in pathogenesis and/or etiology.

Regulation of *MGMT* gene expression has been studied by several groups because of the importance of determining the role of *MGMT* expression in brain tumor resistance to chemotherapeutic agents such as CENUs. Costello *et al.* (1994) demonstrated that methylation of the body and promoter regions of the gene is directly associated with gene expression in a graded, rather that on/off, fashion. Methylation of the body of the *MGMT* gene correlates directly with expression levels, while methylation within the promoter region is inversely related to expression.

Methylation status may explain at least some cases of the Mer$^-$ phenotype in brain and other tissues; however, other possible mechanisms have been suggested. Citron *et al.* (1992) measured levels of MGMT mRNA expression using an RNA protection assay with an antisense probe specific for MGMT mRNA, and the results were correlated with MGMT activity. While a strong correlation between expression levels and protein activity was found for most tissues and tumors, a few samples had moderate levels of MGMT mRNA but no detectable MGMT activity. The authors hypothesize that posttranscriptional control of MGMT mRNA expression may be responsible for these observations. It can also be hypothesized that mutations within the *MGMT* gene may result in the production of an inactive protein form (Edara, Goodtzova and Pegg, 1995).

ROLE OF O^6-METHYLGUANINE-DNA METHYLTRANSFERASE IN DRUG TREATMENT AND RESISTANCE

A number of studies in cell lines and tumors have been directed toward evaluation of the potential role of MGMT activity in drug resistance *in vivo*. Since *N*-nitroso compounds are used in tumor therapy, O^6-methylguanine adducts are of particular concern (Bobola *et al.*, 1995), and it has been postulated that knowledge of MGMT activity, by virtue of its ability to remove O^6-methylguanine adducts and thereby give protection from the lethal effects of CENU chemotherapy, would be critical in the success of this mode of therapy (Mineura *et al.*, 1991; Bobola, Berger and Silber, 1995; Bobola *et al.*, 1995). The primary goal of this work has been to determine whether or not assessment of MGMT activity could be used as a predictive indicator of response to CENU therapy. Human brain tumor cell lines treated *in vitro*, xenografts of human brain tumors treated *in vivo* in mice and results of clinical trials have been evaluated in an effort to achieve this goal (Dolan, Moschel and Pegg, 1990; Dolan *et al.*, 1990; Friedman *et al.*, 1992). While most of this work has focused upon the role of MGMT in CENU chemotherapy success, other alkylating agents, such as temozolomide and procarbazine, have also been studied (Schold *et al.*, 1989; Fong *et al.*, 1992; Baer *et al.*, 1993; Friedman *et al.*, 1995; Russell *et al.*, 1995).

Several investigators have evaluated the relationship between MGMT activity and response to therapy with CENUs in brain tumor specimens removed at surgery and in clinical trials (Mineura *et al.*, 1993; Hotta *et al.*, 1994). In general, MGMT activity serves as a moderately strong indicator of response to therapy when one of the alkylating agents mentioned above is used, although the contribution of MGMT to resistance to alkylation in specific brain tumor cell lines and brain tumors may vary to some degree. The strongest correlation between MGMT activity and response to CENU was seen in glioblastomas, where MGMT activity suggested a refractory tendency (Hotta *et al.*, 1994). Five of 22 gliomas had low levels of MGMT compatible with the Mer$^-$ phenotype. Three of these five patients were treated with 1-(4-amino-2-methyl-5-pyrimidinyl)methyl-3-(2-chloroethyl)-3-nitrosourea (ACNU), and two of the three cases responded well to therapy. Friedman *et al.* (1992) found that depletion of MGMT with O^6-benzylguanine substantially enhanced the response of glioblastoma multiforme and medulloblastoma xenografts to therapy with 1,3-*bis*(2-chloroethyl)-1-nitrosourea (BCNU). In addition, Belanich *et al.* (1996) have shown that, in patients treated with BCNU for high-grade glioma, MGMT levels were inversely related to both time of treatment failure ($P = 0.05$) and death ($P = 0.004$).

With the development of the anti-MGMT antibody MT3.1 by Brent and Bigner (Brent *et al.*, 1993), it has been possible to demonstrate the degree of tumor cell heterogeneity with respect to MGMT status, as well as the relatively small number of MGMT-positive cells that may be present in some tumors. An example is illustrated in Chapter 8. In studies of glioblastomas, the presence of small numbers of neoplastic cells expressing high levels of MGMT protein were readily detectable immunohistochemically, but these cells might have been undetectable in 'grind and measure' biochemical or Western blot analyses. Gerson and his colleagues (Zaidi, Liu and Gerson, 1996) have developed image analysis-based quantitative immunohistochemistry for detection of MGMT protein-expressing neoplastic cells in human brain tumor tissue. Prospective immunohistochemical studies are being conducted by several groups to determine the role of immunohistochemical detection of MGMT in predicting glioma responses to alkylating agents and to determine the effectiveness of depleting MGMT with agents such as O^6-benzylguanine.

The lack of total correlation of MGMT to alkylator resistance suggests that alternate, non-MGMT mechanisms of resistance may be operational in protecting brain tumors from alkylator- and methylator-induced damage. Recent studies with a 3MeA DNA glycosylase repair-deficient cell line provide evidence that other repair proteins or systems are involved in brain tumor resistance to CENU therapy. Engelward *et al.* (1996) have developed a mouse embryonic cell line that has no detectable transcripts for the *TRLP1* gene, which encodes for 3MeA DNA glycosylase and have demonstrated that the loss of *TRLP1* renders the cells significantly more sensitive to DNA damage and cell killing by two methylating agents (one of which produces 3MeA adducts almost exclusively). Strikingly, the absence of *TRLP1* also renders cells more sensitive to the alkylating and cytotoxic effects of BCNU, providing *in vivo* evidence that a mammalian 3MeA DNA glycosylase ameliorates the toxicity of the CENUs. Although these studies did not use nervous tissue cells, they indicate that it will be important to determine the relative contributions of MGMT, 3MeA DNA glycosylase and other repair proteins in protecting cells of the brain and other tissues against the therapeutic actions of CENUs (Engelward *et al.*, 1996). The roles of NER, recombination glutathione-S-transferase or metallothionine in CENU resistance are all potential areas for investigation. Alterations in cell cycle or apoptosis offer another potential mechanism that may be associated with resistance (Bobola, Berger and Silber, 1995).

Future prospects

The foregoing review demonstrates that, in spite of the large body of research addressing DNA damage and repair in mammalian brain, relatively little is known about their precise roles in neuro-oncogenesis. A critical deficiency in our knowledge has to do with the relationships of exogenous versus endogenous sources of DNA adducts and DNA damage to the development of brain tumors in humans. *A priori*, it might be expected that endogenous DNA adducts increase in concentration in association with chemical, dietary or physiological modifications that lead to cancer. If so, quantitation of their levels may provide an estimate of the relative risk of developing certain cancers and could be useful for comparison with levels of adducts resulting from exogenous chemicals (Marnett and Burcham, 1993). Therefore, as sensitive and specific methods for detecting DNA adducts and characterizing DNA damage become available, more studies are needed to investigate the occurrence of specific types of DNA adducts and damage in normal and cancerous brain tissues from people with no significant exposures to exogenous chemicals versus people exposed to environmental agents suspected to be neurocarcinogens in humans or known to be neuro-oncogenic in experimental animals. Additional research is needed to characterize as fully as possible the activities of known and yet to be discovered DNA repair proteins in brain, to define the contribution of defects in specific DNA repair systems and their regulation to the genesis of brain tumors, and to delineate the role of repair in brain cancer chemotherapy (Sancar, 1994). For example, many monoclonal antibodies against a large number of DNA repair enzymes, such as those described for MGMT, will become available in the future. Neuropathologists will play a critical role in determining the usefulness of immunohistochemical analyses of DNA repair enzymes in nervous system neoplasms for predicting response to therapy. Elucidation of the relative contributions of exogenously and endogenously induced DNA damage, as well as the molecular mechanisms leading to repair of the various types of damage, will be crucial to determining the etiology of human brain tumors and to improving brain cancer prevention and treatment.

References

Akbasak, A. and Sunar-Akbasak, B. (1992) Oncogenes: cause or consequence in the development of glial tumors. *Journal of the Neurological Sciences* **111**, 119–33.

Albertini, R.J. (1994) Why use somatic mutations for human biomonitoring? *Environmental and Molecular Mutagenesis* **23** (Suppl. 24), 18–22.

Ames, B.N. and Gold, L.S. (1991) Endogenous mutagens and the causes of aging and cancer. *Mutation Research* **250**, 3–16.

Aquilina, G., Biondo, R., Dogliotto, E., Meuth, M. and Bignami, M. (1992) Expression of the endogenous O^6-methylguanine-DNA-methyltransferase protects Chinese hamster ovary cells from spontaneous G:C to A:T transitions. *Cancer Research* **52**, 6471–5.

Baer, J.C., Freeman, A.A., Newlands, E.S., Watson, A.J., Rafferty, J.A. and Margison, G.P. (1993) Depletion of O^6-alkylguanine-DNA alkyltransferase correlates with potentiation of temoxolomide and CCNU toxicity in human tumour cells. *British Journal of Cancer* **67**, 1299–302.

Bastlová, T., Andersson, B., Lambert, B. and Kolman, A. (1993) Molecular analysis of ethylene oxide-induced mutations at the *HPRT* locus in human diploid fibroblasts. *Mutation Research* **287**, 283–92.

Basu, A.K. and Essigmann, J.M. (1988) Site-specifically modified oligodeoxynucleotides as probes for the structural and biological effects of DNA-damaging agents. *Chemical Research and Toxicology* **1**, 1–18.

Belanich, M., Pastor, M., Randall, T., Guerra, D., Kibitel, J., Alas, L., Li, B., Citron, M., Wasserman, P., White, A., Eyre, H., Jaeckle, K., Schulman, S., Rector, D., Prados, M., Coons, S., Shapiro, W. and Yarosh, D. (1996) Retrospective study of the correlation between the DNA repair protein alkyltransferase and survival of brain tumor patients treated with carmustine. *Cancer Research* **56**, 783–8.

Bergmark, E., Calleman, C.J., He, F. and Costa, L.G. (1994) Determination of hemoglobin adducts in humans occupationally exposed to acrylamide. *Toxicology and Applied Pharmacology* **120**, 45–54.

Berleur, M.-P. and Cordier, S. (1995) The role of chemical, physical, or viral exposures and health factors in neurocarcinogenesis: implications for epidemiologic studies of brain tumors. *Cancer Causes and Control* **6**, 240–56.

Bhanot, O.S., Grevatt, P.C., Donahue, J.M., Grabrielides, C.N. and Solomon, J.J. (1992) *In vitro* DNA replication implicates O^2-ethyldeoxythymidine in transversion mutagenesis by ethylating agents. *Nucleic Acids Research* **20**, 587–94.

Bigner, D.D. and Swenberg, J.A. (1977) *Jänisch and Schreiber's experimental tumors of the central nervous system.* First English edition. Kalamazoo, Mich.: Upjohn.

Bigner, D.D., Bigner, S.H., Burger, P.C., Shelburne, J.D. and Friedman, H.S. (1986) Primary brain tumours in Fischer 344 rats chronically exposed to acrylonitrile in their drinking-water. *Food and Chemical Toxicology* **24**, 129–37.

Bigner, S.H., Vogelstein, B., Mark, J., Friedman, H.S. and Bigner, D.D. (1990) Cytogenetics and molecular genetics: their status and role in understanding the behavior of central nervous system neoplasms. *Monographs in Pathology* **32**, 30–40.

Bishop, J.M. (1991) Molecular themes in oncogenesis. *Cell* **64**, 235–48.

Bobola, M.S., Berger, M.S. and Silber, J.R. (1995) Contribution of O^6-methylguanine-DNA methyltransferase to resistance to 1,3-(2-chloroethyl)-1-nitrosourea in human brain tumor-derived cell lines. *Molecular Carcinogenesis* **13**, 81–8.

Bobola, M.S., Blank, A., Berger, M.S. and Silber, J.R. (1995) Contribution of O^6-methylguanine-DNA methyltransferase to monofunctional alkylating-agent resistance in human brain tumor-derived cell lines. *Molecular Carcinogenesis* **13**, 70–80.

Bodell, W.J., Aida, T., Berger, M.S. and Rosenblum, M.L. (1985) Repair of O^6-(2-chloroethyl)guanine mediates the biological effects of chloroethylnitrosoureas. *Environmental Health Perspectives* **62**, 119–26.

Breimer, L.H. (1988) Ionizing radiation-induced mutagenesis. *British Journal of Cancer* **57**, 6–18.

Brent, T.P., von Wronski, M.A., Edwards, C.C., Bromley, M., Margison, G.P., Rafferty, J.A., Pegram, C.N. and Bigner, D.D. (1993) Identification of nitrosourea-resistant human rhabdomyosarcomas by *in situ* immunostaining of O^6-methylguanine-DNA methyltransferase. *Oncology Research* **5**, 83–6.

Bronstein, S.M., Cochrane, J.E., Craft, T.R., Swenberg, J.A. and Skopek, T.R. (1991) Toxicity, mutagenicity, and mutational spectra of *N*-ethyl-*N*-nitrosourea in human cell lines with different DNA repair phenotypes. *Cancer Research* **51**, 5188–97.

Bronstein, S.M., Hooth, M.J., Swenberg, J.A. and Skopek, T.R. (1992) Modulation of ethylnitrosourea-induced toxicity and mutagenicity in human cells by O^6-benzylguanine. *Cancer Research* **52**, 3851–6.

Bücheler, J. and Kleihues, P. (1977) Excision of O^6-methylguanine from DNA of various mouse tissues following a single injection of *N*-methyl-*N*-nitrosourea. *Chemico-Biological Interactions* **16**, 325–33.

Burch, J.D., Craib, K.J.P., Choi, B.C.K., Miller, A.B., Risch, H.A. and Howe, G.R. (1987) An exploratory case-control study of brain tumors in adults. *Journal of the National Cancer Institute* **78**, 601–9.

Chung, D.C. and Rustgi, A.K. (1995) DNA mismatch repair and cancer. *Gastroenterology* **109**, 1685–99.

Citron, M., Decker, R., Chen, S., Schneider, S., Graver, M., Kleynerman, L., Kahn, L.B., White, A., Schoenhaus, M. and Yarosh, D. (1991) O^6-methylguanine-DNA methyltransferase in human normal and tumor tissue from brain, lung, and ovary. *Cancer Research* **51**, 4131–4.

Citron, M., Graver, M., Schoenhaus, M., Chen, S., Decker, R., Kleynerman, L., Kahn, L.B., White, A., Fornace, A.J. and Yarosh, D. (1992) Detection of messenger RNA from O^6-methylguanine-DNA methyltransferase gene MGMT in human normal and tumor tissues. *Journal of the National Cancer Institute* **84**, 337–40.

Cleaver, J.E. (1968) Defective repair replication of DNA in xeroderma pigmentosum. *Nature* **218**, 652–6.

Cohen, R.J., Wiernik, P.H. and Walker, M.D. (1976) Acute nonlymphocytic leukemia associated with nitrosourea chemotherapy: report of two cases. *Cancer Treatment Reports* **60**, 1257–61.

Collins, A., Johnson, R.T. and Boyle, J.M. (eds) (1987) Molecular biology of DNA repair. *Journal of Cell Science* (Suppl. 6).

Collins, J.J., Swaen, G.M.H., Marsh, G.M., Utidjian, H.M.D., Caporossi, J.C. and Lucas, L.J. (1989) Mortality patterns among workers exposed to acrylamide. *Journal of Occupational Medicine* **31**, 614–17.

Costello, J.F., Futscher, B.W., Tano, K., Graunke, D.M. and Pieper, R.O. (1994) Graded methylation in the promoter and body of the O^6-methylguanine DNA methyltransferase (MGMT) gene correlates with

MGMT expression in human glioma cells. *Journal of Biological Chemistry* **269**, 17228–37.

Cuthbertson, R.A. and Klintworth, G.K. (1988) Biology of disease: transgenic mice–a gold mine for furthering knowledge in pathobiology. *Laboratory Investigation* **58**, 484–502.

Dabholkar, M.D., Berger, M.S., Vionnet, J.A., Egwuagu, C., Silber, J.R., Yu, J.J. and Reed, E. (1995) Malignant and nonmalignant brain tissues differ in their messenger RNA expression patterns for *ERCC1* and *ERCC2*. *Cancer Research* **55**, 1261–6.

Davis, D.L., Ahlbom, A., Hoel, D. and Percy, C. (1991) Is brain cancer mortality increasing in industrial countries? *American Journal of Industrial Medicine* **19**, 421–31.

Den Engelse, L., De Graaf, A., De Brij, R.-J. and Menkveld, G.J. (1987) O^2- and O^4-ethylthymine and the ethylphosphotriester dTp(Et)dT are highly persistent DNA modifications in slowly dividing tissues of the ethylnitrosourea-treated rat. *Carcinogenesis* **8**, 751–7.

Dipple, A. (1995) Commentary: DNA adducts of chemical carcinogens. *Carcinogenesis* **16**, 437–41.

Dolan, M.E., Moschel, R.C. and Pegg, A.E. (1990) Depletion of mammalian O^6-alkylguanine-DNA alkyltransferase activity by O^6-benzylguanine provides a means to evaluate the role of this protein in protection against carcinogenic and therapeutic alkylating agents. *Proceedings of the National Academy of Sciences U.S.A.* **87**, 5368–72.

Dolan, M.E., Stine, L., Mitchell, R.B., Moschel, R.C. and Pegg, A.E. (1990) Modulation of mammalian O^6-alkylguanine-DNA alkyltransferase *in vivo* by O^6-benzylguanine and its effect on the sensitivity of a human glioma tumor to 1-(2-chloroethyl)-3-(4-methylcyclohexyl)-1-nitrosourea. *Cancer Communications* **2**, 371–7.

Dosanjh, M.K., Menichini, P., Eritja, R. and Singer, B. (1993) Both O^4-methylthymine and O^4-ethylthymine preferentially form alkyl T·G pairs that do not block *in vitro* replication in a defined sequence. *Carcinogenesis* **14**, 1915–19.

Dumenco, L.L., Allay, E., Norton, K. and Gerson, S.L. (1993) The prevention of thymic lymphomas in transgenic mice by human O^6-alkylguanine-DNA alkyltransferase. *Science* **259**, 219–22.

Eberhagen, I., Bankmann, M. and Kaina, B. (1995) Detection of O^6-methylguanine-DNA methyltransferase expression in human tumors by means of *in situ* hybridization. *Anticancer Research* **15**, 761–8.

Edara, S., Goodtzova, K. and Pegg, A.E. (1995) The role of tyrosine-158 in O^6-alkylguanine-DNA alkyltransferase activity. *Carcinogenesis* **16**, 1637–42.

Ehrenberg, L. and Hussain, S. (1981) Genetic toxicity of some important epoxides. *Mutation Research* **86**, 1–113.

Engelward, B.P., Dreslin, A., Christensen, J., Huszar, D., Kurahara, C. and Samson, L. (1996) Repair-deficient 3-methyladenine DNA glycosylase homozygous mutant mouse cells have increased sensitivity to alkylation-induced chromosome damage and cell killing. *EMBO Journal* **15**, 945–52.

Evans, D.A.P., Burbach, J.P.H. and van Leeuwen, F.W. (1995) Somatic mutations in the brain: relationship to aging? *Mutation Research* **338**, 173–82.

Fan, C.Y., Potter, P.M., Rafferty, J., Watson, A.J., Cawkwell, L., Searle, P.F., O'Connor, P.J. and Margison, G.P. (1990) Expression of a human O^6-alkylguanine-DNA-alkyl-transferase cDNA in human cells and transgenic mice. *Nucleic Acids Research* **18**, 5723–7.

Fearon, E.R. and Vogelstein, B. (1990) A genetic model for colorectal tumorigenesis. *Cell* **61**, 759–67.

Fedtke, N., Walker, V.E. and Swenberg, J.A. (1989) Determination of 7-(2-oxoethyl)guanine and N^2,3-ethenoguanine in DNA hydrolysates by HPLC. *Archives of Toxicology Supplement* **13**, 214–18.

Focher, P., Mazzarello, P., Verri, A., Hübscher, U. and Spadari, S. (1990) Activity profiles of enzymes that control the uracil incorporation into DNA during neuronal development. *Mutation Research* **237**, 65–73.

Fong, L.Y.Y., Bevill, R.F., Thurmon, J.C. and Magee, P.N. (1992) DNA adduct dosimetry and DNA repair in rats and pigs given repeated doses of procarbazine under conditions of carcinogenicity and human cancer chemotherapy respectively. *Carcinogenesis* **13**, 2153–9.

Föst, U., Marczynski, B., Kasemann, R. and Peter, H. (1989) Determination of 7-(2-hydroxyethyl)guanine with gas chromatography/mass spectrometry as a parameter for genotoxicity of ethylene oxide. *Archives of Toxicology Supplement* **13**, 250–3.

Foulds, L. (1958) The natural history of cancer. *Journal of Chronic Disease* **8**, 2–37.

Frankenberg-Schwager, M. (1990) Induction, repair and biological relevance of radiation-induced DNA lesions in eukaryotic cells. *Radiation and Environmental Biophysics* **29**, 273–92.

Friedberg, E.C. (1985) *DNA repair*. New York: W.H. Freeman.

——(ed.) (1990) The enzymology of DNA repair. *Mutation Research* **236** (2–3).

Friedberg, E.C., Walker, G.C. and Siede, W. (1995) *DNA repair and mutagenesis*. Washington, D.C.: American Society for Microbiology Press.

Friedman, H.S., Dolan, M.E., Moschel, R.C., Pegg, A.E., Felker, G.M., Rich, J., Bigner, D.D. and Schold, S.C. Jr (1992) Enhancement of nitrosourea activity in medulloblastoma and glioblastoma multiforme. *Journal of the National Cancer Institute* **64**, 1926–31.

Friedman, H.S., Dolan, M.E., Pegg, A.E., Marcelli, S., Keir, S., Catino, J.J., Bigner, D.D. and Schold, S.C. Jr (1995) Activity of temozolomide in the treatment of central nervous system tumor xenografts. *Cancer Research* **55**, 2853–7.

Fry, M. and Loeb, L.A. (1986) *Animal cell DNA polymerases*. Boca Raton, Fla.: CRC Press.

Fürst, C.J., Lundell, M., Holm, L.-E. and Silfverswärd, C. (1988) Cancer incidence after radiotherapy for skin hemangioma: a retrospective cohort study in Sweden. *Journal of the National Cancer Institute* **80**, 1387–92.

Garman, R.H., Snellings, W.M. and Maronpot, R.R. (1985) Brain tumors in F344 rats associated with chronic inhalation exposure to ethylene oxide. *Neurotoxicology* **6**, 117–38.

Gerson, S.L., Zaidi, N.H., Dumenco, L.L., Allay, E., Fan, C.Y., Liu, L. and O'Connor, P.J. (1994) Alkyltransferase transgenic mice: probes of chemical carcinogenesis. *Mutation Research* **307**, 541–55.

Golberg, L. (1986) *Hazard assessment of ethylene oxide.* Boca Raton, Fla.: CRC Press.

Goldmacher, V.S., Cuzick, R.A. and Thilly, W.G. (1986) Isolation and partial characterization of human cell mutants differing in sensitivity to killing and mutation by methylnitrosourea and *N*-methyl-*N*'-nitro-nitrosoguanidine. *Journal of Biological Chemistry* **261**, 12462–71.

Gonzaga, P.E., Potter, P.M., Niu, T.Q., Yu, D., Ludlum, D.B., Rafferty, J.A., Margison, G.P. and Brent, T.P. (1992) Identification of the cross-link between human O^6-methylguanine-DNA methyltransferase and chloroethylnitrosourea-treated DNA. *Cancer Research* **52**, 6052–8.

Goodhead, D.T. (1989) The initial physical damage produced by ionizing radiations. *International Journal of Radiation Biology* **56**, 623–34.

Goth, R. and Rajewsky, M.F. (1974) Persistence of O^6-ethylguanine in rat brain DNA. Correlation with nervous system-specific carcinogenesis by ethylnitrosourea. *Proceedings of the National Academy of Sciences U.S.A.* **71**, 639–43.

Habs, M., Eisenbrand, G. and Schmahl, D. (1979) Carcinogenic activity in Sprague-Dawley rats of 2-[3-(2-chloroethyl)-3-nitrosoureido]-D-glucopyranose (chlorozotocin). *Cancer Letters* **8**, 133–7.

Hanahan, D. (1986) Oncogenesis in transgenic mice. In Kahn, P. and Graf, T. (eds), *Oncogenes and growth control.* New York: Springer-Verlag, 349–63.

Hang, B., Chenna, A., Rao, S. and Singer, B. (1996) 1, N^6-Ethenoadenine and 3, N^4-ethenocytosine are excised by separate human DNA glycosylases. *Carcinogenesis* **17**, 155–7.

Haseman, J.K., Crawford, D.D., Huff, J.E., Boorman, G.A. and McConnell, E.E. (1984) Results from 86 two-year carcinogenicity studies conducted by the national toxicology program. *Journal of Toxicology and Environmental Health* **14**, 621–39.

Healy, J.W., Stollar, D., Simon, M.I. and Levine, L. (1963) Characterization of phosphodiesterase from lamb brain. *Archives of Biochemistry and Biophysics* **103**, 461–8.

Herrlich, P., Mallick, U., Ponta, H. and Rahmsdorf, H.J. (1984) Genetic changes in mammalian cells reminiscent of an SOS response. *Human Genetics* **67**, 360–8.

Hogy, L.L. and Guengerich, F.P. (1986) *In vivo* interaction of acrylonitrile and 2-cyanoethylene oxide with DNA in rats. *Cancer Research* **46**, 3932–8.

Hotta, T., Saito, Y., Fujita, H., Mikami, T., Kurisu, K., Kiya, K., Uozumi, T., Isowa, G., Ishizaki, K. and Ikenaga, M. (1994) O^6-alkylguanine-DNA alkyltransferase activity of human malignant glioma and its clinical implications. *Journal of Neuro-Oncology* **21**, 135–40.

Huang, J.C., Hsu, D.S., Kazantsev, A. and Sancar, A. (1994) Substrate spectrum of human excinuclease: repair of abasic sites, methylated bases, mismatches, and bulky adducts. *Proceedings of the National Academy of Sciences U.S.A.* **91**, 12213–17.

Hübscher, U., Kuenzle, C.C. and Spadari, S. (1979) Functional roles of DNA-polymerase β and γ. *Proceedings of the National Academy of Sciences U.S.A.* **76**, 2316–20.

Inoue, N. and Kato, T. (1980) Nuclear DNA ligase and its action on chromatin DNA in neuronal, glial and liver nuclei isolated from adult guinea pigs. *Journal of Neurochemistry* **34**, 1574–83.

Inoue, N., Ono, T. and Kato, T. (1979) Ligation and synthesis of chromatin deoxyribonucleic acid *in vitro* in neuronal, glial, and liver nuclei isolated from adult guinea pig. *Biochemical Journal* **180**, 471–80.

International Agency for Research on Cancer (IARC) Working Group (1994) *IARC monographs on the evaluation of carcinogenic risks to humans. Vol. 60, Some industrial chemicals.* Lyon: World Health Organization, IARC.

Ivanov, V.A., Gaziev, A.I. and Tretyak, T.M. (1983) Exodeoxyribonuclease from rat brain specific for single-stranded DNA. *European Journal of Biochemistry* **137**, 517–22.

Ivanov, V.A., Tretyak, T.M. and Afonin, Y.N. (1988) Excision of apurinic and/or apyrimidinic sites from DNA by nucleolytical enzymes from rat brain. *European Journal of Biochemistry* **172**, 155–9.

Johnson, K.A., Gorzinski, S.J., Bodner, K.M., Campbell, R.A., Wolf, C.H., Friedman, M.A. and Mast, R.W. (1986) Chronic toxicity and oncogenicity study on acrylamide incorporated in the drinking water of Fischer 344 rats. *Toxicology and Applied Pharmacology* **85**, 154–68.

Jones, R.D. (1986) Epidemiology of brain tumours in man and their relationship with chemical agents. *Food and Chemical Toxicology* **24**, 99–103.

Karran, P., Hjelmgren, T. and Lindahl, T. (1982) Induction of a DNA glycosylase for *N*-methylated purines is part of the adaptive response to alkylating agents. *Nature* **296**, 770–3.

Kat, A., Thilly, W.G., Fang W.-H., Longley, M.J., Li, G.-M. and Modrich, P. (1993) An alkylation-tolerant, mutator human cell line is deficient in strand-specific mismatch repair. *Proceedings of the National Academy of Sciences U.S.A.* **90**, 6424–8.

Kaufmann, W.K. (1989) Commentary. Pathways of human cell post-replication repair. *Carcinogenesis* **10**, 1–11.

Kleihues, P. and Margison, G.P. (1974) Carcinogenicity of *N*-methyl-*N*-nitrosourea. Possible role of excision repair of O^6-methylguanine from DNA. *Journal of the National Cancer Institute* **53**, 1839–42.

Kleihues, P. and Rajewsky, M.F. (1984) Chemical neuro-oncogenesis: role of structural DNA modifications, DNA repair and neural target cell population. *Progress in Experimental Tumor Research* **27**, 1–16.

Kleihues, P., Bamborschke, S. and Doerjer, G. (1980) Persistence of alkylated DNA bases in the Mongolian gerbil (*Meriones unguiculatus*) following a single dose of methylnitrosourea. *Carcinogenesis* **1**, 111–13.

Kleihues, P., Lantos, P.L. and Magee, P.N. (1976) Chemical carcinogenesis in the nervous system. *International Review of Experimental Pathology* **15**, 153–232.

Knudson, A.G. Jr (1987) A two-mutation model for human cancer. In Klein, G. (ed.), *Advances in viral oncology*, Vol. 7. New York: Raven Press, 1–17.

Koepke, S.R., Kroeger-Koepke, M.P., Bosan, W., Thomas, B.J., Alvord, W.G. and Michejda, C.J. (1988) Alkylation of DNA in rats by *N*-nitrosomethyl-(2-hydroxyethyl)amine: dose response and persistence of the alkylated lesions *in vivo*. *Cancer Research* **48**, 1537–42.

Kokunai, T., Tamaki, N. and Matsumoto, S. (1987) Promoting effect of 12-*O*-tetradecanoylphorbol-13-acetate on neurogenic microtumors initiated by transplacental exposure to *N*-ethyl-*N*-nitrosourea. *Japanese Journal of Cancer Research (Gann)* **78**, 534–6.

Korr, H. (1980) *Proliferation of different cell types in the brain*. Advances in Anatomical and Embryological Cell Biology 61. Berlin: Springer-Verlag, 5–16.

Korr, H. and Schultze, B. (1989) Unscheduled DNA synthesis in various types of cells of the mouse brain *in vivo*. *Experimental Brain Research* **74**, 573–8.

Krokan, H., Haugen, A., Myrnes, B. and Guddal, P.H. (1983) Repair of premutagenic DNA lesions in human foetal tissues: evidence for low levels of O^6-methylguanine-DNA-methyl transferase and uracil DNA-glycosylase activity in some tissues. *Carcinogenesis* **4**, 1559–64.

Leach, F.S., Polyak, K., Burrell, M., Johnson, K.A., Hill, D., Dunlop, M.G., Wyllie, A.H., Peltomaki, P., de la Chappelle, A., Hamilton, S.R., Kinzler, K.W. and Vogelstein, B. (1996) Expression of the human mismatch repair gene *hMSH2* in normal and neoplastic tissues. *Cancer Research* **56**, 235–40.

Lee, G.S.-F., Blonsky, K.S., Van On, D.L., Savage, E.A., Morgan, A.R. and von Borstel, R.C. (1992) Base alterations in yeast induced by alkylating agents with differing Swain-Scott substrate constants. *Journal of Molecular Biology* **223**, 617–26.

Lee, L.-S., Chou, M.-D., Chi, C.-W., Liu, H.-C., Shih, Y.-H. and Liu, T.-Y. (1993) Aromatic DNA adducts in brain tumors by ^{32}P-postlabeling analysis. *Cancer Letters* **74**, 1–7.

Li, F., Segal, A. and Solomon, J.J. (1992) *In vitro* reaction of ethylene oxide with DNA and characterization of DNA adducts. *Chemico-Biological Interactions* **83**, 35–54.

Lindahl, T. and Nyberg, B. (1972) Rate of depurination of native DNA. *Biochemistry* **11**, 3610–18.

Loeb, L.A. (1989) Endogenous carcinogenesis: molecular oncology into the twenty-first century—presidential address. *Cancer Research* **49**, 5489–96.

Loeb, L.A. and Kunkel, T.A. (1982) Fidelity of DNA synthesis. *Annual Review of Biochemistry* **51**, 429–57.

Ludeke, B.I. and Kleihues, P. (1988) Formation and persistence of O^6-(2-hydroxyethyl)-2'-deoxyguanosine in DNA of various tissues following a single dose of *N*-nitroso-*N*-(2-hydroxyethyl)urea, an immuno-slot-blot study. *Carcinogenesis* **9**, 147–51.

Lukash, L.L., Boldt, J., Pegg, A.E., Dolan, M.E., Maher, V.M. and McCormick, J.J. (1991) Effect of O^6-alkylguanine-DNA alkyltransferase on the frequency and spectrum of mutations induced by *N*-methyl-*N'*-nitro-*N*-nitrosoguanidine in the *HPRT* gene of diploid human fibroblasts. *Mutation Research* **250**, 397–409.

Maekawa, A. and Mitsumori, K. (1990) Spontaneous occurrence and chemical induction of neurogenic tumors in rats – influence of host factors and specificity of chemical structure. *Critical Reviews in Toxicology* **20**, 287–310.

Maher, V.M., Domoradzki, J., Bhattacharyya, N.P., Tsujimura, T., Corner, R.C. and McCormick, J.J. (1990) Alkylation damage, DNA repair and mutagenesis in human cells. *Mutation Research* **233**, 235–45.

Marnett, L.J. and Burcham, P.C. (1993) Endogenous DNA adducts: potential and paradox. *Chemical Research in Toxicology* **6**, 771–85.

Marshall, C.J. (1991) Tumor suppressor genes. *Cell* **64**, 313–26.

Mastrangelo, G., Serena, R. and Marzia, V. (1993) Mortality from tumours in workers in an acrylic fibre factory. *Occupational Medicine* **43**, 155–8.

Matsunaga, T., Mu, D., Park, C.-H., Reardon, J.T. and Sancar, A. (1995) Human DNA repair excision nuclease: analysis of the roles of the subunits involved in dual incisions by using anti-XPG and anti-ERCC1 antibodies. *Journal of Biological Chemistry* **270**, 20862–9.

Mayer, J., Warburton, D., Jeffrey, A.M., Pero, R., Walles, S., Andrews, L., Toor, M., Latriano, L., Wazneh, L., Tang, D., Tsai, W.-Y., Kuroda, M. and Perera, F. (1991) Biologic markers in ethylene oxide-exposed workers and controls. *Mutation Research* **248**, 163–76.

Mazzarello, P., Poloni, M., Spadari, S. and Focher, F. (1992) DNA repair mechanisms in neurological diseases: facts and hypotheses. *Journal of Neurological Sciences* **112**, 4–14.

Melnick, R.L. and Kohn, M.C. (1995) Points of view. Mechanistic data indicate that 1,3-butadiene is a human carcinogen. *Carcinogenesis* **16**, 157–63.

Miller, E.C. and Miller, J.A. (1966) Mechanisms of chemical carcinogenesis: nature of proximate carcinogens and interactions with macromolecules. *Pharmacological Reviews* **18**, 805–38.

——(1974) Biochemical mechanisms of chemical carcinogenesis. In Busch, H. (ed.), *The molecular biology of cancer*. New York: Academic Press, 377–402.

Mineura, K., Izumi, I., Watanabe, K. and Kowada, M. (1991) O^6-alkylguanine-DNA alkyltransferase activity in human brain tumors. *Tohoku Journal of Experimental Medicine* **165**, 223–8.

——(1993) Influence of O^6-methylguanine-DNA methyltransferase activity on chloroethylnitrosourea chemotherapy in brain tumors. *International Journal of Cancer* **55**, 76–81.

Modrich, P. (1991) Mechanisms and biological effects of mismatch repair. *Annual Review of Genetics* **25**, 229–53.

——(1994) Mismatch repair, genetic stability, and cancer. *Science* **266**, 1959–60.

Mueller, B.A. and Gurney, J.G. (1992) Epidemiology of pediatric brain tumors. *Neurosurgery Clinics of North America* **3**, 715–21.

Naito, M., Aoyama, H. and Ito, A. (1985) Inhibitory effect of phenobarbital on the development of gliomas in WF rats treated neonatally with *N*-ethyl-*N*-nitrosourea. *Journal of the National Cancer Institute* **74**, 725–8.

Naito, M., Naito, Y. and Ito, A. (1982) Effect of phenobarbital on the development of tumors in mice treated neonatally with *N*-ethyl-*N*-nitrosourea. *Japanese Journal of Cancer Research* **73**, 111–14.

Nakamura, J., Walker, V.E. and Swenberg, J.A. (1993) DNA adduct formation and persistence in *N*-ethyl-*N*-nitrosourea-treated adult B6C3F1 mice. *Toxicologist* **13**, 108.

Nakaya, N., Sawasaki, Y., Teraoka, H., Nakajima, H. and Tsukada, K. (1977) Changes of DNA ligase in developing rat brain. *Journal of Biochemistry* **81**, 1575–7.

National Toxicology Program (NTP) (1988) *Toxicology and carcinogenesis studies of ethylene oxide (CAS No. 75-21-8) in B6C3F$_1$ mice (inhalation studies)*. Washington, D.C.: U.S. Department of Health and Human Services.

——(1990) *Toxicology and carcinogenesis studies of glycidol (CAS No. 556-52-5) in F344/N rats and B6C3F$_1$ mice (gavage studies)*. Technical report series 374. Washington, D.C.: U.S. Department of Health and Human Services.

Neglia, J.P., Meadows, A.T., Robison, L.L., Kim, T.H., Newton, W.A., Ruymann, F.B., Sather, H.N. and Hammond, G.D. (1991) Second neoplasms after acute lymphoblastic leukemia in childhood. *New England Journal of Medicine* **325**, 1330–6.

Norman, S.A., Berlin, J.A., Soper, K.A., Middendorf, B.F. and Stolley, P.D. (1995) Cancer incidence in a group of workers potentially exposed to ethylene oxide. *International Journal of Epidemiology* **24**, 276–84.

Olinski, R., Zastawny, T., Budzbon, J., Skokowski, J., Zegarski, W. and Dizdaroglu, M. (1992) DNA base modifications in chromatin of human cancerous tissues. *FEBS Letters* **309**, 193–8.

Olsson, M. and Lindahl, T. (1980) Repair of alkylated DNA in *Escherichia coli*. Methyl group transfer from O^6-methylguanine to a protein cysteine residue. *Journal of Biological Chemistry* **255**, 10569–71.

Ono, Y., Watanabe, M., Inoue, Y., Ohmoto, T., Akiyama, K., Tsutsui, K. and Seki, S. (1995) Developmental expression of APEX nuclease, a multifunctional DNA repair enzyme, in mouse brains. *Developmental Brain Research* **86**, 1–6.

Orren, D.K. and Sancar, A. (1987) New discoveries in the enzymology of DNA repair. *Cancer Reviews* **7**, 5–27.

Osterman-Golkar, S.M., MacNeela, J.P., Turner, M.J., Walker, V.E., Swenberg, J.A., Sumner, S.J., Youtsey, N. and Fennell, T.R. (1994) Monitoring exposure to acrylonitrile using adducts with *N*-terminal valine in hemoglobin. *Carcinogenesis* **15**, 2701–7.

Parker, S., Kirk, M.C. and Ludlum, D.B. (1987) Synthesis and characterization of O^6-(2-chloroethyl)guanine: a putative intermediate in the cytotoxic reation of chloroethylnitrosoureas with DNA. *Biochemical and Biophysical Research Communications* **148**, 1124–8.

Parsons, R., Li, G.-M., Longley, M.J., Fang, W.-H., Papadopoulos, N., Jen, J., de la Chapelle, A., Kinzler, K.W., Vogelstein, B. and Modrich, P. (1993) Hypermutability and mismatch repair deficiency in RER$^+$ tumor cells. *Cell* **75**, 1227–36.

Pegg, A.E. (1990) Mammalian O^6-alkylguanine-DNA alkyltransferase: regulation and importance in response to alkylating carcinogenic and therapeutic agents. *Cancer Research* **50**, 6119–29.

Pegg, A.E. and Byers, T.L. (1992) Repair of DNA containing O^6-alkylguanine. *FASEB Journal* **6**, 2302–10.

Peterson, D.L., Sheridan, P.J. and Brown, W.E. Jr (1994) Animal models for brain tumors: historical perspectives and future directions. *Journal of Neurosurgery* **80**, 865–76.

Polednak, A.P. and Flannery, J.T. (1995) Brain, other central nervous system, and eye cancer. *Cancer* **75** (Suppl. 1), 330–7.

Price, A. (1993) The repair of ionising radiation-induced damage to DNA. *Seminars in Cancer Biology* **4**, 61–71.

Purves, D. and Dayan, A. (1992) A preliminary investigation of promotion of brain tumours by hexachlorophane in Sprague-Dawley rats transplacentally exposed to *N*-ethylnitrosourea. *Neuropathology and Applied Neurobiology* **18**, 259–64.

Rajagopal, S.V. and Subba Rao, K. (1992) Purification and properties of a deoxyribonuclease (acid DNase) from rat brain. *Biochemical Archives* **8**, 135–42.

Rakic, P. (1985) Limits of neurogenesis in primates. *Science* **227**, 1054–6.

Randerath, K., Reddy, M.V. and Disher, R.M. (1986) Age- and tissue-related DNA modifications in untreated rats: detection by ^{32}P-postlabeling assay and possible significance for spontaneous tumor induction and aging. *Carcinogenesis* **7**, 1615–17.

Randerath, K., Putman, K.L., Osterburg, H.H., Johnson, S.A., Morgan, D.G. and Finch, C.E. (1993) Age-dependent increases of DNA adducts (I-compounds) in human and rat brain DNA. *Mutation Research* **295**, 11–18.

Riley, P.A. (1994) Free radicals in biology: oxidative stress and the effects of ionizing radiation. *International Journal of Radiation Biology* **65**, 27–33.

Robson, C.N., Hochhauser, D., Craig, R., Rack, K., Buckle, V.J. and Hickson, I.D. (1992) Structure of the human DNA repair gene *HAP1* and its localisation to chromosome 14q 11.2-12. *Nucleic Acids Research* **20**, 4417–21.

Ron, E., Modan, B., Boice, J.D. Jr, Alfandary, E., Stovall, M., Chetrit, A. and Katz, L. (1988) Tumors of the brain and nervous system after radiotherapy in childhood. *New England Journal of Medicine* **319**, 1033–9.

Rubinstein, L.J. (1972) *Tumors of the central nervous system*. Atlas of Tumor Pathology, second series, fascicle 6. Washington, D.C.: Armed Forces Institute of Pathology.

Rupert, C.S. (1975) Enzymatic photoreactivation: overview. In Hanawalt, P.C. and Setlow, R.B. (eds), *Molecular mechanisms for repair of DNA, Part A*. New York: Plenum Press, 73–87.

Russell, S.J., Ye, Y.W., Waber, P.G., Shuford, M., Schold, S.C. and Nisen, P.D. (1995) *p53* mutations, O^6-alkylguanine DNA alkyltransferase activity, and sensitivity to procarbazine in human brain tumors. *Cancer* **75**, 1339–42.

Sancar, A. (1994) Perspectives: mechanisms of DNA excision repair. *Science* **266**, 1954–6.

Sancar, A. and Sancar, G.B. (1988) DNA repair enzymes. *Annual Review of Biochemistry* **57**, 29–67.

Sancar, A. and Tang, M.-S. (1993) Nucleotide excision repair. *Photochemistry and Photobiology* **57**, 905–21.

Schold, S.C. Jr, Brent, T.P., von Hofe, E., Friedman, H.S., Mitra, S., Bigner, D.D., Swenberg, J.A. and Kleihues, P. (1989) O^6-alkylguanine-DNA alkyltransferase and sensitivity to procarbazine in human brain-tumor xenografts. *Journal of Neurosurgery* **70**, 573–7.

Schulte, P.A., Boeniger, M., Walker, J.T., Schober, S.E., Pereira, M.A., Gulati, D.K, Wojciechowski, J.P., Garza, A., Froelich, R., Strauss, G., Halperin, W.E., Herrick, R. and Griffith, J. (1992) Biologic markers in hospital workers exposed to low levels of ethylene oxide. *Mutation Research* **278**, 237–51.

Segal, A., Solomon, J.J. and Mukai, F. (1990) *In vitro* reactions of glycidol with pyrimidine bases in calf thymus DNA. *Cancer Biochemistry Biophysics* **11**, 59–67.

Segerbäck, D. (1990) Reaction products in hemoglobin and DNA after *in vitro* treatment with ethylene oxide and *N*-(2-hydroxyethyl)-*N*-nitrosourea. *Carcinogenesis* **11**, 307–12.

Seki, S., Akiyama, K., Watanabe, S., Hatsushika, M., Ikeda, S. and Tsutsui, K. (1991) cDNA and deduced amino acid sequence of a mouse DNA repair enzyme (APEX nuclease) with significant homology to *Escherichia coli* exonuclease III. *Journal of Biological Chemistry* **266**, 20797–802.

Seki, S., Hatsushika, M., Watanabe, S., Akiyama, K., Nagao, K. and Tsutsui, K. (1992) cDNA cloning, sequencing, expression and possible domain structure of human APEX nuclease homologous to *Escherichia coli* exonuclease III. *Biochimica et Biophysica Acta* **1131**, 287–99.

Silber, J.R., Mueller, B.A., Ewers, T.G. and Berger, M.S. (1993) Comparison of O^6-methylguanine-DNA methyltransferase activity in brain tumors and adjacent normal brain. *Cancer Research* **53**, 3416–20.

Singer, B. and Essigmann, J.M. (1991) Site-specific mutagenesis: retrospective and prospective. *Carcinogenesis* **12**, 949–55.

Singer, B. and Grunberger, D. (1983) *Molecular biology of mutagens and carcinogens*. New York: Plenum Press.

Skopek, T.R., Walker, V.E., Cochrane, J.E., Craft, T.R. and Cariello, N.F. (1992) Mutational spectrum at the *Hprt* locus in splenic T cells of $B6C3F_1$ mice exposed to *N*-ethyl-*N*-nitrosourea. *Proceedings of the National Academy of Sciences U.S.A.* **89**, 7866–70.

Snellings, W.M., Weil, C.S. and Maronpot, R.R. (1984) A two-year inhalation study of carcinogenic potential of ethylene oxide in Fischer 344 rats. *Toxicology and Applied Pharmacology* **75**, 105–17.

Solleveld, H.A., Bigner, D.D., Averill, D.R. Jr, Bigner, S.H., Boorman, G.A., Burger, P.C., Gillespie, G.Y., Hubbard, G.B., Laerum, O.D., McComb, R.D., McGrath, J.T., Morgan, K.T., Peters, A., Rubinstein, L.J., Schoenberg, B.S., Schold, S.C. Jr, Swenberg, J.A., Thompson, M.B., Vandevelde, M. and Vinores, S.A. (1986) Brain tumors in man and animals: a report of a workshop. *Environmental Health Perspectives* **68**, 155–73.

Spadari, S., Focher, F. and Hübscher, U. (1988) Developmental activity profile of DNA polymerases δ and α in rat neurons suggests a coordinated *in vivo* function. *In vivo* **2**, 317–20.

Subba Rao, K. (1993) Genomic damage and its repair in young and aging brain. *Molecular Neurobiology* **7**, 23–48.

Subba Rao, K. and Loeb, L.A. (1992) DNA damage and repair in brain: relationship to aging. *Mutation Research* **275**, 317–29.

Subba Rao, K.V. and Subba Rao, K. (1982) Changes in DNA, RNA and protein and the activities of acid and alkaline deoxyribonucleases in grey and white matter regions of developing and aging rat cerebrum. *Mechanisms of Ageing and Development* **18**, 225–38.

Subba Rao, K., Martin, G.M. and Loeb, L.A. (1985) Fidelity of DNA polymerase-β in neurons from young and very aged mice. *Journal of Neurochemistry* **45**, 1273–8.

Swenberg, J.A. (1982) Neoplasms of the nervous system. In Foster, H.L., Small, J.D. and Fox, J.G. (eds), *The mouse in biomedical research. Vol. IV, Experimental biology and oncology*. New York: Academic Press, 529–37.

Swenberg, J.A., Richardson, F.C., Boucheron, J.A. and Dyroff, M.C. (1985) Relationships between DNA adduct formation and carcinogenesis. *Environmental Health Perspectives* **62**, 177–83.

Swenberg, J.A., Richardson, F.C., Boucheron, J.A., Deal, F.H., Belinsky, S.A., Charbonneau, M. and Short, B.G. (1987) High- to low-dose extrapolation: critical determinants involved in dose response of carcinogenic substances. *Environmental Health Perspectives* **76**, 57–63.

Swenberg, J.A., Fedtke, N., Fennell, T.R. and Walker, V.E. (1990) Relationships between carcinogen exposure, DNA adducts and carcinogenesis. In Clayson, D.B., Munro, I.C., Shubik, P. and Swenberg, J.A. (eds), *Progress in predictive toxicology*. Amsterdam: Elsevier, 161–84.

Szatrowski, T.P. and Nathan, C.F. (1991) Production of large amounts of hydrogen peroxide by human tumor cells. *Cancer Research* **51**, 794–8.

Tan, B.H., Bencsath, F.A. and Gaubatz, J.W. (1990) Steady-state levels of 7-methylguanine increase in nuclear DNA of postmitotic mouse tissues during aging. *Mutation Research* **237**, 229–38.

Tanigawa, H., Ondera, H. and Maekawa, A. (1995) Effects of barbital on neuro-oncogenesis in a transplacental model using F344 rats. *Journal of Toxicological Sciences* **20**(1), 55–65.

Tates, A.D., Grummt, T., Törnqvist, M., Farmer, P.B., van Dam, F.J., van Mossel, H., Schoemaker, H.M., Osterman-Golkar, S., Uebel, Ch., Tang, Y.S., Zwinderman, A.H., Natarajan, A.T. and Ehrenberg, L. (1991) Biological and chemical monitoring of occupational exposure to ethylene oxide. *Mutation Research* **250**, 483–97.

Thompson, L.H., Busch, D.B., Brookman, K., Mooney, C.L. and Glaser, D.A. (1981) Genetic diversity of UV-sensitive DNA repair mutants of Chinese hamster ovary cells. *Proceedings of the National Academy of Sciences U.S.A.* **78**, 3734–7.

Tong, W.P., Kirk, M.C. and Ludlum, D.B. (1981) Molecular pharmacology of the haloethyl nitrosoureas:

formation of 6-hydroxyethylguanine in DNA treated with BCNU (*N,N'*-bis[2-chloroethyl]-*N*-nitrosourea). *Biochemical and Biophysical Research Communications* **100**, 351–7.

——(1982) Formation of the cross-link 1-[N^3-deoxycytidyl],2-[N^1-deoxyguanosinyl]-ethane in DNA treated with *N,N'*-bis(2-chloroethyl)-*N*-nitrosourea. *Cancer Research* **42**, 3102–5.

Törnqvist, M. (1988) Hemoglobin adducts in animals exposed to gasoline and diesel exhausts, 1. Alkenes. *Journal of Applied Toxicology* **8**, 159–70.

Törnqvist, M., Gustafsson, B., Kautiainen, A., Harms-Ringdahl, M., Granath, F. and Ehrenberg, L. (1989) Unsaturated lipids and intestinal bacteria as sources of endogenous production of ethene and ethylene oxide. *Carcinogenesis* **10**, 39–41.

Tsang, R.W., Laperriere, N.J., Simpson, W.J., Brierley, M.B., Panzarella, T. and Smyth, H.S. (1993) Glioma arising after radiation therapy for pituitary adenoma. *Cancer* **72**, 2227–33.

Venugopal, J. and Subba Rao, K. (1993) A broad-specific alkaline DNase from rat brain with a putative role in DNA excision repair. *Biochemistry and Molecular Biology International* **30**, 995–1004.

Verri, A., Verzeletti, S., Mazzarello, P., Spadari, S., Negri, M., Bunone, G., Della Valle, G., Hübscher, U. and Focher, F. (1992) DNA synthesis enzymes and proliferating cell nuclear antigen in normal and neoplastic nerve cells. *Anticancer Research* **12**, 1099–106.

Walker, J.S. and Bigner, D.D. (1985a) Virus-induced brain tumors. In Wilkins, R.H. and Rengachary, S.S. (eds), *Neurosurgery*, Vol. 1. New York: McGraw-Hill, 522–5.

——(1985b) Radiation-induced brain tumors. In Wilkins, R.H. and Rengachary, S.S. (eds), *Neurosurgery*, Vol. 1. New York: McGraw-Hill, 525–8.

——(1985c) Chemically induced brain tumors, primary and transplanted. In Wilkins, R.H. and Rengachary, S.S. (eds), *Neurosurgery*, Vol. 1. New York: McGraw-Hill, 528–31.

Walker, V.E. and Skopek, T.R. (1993) A mouse model for the study of *in vivo* mutational spectra: sequence specificity of ethylene oxide at the *hprt* locus. *Mutation Research* **288**, 151–62.

Walker, V.E. and Swenberg, J.A. (1989) Phenobarbital lacks promoting activity for neurogenic tumors in F344 rats transplacentally exposed to ethylnitrosourea. *Journal of Neuropathology and Experimental Neurology* **48**, 263–9.

Walker, V.E., Fennell, T.R., Boucheron, J.A., Fedtke, N., Ciroussel, F. and Swenberg, J.A. (1990) Macromolecular adducts of ethylene oxide: a literature review and a time-course study on the formation of 7-(2-hydroxyethyl)guanine following exposures of rats by inhalation. *Mutation Research* **233**, 151–64.

Walker, V.E., Fennell, T.R., Upton, P.B., Skopek, T.R., Prevost, V., Shuker, D.E.G. and Swenberg, J.A. (1992) Molecular dosimetry of ethylene oxide: formation and persistence of 7-(2-hydroxyethyl)guanine in DNA following repeated exposures of rats and mice. *Cancer Research* **52**, 4328–34.

Walker, V.E., Fennell, T.R., Upton, P.B., MacNeela, J.P. and Swenberg, J.A. (1993) Molecular dosimetry of DNA and hemoglobin adducts in mice and rats exposed to ethylene oxide. *Environmental Health Perspectives* **99**, 11–17.

Walker, V.E., Morgan, K.T., Zimmerman, H.M. and Innes, J.R.M. (1994) Tumours of the central and peripheral nervous system. In Turusov, V.S. and Mohr, U. (eds), *Pathology of tumours in laboratory animals. Vol. II, Tumours of the mouse.* Second edition. IARC Scientific Publications 111. Lyon: IARC, 731–76.

Walker, V.E., Gorelick, N.J., Andrews, J.L., Craft, T.R., deBoer, J.G., Glickman, B.W. and Skopek, B.W. (1996) Frequency and spectrum of ethylnitrosourea-induced mutation at the *hprt* and *lacI* loci in splenic lymphocytes of exposed *lacI* transgenic mice. *Cancer Research*, **56**, 4654–61.

Walter, C.A., Lu, J., Bhakta, M., Mitra, S., Dunn, W., Herbert, D.C., Weaker, F.J., Hoog, T., Garza, P., Adrian, G.S. and Kamolvarin, N. (1993) Brain and liver targeted overexpression of O^6-methylguanine DNA methyltransferase in transgenic mice. *Carcinogenesis* **14**, 1537–43.

Ward, J.M. and Rice, J.M. (1982) Naturally occurring and chemically induced brain tumors in rats and mice in carcinogenesis bioassays. *Annals of the New York Academy of Sciences* **381**, 304–19.

Waser, J., Hübscher, U., Kuenzle, C.C. and Spadari, S. (1979) DNA polymerase β from brain neurons is a repair enzyme. *European Journal of Biochemistry* **97**, 361–8.

Washington, W.J., Dunn, W.C. Jr, Generoso, W.M. and Mitra, S. (1988) Tissue-specific variation in repair activity for 3-methyladenine in DNA in two stocks of mice. *Mutation Research* **207**, 165–9.

Washington, W.J., Foote, R.S., Dunn, W.C., Generoso, W.M. and Mitra, S. (1989) Age-dependent modulation of tissue-specific repair activity for 3-methyladenine and O^6-methylguanine in DNA in inbred mice. *Mechanisms of Ageing and Development* **48**, 43–52.

Watkins, D. and Rouleau, G.A. (1992) Oncogenes and glial tumors. *Revue Neurologique* **148**, 402–7.

Weisburger, E.K. (1977) Bioassay program for carcinogenic hazards of cancer chemotherapeutic agents. *Cancer* **40**, 1935–49.

Weng, Y. and Sirover, M.A. (1993) Developmental regulation of the base excision repair enzyme uracil DNA glycosylase in the rat. *Mutation Research* **293**, 133–41.

Wu, K.-Y., Ranasinghe, A., Upton, P., Scheller, N. and Swenberg, J.A. (1996) Endogenous formation of the major DNA adduct of ethylene oxide in humans, rats, and mice. (Abstract) *Proceedings of the American Association for Cancer Research* **37**, 102.

Yates, J.M., Sumner, S.C.J., Turner, M.J. Jr, Recio, L. and Fennell, T.R. (1993) Characterization of an adduct and its degradation product produced by the reaction of cyanoethylene oxide with deoxythymidine and DNA. *Carcinogenesis* **14**, 1363–9.

Zaidi, N.H., Liu, L. and Gerson, S.L. (1996) Quantitative immunohistochemical estimates of O^6-alkylguanine-

DNA alkyltransferase expression in normal and malignant human colon. *Clinical Cancer Research* **2**, 577–84.

Zeller, W.J., Fruhauf, S., Chen, G., Eisenbrand, G. and Lijinsky, W. (1989) Biological activity of hydroxylated chloroethylnitrosoureas. *Cancer Research* **49**, 3267–70.

Zimmerman, H.M. (1973) Brain tumors. In Busch, H. (ed.), *Methods in cancer research*, Vol. 10. New York: Academic Press, 105–26.

Zülch, K.J. (1986) *Brain tumors: their biology and pathology*. Third completely revised edition. Berlin: Springer-Verlag.

CHAPTER 6

Experimental tumors and the evaluation of neurocarcinogens

JOHN H. SAMPSON AND DARELL D. BIGNER

This chapter covers an exceptionally broad range of topics and is divided essentially into four parts. It begins with a brief overview of the types of nervous system tumors found in animals, ranging from insects to primates, in order to demonstrate that the peril of nervous system tumors is not solely the property of human beings. In addition, in the same section, more detailed information is provided on the incidence and types of tumors found in common laboratory animals, so that researchers will be able to determine whether, and to what degree, the appearance of spontaneous tumors in these animals might interfere with experimental results. In the second section, the induction of nervous system tumors in animals using physical agents such as ionizing radiation, viruses and chemicals is reviewed. The induction of central and peripheral nervous system (PNS) and pituitary tumors in transgenic mice is also discussed in this section. The third section is devoted to a discussion of the scientific methods used to assess evidence implicating various compounds as neurocarcinogens. The 'weight-of-evidence' approach is outlined in this section and illustrates that theoretical, pathobiologic and statistical evidence must all be incorporated into such assessments. Finally, the last section reviews experimental nervous system tumor models. The transplantation of tumor xenografts from the human nervous system into immunoincompetent animals, such as *nu* or *SCID* mice, is described, as are the more commonly used nervous system tumor models of immunocompetent rodents. The potential pitfalls of artificially induced tumors and the importance of identifying and minimizing the genetic diversity between tumor cell lines and their animal host are emphasized.

Spontaneous nervous system tumors in animals

Tumors of the nervous system are not a manifestation of disease unique in the human being. Evidence for the existence of tumors within the nervous system and the pituitary gland is available in several species, ranging from insects to nonhuman primates (Table 6.1). Although factors such as the age of the animal at autopsy and the completeness of the

Table 6.1 Spontaneous tumors of the nervous system identified in animals

Species	Type of tumor[a]
Fruit flies	Recessively inherited, transplantable nervous system tumor identified in larvae
Oysters	Ganglioneuroma
Bony fish	Astrocytoma, ependymoblastoma, neurofibroma, neurofibrosarcoma, olfactory neuroblastoma, pituitary adenoma, schwannoma
Sharks	Fourth-ventricular choroid plexus papilloma
Reptiles	Olfactory neuroblastoma
Birds	Ependymoma, glioblastoma multiforme, hemangioendothelioma of the choroid plexus, optic glioma, pinealoma and pinealblastoma, pituitary adenoma, teratoma
Mice	Astrocytoma, ependymoma, benign and malignant schwannoma, choriod plexus papilloma, glioblastoma multiforme, granular-cell tumors, lipoma, malignant nerve sheath tumor, medulloblastoma, meningioma, metastatic leukemia and lymphoma, neurofibroma, oligodendroglioma, pituitary adenoma and carcinomasarcoma, teratoma
Rats	Astrocytoma, benign and malignant schwannoma, chordoma, choroid plexus papilloma and carcinoma, craniopharyngioma, ependymoblastoma, ependymoma, glioblastoma multiforme, granular-cell tumor, medulloblastoma, meningioma, neurofibroma, neurofibrosarcoma, oligodendroglioma, optic glioma, optic nerve ganglioneuroma, pinealoma, pituitary adenoma and carcinoma, primary lymphoma
Cats	Astroblastoma, astrocytoma, ependymoma, fibrillary astrocytoma, gangliocytoma, medulloblastoma, meningeal sarcoma, meningioma (usually in third ventricle and occasionally producing metastatic lesions), mixed glioma, pituitary adenoma
Dogs	Angioblastoma, astroblastoma, astrocytoma, chordoma, choroid plexus papilloma and carcinoma, craniopharyngioma, ependymoma, epidermoid and dermoid cyst, gangliocytoma and ganglioglioma, germ-cell tumor, glioblastoma multiforme, granular-cell tumor, hypothalamic hamartoma, infundibuloma, lipoma, medulloblastoma, meningioma, metastatic neoplasms of the brain and spine, microgliomatosis, oligodendroglioma, paraganglioma of the temporal bone and spine, pinealoma, pituitary adenoma and carcinoma, sarcoma of the brain and meninges, schwannomas and neurofibromas of cranial and peripheral nerves, spongioblastoma, teratocarcinoma
Agricultural animals	Angioblastoma, astrocytoma, choroid plexus papilloma, ependymoma, glioblastoma multiforme, granular-cell tumor, lipoma, medulloblastoma, meningeal sarcoma, meningioma, microglioma, nerve sheath tumor, oligodenroglioma, pinealoma, spongioblastoma, trigeminal ganglioglioma, vestibular and vagal schwannoma
Wild and zoo animals	Astrocytoma, ependymoma, gemistocytic astrocytoma, lipoma, meningioma, neurofibroma, oligodendroglioma, pinealoma, schwannoma
Nonhuman primates	Astrocytoma, glioblastoma multiforme, lipoma of the choroid plexus, olfactory neuroblastoma, oligodendroglioma, pituitary adenoma, retinoblastoma

[a] Histologic diagnosis is given as reported by original authors and many do not conform to modern nomenclature systems. Where possible, such reports should be confirmed by direct inspection of original histologic sections.

evaluation do tend to bias statistics on the prevalence of nervous system tumors encountered within a species, the prevalence and histologic type of nervous system tumors do appear to vary considerably across species boundaries.

Reliable data on the existence of central nervous system (CNS) tumors in insects have been presented, and consist of the demonstration by Gateff and Schneiderman (1969) of a transplantable nervous system tumor in *Drosophila* larvae, the tumor being due to the recessively inherited *l(2)gl*[4] gene on the second chromosome. Nervous system tumors have also been identified in invertebrates and lower vertebrates. In this group, PNS tumors

Table 6.2 Incidence of central nervous system tumors in dogs (modified from Bigner and Swenberg, 1977, with permission)

References	No. of cases	No. of CNS tumors	% with CNS tumors	% of CNS tumors of neuroectodermal origin
Hjärre, 1938	3720	23	0.62	100.0
Dahme and Schiefer, 1960	2258	22	0.97	54.5
McGrath, 1962a	6175	118	1.91	69.5
Müller, 1964	5722	4	0.07	75.0
Howard and Nielsen, 1965	1500	11	0.73	63.5
Schiefer *et al.*, 1970	8013	62	0.77	72.0
Overall	27 388	240	0.88	71.7

such as schwannomas, neurofibromas and neurofibrosarcomas are relatively common, whereas CNS tumors are rare, especially in reptiles. The Registry of Tumors in Lower Animals (National Museum of Natural History, Smithsonian Institution, Washington, D.C.) maintains the most comprehensive record of nervous system tumors found in this group of animals (Harshbarger, 1978), and includes the only reported example of a CNS tumor in a reptile, an olfactory neuroblastoma (Harshbarger, J.C., personal communication to J.H.S., 1995). Similarly, sparse reports of nervous system neoplasms in birds can be found in the literature. Pituitary adenomas, however, have been reported quite frequently in parakeets (Schlumberger, 1954), and some of the spontaneous and hormonally induced pituitary tumors in parakeets have been developed into transplantable cell lines (Schlumberger, 1956).

About 1.6% of confirmed tumors in cats originate from the nervous system or its coverings (Hayes, Priester and Pendergrass, 1975). According to most authors mesenchymal tumors, mostly meningiomas (McGrath, 1962b; Luginbühl, 1963; Whitehead, 1967), are the predominant tumor type, and these occur primarily in older cats (Luginbühl, 1961). An unusually high number of these meningiomas are located in the third ventricle (Luginbühl, 1961), but no explanation for this preferential localization has been offered.

Tumors of the CNS have been described only rarely in domestic farm animals, but the paucity of publications on brain tumors in these animal species can probably be explained by the fact that they are autopsied infrequently and, as a rule, do not reach old age. From those cases that have been reported, it appears that PNS tumors are more common than CNS tumors, and mesenchymal tumors are more frequent than gliomas (Vitovec, 1976; Cotchin, 1977). Tumors of the PNS are exceptionally common in horses, and one report indicates that 4.2% of tumors in horses are nerve sheath tumors, making these tumors the fourth most common tumor in the horse (Sundberg *et al.*, 1977). Tumors of the CNS are, however, more frequently reported in cattle than in other domestic farm animals, with glioblastomas multiforme (GBM) and medulloblastoma predominating (Luginbühl, Fankhauser and McGrath, 1968; Bigner and Swenberg, 1977).

Although nervous system tumors of various types have been reported only sporadically in other wild and zoo animals, it is probably no accident that descriptions of brain tumors in nonhuman primates are rare. During autopsies of more than 100 000 young monkeys that were used for vaccination experiments, several nervous system malformations (cavernous hemangioma, tuberous sclerosis and syringomyelia with hyperplastic gliosis), but only a rare CNS tumor, could be found in serial microscopic sections of monkey brains (Newberne and Robinson, 1960). Most of these monkeys, however, would be comparable to a group of healthy young adult humans, where CNS neoplasms would also be expected to be a rare finding. However, the autopsy findings of Lapin and Yakovleva (1963) in 1274 monkeys (macaques, baboons and green long-tailed monkeys) do provide some evidence for the conclusion that CNS tumors are significantly less frequent in nonhuman primates than in humans. Most of the animals in the study by Lapin and Yakovleva died of spontaneous diseases, and some had reached a rather old age (maximum 23 years) for monkeys. The fact that no CNS tumors were found in this study provides much support for such a conclusion.

Human beings and domestic dogs appear to have the highest incidence of nervous system tumors in the animal kingdom. About 1% of autopsied dogs have neoplasms of the CNS (Table 6.2), but since only a very small percentage of the total dog population is completely autopsied, these figures may be biased. A comparison of nervous system tumor data between humans and dogs reveals remarkable similarities. The range and prevalence of tumor types found in dogs is similar to the brain tumor types seen in humans, and metastatic lesions have also been identified (Table 6.1). Immunohistochemical evaluation has also revealed similarities, and canine astrocytomas have been shown to stain positive for vimentin and glial fibrillary acidic protein (GFAP) (Moore, Madewell and Lund, 1989). Also, of the primary CNS tumors in dogs, about 70% are of neuroectodermal origin, which is similar to the proportion of these types of tumors in humans. Dogs, though, do tend to have a higher proportion of undifferentiated gliomas (Solleveld *et al.*, 1986). Some researchers who have examined a high proportion of brachycephalic dogs have reported that oligodendrogliomas are more common in dogs than in humans (Luginbühl, 1963). Others (McGrath, 1960), however, place the proportion of oligodendrogliomas at approximately 15%, which is nearer the proportion reported for humans. The age at which dogs are most at risk for CNS tumors also mirrors that of humans. As in humans (Feldman *et al.*, 1986), the risk of CNS tumors in dogs generally increases with age. The peak risk for glial tumors in dogs occurs at 10–14 years and declines slightly after that time, whereas the risk for meningeal tumors peaks at 7–9 years and then remains constant (Hayes, Priester and Pendergrass, 1975). In addition, young dogs, like children, also have an increased risk of CNS neoplasms. A comparison between dogs ≤6 months of age with those >6 months of age referred to the Veterinary Medical Data Program (National Cancer Institute, College of Veterinary Medicine, Michigan State University) demonstrated that the young dogs had a statistically significant increase in tumors of the brain and hematopoietic system (Keller and Madewell, 1992). Although the tumor types in these young dogs did not mirror the histologic spectrum of CNS tumors found in human infants, other investigators have reported that relatively young dogs do have a predisposition for tumors, such as medulloblastoma, that are more common in children (Luginbühl, Fankhauser and McGrath, 1968).

The breed of dog strongly influences the incidence of certain types of brain tumors. For example, although meningiomas occur relatively frequently in dolichocephalic animals, such as the German shepherd, gliomas occur more frequently in brachycephalic breeds, especially the English bulldog, boxer and Boston terrier (Hjärre, 1938; McGrath, 1960; Luginbühl, 1962; Hayes, Priester and Pendergrass, 1975). The sex of the dog has also been cited as a risk factor; some reports show an increased incidence for gliomas in males (Solleveld *et al.*, 1986), but this has not been seen in all studies (Hayes, Priester and Pendergrass, 1975). Finally, PNS tumors are also not rare in dogs, and a convincing case of neurofibromatosis type 1 has even been reported (Goedegebuure, 1975).

COMMON LABORATORY ANIMALS

Although not intended to be an exhaustive list of nervous system tumors in animals, the examples given above are provided in order to convey the range of tumors observed in diverse animal groups. An attempt was made to convey an approximation of the prevalence of these types of tumors; unfortunately, extracting such information primarily from case reports makes the true prevalence difficult to discern. Specific information on the prevalence and types of spontaneous tumors in common laboratory rodents is available, however. It is provided below in Tables 6.3 and 6.4. This information is provided to make it easier for the reader to decide whether, and to what extent, there is misinterpretation or bias of experimental results due to the occurrence of spontaneous nervous system tumors in common laboratory rodent models of nervous system tumors. Spontaneous brain tumors have been described only rarely in laboratory rodents, although laboratory animals are autopsied more frequently than are wild animals. Of course, the brains of laboratory rodents are not always examined, the spinal cords are rarely examined, and one could easily overlook brain tumors in smaller species. Still, the incidence of spontaneous tumors in laboratory rodents, in general, is much less than that in humans or dogs.

Laboratory mice

With the exception of certain strains, spontaneous CNS tumors in mice are quite rare and generally arise in older animals (Zimmerman and Innes, 1979; Morgan *et al.*, 1984; Solleveld *et al.*, 1986). Excluding the highly susceptible strains, the prevalence of CNS tumors in mice is usually reported as <0.1%. However, in series where thousands of mice have been examined, the prevalence has been reported to be as low as 0.01% (Morgan *et al.*, 1984; Fraser, 1986). The incidence of relevant tumors found in control B6C3F1 mice during the National Toxicology Programs' (NTPs') chronic carcinogenicity testing are given in Table 6.3. The most frequently diagnosed tumors are low-grade gliomas, lipomas, pituitary adenomas and meningiomas (Fraser, 1971, 1986; Morgan *et al.*, 1984; Solleveld *et al.*, 1986). Glial tumors in mice have a morphology similar to that of human gliomas (Zimmerman and

Table 6.3 Nervous system tumor incidences in untreated and corn oil gavage control B6C3F1 mice used in 2-year NTP carcinogenicity studies for a 5-year period ending June 1, 1994[a]

		Male						Female					
		Untreated			Corn oil gavage			Untreated			Corn oil gavage		
Location	Tumor type	Rate	Rate (%)	Range (%)	Rate	Rate (%)	Range (%)	Rate	Rate (%)	Range (%)	Rate	Rate (%)	Range (%)
Cranial	Oligodendroglioma	1/1469	0.1	0–2	0/946	0	–	1/1463	0.1	0–2	0/943	0	–
	Lipoma	1/1469	0.1	0–2	0/946	0	–	0/1463	0	–	0/943	0	–
	Sarcoma	0/1469	0	–	0/946	0	–	1/1463	0.1	0–2	0/943	0	–
Pituitary (pars distalis)	Adenoma	3/1354	0.2	0–6	2/848	0.2	0–2	212/1392	15.2	0–36	126/879	14.3	2–51
	Carcinoma	0/1354	0	–	0/848	0	–	8/1392	0.6	0–4	2/879	0.2	0–2
Pituitary (pars intermedia)	Adenoma	2/1354	0.1	0–2	0/848	0	–	5/1392	0.4	0–2	5/879	0.6	0–4
	Carcinoma	0/1354	0	–	0/848	0	–	1/1392	0.1	0–2	0/879	0	–
Integument/ s.c. tissue[b]	Malignant schwannoma	5/1474	0.3	0–6	0/952	0	–	1/1470	0.1	0–2	1/951	0.1	0–2
	Neurofibrosarcoma	1/1474	0.1	0–2	3/952	0.3	0–4	2/1470	0.1	0–2	1/951	0.1	0–2
Total body	All benign	639/1474	43.4	22–76	469/952	49.3	34–46	607/1470	41.3	22–62	350/951	36.8	12–68
	All malignant	611/1474	41.5	22–60	372/952	39.1	29–58	609/1470	41.3	26–60	332/951	34.9	6–60
	Total tumors	1014/1474	68.8	46–92	669/952	70.3	50–86	984/1470	66.9	48–80	566/951	59.5	18–86

[a] From J.K. Haseman and M.R. Elwell, personal communication to J.H.S., 1996, by permission.

[b] s.c., subcutaneous.

Table 6.4 Nervous system tumor incidences in untreated and corn oil gavage control Fischer 344 rats used in 2-year NTP carcinogenicity studies from 1 January 1977 to 29 April 1987[a]

		Male						Female					
		Untreated			Corn oil gavage			Untreated			Corn oil gavage		
Location	Tumor type	Rate	Rate (%)	Range (%)	Rate	Rate (%)	Range (%)	Rate	Rate (%)	Range (%)	Rate	Rate (%)	Range (%)
Cranial	Astrocytoma	9/1928	0.5	0–4	16/1943	0.8	0–4	18/1969	0.9	0–6	10/1946	0.5	0–4
	Granular-cell tumor	4/1928	0.2	0–2	3/1943	0.2	0–4	0/1969	0	0	5/1946	0.3	0–2
	Meningioma	2/1928	0.1	0–2	2/1943	0.1	0–2	2/1969	0.1	0–2	0/1946	0	0
	Oligodendroglioma	2/1928	0.1	0–2	1/1943	0.1	0–2	3/1969	0.2	0–2	1/1946	0.1	0–2
	Glioma NOS[b]	2/1928	0.1	0–2	3/1943	0.2	0–2	2/1969	0.1	0–2	2/1946	0.1	0–2
	Ependymoma	0/1928	0	0	2/1943	0.1	0–2	0/1969	0	0	1/1946	0.1	0–2
	Medulloblastoma	1/1928	0.1	0–2	0/1943	0	0	1/1969	0.1	0–2	0/1946	0	0
Spinal	Malignant schwannoma	1/1936	0.1	0–3	1/1949	0.1	0–2	0/1983	0	0	0/1950	0	0
Pituitary (pars distalis)	Adenoma	417/1868	22.8	5–52	519/1898	27.3	10–54	869/1934	45.2	18–70	760/1901	40	18–65
	Carcinoma	42/1868	2.3	0–11	38/1898	2.0	0–9	72/1934	3.7	0–16	53/1901	2.8	0–11
Pituitary (pars intermedia)	Adenoma	3/1868	0.2	0–4	6/1898	0.3	0–6	2/1934	0.1	0–2	3/1901	0.2	0–2
Integument/ s.c.[c] tissue	Malignant schwannoma	6/1936	0.3	0–2	8/1949	0.4	0–8	3/1983	0.2	0–4	3/1950	0.2	0–2
	Neurofibroma	2/1936	0.1	0–4	5/1949	0.3	0–4	0/1983	0	0	0/1950	0	0
	Neurofibrosarcoma	7/1936	0.4	0–6	5/1949	0.3	0–2	6/1983	0.3	0–4	3/1950	0.2	0–2
Body cavities	Neurofibrosarcoma	1/1936	0.1	0–2	0/1949	0	0	1/1983	0.1	0–2	0/1950	0	0
Total body	All benign	1816/1936	93.8	82–100	1806/1949	92.7	76–100	1457/1983	73.5	58–86	1408/1950	72.2	52–88
	All malignant	1024/1936	52.9	38–82	729/1949	37.4	18–64	767/1983	38.7	18–56	675/1950	34.6	18–56
	Total tumors	1895/1936	97.9	90–100	1864/1949	95.6	88–100	1725/1983	87.0	64–98	1625/1950	83.3	66–96

[a] Modified from Haseman, Arnold and Eustis, 1990, by permission.
[b] NOS, not otherwise specified.
[c] s.c., subcutaneous.

Innes, 1979), and, when present, can spread via the cerebrospinal fluid pathways, but rarely metastasize extracerebrally. Other less frequently observed CNS tumors in mice include GBMs, medulloblastomas, ependymomas, oligodendrogliomas, choroid plexus papillomas, granular-cell tumors and a third-ventricular teratoma associated with the choroid plexus (Ngowyang, 1930; Slye, Holmes and Wells, 1931; Cottier and Luginbühl, 1961; Morgan *et al.*, 1984; Solleveld *et al.*, 1986). Metastatic CNS tumors are almost exclusively seen in strains, such as BALB/c, with a high incidence of spontaneous leukemias or lymphomas.

A few mice strains have an exceptional incidence of spontaneous gliomas. The VM, VM-derived, and BRVR strains have an incidence of brain or spinal cord infiltrative astrocytomas of 1.27%, 0.62% and 0.9%, respectively, with nearly all of these tumors having the histologic appearance of astrocytomas (Fraser, 1971, 1986; Walker *et al.*, 1994). These neoplasms tend to be less differentiated than those occurring in other strains, have infiltrative margins and occur with equal frequency throughout the brain. About 10% of these astrocytomas occur in the spinal cord as well (Fraser, 1986). The incidence of tumors in VM males is twice that of females, and astrocytomas account for about 10% of the deaths that occur between 200 and 300 days of age in these animals. The inbred VM mouse strain carries the *p7* allele of the *sinc* gene that reduces the latency period in experimental scrapie infection, and this mouse strain has been primarily used in scrapie research. The development of spontaneous astrocytomas in this strain, however, seems to be independent of both this gene and scrapie infection (Fraser, 1971). A transplantable tumor from these spontaneous astrocytomas in VM mice was initially developed by Fraser (Fraser, 1971; 1986; Fraser and McConnell, 1975), but the cell homogenates from this tumor could not be transplanted extracranially, had an unpredictable latency period and were a pleomorphic cell population. These problems were overcome by the establishment of a number of cell lines that are uniformly tumorigenic, both intracranially and subcutaneously, in syngeneic VM mice (Serano, Pegram and Bigner, 1980). These cell lines, confirmed histologically by a number of observers to be glial in origin, were also found to express glutamine synthetase and GFAP *in vitro* (Pilkington *et al.*, 1982, 1983) and *in vivo* (Sampson *et al.*, 1997) (Fig. 6.1). One of these lines (SMA-560) has also been shown to secrete, in a biologically active form, the immunosuppressant, transforming growth factor-β (TGF-β), which is also secreted by a number of human malignant gliomas (Fig. 6.2).

Tumors of the cranial or peripheral nerves, neurofibromas most frequently, are generally rare in mice: an average incidence of between 0.054% (31/57 265) and 0.032% (24/75 070) is reported (Stewart, Kaplan and Bennett, 1950; Stewart *et al.*, 1974; Fraser, 1986). Male mice may have a higher incidence of neurofibromas, but schwannomas seem to have no sex predilection (Walker *et al.*, 1994). In NHO substrains, however, peripheral nerve sheath tumors were found in 8.07% (31/384) of animals. The tumors in NHO mice tend to be malignant tumors with invasive and metastatic properties.

Spontaneous pituitary tumors are also unusual in mice but are found more frequently in female mice, especially of the C57BL strains. The tumors are mostly prolactinomas. In addition, transgenic mice that express a vasopressin-SV40 hybrid oncogene develop tumors of the anterior pituitary gland, as well as of the endocrine pancreas, and are used as a model for human multiple endocrine neoplasia type 1 (Murphy *et al.*, 1987).

Laboratory rats

Examples of almost all types of human nervous system tumors develop spontaneously in the rat or can be induced (Jänisch, 1990). The average incidence of intracranial tumors in all rat strains (excluding pituitary tumors, which are very common in rats) ranges from 0% to 5.8%. In some 2-year chronic bioassays, the incidence of intracranial tumors in Sprague-Dawley rats has been as high as 15%, however. The reported incidence of intracranial tumors in rats depends on age, strain, subtle environmental exposures and completeness of examination. The incidence and types of tumors observed in Fischer 344 (F344) rats at the NTP in 2-year carcinogenicity studies is shown in Table 6.4. Astrocytomas are the most common neuroectodermal CNS tumors in rats, followed by oligodendrogliomas and then ependymomas—a distribution similar to that in humans. Although rat astrocytomas may be anaplastic, most are well-differentiated tumors. Thus, anaplastic astrocytomas and GBMs account for a larger proportion of such tumors in humans. Rat astrocytomas are also often negative when subjected to stains for GFAP (Krinke *et al.*, 1985; Solleveld *et al.*, 1986). Meningiomas, especially if meningeal granular-cell tumors are included, constitute the most common nonglial intracranial tumor in rats (Jänisch, 1990). Overall, meningiomas, including granular-cell tumors, have been reported as the most common intracranial tumors in Sprague-Dawley (Krinke *et al.*, 1985), Wistar (Sumi *et al.*, 1976) and Brown Norway (Burek and Hollander, 1977) rats, whereas the incidence of these tumors seems much lower in F344 rats in which glial tumors are more common. Glial

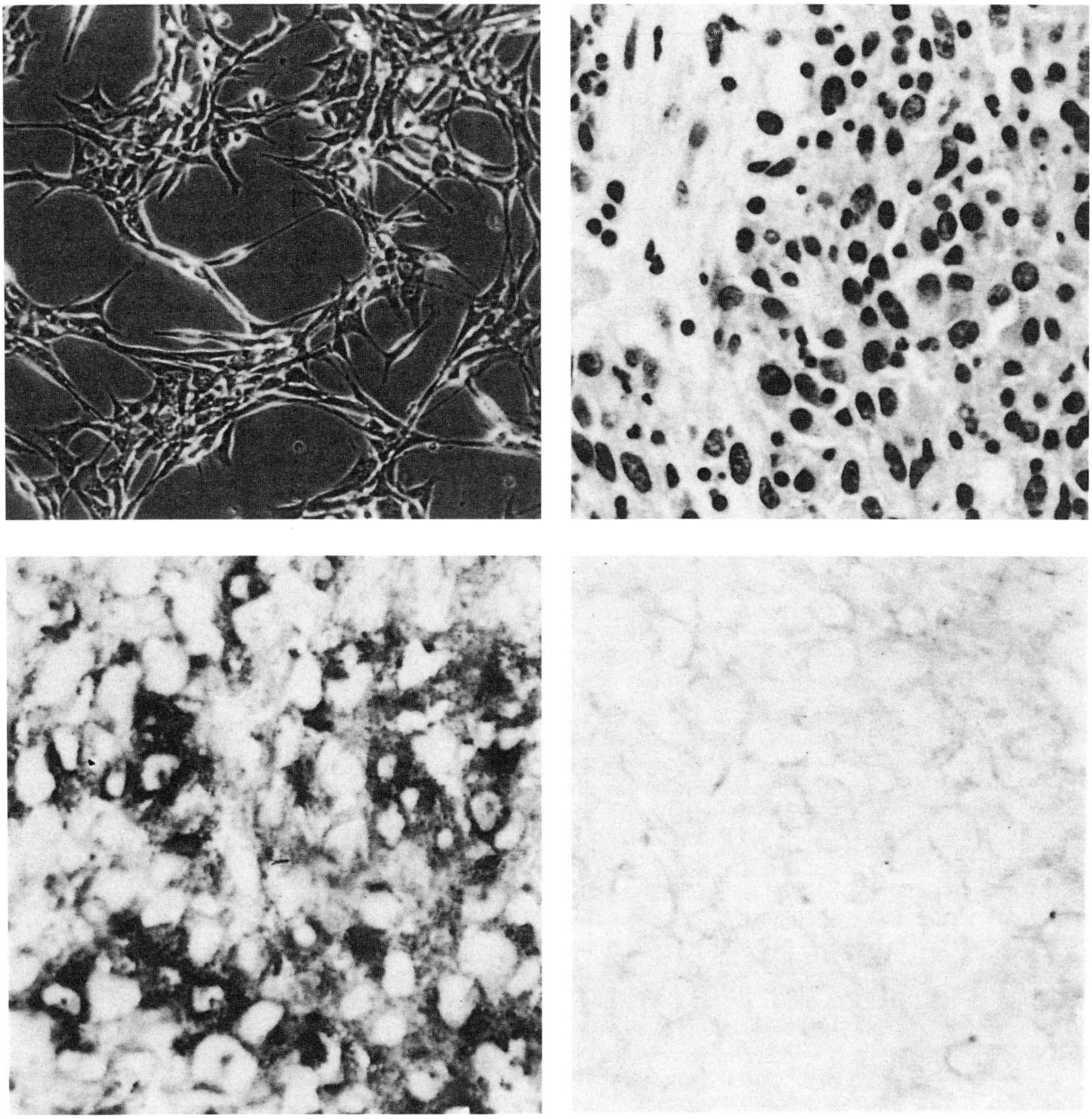

Fig. 6.1 Photomicrographs showing morphology of the 560 spontaneous murine astrocytoma *in vitro* (top left), *in vivo* (top right), with positive immunohistochemical staining for GFAP (bottom left), and negative control (bottom right).

tumors are slightly more common in males, at least in the F344 strain, and the tumors increase in incidence with age, probably reaching a peak incidence at about 2 years of age (Goodman *et al.*, 1979; Maekawa *et al.*, 1984; Solleveld, Haseman and McConnell, 1984; Solleveld and Boorman, 1990).

Individual reports illustrate the number of different types of CNS tumors that can arise spontaneously in rats. Medulloblastomas and choroid plexus papillomas seem to be rare in the rat. Only a few cases of a choroid plexus papilloma (Thompson *et al.*, 1961; Solleveld, Haseman and McConnell, 1984; Solleveld and Boorman, 1990) and one choroid plexus carcinoma (Solleveld and Boorman, 1990) have been reported, and medulloblastomas have been recognized only recently (Solleveld, Haseman and McConnell, 1984; Solleveld and Boorman, 1990). In addition, other

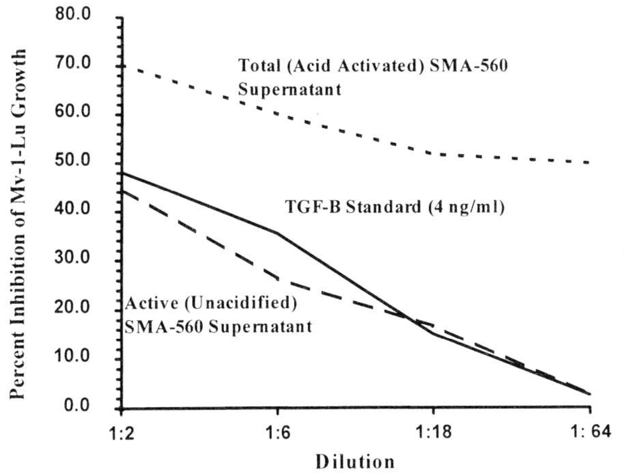

Fig. 6.2 Results of bioassay for TGF-β. (a) Growth of the Mv-1-Lu cell line used in this assay is inhibited by TGF-β. Cell supernatants are collected *in vitro* and activated by acidification. The TGF-β standard is active TGF-β1 at a starting concentration of 4 ng/mL.

types of tumors that have been reported in the rat include ependymoblastomas, GBMs, optic gliomas, pinealomas, craniopharyngiomas, an optic nerve ganglioneuroma, primary malignant lymphomas and chordomas (Bullock and Curtis, 1930; Dagle, Zwicker and Renne, 1979; Al Zubaidy and Malinowski, 1984; Maekawa *et al.*, 1984; Krinke *et al.*, 1985; Gopinath, 1986; Wyand, Zwicker and Pavkov, 1987; Stefanski *et al.*, 1988; Haseman, Arnold and Eustis, 1990; Thurman *et al.*, 1994).

Primary neoplasms affecting the spinal cord (Kaspareit-Rittinghausen and Deerberg, 1989) are extremely rare in rats and not one such tumor has been identified in over 200 carcinogenicity studies at the NTP (Mitsumori and Boorman, 1990). However, rare spinal cord astrocytomas, ependymomas, and oligodendrogliomas have been reported by others (Innes and Borner, 1961; Adams and Crowley, 1987; Frith and Chandra, 1990; Kawaminami *et al.*, 1994).

Tumors of the PNS are certainly thought to be much less common in rats than in humans, and the overall incidence of PNS neoplasms in untreated 2-year-old F344 rats in the NTP data bank is 0.4% (89/22 037) (Mitsumori and Boorman, 1990). However, when Solleveld, Haseman and McConnell (1984) looked at older F344 rats, they found the incidence for neurofibroma to be 16.8% in males and 5.3% in females. The incidence of neurofibrosarcoma in this same group was 6.45% for males and 2.5% for females. Malignant schwannoma had an overall incidence of 0.1%. From several studies, it also appears that male rats have a higher risk of neurofibromas and neurofibrosarcomas than do females, whereas no such sex bias exists for schwannomas.

Pituitary tumors are among the three most common tumors in the rat and often account for the deaths of animals in long-term studies (Ward, 1983). They are much more common in rats than in mice. Rat strains that are particularly susceptible include the F344, Osborne-Medel and Sprague-Dawley strains. The incidence ranges from 0% to 100%, depending on a number of variables but mostly on the adequacy of the pathologic examination and on the sex, age, strain and weight of the rats (Nunziata and Storino, 1982; MacKenzie and Boorman, 1990). Of the F344 rats used at the NTP, approximately 25% of males and ≥40% of females had pituitary tumors, usually benign prolactinomas, by 2 years of age (Table 6.4) (Haseman, Arnold and Eustis, 1990; MacKenzie and Boorman, 1990). A number of rat pituitary cell lines that secrete prolactin or growth hormone have been established for *in vitro* study and *in vivo* transplantation (Bancroft and Tashjian, 1971; Kirkland, Sorrentino and Sirbasku, 1976; McKeel and Hajek, 1981; Dobson and Brown, 1985).

Experimentally induced nervous system tumors in animals

Nervous system tumors can be induced in experimental animals by physical, viral or chemical agents. Although therapeutic ionizing radiation is accepted as the only neurocarcinogen in humans (Brem, Rozental and Moskal, 1995), viruses and chemicals have been successful in inducing nervous system tumors in various species of experimental animals. Attempts to produce nervous system tumors have now been successful for almost half a century. The contributions that have emanated from these approaches command a massive literature and have been summarized in a German language monograph by Jänisch and Schreiber, which has since been translated into English, revised and augmented by Bigner and Swenberg (1977). This monograph includes a bibliography of virtually all the papers on the subject until 1976, and portions of it have been incorporated into this chapter. Relatively little new information on experimentally induced nervous system tumors has been written since that time, and basic research in neuro-oncogenesis has generally shifted to the study of the molecular mechanisms underlying neoplastic transformation and to the investigation of cell lines derived from the original, chemically or virally induced nervous system tumors. Although the induction of animal tumors was initially directed at uncovering the etiology of human brain tumors, the rapid progress that has been made in the last decade in understanding the molecular basis of human nervous system tumors directly may mean that these models will not fulfill their promise in this area.

PHYSICAL CARCINOGENESIS

Ionizing and ultraviolet radiation, low-frequency electric and magnetic fields, and hyperthermia have been considered potential physical neurocarcinogens. Of these, the only established human neurocarcinogen is ionizing radiation. The potential of ionizing radiation as a carcinogen in relation to skin cancer and leukemia was established soon after the discovery of X-rays in 1896 (Von Jagic, Schwarz and von Siebenrock, 1911). Ionizing radiation is that which has sufficient energy to eject an orbital electron from an atom or molecule. This orbital electron may then use its energy to disrupt biochemical bonds, and, in this way, radiation is highly effective at producing deletions and chromosomal translocations. Thus, it has been hypothesized that radiation induces neoplastic transformation, either by the mutation of a proto-oncogene or, more likely, by the inactivation of a tumor suppressor gene. The genetic effects of ionizing radiation are stochastic; that is, no minimal threshold for biologic damage exists, and the severity of the effect is independent of dose, although the probability of genetic damage does increase with dose. For X-rays and γ-rays, the incidence of radiation-induced cancers is nearly proportional to the dose, but levels off at higher doses – where cell death predominates over cell transformation.

Radiation-induced central nervous system tumors in animals

The experimental induction of CNS tumors by radiation has been described in a small number of reports. The techniques used have included the direct intracerebral implantation of ^{60}Co or ^{241}Am, intravenous injection of ^{32}P or ^{90}Sr for transplacental tumor induction in offspring of the recipient, and total body radiation. The animals employed in these attempts have mostly been rats, though nonhuman primates have also been found to be susceptible to glial tumor induction with ionizing radiation. The yield with these techniques has been variable, the best results having been obtained with the intracerebral implantation of radioactive cobalt. Intracerebral implantation of 60 μCi of ^{60}Co into 26- to 30-day-old rats proved to be particularly effective, with GBM being induced in 19/27 animals after a latency period of 365–410 days (McDonald *et al.*, 1973). However, virus-like particles were detected by electron microscopy in several of these gliomas, so oncogenic viruses also might have influenced tumor induction. Less favorable results were achieved when the dose of radioactivity was increased. For example, the intracerebral implantation of 350 μCi of ^{60}Co killed all rats within 192 days and no tumors were found, probably because there was insufficient time for tumors to form prior to death.

Tumors of the CNS can also be induced in animals when radioactive materials are delivered transplacentally. When ^{32}P was injected intravenously into pregnant rats on the second day of gestation, 11/130 offspring born developed neurogenic tumors between 270 and 800 days of life (Druckrey, 1973). Similarly, ^{90}Sr injected intravenously into pregnant rats 18 days after conception produced an intense accumulation of radioactivity at the ossification centers in the skull base, and induced not only primarily pituitary adenomas but also metastasizing meningeal sarcomas. From these experiments, it was postulated that radioactive isotopes, even those like ^{32}P with half-lives as short as 14.4 days, could elicit a neuro-oncogenic effect if fetal tissues were exposed.

Finally, the occurrence of GBM in 3/10 rhesus monkeys (*Macaca mulatta*) that survived dosages of 600 or 800 rad of 55 MeV total body irradiation has been reported (Haymaker, Rubinstein and Miquel, 1972), and this deserves special mention because of the established link between human brain tumors and ionizing radiation (Tsang *et al.*, 1993; Brem, Rozental and Moskal, 1995). Clear evidence that ionizing radiation can induce brain tumors in nonhuman primates has been provided by others as well (Kent and Pickering, 1958; Krupp, 1976). Importantly, these induced tumors possess all the histopathologic features of human GBM. As discussed in the previous section of this chapter, spontaneous gliomas are very rare in nonhuman primates; therefore, it is likely that these GBMs were actually radiation induced. This conclusion is also supported by the similar effects of total body irradiation in rats, as observed by other investigators (Castanera *et al.*, 1968).

VIRAL CARCINOGENESIS

The foundation for the molecular study of carcinogenesis can be attributed to early studies in viral carcinogenesis. The observation by Rous (1911) and others (Ellermann and Bang, 1908) at the turn of the century that, using cell-free extracts, the cancer phenotype could be transferred between animals established the groundwork that led to the discovery of proto-oncogenes and tumor suppressor genes. Through the study of viral oncology, it became clear that genetic disruptions were involved at various stages of tumorigenesis, and this enhanced our understanding of carcinogenesis by other means.

Viruses are basically composed of a minimal genome of nucleic acid encased in a protein shell called 'the capsid'. A lipid envelope may then surround this protein shell. Viruses are classified and grouped into a hierarchical taxonomy of orders (designated by the suffix *-virales*), families (designated by the suffix *-viridae*), genera or groups (designated by the suffix *-virus*), species and strains based on a number of features, including the type of nucleic acid; the morphology and size of the virus particle; the biologic, physical, chemical and immunologic properties; and the pathology or symptomatology induced by the virus. It is helpful to note that the term 'virus' may be used to refer to a species, strain or even variant. Viruses that have been identified as being oncogenic in experimental animals can be divided initially, by nucleic acid type, into two groups: the oncogenic RNA viruses and the oncogenic DNA viruses. The oncogenic RNA viruses are all retroviruses from the family *Retroviridae* and include the avian, murine and simian sarcoma viruses. The oncogenic DNA viruses are a more diverse group and include, from the family *Papovaviridae*, the simian vacuolating virus 40, the human JC and BK papovaviruses and the murine polyomavirus; and from the family *Adenoviridae*, the human, simian and avian adenoviruses.

Vázquez-López (1936) is generally credited with the first induction of an intracranial tumor by a virus. Vázquez-López used cell-free extracts of the Rous sarcoma virus to induce intracranial sarcomas in chickens. Although a number of different viruses have since been used to induce nervous system tumors in lower animals and nonhuman primates, and although some viruses have been implicated in the early carcinogenic steps of certain other human cancers, viruses have not been shown definitively by themselves to induce human nervous system tumors. The local injection of oncogenic viruses has induced intracranial neoplasms in a wide variety of animals, however. In addition to the large number of positive yields, the method has the advantage over chemically induced tumor models (discussed in the next section) of producing tumors within a relatively short time, often within 4 weeks in the case of neonatal dogs (Vick, Bigner and Kvedar, 1971). Newborn animals show the greatest degree of susceptibility, the yield depending on the type of virus used, the exact age of the animal at the time of inoculation, and the precise dose and concentration of the virus injected. The tumors that have been obtained include medulloblastomas and various forms of glial, neural and sarcomal neoplasms.

Work with virus-induced experimental brain tumors is now passing beyond the stage in which various viruses are being surveyed for their ability to induce experimental brain tumors, and the induced tumors are being classified morphologically. A good deal of correlation exists between the type of virus used and the tumor type produced, although this is not absolute. As will be recounted below, anaplastic astrocytomas and GBMs have most often been obtained with the oncogenic RNA viruses such as the avian, murine and simian sarcoma viruses. Choroid plexus papillomas are induced by some of the simian and human types of papovaviruses, and medulloblastomas and pineocytomas by isolates of the human JC papovaviruses. Finally, neuroblastomas and retinoblastomas have been reliably induced with the human adenovirus type 12.

Oncogenic RNA viruses

Family *Retroviridae*, group avian-leukosis-sarcoma

Avian (Rous) sarcoma virus

Among the tumors induced by oncogenic RNA tumor viruses, those produced by the avian (Rous) sarcoma virus (ASV) have been the most thoroughly investigated. Sarcomas of the CNS can be regularly induced in domestic chickens, the species of origin for this virus, when they are inoculated intracerebrally with ASV, but glial tumor production has not been reported in this species. Similarly, only rare sarcomas and no gliomas have been produced in nonhuman primates using this approach (Jänisch *et al.*, 1968). In contrast, both neuroectodermal tumors and sarcomas have been induced in Syrian hamsters, rabbits, guinea pigs and mice, but most frequently in rats and dogs, after the neonates were inoculated intracerebrally with ASV. Rabotti *et al.* (1966) were the first to report glioma and sarcoma induction in dogs using this technique. Tumors obtained by inoculating dogs at birth with the Schmidt-Ruppin strain of this virus have been shown, by light and electron microscopy, to be closely related to the pilocytic astrocytoma of juvenile type found in humans

(Bigner *et al.*, 1969; Haguenau *et al.*, 1971; Vick, Bigner and Kvedar, 1971; Vick and Bigner, 1972). Those produced in rats using either the Schmidt-Ruppin strain (Wilfong *et al.*, 1973) or the Bratislava 77 strain (Copeland, Vogel and Bigner, 1975) include a variety of gliomas that range from low-grade astrocytomas and oligodendrogliomas to GBMs. The gliomas produced in the latter strain, in particular, are morphologically very similar to human cerebral astrocytomas. Immunoperoxidase stains and, in one case, analysis by gel electrophoresis and immunoblot for GFAP have amply confirmed the astrocytic nature of the tumors induced in hamsters and dogs (Nakazato *et al.*, 1981; Britt *et al.*, 1985). Finally, gliosarcomas have also been obtained in dogs following the injection of the Schmidt-Ruppin strain of ASV (Britt *et al.*, 1985, 1987).

A technique for reproducibly inducing glial tumors with a uniform mortality distribution in large numbers of rats has been established by Bigner *et al.* (1975), and a permanent cell line was also derived from an anaplastic astrocytoma induced in a female F344 rat using this technique (Lee *et al.*, 1986). This cell line, S635-clone 5 (S635cl5), has continued to express the glial marker GFAP after repeated passages *in vitro*, and after subcutaneous and intracerebral transplantation in syngeneic rats. It has proven to be a good experimental model for the *in vitro* and *in vivo* study of infiltrating cerebral astrocytomas and is discussed further in the final section of this chapter.

The neurotropicity of these viruses is restricted to glial and mesenchymal cells. No neuronal tumors were obtained when high titers of the Bratislava 77 strain of ASV were injected intracerebrally into fetal F344 rats, even at the time of active neuronal proliferation between 17 and 20 days of gestation (Copeland and Bigner, 1978). As in the case of gliomas induced by other agents, the growths induced by ASV often tend to appear in the region of the subependymal plate of the cerebral hemisphere (Haguenau *et al.*, 1971; Vick, Bigner and Kvedar, 1971). Sequential study of the morphologic events taking place after newborn animals were inoculated with ASV has confirmed the vulnerability of that site to neoplastic transformation in the neonate (Copeland and Bigner, 1977a, 1977b; Vick, Lin and Bigner, 1977). Moreover, in other studies, Bigner *et al.* (1972) showed that whether a homogeneous astrocytic or sarcomatous tumor was induced in a dog could be controlled by the inoculation site. If inoculation was made deep in the periventricular region, only astrocytic tumors were induced. On the other hand, if the ASV inoculum was injected superficially over the meninges or in the vermis of the cerebellum, only sarcomas were induced.

Family *Retroviridae*, group mammalian C-type

Murine sarcoma virus

Moloney murine sarcoma virus (MSV), which causes leukemia and sarcomas when injected subcutaneously into rodents, also induced brain tumors in rats after they were inoculated with it intracerebrally. Ribacchi and Giraldo (1966) reported that, in addition to hemangioendotheliomas and a meningioma of the leptomeninges, numerous GBMs originating in subependymal tissue were also induced. These GBMs demonstrate the vascular endothelial proliferations characteristic of the human growths (Yung, Blank and Vick, 1976).

Simian sarcoma virus

Simian sarcoma virus (SSV), which was originally isolated from a spontaneous fibrosarcoma of a wooly monkey, has also been used to induce intracerebral tumors in animals (Johnson *et al.*, 1975). These SSV-1-induced tumors in neonatal marmosets (*Saguinus nigrocolli*) were composed of variably cellular areas containing pleomorphic cells and abundant neuroglial fibrils, areas of hemorrhage, necrosis, endothelial proliferation and palisading tumor cells. Given these features, morphologically, these tumors resemble human GBMs more closely than any other virally induced tumor.

In vitro transformation by v-*src*

When fetal brain cells that express the v-*src* gene are transplanted, anaplastic astrocytomas and sarcomas can also be induced (Aguzzi *et al.*, 1991).

Oncogenic DNA viruses

Family *Papovaviridae*, group *Polyomavirus*

Simian vacuolating virus 40

Simian vacuolating virus 40 (SV40) is typical of DNA tumor viruses in that it is oncogenic in a non-permissive rodent species, whereas it has not shown any tumor-inducing effect in monkeys, the species from which it was originally isolated. It has also not been possible to induce tumors in dogs, cats, rabbits or rats by using SV40. However, after newborn Syrian hamsters were inoculated intracerebrally with SV40 (Duffell, Hinz and Nelson, 1964; Wilkins and Odom, 1965), and *Mastomys natalensis*, an African mouse-like rodent, was inoculated subcutaneously with the same virus (Rabson *et al.*, 1962), glial and sarcomatous tumors developed in the ventricular wall. Though the glial tumors were initially classified as ependymomas, they were subsequently identified as papillomas of the choroid plexus. The choroid plexi are particularly well developed in rodents at the time of birth and, as the animals were less than 24 hours old at the time of their intracerebral inoculation, it is not unexpected that the choroid plexus should be especially susceptible to the oncogenic virus. Histologically, these tumors contained numerous mitotic figures but were otherwise well differentiated, and electron microscopy of these papillary epithelial-like intraventricular tumors revealed cells with well-developed junctional complexes, tightly packed microvilli and cilia (Duffell, Hinz and Nelson, 1964). There were no virus particles observed, however. Several lines of both the sarcomas and choroid plexus papillomas were transplantable subcutaneously for several passages. While no morphologic change occurred in the sarcomas, a progressive increase in the amount of connective tissue and stromal elements was observed in the choroid plexus papilloma transplants. Furthermore, when examination of these SV40-induced choroid plexus papillomas was carried out for the presence of 2',3'-cyclic nucleotide 3'-phosphohydrolase activity, aldolase C and S-100 protein, no significant activity was found for any of these three glial markers.

JC virus

The JC strain of the human papovavirus is morphologically indistinguishable from, and antigenically and molecularly very similar to, the SV40 virus. Unlike SV40, which does not infect human cells, the JC virus is a common latent infection in humans. This virus can be reactivated in immunosuppressed patients and leads to progressive multifocal leukoencephalopathy (PML). From the experiments described below, it is apparent that the tumor type induced by this virus depends on a combination of variables that include the strain of the inoculum, the animal species inoculated, the route of inoculation and the developmental state of the tissue exposed. However, the relationships between these variables and the cells most vulnerable to neoplastic transformation remain largely unexplained.

The JC virus was first shown by Walker *et al.* (1973) to be highly neuro-oncogenic when injected into the brains of hamsters at birth. The most frequently obtained neoplasms in these experiments were cerebellar medulloblastomas, which occurred in 95% of tumor-bearing animals. These tumors were often multicentric and arose from the internal granular layer (ZuRhein and Varakis, 1979). Matsuda *et al.* (1987) have demonstrated with *in situ* hybridization that the JC virus initially infects the mitotically active cells of the external granular-cell layer in the course of their inward migration. Conversely, injecting the JC virus intraocularly into neonatal hamsters resulted in the production of primarily visceral neuroblastomas (Varakis *et al.*, 1978). The review by ZuRhein (1983) on the tumors induced by this agent in Syrian hamsters details the wide range of neoplasms obtained. These have included anaplastic astrocytoma, GBM, cerebral neuroblastoma, olfactory neuroblastoma and malignant schwannoma. Another notable tumor induced in Syrian hamsters using the JC strain of human papovavirus is a pineocytoma (Varakis and ZuRhein, 1976), the differentiating features having been meticulously confirmed by electron microscopy. Biochemical differentiation in these pineocytomas was also demonstrated by Quay *et al.* (1977), who found various levels of hydroxy-indole-*O*-methyltransferase in the tumor homogenates. The same group of workers subsequently reported an unusually high incidence of such pineal tumors from another isolate of the same virus (Padgett *et al.*, 1977), suggesting that predilection for a particular part of the CNS might be virus strain dependent.

Intracranial injection of the JC virus has also produced nervous system tumors in other animal species besides hamsters. Newborn Sprague-Dawley rats inoculated with the Tokyo-I strain of the JC virus, isolated from a patient with PML (Nagashima *et al.*, 1984; Matsuda *et al.*, 1987), developed poorly differentiated intracerebral neuroepithelial tumors, some of which resembled neuroblastomas while others resembled anaplastic astrocytomas (Ohsumi, Motoi and Ogawa, 1986). In addition, intracerebral inoculation of adult owl and squirrel monkeys with the JC virus produced tumors with the typical features of GBM or anaplastic astrocytoma (London *et al.*, 1978), and infectious JC virus with altered biological activity was subsequently isolated from these tumors (London *et al.*, 1978; Major *et al.*, 1987).

BK virus

Another human papovavirus, the BK strain, was shown to be weakly oncogenic after hamsters were inoculated with it intracerebrally. Two animals developed choroid plexus papillomas only after treatment with antithymocyte serum (Greenlee *et al.*, 1977), and it is apparent that, in this system, the transformed cells are strongly immunogenic. The tumors similarly obtained by Corallini *et al.* (1977) and labeled 'ependymomas' are, from the illustration published, almost certainly anaplastic choroid plexus papillomas. This BK virus was also used to induce a sarcoma in a hamster (Shah, Daniël and Strandberg, 1975).

Polyomavirus

The polyomavirus is a papovavirus whose natural host is the mouse. Tumors induced by the polyomavirus have generally been collagen-forming or anaplastic sarcomas. Polyomavirus has been used to induce meningeal sarcomas in rats (Vandeputte and Brucher, 1962) or rabbits (Postlethwaite *et al.*, 1969) and intracerebral sarcomas in Syrian hamsters (Rabson and Kirschstein, 1960; Romanul, Roizman, and Luttrell, 1961a, 1961b). Although intracerebral inoculation of the animals with this virus induced the highest incidence of intracranial sarcomas, a few leptomeningeal sarcomas were found after subcutaneous or intravenous inoculation as well (Vandeputte and Brucher, 1962).

In vitro transformation by papovaviruses

After cultured fetal or newborn hamster glial cells were transformed by SV40 or polyomavirus, Shein (1968) injected the transformed cells by the subcutaneous or intracerebral route into newborn or adult hamsters and produced astrocytomas or GBMs. Curiously, the astrocytomas produced by polyoma-transformed cells grew more rapidly and metastasized more often, although they were better differentiated than those from cell lines transformed by SV40, an observation that suggested possible differences in viral integration pattern (Duigou *et al.*, 1990). Transformation of trypsinized and minced fragments of whole fetal and neonatal hamster brains induced by SV40 was also achieved by Shein and Pope (1967), who obtained various types of neuroglial and meningeal tumors when the transformed cells were injected subcutaneously into hamsters. It is noteworthy that, in these experiments, GBMs were obtained from the progeny of a single, cloned astrocytoma cell (Shein, 1970), an observation that is clearly significant in the context of the hypothesis that the GBMs developed from less malignant astrocytomas. On the other hand, when similarly transformed human fetal astrocytes were injected, either subcutaneously or intracerebrally, into Syrian hamsters, no tumors were obtained (Shein, 1967). The tumorigenic potential of the hamster brain cells similarly transformed by the polyomavirus was confirmed by Tripier *et al.* (1979b) with the subcutaneous grafting of these cells into syngeneic animals, producing poorly differentiated astrocytic gliomas. Similar tumors have also been obtained after hamster brain cells were transformed by the human BK papovavirus (Tanaka *et al.*, 1978). In addition, cell suspensions, derived from day-14 fetal rat brains and transfected with the SV40 large T antigen by a retroviral vector, were also tumorigenic, though only after a considerable latency period, suggesting that additional genetic alterations may have played a role. These tumors closely resembled human medulloblastomas (Eibl *et al.*, 1994; Fung *et al.*, 1994; Fung and Trojanowski, 1995). A series of experiments in which hamster pineal gland cultures were transformed *in vitro* by polyomavirus and SV40 has also been reported (Wells, Wurtman and Rabson, 1966; Orme *et al.*, 1968). The resultant transformed cells produced progressively growing tumors when the cells were injected into sublethally irradiated hamsters. Both the transformed cells in culture and the transplanted tumors have high levels of ortho-methyltransferase, an enzyme specific to the pineal gland. Finally, although most rats that were transplanted with brain elements expressing the polyomavirus middle T antigen developed early endothelial hemangiomas and died of intracerebral hemorrhage, some demonstrated delayed growth of anaplastic gliomas after a prolonged latency period. Again, the delayed growth of these gliomas may imply the need for an accumulation of genetic changes in addition to those provided directly by the middle T antigen (Aguzzi *et al.*, 1991).

Family *Adenoviridae*, group *Mastadenovirus/Aviadenovirus*

Human adenoviruses

Huebner, Rowe and Lane (1962) were the first to show that human adenoviruses could induce experimental intracranial tumors. Malignant mesenchymal tumors that originated in the meninges were found in two Syrian hamsters 35–40 days after the animals were inoculated intracerebrally with human adenovirus 12. Most tumors induced *in vivo* after intraperitoneal, intraocular or intracerebral inoculation of neonatal hamsters, rats and mice with human adenovirus type 12, however, are composed of neuroblastic cells. This virus seems to have a special affinity for primitive neuronal and photosensory elements. When the agent is introduced intracerebrally into the rat or hamster, the tumors are, from their cytological architecture and some of their electron microscopic features, similar to neuroblastomas, although they were first regarded by their observers as embryonic gliomas in hamsters and as medulloepitheliomas in rats (Mukai and Kobayashi, 1973a, 1973b). When injected intraocularly, the virus induces retinoblastomas that are relatively poorly differentiated (Mukai, Kobayashi and Oguri, 1974; Mukai and Murao, 1975). Cell lines have been derived from these retinoblastomas, and one of them, designated EXP-5, predictably reproduces retinoblastomas when it is injected into the vitreous humor of newborn, inbred CDF rats (Kobayashi *et al.*, 1982). Multicentric visceral and subcutaneous neuroblastomas have also been obtained after this agent was introduced, respectively, into the peritoneal cavities and subcutaneous tissues of newborn hamsters (Mukai, 1976; Nakajima and Mukai, 1979). In addition, a human embryo retinoblast cell line transfected with cloned adenovirus 12 DNA was tumorigenic when injected subcutaneously or intracranially into 6- to 10-day old athymic mice, and the tumors produced had the features of neuroblastomas (Byrd, Brown and Gallimore, 1982). Other neoplasms induced by Ogawa (1979) in a wide range of experiments with this agent included tumors identical with medulloblastomas, some of which showed typical Homer-Wright rosettes or a rhythmical arrangement of spongioblastoma-like cells; tumors similar to the human ependymoblastoma and to cerebral and sympathetic neuroblastomas; and highly anaplastic and pleomorphic gliomas resembling GBMs. In addition, typical medulloepitheliomas have been obtained in the subpleural and subserosal tissues, as well as in the lung and liver, after adenovirus type 12 was injected into the peritoneal cavities of mice. Similar tumors, which have been designated peripheral neuroepitheliomas, were also obtained along peripheral nerves of immunocompetent mice and hamsters, but not rats, after the animals were inoculated intraperitoneally with virus (Ogawa, 1989). Finally, injection of the human adenovirus type 31 into the peritoneal or cranial cavities of newborn Syrian hamsters has also produced undifferentiated neuroepithelial cell tumors showing differentiation features along glial lines (Mizobuchi, Motoi and Ogawa, 1984). These experiments indicate that, with oncogenic human adenoviruses, the viral target is not exclusively neuronal, but a high degree of neuronal tropicity is expressed. The potential of human adenoviruses to induce other embryonal neuroepithelial tumors displaying different lines of cellular differentiation needs to be further explored.

Simian and avian adenoviruses

Simian adenoviruses have induced undifferentiated tumors of the choroid plexus, trigeminal nerve and dura mater in Syrian hamsters (Merkow *et al.*, 1970). Similarly, the avian adenoviruses, which are antigenically different from the primate adenoviruses, have also induced tumors in Syrian hamsters (Mancini *et al.*, 1969). The morphology of the tumors induced by the avian adenoviruses was, however, distinctly different from the neuroblastic tumors induced with the human adenoviruses and the undifferentiated tumors induced with the simian adenoviruses. These avian adenovirus-induced tumors were composed of cuboidal and columnar cells arranged in a papillary pattern that had a connective tissue stroma and could be traced to a beginning point in the ependymal cell layer. Morphologically, however, these tumors could be classified as choroid plexus papillomas.

PRODUCTION OF NERVOUS SYSTEM TUMORS IN TRANSGENIC MICE

In addition to morphologic classification, the genetic alterations responsible for tumor induction by viruses are now being investigated through 'transgenic' and 'knockout' mouse technology (Table 6.5) and by direct oncogene transfer to fetal brain cells by *ex vivo* or *in situ* infection with retroviruses expressing various oncogenes (Table 6.6). Transgenes are usually under the control of viral promoter and enhancer elements and are, therefore, expressed ubiquitously. Tissue-specific expression is possible, however, and can be used to direct tumor induction to specific organs. More recently, specific control sequences, such as the native promoters for myelin basic protein (Kimura *et al.*, 1989; Hayes *et al.*, 1992) or GFAP (Mucke *et al.*, 1991; Danks *et al.*, 1995), have been used for this purpose in the nervous system. These glial-specific promoters are currently being tested in transgenic mice that express oncogenes commonly amplified in human brain tumors, such as the wild-type and mutant forms of the epidermal growth factor receptor and *MYC*.

Oncogenic RNA viruses

Family *Retroviridae*, group human T-cell leukemia virus

Human T-cell lymphotropic virus type 1 *TAT* gene

Transgenic mice bearing the human T-cell lymphotrophic virus type 1 (HTLV-1) *TAT* gene under the control of its own long terminal repeat (LTR) sequence simultaneously develop multiple tumors at about 3 months of age. These tumors consist of fibroblasts and perineural cells and closely resemble the characteristic tumors found in human neurofibromatosis type 1 (Hinrichs *et al.*, 1987).

***MYC* and *TAX* Double transgenic mice**

Although transgenic mice expressing either the *MYC* gene under control of the HTLV-1 LTR, or

Table 6.5 Transgenic and knockout mice as models for nervous system tumors[a]

Gene	Regulatory sequence	Tumor type	Reference(s)
SV40[b] large T antigen	Rat tyrosine hydroxylase promoter-enhancer	PNETs[b] (brainstem)	Suri *et al.*, 1993
	MSV[b] enhancer–natural promoter of SV40 large T antigen	PNETs (pineal gland)	Theuring *et al.*, 1990; Götz *et al.*, 1992; Korf *et al.*, 1990
	Human luteinizing hormone β-subunit promoter	PNETs (mesencephalon), retinoblastoma	Marcus *et al.*, 1991; Windle *et al.*, 1990
	Human interphotoreceptor retinoid-binding protein promoter	PNETs (brain and retina)	Al Ubaidi *et al.*, 1992
	Human PNMT[b] promoter	Retinoblastoma	Hammang *et al.*, 1993; Baetge *et al.*, 1988
	Schwann cell-specific rat P_0	Schwannoma	Messing *et al.*, 1994
	LPV[b] or SV40 enhancer–promoter	Choroid plexus tumor	Chen and Van Dyke, 1991
	Human cystic fibrosis transmembrane conductance regulator promoter	Malignant intraventricular ependymomas and choroid plexus carcinomas	Perraud *et al.*, 1992
	Gonadotropin-releasing hormone promoter	Hypothalamic tumors with neuronal markers (neuroblastomas)	Mellon *et al.*, 1990; Radovick *et al.*, 1991
	Olfactory marker protein regulatory elements	Neuroblastoma	Largent, Sosnowski and Reed, 1993
	Murine GFAP[b] promoter	Anaplastic astrocytomas	Danks *et al.*, 1995
	Human glycoprotein hormone α-subunit promoter–enhancer	Gonadotrope anterior pituitary adenomas	Windle, Weiner and Mellon, 1990
SV40 early region	Metallothionein promoter	Choroid plexus carcinoma	Brinster *et al.*, 1984; Palmiter *et al.*, 1985
JC virus T antigen	SV40 regulatory region	Choroid plexus papilloma	Ressetar *et al.*, 1993
LPV[b] T antigen	LPV or SV40 enhancer–promoter	Choroid plexus tumor	Chen and Van Dyke, 1991
Adenovirus E1A and E1B	MMTV LTR[b]	Neuroblastoma	Koike *et al.*, 1990
Polyomavirus large T antigen	Polyoma early region promoter	Pituitary adenoma	Helseth *et al.*, 1995
Polyomavirus middle T antigen	Polyoma early region promoter	Pituitary adenoma	Bautch *et al.*, 1987
	Thymidine kinase promoter	Neuroblastoma (rare)	Aguzzi *et al.*, 1990
Papillomavirus 16 E6, E7 and ORF	Human β-actin promoter	Ependymoma, pituitary carcinoma, choroid plexus carcinoma	Arbeit *et al.*, 1993
HTLV-1[b] *TAT* gene	HTLV-1 LTR	Peripheral nerve sheath tumors	Hinrichs *et al.*, 1987
ERBB2	Myelin basic protein promoter	Oligodendroglioma	Hayes *et al.*, 1992
RB1	Knockout	Pituitary carcinoma	Jacks *et al.*, 1992
TP53	Heterozygous knockout	Ependymoma (rare)	Jacks *et al.*, 1994
	Homozygous knockout	No brain tumors	Jacks *et al.*, 1994
Nerve growth factor	Rat prolactin promoter	Pituitary hyperplasia	Borrelli, Sawchenko and Evans, 1992
MYC and *TAX*	HTLV-1 LTR Immunoglobin promoter–enhancer	Brain tumors not otherwise specified	Benvenisty *et al.*, 1992

[a] Modified from Lantos, VandenBerg and Kleihues, 1997, by permission.

[b]GFAP, glial fibrillary acidic protein; HTLV-1, human T lymphotropic virus type 1; LPV, lymphotropic papoma virus; LTR, long terminal repeat; MMTV, mouse mammary tumor virus; MSV, Maloney murine sarcoma virus; PNET, primitive neuroectodermal tumor; PNMT, phenylethanolamine *N*-methyltransferase; SV40, Sirian virus 40.

Table 6.6 Nervous system tumors induced by *ex vivo* or *in situ* by oncogene transfer[a]

Oncogene	Tumor type	Latency	Reference(s)
SV40 large T	PNET	5–9 months	Eibl *et al.*, 1994
Polyomavirus medium T	Hemangioma Anaplastic glioma	2–6 weeks 9–15 months	Aguzzi *et al.*, 1991 Aguzzi *et al.*, 1991
HRAS	Anaplastic glioma	4–6 months	Wiestler *et al.*, 1992, 1994
SRC	Glioma, sarcoma	3–6 months	Aguzzi *et al.*, 1991
MYC	PNET (rare)	~2 months	Wiestler *et al.*, 1992, 1994
HRAS and *MYC*	Anaplastic glioma	2–8 weeks	Wiestler *et al.*, 1992, 1994
MYC and *ENU*	Anaplastic glioma	3–6 months	Brüstle *et al.*, 1993

[a] From Kleihues *et al.*, 1997, with permission.

the *TAX* gene (HTLV-1 transcription activator) with the immunoglobulin promoter/enhancer complex, do not develop nervous system tumors, double transgenic mice with both of these complexes develop brain tumors and T-cell lymphomas (Benvenisty *et al.*, 1992).

Oncogenic DNA viruses

Family *Papovaviridae*, group *Polyomavirus*

Simian vacuolating virus 40 large T antigen

Transgenic mice have been developed that carry the SV40 large T antigen—the major transcriptional regulator of the SV40 viral gene products (Brinster *et al.*, 1984; Palmiter *et al.*, 1985). Adult transgenic mice expressing the SV40 large T antigen may develop anaplastic astrocytomas, ependymomas, choroid plexus tumors, retinoblastomas, neuroblastomas, hypothalamic tumors that express neuronal markers, pituitary adenomas or schwannomas, depending on the promoter sequence associated with the oncogene (Table 6.5). Those that carry the SV40 large T antigen under the control of the tissue-specific GFAP promoter develop anaplastic astrocytomas that originate near the subependymal plate (Danks *et al.*, 1995). Those mice with other transgene promoter sequences that develop choroid plexus carcinomas often have tumors which increase in number and size with age and show a progressive tendency toward invasion of the local neural parenchyma, and even toward metastatic dissemination (Van Dyke *et al.*, 1987). However, only some of the choroid cells that express the large T antigen progress to neoplastic transformation, an outcome suggesting that secondary events are necessary in the transformation process (Messing *et al.*, 1988). The large T antigen protein has been shown to inactivate a number of growth-regulating proteins, including *TP53*, *RB1* and p107 proteins, and the antigenic protein probably serves its oncogenic function in this way (Green, 1989; Marks *et al.*, 1989). The induction of choroid plexus tumors in these mice, while not dependent on T antigen binding to *TP53* protein, does require binding to the other two growth-regulating proteins (Chen *et al.*, 1992).

The SV40 viral genome is the only one that has been implicated in human brain tumors. Even though the SV40 virus does not infect human cells, DNA sequences similar to those of the SV40 virus have been detected in childhood ependymomas and choroid plexus papillomas (Bergsagel *et al.*, 1992). The possible association of these human tumors with SV40-contaminated polio vaccines during the late 1950s and early 1960s, or with exposure of scientists to this virus in the laboratory, has not been established by epidemiologic studies, however (Howley *et al.*, 1991).

JC virus large T antigen

Despite ample gene expression in the brain, transgenic mice expressing the JC large T antigen under the control of the SV40 regulatory region do not consistently develop brain tumors, although they do develop B-cell lymphomas and osteosarcomas (Ressetar *et al.*, 1993).

Polyomavirus

In transgenic mice, expression of the polyomavirus large (Helseth *et al.*, 1995) or middle (Bautch *et al.*,

1987) T antigen, when linked to the early region promoter, has produced some pituitary adenomas. In one transgenic mouse, expression of the middle T antigen, which complexes with and increases the tyrosine kinase activity of the *SRC*, *YES* and *FYN* oncogenes, resulted in the development of a heritable syndrome of multiple neuroblastomas (Aguzzi *et al.*, 1990). These neuroblastomas develop in typical locations, such as the adrenal medulla and sympathetic trunk, and progress from preneoplastic lesions to malignant tumors. Homer-Wright rosettes and immunoreactivity for synaptophysin are typical in these lesions. It should be noted that most of the middle T antigen transgenic mice in this series actually developed hemangiomas at multiple sites rather than neuroblastomas; therefore, the development of neuroblastomas in the descendants of this one mouse may be more related to the position of integration of the transgene than to the action of the transgene itself.

Family *Papovaviridae*, group *Papillomavirus*

Human papillomavirus 16, E6 and E7 oncoproteins
Transgenic mice expressing the E6 and E7 oncoproteins of the human papillomavirus 16 under the β-actin promoter develop third ventricular ependymal anaplastic neuroepithelial tumors (Arbeit *et al.*, 1993). These mice are also prone to develop choroid plexus tumors and pituitary carcinomas.

Family *Adenoviridae*, group *Mastadenovirus/Aviadenovirus*

Human adenovirus type 12, *E1A* and *E1B* genes
Koike *et al.* (1990) have developed transgenic mice that express the *E1A* and *E1B* genes of the human adenovirus type 12 under the control of the mouse mammary tumor virus LTR. These transgenic mice consistently develop olfactory neuroblastomas.

Other oncogenes
A number of other genes have been associated with neoplastic transformation in transgenic models. For example, the oncogene *ERBB2*, under the same control as the myelin basic protein genes, results in oligodendrogliomas (Hayes *et al.*, 1992). In addition, although mice with homozygous *RB1* gene deletions are not viable (Lee *et al.*, 1992), heterozygous *RB1* gene disruption results in the development of pituitary adenocarcinomas (Jacks *et al.*, 1992). Finally, despite the frequency of *TP53* mutations in human gliomas (Louis, 1994) and in heritable genetic syndromes that predispose to the development of gliomas, heterozygous *TP53* knockout mice develop only rare ependymomas, and homozygous knockout mice develop no brain tumors at all (Jacks *et al.*, 1994). Recently, however, Oda *et al.* (1997) have demonstrated that transplacental administration of ethylnitrosourea (ENU) to heterozygous *TP53* knockout mice induced rapid development of brain tumors resembling GBMs in the majority of *TP53*-null offspring. These data suggest that *TP53* gene loss may indeed be an important early event in brain tumorigenesis.

Induction of nervous system tumors by in vitro *or* in situ *transfection of oncogenes*

Replication-incompetent retroviral vectors encoding the oncogenes *HRAS* and *MYC* have been used cooperatively to transform fetal F344 rat brain cells *in vitro*. These transformed cells can then be transplanted into the brains of syngeneic rats and can form poorly differentiated malignant tumors that, based on their immunoreactivity for GFAP, are derived from glial precursors (Wiestler *et al.*, 1992, 1994). Infection of mouse embryos with similar retroviral constructs have induced vascular meningeal neoplasms and malignant neoplasms in other tissues, but not gliomas (Compere *et al.*, 1989). Similarly, *in situ* injection of plasmids encoding the BK virus early region, including the large T antigen along with the activated *HRAS* oncogene, into newborn hamsters has induced intracranial sarcomas (Corallini *et al.*, 1988).

CHEMICAL CARCINOGENESIS

Early epidemiologic studies, such as those that associated use of tobacco snuff with oral cancers (Hill, 1761) and chimney sweeping with scrotal cancer (Potts, 1775), laid the foundation for the study of chemical carcinogenesis. Since that time, in an effort to establish models for testing brain tumor therapies, a number of different compounds that consistently induce nervous system tumors in experimental animals have been identified. The relative ease with which nervous system tumors could be selectively obtained in experimental animals after the administration of these agents, particularly polycyclic aromatic hydrocarbons (PAHs) and the *N*-nitroso compounds, resulted in a vigorous exploration of these animal models in various basic and applied aspects of neuro-oncology research. Many of these tumors have been subsequently passaged *in vitro* and *in vivo* and are now widely used to evaluate potential therapeutic agents.

More recently, a relatively small number of additional neurocarcinogens have been identified using the 'weight-of-evidence' approach to evaluate data obtained from *in vitro* mutagenicity assays and *in vivo* bioassays that are usually initiated because of epidemiologic concerns based on environmental or occupational exposure of humans. The scientific methods involved in the evaluation of potential human neurocarcinogens and the application of the 'weight-of-evidence' approach is detailed at the end of this section.

Polycyclic aromatic hydrocarbons and derivatives

The PAHs and their derivatives, notably fluorenylacetamides, were the first chemicals successfully used to induce nervous system tumors in experimental animals. Such compounds have been used to induce gliomas, sarcomas and meningiomas, intracranially, and malignant schwannomas, both intracranially and peripherally. It is also believed that PAHs are capable of transforming fetal mouse brain cells *in vitro* (Markovits *et al.*, 1979; Tripier *et al.*, 1979a). It should be mentioned, however, that murine glial cells maintained in long-term cultures may occasionally undergo spontaneous neoplastic transformation (Coulomb *et al.*, 1979).

Intracranial tumors induced by polycyclic aromatic hydrocarbons in experimental animals

Several chemicals from this large group of compounds have shown a carcinogenic effect intracranially. Benzo[a]pyrene, 3- and 20-methylcholanthrene (MCA), or dimethylbenz[a]anthracene (DMBA) have been the most effective and widely studied, however (Bigner and Swenberg, 1977). Tumor induction generally requires direct implantation of these compounds in the form of powder or pellets into the brain (Seligman and Shear, 1939), though intravenous DMBA, which has been shown to cross the placenta and enter the fetal CNS (Kleihues, Patzschke and Doerjer, 1982), was used successfully in pregnant animals to induce tumors in offspring (Hosobuchi and Ishii, 1967; Napalkov and Alexandrov, 1974). Mice, rats and Syrian hamsters are generally the only animal species vulnerable to this form of neuro-oncogenesis, though occasional tumors have been induced in ferrets, cats, rhesus monkeys, guinea pigs, rabbits and dogs (Mulligan *et al.*, 1946; Yablonovskya and Avtsyn, 1963). In addition, the successful attempts of Caputo and Giovanella (1957) to use PAHs to induce brain tumors in amphibians deserve special mention, given the rarity of spontaneous nervous system tumors in these animals.

The incidence, histology and latency of the intracranial tumors induced by PAHs were found to depend on a number of variables. The incidence of induced tumors was influenced by the PAH tested and the animal species and strain used (Zimmerman and Arnold, 1944). C3H/St mice were found to be especially susceptible to MCA (Zimmerman and Arnold, 1944) and Sprague-Dawley rats to be particularly susceptible to benzo[a]pyrene (Hopewell and Wright, 1969). The specific site of implantation of the pellet also has been found to influence the incidence of tumors, and gliomas were selectively induced in rats when the pellet was implanted in the periventricular region (Hopewell and Wright, 1969). This preferential induction of gliomas has been attributed to the selective involvement of the subependymal plate in glial tumorigenesis (Hopewell, 1975), a phenomenon that can also be seen in transplacental carcinogenesis that is caused by alkylating agents and also after the local introduction of oncogenic viruses. The susceptibility is reasonably attributable to the fact that this region remains as a pool for the further migration and replication of glial cells, a number of which may still be intermitotic at the time of implantation.

The latency period, usually slightly shorter for sarcomas than gliomas, varies considerably, with a range from 68 to 750 days reported in one experiment (Perese and Moore, 1960). Latency period also varies with the position of the implantation and with the form of administration. Shorter latency periods are generally associated with superficial implantation of pellets rather than the deeper implantation of powders. Russell (1945) also discovered that a vitamin-deficient diet reduced the latency period.

Fluorenylacetamides, which are derivatives of aromatic hydrocarbons, induce a variety of intracranial tumors in addition to tumors in various other organs and tissues of the rat, especially the liver, mammary glands, urinary bladder and ear duct. The oral administration of *N*-acetyl-2-acetylaminofluorene and of *N,N'*-diacetyl-2,7-diaminofluorene to these animals has resulted in a small number of malignant gliomas, including GBMs, oligodendrogliomas, meningiomas and malignant intracranial schwannomas (Vázquez-López, 1945; Hoch-Ligeti and Russell, 1950; Symeonidis, 1954; Snell *et al.*, 1961).

Pathology of polycyclic aromatic hydrocarbon-induced intracranial tumors in experimental animals

Both the gliomas and sarcomas induced by PAHs develop adjacent to the implanted pellet (Fig. 6.3).

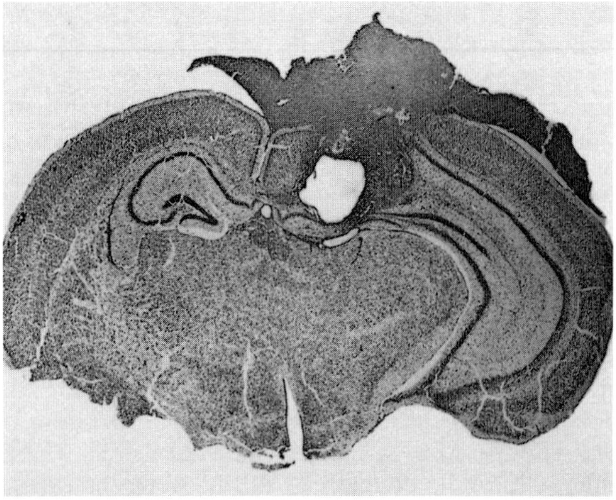

Fig. 6.3 Intracranial sarcoma produced by implanting a polycyclic aromatic hydrocarbon pellet in a mouse. Note the eccentric development of the tumor around the pellet site with meningeal spreading. Cresyl violet stain, magnifying glass. (From Bigner and Swenberg, 1977, with permission)

Preneoplastic lesions consist of multinucleated giant cells with narrow processes that stretch into the fissures and cracks in the pellet. These giant cells are surrounded by two or three layers of elongated, flat cells that contain round, hyperchromatic nuclei (Fig. 6.4). This appearance is stable for several months, and then tumor development proceeds very rapidly. Intracerebral tumors grow as nodules that are poorly demarcated and that often do not remain restricted to one hemisphere or to the cerebrum, but also spread into the midbrain, cerebellum or pons. These tumors are continuous from the pellet implantation site to distant parts of the brain. No tumor foci are observed that are not contiguous with the carcinogenic pellet. Large tumors often infiltrate or totally obliterate the ventricles and invade the leptomeninges; however, no metastases along the neuraxis or tumors of the spinal cord are found. Gliomas usually remain intracranial, whereas sarcomas often infiltrate extracranially into the soft tissues. Gliomas often exhibit extensive necrosis and hemorrhage on the cut surface of the brain, with only a small strip of glassy gray tumor tissue remaining at the border. In contrast, sarcomas are usually grayish-white and homogeneous, and necrosis and hemorrhage are rarely found in the intracranial sarcomas induced with PAHs.

Peripheral nervous system tumors induced by polycyclic aromatic hydrocarbons in experimental animals

Malignant tumors of the sciatic nerve in mice have also been produced by injecting PAHs locally (Causey, 1960). The tumor incidence is appreciably

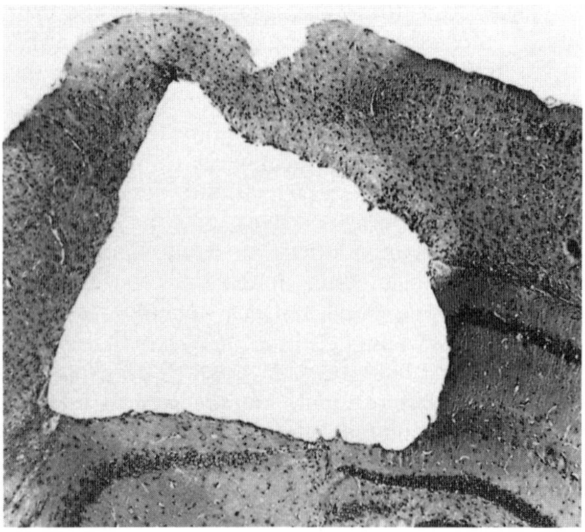

a

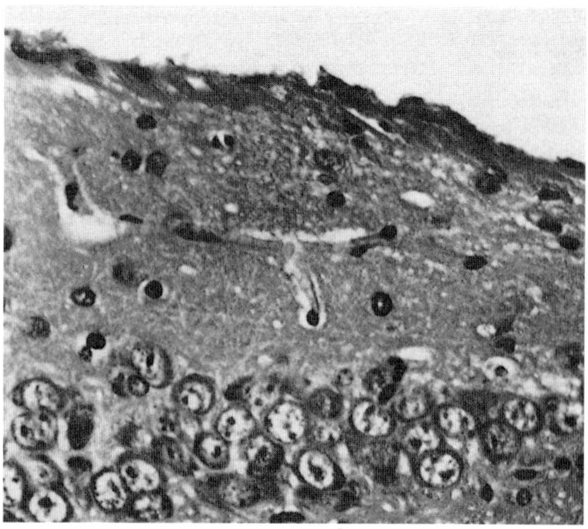

b

Fig. 6.4 Region surrounding a methylcholanthrene pellet in a mouse cerebrum 8 months after the pellet was implanted. (a) Pellet lodged in the cerebral cortex and in the bordering part of Ammon's horn (the pellet is dissolved). Hematoxylin and eosin (H&E), × 45 (b) Higher magnification of a narrow rim of flat cells around the pellet. No proliferative or inflammatory reaction is evident. H&E, × 410 (From Bigner and Swenberg, 1977, with permission) increased by crushing the nerve proximal to the site of injection of the carcinogen, an observation that supports Causey's contention that a neoplastic proliferation of Schwann cells accounted for these intraneural growths, as distinct from those that arose outside the intact perineurium, which he interpreted as fibrosarcomas; the latter being more apt to arise when the nerve had not been crushed.

Mechanism of action of polycyclic aromatic hydrocarbons

The precise mode of action of the PAHs in the genesis of brain tumors in experimental animals remains incompletely understood. It is, however, apparent that the factor of constitutional susceptibility in different species and strains is as important here as in experimental neoplasms induced by other techniques. The significance to be attached to the demonstration of cylindrical or filamentous virus-like particles in the cytoplasm of reactive cells in the precancerous stage that follows the local implantation of the PAHs is unclear (Ikuta and Zimmerman, 1965). The pathogenic implications of such findings are limited because many chemically induced tumors in mice express endogenous oncogenic retroviruses, including those obtained with nitrosourea derivatives (Denlinger, Koestner and Wechsler, 1974). An infectious murine mammary tumor virus is, apparently, constantly present in a transplantable primitive MCA-induced neuroepithelial mouse tumor (Rubin and Ames, 1973). Collectively, these observations may simply represent the morphological unmasking of passenger virus-related genetic material, which may be partially activated in a variety of experimental circumstances.

Interest in the local implantation of PAHs, however, has receded with the advent of the N-nitroso compounds as simple, reliable, dose-dependent and quantitatively assessable oncogenic agents. Still, most murine glioma cell lines were developed from PAH-induced tumors and have been maintained by serial passage. They are still used in a variety of experimental protocols and are discussed in the last section of this chapter.

N-nitroso compounds and other alkylating agents

Alkylating agents, like the nitrosourea derivatives, are more reliable inducers of experimental nervous system tumors than are PAHs. This is due, in part, to the striking neurotropicity of some of these powerful neurocarcinogens. Through a systematic testing of the oncogenic characteristics of 65 different

MNU *N*-methyl-*N*-nitrosourea

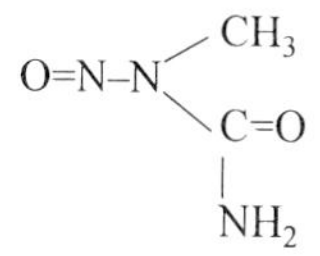

ENU Ethyl-nitrosourea

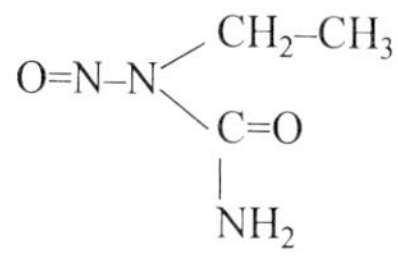

Fig. 6.5 Chemical structure of MNU and ENU.

N-nitroso compounds, Druckrey and colleagues (Druckrey, Ivankovic and Preussmann, 1964, 1965, 1966, 1967; Druckrey *et al.*, 1967) first established this neurotropicity. These workers found that neoplasms induced by *N*-methyl-*N*-nitrosourea (MNU) (Fig. 6.5), ethylnitrosourea (ENU), *N,N*-dimethyl-*N*-nitrosourea (DMNU), and *N,N',N'*-trimethyl-*N*-nitrosourea arose almost exclusively in the nervous system, whereas other *N*-nitroso compounds produced tumors in different organs but almost never in the brain or spinal cord. Since then, a vast number of additional neurotropic carcinogens have been found, and these compounds have been widely used for producing an impressive variety of tumors of the CNS and PNS. Although a large number of different alkylating agents have been employed for inducing nervous system neoplasms in experimental animals, their effectiveness has varied greatly. However, MNU, and especially ENU, remain the most widely used of the nitroso compounds for the production of nervous system tumors in experimental animals, especially rats.

Whether they are administered via the oral, subcutaneous, intramuscular, intravenous, intraperitoneal, intracerebral or transplacental route, MNU and ENU maintain their neurotropicity. Not all animals are equally susceptible to these neurocarcinogenic agents, however. Although animals such as the mouse, hamster, gerbil and dog have been used successfully, the laboratory rat, from various strains, has been the experimental animal of choice, though the rabbit is also highly susceptible to these agents. Importantly, nonhuman primates are also susceptible to the carcinogenic action of these substances. Rhesus (*M. mulatta*) or patas (*Erythrocebus patas*) monkeys exposed transplacentally to ENU early in gestation develop a disproportionate number of CNS tumors (Rice and Ward, 1982; Rice *et al.*, 1989). A ganglioglioma, an oligodendroglioma, an astrocytoma and a GBM have all been reported. However, PNS tumors have not been observed, and exposure of nonhuman primates to these agents after birth fails to induce CNS neoplasms, even after prolonged periods of observation (Bigner and Swenberg, 1977; Rice and Ward, 1982). In contrast, mice are relatively resistant to the neuro-oncogenic action of these compounds at any stage (Wechsler, Rice and Vesselinovitch, 1979). Central nervous system tumors in mice are especially difficult to obtain with these agents, and the mean latency is much longer than in rats. Tumors can generally only be obtained in mice when these compounds are given prenatally or neonatally. Nitrosourea-induced tumors in mice are almost always found singly and as an incidental accompaniment of multiple visceral tumors, which are usually the cause of death.

The activity of MNU and ENU in the rat is highly dependent on the age of the animal at the time of injection. In adult animals, MNU is the most active neuro-oncogenic substance. Repeated intravenous injections of MNU to young adult rats results in neurogenic tumors in 97% of animals, with a latency period of about 250 days (Swenberg, Koestner and Wechsler, 1972). Higher alkyl homologs, including ENU, however, are significantly less effective in adult rats. An exception is the strong oncogenic effect seen with butylnitrosourea in adult rats (Takizawa and Nishihara, 1971). In very young animals, on the other hand, the relative oncogenicity of MNU and ENU is curiously reversed. A very high incidence of nervous system tumors is induced by a single subcutaneous or intracerebral injection of ENU in newborn animals (Grossi-Paoletti *et al.*, 1972; Gerlach, Wessel and Musil, 1974). The tumor incidence attained with MNU in this age group is, in contrast, significantly lower (Warzok *et al.*, 1972; Gerlach, Wessel and Musil, 1974). In addition, it has been found that brain tumors could also be induced with intraportal injection of ENU, but not with MNU (Lijinsky *et al.*, 1972).

This marked susceptibility of younger animals to tumor induction with ENU eventually led to the establishment of the highly successful and convenient transplacental approach to nervous system tumor induction using ENU. In this protocol, a single low-dose intravenous injection of ENU is given to gravid rats on the 15th or 16th day of gestation. This technique produces tumors in virtually 100% of the offspring, with a latency period of approximately 300 days (Ivankovic and Druckrey, 1968; Koestner, Swenberg and Wechsler, 1971). Advantages of this model include the low level of exposure of laboratory personnel to the carcinogen, its technical simplicity, and the convenient production of tumors simultaneously in a large number of age-matched animals. In addition to brain tumors, tumors of the trigeminal nerve, spinal cord and PNS are also induced (Koestner, Swenberg and Wechsler, 1972; Schiffer, 1973). The time of ENU administration influences not only the tumor incidence (Ivankovic and Druckrey, 1968), but also the tumor location. A single ENU injection in rats on the 15th day of gestation induces mainly brain tumors in the offspring, while on the 21st day, the same dosage predominantly induces spinal cord tumors (Kahle, 1970). The search for additional neurotropic carcinogens revealed substances that are equal to ENU in transplacental effectiveness. These include azoethane, azoxyethane, diethylhydrazine, ethylnitrosobiuret, several triazene compounds and procarbazine (Bigner and Swenberg, 1977). With these substances, a neurogenic tumor incidence of over 80% is usually achieved.

The amazing neuro-oncogenic potential of these compounds is especially important in light of evidence that MNU and ENU can be synthesized in the digestive tract from inactive precursors given orally (Sander, 1970). Mirvish and Chu (1973) have demonstrated endogenous nitrosourea formation in the stomach of rats, and the oncogenic potential of this endogenous synthesis was demonstrated by adding nitrate to the dry food and methyl- or dimethylurea to the drinking water for long periods. The acid medium of the stomach favors the formation of MNU or DMNU from these additives. Most of the rats tested in this study developed tumors, predominantly in the nervous system. Nervous system tumors also developed in rats when ethylurea combined with sodium nitrite was given intragastrically to pregnant rats during the third week of their pregnancy. Since neither of these two chemicals produces neurogenic tumors on its own, these findings suggest that ENU is synthesized from these precursor substances under the influence of the gastric juice (Ramadan and Wechsler, 1975).

Central nervous system tumors induced by the *N*-nitrosoureas in experimental animals

Nitrosourea administration usually results in multiple subependymal tumors that morphologically resemble mixed gliomas, usually with a mixture of oligodendroglia and astrocytes, which may involve the cerebrum, cerebellum or spinal cord. Although the different cellular components of these mixed gliomas cannot always be identified with certainty, Conley (1979) found that a positive reaction for GFAP was present in the astrocytic portion of these tumors, and this observation

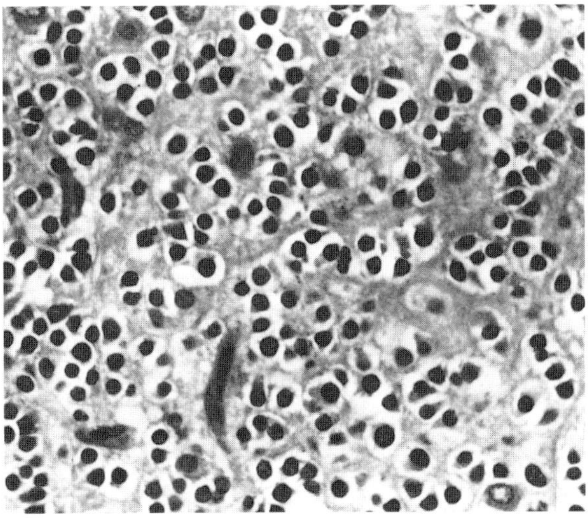

Fig. 6.6 Oligodendroglioma in a rat after MNU injections. H&E, × 420 (From Bigner and Swenberg, 1977, with permission)

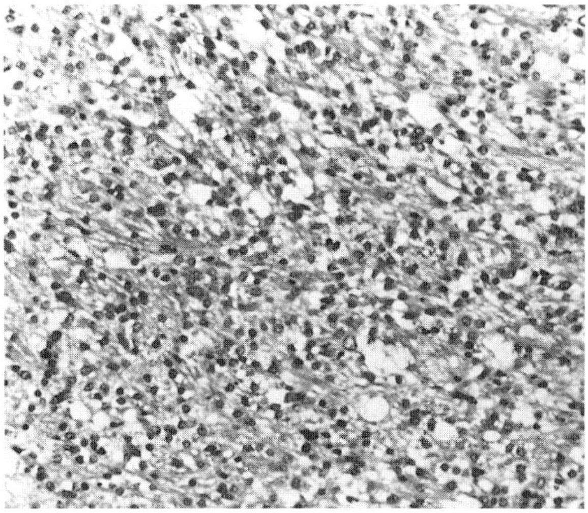

Fig. 6.7 Astrocytoma in a rat after MNU injections. Medium-sized, regular cells are present with no mitoses. H&E, × 175 (From Bigner and Swenberg, 1977, with permission)

was confirmed by Yoshino, Motoi and Ogawa (1985). Typical oligodendrogliomas, which more frequently appear in the hemispheric subcortical white matter (Fig. 6.6), and also typical astrocytomas (Fig. 6.7) are produced with these compounds (Sipe *et al.*, 1974; Bigner and Swenberg, 1977; Lantos, 1977), but these gliomas hardly ever show the typical histologic features of GBMs. Medulloblastomas, on the other hand, have been obtained only exceptionally, and then preferentially in mice rather than in rats. In addition, a type of tumor characteristically obtained is one in which the cells tend to be arranged in solid groups and cords with pseudorosette formation; it has often been called ependymoma, but shows no evidence of ependymal differentiation when examined by electron microscopy (Goebel and Cravioto, 1972). This was confirmed in a more recent fine structural study by Mandybur and Alvira (1982), who concluded that this neoplasm may represent a more primitive type of neuroepithelial tumor, perhaps a form of poorly differentiated oligodendroglioma. Recently, a number of these ENU-induced 'ependymomas' have been shown by immunohistochemical studies to express synaptophysin, a neuronal marker, suggesting that these tumors may be best classified as primitive neuroectodermal tumors (PNETs) with neuronal differentiation (Vaquero *et al.*, 1992). Finally, even neuronal neoplasms have been induced with these compounds, though only exceptionally (Brucher and Ermel, 1974).

This vast diversity of tumor histopathology, along with the high incidence of tumors with mixed morphologic and immunohistochemical features that arise in the subependymal region after administration of these chemicals, has led some to suggest that these tumors derive from the pluripotent neuroepithelial cells in the periventricular subependymal matrix (Shibutani *et al.*, 1994). The exclusive development of oligodendrogliomas from fetal brain transplants exposed to ENU pre- and postnatally, however, suggests that neoplastic transformation can be induced in a cell committed to oligodendrocyte differentiation (Burger *et al.*, 1988). Thus, pluripotent stem cells may not be required for tumor induction in the brain by these compounds.

Olfactory neuroblastomas in rats have also been induced following the repeated subcutaneous injection of nitrosopiperidine and nitrosopiperazine compounds (Vollrath *et al.*, 1986). Somewhat similar olfactory tumors may be obtained by adding the compound to the drinking water (Reznik-Schüller, 1983), or may be induced in Syrian hamsters by subcutaneous injection with *N*-diethylnitrosamine (Reznik-Schüller, 1978). Their differentiating features are complex: areas of squamous metaplasia may be found, and these may progress to squamous-cell carcinoma. Thus, the morphologic patterns may in places be neuroendocrine, in others neuroblastic and in others adenoid or squamous. Both neuroblastic and Flexner rosettes may be found, and a few cells express neurofilament protein.

Pathology of *N*-nitroso-induced intracranial tumors in experimental animals

Many of the tumors induced by these compounds are partially visible on external examination of the brain (Fig. 6.8). In other cases, an intracranial tumor is suggested by asymmetrical enlargement of one hemisphere, with contralateral displacement of the interhemispheric fissure (Fig. 6.9). The ventricles are often narrowed or filled by tumor, and dilatation of the ventricles is seldom found. Large hemorrhages in intracerebral tumors can be seen as areas of discoloration if the tumors are sufficiently superficial. Tumors are usually not sharply delineated on cut surfaces (Fig. 6.10) and are reddish-gray or yellowish in color. Some tumors are noticeable only because of an indistinct pattern of

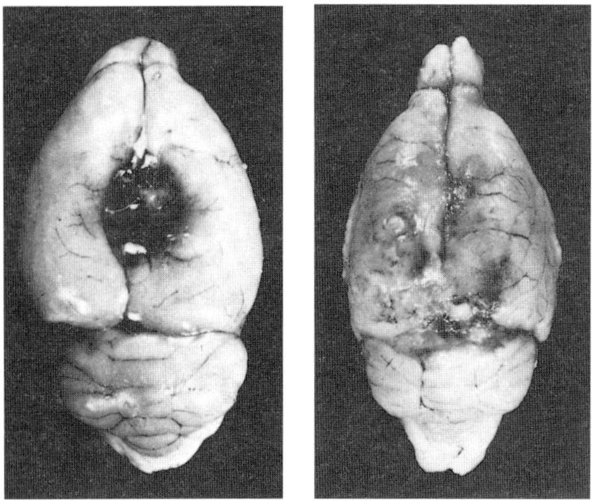

a b

Fig. 6.8 Rat tumors induced by nitrosamides. (a) Hemorrhagic tumor in the right cerebral hemisphere. The interhemispheric fissure is displaced contralaterally. (b) Intracerebral tumor, with infiltration of the leptomeninges. (From Bigner and Swenberg, 1977, with permission)

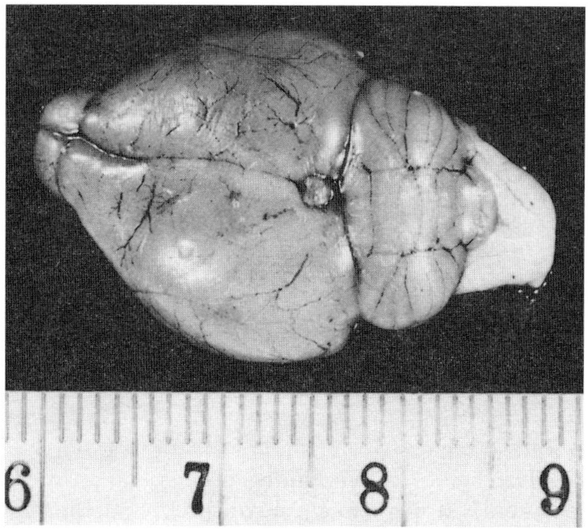

Fig. 6.9 Rat tumor induced by nitrosamides. Swelling of the left cerebral hemisphere with contralateral displacement of the interhemispheric fissure due to a tumor in the central portion of the hemisphere. (From Bigner and Swenberg, 1977, with permission)

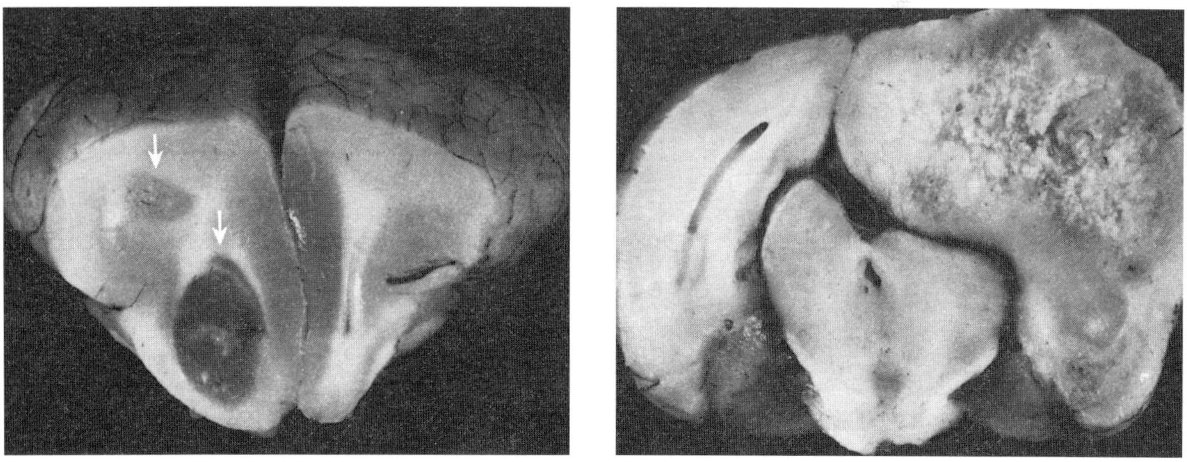

a b

Fig. 6.10 Rabbit tumors induced by nitrosamides. (a) Two different-sized tumor foci (white arrows) in the right frontal lobe after intravenous MNU injections. (b) Intracerebral sarcoma in the right occipital lobe after intravenous MNU injections. (From Bigner and Swenberg, 1977, with permission) brain tissue, or are only detected by histologic examination although they are actually quite large. In addition to various degrees of hemorrhage (Fig. 6.11), occasional yellowish necrosis and pseudocysts are also observed (Fig. 6.12).

Tumor induction with nitrosamides provides an opportunity to evaluate early stages of tumor development. Within a short period of time, several tumors develop independently at various points in the CNS. Therefore, one can sometimes find tumors that are in the early stages of development

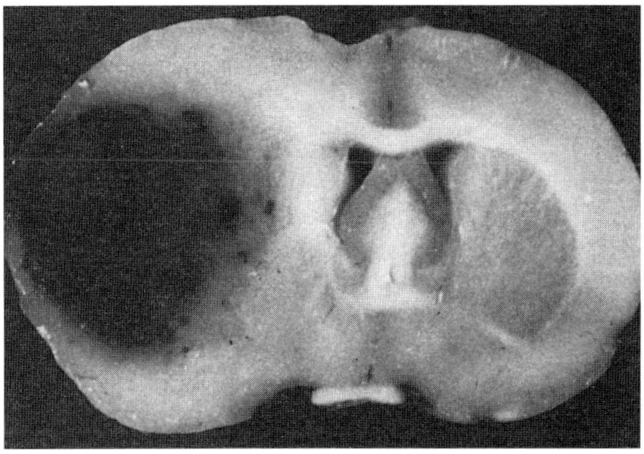

Fig. 6.11 Poorly demarcated, hemorrhagic glioblastoma in the cerebrum of a rat after MNU administration. (From Bigner and Swenberg, 1977, with permission)

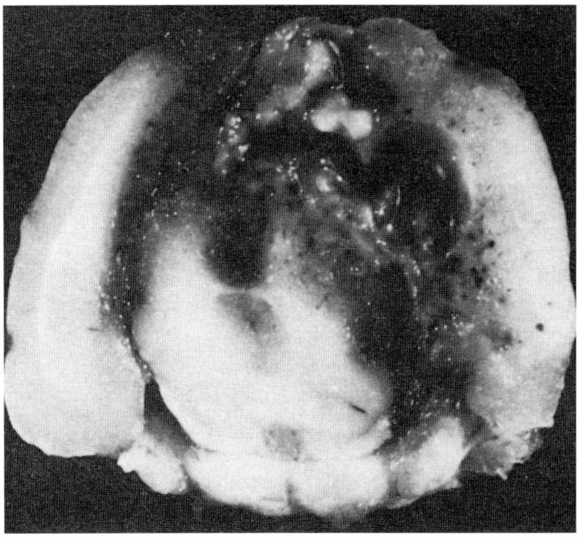

Fig. 6.12 Pseudocysts in a largely necrotic glioblastoma multiforme of the occipital lobe of the cerebrum and midbrain of a rat after MNU injections. (From Bigner and Swenberg, 1977, with permission)

and are independent of the larger tumors causing neurologic symptoms or death. Thus, several stages of tumor development may exist side by side in one animal, facilitating a better understanding of the neoplastic process. Two distinct patterns can be observed. In the first pattern, which can be observed 2 months after tumor induction, abnormal clusters of undifferentiated cells proliferate as single or multiple lesions in the periventricular subependymal plate (Lantos and Pilkington, 1979). Later, these proliferations increase in size and form small tumors, most often in the angles of the lateral ventricles between the corpus callosum and the caudate nucleus, but also over the lateral aspect of the ventricles (Pilkington and Lantos, 1979). The cellular nature of these early microtumors has been variously interpreted. Some regarded them as oligodendroglial (Schiffer *et al.*, 1978), whereas others (Bigner and Swenberg, 1977; Mennel and Simon, 1985) considered that they were of two kinds: purely oligodendroglial, and mixed oligodendrocytic and astrocytic (Figs 6.13 and 6.14). On the basis of the lack of cellular immunoreactivity for GFAP and with the Leu 7 monoclonal antibody, Yoshino, Motoi and Ogawa (1985) regarded the cells forming these early tumors as undifferentiated glial precursor cells. In the white matter, these cells are found as isolated cells or as short chains among the myelinated fibers. In the gray matter, they are grouped around neurons, thus resembling the satellitosis that occurs in human oligodendroglioma. At this stage, the neoplastic cells can hardly be differentiated from normal cells morphologically, and mitoses are rarely visible. The blood vessels of these early stages are thin walled and lack proliferation of endothelial or adventitial cells. Giant cells and atypical cells are not found in the early stages of glioma development. These scattered neoplastic cells progressively proliferate to form larger nodules of tumor tissue that increase in size and develop into mixed gliomas and PNETs.

A second pattern of tumor development can also be discerned. Here, small foci of hyperplastic astrocytes primarily develop subcortically in the white matter of the cerebrum (Schiffer *et al.*, 1978) or just under the internal granular layer of the cerebellum (Naito *et al.*, 1986). After several months, these proliferations can be seen to enlarge into microtumors that stain with Alcian blue and ultimately develop into pure anaplastic oligodendrogliomas.

Peripheral nervous system tumors induced by nitrosoureas in experimental animals

The PNS tumors that most frequently develop after administration of the *N*-nitroso compounds are schwannomas, which exhibit various degrees of

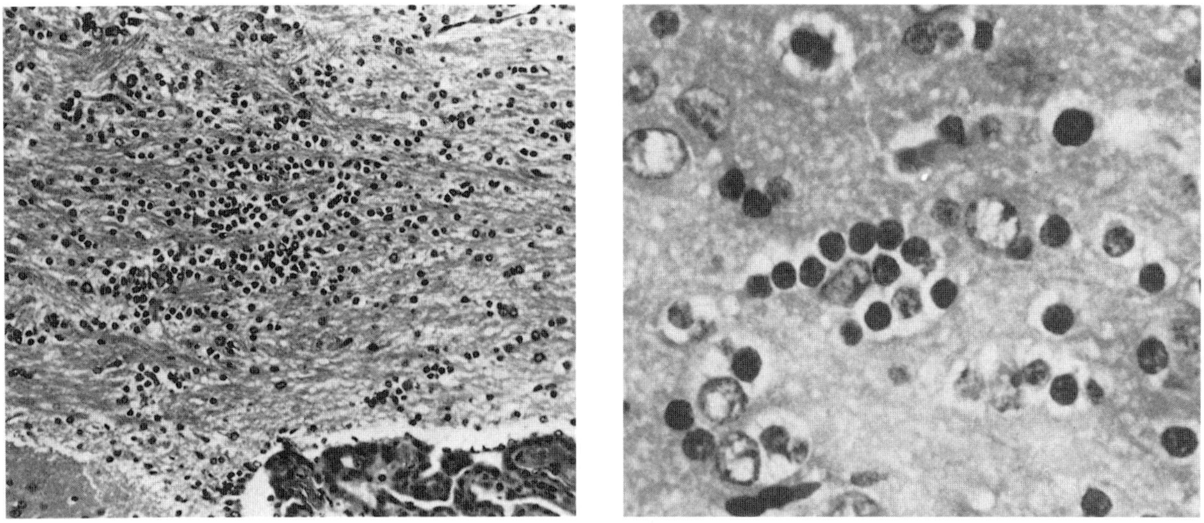

a b

Fig. 6.13 Early stages of intracerebral gliomas in rats that have received an intravenous MNU injection. (a) Proliferation of oligodendroglia in the vicinity of the lateral ventricle. H&E, × 175 (b) Proliferation of oligodendroglia in the cerebral cortex with satellitosis around a neuron. H&E, × 685 (From Bigner and Swenberg, 1977, with permission)

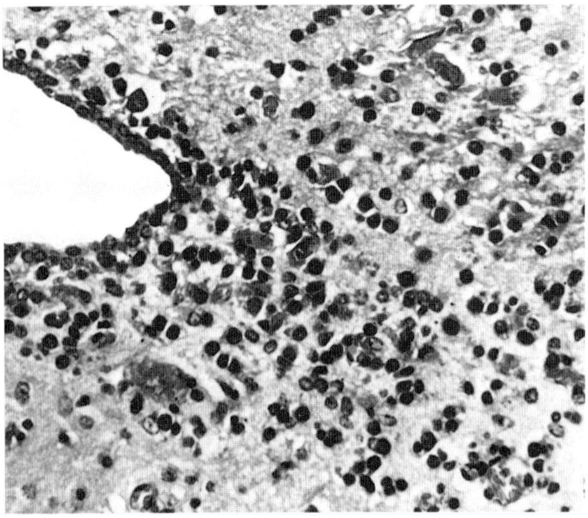

Fig. 6.14 Early stage of a glioma in a rat that has received an MNU injection. Note the proliferation of astrocytic cells in the vicinity of the lateral ventricle. H&E, × 260 (From Bigner and Swenberg, 1977, with permission)

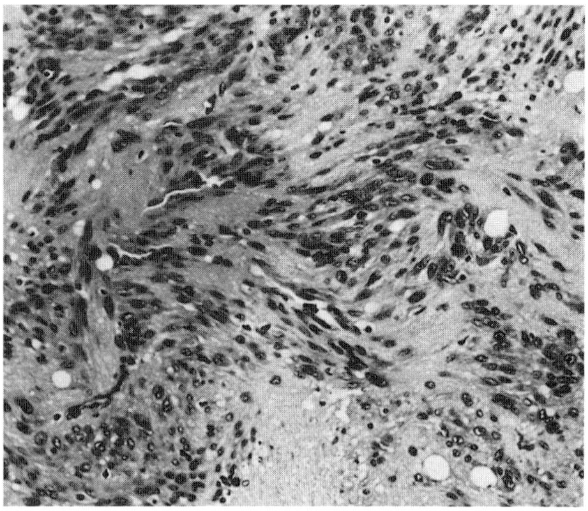

Fig. 6.15 Nerve root tumor in a rat that received intravenous MNU injections. The neurinoma-like histostructure is composed of regular cells, partly arranged in a row and containing small hyalinized areas within the tumor. H&E, × 175 (From Bigner and Swenberg, 1977, with permission)

anaplasia, depending on the compound used, the technique of administration and the strain of the animal. The less differentiated examples are usually obtained following transplacental ENU in Sprague-Dawley or Long-Evans rats, whereas more differentiated schwannomas are more often produced after repeated intravenous MNU injection in Fischer rats (Fig. 6.15). The trigeminal nerve root or cranial nerve roots within the cerebellopontine angle (Fig. 6.16) are most frequently involved by growth, followed by the spinal nerve roots (Fig. 6.17). When these neoplasms are induced, transplacentally, with

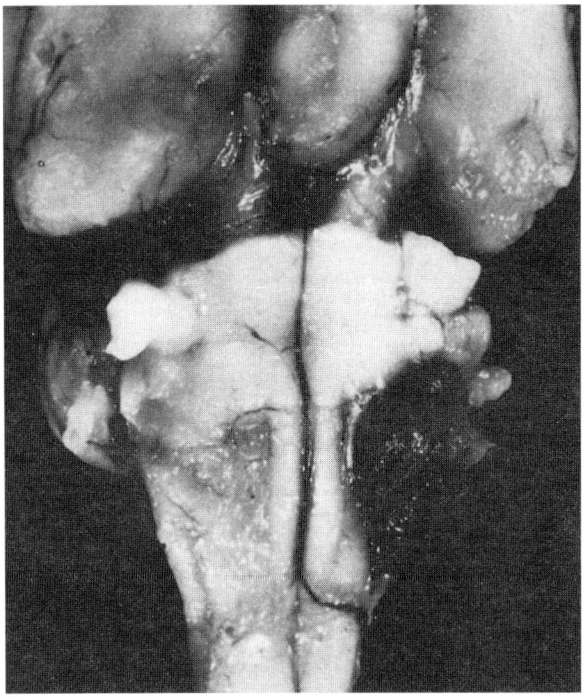

a

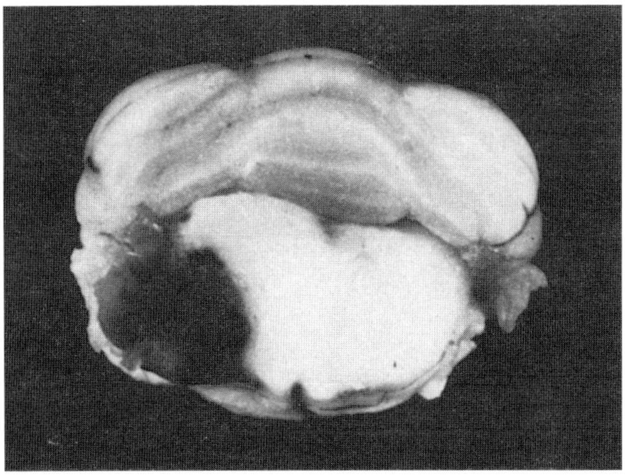

b

Fig. 6.16 Nerve root tumor in the left cerebellopontine angle of a rat that has received intravenous MNU injections. (a) Anterior view of the base of the brain. (b) Cut surface of the same tumor compressing the medulla. (From Bigner and Swenberg, 1977, with permission)

ENU, they generally appear in the offspring after approximately 200 days, whereas the latent interval is approximately 265 days after a single injection of ENU in the neonate. The Schwann cell origin of these tumors has been well established from electron microscopic examination of very early examples, and their behavior *in vitro* convincingly aligns them with the more differentiated schwannomas found in humans (Conley, Rubinstein and Spence, 1976). In the offspring of Wistar rats that have been treated intraperitoneally with a single dose of ENU on the 15th day of pregnancy, the Schwann cell tumors are more complex. They frequently involve the maxillary region as well as the Gausserian ganglion, and often display, in places, the structure of a plexiform neurofibroma (Cardesa *et al.*, 1983, 1989).

Mechanism of action of *N*-nitrosoureas

The neurotropicity of these compounds is generally believed to be due primarily to the guiding action of their urea radical, which facilitates their diffusibility into the nervous system, thus compensating for their instability as carcinogens. Their small molecular weight and their lipid solubility may also play a part, however. Like other alkylating agents, the nitrosoureas are both mutagenic and teratogenic, the deleterious action in each case being due to the reaction of the alkyl radical with one or more bases in the DNA chain. The ability of various carcinogens of this class to cause nucleophilic substitutions that occur at the extranuclear oxygen of nucleic acids, usually guanine but less frequently also thymine and cytosine, correlates well with their carcinogenic potential (Singer and Grunberger, 1983). Therefore, the carcinogenic action of the nitrosoureas should be linked to a defect in DNA excision repair within brain tissue. In most tissues, the O^6-alkylguanines produced by these nucleophilic substitutions would be readily repaired by the enzyme O^6-alkylguanine-DNA alkyltransferase (Pegg, 1990). Brain cells, however, eliminate O^6-alkylated bases much less efficiently than do other tissues (Goth and Rajewsky, 1974a; Margison and Kleihues, 1975). A failure to repair these changes produces anomalous base-pairing of the alkylated guanine with thymine, resulting in a G:C $\rightarrow$ A:T transition mutation (Goth and Rajewsky, 1974b; Margison and Kleihues, 1975). On the other hand, whereas there is fairly general acceptance that the O^6 position of guanine is the critical target in the initiation of tumors by these carcinogenic agents, species and strain-related differences in the response to alkylating agents have not been paralleled by differences in the excision repair capacity of O^6-alkylguanine adducts (Kleihues *et al.*, 1979). For example, although mice and gerbils are similarly deficient in O^6-alkylguanine repair, these species are considerably more resistant than rats to tumor induction with ENU and related alkylators (Kleihues and Rajewsky, 1984) (see Chapter 5).

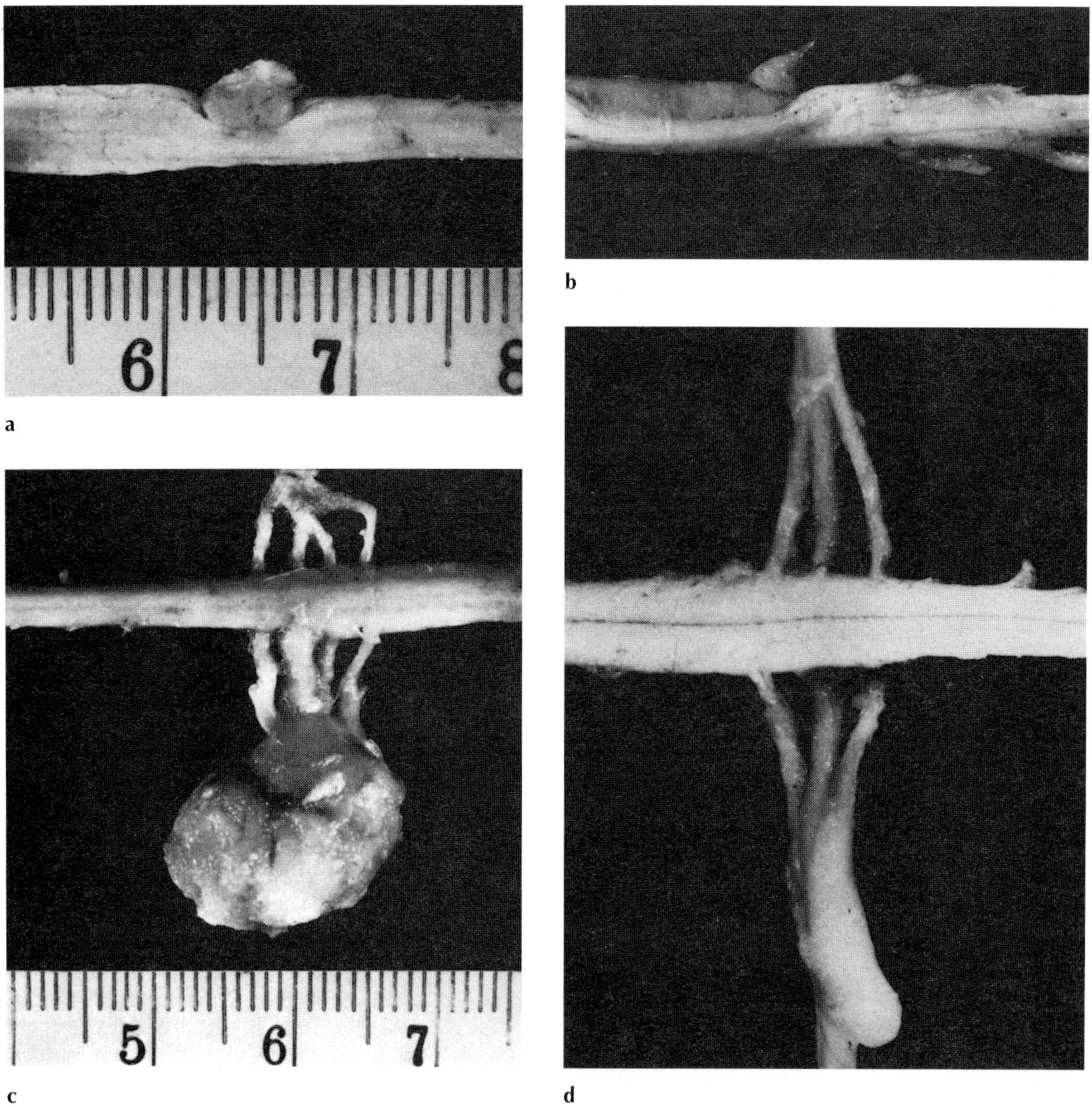

Fig. 6.17 Nerve root tumors in rats following MNU administration. (a) Oval-shaped nerve root tumor with compression of the spinal cord in a rat after intravenous MNU injections. (b) Elongated nerve root tumor causing depression of the conus medullaris in a rat after MNU administration. (c) Cherry-sized tumor of the brachial plexus and accompanying spinal cord nerve roots in a rat after intragastric MNU administration. (d) Neoplastic thickening of several nerve roots in a rat after intravenous MNU injections. (From Bigner and Swenberg, 1977, with permission)

It is well recognized that in transplacental carcinogenesis the rat nervous system is maximally vulnerable to neoplastic transformation during the last days before birth and shortly thereafter. When given before or around the 12th day of gestation, ENU does not cause any nervous system tumors, and its effects are solely toxic and teratogenic. One factor that may preclude the neuro-oncogenicity of ENU before the 12th day of gestation could be the insufficient critical size of the target cell population in demonstrating a carcinogenic effect (Kleihues and Rajewsky, 1984). In the later stages of pregnancy, the subependymal cells of the cerebral hemispheres of the fetus are the CNS cells that are especially susceptible to neoplastic transformation, the target cells being the still-cycling glioblasts in the course of their migration from the primitive ventricular zone. The nitrosoureas have been shown to inhibit the mitotic activity of these proliferating cells, resulting in temporary cell cycle arrest in, or shortly before, the S phase (Bosch, 1979). Re-entry into the cell cycle takes place, however, long before the chemically induced alterations in the cellular macromolecules have been repaired, and this effect will be especially notable if, in addition, excision repair mechanisms are deficient in the target cells. In contrast, when ENU is given in the earlier stages of pregnancy, the subependymal cells and the external granular matrices experience the cytotoxic effects alone (Bosch, Gerrits and Ebels, 1972). The apparent lack of vulnerability of the external fetal granular layer to neoplastic transformation and the almost total failure to obtain medulloblastomas with these compounds, however, remain an enigma. The last observation is puzzling because various strains of rats that were given ENU in the neonatal period were found to be vulnerable to neuro-oncogenic action at the cerebellum, but most of the tumors produced in that part of the central neuraxis have been oligodendrogliomas in the subcortical white matter just under the internal granular-cell layer (Naito *et al.*, 1986).

From a molecular perspective, no specific genetic alteration has been definitively associated with CNS tumors induced by MNU or ENU. Some evidence from cell lines obtained from ENU-induced tumors, however, demonstrate nonrandom abnormalities, especially in chromosome 4, but also in chromosomes 1, 2, 3 and 7 (Haag and Soukup, 1984). These may be late changes in tumor development, however. In addition, mutations have been observed in the tumor suppressor gene *TP53*, but they are rare (Calvert *et al.*, 1994), and no mutations in the *RAS* oncogene have been reported for brain tumors induced with these compounds, despite the frequent occurrence of *RAS* mutations in similarly induced mammary tumors (Sukumar, 1989).

More is known regarding tumors induced in the PNS, however. Activation of the *ERBB2* oncogene has been reported in ENU-induced rat schwannomas obtained by the transplacental route. This gene appears to be related to human epidermal growth factor receptor gene (Bargmann *et al.*, 1986a) and, when mutated, invariably contains a T:A $\rightarrow$ A:T transversion mutation at nucleotide 2012 of codon 664 (Bargmann *et al.*, 1986b; Perantoni *et al.*, 1987). Similarly, in the ENU-induced neurofibromas in Syrian hamsters, T:A $\rightarrow$ A:T transversions have also been identified in codons 658 and 659 (Nakamura *et al.*, 1994). Similar mutations have not been identified in human PNS tumors, however (Saya *et al.*, 1990).

Assessment of potential human neurocarcinogens

As discussed in Chapter 1 of this textbook, a number of agents have been implicated in the etiology of primary brain tumors. Methodological inconsistencies and conflicting results have prevented the establishment of firm connections between almost all of these factors and brain tumors, however. As a result, ionizing radiation remains the only established cause of human primary CNS tumors (Jänisch *et al.*, 1984; Preston-Martin, 1989; Hochberg *et al.*, 1990; Kuijten and Bunin, 1993; Preston-Martin *et al.*, 1993; Wrensch *et al.*, 1993; Bondy *et al.*, 1994; Bunin *et al.*, 1994; Brem, Rozental and Moskal, 1995). High-dose therapeutic ionizing radiation that covers the area of the brain in which the induced tumor later arises has been shown, using the original criteria established by Cahan *et al.* (1948) for radiation-induced bone sarcoma, to induce brain tumors. These criteria require evidence that the initial and second neoplastic disorders are of a different cell lineage, that the second neoplastic disorder arose within an area incorporated by the radiation beam and that an appropriate latent period elapsed before the appearance of the new tumor. In a long-term follow-up study of patients irradiated for pituitary adenoma, Tsang *et al.* (1993) found that the risk for developing malignant gliomas in those patients was 16 times greater than the risk of such tumors in the general population. The study results were statistically significant. Other tumor types that have been reported in association with ionizing radiation include meningiomas, medulloblastomas, cerebellar GBMs and brainstem gliomas (Lubetzki *et al.*, 1991; Brüstle *et al.*, 1992; Zagzag *et al.*, 1992; Mack and Wilson, 1993). Aside from radiation, the initiating events for causing genetic damage that leads to primary brain tumors in humans remain unknown. The mutational events that begin the process may very well be random background events, such as low-level cosmic rays or endogenous (i.e., not caused by genotoxic environmental carcinogens) DNA adducts (Louis, 1994; Ohgaki *et al.*, 1995), since there is a background incidence of primary brain tumors, as discussed in the first section of this chapter, in virtually all mammalian and most other species, including nonhuman primates.

The potential for some chemicals to promote tumor growth, although incapable of inducing tumors themselves, has undergone very limited study with regard to brain tumors. Phenobarbital has been implicated in this process, but several studies have shown that phenobarbital has no promotional activity (Walker and Swenberg, 1989; Purves and Dayan, 1992). In fact, until recently, no scientific studies were able to show that any chemical could promote growth of primary brain tumors that had been initiated by other causes. However, Burger *et al.* (1988) have now provided some evidence that brain tumor development *in vivo* may be a multistep process. They demonstrated that adult rats, harboring fetal brain transplants derived from donors exposed to ENU *in utero* and themselves exposed to ENU postnatally, grew oligodendrogliomas, selectively, within the grafts. Eliminating either the prenatal exposure of the donors or the postnatal exposure of the transplanted rats to ENU, however, significantly reduced the incidence of tumors, suggesting that both an initiation and a promotion step had occurred.

To establish that an agent may increase the risk to humans of a given type of cancer, for example brain tumors, two broad criteria must be fulfilled. First, significant human exposure must be documented, and, second, the agent must be found to be carcinogenic in the tissue of interest. Epidemiologic studies can provide the only real data on the risk of carcinogens to humans. These studies have been able to identify, for testing, potential carcinogens that had not previously been considered suspect. For example, such studies were able to identify the risk of mesothelioma from asbestos exposure, leukemia from benzene exposure, bladder cancer in dye workers and lung cancer from cigarette smoking. Still, such studies cannot directly establish causation as a result of the innumerable uncontrolled factors that may bias such assessments. The Hill criteria (Table 6.7) have been widely accepted by the scientific community and, traditionally, have been recommended by prominent agencies, including the World Health Organization (WHO), the International Agency for Research Cancer (IARC) and the U.S. Environmental Protection Agency (EPA), as suitable criteria for the assessment of causation (Hill, 1965).

Table 6.7 Hill's criteria of causation

1. Strength of the association
2. Consistency of the association
3. Specificity of the association
4. Temporality of the association
5. Biologic gradient relating exposure to disease
6. Biologic plausibility of the association
7. Coherence of the evidence
8. Experiment evidence for the association
9. An analogy for the relationship between the exposure and the association

[a] From Hill, 1965.

Demonstration that an agent is carcinogenic within the brain begins with a summation of evidence from a number of different sources regarding the ability of the compound to act as a carcinogen within the nervous system. Sources of data used in the assessment of carcinogenicity primarily include *in vitro* mutagenesis assays and *in vivo* chronic bioassays.

The Ames' *in vitro* mutagenesis assay (Ames, McCann and Yamasaki, 1975), is a widely used and sensitive assay in which frameshift mutations or base-pair substitutions are measured in *Salmonella typhimurium* bacteria. Other similar mutagenesis assays use *in vitro* culture of various mammalian cell lines to detect forward mutations, sister chromatid exchanges and unscheduled DNA synthesis. These assays provide efficient and economical screening tests for potential carcinogens, but lack specificity.

In contrast, chronic bioassays in animals are expensive and lengthy, but few better alternatives exist for the prediction of potential human carcinogenic risk. Such studies employ designated strains of rats and mice that undergo lifetime exposure to a carcinogen at the maximal dose that does not produce clinical toxicity, defined as the maximum tolerated dose (MTD), in addition to one or more lower doses that represent a significant fraction of the MTD—usually 50% and 30%. These relatively high doses are used so that an increase in cancer incidence will be detectable in a reasonably sized population of about 50 male and 50 female test animals per exposure dose. Although use of the MTD in these studies is intended to increase the sensitivity of such assays, the tests suffer from certain biases associated with the use of very high doses, which may increase the endogenous mutation rate and often exceed practical levels of human exposure. On the other hand, even conservative extrapolations from these high doses to much lower doses have been shown in a small, but significant, number of cases to *underestimate* the carcinogenic risk significantly (Bailar *et al.*, 1988). Furthermore, some known human carcinogens are not carcinogenic in common laboratory animals, carcinogens identified in one animal species will not always be carcinogenic in another, and many carcinogens identified in chronic bioassays have different organ targets in humans (Purchase, 1980).

THE NEED FOR THE 'WEIGHT-OF-EVIDENCE' APPROACH IN ASSESSING CARCINOGENICITY THROUGH CHRONIC BIOASSAYS

In assessing carcinogenicity, although concordance among different methods of evaluation and among different studies is usually high, it is not absolute. Inference of a carcinogenic effect in animals, then, should be based on several factors and not just on a statistically significant increase in tumors in a given test group. Factors such as differences between concurrent control populations and historically used controls, uncontrollable variables and statistical methods can influence such results greatly. Therefore, statistical measures of an increased incidence of certain tumors, such as brain tumors, in an exposed population, either humans or laboratory animals, should not in itself ever be regarded as irrefutable evidence that an agent is a potential neurocarcinogen. Instead a 'weight-of-evidence' approach, which takes into consideration pathobiologic parameters and biologic variability, must be used to evaluate the evidence (Koestner, 1986; Swenberg, 1986).

To illustrate this point, consider spontaneous tumor incidence and the variation in its occurrence across control groups of experimental animals, as discussed in the first section of this chapter (Tables 6.3 and 6.4). In some cases, these differences can be statistically significant. Such variation, then, creates a problem with the interpretation of chronic bioassays when it results, by chance, in a statistically significant increase in specific tumor types in a test group for a given agent in a given experiment. In this regard, Koestner (1986) has emphasized the necessity, in such assays, of using a strain of animals that have a low variability in their incidence of spontaneous primary brain tumors. As a result, the NTP uses the F344 rat strain in its chronic bioassays because this rat strain has a fairly stable incidence of such tumors. This is in sharp contrast to the Sprague-Dawley rat strain, which is known to have great variability in its incidence of spontaneous primary brain tumors and, as a result, is really an inappropriate animal strain for use in these assays. Still, it should be noted that even in the life-span studies of Solleveld, Haseman and McConnell (1984) with F344 rats, a statistically significant intergroup variability was observed for the incidence of astrocytomas in male rats. This type of problem has been encountered several times in recent years by a number of regulatory agencies, and has been dealt with by their application of weight-of-evidence guidelines. Given the low and variable incidence of spontaneous nervous system tumors in animals used in even the most well-controlled chronic bioassays, a statistical analysis alone cannot substantiate a conclusion of carcinogenicity without collaborative biologic evidence of neurocarcinogenicity. The weight-of-evidence approach takes into consideration biologic variation and pathobiologic parameters, and uses a biologic as well as a statistical analysis to determine carcinogenicity. It has been used successfully by the U.S. Food and Drug Administration in evaluating aspartame, FD&C blue #2 dye, and 18 color dyes tested by the Certified Color Manufacturers' Association. The general criteria used in this approach when applied to brain tumors are given in Table 6.8.

The pathobiologic parameters evaluated in the weight-of-evidence approach can be validated if one considers that all of the relatively small number of already established animal neurocarcinogens share a number of the features included in this type of assessment. First, ionizing radiation, the only established human neurocarcinogen, and all chemicals known to be neurocarcinogenic in animals are strongly and unequivocally genotoxic; that is, they exert DNA damage detectable by DNA adduct formation or other tests of DNA damage in the target organ, namely the PNS or the CNS. This includes PAHs, such as MCA, benzopyrene and DMBA when they are implanted into the CNS; systemically administered *N*-nitroso chemicals, such as MNU and ENU; hydrazines, such as ethylhydrazine; aryl diakyltrazines, such as 1-phenyl-3,3-dimethyltriazine; alkylating agents, such as propane sultone; other agents, such as 2-acetylaminofluorene and methyl methane sulfonate; and the most recently tested industrial compounds shown to be neurocarcinogenic, namely acrylonitrile (Bigner *et al.*, 1986), ethylene oxide (Garman, Snellings and Maronpot, 1986) and glycidol. Oncogenic viruses are the only class of substances that induce brain tumors in animals but are not directly genotoxic. They do, however, cause brain cancer through a genetic mechanism, in this case through the overexpression of a transforming oncogene. All known animal neurocarcinogens also demonstrate a dose response. This means that, with increasing dose, an increase in nervous system tumor incidence and multiplicity and a decrease in tumor latency and survival are observed. In addition, none of the proven animal neurocarcinogens produce only microtumors. That is, all of the known and accepted neurocarcinogens produced mostly macroscopic brain tumors of $\geqslant$5 mm in chronic bioassays. Finally, all known animal neurocarcinogens induce tumors in both sexes with an increased frequency of tumors in organ sites other than the nervous system. For

Table 6.8 'Weight-of-evidence' criteria used to establish that an agent is a neurocarcinogen in animals

	Neurocarcinogen[a]						
Criteria	RAD	MNU	ENU	ASV	ACN	ETO	GLY
Genotoxicity	+	+	+	NA	+	+	+
Dose–response relationship:							
(a) increasing dose increases tumor incidence and multiplicity compared with controls at each effective dose level	+	+	+	+	+	+	+
(b) increasing dose decreases tumor latency and survival, and increases size and progression of tumor	+	+	+	+	+	+	+
Uniform increase in the induction of neoplasia:							
(a) in the spinal cord and peripheral nerves	NT	+	+	+	+	+	NT
(b) at other systemic sites	+	+	+	+	+	+	+
(c) in both sexes	+	+	+	+	+	+	+
(d) in more than one species	+	+	+	+	NT	NT	NT
Histologic features:							
(a) evidence of preneoplastic lesions in interim kill animals	NT	+	+	+	+	+	+
(b) predominantly macroscopic ($\geq$5 mm) tumors in chronic bioassay animals	+	+	+	+	+	+	+
(c) increasing tumor grade or distinctive tumor morphology	+	+	–	–	–	–	–
Statistically significant increase in brain tumor incidence over internal controls in experimental animal chronic bioassays	+	+	+	+	+	+	+
Statistically significant increase in brain tumor incidence over internal controls in human epidemiologic studies	+	–	–	–	–	–	–

[a] RAD, ionizing radiation; MNU, *N*-methyl-*N*-nitrosourea; ENU, ethylnitrosourea; ASV, avian sarcoma virus; ACN, acrylonitrile; ETO, ethylene oxide; GLY, glycidol.

[b] NA, not applicable; NT, not tested.

example, acrylonitrile also produces Zymbal gland tumors and papillomas of the stomach and skin, and ethylene oxide produces a dose-related increase in mononuclear cell leukemia in female rats and in peritoneal mesotheliomas in male rats. These criteria, then, can be used to substantiate that an increased incidence of brain tumors observed in experimental animal chronic bioassays or in human epidemiologic studies is, in fact, due to a carcinogenic effect and not simply to a confounding variable or a chance occurrence.

In summary, then, any attempt to establish a substance as an animal neurocarcinogen should address a number of specific questions, as follows:

1. Is the test substance genotoxic?
2. Is there a statistically significant increase in the incidence of primary brain tumors in exposed animals relative to both unexposed internal controls and historically used controls? Does this occur in both sexes? Can the same increase be seen in more than one species?
3. Is there an increase in the incidence of primary tumors with increasing exposure dose? Is there an associated increase in the number of primary brain tumors in a single animal? Do the tumors occur earlier in the animals' lifespan, and is the appearance of the tumors associated with a decrease in survival?

4. Are tumors also 'induced' in the spinal cord, peripheral nerves or at other extraneural organ sites?
5. Are the induced brain tumors macroscopic (≥5 mm)? Can characteristic, coexisting preneoplastic lesions be identified? Do the induced tumors have a morphology that is distinct from that of tumors arising spontaneously in the same species?

When a substance meets most of the criteria outlined above, the biologic plausibility of its potential as a neurocarcinogen has been reasonably well established. Such findings identify it as a *potential* risk to humans. This should not be misconstrued to mean that such a substance is a human neurocarcinogen, however. This conclusion would need further evidence, as discussed above, including the establishment, by epidemiologic studies, of a consistent relationship between exposure to the substance and a specific primary brain tumor histiotype in humans. In light of the weight-of-evidence criteria outlined above, chemicals for which chronic bioassays have demonstrated clear evidence of carcinogenicity in the brain include the nitrosoureas, such as ENU, given orally, subcutaneously, intraperitoneally, intravenously or transplacentally in rats, orally in opossums and prenatally in mice; MNU, given in the diet, drinking water, or subcutaneously or intravenously in rats, in the drinking water of guinea pigs and intravenously in dogs; lead subacetate, given in the diet of Sprague-Dawley CD rats of both sexes (Oyasu *et al.*, 1970); 1,3-propane sultone, given by gavage in Charles River CD rats of both sexes (Ulland *et al.*, 1971); propylene imine, given by gavage in Charles River CD rats of both sexes (Ulland *et al.*, 1971); and acrylamide, given in the drinking water of F344 rats (Johnson *et al.*, 1986). More recently, a number of additional neurocarcinogenic industrial compounds have been identified in chronic bioassays as potential neurocarcinogens (Table 6.9). They are discussed in the paragraphs that follow.

In addition, chemicals for which chronic bioassays have concluded that there was clear evidence for the induction of olfactory neuroblastomas included procarbazine injected intraperitoneally into Sprague-Dawley rats of both sexes and B6C3F1 mice of both sexes, *p*-cresidine given in the food of male and female F344 rats but not B6C3F1 mice of either sex, and bis(chloromethyl) ether inhaled by male Sprague-Dawley rats (Kuschner and Laskin, 1975).

Table 6.9 Some known animal chemical neurocarcinogens with potential for human exposure[a]

Specific chemicals	Chemical classes
Acrylamide (2-propenamide)	Alkylsulfates
Acrylonitrile (vinyl cyanide)	Hydrazines
Cyclophosphamide (peripheral neurogenic sarcomas)	*N*-Nitrosourea derivatives
Ethylene oxide (1,2-epoxyethane)	Polycyclic aromatic hydrocarbons
Glycidol (2,3-epoxy-1-propanol)	Triazenes
Lead subacetate	
Procarbazine hydrochloride (olfactory neuroblastomas)	
Propane sultone	
Propylene imine	

Modified from Berleur and Cordier, 1995, with permission.

Acrylonitrile

Acrylonitrile, also know as vinyl cyanide (CH_2=CHCN), is used as a bulk chemical commodity in the textile, plastics and rubber industries. In 1977, the National Institute for Occupational Safety and Health estimated that 1.5 $\times 10^7$ lbs of this compound was produced annually in the United States and that an estimated 125 000 workers came into contact with this compound annually during its manufacture or use.

An increased incidence of brain tumors was observed after male and female F344 rats were exposed to acrylonitrile in their drinking water (Bigner *et al.*, 1986). These tumors were uniformly densely cellular and infiltrative at their margins, with focal areas of necrosis. Many of these tumors exceeded 5 mm in size. They did not stain with GFAP, however.

Ethylene oxide

Ethylene oxide, also known as 1,2-epoxyethane (C_2H_4O), is an alkylating agent primarily used as an intermediate in producing ethylene glycol and some nonionic surfactants. A relatively small amount of this compound is also used as a sterilant in the health care industry, where the potential for human exposure is greatest. In 1977, the National Institute for Occupational Safety and Health estimated that 150 000 workers were exposed to ethylene oxide annually.

When ethylene oxide was given to F344 rats, a statistically significant increase was observed in gliomas of the brain and tumors in other organs (Lynch *et al.*, 1984; Garman, Snellings and Maronpot, 1985, 1986). The gliomas were primarily astrocytomas or tumors of mixed cell type and were similar to those observed spontaneously in this rat strain. However, the incidence was dose related, tumors were consistently larger in dosed animals, and these tumors were frequently the cause of death. In NTP studies, when ethylene oxide was administered to B6C3F1 mice by inhalation, dose-related increases in tumors of other organ systems, but not the brain, were observed. This may not be significant, however, in light of the almost routine failure of many potent carcinogenic agents to induce CNS tumors in mice.

Glycidol

Glycidol, also known as 2,3-epoxy-1-propanol ($C_3H_6O_2$), is a multipurpose viscous liquid used primarily as a stabilizer during the manufacture of vinyl polymers, but also as an additive for hydraulic fluids and as an epoxy resin diluent. In 1983, over 10×10^6 lbs of glycidyl compounds were produced or imported into the United States. In NTP studies (1990), an increased incidence of gliomas of the brain and tumors in other tissues was observed after glycidol in water was given by gavage for 2 years in male and female F344/N rats. Also, the carcinogenicity of glycidol was clearly evident, based on an increase in the incidence of tumors in multiple organ systems of B6C3F1 mice of both sexes, despite the lack of increase in the incidence of brain tumors in mice.

Vinyl chloride

The case of vinyl chloride (VC) illustrates the impact that the misclassification of tumors induced by a carcinogen can have on establishing the cause of brain tumors (see Chapter 1). The fact that VC is a carcinogen is clear from several animal studies. Chronic exposure of rats, mice and other rodents to VC has consistently demonstrated a dose-related induction of angiosarcomas in liver and carcinomas in various other organs (Maltoni and Lefemine, 1975; Maltoni, 1976; Lee *et al.*, 1977, 1978; Feron and Kroes, 1979; Drew *et al.*, 1983; Bi *et al.*, 1985; Maltoni and Cotti, 1988). Certain animal studies indicate that VC is also capable of inducing tumors in the olfactory sensory epithelium (see below). Nevertheless, VC has not been shown to induce primary brain tumors in either animals or humans.

While animal studies of VC exposure plainly reveal that tumors may be induced in the liver and other organs of several species, intracranial tumors have been observed in only one species, the rat. Even then, exposure levels are many times higher than the level needed to induce angiosarcoma of the liver (Maltoni and Lefemine, 1975). Furthermore, Ward and Rice (1982) stated what is now the belief of many: that 'some investigators have described [the rat VC-induced brain tumors] as neuroblastomas arising in the olfactory lobes of the brain when in fact they may have arisen in the nasal epithelium'. These tumors, then, arise from the olfactory sensory epithelium, and they are either olfactory neuroblastomas or, as reported by Feron and Kroes (1979), adenocarcinomas. Both the olfactory neuroblastomas and nasal cavity carcinomas metastasize to the forebrain through the floor of the skull. It is our opinion (J.H.S. and D.D.B.), then, that VC-induced 'brain' tumors are *metastatic* and not primary brain tumors.

Unfortunately, fundamental errors in interpreting chronic bioassays in which a carcinogen is deemed capable of inducing primary brain tumors in animals can lead to false assumptions in human epidemiologic studies. Because early reports labeled VC-induced animal brain tumors as 'primary brain tumors', many subsequent epidemiologic studies investigated VC as a cause of primary human brain tumors, when such a conclusion was not biologically plausible. The lack of consistent or reproducible epidemiologic studies for establishing significant associations between VC exposure and human brain tumors is discussed in Chapter 1.

The biologic implausibility of VC as a cause of primary brain tumors is supported, additionally, by other evidence. Neoplasia resulting from carcinogenic exposure requires that target cells or organs must be able to activate a carcinogen to its reactive metabolites, and the reactive metabolites must be able to initiate carcinogenesis, for example, by forming promutagenic DNA adducts. The reactive epoxide intermediate of VC, 2-chloroethylene oxide, is formed when VC is oxidized by P-450 isoenzymes (ATSDR, 1995). Ravindranath and colleagues (Ravindranath, Anandatheerthavarada and Shankar, 1990; Anandatheerthavarada, Boyd and Ravindranath, 1992) reported that rat brain has approximately one-tenth the amount of P-450 isoenzymes as rat liver. Liver is a target organ for VC carcinogenesis, while brain is not. The low levels of P-450 isoenzymes in brain relative to liver constitute a further argument against the biologic plausibility of VC as a carcinogen that is capable of inducing primary brain tumors.

In rat liver, the initiating mechanism of VC-induced angiosarcomas is thought to be the VC exposure-related production of promutagenic DNA adducts by the reactive intermediate 2-chloroethylene oxide. The four well-described VC DNA adducts are: (1) OEG, or 7-(2-oxoethyl)guanine, accounting for 98% of the total adducts, but not actively causing incorporation of the wrong nucleotides; (2) EG, or N^2,3-ethenoguanine, accounting for 1%; (3) εdA, or 1,N^6-ethenodeoxyadenosine, accounting for 0.4%; and (4) εdC, or 1,N^4-ethenodeoxycytosine, accounting for 0.6%. The latter three VC DNA adducts are thought to be capable of causing miscoding. Despite the formation of these adducts in liver after it is exposed to VC, levels of VC adducts in the brain are consistently either undetectable or significantly less than in liver (Singer *et al.*, 1987; Ciroussel *et al.*, 1990; Fedtke *et al.*, 1990; Swenberg *et al.*, 1992; Miller, 1994; Mitro *et al.*, 1995; Nair *et al.*, 1995). Moreover, it has been shown that VC-induced adducts are repaired by the enzyme 3-methyladenine DNA glycosolase, a DNA repair enzyme present in brain (Washington *et al.*, 1989; Hang *et al.*, 1996). The capability of VC to induce primary brain tumors is made less likely by these facts.

Finally, the location (molecular) and types of genetic changes that occur with VC-associated cancers in human liver, such as changes in the *TP53* tumor suppressor gene and the *RAS* oncogenes, are not like the genetic changes observed in human astrocytic brain tumors. Hollstein *et al.* (1994) report that *TP53* mutations in human VC-related angiosarcomas of the liver consistently occur in codons 249 and 255. In primary human astrocytic brain tumors, however, *TP53* mutations are mainly located in highly conserved clusters at codons 175, 248 and 273 (Louis, 1994; Rasheed *et al.*, 1994; Ohgaki *et al.*, 1995). The other consistent, VC-related genetic change in human liver angiosarcomas appears in the *KRAS* gene (Marion, Froment and Trépo, 1991), but primary brain tumors virtually never show *KRAS* mutations (see Chapter 2).

Five lines of evidence challenging the biologic plausibility of VC as a carcinogenic inducer of primary brain tumors have been discussed as follows.

1. VC causes only metastatic tumors to brain, and even that induction requires much higher exposures than do liver angiosarcomas.
2. Metastatic brain tumors from the nasal sensory epithelium are observed in only one species, the rat, and are likely to be a species-specific effect.
3. P-450 isoenzymes, which are necessary for formation of the DNA-reactive VC metabolite, 2-chloroethylene oxide, occur at low levels in brain.
4. The VC promutagenic DNA adducts are present at low-to-undetectable levels in brain, and the repair enzyme for these adducts is present in brain.
5. The genetic changes in human VC-induced liver angiosarcomas are not like those observed in primary brain tumors.

Thus, if one applied a weight-of-evidence approach to VC-induced angiosarcoma of the liver, there is overwhelming evidence for VC as the causative agent of liver angiosarcomas in multiple animal species and exposed humans. On the other hand, a weight-of-evidence approach from the standpoint of chronic animal exposure bioassays, genetic or other mechanisms and human epidemiology would not support VC as a primary brain tumor carcinogen in either animals or humans. The evidence, therefore, does not support a conclusion that VC is a carcinogenic inducer of primary brain tumors in animals or humans.

Recently, the U.S. Environmental Protection Agency (EPA, 1996) proposed a set of new guidelines for assessing cancer risk. The guidelines differ from those published in 1986 by introducing a broader range of evidence, from a variety of sources, into the assessment of cancer risk, rather than relying substantially on chronic rodent bioassays. Recognizing that chronic bioassays may be more accurate in the assessment of some agents than others, the EPA proposed new guidelines that will emphasize the use of genetic data as an important supplement to chronic bioassays in determining how an agent might cause cancer. Thus, the EPA advocates that a 'weight-of-evidence' approach be applied to all available data regarding a substance that is being assessed for cancer risk. The genetic changes discussed above, whereby promutagenic DNA adducts are produced, are an example of the genetic data advocated as criteria by the EPA, as is the genetic data for human brain tumors.

Experimental models of nervous system tumors

MULTICELLULAR TUMOR SPHEROIDS

Although standard cell culture techniques have been used extensively to study various aspects of nervous system tumors, another approach designed to obtain an *in vitro* model that more closely resembles the architectural pattern of human gliomas *in situ* is the use of *multicellular spheroids*, prepared either directly from biopsies digested with collagenase and plated onto agar-coated flasks (Darling, Oktar and Thomas, 1983; Bjerkvig *et al.*, 1990), or from cell lines (Carlsson *et al.*, 1983; Bradford *et al.*, 1990). The technique, as applied to human gliomas, is still in its infancy, but the growth characteristics of these preparations suggest that they may be a promising tool for appropriate laboratory manipulation, including the testing of cytotoxic and cytostatic drugs. In addition, the production of extracellular matrix glycoproteins (laminin, fibronectin, collagens and glycosaminoglycans) has been found to be promoted in this system (Nederman *et al.*, 1984). Not unexpectedly, as in other three-dimensional *in vitro* systems, proliferation rates vary according to the culture conditions that determine the diffusion of oxygen and nutrients from the spheroid surface. These conditions will have to be optimized and controlled before the technique can be employed routinely in chemosensitivity and radiosensitivity experiments.

XENOGRAFT TRANSPLANTATION INTO 'IMMUNOLOGICALLY PRIVILEGED' SITES

Although *in vitro* systems can assess a number of aspects of cancer therapy, some aspects can only be assessed with *in vivo* models of human neoplasms. In the 1940s, it was established that human tumors, including nervous system tumors, could be grown in 'immunologically privileged' compartments of normal heterologous hosts. The first report of a successful xenotransplantation of human nervous system tumors appeared in 1945. Greene and Arnold (1945) successfully transplanted human GBM into the anterior chamber of the eye of an immunocompetent guinea pig. In these studies at Yale University, the anterior chamber of the guinea pig eye was successfully used as an initial site for the implantation of human glioblastoma, with subsequent transfer of the tumor to the brains of experimental animals. As recounted by Greene (1951), in guinea pigs the cerebral growths recapitulated histologically the features of the parent tumor, but in mice the transplants became more undifferentiated and sarcomatous in appearance. In subsequent trials, Greene (1953) successfully transferred three human GBMs directly to the brains of guinea pigs and mice, with similar histologic results. Further work at Yale by Manuelidis (1961) on the heterologous transplantation of tissue culture cell lines from human GBMs into the subcutaneous tissue of cortisone-treated hamsters yielded the interesting observation that, occasionally, the tumors thus derived acquire an epithelial appearance indistinguishable from carcinoma. This morphologic alteration was maintained on subsequent transfer of these transplants to the brain and eye of unconditioned guinea pigs, thus suggesting that the conditions of tissue culture may play a role in bringing about this transformation. On the other hand, after serial transfers for many years, the fine structure of human glioblastoma-derived tumors, heterologously transplanted to the guinea pig eye and brain, preserves its identity with human neoplastic astrocytes (Herman, Adams and Manuelidis, 1967). Transplantation of other nervous system tumor histiotypes, notably medulloblastomas, into the anterior chamber of the eye or the brain (Greene, 1953) and, rarely, into the intrathecal space (Wilson and Barker, 1968) has also been reported. Overall, however, attempts to transplant human nervous system tumors into *immunocompetent* hosts have, with the exception of those described by Greene and his collaborators, been generally disappointing. Subsequent attempts at heterologous transplantation of 22 human cerebral and cerebellar astrocytomas into the guinea pig eye or brain led to failure in all instances, except for one successful intracerebral transplantation of a cerebellar astrocytoma from a child (Manuelidis, 1972). It has been pointed out (Schold and Friedman, 1984) that Greene's success in the transplantation of human tumors into immunocompetent heterologous hosts has so far never been achieved in another laboratory.

A somewhat different approach to the heterotransplantation of human nervous system tumors has been attempted in some laboratories by isolating small fragments of tumor in diffusion chambers incorporating a Millipore filter; this allows the passage of metabolites, but restricts the interchange of cells between the host and the graft (Conley, 1974). Implantation of the chambers in rats has permitted the preservation, usually from 1 to 2 weeks, of viable transplants from four GBMs, one astrocytoma, one oligodendroglioma and one meningioma. Experimentally induced nervous system tumors can also be maintained for periods of up to 3 weeks by this method.

IMMUNOINCOMPETENT RODENT MODELS

The desire to experiment on human neoplasms within a convenient *in vivo* system eventually led to the use of immunosuppressed animals that can serve as tolerant hosts for human neoplastic tissue. Growth of human tumor xenografts in such animals provides a convenient source of large numbers of tumor cells, while permitting assessment of the toxicity of various therapeutic modalities in a mammalian species. Initially, immunologically incompetent animals were created through the use of irradiation, immunotoxic drug therapy or thymectomy. More recently, however, spontaneous genetic mutations resulting in different immunodeficient phenotypes have been used to establish inbred mouse and rat strains with various immunologic deficiencies. For example, nude mice are deficient in T-cell function, severe combined immunodeficiency (SCID) mice are deficient in B- and T-cell function, beige mice have subnormal natural killer (NK) cell function (Roder and Duwe, 1979) and osteopetrosis mice are deficient in growth factors necessary for macrophage differentiation. In addition, many combinations of these different phenotypes have been established. Finally, specific genes, such as *RAG1* and *RAG2*, that play a role in the development or function of the immune system have been 'knocked out' in mice, and these animals are now also becoming available as immunodeficient models. It is important to remember, however, that none of these animals is absolutely without an immune system, and each has specific immunologic parameters that must be kept in mind. The most commonly used immunodeficient genetic mutants are the SCID mice and the athymic or nude mice or rats. These are discussed in detail below.

Athymic (nude) rodents

In 1953, the so-called 'nude' rat was first recognized in an outbred hooded rat colony at the Rowett Research Institute in the United Kingdom (Festing *et al.*, 1978). A breeding colony was briefly established, but ultimately died out. This phenotype reappeared, though, in 1975, and a successful breeding colony was established. A similar phenotype in the rat was independently identified at Victoria University in New Zealand at about the same time (McNeilage, Heslop and Berridge, 1979). Nude mice were also recognized in the interim (Flanagan, 1966). The genetic mutation in these animals produces a phenotypic triad of hairlessness, thymic aplasia and T-cell deficiency, which is transmitted in an autosomal recessive manner. The gene product has not been identified, but the rat *rnu* gene has been mapped to rat chromosome 10 (Cash *et al.*, 1993) and seems to be homologous with the murine *nu* gene on mouse chromosome 11 (Takahashi *et al.*, 1992; Blackburn, Griffith and Morahan, 1995). Since their discovery, the *rnu* and *nu* genes have been introduced into a number of inbred rat and mouse strains, thus producing various strains of inbred or outbred immunodeficient mice and rats.

Phenotypically, the most striking feature of these animals is their almost complete lack of hair. Some hair is characteristically present on the head of nude rats, and hair on the rest of the body varies with individual animals, even in inbred colonies. Another characteristic physical feature is the presence of bent vibrissae, which can be used to identify homozygous animals soon after birth. Histologically, the hair follicles initially appear normal, but the hairs are abnormal and fail to erupt through the dermis (Flanagan, 1966). The thymus is replaced by brown fat, leaving only an abnormal thymus rudiment consisting primarily of undifferentiated epithelial cells. Homozygous nude rodents of both sexes usually obtain only approximately 75% of the weight of their heterozygous litter mates, and preweaning mortality is slightly higher. Nude rodents housed under conventional conditions also have a life-span drastically shortened to about 6 months, depending on the strain. This can easily be extended to between 18 and 24 months in pathogen-free conditions, however. Although most homozygous athymic mice and rats of both sexes are fertile, and homozygous females have normally sized litters, homozygous females cannot rear such litters successfully. Therefore, heterozygous females are usually bred with homozygous males to increase animal production. The nude rat is perhaps more useful than the nude mouse in neuro-oncology research because its larger size is more adaptable to surgical or stereotactic procedures in the brain. In addition, the nude rat is less sensitive to common murine viral infections with agents such as murine hepatitis or Sendai viruses, which can be life threatening in the nude mouse.

Immunologically, these athymic animals have a number of abnormalities that are generally more pronounced in younger animals, resulting in some increased resistance to xenograft transplantation in older animals, especially in rats (Salomon and Fogh, 1982; Bubeník *et al.*, 1992; Schuurman, 1995). The main deficiency is a congenital aplasia of the thymus (Pantelouris, 1968), which produces cell-mediated immunologic incompetence. In 3- to 10-week-old rats, the thymic rudiment is populated by undifferentiated epithelial cells and fat tissue, without significant numbers of lymphocytes (Vos, Berkvens and Kruijt, 1980). As a result, T-cell-mediated immune responses tend to be diminished or absent in these animals, while T-cell-independent B-cell function appears to be normal. Perhaps as a compensatory response, both nude mice and rats appear to have higher NK cell activity that increases with age (de Jong *et al.*, 1980).

The lymphoid organs in these athymic animals generally lack lymphocytes in areas that are thymus dependent. In almost all cases, this depletion seems to be more prominent in the nude mouse than in the nude rat (Vos, Berkvens and Kruijt, 1980). The lymph nodes in these animals tend to be smaller, with the paracortical area virtually free of lymphocytes, and only occasional germinal centers can be identified (Brooks *et al.*, 1980; Vos, Berkvens and Kruijt, 1980). Similarly, the thymus-dependent periarteriolar area of the normally sized spleen is also depleted of lymphocytes, though less significantly than are the lymph nodes. Finally, very few Peyer's patches can be seen along the small intestines of these animals, and those that are seen lack lymphocytes in the interfollicular areas. As expected, there is also a lower number of peripheral lymphocytes in these animals.

Immune functions not dependent on the thymus, such as macrophage or NK cell activity and IgM antibody production against T-cell-independent antigens, are normal or enhanced. Antibody production of IgG or IgA may also be present at low levels in older animals, and the B-cell count—and response to B-cell mitogens—is normal. Despite the reduced number of lymphocytes, the overall white blood cell count is usually elevated due to the increased numbers of neutrophils, eosinophils and monocytes, which may be solely a manifestation of occult concurrent infections.

Overall, the response to T-cell-specific mitogens is diminished or absent, and delayed-type hypersensitivity reactions to tuberculin purified protein derivative cannot be elicited in nude animals (Vos *et al.*, 1980). Although mature nude mice and rats are lymphopenic, lymphocytes that morphologically and antigenically resemble T cells with αβ-T-cell receptors can be detected in these animals. Nevertheless, at least in nude mice, these T cells have been shown to be oligoclonal and incapable of generating a significant antigen-specific immune response, though if isolated they can be stimulated to produce interleukin-2 by nonspecific mitogens. Conversely, T-cell-independent B-cell function appears normal. For example, responses to B-cell mitogens such as *Staphylococcus aureus* are normal, and, in nude rats, IgM, IgD and IgG_{2b} serum levels are normal. Levels of IgG_{2a} and IgE in nude rats are found to be diminished, while IgG_1 and IgG_{2c} levels are slightly elevated. In contrast, in nude mice, levels of IgG_1 and IgA are low (Bazin *et al.*, 1980). As expected, no antibody production is observed when these animals are immunized with T-cell-dependent antigens.

Severe combined immunodeficiency mice

Bosma, Custer and Bosma (1983) were the first to report the murine *scid* mutation. This mutation is inherited in an autosomal recessive fashion and segregates independently of the major histocompatibility locus or the immunoglobulin heavy-chain locus (Bosma, Custer and Bosma, 1983). It maps to chromosome 16 in the mouse (Bosma and Caroll, 1991) and apparently causes a defect in DNA repair that has its greatest effect during the resolution of immunoglobulin and T-cell receptor gene rearrangements (Fulop and Philips, 1990). This defect has been shown to be different from that produced in *RAG1* (Mombaerts *et al.*, 1992) and *RAG2* (Shinkai *et al.*, 1992) knock-out mice, but the knock-out mice have defects in B- and T-cell function that are similar to those found in *scid* mice and are related to an inability to initiate immunoglobulin and T-cell-receptor gene rearrangements.

Examination of SCID mice reveals severe lymphopenia in the blood and all lymphoid organs, which are also drastically reduced in size. In addition, their spleen cells fail to respond to either allogeneic lymphocytes or to B- or T-cell nonspecific mitogens, and the serum immunoglobulin fraction is also drastically reduced or absent. The bone marrow and splenic red pulp, however, appear normal, and these mice can support the differentiation of lymphocyte stem cells adoptively transferred from normal animals. The NK cells also appear to be present and functioning normally in *scid* mice.

The *scid* mice have at least two specific advantages over nude mice for the study of human nervous system tumor xenografts. First, many tumors and their accompanying tumor infiltrating lymphocytes that will not grow in nude mice can be successfully engrafted into *scid* mice. It has been postulated that this difference between *scid* and nude mice may be due to the production of xenoreactive antibodies against T-cell-independent antigens in nude mice (Fidler, 1986). Second, *scid* mice can be reconstituted with human peripheral blood leukocytes (PBLs), providing a unique potential opportunity to test a human immune response *ex vivo* (Mueller and Reisfeld, 1991). However, *scid* mice reconstituted with human PBLs do not produce a long-term system in which human immune responses can be tested. Although most of the injected human cells die, within a few weeks of intraperitoneal transfer most of the injected human peripheral blood cell lineages can be detected intraperitoneally (Hoffmann-Fezer *et al.*, 1992). By 1 month, although human leukocytes have disseminated to other organs, mostly to extralymphoid tissues such as the lung, liver and spleen, almost all of these cells are anergic xenoreactive memory T cells (Tary-Lehmann *et al.*, 1994), with only a few oligoclonal B-cell clones (Saxon *et al.*, 1991) and no detectable human macrophages or accessory cells. Thus, it appears that the *scid* mouse does not provide an appropriate environment for the persistence of naive human leukocytes. In fact, even injection of human bone marrow cells fails to produce long-term engraftment of naive human lymphocytes (Tary-Lehmann and Saxon, 1992). On the other hand, specific T-cell responses can be generated early on in the peritoneal cavity, and these cells will then proliferate and disseminate, providing a long-term system of specific systemic immunity. Though such techniques have not been applied in the investigation of human nervous system tumors, both human (Huang *et al.*, 1995) and nonsyngeneic murine gliomas (Chambers *et al.*, 1995) have been successfully grown in SCID mice.

XENOTRANSPLANTATION OF HUMAN NERVOUS SYSTEM TUMORS

Human tumors of nearly every histiotype can be serially transplanted in immunodeficient animals. Rana *et al.* (1977) were the first to demonstrate that human nervous system tumors could be grown in nude mice. Since that time, a vast number of human nervous system tumor xenografts, primarily GBMs with some medulloblastomas and very few ependymomas, have been established, either subcutaneously or intracranially, and propagated (Bradley *et al.*, 1978; Shapiro *et al.*, 1979; Horten, Basler and Shapiro, 1981; Jones *et al.*, 1981, 1982; Schold *et al.*, 1983; Mandybur, Sawaya and Ormsby, 1986; McLendon *et al.*, 1996). It appears that, with the more malignant forms of astrocytic tumor, a high rate of success can be achieved; that valuable quantitative data can be gathered on the growth characteristics of the serially passaged tumors; and that the experimental model is histologically valid inasmuch as it maintains many morphologic and immunohistochemical similarities with the originally transplanted glioma. However, as pointed out by Horten, Basler and Shapiro (1981), there is also evidence that cellular subpopulations from the initial tumor may be preferentially selected for growth in the heterotransplants. This is supported by the observation that ependymal differentiation has been reported after xenogeneic transplantation of a GBM (Jacobsen, Parker and Papadimitriou, 1987). This places limitations on the clinical inferences that may be drawn from these models.

Factors that have been found to affect the success of xenotransplantation of tumors into immunologically deficient rodents include the age and immunologic status of the animal, the histiotype and malignant grade of the tumor, the site of injection and factors in the environment. Specifically, direct antitumor activity may be initiated by NK cells or macrophages and may be assisted by antigen-specific IgM antibodies against the xenografts, even in relatively immunoincompetent athymic animals. Although some xenografts will grow immediately after transplantation, most have a considerable latency period that may be as long as 1 year.

Morphologically, these xenografts usually form discrete lobulated masses when grown subcutaneously. They may be more infiltrative when grown in the brain, but, like xenografts of other histiotypes, seldom metastasize. The morphologic features of the original tumor, including reactivity for GFAP and expression of tumor-associated antigens (unpublished data from our laboratory), are usually maintained by the xenograft, and all of the morphologic features that characterize human GBMs, including necrosis, can be seen in these transplanted tumors, though endothelial proliferation is less common. Although most of these xenografts maintain karyotypes similar to the original tumor (Bigner *et al.*, 1989), the tumors often progress toward a more uniform histologic appearance, after serial passage, and may then appear more 'sarcomatous'. This may result from a preferential selection of a certain cell subpopulation, or it may represent factors contributed by the surrounding murine stroma. As a result, it is always important to confirm routinely that the tumors arising in animals receiving a neoplastic xenograft are, in fact, of human origin, as some murine tumors have been induced after xenotransplantation (Houghton and Taylor, 1978). Fortunately, this differentiation can be easily achieved by morphologic analysis, karyotyping, lactate dehydrogenase isoenzyme typing or restriction fragment length polymorphism analysis. In this regard, it has been well demonstrated that the endothelium of a xenograft is composed of murine cells, and this must be taken into consideration when using xenografts to study therapies in which vascular supply plays a crucial role (Warenius, 1980).

Human nervous system tumor xenografts can be grown in a variety of locations in immunoincompetent rodents. Although intracranial growth, after stereotactic injection of cells into the cerebrum or carotid artery (Schuster *et al.*, 1993; Kurpad *et al.*, 1995), better simulates the clinical situation, it usually requires that therapeutic efficacy be evaluated solely on the basis of animal survival, which may not directly correlate with tumor growth. On the other hand, subcutaneous growth can be used to evaluate some of these additional parameters, and it provides an assessment of tumor susceptibility to a specific therapy without other confounding variables that are related to delivery and may inhibit therapeutic efficacy in the CNS. More recently, these xenografts have been successfully grown in the intrathecal space of the rat and provide an excellent and now well-characterized model of neoplastic meningitis (Fuchs *et al.*, 1990; Friedman *et al.*, 1994; Pastan *et al.*, 1995) (Fig. 6.18).

A large number of well-characterized human nervous system tumor cell lines and xenografts are now available for use in these models. Almost all of these have been derived from GBMs or other undifferentiated, highly malignant gliomas, and although relatively few human GBMs have been

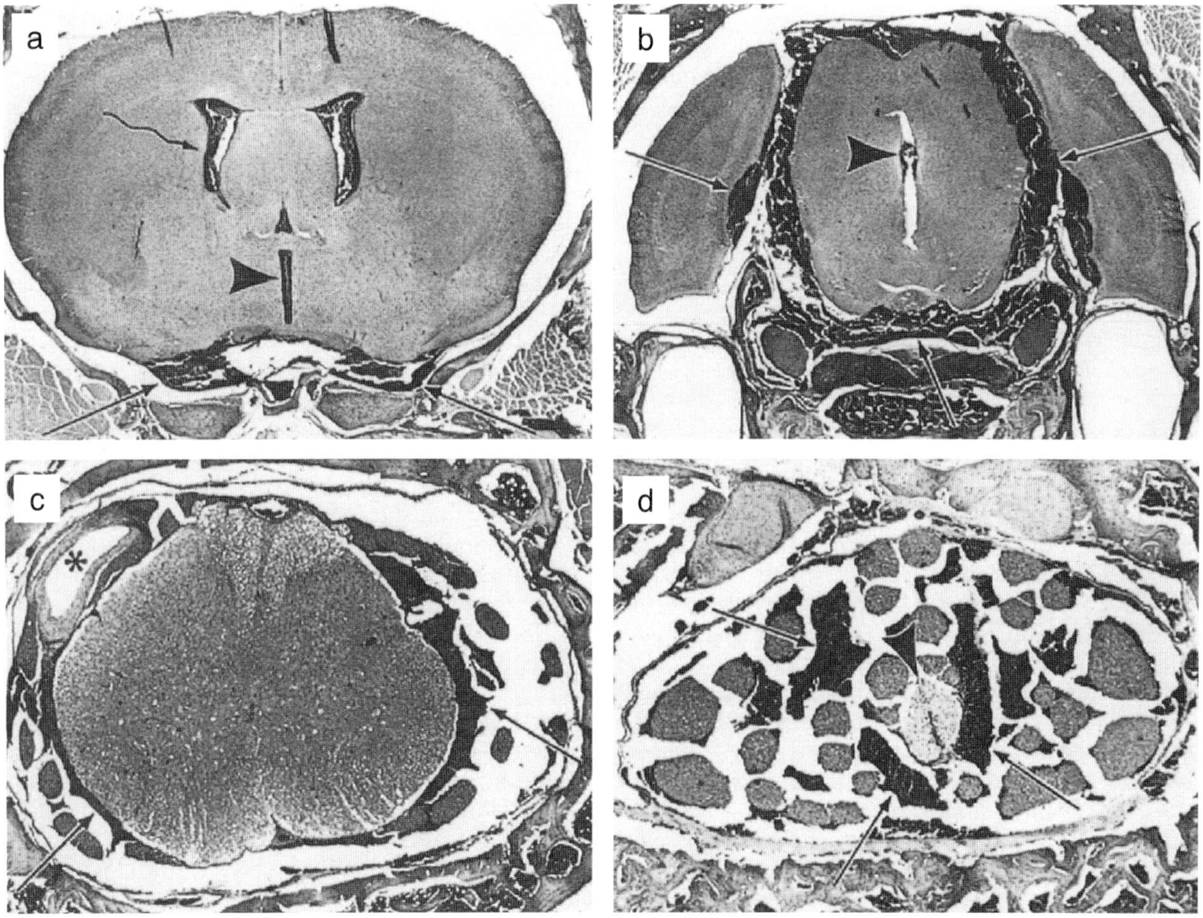

Fig. 6.18 Whole-mount cross sections of a xenograft grown in a rat given injections of D341 Med cells. (a) Cerebrum: tumor is present in the basilar subarachnoid space (→), third ventricle (▶) and lateral ventricles (⤳). × 9.5 (b) Brainstem: tumor is in the cerebral aqueduct (▶) and in the subarachnoid space encircling the brainstem (→). × 8.5 (c) Lumbar spinal cord: tumor is seen in the spinal subarachnoid space (→); catheter site (*). × 32 (d) Lumbar cistern: tumor (→) surrounds the nerve roots of the cauda equina and the filum terminale (▶). × 40 (From Friedman *et al.*, 1991, with permission)

established as permanent cell lines *in vitro*, more than 50% of human GBMs can usually be serially passed in athymic mice. The number of bizarre multinucleated giant cells and the efficiency of colony formation in soft agar correlate best with ability of these tumors to grow as xenografts (Bigner *et al.*, 1981).

In addition to the large number of human GBM xenografts available, a few human medulloblastomas have also been established as permanent cell lines and xenografts (Friedman *et al.*, 1983a, 1983b, 1984). The first human cell line designated as a medulloblastoma was TE-671 (McAllister *et al.*, 1977), but this was subsequently shown to be a rhabdomyosarcoma (Stratton *et al.*, 1989). The human medulloblastoma cell line designated D283 Med was established after successful intracranial and subcutaneous transplantation in athymic mice (Friedman *et al.*, 1985). The intracranial, but not the subcutaneous, transplants of this cell line show rosette formation. Transplants of D283 Med also express glutamine synthetase and neuron-specific enolase, but not GFAP or S-100 protein. All three subunits of the neurofilament protein triplet are also expressed by this cell line (Trojanowski *et al.*, 1987). Another established line, termed Daoy, obtained from a desmoplastic medulloblastoma and less differentiated than D283 Med, has been described by Jacobsen, Jenkyn and Papadimitriou (1985). When injected intracerebrally in nude mice, it results in a diffuse infiltration of the brain parenchyma rather than a circumscribed mass. A pattern of rather extensive intraventricular and subarachnoid dissemination was similarly obtained on xenogeneic transplantation of a fourth line (D341 Med), recently established and characterized by Friedman *et al.* (1988). The line, like D283 Med, expresses neurofilament proteins, but mostly the high- and middle-molecular-weight triplets, as well as neuron-specific enolase and glutamine synthetase, but it is, again, negative for GFAP and S-100 protein. Karyotypic study reveals a large number of double minute chromatin bodies in the tumor cells, a finding that is consonant with the demonstration of a modest amplification (20-fold) of the *MYC* oncogene. More recently, additional medulloblastoma cell lines, including D384 Med, D425 Med and D458 Med – which express neurofilament proteins and synaptophysin in the absence of GFAP – and ONS-76 and ONS-81, have been established (Tamura *et al.*, 1989; He *et al.*, 1991). Some of these lines were even derived from surgical resections by using an ultrasonic surgical aspirator (D384 Med and D-425 Med) (Oakes *et al.*, 1990).

Finally, a very few ependymomas have been established *in vivo* and *in vitro* along with a myxopapillary ependymoma (Batzdorf and Pokress, 1968; Rawlinson, Rubinstein and Herman, 1974; Vraa-Jensen *et al.*, 1976; Horowitz *et al.*, 1987; McLendon *et al.*, 1996).

COMMONLY USED IMMUNOCOMPETENT RODENT MODELS AND EXPERIMENTAL RODENT TUMOR CELL LINES

Xenografts permit experiments with tumor cells derived from actual human brain tumors, but use of immunoincompetent animals not only requires special facilities, but also limits the types of experimental questions that can be asked. Thus, rodent tumors and permanent cell lines derived from these tumors remain invaluable models of human brain tumors (Table 6.10).

Mouse models

Ependymoblastoma series

The GL261, GL26, Ep and EpA murine gliomas (Ausman, Shapiro and Rall, 1970) are the most widely used models of murine primary intracranial glial neoplasms. These tumors can all be grown subcutaneously and intracranially *in vivo*, and some have been established as cell lines *in vitro* (Rubin and Ames, 1973; Naidu *et al.*, 1993). These four tumors have similar histologic appearances, consisting of compact sheets of poorly differentiated, uniform, small cuboidal cells with little cytoplasm and darkly staining nuclear chromatin. Mitotic figures are usually visible at the tumor periphery, and the cells are found frequently arranged in cords or pseudorosettes. This histologic picture is similar to the rare childhood human ependymoblastoma, but these murine tumor cells demonstrate no signs of ependymal differentiation on closer examination, and really consist of undifferentiated cells of uncertain origin (Rubin, Sutton and Zimmerman, 1968; Herman *et al.*, 1975). Microscopic areas of necrosis can be seen in all these tumors, but GL26 tends to be exceptionally vascular and hemorrhage can usually be seen within these tumors without microscopic examination.

Despite their histologic similarity, however, these tumors grow at different rates. The standard technique for injecting tumor intracerebrally consists of harvesting tumor passaged subcutaneously and implanting 1 mm^3 of minced tumor tissue into the cerebrum. The median survival time of mice given EpA tumor injections in this way is usually shortest, followed by mice given GL26 and GL261, which are fairly similar, and then mice given Ep tumor cells, which usually produce the longest survival times (Ausman, Shapiro and Rall, 1970). The *in vivo* population doubling times of the Ep, GL261 and EpA tumors have been estimated at 69, 57 and 45 hours, respectively (Shapiro, 1974), while the *in vitro* doubling time of GL26 cells was about 36 hours (Albright *et al.*, 1975). These tumors have also been found to have different chemotherapeutic drug sensitivities (Shapiro, Ausman and Rall, 1970), but overall have generally overpredicted the response to the same drugs in human tumors.

Unfortunately, despite their extensive use, these tumors have been poorly characterized, and their derivation is not well documented in the literature. For example, induction of the Ep tumor is generally attributed to Zimmerman and Arnold (1941). In this paper, Zimmerman and Arnold injected 20-methylcholanthrene pellets into the parietal lobe, cerebellum or subdural space of male C3H mice with the (H-2^k) major histocompatibility complex (MHC) and successfully obtained a number of tumors—of the cerebrum, cerebellum and meninges—with different histologies. None of these tumors was initially classified as ependymoblastoma, and so it is unclear from this paper which tumor ultimately became referred to as Ep. Apparently, one of the mixed gliomas induced in these experiments emerged with the histologic appearance of ependymoblastoma after serial subcutaneous passage (Netsky *et al.*, 1956). Subsequent authors (Ausman, Shapiro and Rall, 1970), using the Ep cell line from Zimmerman and referencing this

Table 6.10 Frequently used rodent brain tumor models

Cell lines	Species	Syngeneic strain	Induction technique	Histologic type	GFAP staining	Reference(s)
SMA 560	Mouse	Inbred VM/Dk	Spontaneous[a]	Anaplastic astrocytoma	++	Serano, Pegram and Bigner, 1980; Sampson *et al.*, 1997
S635-clone 5	Rat	Inbred Fischer 344 CD	ASV (Schmidt -Ruppin)	Anaplastic astrocytoma	++	Lee *et al.*, 1986
9L	Rat	Inbred Fischer 344 CD[e]	MNU	Gliosarcomas	–	Barker *et al.*, 1973; Benda *et al.*, 1971
RG-2	Rat	Inbred Fischer 344 CD	ENU	Glioma	–[b]	Wechsler, Ramadan and Gieseler, 1972
CNS-1	Rat	Inbred Lewis	MNU	Glioma	+	Kruse *et al.*, 1994
GL261	Mouse	Unclear	MCA[c]	Ependymoblastoma		Seligman and Shear, 1939
GL26	Mouse	Unclear	MCA	Ependymoblastoma	+	Wiranowska *et al.*, 1992
Ep, EpA	Mouse	Unclear	MCA	Ependymoblastoma		Ausman, Shapiro and Rall, 1970; Zimmerman and Arnold, 1941, 1944
C6	Rat	None (random-bred Wistar-Furth)	MNU	Glioma	+[d]	Benda *et al.*, 1968

[a] VM/Dk mice have a high incidence of spontaneous CNS tumors. These lines were derived from spontaneous astrocytomas in this mouse strain.
[b] Some GFAP-positive cells have been noted in intracerebral xenografts (Reifenberger *et al.*, 1989), but these could be reactive cells only.
[c] MCA, 3- and 20-methylcholanthrene.
[d] Inducable by dbcAMP, norepinephrine and organ culture.
[e] The significant genetic drift of this cell line may mean that no syngeneic strain exists for some cell stocks.

original paper (Zimmerman and Arnold, 1941), have usually transplanted this tumor into C57BL/6 mice (H-2^b) (which have a different MHC) instead of C3H (H-2^k) mice, however. Even Zimmerman himself, when referring to this ependymoblastoma, references this original paper (Zimmerman and Arnold, 1941), which used C3H mice (H-2^k) exclusively, but states that the tumor has been propagated in C57BL/6 mice (Rubin *et al.*, 1969). Although some reference is made to the induction of tumors by Zimmerman in strains of mice other than C3H, and including C57BL mice (Zimmerman and Arnold, 1944; Netsky *et al.*, 1956), the documentation for the derivation and ultimate propagation of these lines is not available. Because the EpA tumor was derived as a subline from the Ep tumor, it suffers from the same problems. The derivation of the GL26 tumor, also induced by Zimmerman, is similarly unclear. Finally, the GL261 line was also established in C3H mice by the implantation of 20-methylcholanthrene pellets (Seligman and Shear, 1939). From this paper, it appears that GL261 was originally derived from mouse no. 17 and serially transplanted subcutaneously. Again, the details are unclear.

Although these tumors have been widely used to test therapeutic responses, a number of potential pitfalls exist regarding the appropriate interpretation of results obtained from therapeutic studies conducted with these tumors (Rubinstein, 1977). First, their histologic appearance as an ependymoblastoma suggests that, if they model human gliomas at all, they best represent a rare form of childhood glioma and not the more common malignant astrocytic tumors generally seen in humans. Furthermore, the problems created by the lack of clear lineage documentation for most of these cell lines and the mice from which they were derived cannot be overemphasized. The failure to document stringently that the tumor lines used by a particular investigator are syngeneic with the inbred mouse strain used will allow potential histocompatibility differences to influence experimental results greatly, especially in cell-mediated immunotherapy protocols. In fact, these cell lines have been clearly shown to be highly immunogenic (Scheinberg *et al.*, 1963). Furthermore, the known expression of mammary tumor virus and other endogenous murine oncogenic retroviruses may significantly affect studies dependent on cell membrane antigen expression (Rubin *et al.*, 1969; Rubin and Ames, 1973). Finally, because all these tumors did not arise spontaneously, but were chemically induced, these artificially induced tumors cannot, by virtue of their origin, accurately portray the intrinsic qualities of spontaneous human tumors (Hewitt, Blake and Walder 1976). Favorable responses to various therapeutic modalities using these cell lines must, therefore, always be interpreted with caution.

Spontaneous murine astrocytomas

As discussed previously in this chapter, mice from the inbred VM strain and the inbred VM/Dk (Dickinson) subline (H-2^b) have a remarkable propensity for the spontaneous development of brain and spinal cord astrocytomas, which are otherwise extraordinarily rare in mice. A transplantable astrocytic tumor from one of these spontaneous astrocytomas in VM/Dk mice was initially developed by Fraser (Fraser, 1971, 1986; Fraser and McConnell, 1975), but cell homogenates from this tumor could not be transplanted extracranially, had an unpredictable latency period and were a pleomorphic cell population. Subsequently, a number of cell lines were derived directly from the original tumors propagated by Fraser (Serano, Pegram and Bigner, 1980). Two of these cell lines have been extensively characterized. The SMA-497-P(1) cell line (Bradford, Darling and Thomas, 1990) is a subline developed from intracerebral tumor transplants of the SMA-497 cell line of Serano, Pegram and Bigner (1980) and has been extensively studied in chemotherapeutic assays, both *in vitro* as multicellular tumor spheroids (Bradford *et al.*, 1990) and *in vivo* in syngeneic VM mice (Bradford, Darling and Thomas, 1990). The other cell line, SMA-560, was originally developed by Serano, Pegram and Bigner (1980) from spontaneous astrocytomas discovered by Fraser, as described above. Both of these cell lines are uniformly tumorigenic intracranially and subcutaneously, appear to be glial in origin to a number of observers and express glial markers such as GFAP and glutamine synthetase (Pilkington *et al.*, 1982, 1983; Sampson *et al.*, 1997). In addition, the SMA-560 cell line has recently been shown to secrete biologically active transforming growth factor-β, an immunosuppressant secreted by many human malignant gliomas (Sampson *et al.*, 1997). Because these tumors arose spontaneously in an inbred mouse strain, are highly tumorigenic, are clearly of astrocytic lineage, are not derived from a single cell clone and because SMA-560 secretes an immunosuppressant commonly secreted by human gliomas, they are excellent animal models of human gliomas, especially when immunotherapeutic protocols are being assessed.

Neuroblastoma (C1300)

The C1300 cell line originated spontaneously in the abdominal cavity of an A-strain mouse at Jackson Laboratories (Snell, Cloudman and Woodworth, 1948; Moore, 1951). It can be grown intraperitoneally or subcutaneously in syngeneic A/J strain mice and has a typical neuroblastic appearance consisting of round cells that are densely packed

(Watanabe *et al.*, 1989). Although adequate as a tumor line, C1300's primary use is in the study of neuronal differentiation and function and in neuroelectrophysiology (Schubert *et al.*, 1969; Amano, Richelson and Nirenberg, 1972). These cells are fairly unique in that they can be induced to develop neuritic extensions in response to cyclic adenosine monophosphate (cAMP) (Prasad and Hsie, 1971) and prostaglandins (Prasad, 1972).

Extracerebrally derived tumors transplanted intracerebrally

A number of cell lines derived from tumors that arose extracerebrally have been used as brain tumor models. The main advantage of using such tumors is that their growth and therapeutic response characteristics are well established outside the CNS; therefore, the specific effect of the environment within the brain can be isolated. Some of the better characterized extracerebral tumor cell lines that have been transplanted directly into the CNS in experimental models (Sampson *et al.*, 1997) are the poorly immunogenic B16 murine melanoma cell lines that have been well characterized elsewhere (Fidler, 1975). Alternatively, cell lines such as the P388 and L1210 leukemias can be injected systemically and will spread to the nervous system secondarily. The L1210 leukemia cell line was induced in an inbred female DBA mouse (subline 212) by the cutaneous application of 0.2% methylcholanthrene in ethyl ether (Law *et al.*, 1949). This tumor can be carried in DBA mice by repeated injections subcutaneously, intramuscularly, intravenously or intraperitoneally. After systemic injections, these leukemic cells disseminate and infiltrate peripheral blood, lymph nodes, liver, spleen and brain (Skipper *et al.*, 1961). The latency before the appearance of leukemic cells in the brain after systemic injection depends on the number of cells injected. For example, after 1×10^6 cells are injected intraperitoneally, L1210 cells can be detected in the brain usually within 2–4 days (Skipper *et al.*, 1961). Alternatively, as few as 10 cells can be injected directly into the brain for a more precise tumor location and a more predictable death rate. At this cell dose intracerebrally, the median survival in one study was still only 12.8 days (Skipper, Schabel and Wilcox, 1967). This cell line obviously proliferates rapidly and has a doubling time of about 12 hours, both *in vitro* and *in vivo* (Skipper, Schabel and Wilcox, 1967). The tumor grows primarily along the leptomeninges, as in humans with CNS leukemia. The L1210 leukemia cell line has been used to demonstrate the efficacy of a number of chemotherapeutic agents and has been extensively used to demonstrate the protective barrier that the brain provides against many of these agents (Skipper *et al.*, 1961).

Mouse teratoma: models of embryonal tumors and divergent differentiation

A model for the study of divergent differentiation in embryonal central neuroepithelial tumors has been developed from the transplantable mouse teratoma, of which various lines are available. These experimental tumors can be produced by grafting pregastrulation embryos into the testis or beneath the renal capsule of susceptible inbred strains of adult mice. The teratomas are multipotential and malignant, and the progeny of the undifferentiated stem cells that are injected into syngeneic animals form either ascitic or solid tumor implants, depending on the site of the injection, and differentiate into derivatives of the three classic germ layers. The solid tumors derived from the OTT-6050 line, originally developed by Stevens (1970), contain a high percentage of neuroepithelial cells, estimated from serial section of one entire transplant at 80–90% of the cell population in some instances (VandenBerg *et al.*, 1975). The study of this model by using light and electron microscopy (Herman *et al.*, 1975) permitted a detailed morphologic analysis of its progressive stages of neuroepithelial differentiation. The study demonstrated convincing equivalences with the cytogenic stages postulated for the developing avian and mammalian CNS and with the stages encountered in embryonal tumors of the human CNS. These stages range from areas, on the one hand, that are still undifferentiated but contain multipotential medullary epithelium that mimics the primitive neural tube and corresponds to the cerebral medulloepithelioma, to areas, on the other hand, of neuroblastic and mature ganglion cells, of ependymoblastic and ependymal areas, or of divergent terminal states of neuroglial differentiation. Similar observations have been made on other mouse teratoma models (Damjanov, Solter and Šerman, 1973; Tresman and Evans, 1975; Gaillard *et al.*, 1984). The various cellular arrangements and cytologic types can be identified with considerable precision, including the distinction between primitive medullary, ependymoblastic and ependymal rosettes.

Biochemical differentiation is expressed by the presence of GFAP (VandenBerg *et al.*, 1975), of significant serotonin concentrations, of cAMP and of enzymes involved in the metabolism of biogenic amines or acetylcholine (Orenberg *et al.*, 1976). Brain-associated cell surface antigens, which can be demonstrated both *in vivo* and *in vitro*, appear early on the neural cells that differentiate from the nonneural stem-cell population (VandenBerg, Hickey and Herman, 1977; Ramsay *et al.*, 1982). Divergent differentiation also occurs early *in vitro*, with the expression of GFAP (VandenBerg *et al.*, 1976) and the subsequent appearance of biogenic amines as shown by histochemical fluorescence. The latter have the emission characteristics and fading kinetics of serotonin, and their demonstration is increased after tryptophan loading (Herman and VandenBerg, 1978). Both serotonin and 5-hydroxyindole acetic acid were also reported in another transplantable teratoma (of the C3H mouse strain) in which exclusive neural differentiation was established (Jakupevic *et al.*, 1974).

Of interest in this model is the presence of a primitive neural stem-cell population that can sustain repeated transplantation, in addition to the existence of undifferentiated embryonal stem cells. The production of transplantable tumors, restricted to undifferentiated stem cells and their neuroepithelial derivatives, is made possible because of the persistence of these primitive neural cells (Damjanov, Solter and Šerman, 1973; VandenBerg *et al.*, 1981a). These cells exhibited divergent glial and neuronal differentiation. Further potential of this model for experimental study of embryonal neoplasms is suggested by the expression of the oncogene N-*myc* in related tumor cell lines and by the variation of this expression with changes in growth potential and cellular maturation (Dony, Kessel and Gruss, 1985; Jakobovits *et al.*, 1985; Griep and DeLuca, 1986). The model has also shown that protein kinase C and phorbol ester expression could be correlated with growth and differentiation of related teratoma cell lines (Snoek *et al.*, 1986).

Finally, this tumor has permitted the study of melanogenesis in primitive central neuroepithelial cells and has shown that melanosomal melanin is not restricted to cells of neural crest derivation (VandenBerg *et al.*, 1981b). Enzyme assays of a pigmented fraction of the tumor for the presence of tyrosinase and tyrosine hydroxylase, supplemented by immunofluorescence histochemistry, indicated that melanosomal pigment results from tyrosinase activity and is unrelated to the metabolic pathways involved in catecholamine synthesis and degradation as expressed by tyrosine hydroxylase activity (Erdelyi *et al.*, 1981). The relevance of this observation is apparent when the significance of melanosomal melanin pigment in human central neuroepithelial tumors is considered.

Beyond the potential of the mouse teratoma model for the study of embryonal tumors of the CNS, its significance is linked to the concept that faulty expression of developmentally relevant genes, whether due to mutational, viral or other causes, may accompany all forms of neoplasia and that the genes involved could be any of those concerned with cell growth and differentiation (Mintz and Fleischman, 1981). In neuro-oncology, the importance of epigenetic phenomena is illustrated by the experiments of Artzt and Bennett (1972) on mice bearing a specific allele that causes defective primitive streak formation and its subsequent overgrowth in homozygous animals (t^{w18}). Implanting these genetically aberrant embryos into the testes of adult mice results in an appreciable incidence, in the recipients, of tumors comprising extensive areas of embryonal neuroepithelial tissue that are equivalent to the medulloepithelioma, the medulloblastoma and the neuroblastoma in humans. However, the transplantability of these tumors is limited, and, after one passage, they develop into well-differentiated teratomas that can no longer be transplanted. These experiments nevertheless suggest that a specific genetic factor that normally codes for a block in early development can be made to express an error of differentiation in the form of a largely embryonal tumor of neuroepithelial cell type. The characterization of endogenous factors that could modulate the growth, differentiation and maturation potential of such embryonal tumors is virtually unknown territory that awaits exploration.

Rat models

Most of the commonly used rat glioma cell lines have been induced by systemic or transplacental injection of nitrosoureas. The most commonly used lines that were induced using such techniques include the 9L gliosarcoma and the C6 glioma. These cell lines, and the popular, virally induced S635-clone 5 cell line, are discussed in detail below. Another less frequently used cell line is the RG-2 glioma induced in F344 rats by ENU administration (Wechsler, Ramadan and Gieseler, 1972).

9L gliosarcoma

The 9L cell line was derived from one originally induced by weekly intravenous injections of 5 mg/kg MNU in inbred male F344 rats (Benda *et al.*, 1971). The 9L cell line, however, because of its extensive sarcomatous component that was acquired after serial passage (Barker *et al.*, 1973), differs considerably from the original tumor, which had the histologic appearance of an anaplastic astrocytoma. Intracerebral transplants of 9L cells are well circumscribed, lack significant necrosis and tend to encircle blood vessels at the tumor margin in a manner characteristic of sarcomas. Although the origin of the sarcomatous component cannot be determined with certainty, these changes demonstrate the phenotypic and genetic instability associated with this cell line and sublines derived from it (Rubinstein, 1977). Thus, this cell line should be obtained from the original source when possible, and the source of any sublines should always be identified.

The 9L cell line can be grown *in vitro* and *in vivo*. As a monolayer culture *in vitro* it has a population doubling time of between 18 and 20 hours (Barker *et al*., 1973). 9L cells can also be grown *in vitro* as multicellular spheroids and have been shown to approximate the properties of *in vivo* tumors. It has also been used to produce subcutaneous or intracerebral tumors that morphologically resemble human gliosarcomas (Rubinstein, 1977). Subcutaneous implantation of 1×10^6 cells can produce tumors greater than 2 cm in diameter in 3–4 weeks (Weizsaecker *et al*., 1981), and intracerebral injection of 4×10^4 cells should be tumorigenic in all syngeneic animals, resulting in a median survival of 23 days, which is usually preceded by a 5- to 6-day symptomatic period (Barker *et al*., 1973). Finally, the 9L line has been useful in demonstrating the efficacy of a number of therapeutic agents (Culver *et al*., 1992), but favorable therapeutic outcomes must always be viewed in light of its genetic instability, which potentially could produce confounding immune responses against this tumor even in inbred F344 rats (Tapscott *et al*., 1994).

C6 glioma

This cell line was induced by weekly intravenous injections of 5 mg/kg MNU in random-bred male Wistar-Furth rats (Benda *et al*., 1968, 1971). The C6 cell line is best used for evaluating the composition and function of glia; the presence of specific surface antigens, such as β-adrenergic receptors; the response to β-agonists, such as norepinephrine; and the expression of various enzymes implicated in active transport and cAMP metabolism (Bissell *et al*., 1974). Morphologically, the C6 line appears as a poorly differentiated glial cell type with a potential to differentiate structurally, and in certain well-defined situations biochemically, into astrocytes, and to produce GFAP. The level of expression of this marker protein can be enhanced by dibutyryl cAMP (Raju, Bignami and Dahl, 1980), norepinephrine (Browning and Ruina, 1984), high cell density (Frame *et al*., 1984) and organ culture (Liao *et al*., 1978). These cells also appear to be capable of transdifferentiating *in vitro* (Parker, Norenberg and Vernadakis, 1980). For example, in early passages, 2',3'-cyclic nucleotide 3'-phosphohydrolase, a marker for myelin and oligodendroglia, is high, whereas reactivity for glutamine synthetase, an astrocytic marker, is low. These characteristics are reversed in later passages, however.

The major limitation to using the C6 cell line as a model of human gliomas stems from its uncertain genetic background and, therefore, the lack of a syngeneic host that can be used for transplantation. Because the C6 line was derived from random-bred rats, therapeutic responses must always be evaluated in the context of the allogeneic responses that may be stimulated against this line, even in inbred Wistar-Furth rats, because they are not syngeneic with the cell line itself. Because this cell line has well-characterized glial differentiation features, it has been grown as a xenograft in neonatal and adult immunoincompetent mice of various strains (Kaye *et al*., 1986) and neonatal Wistar rats (Auer, Del Maestro and Anderson, 1981). These models were initially quite valuable because they circumvented the variability encountered with the earlier methods of direct chemical or viral CNS tumor induction, and provided a way of studying therapeutic responses based on the intrinsic properties of a glioma cell line and the surrounding environment of the brain. With the subsequent advent of human glioma xenograft models in immunoincompetent animals (see above) and the cloning of syngeneic, spontaneously arising rodent glioma cell lines, the specific usefulness of such models needs to be carefully evaluated. In conclusion, the C6 cell line expresses a number of glial differentiation markers, including GFAP, and remains a good model for *in vitro* glioma studies; but for *in vivo* studies, especially ones where immunologic responses may play an important role, results should always be confirmed in more appropriate model systems.

S635-clone 5 anaplastic astrocytoma

The S635cl5 cell line was derived from an anaplastic astrocytoma induced in an inbred neonatal female F344 rat by intracerebral inoculation with concentrated Schmidt-Ruppin-D strain ASV (Lee *et al*., 1986). Cells cultured *in vitro* and tumors grown *in vivo* using this cell line have a consistent architecture composed of interlaced, elongated cells that express GFAP, even after more than 100 passages *in vitro*. This cell line, *in vitro*, has a population doubling time of 18.82 hours and a colony formation efficiency of 90.8%. *In vivo*, these cells are highly tumorigenic, with as few as 100 cells being uniformly lethal within 1 month when injected intracerebrally into syngeneic rats (unpublished data from our laboratory). This cell line may be particularly useful for some immunologic studies because it has been shown to express a common antigen (Harwood *et al*., 1976), as well as a glioma-associated antigen (Lee, Wikstrand and Bigner, 1986). In addition, syngeneic rats bearing ASV-induced tumors have exhibited a depression in their cell-mediated immune responses (Roszman *et al.*, 1978), but remain susceptible to the induction of experimental allergic encephalomyelitis (Strauss, Bigner and Bigner, 1982). A more extensive description of this tumor model has been published elsewhere (Lee *et al.*, 1986).

CNS-1 glioma

The CNS-1 cell line was induced in inbred Lewis rats by weekly injection of MNU (Kruse *et al.*, 1994). Although chemically induced, this cell line has a number of desirable features, including infiltrative growth and GFAP reactivity, both *in vivo* and *in vitro*. The line is tumorigenic when injected either subcutaneously or intracerebrally. Intracerebral injection, with $>1 \times 10^4$ CNS-1 cells is uniformly lethal and produces survival times greater than 2 weeks, depending on dose. Perhaps most importantly, however, this cell line permits more extensive evaluation of the safety of experimental immunotherapeutic protocols. Because Lewis rats are highly susceptible to the induction of experimental allergic encephalomyelitis, this model seems well suited to detecting the potential for inducing such detrimental autoimmune responses that could be stimulated by cell-mediated immunotherapy protocols. In light of the documented expression of normal and fetal CNS antigens on glioma cell lines and brain tumor tissues (Wikstrand and Bigner, 1979) and the ability of human GBM tissue to induce lethal experimental allergic encephalomyelitis in nonhuman primates (Bigner, Pitts and Wikstrand, 1981), formally evaluating the risk of immunologically based therapies using this model should be considered in the preclinical testing of all such agents.

Summary

In summary, a number of transplantable animal brain tumor models are available, and each has unique qualities that may make it more or less useful for answering specific experimental questions. Appropriate criteria to use in evaluating the suitability of a brain tumor model might include the following: a tumor that arose spontaneously, one that displays evidence of glial differentiation histologically and at a molecular level, one that is biologically and genetically stable, and one that requires few tumor cells to initiate predictable tumor growth *in vitro* and reproducible and fatal growth intracranially and subcutaneously *in vivo* in syngeneic animals. The primary use of experimental models, however, is to predict therapeutic responses in human tumors. In this sense, because very few treatment modalities have shown efficacy against human primary brain tumors clinically, it is difficult to prove that one model is necessarily better than another. Nevertheless, it is probably prudent to avoid basing clinical decisions on information obtained using models that can be predicted to provide potentially misleading results; for example, models with inherent histoincompatibilities.

References

Adams, S.W. and Crowley, A.M. (1987) Posterior paralysis due to spontaneous oligodendroglioma in the spinal cord of a rat. *Laboratory Animal Science* **37**, 345–7.

Aguzzi, A., Wagner, E.F., Williams, R.L. and Courtneidge, S.A. (1990) Sympathetic hyperplasia and neuroblastomas in transgenic mice expressing polyoma middle T antigen. *New Biologist* **2**, 533–43.

Aguzzi, A., Kleihues, P., Heckl, K. and Wiestler, O.D. (1991) Cell type-specific tumor induction in neural transplants by retrovirus-mediated oncogene transfer. *Oncogene* **6**, 113–18.

Albright, L., Madigan, J.C., Gaston, M.R. and Houchens, D.P. (1975) Therapy in an intracerebral murine glioma model, using Bacillus Calmette-Guerin, neuraminidase-treated tumor cells, and 1-(2-chloroethyl)-3-cyclohexyl-1-nitrosourea. *Cancer Research* **35**, 658–65.

Al Ubaidi, M.R., Font, R.L., Quiambao, A.B., Keener, M.J., Liou, G.I., Overbeek, P.A. and Baehr, W. (1992) Bilateral retinal and brain tumors in transgenic mice expressing simian virus 40 large T antigen under control of the human interphotoreceptor retinoid-binding protein promoter. *Journal of Cell Biology* **119**, 1681–7.

Al Zubaidy, A.J. and Malinowski, W. (1984) Spontaneous pineal body tumors (pinealomas) in Wistar rats: a histological and ultrastructural study. *Laboratory Animals* **18**, 224–9.

Amano, T., Richelson, E. and Nirenberg, M. (1972) Neurotransmitter synthesis by neuroblastoma clones. *Proceedings of the National Academy of Sciences U.S.A.* **69**, 258–63.

Ames, B.N., McCann, J. and Yamasaki, E. (1975) Methods for detecting carcinogens and mutagens with the Salmonella/mammalian-microsome mutagenicity test. *Mutation Research* **31**, 347–64.

Anandatheerthavarada, H.K., Boyd, M.R. and Ravindranath, V. (1992) Characterization of a phenobarbital-inducible cytochrome P-450, NADPH-cytochrome P-450 reductase and reconstituted cytochrome P-450 mono-oxygenase system from rat brain. Evidence for constitutive presence in rat and human brain. *Biochemical Journal* **288**, 483–8.

Arbeit, J.M., Münger, K., Howley, P.M. and Hanahan, D. (1993) Neuroepithelial carcinomas in mice transgenic with human papillomavirus type 16 E6/E7 ORFs. *American Journal of Pathology* **142**, 1187–97.

Artzt, K. and Bennett, D. (1972) A genetically caused embryonal ectodermal tumor in the mouse. *Journal of the National Cancer Institute* **48**, 141–58.

ATSDR [Agency for Toxic Substances and Disease Registry (U.S.)] (1995) *Toxicological profile for vinyl chloride*. Draft for public comment (update). Atlanta, Ga.: U.S. Department of Health and Human Services; Public Health Service; ATSDR.

Auer, R.N., Del Maestro, R.F. and Anderson, R. (1981) A simple and reproducible experimental *in vivo* glioma model. *Canadian Journal of Neurological Sciences* **8**, 325–31.

Ausman, J.I., Shapiro, W.R. and Rall, D.P. (1970) Studies on the chemotherapy of experimental brain tumors: development of an experimental model. *Cancer Research* **30**, 2394–400.

Baetge, E.E., Behringer, R.R., Messing, A., Brinster, R.L. and Palmiter, R.D. (1988) Transgenic mice express the human phenylethanolamine *N*-methyltransferase gene in adrenal medulla and retina. *Proceedings of the National Academy of Sciences U.S.A.* **85**, 3648–52.

Bailar, J.C. III, Crouch, E.A.C., Shaikh, R. and Spiegelman, D. (1988) One-hit models of carcinogenesis: conservative or not? *Risk Analysis* **8**, 485–97.

Bancroft, F.C. and Tashjian, A.H. Jr (1971) Growth in suspension culture of rat pituitary cells which produce growth hormone and prolactin. *Experimental Cell Research* **64**, 125–8.

Bargmann, C.I., Hung, M.-C. and Weinberg, R.A. (1986a) The *neu* oncogene encodes an epidermal growth factor receptor-related protein. *Nature* **319**, 226–30.

——(1986b) Multiple independent activations of the *neu* oncogene by a point mutation altering the transmembrane domain of p185. *Cell* **45**, 649–57.

Barker, M., Hoshino, T., Gurcay, O., Wilson, C.B., Nielsen, S.L., Downie, R. and Eliason, J. (1973) Development of an animal brain tumor model and its response to therapy with 1,3-bis(2-chloroethyl)-1-nitrosourea. *Cancer Research* **33**, 976–86.

Batzdorf, U. and Pokress, S.M. (1968) Architectural features of ependymomas in tissue culture. *Journal of Neuropathology and Experimental Neurology* **27**, 333–47.

Bautch, V.L., Toda, S., Hassell, J.A. and Hanahan, D. (1987) Endothelial cell tumors develop in transgenic mice carrying polyoma virus middle T oncogene. *Cell* **51**, 529–37.

Bazin, H., Platteau, B., Pauwels, R. and Capron, A. (1980) Immunoglobulin production in nude rats with special attention to the IgE isotype. *Annales d'Immunologie* **131C**, 31–7.

Benda, P., Lightbody, J., Sato, G., Levine, L. and Sweet, W. (1968) Differentiated rat glial cell strain in tissue culture. *Science* **161**, 370–1.

Benda, P., Someda, K., Messer, J. and Sweet, W.H. (1971) Morphological and immunochemical studies of rat glial tumors and clonal strains propagated in culture. *Journal of Neurosurgery* **34**, 310–23.

Benvenisty, N., Ornitz, D.M., Bennett, G.L., Sahagan, B.G., Kuo, A., Cardiff, R.D. and Leder, P. (1992) Brain tumours and lymphomas in transgenic mice that carry HTLV-I LTR/c-*myc* and Ig/*tax* genes. *Oncogene* **7**, 2399–405.

Bergsagel, D.J., Finegold, M.J., Butel, J.S., Kupsky, W.J. and Garcea, R.L. (1992) DNA sequences similar to those of simian virus 40 in ependymomas and choroid plexus tumors of childhood. *New England Journal of Medicine* **326**, 988–93.

Berleur, M.-P. and Cordier, S. (1995) The role of chemical, physical, or viral exposures and health factors in neurocarcinogenesis: implications for epidemiologic studies of brain tumors. *Cancer Causes and Control* **6**, 240–56.

Bi, W.F., Wang, Y.S., Huang, M.Y. and Meng, D.S. (1985) Effect of vinyl chloride on testis in rats. *Ecotoxicology and Environmental Safety* **10**, 281–9.

Bigner, D.D. and Swenberg, J.A. (1977) *Jänisch and Schreiber's Experimental tumors of the central nervous system*. First English edition. Kalamazoo: The Upjohn Company.

Bigner, D.D., Pitts, O.M. and Wikstrand, C.J. (1981) Induction of lethal experimental allergic encephalomyelitis in nonhuman primates and guinea pigs with human glioblastoma multiforme tissue. *Journal of Neurosurgery* **55**, 32–42.

Bigner, D.D., Odom, G.L., Mahaley, M.S. Jr and Day, E.D. (1969) Brain tumors induced in dogs by the Schmidt-Ruppin strain of Rous sarcoma virus. *Journal of Neuropathology and Experimental Neurology* **28**, 648–80.

Bigner, D.D., Kvedar, J.P., Thomas, B.A., Shaffer, C., Vick, N.A., Engel, W.K. and Day, E.D. (1972) Factors influencing the cell type of brain tumors induced in dogs by Schmidt-Ruppin Rous sarcoma virus. *Journal of Neuropathology and Experimental Neurology* **31**, 583–95.

Bigner, D.D., Self, D.J., Frey, J., Ishizaki, R., Langlois, A.J. and Swenberg, J.A. (1975) Refinement of the avian oncornavirus-induced primary rat brain tumor model and its potential for therapeutic screening. *Recent Results in Cancer Research* **51**, 20–34.

Bigner, D.D., Bigner, S.H., Burger, P.C., Shelburne, J.D. and Friedman, H.S. (1986) Primary brain tumours in Fischer 344 rats chronically exposed to acrylonitrile in their drinking-water. *Food and Chemical Toxicology* **24**, 129–37.

Bigner, S.H., Bullard, D.E., Pegram, C.N., Wikstrand, C.J. and Bigner, D.D. (1981) Relationship of *in vitro* morphologic and growth characteristics of established human glioma-derived cell lines to their tumorigenicity in athymic nude mice. *Journal of Neuropathology and Experimental Neurology* **40**, 390–409.

Bigner, S.H., Schold, S.C., Friedman, H.S., Mark, J. and Bigner, D.D. (1989) Chromosomal composition of malignant human gliomas through serial subcutaneous transplantation in athymic mice. *Cancer Genetics and Cytogenetics* **40**, 111–20.

Bissell, M.G., Rubinstein, L.J., Bignami, A. and Herman, M.M. (1974) Characteristics of the rat C-6 glioma maintained in organ culture systems. Production of glial fibrillary acidic protein in the absence of gliofibrillogenesis. *Brain Research* **82**, 77–89.

Bjerkvig, R., Tonnesen, A., Laerum, O.D. and Backlund, E.O. (1990) Multicellular tumor spheroids from human gliomas maintained in organ culture. *Journal of Neurosurgery* **72**, 463–75.

Blackburn, C.C., Griffith, J. and Morahan, G. (1995) A high-resolution map of the chromosomal region surrounding the *nude* gene. *Genomics* **26**, 308–17.

Bondy, M., Wiencke, J., Wrensch, M. and Kyritsis, A.P. (1994) Genetics of primary brain tumors: a review. *Journal of Neuro-Oncology* **18**, 69–81.

Borrelli, E., Sawchenko, P.E. and Evans, R.M. (1992) Pituitary hyperplasia induced by ectopic expression of nerve growth factor. *Proceedings of the National Academy of Sciences U.S.A.* **89**, 2764–8.

Bosch, D.A. (1979) Chemical neuro-oncogenesis. An experimental study on some effects of *N*-methyl- and *N*-ethyl-*N*-nitrosourea on the developing nervous system of the rat. *Acta Neurochirurgica* **50**, 43–7.

Bosch, D.A., Gerrits, P.O. and Ebels, E.J. (1972) The cytotoxic effect of ethylnitrosourea and methylnitrosourea on the nervous system of the rat at different stages of development. *Zeitschrift für Krebsforschung und Klinische Onkologie – Cancer Research and Clinical Oncology* **77**, 308–18.

Bosma, G.C., Custer, R.P. and Bosma, M.J. (1983) A severe combined immunodeficiency mutation in the mouse. *Nature* **301**, 527–30.

Bosma, M.J. and Carroll, A.M. (1991) The SCID mouse mutant: definition, characterization, and potential uses. *Annual Review of Immunology* **9**, 323–50.

Bradford, R., Darling, J.L. and Thomas, D.G. (1990) The chemotherapeutic response of a murine (VM) model of human glioma. *British Journal of Cancer* **61**, 46–50.

Bradford, R., Darling, J.L., Sier, N. and Thomas, D.G. (1990) The VM model of glioma: preparation of multicellular tumour spheroids (MTS) and their response to chemotherapy. *Journal of Neuro-Oncology* **9**, 105–14.

Bradley, N.J., Bloom, H.J.G., Davies, A.J.S. and Swift, S.M. (1978) Growth of human gliomas in immune-deficient mice: a possible model for pre-clinical therapy studies. *British Journal of Cancer* **38**, 263–72.

Brem, S., Rozental, J.M. and Moskal, J.R. (1995) What is the etiology of human brain tumors? A report of the First Lebow Conference. *Cancer* **76**, 709–13.

Brinster, R.L., Chen, H.Y., Messing, A., van Dyke, T., Levine, A.J. and Palmiter, R.D. (1984) Transgenic mice harboring SV40 T-antigen genes develop characteristic brain tumors. *Cell* **37**, 367–79.

Britt, R.H., Lyons, B.E., Eng, L.F., Bigner, S.H. and Bigner, D.D. (1985) Immunohistochemical study of glial fibrillary acidic protein in avian sarcoma virus-induced gliomas in dogs. *Journal of Neuro-Oncology* **3**, 53–9.

Britt, R.H., Lyons, B.E., Enzmann, D.R., Saxer, E.L., Bigner, S.H. and Bigner, D.D. (1987) Correlation of neuropathologic findings, computerized tomographic and high-resolution ultrasound scans of canine avian sarcoma virus-induced brain tumors. *Journal of Neuro-Oncology* **4**, 243–68.

Brooks, C.G., Webb, P.J., Robbins, R.A., Robinson, G., Baldwin, R.W. and Festing, M.F.W. (1980) Studies on the immunobiology of *rnu/rnu* 'nude' rats with congenital aplasia of the thymus. *European Journal of Immunology* **10**, 58–65.

Browning, E.T. and Ruina, M. (1984) Glial fibrillary acidic protein: norepinephrine stimulated phosphorylation in intact C-6 glioma cells. *Journal of Neurochemistry* **42**, 718–26.

Brucher, J.M. and Ermel, A.E. (1974) Central neuroblastoma induced by transplacental administration of methylnitrosourea in Wistar-R rats. An electron microscopic study. *Journal of Neurology* **208**, 1–16.

Brüstle, O., Ohgaki, H., Schmitt, H.P., Walter, G.F., Ostertag, H. and Kleihues, P. (1992) Primitive neuroectodermal tumors after prophylactic central nervous system irradiation in children. Association with an activated K-*ras* gene. *Cancer* **69**, 2385–92.

Brüstle, O., Petersen, I., Radner, H., Höll, T., Plate, K.H., Kleihues, P. and Wiestler, O.D. (1993) Complementary tumor induction in neural grafts exposed to *N*-ethyl-*N*-nitrosourea and an activated *myc* gene. *Carcinogenesis* **14**, 1715–18.

Bubeník, J., Kieler, J., Jandlová, T. and Šímova, J. (1992) Age-related decrease in transplantability of human tumors in *nu/nu* mice. *Anticancer Research* **12**, 1695–8.

Bullock, F.D. and Curtis, M.R. (1930) Spontaneous tumors of the rat. *Journal of Cancer Research* **14**, 1–115.

Bunin, G.R., Buckley, J.D., Boesel, C.P., Rorke, L.B. and Meadows, A.T. (1994) Risk factors for astrocytic glioma and primitive neuroectodermal tumor of the brain in young children: a report from the Children's Cancer Group. *Cancer Epidemiology, Biomarkers and Prevention* **3**, 197–204.

Burek, J.D. and Hollander, C.F. (1977) Incidence patterns of spontaneous tumors in BN/Bi rats. *Journal of the National Cancer Institute* **58**, 99–105.

Burger, P.C., Shibata, T., Aguzzi, A. and Kleihues, P. (1988) Selective induction by *N*-nitrosoethylurea of oligodendrogliomas in fetal forebrain transplants. *Cancer Research* **48**, 2871–5.

Byrd, P., Brown, K.W. and Gallimore, P.H. (1982) Malignant transformation of human embryo retinoblasts by cloned adenovirus 12 DNA. *Nature* **298**, 69–71.

Byrén, D., Engholm, G., Englund, A. and Westerholm, P. (1976) Mortality and cancer morbidity in a group of Swedish VCM and PCV production workers. *Environmental Health Perspectives* **17**, 167–70.

Cahan, W.G., Woodward, H.Q., Higinbotham, N.L., Stewart, F.W. and Coley, B.L. (1948) Sarcoma arising in irradiated bone. *Cancer* **1**, 3–29.

Calvert, R.J., Hongyo, T., Buzard, G.S., Weghorst, C.M., Diwan, B.A. and Rice, J.M. (1994) Mutations in the *p53* gene of transplacentally induced rat gliomas. (Abstract) *Proceedings of the American Association for Cancer Research* **35**, 173.

Caputo, A. and Giovanella, B. (1957) Chemical carcinogenesis of CNS tumors in anura. *Neoplasie* **10**, 245–66.

Cardesa, A., Llanes, F., Merchan, J., Alvarez, T., Ludeña, M.D. and Mohr, U. (1983) Plexiform structures in malignant schwannomas after prenatal exposure to ethylnitrosourea. *Experimental Pathology* **24**, 103–15.

Cardesa, A., Ribalta, T., Von Schilling, B., Palacin, A. and Mohr, U. (1989) Experimental model of tumors associated with neurofibromatosis. *Cancer* **63**, 1737–49.

Carlsson, J., Nilsson, K., Westermark, B., Pontén, J., Sundström, C., Larsson, E., Bergh, J., Pahlman, S., Busch, C. and Collins, V.P. (1983) Formation and growth of multicellular spheroids of human origin. *International Journal of Cancer* **31**, 523–33.

Cash, J.M., Remmers, E.F., Goldmuntz, E.A., Crofford, L.J., Zha, H., Hansen, C.T. and Wilder, R.L. (1993) Genetic mapping of the athymic nude (*RNU*) locus in the rat to a region on chromosome 10. *Mammalian Genome* **4**, 37–42.

Castanera, T.J., Jones, D.C., Kimeldorf, D.J. and Rosen, V.J. (1968) The influence of whole-body exposure to X-rays or neutrons on the life span distribution of tumors among male rats. *Cancer Research* **28**, 170–82.

Causey, G. (1960) *The cell of Schwann*. London: Livingstone.

Chambers, R., Gillespie, G.Y., Soroceanu, L., Andreansky, S., Chatterjee, S., Chou, J., Roizman, B. and Whitley, R.J. (1995) Comparison of genetically engineered herpes simplex viruses for the treatment of brain tumors in a scid mouse model of human malignant glioma. *Proceedings of the National Academy of Sciences U.S.A.* **92**, 1411–15.

Chen, J.D. and Van Dyke, T. (1991) Uniform cell-autonomous tumorigenesis of the choroid plexus by papovavirus large T antigens. *Molecular and Cellular Biology* **11**, 5968–76.

Chen, J., Tobin, G.J., Pipas, J.M. and Van Dyke, T. (1992) T-antigen mutant activities *in vivo*: roles of p53 and pRB binding in tumorigenesis of the choroid plexus. *Oncogene* **7**, 1167–75.

Ciroussel, F., Barbin, A., Eberle, G. and Bartsch, H. (1990) Investigations on the relationship between DNA ethenobase adduct levels in several organs of vinyl chloride-exposed rats and cancer susceptibility. *Biochemical Pharmacology* **39**, 1109–13.

Compere, S.J., Baldacci, P., Sharpe, A.H., Thompson, T., Land, H. and Jaenisch, R. (1989) The *ras* and *myc* oncogenes cooperate in tumor induction in many tissues when introduced into midgestation mouse embryos by retroviral vectors. *Proceedings of the National Academy of Sciences U.S.A.* **86**, 2224–8.

Conley, F.K. (1974) Transplantation of nervous system tumors in diffusion chambers. *Journal of Neurosurgery* **41**, 332–8.

——(1979) The immunocytochemical localization of GFA protein in experimental murine CNS tumors. *Acta Neuropathologica* **45**, 9–16.

Conley, F.K., Rubinstein, L.J. and Spence, A.M. (1976) Studies on experimental malignant nerve sheath tumors maintained in tissue and organ culture systems. II. Electron microscopy observations. *Acta Neuropathologica* **34**, 293–310.

Copeland, D.D. and Bigner, D.D. (1977a) The role of the subependymal plate in avian sarcoma virus brain tumor induction: comparison of incipient tumors in neonatal and adult rats. *Acta Neuropathologica* **38**, 1–6.

——(1977b) Influence of age at inoculation on avian oncornavirus-induced brain tumor incidence, tumor morphology, and postinoculation survival in F344 rats. *Cancer Research* **37**, 1657–61.

——(1978) Glial-mesenchymal tropism of *in vivo* avian sarcoma virus neuro-oncogenesis in rats. *Acta Neuropathologica* **41**, 23–5.

Copeland, D.D., Vogel, F.S. and Bigner, D.D. (1975) The induction of intracranial neoplasms by the inoculation of avian sarcoma virus in perinatal and adult rats. *Journal of Neuropathology and Experimental Neurology* **34**, 340–58.

Corallini, A., Barbanti-Brodano, G., Bortoloni, W., Nenci, I., Cassai, E., Tampieri, M., Portolani, M. and Borgatti, M. (1977) High incidence of ependymomas induced by BK virus, a human papovavirus: brief communication. *Journal of the National Cancer Institute* **59**, 1561–4.

Corallini, A., Pagnani, M., Caputo, A., Negrini, M., Altavilla, G., Catozzi, L. and Barbanti-Brodano, G. (1988) Cooperation in oncogenesis between BK virus early region gene and the activated human c-Harvey *ras* oncogene. *Journal of General Virology* **69**, 2671–9.

Cotchin, E. (1977) A general survey of tumors in the horse. *Equine Veterinary Journal* **9**, 16–21.

Cottier, H. and Luginbühl, H. (1961) Oligodendroglioma in a white mouse. *Acta Neuropathologica* **1**, 198–200.

Coulomb, B., Levy, S., Maunoury, R: and Markovits, P. (1979) Transformation spontanée et maintien prolongé *in vitro* de cellules gliales d'embryons de souris. *Bulletin du Cancer* **66**, 229–34.

Culver, K.W., Ram, Z., Wallbridge, S., Ishii, H., Oldfield, E.H. and Blaese, R.M. (1992) *In vivo* gene transfer with retroviral vector-producer cells for treatment of experimental brain tumors. *Science* **256**, 1550–2.

Dagle, G.E., Zwicker, G.M. and Renne, R.A. (1979) Morphology of spontaneous brain tumors in the rat. *Veterinary Pathology* **16**, 318–24.

Dahme, E. and Schiefer, B. (1960) Intracranial tumors in animals. *Zentralblatt Veterinärmedizin* **7**, 341–63.

Damjanov, I., Solter, D. and Šerman, D. (1973) Teratocarcinoma with the capacity for differentiation restricted to neuro-ectodermal tissue. *Virchows Archiv B, Cell Pathology* **13**, 179–95.

Danks, R.A., Orian, J.M., Gonzales, M.F., Tan, S.S., Alexander, B., Mikoshiba, K. and Kaye, A.H. (1995) Transformation of astrocytes in transgenic mice expressing SV40 T antigen under the transcriptional control of the glial fibrillary acidic protein promoter. *Cancer Research* **55**, 4302–10.

Darling, J.L., Oktar, N. and Thomas, D.G.T. (1983) Multicellular tumour spheroids derived from human brain tumours. *Cell Biology International Reports* **7**, 23–30.

de Jong, W.H., Steerenberg, P.A., Ursem, P.S., Osterhaus, A.D.M.E., Vos, J.G. and Ruitenberg, E.J. (1980) The athymic nude rat. III. Natural cell-mediated cytotoxicity. *Clinical Immunology and Immunopathology* **17**, 163–72.

Denlinger, R.H., Koestner, A. and Wechsler, W. (1974) Induction of neurogenic tumors in C3HeB/FeJ mice by nitrosourea derivatives: observations by light microscopy, tissue culture, and electron microscopy. *International Journal of Cancer* **13**, 559–71.

Dobson, P.R.M. and Brown, B.L. (1985) The preparation, culture, and incubation of rat anterior pituitary cells for static and dynamic studies of secretion. *Methods in Enzymology* **109**, 293–8.

Dony, C., Kessel, M. and Gruss, P. (1985) Post-transcriptional control of *myc* and *p53* expression during differentiation of the embryonal carcinoma cell line F9. *Nature* **317**, 636–9.

Drew, R.T., Boorman, G.A., Haseman, J.K., McConnell, E.E., Busey, W.M. and Moore, J.A. (1983) The effect of age and exposure duration on cancer induction by a known carcinogen in rats, mice, and hamsters. *Toxicology and Applied Pharmacology* **68**, 120–30.

Druckrey, H. (1973) Chemical structure and action in transplacental carcinogenesis and teratogenesis. In Tomatis, L., Mohr, U. and Davis, W. (eds), *Transplacental carcinogenesis*. Lyon: International Agency for Research on Cancer, 45–58.

Druckrey, H., Ivankovic, S. and Preussmann, R. (1964) Selective induction of brain tumors in rats with MNU. *Naturwissenschaften* **51**, 144.

——(1965) Selective induction of malignant tumors in the brain and spinal cord of rats with MNU. *Zeitschrift für Krebsforschung* **66**, 389–408.

——(1966) Teratogenic and carcinogenic effects in the offspring after single injection of ethylnitrosourea to pregnant rats. *Nature* **210**, 1378–9.

——(1967) Neurotropic carcinogenic effect of phenyl-dimethyl-triazene on rats. *Naturwissenschaften* **54**, 171.

Druckrey, H., Preussmann, R., Ivanković, S. and Schmähl, D. (1967) Organotropic carcinogenic effects of 65 different *N*-nitroso compounds in BD rats. *Zeitschrift für Krebsforschung* **69**, 103–201.

Duffell, D., Hinz, R. and Nelson, E. (1964) Neoplasms in hamsters induced by simian virus 40. Light and electron microscopic observations. *American Journal of Pathology* **45**, 59–73.

Duigou, G.J., Walsh, J.W., Oeltgen, J. and Zimmer, S.G. (1990) Alterations in SV40 DNA integration patterns are associated with acquisition of the invasive phenotype in hamster brain tumors. *Anticancer Research* **10**, 1683–92.

Eibl, R.H., Kleihues, P., Jat, P.S. and Wiestler, O.D. (1994) A model for primitive neuroectodermal tumors in transgenic neural transplants harbouring the SV40 large T antigen. *American Journal of Pathology* **144**, 556–64.

Ellermann, V. and Bang, O. (1908) Experimentelle leukämie bei hühnern. *Zentralblatt Bakteriologie Parasitenkunde und Infektion Skrankheiten* **46**, 595–609.

EPA [Environmental Protection Agency (U.S.)] (1996) Notice. Proposed guidelines for carcinogen risk assessment. *Federal Register* **61**(79), 17959–8011.

Erdelyi, E., VandenBerg, S.R., Raese, J., Barchas, J.D., Rubinstein, L.J. and Herman, M.M. (1981) Neural differentiation in the OTT-6050 mouse teratoma: enzymatic and immunofluorescence characterization of a tumor fraction showing melanogenesis in neuroepithelial cells. *Virchows Archiv A, Pathological Anatomy and Histology* **393**, 27–37.

Fedtke, N., Boucheron, J.A., Walker, V.E. and Swenberg, J.A. (1990) Vinyl chloride-induced DNA adducts. II: Formation and persistence of 7-(2'oxoethyl)guanine and N^2,3-ethenoguanine in rat tissue DNA. *Carcinogenesis* **11**, 1287–92.

Feldman, A.R., Kessler, L., Myers, M.H. and Naughton, M.D. (1986) The prevalence of cancer. Estimates based on the Connecticut Tumor Registry. *New England Journal of Medicine* **315**, 1394–7.

Feron, V.J. and Kroes, R. (1979) One-year time-sequence inhalation toxicity study of vinyl chloride in rats. II. Morphological changes in the respiratory tract, ceruminous glands, brain, kidneys, heart and spleen. *Toxicology* **13**, 131–41.

Festing, M.F.W., May, D., Connors, T.A., Lovell, D. and Sparrow, S. (1978) An athymic nude mutation in the rat. *Nature* **274**, 365–6.

Fidler, I.J. (1975) Biological behavior of malignant melanoma cells correlated to their survival *in vivo*. *Cancer Research* **35**, 218–24.

——(1986) Rationale and methods for use of nude mice to study the biology and therapy of human cancer metastasis. *Cancer and Metastasis Reviews* **5**, 29–49.

Flanagan, S.P. (1966) '*Nude*', a new hairless gene with pleiotropic effects in the mouse. *Genetical Research* **8**, 295–309.

Frame, M.C., Freshney, R.I., Vaughan, P.F., Graham, D.I. and Shaw, R. (1984) Interrelationship between differentiation and malignancy-associated properties in glioma. *British Journal of Cancer* **49**, 269–80.

Fraser, H. (1971) Astrocytomas in an inbred mouse strain. *Journal of Pathology* **103**, 266–70.

——(1986) Brain tumors in mice, with particular reference to astrocytoma. *Food and Chemical Toxicology* **24**, 105–11.

Fraser, H. and McConnell, I. (1975) Experimental brain tumors. *Lancet* **1**, 44.

Friedman, H.S., Bigner, S.H., McComb, R.D., Schold, S.C. Jr, Pasternak, J.F., Groothuis, D.R. and Bigner, D.D. (1983a) A model for human medulloblastoma. Growth, morphology, and chromosomal analysis *in vitro* and in athymic mice. *Journal of Neuropathology and Experimental Neurology* **42**, 485–503.

Friedman, H.S., Schold, S.C. Jr, Varia, M. and Bigner, D.D. (1983b) Chemotherapy and radiation therapy of human medulloblastoma in athymic nude mice. *Cancer Research* **43**, 3088–93.

Friedman, H.S., Schold, S.C. Jr, Muhlbaier, L.H., Bjornsson, T.D. and Bigner, D.D. (1984) *In vitro* versus *in vivo* correlations of chemosensitivity of human medulloblastoma. *Cancer Research* **44**, 5145–9.

Friedman, H.S., Burger, P.C., Bigner, S.H., Trojanowski, J.Q., Wikstrand, C.J., Halperin, E.C. and Bigner, D.D. (1985) Establishment and characterization of the human medulloblastoma cell line and transplantable xenograft D283 Med. *Journal of Neuropathology and Experimental Neurology* **44**, 592–605.

Friedman, H.S., Burger, P.C., Bigner, S.H., Trojanowski, J.Q., Brodeur, G.M., He, X.M., Wikstrand, C.J., Kurtzberg, J., Berens, M.E., Halperin, E.C. and Bigner, D.D. (1988) Phenotypic and genotypic analysis of a human medulloblastoma cell line and transplantable xenograft (D341 Med) demonstrating amplification of c-*myc*. *American Journal of Pathology* **130**, 472–84.

Friedman, H.S., Oakes, W.J., Bigner, S.H., Wikstrand, C.J. and Bigner, D.D. (1991) Medulloblastoma: tumor biological and clinical perspectives. *Journal of Neuro-Oncology* **11**, 1–15.

Friedman, H.S., Archer, G.E., McLendon, R.E., Schuster, J.M., Colvin, O.M., Guaspari, A., Blum, R., Savina, P.A., Fuchs, H.E. and Bigner, D.D. (1994) Intrathecal melphalan therapy of human neoplastic meningitis in athymic nude rats. *Cancer Research* **54**, 4710–14.

Frith, C.H. and Chandra, M. (1990) Spontaneous primary astrocytoma in the spinal cord of a mouse and a rat. *Toxicologic Pathology* **18**, 427–9.

Fuchs, H.E., Archer, G.E., Colvin, O.M., Bigner, S.H., Schuster, J.M., Fuller, G.N., Muhlbaier, L.H., Schold, S.C. Jr, Friedman, H.S. and Bigner, D.D. (1990) Activity of intrathecal 4-hydroperoxycyclophosphamide in a nude rat model of human neoplastic meningitis. *Cancer Research* **50**, 1954–9.

Fulop, G.M. and Philips, R.A. (1990) The *scid* mutation in mice causes a general defect in DNA repair. *Nature* **347**, 479–82.

Fung, K.M. and Trojanowski, J.Q. (1995) Animal models of medulloblastomas and related primitive neuroectodermal tumors. A review. *Journal of Neuropathology and Experimental Neurology* **54**, 285–96.

Fung, K.M., Chikaraishi, D.M., Suri, C., Theuring, F., Messing, A., Albert, D.M., Lee, V.M. and Trojanowski, J.Q. (1994) Molecular phenotype of simian virus 40 large T antigen-induced primitive neuroectodermal tumors in four different lines of transgenic mice. *Laboratory Investigation* **70**, 114–24.

Gaillard, J.A., Caillaud, J.-M., Maunoury, R., Ohayon, H. and Trojan, J. (1984) Expression du neuro-ectoblaste dans les tératocarcinomes et les tératomes de la souris: étude microscopique, ultrastructurale et immuno-histochimique, et applications à l'embryologie, à la pathologie tumorale du système nerveux central. *Bulletin de l'Institute Pasteur* **82**, 335–85.

Garman, R.H., Snellings, W.M. and Maronpot, R.R. (1985) Brain tumors in F344 rats associated with chronic inhalation exposure to ethylene oxide. *Neurotoxicology* **6**, 117–37.

——(1986) Frequency, size and location of brain tumors in F-344 rats chronically exposed to ethylene oxide. *Food and Chemical Toxicology* **24**, 145–53.

——(1967) Murine neuropathology. In Cotchin, E. and Roe, F.J.C. (eds), *Pathology of laboratory rats and mice*. Oxford: Blackwell, 295–348.

Gateff, E. and Schneiderman, H.A. (1969) Neoplasms in mutant and cultured wild-type tissues of Drosophila. *National Cancer Institute Monographs* **31**, 365–97.

Gerlach, H., Wessel, H. and Musil, A. (1974) Comparative investigation of the neuro-oncogenic effect of MNU and ENU after postnatal administration. *Zentralblatt für Allgemeine Pathologie und Pathologische Anatomie* **118**, 278.

Goebel, H.H. and Cravioto, H. (1972) Ultrastructure of human and experimental ependymomas. *Journal of Neuropathology and Experimental Neurology* **31**, 54–71.

Goedegebuure, S.A. (1975) A case of neurofibromatosis in the dog. *Journal of Small Animal Practice* **16**, 329–35.

Goodman, D.G., Ward, J.M., Squire, R.A., Chu, K.C. and Linhart, M.S. (1979) Neoplastic and nonneoplastic lesions in aging F344 rats. *Toxicology and Applied Pharmacology* **48**, 237–48.

Gopinath, C. (1986) Spontaneous brain tumors in Sprague-Dawley rats. *Food and Chemical Toxicology* **24**, 113–20.

Goth, R. and Rajewsky, M.F. (1974a) Persistence of O^6-ethylguanine in rat-brain DNA: correlation with nervous system-specific carcinogenesis by ethylnitrosourea. *Proceedings of the National Academy of Sciences U.S.A.* **71**, 639–43.

——(1974b) Molecular and cellular mechanisms associated with pulse-carcinogenesis in the rat nervous system by ethylnitrosourea: ethylation of nucleic acids and elimination rates of ethylated bases from the DNA of different tissues. *Zeitschrift für Krebsforschung und Klinische Onkologie–Cancer Research and Clinical Oncology* **82**, 37–64.

Götz, W., Theuring, F., Schachenmayr, W. and Korf, H.-W. (1992) Midline brain tumors in MSV-SV 40-transgenic mice originate from the pineal organ. *Acta Neuropathologica* **83**, 308–14.

Green, M.R. (1989) When the products of oncogenes and anti-oncogenes meet. *Cell* **56**, 1–3.

Greene, H.S.N. (1951) The transplantation of tumors to the brains of heterologous species. *Cancer Research* **11**, 529–34.

——(1953) The transplantation of human brain tumors to the brains of laboratory animals. *Cancer Research* **13,** 422–6.

Greene, H.S.N. and Arnold, H. (1945) The homologous and heterologous transplantation of brain and brain tumors. *Journal of Neurosurgery* **2**, 315–31.

Greenlee, J.E., Narayan, O., Johnson, R.T. and Herndon, R.M. (1977) Induction of brain tumors in hamsters with BK virus, a human papovavirus. *Laboratory Investigation* **36**, 636–41.

Griep, A.E. and DeLuca, H.F. (1986) Decreased c-*myc* expression is an early event in retinoic acid-induced differentiation of F9 teratocarcinoma cells. *Proceedings of the National Academy of Sciences U.S.A.* **83**, 5539–43.

Grossi-Paoletti, E., Paoletti, P., Pezzotta, S., Schiffer, D. and Fabiani, A. (1972) Tumors of the nervous system induced by ethylnitrosourea administered either intracerebrally or subcutaneously to newborn rats. Morphological and biochemical characteristics. *Journal of Neurosurgery* **37**, 580–90.

Haag, M.M. and Soukup, S.W. (1984) Association of chromosome 4 abnormalities with ethylnitrosourea-induced neuro-oncogenesis in the rat. *Cancer Research* **44**, 784–90.

Haguenau, F., Rabotti, G.F., Lyon, G. and Moraillon, A. (1971) Gliomas induced by Rous sarcoma virus in the dog–an ultrastructural study. *Journal of the National Cancer Institute* **46**, 539–45.

Hammang, J.P., Behringer, R.R., Baetge, E.E., Palmiter, R.D., Brinster, R.L. and Messing, A. (1993) Oncogene expression in retinal horizontal cells of transgenic mice results in a cascade of neurodegeneration. *Neuron* **10**, 1197–209.

Hang, B., Chenna, A., Rao, S. and Singer, B. (1996) 1,N^6-ethenoadenine and 3,N^4-ethenocytosine are excised by separate human DNA glycosylases. *Carcinogenesis* **17**, 155–7.

Harshbarger, J.C. (1978) Role of the Registry of Tumors in Lower Animals in the study of environmental carcinogenesis in aquatic animals. *Annals of the New York Academy of Sciences* **298**, 280–9.

Harwood, S.E., Bigner, D.D., Wechsler, W. and Day, E.D. (1976) Sequential adsorption analysis of antibodies to neuroectodermal cells by an indirect quantitative method. *Journal of the National Cancer Institute* **56**, 1201–5.

Haseman, J.K., Arnold, J. and Eustis, S.L. (1990) Tumor incidences in Fischer rats: NTP historical data. In Boorman, G.A., Eustis, S.L., Elwell, M.R., Montgomery, C.A. Jr and MacKenzie, W.F. (eds), *Pathology of the Fischer rat. Reference and atlas*. San Diego: Academic Press, 555–64.

Hayes, C., Kelly, D., Murayama, S., Komiyama, A., Suzuki, K. and Popko, B. (1992) Expression of the *neu* oncogene under the transcriptional control of the myelin basic protein gene in transgenic mice: generation of transformed glial cells. *Journal of Neuroscience Research* **31**, 175–87.

Hayes, H.M. Jr, Priester, W.A. and Pendergrass, T.W. (1975) Occurrence of nervous-tissue tumors in cattle, horses, cats and dogs. *International Journal of Cancer* **15**, 39–47.

Haymaker, W., Rubinstein, L.J. and Miquel, J. (1972) Brain tumors in irradiated monkeys. *Acta Neuropathologica* **20**, 267–77.

He, X.M., Wikstrand, C.J., Friedman, H.S., Bigner, S.H., Pleasure, S., Trojanowski, J.Q. and Bigner, D.D. (1991) Differentiation characteristics of newly established medulloblastoma cell lines (D384 Med, D425 Med, and D458 Med) and their transplantable xenografts. *Laboratory Investigation* **64**, 833–43.

Helseth, A., Haug, E., Nesland, J.M., Siegal, G.P., Fodstad, Ø. and Bautch, V.L. (1995) Endocrine and metabolic characteristics of polyoma large T transgenic mice that develop ACTH-producing pituitary tumors. *Journal of Neurosurgery* **82**, 879–85.

Herman, M.M. and VandenBerg, S.R. (1978) Neoplastic neuroepithelial differentiation in an experimental transplantable teratoma. In Saunders, G.F. (ed.), *Cell differentiation and neoplasia*. New York: Raven Press, 93.

Herman, M.M., Adams, W.R. and Manuelidis, E.E. (1967) The ultrastructure of a human glioblastoma multiforme-derived tumor heterologously transplanted to guinea pig eye and brain. *Acta Neuropathologica* **8**, 321–30.

Herman, M.M., Sipe, J.C., Rubinstein, L.J., VandenBerg, S.R., Spence, A.M. and Vraa-Jensen, J. (1975) An experimental mouse testicular teratoma as a model for neuroepithelial neoplasia and differentiation. II. Electron microscopy. *American Journal of Pathology* **81**, 421–44.

Hewitt, H.B., Blake, E.R. and Walder, A.S. (1976) A critique of the evidence for active host defence against cancer, based on personal studies of 27 murine tumours of spontaneous origin. *British Journal of Cancer* **33**, 241–59.

Hill, A.B. (1965) The environment and disease: association or causation? *Proceedings of the Royal Society of Medicine* **58**, 295–300.

Hill, J. (1761) *Cautions against the immoderate use of snuff*. London: R. Baldwin and J. Jacobson.

Hinrichs, S.H., Nerenberg, M., Reynolds, R.K., Khoury, G. and Jay, G. (1987) A transgenic mouse model for human neurofibromatosis. *Science* **237**, 1340–3.

Hjärre (1938) Cited by Henchen, F. (1955) Tumors of the CNS and its coverings (membranes). In Lubarsch, O., Henke, F. and Rössle, R. (eds), *Handbook of special pathology, anatomy, and histology*, Vol. 13, Pt 3. Berlin: Springer-Verlag, 639.

Hochberg, F., Toniolo, P., Cole, P, and Salcman, M. (1990) Nonoccupational risk indicators of glioblastoma in adults. *Journal of Neuro-Oncology* **8**, 55–60.

Hoch-Ligeti, C. and Russell, D.S. (1950) Primary tumors of the brain and meninges in rats fed 2-acetylaminofluorene. *Acta Unio Internationalis Contra Cancrum* **7**, 126–9.

Hoffmann-Fezer, G., Kranz, B., Gall, C. and Thierfelder, S. (1992) Peritoneal sanctuary for human lymphopoiesis in SCID mice injected with human peripheral blood lymphocytes from Epstein-Barr virus-negative donors. *European Journal of Immunology* **22**, 3161–6.

Hollstein, M., Marion, M.-J., Lehman, T., Welsh, J., Harris, C.C., Martel-Planche, G., Kusters, I. and Montesano, R. (1994) *p53* Mutations at A:T base pairs in angiosarcomas of vinyl chloride-exposed factory workers. *Carcinogenesis* **15**, 1–3.

Hopewell, J.W. (1975) The subependymal plate and the genesis of gliomas. *Journal of Pathology* **117**, 101–3.

Hopewell, J.W. and Wright, E.A. (1969) The importance of implantation site in cerebral carcinogenesis in rats. *Cancer Research* **29**, 1927–31.

Horowitz, M.E., Parham, D.M., Douglass, E.C., Kun, L.E., Houghton, J.A. and Houghton, P.J. (1987) Development and characterization of human ependymoma xenograft HxBr5. *Cancer Research* **47**, 499–504.

Horten, B.C., Basler, G.A. and Shapiro, W.R. (1981) Xenograft of human malignant glial tumors into brains of nude mice. A histopathological study. *Journal of Neuropathology and Experimental Neurology* **40**, 493–511.

Hosobuchi, Y. and Ishii, S. (1967) A new approach to hydrocarbon-induced brain tumors. *Archives of Neurology* **16**, 664–75.

Houghton, J.A. and Taylor, D.M. (1978) Maintenance of biological and biochemical characteristics of human colorectal tumours during serial passage in immune-deprived mice. *British Journal of Cancer* **37**, 199–212.

Howard, E.B. and Nielsen, S.W. (1965) Neoplasia of the boxer dog. *American Journal of Veterinary Research* **26**, 1121–31.

Howley, P.M., Levine, A.J., Li, F.P., Livingston, D.M. and Rabson, A.S. (1991) Lack of SV40 DNA in tumors from scientists working with SV40 virus. *New England Journal of Medicine* **324**, 494.

Huang, P., Allam, A., Taghian, A., Freeman, J., Duffy, M. and Suit, H.D. (1995) Growth and metastatic behavior of five human glioblastomas compared with nine other histological types of human tumor xenografts in SCID mice. *Journal of Neurosurgery* **83**, 308–15.

Huebner, R.J., Rowe, W.P. and Lane, W.T. (1962) Oncogenic effects in hamsters of human adenovirus types 12 and 18. *Proceedings of the National Academy of Sciences U.S.A.* **48**, 2051–8.

Ikuta, F. and Zimmerman, H.M. (1965) The viral particles in the reactive cells of the brain induced by chemical carcinogens. *International Journal of Neurology* **5**, 10–28.

Innes, J.R.M. and Borner, G. (1961) Tumors of the central nervous system of rats: with report of two tumors of the spinal cord and comments on posterior paralysis. *Journal of the National Cancer Institute* **26**, 719–35.

Ivankovic, S. and Druckrey, H. (1968) Transplacental induction of malignant tumors of the nervous system. I. Ethyl-nitroso-urea (ENU) in BD IX rats. *Zeitschrift für Krebsforschung* **71**, 320–60.

Jacks, T., Fazeli, A., Schmitt, E.M., Bronson, R.T., Goodell, M.A. and Weinberg, R.A. (1992) Effects of an *Rb* mutation in the mouse. *Nature* **359**, 295–300.

Jacks, T., Remington, L., Williams, B.O., Schmitt, E.M., Halachmi, S., Bronson, R.T. and Weinberg, R.A. (1994) Tumor spectrum analysis in *p53*-mutant mice. *Current Biology* **4**, 1–7.

Jacobsen, P.F., Jenkyn, D.J. and Papadimitriou, J.N. (1985) Establishment of a human medulloblastoma cell line and its heterotransplantation into nude mice. *Journal of Neuropathology and Experimental Neurology* **44**, 472–85.

Jacobsen, P.F., Parker, T.J. and Papadimitriou, J.M. (1987) Ependymal differentiation of a glioblastoma multiforme after heterotransplantation into nude mice. *Journal of the National Cancer Institute* **79**, 771–9.

Jakobovits, A., Schwab, M., Bishop, J.M. and Martin, G.R. (1985) Expression of N-*myc* in teratocarcinoma stem cells and mouse embryos. *Nature* **318,** 188–91.

Jakupevic, M., Lackovic, Z., Damjanov, I. and Bulat, M. (1974) Biogenic amines in a retransplantable neurogenic teratocarcinoma. *Experientia* **30**, 652–3.

Jänisch, W. (1990) Tumors of the central nervous system. In Turusov, V. and Mohr, U. (eds), *Pathology of tumours of laboratory animals. Vol. 1, Tumours of the rat.* Second edition. Lyon: International Agency for Research on Cancer Scientific Publications, 677–98.

Jänisch, W., Horn, K.H., Scholtze, P. and Schreiber, D. (1968) Experimental induction of brain tumors by intracerebral inoculation of Rous sarcoma virus in newborn Rhesus monkeys. *Experimentelle Pathologie* **2**, 226–35.

Jänisch, W., Haas, J.F., Schreiber, D. and Gerlach, H. (1984) Primary central nervous system tumors in stillborns and infants: epidemiological considerations. *Journal of Neuro-Oncology* **2**, 113–16.

Johnson, K.A., Gorzinski, S.J., Bodner, K.M., Campbell, R.A., Wolf, C.H., Friedman, M.A. and Mast, R.W. (1986) Chronic toxicity and oncogenicity study on acrylamide incorporated in the drinking water of Fischer 344 rats. *Toxicology and Applied Pharmacology* **85**, 154–68.

Johnson, L. Jr, Wolfe, L.G., Whisler, W.W., Norton, T., Thakkar, B. and Deinhardt, F. (1975) Induction of gliomas in marmosets with simian sarcoma virus, type 1 (SSV-1). (Abstract) *Proceedings of the American Association for Cancer Research* **16**, 119.

Jones, T.R., Bigner, S.H., Schold, S.C. Jr, Eng, L.F. and Bigner, D.D. (1981) Anaplastic human gliomas grown in athymic mice. Morphology and glial fibrillary acidic protein expression. *American Journal of Pathology* **105**, 316–27.

Jones, T.R., Ruoslahti, E., Schold, S.C. and Bigner, D.D. (1982) Fibronectin and glial fibrillary acidic protein expression in normal human brain and anaplastic human gliomas. *Cancer Research* **42**, 168–77.

Kahle, W. (1970) Embryogenetic aspects of diaplacental induction of gliomata. *Proceedings of the VI International Congress of Neuropathology*. Paris: Masson et Cie, 556–7.

Kaspareit-Rittinghausen, J. and Deerberg, F. (1989) Spontaneous tumours of the spinal cord in laboratory rats. *Journal of Comparative Pathology* **100**, 209–15.

Kawaminami, A., Yoshida, M., Ide, Y., Tawaratani, T., Nakazawa, M., Uchimoto, H. and Sumi, N. (1994) Forelimb paralysis due to spontaneously developed astrocytoma in the spinal cord of a Sprague Dawley rat. *Laboratory Animal Science* **44**, 175–6.

Kaye, A.H., Morstyn, G., Gardner, I. and Pyke, K. (1986) Development of a xenograft glioma model in mouse brain. *Cancer Research* **46**, 1367–73.

Keller, E.T. and Madewell, B.R. (1992) Locations and types of neoplasms in immature dogs: 69 cases (1964–1989). *Journal of the American Veterinary Medical Association* **200**, 1530–2.

Kent, S.P. and Pickering, J.E. (1958) Neoplasms in monkeys (*Macaca mulatta*): spontaneous and radiation induced. *Cancer* **11**, 138–47.

Kimura, M., Sato, M., Akatsuka, A., Nozawa-Kimura, S., Takahashi, R., Yokoyama, M., Nomura, T. and Katsuki, M. (1989) Restoration of myelin formation by a single type of myelin basic protein in transgenic shiverer mice. *Proceedings of the National Academy of Sciences U.S.A.* **86**, 5661–5.

Kirkland, W.L., Sorrentino, J.M. and Sirbasku, D.A. (1976) Control of cell growth. III. Direct mitogenic effect of thyroid hormones on an estrogen-dependent rat pituitary tumor cell line. *Journal of the National Cancer Institute* **56**, 1159–64.

Kleihues, P. and Rajewsky, M.F. (1984) Chemical neuro-oncogenesis: role of structural DNA modifications, DNA repair and neural target cell population. *Progress in Experimental Tumor Research* **27**, 1–16.

Kleihues, P., Patzschke, K. and Doerjer, G. (1982) DNA modification and repair in the experimental induction of nervous system tumors by chemical carcinogens. *Annals of the New York Academy of Sciences* **381**, 290–303.

Kleihues, P., Doerjer, G., Swenberg, J.A., Hauenstein, E., Bücheler, J. and Cooper, H.K. (1979) DNA repair as regulatory factor in the organotropy of alkylating carcinogens. *Archives of Toxicology* (Suppl.) **2**, 253–61.

Kleihues, P., Wiestler, O.D., Ohgaki, H. and Aguzzi, A. (1997) Animal models of tumors of the nervous system. In Berger, M. and Wilson, C. (eds), *Gliomas*. Cambridge: W.B. Saunders, in press.

Kobayashi, M., Mukai, N., Solish, S.P. and Pomeroy, M.E. (1982) A highly predictable animal model of retinoblastoma. *Acta Neuropathologica* **57**, 203–8.

Koestner, A. (1986) The brain-tumour issue in long-term toxicity studies in rats. *Food and Chemical Toxicology* **24**, 139–43.

Koestner, A., Swenberg, J.A. and Wechsler, W. (1971) Transplacental production with ethylnitrosourea of neoplasms of the nervous system in Sprague-Dawley rats. *American Journal of Pathology* **63**, 37–56.

——(1972) Experimental tumors of the nervous system induced by resorptive *N*-nitrosourea compounds. *Progress in Experimental Tumor Research* **17**, 9–30.

Koike, K., Jay, G., Hartley, J.W., Schrenzel, M.D., Higgins, R.J. and Hinrichs, S.H. (1990) Activation of retrovirus in transgenic mice: association with development of olfactory neuroblastoma. *Journal of Virology* **64**, 3988–91.

Korf, H.-W., Götz, W., Herken, R., Theuring, F., Gruss, P. and Schachenmayr, W. (1990) S-antigen and rod-opsin immunoreactions in midline brain neoplasms of transgenic mice: similarities to pineal cell tumors and certain medulloblastomas in man. *Journal of Neuropathology and Experimental Neurology* **49**, 424–37.

Krinke, G., Naylor, D.C., Schmid, S., Fröhlich, E. and Schnider, K. (1985) The incidence of naturally-occurring primary brain tumors in the laboratory rat. *Journal of Comparative Pathology* **95**, 175–92.

Krupp, J.H. (1976) Nine-year-mortality experience in proton exposed *Macaca mulatta*. *Radiation Research* **67**, 244–51.

Kruse, C.A., Molleston, M.C., Parks, E.P., Schiltz, P.M., Kleinschmidt-DeMasters, B.K. and Hickey, W.F. (1994) A rat glioma model, CNS-1, with invasive characteristics similar to those of human gliomas: a comparison to 9L gliosarcoma. *Journal of Neuro-Oncology* **22**, 191–200.

Kuijten, R.R. and Bunin, G.R. (1993) Risk factors for childhood brain tumors. *Cancer Epidemiology, Biomarkers and Prevention* **2**, 277–88.

Kurpad, S.N., Friedman, H.S., Archer, G.E., McLendon, R.E., Petros, W.M., Fuchs, H.E., Guaspari, A. and Bigner, D.D. (1995) Intraarterial administration of melphalan for treatment of intracranial human glioma xenografts in athymic rats. *Cancer Research* **55**, 3803–9.

Kuschner, M. and Laskin, S. (1975) Inhalation carcinogenicity of alpha halo ethers. III. Lifetime and limited period inhalation studies with bis(chloromethyl) ether at 0.1 ppm. *Archives of Environmental Health* **30**, 73–7.

Lantos, P.L. (1977) The distribution and role of microtubules and filaments in the neoplastic astrocytes of experimental gliomas. *Neuropathology and Applied Neurobiology* **3**, 281–96.

Lantos, P.L. and Pilkington, G.J. (1979) The development of experimental brain tumors. A sequential light and electron microscope study of the subependymal plate. I. Early lesions (abnormal cell clusters). *Acta Neuropathologica* **45**, 167–75.

Lantos, P.L., VandenBerg, S. and Kleihues, P. (1997) Tumours of the nervous system. In Graham, D.I. and Lantos, P.L. (eds), *Greenfield's neuropathology*, Vol. 2. Sixth edition. London: Arnold, pp. 583–881.

Lapin, B.A. and Yakovleva, L.A. (1963) *Comparative pathology in monkeys*. Springfield: C. Thomas.

Largent, B.L., Sosnowski, R.G. and Reed, R.R. (1993) Directed expression of an oncogene to the olfactory neuronal lineage in transgenic mice. *Journal of Neuroscience* **13**, 300–12.

Law, L.W., Dunn, T.B., Boyle, P.J. and Miller, J.H. (1949) Observations on the effect of a folic-acid antagonist on transplantable lymphoid leukemias in mice. *Journal of the National Cancer Institute* **10**, 179–92.

Lee, C.C., Bhandari, J.C., Winston, J.M., House, W.B., Peters, P.J., Dixon, R.L. and Woods, J.S. (1977) Inhalation toxicity of vinyl chloride and vinylidene chloride. *Environmental Health Perspectives* **21**, 25–32.

Lee, C.C., Bhandari, J.C., Winston, J.M., House, W.B., Dixon, R.L. and Woods, J.S. (1978) Carcinogenicity of vinyl chloride and vinylidene chloride. *Journal of Toxicology and Environmental Health* **4**, 15–30.

Lee, E.Y., Chang, C.Y., Hu, N., Wang, Y.C., Lai, C.C., Herrup, K., Lee, W.H. and Bradley, A. (1992) Mice deficient for Rb are nonviable and show defects in neurogenesis and haematopoiesis. *Nature* **359**, 288–94.

Lee, Y.S., Wikstrand, C.J. and Bigner, D.D. (1986) Glioma-associated antigens defined by monoclonal antibodies against an avian sarcoma virus-induced rat astrocytoma. *Journal of Neuroimmunology* **13**, 183–202.

Lee, Y.S., Bigner, S.H., Eng, L.F., Molnar, P., Kuruvilla, A., Groothuis, D.R. and Bigner, D.D. (1986) A glial fibrillary acidic protein-expressing and tumorigenic cell line derived from an avian sarcoma virus-induced rat astrocytoma. *Journal of Neuropathology and Experimental Neurology* **45**, 704–20.

Liao, C.L., Eng, L.F., Herman, M.M. and Bensch, K.G. (1978) Glial fibrillary acidic protein-solubility characteristics, relation to cell growth phases and cellular localization in the rat C-6 glioma cells: an immunoradiometric and immunohistologic study. *Journal of Neurochemistry* **30**, 1181–6.

Lijinsky, W., Garcia, H., Keefer, L., Loo, J. and Ross, A.E. (1972) Carcinogenesis and alkylation of rat liver nucleic acids by nitrosomethylurea and nitrosoethylurea administered by intraportal injection. *Cancer Research* **32**, 893–7.

London, W.T., Houff, S.A., Madden, D.L., Fuccillo, D.A., Gravell, M., Wallen, W.C., Palmer, A.E., Sever, J.L., Padgett, B.L., Walker, D.L., ZuRhein, G.M. and Ohashi, T. (1978) Brain tumors in owl monkeys inoculated with a human polyomavirus (JC virus). *Science* **201**, 1246–9.

Louis, D.N. (1994) The *p53* gene and protein in human brain tumors. *Journal of Neuropathology and Experimental Neurology* **53**, 11–21.

Lubetzki, C., Mercier, B., Duyckaerts, C., Lebiez, E. and Lyon-Caen, O. (1991) Glioblastome après radiothérapie d'un méningiome. *Revue Neurologique* **147**, 151–5.

Luginbühl, H. (1961) Studies on meningiomas in cats. *American Journal of Veterinary Research* **22**, 1030–40.

——(1962) Tumors of the CNS in animals. *Acta Neuropathologica* **1**, 9–18.

——(1963) Comparative aspects of tumors of the nervous system. *Annals of the New York Academy of Sciences* **108**, 702–21.

Luginbühl, H., Fankhauser, R. and McGrath, J.T. (1968) Spontaneous neoplasms of the nervous system in animals. *Progress in Neurological Surgery* **2**, 85–164.

Lynch, D.W., Lewis, T.R., Moorman, W.J., Burg, J.R., Groth, D.H., Khan, A., Ackerman, L.J and Cockrell, B.Y. (1984) Carcinogenic and toxicologic effects of inhaled ethylene oxide and propylene oxide in F344 rats. *Toxicology and Applied Pharmacology* **76**, 69–84.

Mack, E.E. and Wilson, C.B. (1993) Meningiomas induced by high-dose cranial irradiation. *Journal of Neurosurgery* **79**, 28–31.

MacKenzie, W.F. and Boorman, G.A. (1990) Pituitary gland. In Boorman, G.A., Eustis, S.L., Elwell, M.R., Montgomery, C.A. Jr and MacKenzie, W.F. (eds), *Pathology of the Fischer rat. Reference and atlas*. San Diego: Academic Press, 485–500.

Maekawa, A., Onodera, H., Tanigawa, H., Furuta, K., Takahashi, M., Kurokawa, Y., Kokubo, T., Ogiu, T., Uchida, O., Kobayashi, K. and Hayashi, Y. (1984) Spontaneous tumors of the nervous system and associated organs and/or tissues in rats. *Gann* **75**, 784–91.

Major, E.O., Vacante, D.A., Traub, R.G., London, W.T. and Sever, J.L. (1987) Owl monkey astrocytoma cells in culture spontaneously produce infectious JC virus which demonstrates altered biological properties. *Journal of Virology* **61**, 1435–41.

Maltoni, C. (1976) Occupational carcinogenesis. Predictive value of carcinogenesis bioassays. *Annals of the New York Academy of Sciences* **271**, 431–43.

Maltoni, C. and Cotti, G. (1988) Carcinogenicity of vinyl chloride in Sprague-Dawley rats after prenatal and postnatal exposure. *Annals of the New York Academy of Sciences* **534**, 145–59.

Maltoni, C. and Lefemine, G. (1975) Carcinogenicity bioassays of vinyl chloride: current results. *Annals of the New York Academy of Sciences* **246**, 195–218.

Mancini, L.O., Yates, V.J., Jasty, V. and Anderson, J. (1969) Ependymomas induced in hamsters inoculated with an avian adenovirus (CELO). *Nature* **222**, 190–1.

Mandybur, T.I. and Alvira, M.M. (1982) Ultrastructural findings in so-called ependymal rat tumors induced by transplacental administration of ethylnitrosourea (ENU). *Acta Neuropathologica* **57**, 51–8.

Mandybur, T.I., Sawaya, R. and Ormsby, I. (1986) The morphology and biologic behavior of human glioblastoma growing in nude mice. *Cancer* **58**, 1061–9.

Manuelidis, E.E. (1961) Heterologous transplantation of two tissue culture lines of glioblastoma multiforme (TC 178 and TC 224). *Proceedings of the Society for Experimental Biology and Medicine* **107**, 636–9.

——(1972) Heterologous transplantation of cerebral and cerebellar astrocytomas. *Acta Neuropathologica* **20**, 160–70.

Marcus, D.M., Carpenter, J.L., O'Brien, J.M., Kivela, T., Brauner, E., Tarkkanen, A., Virtanen, I. and Albert, D.M. (1991) Primitive neuroectodermal tumor of the midbrain in a murine model of retinoblastoma. *Investigative Ophthalmology and Visual Science* **32**, 293–301.

Margison, G.P. and Kleihues, P. (1975) Chemical carcinogenesis in the nervous system. Preferential accumulation of O^6-methylguanine in rat brain deoxyribonucleic acid during repetitive administration of *N*-methyl-*N*-nitrosourea. *Biochemical Journal* **148**, 521–5.

Marion, M.-J., Froment, O. and Trépo, C. (1991) Activation of Ki-*ras* gene by point mutation in human liver angiosarcoma associated with vinyl chloride exposure. *Molecular Carcinogenesis* **4**, 450–4.

Markovits, P., Maunoury, R., Tripier, M.F., Coulomb, B., Levy, S., Papadopoulo, D., Vedrenne, C. and Benda, P. (1979) Normal and benzo(a)pyrene-transformed fetal mouse brain cells. I. Tumorigenicity and immunochemical detection of glial fibrillary acidic protein. *Acta Neuropathologica* **47**, 197–203.

Marks, J.R., Lin, J., Hinds, P., Miller, D. and Levine, A.J. (1989) Cellular gene expression in papillomas of the choroid plexus from transgenic mice that express the simian virus 40 large T antigen. *Journal of Virology* **63**, 790–7.

Matsuda, M., Yasui, K., Nagashima, K. and Mori, W. (1987) Origin of the medulloblastoma experimentally induced by human polyomavirus JC. *Journal of the National Cancer Institute* **79**, 585–91.

McAllister, R.M., Isaacs, H., Rongey, R., Peer, M., Au, W., Soukup, S.W. and Gardner, M.B. (1977) Establishment of a human medulloblastoma cell line. *International Journal of Cancer* **20**, 206–12.

McDonald, L.W., Lippert, W., Brownson, R.H. and McDougal, H.D. (1973) Induction of neuroglial tumors by implanted ^{60}cobalt radionuclides. In Sanders, C.L., Busch, R.H., Ballou, J.E. and Mahlum, D.D. (eds), *Proceedings of the XII Annual Hanford Biology Symposium*. AEC Office of Technical Information, No. 720505. Richland, Wash.: Battelle-Northwest, 391–405.

McGrath, J.T. (1960) *Neurologic examination of the dog*. Second edition. Philadelphia: Lea and Febiger.

——(1962a) Intracranial pathology in the dog. *Acta Neuropathologica* (Suppl.) **1**, 3–4.

——(1962b) Meningiomas in animals. *Journal of Neuropathology and Experimental Neurology* **21**, 327–8.

McKeel, D.W. Jr and Hajek, S.A. (1981) Characterization of long term hormonal cell cultures from the MtT/W15 prolactin- and growth hormone-secreting rat pituitary tumor. *Endocrinology* **108**, 1571–86.

McLendon, R.E., Fung, K.-M., Bentley, R.C., Rasheed, B.K.A., Trojanowski, J.Q., Bigner, S.H., Bigner, D.D. and Friedman, H.S. (1996) Production and characterization of two ependymoma xenografts. *Journal of Neuropathology and Experimental Neurology* **55**, 540–8.

McNeilage, L.J., Heslop, B.F. and Berridge, M.V. (1979) Nude (athymic) rats maintained in conventional conditions: a progress report. *Proceedings of the University of Otago Medical School* **57**, 47–8.

Mellon, P.L., Windle, J.J., Goldsmith, P.C., Padula, C.A., Roberts, J.L. and Weiner, R.I. (1990) Immortalization of hypothalamic GnRH neurons by genetically targeted tumorigenesis. *Neuron* **5**, 1–10.

Mennel, H.D. and Simon, H. (1985) Morphology of early stages of ENU-induced brain tumors in rats. *Experimental Pathology* **28**, 207–14.

Merkow, L.P., Slifkin, M., Pardo, M. and Rapoza, N.P. (1970) Pathogenesis of oncogenic simian adenoviruses.

VIII. The histopathology and ultrastructure of simian adenovirus 7-induced intracranial neoplasms. *Experimental and Molecular Pathology* **12**, 264–74.

Messing, A., Pinkert, C.A., Palmiter, R.D. and Brinster, R.L. (1988) Developmental study of SV40 large T antigen expression in transgenic mice with choroid plexus neoplasia. *Oncogene Research* **3**, 87–97.

Messing, A., Behringer, R.R., Wrabetz, L., Hammang, J.P., Lemke, G., Palmiter, R.D. and Brinster, R.L. (1994) Hypomyelinating peripheral neuropathies and schwannomas in transgenic mice expressing SV40 T-antigen. *Journal of Neuroscience* **14**, 3533–9.

Miller, J.A. (1994) Recent studies on the metabolic activation of chemical carcinogens. *Cancer Research* (Suppl.) **54**, 1879s–81s.

Mintz, B. and Fleischman, R.A. (1981) Teratocarcinomas and other neoplasms as developmental defects in gene expression. *Advances in Cancer Research* **34**, 211–78.

Mirvish, S.S. and Chu, C. (1973) Chemical determination of methylnitrosourea and ethylnitrosourea in stomach contents of rats, after intubation of alkylureas plus sodium nitrite. *Journal of the National Cancer Institute* **50**, 745–50.

Mitro, K.L., Scheller, N.A., Ranasinghe, A. and Swenberg, J.A. (1995) Quantitation of endogenous N^2,3-ethenoguanine in human and rat liver DNA using high resolution mass spectrometry. (Abstract) *Proceedings of the American Association for Cancer Research* **36**, 142.

Mitsumori, K. and Boorman, G.A. (1990) Spinal cord and peripheral nerves. In Boorman, G.A., Eustis, S.L., Elwell, M.R., Montgomery, C.A. Jr and MacKenzie, W.F. (eds), *Pathology of the Fischer rat. Reference and atlas.* San Diego: Academic Press, 179–91.

Mizobuchi, K., Motoi, M. and Ogawa, K. (1984) Undifferentiated neuroectodermal tumors induced by human adenovirus type 31 in Syrian hamsters. *Acta Pathologica Japonica* **34**, 1313–26.

Mombaerts, P., Iacomini, J., Johnson, R.S., Herrup, K., Tonegawa, S. and Papaioannou, V.E. (1992) RAG-1-deficient mice have no mature B and T lymphocytes. *Cell* **68**, 869–77.

Moore, A.E. (1951) Inhibition of growth of five transplantable mouse tumors by the virus of Russian far east encephalitis. *Cancer* **4**, 375–82.

Moore, A.S., Madewell, B.R. and Lund, J.K. (1989) Immunohistochemical evaluation of intermediate filament expression in canine and feline neoplasms. *American Journal of Veterinary Research* **50**, 88–92.

Morgan, K.T., Frith, C.H., Swenberg, J.A., McGrath, J.T., Zulch, K.J. and Crowder, D.M. (1984) A morphologic classification of brain tumors found in several strains of mice. *Journal of the National Cancer Institute* **72**, 151–60.

Mucke, L., Oldstone, M.B.A., Morris, J.C. and Nerenberg, M.I. (1991) Rapid activation of astrocyte-specific expression of GFAP-*lacZ* transgene by focal injury. *New Biologist* **3**, 465–74.

Mueller, B.M. and Reisfeld, R.A. (1991) Potential of the SCID mouse as a host for human tumors. *Cancer and Metastasis Reviews* **10**, 193–200.

Mukai, M., Kobayashi, S. and Oguri, M. (1974) Ultrastructural studies of human adenovirus-produced retinoblastoma-like neoplasms in Sprague-Dawley rats. *Investigative Ophthalmology* **13**, 593–601.

Mukai, N. (1976) Human adenovirus-induced embryonic neuronal tumor phenotype in rodents. *Progress in Neuropathology* **3**, 89–128.

Mukai, N. and Kobayashi, S. (1973a) Human adenovirus-induced medulloepitheliomatous neoplasms in Sprague-Dawley rats. *American Journal of Pathology* **73**, 671–90.

——(1973b) Primary brain and spinal cord tumors induced by human adenovirus type 12 in hamsters. *Journal of Neuropathology and Experimental Neurology* **32**, 523–41.

Mukai, N. and Murao, T. (1975) Retinal tumor induction by ocular inoculation of human adenovirus in 3-day-old rats. *Journal of Neuropathology and Experimental Neurology* **34**, 28–35.

Müller, D. (1964) *Contribution to tumor statistics in the dog.* Thesis, University of Hannover, Germany.

Mulligan, R.M., Neubuerger, K.T., Lucas, Jr, J.T. and Lewis, W.B. (1946) Intracranial neoplasms produced in dogs by methylcholanthrene. *Experimental Medicine and Surgery* **4**, 7–19.

Murphy, D., Bishop, A., Rindi, G., Murphy, M.N., Stamp, G.W.H., Hanson, J., Polak, J.M. and Hogan, B. (1987) Mice transgenic for vasopression-SV40 hybrid oncogene develop tumors of the endocrine pancreas and the anterior pituitary. A possible model for human multiple endocrine neoplasia type 1. *American Journal of Pathology* **129**, 552–66.

Nagashima, K., Yasui, K., Kimura, J., Washizu, M., Yamaguchi, K. and Mori, W. (1984) Induction of brain tumors by a newly isolated JC virus (Tokyo-1 strain). *American Journal of Pathology* **116**, 455–63.

Naidu, A.K., Wiranowska, M., Kori, S.H., Roetzheim, K.C. and Kulkarni, A.P. (1993) Inhibition of cell proliferation and glutathione *S*-transferase by ascorbyl esters and interferon in mouse glioma. *Journal of Neuro-Oncology* **16**, 1–10.

Nair, J., Barbin, A., Guichard, Y. and Bartsch, H. (1995) 1,N^6-ethenodeoxyadenosine and 3,N^4-ethenodeoxycytidine in liver DNA from humans and untreated rodents detected by immunoaffinity/^{32}P-postlabeling. *Carcinogenesis* **16**, 613–17.

Naito, M., Aoyama, H., Naito, Y., Fujioka, Y. and Ito, A. (1986) Morphological and immunohistochemical evidence for the presence of subcortical target cells of *N*-ethyl-*N*-nitrosourea-induced cerebellar tumors in rats. *Cancer Research* **46**, 5836–41.

Nakajima, T. and Mukai, N. (1979) Cell origin of human adenovirus type 12-induced subcutaneous tumor in Syrian hamsters. *Acta Neuropathologica* **45**, 187–94.

Nakamura, T., Ushijima, T., Ishizaka, Y., Nagao, M., Nemoto, T., Hara, M. and Ishikawa, T. (1994) neu Proto-oncogene mutation is specific for the neurofibromas in a *N*-nitroso-*N*-ethylurea-induced hamster neurofibromatosis model but not for hamster melanomas and human Schwann cell tumors. *Cancer Research* **54**, 976–80.

Nakazato, Y., Yamaguchi, H., Takahashi, K. and Ishida, Y. (1981) The localization of glial fibrillary acidic protein in brain tumors induced in hamsters with avian sarcoma virus. *Acta Neuropathologica* **55**, 293–5.

Napalkov, N.P. and Alexandrov, V.A. (1974) Neurotropic effect of 7,12-dimethylbenz(a)anthracene in transplacental carcinogenesis. *Journal of the National Cancer Institute* **52**, 1365–6.

Nederman, T., Norling, B., Glimelius, B., Carlsson, J. and Brunk, U. (1984) Demonstration of an extracellular matrix in multicellular tumor spheroids. *Cancer Research* **44**, 3090–7.

Netsky, M.G., Shapiro, J., Hoffman, M., Corsentino, B., Fried, J.R. and Zimmerman, H.M. (1956) The effect of single doses of Roentgen radiation on experimentally induced gliomas: with a critical review of the effects of Roentgen radiation on gliomas in man. *American Journal of Roentgenology, Radium Therapy and Nuclear Medicine* **76**, 351–66.

Newberne, J.W. and Robinson, V.B. (1960) Spontaneous tumors in primates—a report of two cases with notes on the apparent low incidence of neoplasms in subhuman primates. *American Journal of Veterinary Research* **21**, 150–5.

Ngowyang, M.G. (1930) A tumor in Ammon's horn in the white mouse. *Revue Neurologique* **2**, 584–8.

NTP (National Toxicology Program) (1990) *Toxicology and carcinogenesis studies of glycidol (CAS No. 556–52–5) in F344/N rats and B6C3F$_1$ mice (gavage studies).* NTP Technical Report Series 374, NIH Publication No. 90–2829. Research Triangle Park, N.C.: NTP, U.S. Department of Health and Human Services.

Nunziata, A. and Storino, A.A. (1982) Spontaneous neoplastic pathology in control rats—a review. *Veterinary and Human Toxicology* **24**, 243–7.

Oakes, W.J., Friedman, H.S., Bigner, S.H., Bullock, N.H. and Bigner, D.D. (1990) Successful laboratory growth and analysis of CUSA-obtained medulloblastoma samples. *Journal of Neurosurgery* **72**, 821–3.

Oda, H., Zhang, S., Tsurutani, N., Shimizu, S., Nakatsuru, Y., Aizawa, S. and Ishikawa, T. (1997) Loss of *p53* is an early event in induction of brain tumors in mice by transplacental carcinogen exposure. *Cancer Research* **57**, 646–50.

Ogawa, K. (1979) Adenovirus 12-induced tumors—especially on the approach to experimental brain tumors. *Transactions of the Pathology Society of Japan* **68**, 35.

——(1989) Embryonal neuroepithelial tumors induced by human adenovirus type 12 in rodents. 1. Tumor induction in the peripheral nervous system. *Acta Neuropathologica* **77**, 244–53.

Ohgaki, H., Schäuble, B., zur Hausen, A., von Ammon, K. and Kleihues, P. (1995) Genetic alterations associated with the evolution and progression of astrocytic brain tumours. *Virchows Archiv* **427**, 113–18.

Ohsumi, S., Motoi, M. and Ogawa, K. (1986) Induction of undifferentiated tumors by JC virus in the cerebrum of rats. *Acta Pathologica Japonica* **36**, 815–25.

Orenberg, E.K., VandenBerg, S.R., Barchas, J.D. and Herman, M.M. (1976) Neurochemical studies in a mouse teratoma with neuroepithelial differentiation. Presence of cyclic AMP, serotonin and enzymes of the serotonergic, adrenergic and cholinergic systems. *Brain Research* **101**, 273–81.

Orme, S.K., Wells, S.A., Rabson, A.S. and Wurtman, R.J. (1968) *In vitro* neoplastic transformation of hamster pineal cells by three oncogenic DNA viruses. *Cancer* **21**, 477–82.

Oyasu, R., Battifora, H.A., Clasen, R.A., McDonald, J.H. and Hass, G.M. (1970) Induction of cerebral gliomas in rats with dietary lead subacetate and 2-acetylaminofluorene. *Cancer Research* **30**, 1248–61.

Padgett, B.L., Walker, D.L., ZuRhein, G.M. and Varakis, J.N. (1977) Differential neurooncogenicity of strains of JC virus, a human polyoma virus, in newborn Syrian hamsters. *Cancer Research* **37**, 718–20.

Palmiter, R.D., Chen, H.Y., Messing, A. and Brinster, R.L. (1985) SV40 enhancer and large-T antigen are instrumental in development of choroid plexus tumors in transgenic mice. *Nature* **316**, 457–60.

Pantelouris, E.M. (1968) Absence of thymus in a mouse mutant. *Nature* **217**, 370–1.

Parker, K.K., Norenberg, M.D. and Vernadakis, A. (1980) 'Transdifferentiation' of C6 glial cells in culture. *Science* **208**, 179–81.

Pastan, I.H., Archer, G.E., McLendon, R.E., Friedman, H.S., Fuchs, H.E., Wang, Q.-C., Pai, L.H., Herndon, J. and Bigner, D.D. (1995) Intrathecal administration of single-chain immunotoxin, LMB-7 [B3(Fv)-PE38], produces cures of carcinomatous meningitis in a rat model. *Proceedings of the National Academy of Sciences U.S.A.* **92**, 2765–9.

Pegg, A.E. (1990) Mammalian O^6-alkylguanine-DNA-alkyltransferase: regulation and importance in response to alkylating carcinogenic and therapeutic agents. *Cancer Research* **50**, 6119–29.

Perantoni, A.O., Rice, J.M., Reed, C.D., Watatani, M. and Wenk, M.L. (1987) Activated *neu* oncogene sequences in primary tumors of the peripheral nervous system induced in rats by transplacental exposure to ethylnitrosourea. *Proceedings of the National Academy of Sciences U.S.A.* **84**, 6317–21.

Perese, D.M. and Moore, G.E. (1960) Methods of induction and histogenesis of experimental brain tumors. *Journal of Neurosurgery* **17**, 677–97.

Perraud, F., Yoshimura, K., Louis, B., Dalemans, W., Ali-Hadji, D., Schultz, H., Claudepierre, M.-C., Chartier, C., Danel, C., Bellocq, J.-P., Crystal, R.G., Lecocq, J.-P. and Pavirani, A. (1992) The promoter of the human cystic fibrosis transmembrane conductance regulator gene directing SV40 T antigen expression induces malignant proliferation of ependymal cells in transgenic mice. *Oncogene* **7**, 993–7.

Pilkington, G.J. and Lantos, P.L. (1979) The development of experimental brain tumors. A sequential light and electron microscope study of the subependymal plate. II. Microtumors. *Acta Neuropathologica* **45**, 177–85.

Pilkington, G.J., Lantos, P.L., Darling, J.L. and Thomas, D.G.T. (1982) Three cell lines from a spontaneous murine astrocytoma show variation in astrocytic differentiation. *Neuroscience Letters* **34**, 315–20.

Pilkington, G.J., Darling, J.L., Lantos, P.L. and Thomas, D.G.T. (1983) Cell lines (VMDk) derived from a spontaneous murine astrocytoma. *Journal of Neurological Sciences* **62**, 115–39.

Postlethwaite, R., Best, P.V., Porteous, I.B. and Blair, D.W. (1969) Growth and regression of rabbit tumors induced by polyoma virus. *British Journal of Cancer* **23**, 116–24.

Potts, P. (1775) *Chirurgical observations relative to the cataract, the polypus of the nose, the cancer of the scrotum, the different kinds of ruptures, and the mortification of the toes and feet.* London: L. Hawes, W. Clark and R. Collins.

Prasad, K.N. (1972) Morphological differentiation induced by prostaglandin in mouse neuroblastoma cells in culture. *Nature, New Biology* **236**, 49–52.

Prasad, K.N. and Hsie, A.W. (1971) Morphologic differentiation of mouse neuroblastoma cells induced *in vitro* by dibutyryl adenosine 3':5'-cyclic monophosphate. *Nature, New Biology* **233**, 141–2.

Preston-Martin, S. (1989) Descriptive epidemiology of primary tumors of the brain, cranial nerves and cranial meninges in Los Angeles County. *Neuroepidemiology* **8**, 283–95.

Preston-Martin, S., Lewis, S., Winkelmann, R., Borman, B., Auld, J. and Pearce, N. (1993) Descriptive epidemiology of primary cancer of the brain, cranial nerves, and cranial meninges in New Zealand, 1948–1988. *Cancer Causes and Control* **4**, 529–38.

Purchase, I.F.H. (1980) Range of experimental evidence in assessing potential human carcinogenicity. *Archives of Toxicology Supplement* **3**, 283–93.

Purves, D. and Dayan, A. (1992) A preliminary investigation of promotion of brain tumours by hexachlorophane in Sprague-Dawley rats transplacentally exposed to *N*-ethylnitrosourea. *Neuropathology and Applied Neurobiology* **18**, 259–64.

Quay, W.B., Ma, Y.-H., Varakis, J.N., ZuRhein, G.M., Padgett, B.L. and Walker, D.L. (1977) Modification of hydroxyindole-*O*-methyltransferase activity in experimental pineocytomas induced in hamsters by a human papovavirus (JC). *Journal of the National Cancer Institute* **58**, 123–7.

Rabotti, G.F., Grove, A.S., Jr, Sellers, R.L. and Anderson, W.R. (1966) Induction of multiple brain tumors (gliomata and leptomeningeal sarcomata) in dogs by Rous sarcoma virus. *Nature* **209**, 884–6.

Rabson, A.S. and Kirschstein, R.L. (1960) Intracranial sarcomas produced by Polyoma virus in Syrian hamsters. *Archives of Pathology* **69**, 663–71.

Rabson, A.S., O'Connor, G.T., Kirschstein, R.L. and Branigan, W.J. (1962) Papillary ependymomas produced in *Rattus (Mastomys) natalensis* inoculated with vacuolating virus (SV40). *Journal of the National Cancer Institute* **29**, 765–87.

Radovick, S., Wray, S., Lee, E., Nicols, D.K., Nakayama, Y., Weintraub, B.D., Westphal, H., Cutler, G.B. Jr and Wondisford, F.E. (1991) Migratory arrest of gonadotropin-releasing hormone neurons in transgenic mice. *Proceedings of the National Academy of Sciences U.S.A.* **88**, 3402–6.

Raju, T.R., Bignami, A. and Dahl, D. (1980) Glial fibrillary acidic protein in monolayer cultures of C-6 glioma cells: effect of aging and dibutyryl cyclic AMP. *Brain Research* **200**, 225–30.

Ramadan, M.A. and Wechsler, W. (1975) Transplacental induction of neurogenic tumors in BD IX rats by intragastric administration of ethylnitrosourea precursors. *Zeitschrift für Krebsforschung und Klinische Onkologie–Cancer Research and Clinical Oncology* **84**, 177–87.

Ramsay, P.B., VandenBerg, S.R., Eng, L.F., Herman, M.M. and Rubinstein, L.J. (1982) Immunologic recognition of cell surface antigens in normal mouse neural tissues and neuroepithelial cells of the OTT-6050 mouse teratoma. A radiometric, gel electrophoretic, and morphologic (immunofluorescence and immunoperoxidase) study. *Acta Neuropathologica* **56**, 214–24.

Rana, M.W., Pinkerton, H., Thornton, H. and Nagy, D. (1977) Heterotransplantation of human glioblastoma multiforme and meningioma to nude mice. *Proceedings of the Society for Experimental Biology and Medicine* **155**, 85–8.

Rasheed, B.K.A., McLendon, R.E., Herndon, J.E., Friedman, H.S., Friedman, A.H., Bigner, D.D. and Bigner, S.H. (1994) Alterations of the *TP53* gene in human gliomas. *Cancer Research* **54**, 1324–30.

Ravindranath, V., Anandatheerthavarada, H.K. and Shankar, S.K. (1990) NADPH cytochrome P-450 reductase in rat, mouse, and human brain. *Biochemical Pharmacology* **39**, 1013–18.

Rawlinson, D.G., Rubinstein, L.J. and Herman, M.M. (1974) *In vitro* characteristics of a myxopapillary ependymoma of the filum terminale maintained in tissue and organ culture systems. Light and electron microscopic observations. *Acta Neuropathologica* **27**, 185–200.

Reifenberger, G., Bilzer, T., Seitz, R.J. and Wechsler, W. (1989) Expression of vimentin and glial fibrillary acidic protein in ethylnitrosourea-induced rat gliomas and glioma cell lines. *Acta Neuropathologica* **78**, 270–82.

Ressetar, H.G., Prakash, O., Frisque, R.J., Webster, H.D., Re, R.N. and Stoner, G.L. (1993) Expression of viral T-antigen in pathological tissues from transgenic mice carrying JC-SV40 chimeric DNAs. *Molecular and Chemical Neuropathology* **20**, 59–79.

Reznik-Schüller, H. (1978) Ultrastructure of N-diethylnitrosamine induced tumors in the nasal olfactory region of the Syrian golden hamster. *Journal of Pathology* **124**, 161–4.

Reznik-Schüller, H.M. (1983) Pathogenesis of tumors induced with *N*-nitrosomethylpiperazine in the olfactory region of the rat nasal cavity. *Journal of the National Cancer Institute* **71**, 165–72.

Ribacchi, R. and Giraldo, G. (1966) Intracranial tumors in rats injected intracerebrally with murine sarcoma virus (MSV), Moloney's strain. Preliminary report. *Lavori dell Istituto di Anatomia e Istologia Patologica, Universita degli Studi Perugia* **26**, 141–8.

Rice, J.M. and Ward, J.M. (1982) Age dependence of susceptibility to carcinogenesis in the nervous system. *Annals of the New York Academy of Sciences* **381**, 274–89.

Rice, J.M., Rehm, S., Donovan, P.J. and Perantoni, A.O. (1989) Comparative transplacental carcinogenesis by directly acting and metabolism-dependent alkylating agents in rodents and nonhuman primates. In

Napalkov, N.P., Rice, J.M., Tomatis, L. and Yamasaki, H. (eds), *Perinatal and multigeneration carcinogenesis*. Lyon: International Agency for Research on Cancer, 17–34.

Roder, J. and Duwe, A. (1979) The *beige* mutation in the mouse selectively impairs natural killer cell function. *Nature* **278**, 451–3.

Romanul, F.C.A., Roizman, B. and Luttrell, C.N. (1961a) Studies of polyoma virus. Pathology and distribution of tumors produced in Syrian hamsters following intracranial or subcutaneous inoculation. *Bulletin of the Johns Hopkins Hospital* **108**, 1–15.

——(1961b) Intracranial sarcomas in hamsters induced by intracerebral injection of Se polyoma virus. *Journal of Neuropathology and Experimental Neurology* **20**, 299–300.

Roszman, T.L., Brooks, W.H., Markesbery, W.R. and Bigner, D.D. (1978) General immunocompetence of rats bearing avian sarcoma virus-induced intracranial tumors. *Cancer Research* **38**, 74–7.

Rous, P. (1911) A sarcoma of the fowl transmissible by an agent separable from the tumor cells. *Journal of Experimental Medicine* **13**, 397–411.

Rubin, R.C. and Ames, R.P. (1973) Mammary tumor virus in experimental ependymoblastoma. *Progress in Neuropathology* **2**, 335–49.

Rubin, R., Sutton, C.H. and Zimmerman, H.M. (1968) Experimental ependymoblastoma (fine structure). *Journal of Neuropathology and Experimental Neurology* **27**, 421–38.

Rubin, R., Ames, R.P., Sutton, C.H. and Zimmerman, H.M. (1969) Virus-like particles in murine ependymoblastoma. *Journal of Neuropathology and Experimental Neurology* **28**, 371–87.

Rubinstein, L.J. (1977) Correlation of animal brain tumor models with human neuro-oncology. *National Cancer Institute Monographs* **46**, 43–9.

Russell, W.O. (1945) The response of the central nervous system of the rat to methylcholanthrene. II. The effect of a diet deficient in thiamine and riboflavin on the induction of tumors derived from nervous tissue. *Cancer Research* **5**, 152–6.

Salomon, J.-C. and Fogh, J. (1982) The nude rat. In Fogh, J. and Giovanella, B.C. (eds), *The nude mouse in experimental and clinical research*, Vol. 2. New York: Academic Press, 229–45.

Sampson, J.H., Archer, G.E., Ashley, D.M., Fuchs, H.E., Hale, L.P., Dranoff, G. and Bigner, D.D. (1996) Subcutaneous vaccination with irradiated, cytokine-producing tumor cells stimulates CD8+ cell-mediated immunity against tumors located in the 'immunologically privileged' central nervous system. *Proceedings of the National Academy of Sciences U.S.A.* **93**, 10399–404.

Sampson, J.H., Ashley, D.M., Archer, G.E., Fuchs, H.E., Dranoff, G., Hale, L.P. and Bigner, D.D. (1997) Characterization of a spontaneous murine astrocytoma model and abrogation of its tumorigenicity by cytokine secretion. *Neurosurgery* in press.

Sander, J. (1970) Induction of malignant tumors in rats by oral administration of *N,N'*-dimethylurea and nitrite. *Arzneimittel-Forschung* **20**, 418–19.

Saxon, A., Macy, E., Denis, K., Tary-Lehmann, M., Witte, O. and Braun, J. (1991) Limited B cell repertoire in severe combined immunodeficient mice engrafted with peripheral blood mononuclear cells derived from immunodeficient or normal humans. *Journal of Clinical Investigation* **87**, 658–65.

Saya, H., Ara, S., Lee, P.S., Ro, J. and Hung, M.C. (1990) Direct sequencing analysis of transmembrane region of human *Neu* gene by polymerase chain reaction. *Molecular Carcinogenesis* **3**, 198–201.

Scheinberg, L.C., Suzuki, K., Edelman, F. and Davidoff, L.M. (1963) Studies in immunization against a transplantable cerebral mouse glioma. *Journal of Neurosurgery* **20**, 312–17.

Schiefer, B., Stavrou, D., Shadduck, J., Kaiser, E. and Dahme, E. (1970) Tumors of the CNS in the dog. *Tierärztliene Umschan* **25**, 297–9.

Schiffer, D. (1973) On the occurrence of oligodendroglia-like areas in neurinomas experimentally induced in the rat by nitrosourea derivatives. *Journal of the Neurological Sciences* **19**, 45–52.

Schiffer, D., Giordana, M.T., Pezzotta, S., Lechner, C. and Paoletti, P. (1978) Cerebral tumors induced by transplacental ENU: study of different tumoral stages, particularly of early proliferations. *Acta Neuropathologica* **41**, 27–31.

Schlumberger, H.G. (1954) Neoplasia in the parakeet. I. Spontaneous chromophobe pituitary tumors. *Cancer Research* **14**, 237–45.

——(1956) Neoplasia in the parakeet. II. Transplantation of the pituitary tumor. *Cancer Research* **16**, 149–53.

Schold, S.C. Jr and Friedman, H.S. (1984) Human brain tumor xenografts. *Progress in Experimental Tumor Research* **28**, 18–31.

Schold, S.C. Jr, Bullard, D.E., Bigner, S.H., Jones, T.R. and Bigner, D.D. (1983) Growth, morphology, and serial transplantation of anaplastic human gliomas in athymic mice. *Journal of Neuro-Oncology* **1**, 5–14.

Schubert, D., Humphreys, S., Baroni, C. and Cohn, M. (1969) *In vitro* differentiation of a mouse neuroblastoma. *Proceedings of the National Academy of Sciences U.S.A.* **64**, 316–23.

Schuster, J.M., Friedman, H.S., Archer, G.E., Fuchs, H.E., McLendon, R.E., Colvin, O.M. and Bigner, D.D. (1993) Intraarterial therapy of human glioma xenografts in athymic rats using 4-hydroperoxycyclophosphamide. *Cancer Research* **53** (Suppl. 10), 2338–43.

Schuurman, H.-J. (1995) The nude rat. *Human and Experimental Toxicology* **14**, 122–5.

Seligman, A.M. and Shear, M.J. (1939) Studies in carcinogenesis. VIII. Experimental production of brain tumors in mice with methylchoanthrene. *American Journal of Cancer* **37**, 364–95.

Serano, R.D., Pegram, C.N. and Bigner, D.D. (1980) Tumorigenic cell culture lines from a spontaneous VM/Dk murine astrocytoma (SMA). *Acta Neuropathologica* **51**, 53–64.

Shah, K.V., Daniel, R.W. and Strandberg, J.D. (1975) Sarcoma in a hamster inoculated with BK virus, a human papovavirus. *Journal of the National Cancer Institute* **54**, 945–50.

Shapiro, W.R. (1974) The chemotherapy of intacerebral vs. subcutaneous murine gliomas. A comparative study of the effect of VM 26. *Archives of Neurology* **30**, 222–6.

Shapiro, W.R., Ausman, J.I. and Rall, D.P. (1970) Studies on the chemotherapy of experimental brain tumors: evaluation of 1,3-bis(2-chloroethyl)-l-nitrosourea, cyclophosphamide, mithramycin, and methotrexate. *Cancer Research* **30**, 2401–13.

Shapiro, W.R., Basler, G.A., Chernik, N.L. and Posner, J.B. (1979) Human brain tumor transplantation into nude mice. *Journal of the National Cancer Institute* **62**, 447–53.

Shein, H.M. (1967) Transformation of astrocytes and destruction of spongioblasts induced by a simian tumor virus (SV40) in cultures of human fetal neuroglia. *Journal of Neuropathology and Experimental Neurology* **26**, 60–76.

——(1968) Neoplastic transformation of hamster astrocytes *in vitro* by Simian virus 40 and Polyoma virus. *Science* **159**, 1476–7.

——(1970) Neoplastic transformation of hamster astrocytes and choroid plexus cells in culture by polyoma virus. *Journal of Neuropathology and Experimental Neurology* **29**, 70–88.

Shein, H.M. and Pope, A. (1967) Viral induction of brain tumors *in vitro*. *Transactions of the American Neurological Association* **92**, 94–8.

Shibutani, M., Mitsumori, K., Okeda, R., Imazawa, T., Maekawa, A., Hatanaka, H., Takahashi, M., Inoue, K. and Hayashi, Y. (1994) Evidence for an origin of ethylnitrosourea-induced rat central nervous system tumors from pluripotent germinal neuroepithelium. *Acta Neuropathologica* **87**, 293–301.

Shinkai, Y., Rathbun, G., Lam, K.P., Oltz, E.M., Stewart, V., Mendelsohn, M., Charron, J., Dalta, M., Young, F., Stall, A.M. and Alt, F.W. (1992) RAG-2-deficient mice lack mature lymphocytes owing to inability to initiate V(D)J rearrangement. *Cell* **68**, 855–67.

Singer, B. and Grunberger, D. (1983) *Molecular biology of mutagens and carcinogens*. New York: Plenum Press.

Singer, B., Spengler, S.J., Chavez, F. and Kusmierek, J.T. (1987) The vinyl chloride-derived nucleoside, N^2,3-ethenoguanosine, is a highly efficient mutagen in transcription. *Carcinogenesis* **8**, 745–7.

Sipe, J.C., Rubinstein, L.J., Herman, M.M. and Bignami, A. (1974) Ethylnitrosourea-induced astrocytomas. Morphologic observations on rat tumors maintained in tissue and organ culture systems. *Laboratory Investigation* **31**, 571–9.

Skipper, H.E., Schabel, F.M. Jr and Wilcox, W.S. (1967) Experimental evaluation of potential anticancer agents. XXI. Scheduling of arabinosylcytosine to take advantage of its S-phase specificity against leukemia cells. *Cancer Chemotherapy Reports–Part 1* **51**, 125–65.

Skipper, H.E., Schabel, F.M. Jr, Trader, M.W. and Thomson, J.R. (1961) Experimental evaluation of potential anticancer agents. VI. Anatomical distribution of leukemic cells and failure of chemotherapy. *Cancer Research* **21**, 1154–64.

Slye, M., Holmes, H.F. and Wells, H.G. (1931) Intracranial neoplasms in lower animals. Studies in the incidence and inheritability of spontaneous tumors in mice. *American Journal of Cancer* **15**, 1387–400.

Snell, G.D., Cloudman, A.M. and Woodworth, E. (1948) Tumor immunity in mice, induced with lyophilized tissue, as influenced by tumor strain, host strain, source of tissue, and dosage. *Cancer Research* **8** 429–37.

Snell, K.C., Stewart, H.L., Morris, H.P., Wagner, B.P. and Ray, F.E. (1961) Intracranial neurilemmoma and medulloblastoma induced in rats by the dietary administration of *N,N'*-2,7-fluorenylene-bisacetamide. *National Cancer Institute Monographs* **5**, 85–104.

Snoek, G.T., Mummery, C.L., van den Brink, C.E., van der Saag, P.T. and de Laat, S.W. (1986) Protein kinase C and phorbol ester receptor expression related to growth and differentiation of nullipotent and pluripotent embryonal carcinoma cells. *Developmental Biology* **115**, 282–92.

Solleveld, H.A. and Boorman, G.A. (1990) Brain. In Boorman, G.A., Eustis, S.L., Elwell, M.R., Montgomery, C.A. Jr and MacKenzie, W.F. (eds) *Pathology of the Fischer rat. Reference and atlas*. San Diego: Academic Press, 155–77.

Solleveld, H.A., Haseman, J.K. and McConnell, E.E. (1984) Natural history of body weight gain, survival, and neoplasia in the F344 rat. *Journal of the National Cancer Institute* **72**, 929–40.

Solleveld, H.A., Bigner, D.D., Averill, D.R. Jr, Bigner, S.H., Boorman, G.A., Burger, P.C., Gillespie, Y., Hubbard, G.B., Laerum, O.D., McComb, R.D., McGrath, J.T., Morgan, K.T., Peters, A., Rubinstein, L.J., Schoenberg, B.S., Schold, S.C., Swenberg, J.A., Thompson, M.B., Vandevelde, M. and Vinores, S.A. (1986) Brain tumors in man and animals: report of a workshop. *Environmental Health Perspectives* **68**, 155–73.

Stefanski, S.A., Elwell, M.R., Mitsumori, K., Yoshitomi, K., Dittrich, K. and Giles, H.D. (1988) Chordomas in Fischer 344 rats. *Veterinary Pathology* **25**, 42–7.

Stevens, L.C. (1970) The development of transplantable teratocarcinomas from intratesticular grafts of pre- and postimplantation mouse embryos. *Developmental Biology* **21**, 364–82.

Stewart, H.L., Kaplan, H.S. and Bennett, J.G. (1950) Report of two cases of identical primary tumors involving spinal nerve roots and meninges in strain NHO mice. *Journal of the National Cancer Institute* **11**, 177–97.

Stewart, H.L., Deringer, M.K., Dunn, T.B. and Snell, K.C. (1974) Malignant schwannomas of nerve roots, uterus, and epididymis in mice. *Journal of the National Cancer Institute* **53**, 1749–58.

Stratton, M.R., Darling, J., Pilkington, G.J., Lantos, P.L., Reeves, B.R. and Cooper, C.S. (1989) Characterization of the human cell line TE671. *Carcinogenesis* **10**, 899–905.

Strauss, M.M., Bigner, S.H. and Bigner, D.D. (1982) Experimental allergic encephalomyelitis in Lewis rats bearing avian sarcoma virus induced brain tumors. *Journal of Neuroimmunology* **2**, 283–94.

Sukumar, S. (1989) *Ras* oncogenes in chemical carcinogenesis. *Current Topics in Microbiology and Immunology* **148**, 93–114.

Sumi, N., Stavrou, D., Frohberg, H. and Jochmann, G. (1976) The incidence of spontaneous tumors of the central nervous system of Wistar rats. *Archives of Toxicology* **35**, 1–13.

Sundberg, J.P., Burnstein, T., Page, E.H., Kirkham, W.W. and Robinson, F.R. (1977) Neoplasms of Equidae. *Journal of the American Veterinary Medical Association* **170**, 150–2.

Suri, C., Fung, B.P., Tischler, A.S. and Chikaraishi, D.M. (1993) Catecholaminergic cell lines from the brain and adrenal glands of tyrosine hydroxylase-SV40 T antigen transgenic mice. *Journal of Neuroscience* **13**, 1280–91.

Swenberg, J.A. (1986) Brain tumours–problems and perspectives. *Food and Chemical Toxicology* **24**, 155–8.

Swenberg, J.A., Koestner, A. and Wechsler, W. (1972) The induction of tumors of the nervous system with intravenous methylnitrosourea. *Laboratory Investigation* **26**, 74–85.

Swenberg, J.A., Fedtke, N., Ciroussel, F., Barbin, A. and Bartsch, H. (1992) Etheno adducts formed in DNA of vinyl chloride-exposed rats are highly persistent in liver. *Carcinogenesis* **13**, 727–9.

Symeonidis, A. (1954) Tumors induced by 2-acetylaminofluorene in virgin and breeding females of five strains of rats and in their offspring. *Journal of the National Cancer Institute* **15**, 539–49.

Takahashi, T., Shimizu, A., Sakai, T., Endo, Y., Osowa, N., Shisa, H. and Honjo, T. (1992) Mapping of the *nu* gene using congenic nude strains and *in situ* hybridization. *Journal of Experimental Medicine* **175**, 873–6.

Takizawa, S. and Nishihara, H. (1971) Induction of tumors in the brain, kidney, and other extra-mammary gland organs by a continuous oral administration of *N*-nitrosobutylurea in Wistar/Furth rats. *Gann* **62**, 495–503.

Tamura, K., Shimizu, K., Yamada, M., Okamoto, Y., Matsui, Y., Park, K.C., Mabuchi, E., Moriuchi, S. and Mogami, H. (1989) Expression of major histocompatibility complex on human medulloblastoma cells with neuronal differentiation. *Cancer Research* **49**, 5380–4.

Tanaka, R., Sekiguchi, K., Ueki, K., Gilden, D.H. and Koprowski, H. (1978) Morphological studies of hamster brain cells transformed *in vitro* by a human papovavirus BK. *Acta Neuropathologica* **41**, 235–9.

Tapscott, S.J., Miller, A.D., Olson, J.M., Berger, M.S., Groudine, M. and Spence, A.M. (1994) Gene therapy of rat 9L gliosarcoma tumors by transduction with selectable genes does not require drug selection. *Proceedings of the National Academy of Sciences U.S.A.* **91**, 8185–9.

Tary-Lehmann, M. and Saxon, A. (1992) Human mature T cells that are anergic *in vivo* prevail in SCID mice reconstituted with human peripheral blood. *Journal of Experimental Medicine* **175**, 503–16.

Tary-Lehmann, M., Lehmann, P.V., Schols, D., Roncarolo, M.G. and Saxon, A. (1994) Anti-SCID mouse reactivity shapes the human CD4+ T cell repertoire in hu-PBL-SCID chimeras. *Journal of Experimental Medicine* **180**, 1817–27.

Theuring, F., Götz, W., Balling, R., Korf, H.-W., Schulze, F., Herken, R. and Gruss, P. (1990) Tumorigenesis and eye abnormalities in transgenic mice expressing MSV-SV40 large T-antigen. *Oncogene* **5**, 225–32.

Thompson, S.W., Huseby, R.A., Fox, M.A., Davis, C.L. and Hunt, R.D. (1961) Spontaneous tumors in the Sprague-Dawley rat. *Journal of the National Cancer Institute* **27**, 1037–57.

Thurman, J.D., Bucci, T.J., Hart, R.W. and Turturro, A. (1994) Survival, body weight, and spontaneous neoplasms in *ad libitum*-fed and food-restricted Fischer-344 rats. *Toxicologic Pathology* **22**, 1–9.

Tresman, R.L. and Evans, M.J. (1975) A light and electron microscopical study of the nervous tissue of mouse teratomas. *Journal of Neurocytology* **4**, 310–14.

Tripier, M.F., Markovits, P., Papadopoulo, D. and Toga, M. (1979a) Normal and benzo(a)pyrene-transformed fetal mouse brain cells. II. Ultrastructural study. *Acta Neuropathologica* **47**, 205–11.

Tripier, M.F., Hassoun, J., de Micco, C., Meyer, G. and Toga, M. (1979b) Tumorigenic clones of hamster brain cells transformed *in vitro* by polyoma virus. Ultrastructural and immunohistochemical study. *Acta Neuropathologica* **48**, 189–97.

Trojanowski, J.Q., Friedman, H.S., Burger, P.C. and Bigner, D.D. (1987) A rapidly dividing human medulloblastoma cell line (D283 MED) expresses all three neurofilament subunits. *American Journal of Pathology* **126**, 358–63.

Tsang, R.W., Laperriere, N.J., Simpson, W.J., Brierley, J., Panzarella, T. and Smyth, H.S. (1993) Glioma arising after radiation therapy for pituitary adenoma. A report of four patients and estimation of risk. *Cancer* **72**, 2227–33.

Ulland, B., Finkelstein, M., Weisburger, E.K., Rice, J.M. and Weisburger, J.H. (1971) Carcinogenicity of industrial chemicals propylene imine and propane sultone. *Nature* **230**, 460–1.

VandenBerg, S.R., Hickey, J.E. and Herman, M.M. (1977) Brain-associated cell surface antigens on neuroepithelial cells in a transplantable mouse teratoma. *Acta Neuropathologica* **39**, 281–7.

VandenBerg, S.R., Herman, M.M., Ludwin, S.K. and Bignami, A. (1975) An experimental mouse testicular teratoma as a model for neuroepithelial neoplasia and differentiation. I. Light microscopic and tissue and organ culture observations. *American Journal of Pathology* **79**, 147–69.

VandenBerg, S.R., Ludwin, S.K., Herman, M.M. and Bignami, A. (1976) *In vitro* astrocytic differentiation from embryoid bodies of an experimental mouse testicular teratoma. *American Journal of Pathology* **83**, 197–212.

VandenBerg, S.R., Chatel, M., Griffiths, O.M., DeArmond, S.J., Pappas, C. and Herman, M.M. (1981a) Neural differentiation in the OTT-6050 mouse teratoma. Production of a tumor fraction restricted to stem cells and neural cells after centrifugal elutriation. *Virchows Archiv A, Pathological Anatomy and Histology* **392**, 281–94.

VandenBerg, S.R., Hess, J.R., Herman, M.M., DeArmond, S.J., Halks-Miller, M. and Rubinstein, L.J. (1981b) Neural differentiation in the OTT-6050 mouse teratoma. Production of a tumor fraction showing melanogenesis in neuroepithelial cells after centrifugal elutriation. *Virchows Archiv A, Pathological Anatomy and Histology* **392**, 295–308.

Vandeputte, M.C. and Brucher, J.M. (1962) Experimental meningeal sarcomatosis provoked in newborn rats by the polyoma virus. *Acta Neuropathologica* **1**, 397–405.

Van Dyke, T.A., Finlay, C., Miller, D., Marks, J., Lozano, G. and Levine, A.J. (1987) Relationship between simian virus 40 large tumor antigen expression and tumor formation in transgenic mice. *Journal of Virology* **61**, 2029–32.

Vaquero, J., Coca, S., Zurita, M., Oya, S., Arias, A., Moreno, M. and Morales, C. (1992) Synaptophysin expression in 'ependymal tumors' induced by ethylnitrosourea in rats. *American Journal of Pathology* **141**, 1037–41.

Varakis, J.N. and ZuRhein, G.M. (1976) Experimental pineocytoma of the Syrian hamster induced by human papovavirus (JC). A light and electron microscopic study. *Acta Neuropathologica* **35**, 243–64.

Varakis, J., ZuRhein, G.M., Padgett, B.L. and Walker, D.L. (1978) Induction of peripheral neuroblastomas in Syrian hamsters after injection as neonates with JC virus, a human polyoma virus. *Cancer Research* **38**, 1718–22.

Vázquez-López, E. (1936) On the growth of Rous sarcoma inoculated into the brain. *American Journal of Cancer* **26**, 29–55.

—— (1945) Glioma in a rat fed with 2-acetyl-amino-fluorene. *Nature* **156**, 296–7.

Vick, N.A. and Bigner, D.D. (1972) Some structural aspects of dog brain tumors induced with the Schmidt-Ruppin strain of the Rous sarcoma virus. *Progress in Experimental Tumor Research* **17**, 59–73.

Vick, N.A., Bigner, D.D. and Kvedar, J.P. (1971) The fine structure of canine gliomas and intracranial sarcomas induced by the Schmidt-Ruppin strain of the Rous sarcoma virus. *Journal of Neuropathology and Experimental Neurology* **30**, 354–67.

Vick, N.A., Lin, M.-J. and Bigner, D.D. (1977) The role of the subependymal plate in glial tumorigenesis. *Acta Neuropathologica* **40**, 63–71.

Vitovec, J. (1976) Statistical data on 370 cattle tumors collected over the years 1964–1973 in South Bohemia. *Zentralblatt für Veterinarmedizin – Reihe A* **23**, 445–53.

Vollrath, M., Altmannsberger, M., Weber, K. and Osborn, M. (1986) Chemically induced tumors of rat olfactory epithelium: a model for human esthesioneuroepithelioma. *Journal of the National Cancer Institute* **76**, 1205–16.

Von Jagic, N., Schwarz, G. and von Siebenrock (1911) Blutbefunde bei Röntgenologen. *Berliner Klinische Wochenschrift* **48**, 1220–2.

Vos, J.G., Berkvens, J.M. and Kruijt, B.C. (1980) The athymic rat. I. Morphology of lymphoid and endocrine organs. *Clinical Immunology and Immunopathology* **15**, 213–28.

Vos, J.G., Kreeftenberg, J.G., Kruijt, B.C., Kruizinga, W. and Steerenberg, P. (1980) The athymic nude rat. II. Immunological characteristics. *Clinical Immunology and Immunopathology* **15**, 229–37.

Vraa-Jensen, J., Herman, M.M., Rubinstein, L.J. and Bignami, A. (1976) *In vitro* characteristics of a fourth ventricle ependymoma maintained in organ culture systems: light and electron microscopic observations. *Neuropathology and Applied Neurobiology* **2**, 349–64.

Walker, D.L., Padgett, B.L., ZuRhein, G.M., Albert, A.E. and Marsh, R.F. (1973) Human papovavirus (JC): induction of brain tumors in hamsters. *Science* **181**, 674–6.

Walker, V.E. and Swenberg, J.A. (1989) Phenobarbital lacks promoting activity for neurogenic tumors in F344 rats transplacentally exposed to ethylnitrosourea. *Journal of Neuropathology and Experimental Neurology* **48**, 263–9.

Walker, V.E., Morgan, K.T., Zimmerman, H.M. and Innes, J.R.M. (1994) Tumors of the central and peripheral nervous system. In Turusov, V.S. and Mohr, U. (eds), *Pathology of tumors in laboratory animals*. Second edition. Lyon: International Agency for Research on Cancer, 731–76.

Ward, J.M. (1983) Background data and variations in tumor rates of control rats and mice. *Progress in Experimental Tumor Research* **26**, 241–58.

Ward, J.M. and Rice, J.M. (1982) Naturally occurring and chemically induced brain tumors of rats and mice in carcinogenesis bioassays. *Annals of the New York Academy of Sciences* **381**, 304–19.

Warenius, H.M. (1980) Identification and separation of mouse and human components of heterotransplanted human tumors. In Sparrow, S. (ed.), *Immunodeficient animals for cancer research*. London: MRC Laboratory Animals Centre, 207–20.

Warzok, R., Pötzsch, D., Henning, F. and Heiderstädt, R. (1972) Induction of nervous system tumors by administration of MNU and ENU in newborn rats. Comparative investigation. *Zentralblatt für Allgemeine Pathologie und Pathologische Anatomie* **116**, 551–5.

Washington, W.J., Foote, R.S., Dunn, W.C., Generoso, W.M. and Mitra, S. (1989) Age-dependent modulation of tissue-specific repair activity for 3-methyladenine and O^6-methylguanine in DNA in inbred mice. *Mechanisms of Ageing and Development* **48**, 43–52.

Watanabe, Y., Kuribayashi, K., Miyatake, S., Nishihara, K., Nakayama, E., Taniyama, T. and Sakata, T. (1989) Exogenous expression of mouse interferon γ cDNA in mouse neuroblastoma C1300 cells results in reduced tumorigenicity by augmented anti-tumor immunity. *Proceedings of the National Academy of Sciences U.S.A.* **86**, 9456–60.

Wechsler, W., Ramadan, M.A. and Gieseler, A. (1972) Isogenic transplantation of ethylnitrosourea-induced tumors of the central and peripheral nervous system in two different inbred rat strains. *Naturwissenschaften* **59**, 474.

Wechsler, W., Rice, J.M. and Vesselinovitch, S.D. (1979) Transplacental and neonatal induction of neurogenic tumors in mice: comparison with related species and with human pediatric neoplasms. *National Cancer Institute Monographs* **51**, 219–26.

Weizsaecker, M., Deen, D.F., Rosenblum, M.L., Hoshino, T., Gutin, P.H. and Barker, M. (1981) The 9L rat brain tumor: description and application of an animal model. *Journal of Neurology* **224**, 183–92.

Wells, S.A. Jr, Wurtman, R.J. and Rabson, A.S. (1966) Viral neoplastic transformation of hamster pineal cells *in vitro*: retention of enzymatic function. *Science* **154**, 278–9.

Whitehead, J.E. (1967) Neoplasia in the cat. *Veterinary Medicine Small Animal Clinician* **62**, 357–8.

Wiestler, O.D., Aguzzi, A., Schneemann, M., Eibl, R., von Deimling, A. and Kleihues, P. (1992) Oncogene complementation in fetal brain transplants. *Cancer Research* **52**, 3760–7.

Wiestler, O.D., Brüstle, O., Eibl, R.H., Radner, H., Aguzzi, A. and Kleihues, P. (1994) Oncogene transfer into the brain. *Recent Results in Cancer Research* **135**, 55–66.

Wikstrand, C.J. and Bigner, D.D. (1979) Surface antigens of human glioma cells shared with normal adult and fetal brain. *Cancer Research* **39**, 3235–43.

Wilfong, R.F., Bigner, D.D., Self, D.J. and Wechsler, W. (1973) Brain tumor types induced by the Schmidt-Ruppin strain of Rous sarcoma virus in inbred Fischer rats. *Acta Neuropathologica* **25**, 196–206.

Wilkins, R.H. and Odom, G.L. (1965) Attempted induction of gliomas utilizing simian virus 40. *Archives of Neurology* **13**, 149–54.

Wilson, C.B. and Barker, M. (1968) Intrathecal transplantation of human neural tumors to the guinea pig. *Journal of the National Cancer Institute* **41**, 1229–40.

Windle, J.J., Weiner, R.I. and Mellon, P.L. (1990) Cell lines of the pituitary gonadotrope lineage derived by targeted oncogenesis in transgeneic mice. *Molecular Endocrinology* **4**, 597–603.

Windle, J.J., Albert, D.M., O'Brien, J.M., Marcus, D.M., Disteche, C.M., Bernards, R. and Mellon, P.L. (1990) Retinoblastoma in transgenic mice. *Nature* **343**, 665–9.

Wiranowska, M., Gonzalvo, A.A., Saporta, S., Gonzalez, O.R. and Prockop, L.D. (1992) Evaluation of blood-brain barrier permeability and the effect of interferon in mouse glioma model. *Journal of Neuro-Oncology* **14**, 225–36.

Wrensch, M., Bondy, M.L., Wiencke, J. and Yost, M. (1993) Environmental risk factors for primary malignant brain tumors: a review. *Journal of Neuro-Oncology* **17**, 47–64.

Wyand, D.S., Zwicker, G.M. and Pavkov, K. (1987) Spontaneous glioblastoma multiforme in a Charles River CD rat. *Toxicologic Pathology* **15**, 474–8.

Yablonovskya, L.Y. and Avtsyn, A.P. (1963) Malignant glioma in a rabbit induced by MCA. *Arkhiv Patologii* **25**(10), 28–34.

Yoshino, T., Motoi, M. and Ogawa, K. (1985) Morphological maturation of tumor cells induced by ethylnitrosourea (ENU) in rat brains. I. On the tumors by administration of ENU in the late gestational stage. *Acta Pathologica Japonica* **35**, 1385–96.

Yung, W.K., Blank, N.K. and Vick, N.A. (1976) 'Glioblastoma'. Induction of a reproducible autochthonous tumor in rats with murine sarcoma virus. *Neurology* **26**, 76–83.

Zagzag, D., Miller, D.C., Cangiarella, J., Allen, J.C. and Greco, M.A. (1992) Brainstem glioma after radiation therapy for acute myeloblastic leukemia in a child with Down syndrome. Possible pathogenetic mechanisms. *Cancer* **70**, 1188–93.

Zimmerman, H.M. and Arnold, H. (1941) Experimental brain tumors. I. Tumors produced with methylcholanthrene. *Cancer Research* **12**, 919–38.

——(1944) Experimental brain tumors. IV. The incidence in different strains of mice. *Cancer Research* **4**, 98–101.

Zimmerman, H.M. and Innes, J.R.M. (1979) Tumors of the central and peripheral nervous system. In Turusov, V.S. (ed.), *Tumors of the mouse*. Lyon: International Agency for Research on Cancer, 629–54.

ZuRhein, G.M. (1983) Studies of JC virus-induced nervous system tumors in the Syrian hamster: a review. In Sever, J.L. and Madden, D.L. (eds), *Polyomaviruses and human neurological diseases*. New York: Alan R. Liss, 205.

ZuRhein, G.M. and Varakis, J.N. (1979) Perinatal induction of medulloblastomas in Syrian golden hamsters by a human polyoma virus (JC). *National Cancer Institute Monographs* **51**, 205–8.

CHAPTER 7

Cellular immunology

Lymphocyte populations, cytokines and target–effector systems

CAROL J. WIKSTRAND, DAVID M. ASHLEY, DARELL D. BIGNER AND LAURA P. HALE

Introduction

CELLULAR IMMUNE RESPONSE TO TUMORS: GENERAL PRINCIPLES

Classic immune functions that are regarded as cellular include delayed-type hypersensitivity and the rejection of foreign tissue (grafts or tumors) (Restifo and Wunderlich, 1995). The thymus-derived lymphocytes, or T cells, are the major specific effector cells of the cellular immune system. Although there is a degree of overlap in their function, in general terms, T lymphocytes can be divided into two separate groups: $CD8^+$ lymphocytes, or 'cytotoxic T cells' (cytotoxic T lymphocytes: CTLs), so termed because they are capable of direct lysis of target cells; and $CD4^+$ lymphocytes, called 'helper T cells' because of their ability to enhance and orchestrate the immune response toward either cellular (T_H1) or humoral, antibody-mediated (T_H2) mechanisms (Fitch *et al.*, 1993). Fundamental to cellular immune mechanisms, in contrast to humoral responses, is the fact that T cells can only recognize protein-derived antigens in the context of other cell surface molecules, specifically those of the major histocompatibility complex (MHC). When MHC class I and class II molecules are noncovalently linked to antigenic peptides, the molecules serve as ligands for the T-cell receptors (TCRs) expressed by $CD8^+$ and $CD4^+$ T cells, respectively (Restifo and Wunderlich, 1995).

The CD8 and CD4 molecules that distinguish the T-cell subsets are cell surface glycoproteins, which, along with TCRs, serve as coreceptors for MHC molecules. The $CD8^+$ cells recognize the MHC I complex, which is expressed on most nucleated mammalian cells. The $CD4^+$ cells interact with MHC II molecules, which are normally found on only a subset of cells, including antigen-presenting cells such as dendritic cells and macrophages, B cells, some T cells and some epithelial cells. The MHC II molecules also may be up regulated on other cell types in response to inflammatory or various activation stimuli. Interaction between the antigen-specific TCR and the corresponding MHC/peptide complex provides the initial signal required for activation of the T cell. Essential second signals for T-cell activation include the interaction of cell-surface molecules such as CD28 and B7, lymphocyte function-associated antigen (LFA)-1 (CD11a/CD18) and intracellular adhesion molecule (ICAM)-1 (CD54), CD2 and LFA-3 (CD58) or CD5 and CD72. Signals are also provided by a variety of cytokines, including interleukin (IL)-2, IL-4, IL-5, IL-6, IL-7, IL-12, IL-15, interferon (IFN)-α and IFN-γ. Both initial and secondary signals for T-cell activation may be provided by antigen-presenting cells (Shimizu and Shaw, 1989–90; Romagnani, 1992; Fitch *et al.*, 1993; Fraser, Straus and Weiss, 1993; Mosmann, 1995). The $CD4^+$ T cells usually require that tumor antigens be presented to them by antigen-presenting cells, such as macrophages or dendritic cells, that have taken in the antigenic substrates. The antigen-presenting cells have excised the peptides from the antigenic substrates and presented them on the cell surface, bound to MHC class II molecules. Once stimulated by the antigen, the $CD4^+$ cells then differentiate either into T_H1 cells, which promote the cellular immune response by secreting cytokines such as IL-2, IFN-γ and tumor necrosing factor (TNF)-α, or into T_H2 cells, which stimulate B cells to proliferate and elaborate antigen-specific antibody by secreting cytokines such as IL-4, IL-5, IL-6 and IL-10. Some tumor cells, for example melanoma and glial tumors (Romagnani, 1992), express MHC II antigens as well, and thus are also capable of directly stimulating $CD4^+$ T cells.

The $CD8^+$ T cells are activated by antigens presented in association with MHC I molecules. Such antigens arise predominantly from synthesized endogenous proteins; however, recent evidence suggests that extracellular antigens can also be processed by antigen-presenting cells and presented in the context of MHC I (Kovacsovics-Bankowski and Rock, 1995). Thus, an initial signal for activation of $CD8^+$ T cells may potentially come from antigens processed and presented on MHC I molecules, on tumor cells, or on other 'professional' antigen-presenting cells. The second activation signals described above are then provided by either $CD4^+$ helper T cells or antigen-presenting cells. Because of the requirement that antigen be complexed with self-MHC I molecules before $CD8^+$ CTLs are activated, the killing of target cells by $CD8^+$ CTLs is termed 'MHC I restricted'. Stated in simple terms, this means that the association of tumor antigen with MHC I molecules is an essential prerequisite for killing of those tumor cells by $CD8^+$ CTLs.

A variety of cellular defense mechanisms that are innate and nonspecific exist in addition to the specific arm of the cellular immune system represented by T cells. Natural killer (NK) cells are a small population of cells that can be distinguished from T cells by their lack of TCR expression and by their expression of CD56 and receptors for Fc portions of immunoglobulin molecules (FcR^+). Killing of target cells by NK cells is apparently mediated by a mechanism similar to that used by CTLs; however, killing is not MHC class I restricted. Some specificity exists, however, as tumor cells are more vulnerable targets for NK killing than are normal cells (Frey *et al.*, 1991; Moretta *et al.*, 1994; Ortaldo, Mason and O'Shea, 1995). Lymphokine-activated killer (LAK) cells are derived from lymphocytes stimulated *in vitro* with IL-2. The LAK cells consist of a heterogeneous population of CTLs and NK cells and seemingly mediate killing in an MHC-independent fashion (Ortaldo, Mason and Overton, 1986). Finally, both activated macrophages and polymorphonuclear leukocytes (neutrophils) can have antitumor effects, either directly or through antibody-dependent mechanisms (Fidler and Schroit, 1988; Shau and Roberts, 1992).

Unique features of brain tumors and the concept of immunologic privilege in the central nervous system

Shirai (1921) and Murphy and Sturm (1923) reported a series of experiments based upon the premise that the brain lacked lymphatic drainage. In these studies, tumors transplanted into the brains of outbred rats were often successfully established, whereas the same tumor transplanted subcutaneously was frequently rejected. Medawar (1948) extended and updated these observations by demonstrating that histoincompatible skin grafts that were vigorously rejected when applied orthotopically, grew successfully when implanted within the brain away from the ventricular system. These observations led to an initial concept of the brain as an immunologically privileged site. However, classic transplantation studies performed by Scheinberg *et al.* (1963), with an intracerebrally transplantable methylcholanthrene-induced ependymoblastoma, demonstrated that tumor cells injected intracerebrally could elicit first-set rejection in allogeneic hosts and second-set rejection of subcutaneous or intracerebral tumor cell implants in syngeneic hosts. Multiple studies also demonstrated that primary subcutaneous tumor transplants could confer resistance to subsequent intracerebral or subcutaneous challenge (Scheinberg *et al.*, 1963, 1966; Scheinberg, Edelman and Levy, 1964; Scheinberg, Levy and Edelman, 1965). Accordingly, the original concept of immune privilege of the central nervous system (CNS) was modified, in the 1960s, to one of partial privilege.

A variety of anatomic studies have now demonstrated that both afferent and efferent immune pathways are present in the normal CNS. As summarized recently by Knopf *et al.* (1995), in normal animals, efflux pathways from the cranial and spinal subarachnoid space include passage through the arachnoid villi into blood of the dural sinus and drainage into lymph along routes that are adjacent to cranial and spinal nerves and that lead to regional (cervical) lymph nodes. Injecting radiolabeled protein into rabbit cerebrospinal fluid results in significant levels (30% injected dose) in the cervical lymph within 6 hours (Yamada *et al.*, 1991). Knopf *et al.* (1995) demonstrated that antigens, both those requiring T-cell help for generation of an antibody response (T-dependent; e.g., serum albumin) and those independent of it (T-independent; e.g., tri-nitrophenol-Ficoll), are capable of stimulating humoral immune responses in the cervical lymph nodes and spleen when the antigens are injected into the cerebrospinal fluid. The time course of IgM and IgG appearance is identical to conventionally immunized hosts. In this study, removing cervical lymph nodes before infusing the antigen into the cerebrospinal fluid significantly diminished the humoral response, suggesting that trafficking of activated B cells from the cervical nodes to the spleen might occur, as well as stimulation of splenic T cells by direct blood-borne antigen. Several lines of evidence suggest that similar lymphatic drainage of the brain does exist in man, and they are outlined by Kida *et al.* (1995) as follows: (1) noniatrogenic metastasis of glial tumors to cervical lymph nodes occurs; (2) perivascular spaces in cerebral gray matter are continuous with leptomeningeal perivascular spaces; and (3) perivascular cells exist in human brains, and the cells serve as scavengers or antigen-presenting cells, as do similar cells in rats.

The presence of brain tumor may lead to enhanced connections between the CNS and the systemic immune system. Salcman and Broadwell (1991) demonstrated that the routine localization of labeled serum albumin and contrast agents in computed tomography and magnetic resonance imaging depends on the relative leakiness of brain tumor endothelial cells. Anomalies observed by electron microscopy in the vascular endothelium of glioma capillaries, as opposed to those in normal brain, include tight junctions lacking normal pentalaminar structure, vesicular formations and fenestrations (Long, 1970; Vick, Bigner and Kvedar, 1971; Shuttleworth, 1972). This potential for vascular 'leakiness' was also observed in peritumoral endothelium, and it decreased progressively in normal brain adjacent to brain tumor, with blood-to-tumor transfer constants of tracer compounds 15-fold higher in human glioblastoma multiforme than in normal brain (Groothuis *et al.*, 1991; Salcman and Broadwell, 1991).

The documentation that experimental allergic encephalomyelitis can be directly induced by systemic immunization or by passive transfer of immune effectors (Paterson, 1960; Levine, 1973), that rejection of virally induced experimental gliomas occurs in the brains of dogs (Bigner, Fritz and Day, 1969) and that perivascular accumulations of small lymphocytes are frequently observed in human gliomas (Ridley and Cavanagh, 1971) has also established that effector cells originating systemically can enter the brain.

A number of studies have addressed the role of immunosurveillance on the pathogenesis of brain tumors. In the 1970s, Morantz, Shain and Cravioto (1978) claimed that the immune privilege of the brain prevented immunosuppressive or immunoenhancement protocols from altering the incidence of brain tumors in rats exposed intrauterinely to ethylnitrosourea. Denlinger *et al.* (1973) found that immunosuppression with heterologous antilymphocyte serum affected neither the incidence of *N*-methyl *N*-nitrosourea-induced central or peripheral nervous system tumors in F344 rats, nor their survival. Identical results were obtained when the primary brain tumor induction was by intracerebral inoculation of the B77-avian sarcoma virus (Bigner *et al.*, 1975).

In contradistinction to these laboratory studies are the recent observations that patients who are immunocompromised by iatrogenic procedures, inherited immunodeficiencies or acquired immunodeficiency syndrome (AIDS) have an increased incidence of both systemic and primary CNS lymphoma (Eby *et al.*, 1988; Jellinger and Paulus, 1992; Miller *et al.*, 1994). While little is known about the origin of primary CNS lymphoma, the EBV (Epstein-Barr virus) genome is detectable in most lesions. One inference that may be drawn from the frequent observation of primary CNS lymphoma in this group of patients is that immunosuppression creates a breakdown in immune surveillance, which

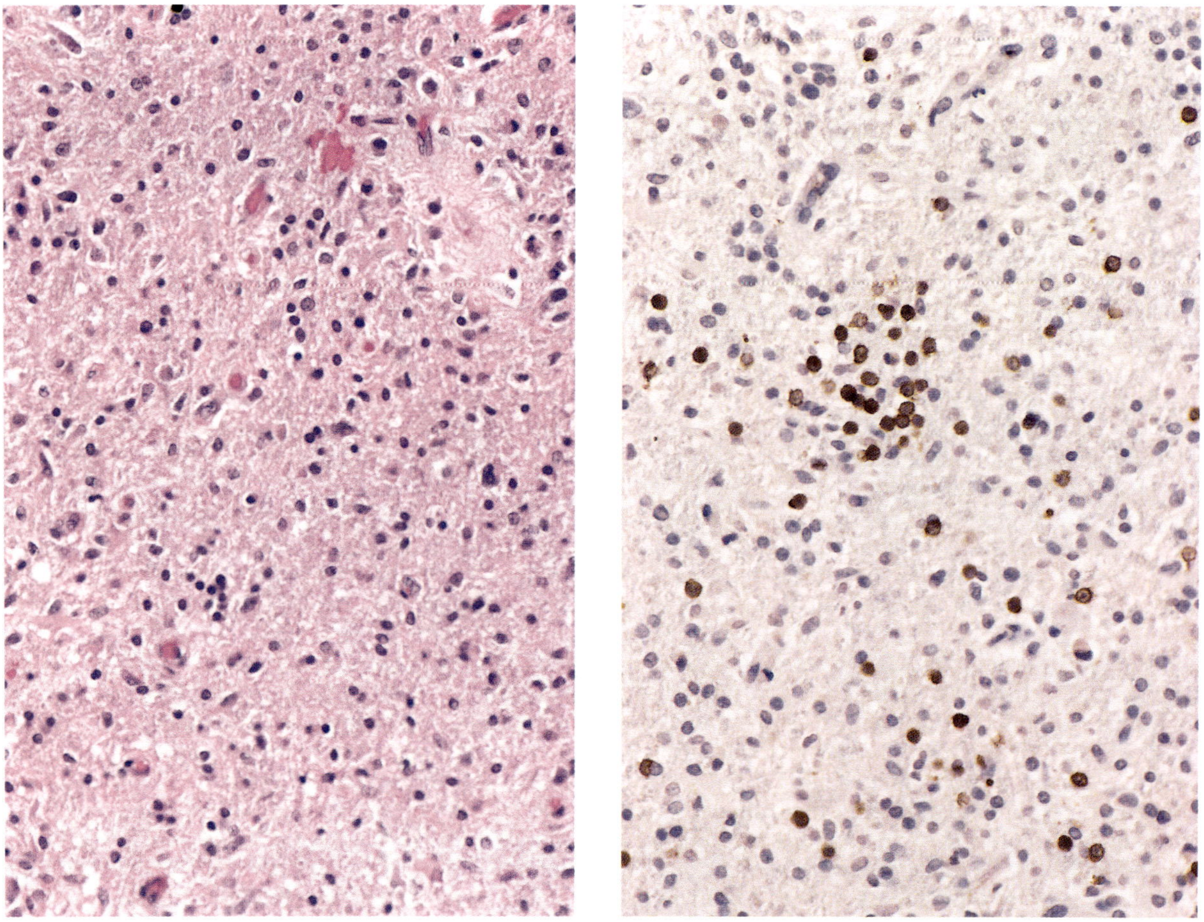

a b

Fig. 7.1 Lymphocytic infiltrate in a high-grade malignant glioma. There are T cells scattered throughout the tumor. (a) Hematoxylin and eosin stain; (b) CD3 (pan T cell) antibody, immunoperoxidase method, hematoxylin counterstain; × 66

may lead to an overt malignancy in the setting of polyclonal B-cell proliferation caused by Epstein-Barr virus. Therefore, these data implicate a normally functioning CNS surveillance response in preventing such lymphomas.

In summary of immunologic privilege, both afferent and efferent arcs of immune response within the CNS have been established as functional by the following evidence: (1) antigen infusion into the cerebrospinal fluid can induce systemic humoral response; (2) graft rejection, albeit slow and possibly via nonclassic cell populations or interactions, does occur intracerebrally; (3) intracerebral transplants can induce a systemic response; and (4) effector cells and antibodies of systemic origin can enter the brain's parenchyma. It is also probable that the loss of the immune privilege presumed to exist in the normal brain occurs in nonnormal brain as the result of barrier compromise from neovascularity associated with neoplastic transformation, or as the result of an inflammatory process, as in experimental allergic encephalomyelitis.

CHARACTERISTICS OF THE INFLAMMATORY RESPONSE TO BRAIN TUMORS

Early observations estimated that focal, perivascular accumulations of tumor-infiltrating lymphocytes (TILs) occurred in 28–52% of human gliomas as determined in surgical biopsy material (Schiffer, Croveri and Pautasso, 1974; Takeuchi and Barnard, 1976), or in as high as 65% in postmortem

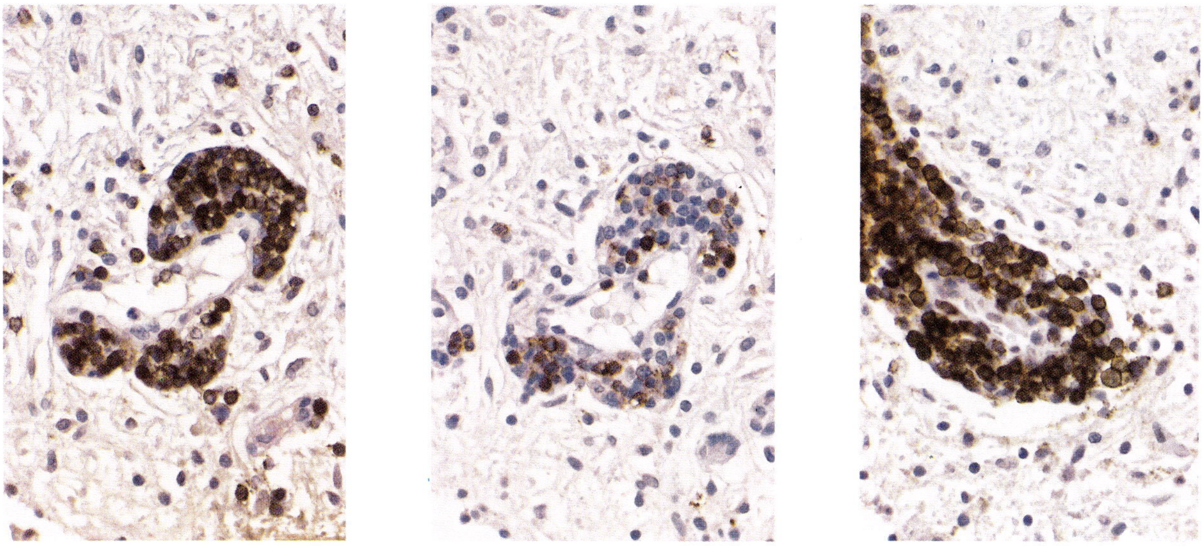

a b c

Fig. 7.2 Perivascular cellular infiltrates in high-grade malignant glioma. Predominant cell types present are CD3$^+$, CD8$^+$ and CD45RO$^+$ T lymphocytes. Sections were reacted with (a) CD3 (pan T cell), (b) CD8 (cytotoxic T cell) and (c) CD45RO (previously activated or memory T cells) antibodies. Immunoperoxidase method, hematoxylin counterstain; × 132

material (Ridley and Cavanagh, 1971). As reviewed by Hayes (1992), marked perivascular cuffing is usually associated with the less differentiated grades III and IV gliomas. However, diffuse infiltration throughout the tumor is confirmed in only a minority of cases (Fig. 7.1) and is generally only found within necrotic areas. Approximately one-fifth of anaplastic astrocytomas (Brooks *et al.*, 1978) exhibit clear infiltration, rarely deemed 'marked' cuffing. However, far fewer TILs are observed in gliomas as compared with other tumors, both systemic tumors and those metastatic to the CNS (Sawamura *et al.*, 1989; Morioka *et al.*, 1992). In a retrospective study of 149 cases of anaplastic astrocytoma or glioma, overall survival did not correlate with the presence of lymphocytic infiltration (Brooks *et al.*, 1978).

Inflammatory cell populations observed in brain tumors are predominantly T cells, and varying numbers of macrophages may be represented. Populations of NK and B cells are infrequent but have been documented (Black *et al.*, 1992; Sawamura and de Tribolet, 1995). Most studies characterizing brain TILs were performed on biopsy specimens. In these studies, TILs are generally small, nonblastic and negative for activation antigens (Miescher *et al.*, 1988; Sawamura and de Tribolet, 1995). The predominant class of TIL detected in multiple studies of primary brain tumors is the CD3$^+$, CD8$^+$ subset (Fig. 7.2) (Stevens, Klöter and Roggendorf, 1988; Kuppner, Hamou and de Tribolet, 1990; Hayes, 1992). This contrasts with the predominance of CD4$^+$ T cells and B cells found in intracranial carcinoma metastases to the CNS (Paine *et al.*, 1986; Stevens, Klöter and Roggendorf, 1988; Hayes, 1992). Some activation-associated antigens that have been identified *in situ*, and are expressed on most glioma-associated TILs, include CD58 and the 'activated' form of CD45R, CD45RO (Schwinzer, 1989), which identifies previously activated or memory T cells (Kuppner, Hamou and de Tribolet, 1990). In contrast to TILs, peritumoral lymphocytes examined in tissue sections are frequently 2- to 15-fold higher in number and express class II major histocompatibility and activation antigens (Black *et al.*, 1992).

Many groups have extended the immunophenotypic analysis of TILs by enzymatically digesting brain tumor specimens. These studies confirm that TILs are predominantly CD2$^+$ and CD3$^+$ T cells and do not express HLA-DR (histocompatibility antigens) or the IL-2 receptor (Miescher *et al.*, 1988). Interestingly, recent studies of TILs from disaggregated brain tumors with TCR-β chain analysis demonstrate that TILs are primarily oligoclonal (Fishleder *et al.*, 1990). Ebato *et al.* (1993, 1994) detected limited expression of the TCR-α variable region (*V*α) genes, with predominant usage of *V*α 7 within TILs. The TCR-β gene usage, while more diverse than that for *V*α, still demonstrated restriction, with 9/12 patients studied found to express TCR Vβ13.1 dominantly. This analysis was extended (Ebato *et al.*, 1994) to demonstrate that 84% of TIL clones obtained from 12 glioma patients expressed a shared Vβ13.1 sequence, whereas only 12.1% of similarly obtained peripheral blood lymphocyte clones from the same panel were committed to this sequence. While the authors did not assess these Vα7 and Vβ13.1 T cells for functional glioma-reactivity, the data suggest that clonal expansion of such lineage-specific T cells has occurred and that they may be recognizing glioma-specific antigens.

Another measure of brain TIL phenotype, although complicated by the provision of exogenous cytokines, is obtained by isolation of TILs from disaggregated brain tumor material after *in vitro* stimulation with IL-2. Sawamura *et al.* (1989) isolated TILs from human gliomas and anaplastic astrocytomas and expanded them in the presence of rIL-2 for 20–40 days. Subsequent phenotyping revealed, in keeping with other reports, that most cells (89%) were mature $CD3^+$ T cells. In contrast, however, virtually all of these IL-2-stimulated cells expressed MHC class II HLA-DRs, and there was an increase in $CD8^+$ cells along with a concomitant decrease in $CD4^+$ cells. Bosnes and Hirschberg (1989) also reported on TILs that were expanded in a similar fashion from 5/7 glioma specimens, and found they were not cytotoxic against autologous brain tumor, K562 or Daudi cells, ruling out not only the induction of cytotoxic TILs, but also the presence of NKs or recruited LAK activity from *in vivo*-activated cells. Similarly, Sawamura *et al.* (1989) could not demonstrate the low affinity IgG Fc receptor, which correlates with cytotoxic NK and LAK cell killing, on more than 1–6% of isolated, cultured TILs.

A variety of receptor–ligand systems have now been described on lymphocytes infiltrating brain tumors and on the brain tumor tissues. Most striking in terms of incidence is the demonstration of LFA-1 (CD11a/CD18) on perivascular brain TILs. The LFA-1 mediates nonspecific leukocyte adhesion by binding to ICAM-1 (CD54), which is prominently displayed on target glioma cells or on the endothelial cells of intratumoral vessels (Kuppner, Hamou and de Tribolet, 1990). Also found were LFA-1-positive intraparenchymal lymphocytes, present in 12/14 sections from human gliomas, suggesting that LFA-1 may play a role in the binding and migration of TILs in brain tumor tissue.

Originally described as a T-cell activation antigen, CD29 is the β-chain of the VLA (very late activation antigen) family of integrins, which function as leukocyte/cell matrix adhesion receptors. The CD29 molecule has been reported to be strongly expressed by endothelial cells of both normal and tumor-containing brain. In cases in which positive endothelial staining in brain tumor vessels was demonstrated, there was no evidence of glioma TIL staining for CD29 (Kuppner, Hamou and de Tribolet, 1990). The LFA-3/CD58 molecule has been demonstrated on glioma cells, and its ligand, the T-cell activation molecule CD2, has been demonstrated on brain TILs in the same biopsy sample (Kuppner, Hamou and de Tribolet, 1990). The CD44 molecules implicated in lymphocyte trafficking and in cellular interactions with the extracellular matrix are present on multiple cell types in normal and tumor-containing brain, including glial cells (Picker, Nakache and Butcher, 1989). Standard forms of the CD44 hyaluronate receptor are strongly expressed on high-grade gliomas and weakly expressed in meningiomas, medulloblastomas and cells in normal brain (Kuppner, Hamou and de Tribolet, 1990; Asher and Bignami, 1992; Kuppner *et al.*, 1992) (Fig. 7.3). However, CD44 splice variants associated with metastatic capacity are not detected immunohistochemically in gliomas, although they are abundantly present on extraneural tumor cells metastatic to the CNS (Li *et al.*, 1993; Ariza *et al.*, 1995).

CYTOKINE EXPRESSION ASSOCIATED WITH BRAIN TUMORS

The scant and apparently ineffective brain TIL population within gliomas undoubtedly results from a combination of immunomodulatory factors. Such factors may include a number of cytokines that have been identified as being produced either by glioma cells themselves or by inflammatory cells present in brain tumor tissue (Black *et al.*, 1992; Kurpad, Wikstrand and Bigner, 1994).

Immunosuppressive and growth-promoting cytokines

The variety of immunosuppressive or brain tumor-promoting cytokines suggests that this role of cytokines may be more extensive than that of immunostimulator. The most important of the immunosuppressive factors identified to date are the transforming growth factors-β (TGF-β1, TGF-β2 and TGF-β3). The TGF-βs are expressed by both glioma cells and normal brain, and exert a brain tumor-promoting effect via multiple

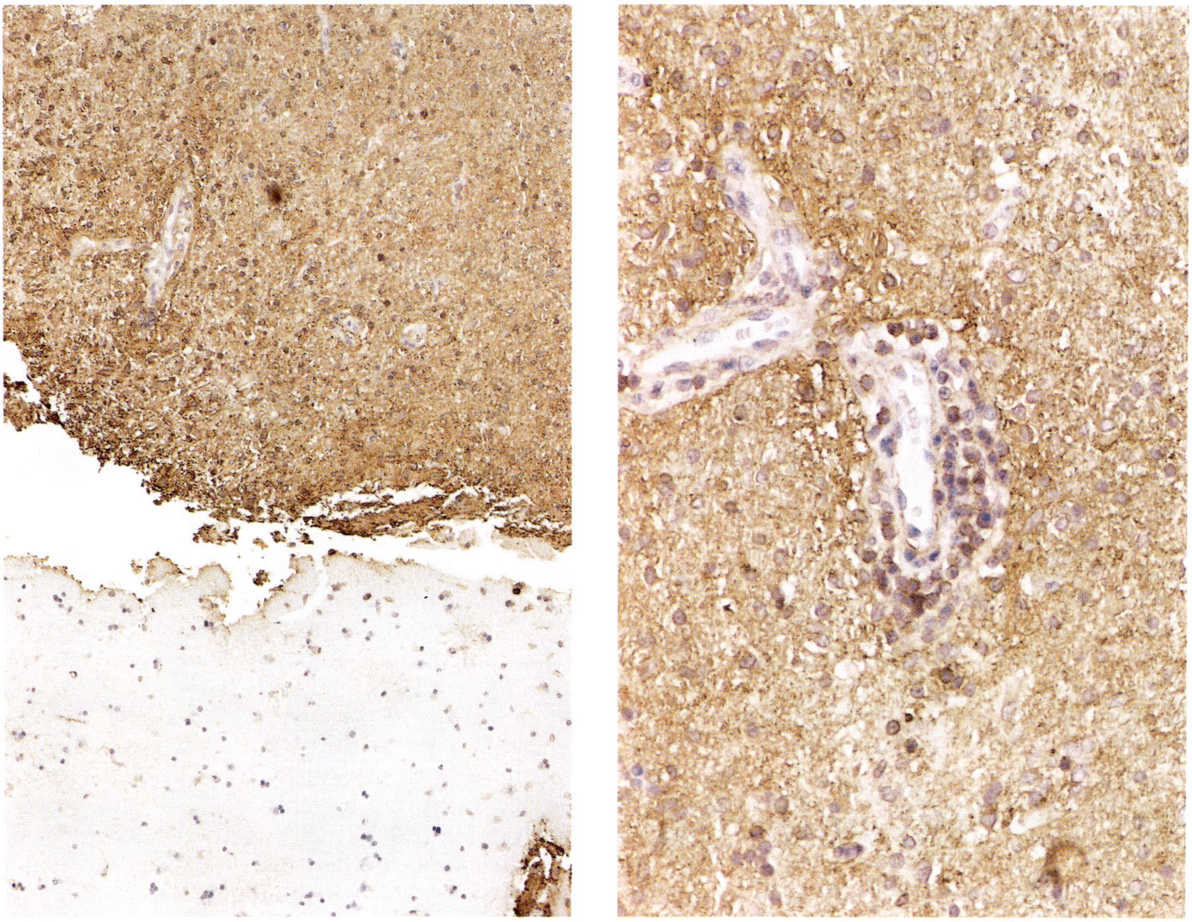

a b

Fig. 7.3 Expression of CD44 in high-grade malignant glioma. (a) Tumor (left) is highly reactive with CD44 antibody as compared with normal brain (right) in this fragmented biopsy. (b) Higher magnification shows strong fibrillar reactivity in tumor, as well as membrane reactivity of infiltrating lymphocytes and endothelial cells. Immunoperoxidase method, hematoxylin counterstain; (a) × 33, (b) × 66

immunoregulatory functions (Ashley *et al.*, 1997a). The TGF-βs most importantly act by inhibiting the proliferation and cytotoxic activity of brain tumor TILs, with additional inhibitory effects on B cells, NK cells, LAK cells and macrophages (Tada and de Tribolet, 1993). The TGF-βs also promote brain tumor growth by contributing to angiogenesis and possibly by serving as autocrine tumor cell growth factors (Kuppner *et al.*, 1989; Couldwell *et al.*, 1991; Yamanaka *et al.*, 1994). Whelan *et al.* (1993) have shown that an autocrine loop involving TGF-β on the *in vitro* growth of canine glioma cells may exist. This may provide a growth advantage early in the process of neoplastic transformation. In addition to stimulating cell growth, TGF-β1 has been characterized as a potent modulator of interactions between the extracellular matrix and the cell, including diffuse brain invasion by glioma cells, virtual lack of extracranial metastasis and invasion, and marked production of extracellular matrix components (collagens, integrins, fibronectin, laminin and tenascin) by glioma cells *in vitro* (Bourdon *et al.*, 1983; Paulus *et al.*, 1995.). Paulus *et al.* (1995) demonstrated that supplementing endogenous TGF-β1 production by the U-138 MG and U-373 MG human glioma cell lines with exogenous TGF-β1 increased collagen and α5-integrin chain synthesis, and augmented adhesion to extracellular matrix substrates.

The ILs have long been implicated in glioma growth. Interleukin-1 is variably expressed by many glioma cell lines tested (Elliott, Brooks and

Roszman, 1990; Ross *et al.*, 1994) and stimulates the production of IL-6 (Cinque *et al.*, 1992). Interleukin-6 is produced by glioma cells (Couldwell *et al.*, 1991) and both peritumoral and infiltrating lymphocytes (Black *et al.*, 1992), and is thought to facilitate tumor growth and inhibit immune recognition by reducing MHC class II HLA-DR expression. Expression of IL-10 by cultured glioma cells has recently been reported (Tada and de Tribolet, 1993). Interleukin-10 is a potent suppressor of the T_H1 response and, if produced *in vivo*, may act as an important immunosuppressive factor. A relationship between IL-6 and IL-10 expression was established by Huettner, Paulus and Roggendorf (1995) in human glioma tissue, by reverse transcriptase-polymerase chain reaction. Interleukin-10 mRNA was demonstrable in 37/37 glioma tissues sampled, with IL-6 mRNA in 30/37 tissues. The authors suggested that IL-6 provided a growth advantage to glioma cells, and that IL-10 contributed to brain tumor progression by suppressing the local immune response.

Tumor necrosis factor-α (TNF-α) is also produced by glioma cells and macrophages (Black *et al.*, 1992; Kurpad, Wikstrand and Bigner, 1994), and promotes brain tumor growth by angiogenic effects. The expression of TNF-α receptors by glioma cells suggests an autocrine loop effect, a theory supported by the work of Adachi *et al.* (1992), demonstrating that exogenous TNF-α significantly increases the density of epidermal growth factor receptors on cultured glioma cells, which may result in growth advantage.

Immunoenhancing and growth-suppressive cytokines

Peritumoral lymphocytes and TILs produce cytokines that are presumed to facilitate an effective *in situ* antitumor response (Black *et al.*, 1992). The T-cell proliferative and maturation factor IL-2, secreted by $CD4^+$ cells or derived from exogenous sources, has been demonstrated to antagonize the brain tumor-promoting effects of TGF-β (Sedlacek, 1994). Although conflicting data exist, it appears that the effect of IL-2 within gliomas may be compromised by the expression of an impaired p55 IL-2 receptor subunit in glioma-derived brain TILs (Roszman, Elliott and Brooks, 1991). The presence of such impaired receptors possibly underlies the generally reduced ability of glioma-derived brain TILs to proliferate *in vitro* after IL-2 stimulation (Sawamura *et al.*, 1989; Elliott, Brooks and Roszman, 1990; Roszman, Elliott and Brooks, 1991).

Interferon-γ is expressed by lymphocytes infiltrating into gliomas (Black *et al.*, 1992), and has also been demonstrated to counteract the effects of TGF-β and to increase MHC class II HLA-DR, neural cell adhesion molecule (NCAM/CD56) and ICAM-1/CD54 expression by glioma cells (Hong, Johannsen, and Krueger, 1991; Schneider *et al.*, 1992; Yamanaka *et al.*, 1994). Expression of MHC class I and class II antigens by murine glioma cell lines is enhanced after IFN-γ stimulation (Akbasak, Oldfield and Saris, 1991). Similarly, increased expression of MHC class I and ICAM-1 is found in the human glioma cell lines U-87 MG and U-251 MG after IFN-γ stimulation (Yin *et al.*, 1994). Intriguingly, however, these authors found that the increase in MHC class I antigen resulted in a decreased susceptibility of these cells to lysis by LAK cells *in vitro*. Conversely, the up regulation of MHC class II HLA-DR expression observed in glioma cells after exposure to TNF-α may well promote T-cell recognition (Kasahara *et al.*, 1991).

In summary, TILs are present in approximately half of human gliomas, predominantly in a perivascular location, with rare intraparenchymal extension. The predominant classes of brain TIL cells are $CD3^+$ and $CD8^+$ cytotoxic/suppressor T cells, with little evidence of NK or activated B cell involvement. Macrophages, though frequently observed, do not appear to be activated. In addition, the production, by glioma cells and brain tumor-associated inflammatory cells, of many cytokines with demonstrable brain tumor-enhancing and lymphocyte-suppressing activity, may contribute to a lack of effective host T-cell-mediated immune detection and response to these brain tumors.

Cell-mediated immunotherapy in brain tumors

Many studies have evaluated the efficacy of the infusion of immunocompetent cells as cytotoxic or cytostatic therapy for gliomas in both experimental systems and patient trials. Extensive reviews of such approaches to immunotherapy, involving nonspecific immunoadjuvants, biologic response modifiers and specific active immunization, have been published (Packer, Kramer and Ryan, 1991; Hayes, 1992; Sedlacek, 1994; Wikstrand and Bigner, 1996).

ANIMAL MODEL SYSTEMS

Two major classes of potential lymphocyte effectors were investigated in experimental model systems before the results were translated to patient studies. As described earlier, these classes consist of antigen-specific CTLs, of which brain TILs may be considered a subset, and nonantigen-specific LAK cells.

Cytotoxic T lymphocytes

Cytotoxic T lymphocytes have been obtained by priming lymphocytes *in vivo* with brain tumor cells, then restimulating these lymphocytes *in vitro* with the same or antigenically related brain tumor cells (Kurpad, Wikstrand and Bigner, 1994). Including IL-2 in the *in vitro* step considerably facilitates the induction of reactive CTLs, which are class I MHC restricted in target recognition (Townsend and Bodmer, 1989; Sakai, Chang and Shu, 1990). Several studies have claimed *in vivo* therapeutic efficacy of such CTLs in rodent systems (Sakai, Chang and Shu, 1990; Holladay, Heitz and Wood, 1992). Recently, Holladay *et al.* (1994) summarized their earlier investigations of the intracerebrally transplantable model based on RT-2, an anaplastic rat glioma. Briefly, lymphocytes isolated from rats bearing intracerebral RT-2 gliomas generally did not proliferate *in vitro* in response to exposure to RT-2 cells and IL-2, indicating that *in vivo* priming had not occurred. In the few instances in which proliferation did occur, the lymphocytes were not cytotoxic for autologous glioma. Conversely, lymphocytes isolated from rats bearing subcutaneous RT-2 tumors proliferated under the same conditions and exhibited RT-2-specific toxicity. Effector CTLs so generated, when administered in conjunction with IL-2, caused extended survival and potential cures in rats bearing intracerebral RT-2 gliomas. Cytotoxic T lymphocytes or IL-2 alone were ineffective. Similarly, Saris *et al.* (1992), using the GL261 primary murine brain tumor model, generated IL-2-stimulated TILs from subcutaneously grown tumor. The tumor-TILs were cytotoxic against target tumor cells *in vitro* and against liver metastases *in vivo* after the TILs were given intravenously, combined with daily intraperitoneal IL-2. They were ineffective against intracerebral tumor as assessed by comparing them with survival curves of animals receiving irradiation, IL-2 or various combinations thereof.

Recently, it was demonstrated that treating severe combined immunodeficient mice with a killer T-cell clone that was nonrestricted to the MHC, dependent on IL-2 and isolated from a patient with acute T-lymphoblastic leukemia (TALL-104 cells), resulted in a 50–70% reduction in the human glioma (U-87 MG) subcutaneously engrafted onto the mice. The T-cell clone was lethally irradiated and administered to the brain tumor site on multiple occasions. Although the *in vitro* IL-2-dependent TALL-104 line was active *in vivo* after irradiation and removal from IL-2, the cytocidal activity *in vivo* was definitely enhanced by stimulation with IL-2 or IL-12 immediately before transfer.

Lymphokine-activated killer cells

Extensive model therapy trials have been conducted with LAK cells. As described earlier, LAK cells are generated by *in vitro* stimulation of peripheral blood leukocytes with IL-2. The LAK cells are heterogeneous, exhibiting surface phenotypes of both T lymphocyte (T-LAK) and NK (NK-LAK) cells. Short-term cultured LAK cells (<1 week) are primarily T-LAKs and induce contact-mediated tumor cell lysis, with little or no tumor specificity (Barba *et al.*, 1989; Iwasaki *et al.*, 1990). After adhering to tumor targets, T-LAKs extend cellular processes into target cell cytoplasm, inducing a degenerative change similar to that seen with CTLs (Iwasaki *et al.*, 1990). Jääskelainen *et al.* (1990, 1992) have demonstrated that CD16 and $CD56^+$ LAK cells (NK-LAKs) are highly effective in migrating into glioma spheroids and lysing them, *in vitro*. The LAK cells obtained after longer culture periods are capable of mediating target cell lysis by contact or noncontact, and have been implicated in antibody-dependent cellular cytotoxicity systems (Iwasaki *et al.*, 1990; Kurpad, Wikstrand and Bigner 1994). The immediate effectors of target cell lysis may be the well-defined secretory granules present in these LAK cells.

Despite the ready demonstration of LAK cell effectiveness in *in vitro* cytotoxicity assays, there have been few studies of the *in vivo* administration of LAK cells in intracerebral tumor model systems. Tzeng *et al.* (1990) reported that administration of adherent, IL-2-generated LAK cells (A-LAKs) with systemic administration of IL-2 temporarily increased the survival time of Fischer rats bearing intracerebral F98 gliomas. However, all brain tumor-bearing animals treated with A-LAK died within 21 days of those receiving no treatment, suggesting that transient suppression, at best, was achieved, with eventual outgrowth of tumor. Although Nakagawa *et al.* (1992) reported that administering 5 Gy of irradiation in a similar rat intracerebral tumor model enhanced the brain tumor killing by LAK or NK cells, presumably by increasing the release of cytotoxic factors, no clear efficacy of effector cell administration was claimed. Surprisingly, most studies of *in vivo* efficacy of adoptively transferred cells were conducted in human patients.

In an attempt to increase the recognition by, and potential cytotoxic effect of, LAK cells, studies were also performed to facilitate the cross-linking of effector and target by using bispecific hybrid antibodies. Nitta *et al.* (1990) chemically conjugated CD3 MAb with an antiglioma-reactive monoclonal antibody (MAb) and administered this construct intralesionally to glioma patients; the authors claimed this gave brain tumor regression and/or eradication. Obukhov *et al.* (1992) used bispecific MAbs containing either CD3 or CD16 with CD56 to stimulate LAK cell activity versus CD56-positive brain tumor cell targets. The CD-16/CD56 conjugates were most effective, notably in $F(ab')_2$ format as compared with intact IgG. Although this enhancing effect was not observed *in vitro* when IL-2 concentration was optimal, the antibody treatment enhanced killing under suboptimal IL-2 concentration, which may be promising for human intracavitary administration.

CELL-MEDIATED IMMUNOTHERAPY IN HUMAN PATIENTS

Extensive summaries of adoptive cellular immunotherapy trials in brain tumor patients through 1992 were published by Merchant, Ellison and Young (1990), Hayes (1992) and Wen (1993). Although additional studies have been reported since these reviews, none has reported significant effects (Nakagawa *et al.*, 1995). Also, potential adverse effects, including the formation of granulation tissue with hypervascularization leading to hemorrhage, have been reported (Nagane *et al.*, 1993).

Adoptive cellular replacement therapy in glioma patients began in the early 1970s with intravenous, intracavitary or intralesional administration of non-activated peripheral blood lymphocytes or bone marrow cells (Takakura *et al.*, 1972; Takakura, Miki and Kubo, 1975; Young, Kaplan and Regelson 1977; Neuwelt *et al.*, 1978; Steinbok *et al.*, 1984). None of these studies demonstrated a significant extension of survival beyond that achieved by conventional therapy. Administration of IL-2-stimulated LAK cells dominated clinical trials in the 1980s and early 1990s. The intracavitary administration of IL-2 and LAK cells was most extensively investigated. Yoshida, Takai and Tanaka (1987) reported partial responses in 6/23 patients and clinical improvement in an additional 9/23. In a similar study of 17 patients with glioblastoma multiforme, Merchant *et al.* (1988a, 1988b) could demonstrate no difference in median survival between IL-2/LAK-treated patients and historical controls. The morbidity of intracavitary administration of IL-2 and LAK was revealed by Barba *et al.* (1989) in a study of nine patients treated with LAK cells and IL-2, delivered intralesionally by an intracavitary reservoir and catheter system. Only one partial response was seen, and neurologic side effects thought to be related to cerebral edema were seen in all patients. An adverse median survival of 9 weeks after reoperation was reported, as opposed to 22–30 weeks in historical controls. More importantly, the study was discontinued due to irreversible neurologic deficit that was unresponsive to additional steroid therapy and was attributed to dose-limiting toxicity of intracavitary IL-2. A more promising study involving intracavitary LAK cell and IL-2 treatment has been reported (Hayes *et al.*, 1995). In this study, the author claims that the median survival of 19 treated patients increased to 53 weeks. Lower doses of IL-2 were used in this study than were previously administered. Once again, the dose-limiting toxicity was neurologic and was seen in 2/3 patients at 2.4 million IU IL-2. Pericavitary necrosis and the presence of predominant eosinophilic infiltrates and perivascular lymphocytes were observed in five tissue samples examined; viable tumor cells were also present.

Studies with LAK cells variously stimulated or selected *ex vivo* with mitogens such as phytohemagglutinin (PHA), cytokines (TNF-α) or anti-receptor antibodies (OKT3) have not improved upon standard IL-2/LAK therapy (Lillehei *et al.*, 1991; Koberda, Grimm and Moser, 1993; Koberda *et al.*, 1994). Although OKT3 activation of LAK cells resulted in a $CD8^+$ lytic population *in vitro* (Yang *et al.*, 1990), no significant effect was seen *in vivo*. Finally, Kitahara *et al.* (1987) established IL-2-dependent CTL lines from the peripheral blood of five patients with brain tumors and administered these cell lines without the maintenance IL-2 intracavitarily. Responses were seen in two patients but, unfortunately, the small number of patients in this study precluded meaningful evaluation.

Conventional adoptive transfer experiments with CTLs (including TILs) and LAK cells in patient trials have not been encouraging. While both CTLs and TILs could be administered intravenously (Ratner and Heppner, 1988; Kasid *et al.*, 1990), the technical difficulties in generation of CTLs and expansion of sufficient brain TILs in glioma patients (Sawamura and de Tribolet, 1995) produced both treatment delays and poor expansion of effector populations. In addition, in a series of four patients, CD3-selected TILs expanded with IL-2 were not necessarily more cytotoxic than were autologous LAK cells (Kikuchi, Watanabe and Ohno 1991). Although LAK cells were readily generated in sufficient numbers for rapid therapy, they did not traffic well to the site of the brain tumor when administered intravenously (Lotze *et al.*, 1980), and they required exogenous IL-2 for delivery to the brain tumor site. Even local delivery did not accomplish extension of LAK cells throughout an infiltrative tumor, and lack of sufficient IL-2 resulted in loss of a LAK-mediated tumor kill (Hayes, 1992). On the other hand, continued maintenance of sufficient IL-2 levels might result in toxicity due to vascular leak syndrome leading to cerebral edema (Rosenberg *et al.*, 1987; Kurpad, Wikstrand and Bigner, 1994).

In summary of cell-mediated therapy, 20 years of study, employing both model systems and patient trials of adoptive cell transfer in brain tumors, have failed to show clear efficacy and have been hampered by substantial toxicity (List *et al.*, 1992). Clearly, novel approaches are required if the immunologic response in brain tumor patients is to be rendered an effective therapeutic tool.

The efficacy of allogeneic tumor cell vaccines for brain tumors has been examined (Bullard *et al.*, 1985). In a phase II study, 20 patients with malignant gliomas were actively immunized monthly with one of two tissue culture cell lines (D-54 MG or U-251 MG), the first injection of which included 500 μg of bacillus Calmette-Guerin cell wall. Each patient also received levamisole, 2.5 mg/kg, for 3 days per week, every other week. Radiotherapy and chemotherapy with BCNU [1,3-bis(2-chloroethyl)-1-nitrosourea] were begun after the first month of immunization. No evidence of allergic encephalomyelitis was noted clinically, nor was any gross or microscopic evidence of such pathology obtained upon autopsy of three of these patients. Serial studies of general immune competence showed no alterations from those previously described with nonimmunized patients. Most patients mounted a significant serum reaction to HLAs, as well as an antibody response to fetal bovine serum, which was added to the glioma-cell inoculum. Further to these studies, a larger phase III study was performed. Patients who were inoculated with allogeneic vaccines had a longer survival time compared with historical cases of glioma patients treated with levamisole, radiation therapy and chemotherapy alone. However, strict entry criteria for the study, including the following, may have heavily biased such comparisons: a Karnofsky Functional Rating equal to or greater than 70, a peripheral blood lymphocyte count equal to or greater than 1000 cells/mm^3, skin test responses to one or more of four recall antigens, peripheral blood T cells equal to or greater than half that of control, and not receiving steroid therapy at the time of entry into the study (G.Y. Gillespie, personal communication, 1996).

New approaches to cell-mediated immunotherapy in brain tumors

As outlined above, a variety of factors are believed to lead to a deficient host immune response to brain tumors. These may include: (1) production of lymphocyte-suppressive cytokines or other substances by gliomas (Wrann *et al.*, 1987; Roszman, Elliott and Brooks, 1992), (2) decreased expression of MHC molecules by glioma cells (Sedlacek, 1994) and (3) paucity of activation and/or activation potential of TILs in human gliomas (Miescher *et al.*, 1988; Roszman, Elliott and Brooks, 1992; Sawamura and de Tribolet, 1995). Moreover, the poor efficacy of systemically administered TILs or CTLs against intracerebral tumor (Saris *et al.*, 1992; Holladay *et al.*, 1994), combined with the CNS toxicity of the necessary adjunctive cytokine concentrations, have led investigators to explore novel approaches toward modifying or abrogating these brain tumor-promoting effects through the alterations of the target cells, effector cells or both.

ALTERATIONS OF BRAIN TUMOR TARGET CELLS

The effects of cytokine secretion by tumor cells upon their growth and susceptibility to cell-mediated killing have been examined by either transfection of transplantable tumor cell lines, *ex vivo*, or coadministration of target tumor and cytokine-secreting cells. These approaches were undertaken potentially to increase the presentation of covert tumor-associated antigens and their interactions with the immune system. It has long been established that administration of IFN-γ results in the reduction of tumorigenicity through the up regulation of MHC I and recognition by MHC-restricted cytotoxic lymphocytes (Goodenow, Vogel and Linsk, 1985). Furthermore, Watanabe *et al.* (1989) reported on a series of murine C1300 neuroblastoma cell lines transfected with mouse IFN-γ cDNA, in which outgrowth of tumor cells, upon transplantation to syngeneic A/J mice, was inversely proportional to the level of IFN-γ expressed. The outgrowth of high-producing tumors was strongly suppressed, independent of the level of MHC expression. As administration of anti-IFN-γ MAb reversed this effect, it was hypothesized that an augmented antitumor T-cell response elicited by secreted IFN-γ was responsible for the tumor suppression. In a similar study, Mizuno *et al.* (1994) determined that the up regulation of ICAM-1 was responsible for the enhanced susceptibility of IFN-γ-transfected cells to LAK cells. Similar up regulation of ICAM-1 after tumor cell transfection with the TNF-α gene was also reported to result in increased susceptibility of the transfected targets to LAK cell cytolysis *in vitro* (Takaoka *et al.*, 1994).

Several groups have transfected brain tumor cell targets with genes encoding the interleukins in an attempt to increase brain tumor cell immunogenicity. Transfection of the murine 203 ependymoblastoma with the IL-7 gene resulted in IL-7 dose-dependent suppression of tumor outgrowth. This study implicated CD8$^+$ T-lymphocyte-mediated rejection of tumors. Increased expression of MHC antigens was not observed and was assumed not to be contributing to the enhanced T-cell reactivity (Aoki *et al.*, 1992). We have also recently investigated such a cytokine transfection strategy in an astrocytoma that arose spontaneously in inbred VM mice and that naturally produces active TGF-β. Retroviral vectors were used to transfect the astrocytoma cells *in vitro* with the genes encoding a variety of murine cytokines, including IL-2, IL-3, IL-4, IL-6, TNF-α, IFN-γ or granulocyte-macrophage colony-stimulating factor (GM-CSF). Although cytokine production from transfected cells failed to reduce the astrocytoma cell growth *in vitro* and failed to abrogate TGF-β production, in reproducible experiments, most mice given injections of 560 cells producing IL-2 (n = 15), IL-4 (n = 15) or TNF-α (n = 5) failed to develop tumors. In these groups, 80%, 66.6% and 60% of the mice, respectively, remained alive without evidence of tumor at 100 days. This survival rate was significantly better than that for mice given injections of untransfected cells; their median survival was only 26 ± 2 days ($P < 0.025$). All other cytokines tested failed to increase survival (Sampson *et al.*, 1996a).

Several investigators have examined the cotransplantation of tumor cells with cytokine-secreting cells. Intracerebral cotransplantation of IL-4-secreting LT-1 plasmacytoma cells with the U-87 MG human glioma line into athymic mice effected prolonged survival compared with U-87 MG alone. The absence of viable brain tumor cells and presence of necrosis and an eosinophilic infiltrate 19–50 days after treatment suggested complete brain tumor regression (Yu *et al.*, 1993). Coimplantation of RG-2 glioma cells and retrovirally infected cell lines producing IL-2 or IFN-γ generated a cell-mediated antitumor response. However, this response was short lived, and animals suffered the effects of severe toxicity, including vasogenic brain edema and early demise, similar to those observed in human studies with IL-2 (Tjuvajev *et al.*, 1995). Finally, coimplantation of IL-2 and IFN-γ-producing allogeneic fibroblasts with the G1261 glioma (Glick *et al.*, 1995) produced increased survival as compared with G1261 alone. Differences in these studies underscore the difficulties in establishing optimum conditions for this type of therapy with such a narrow therapeutic window, and the potentially detrimental consequences should toxicity be observed.

A number of groups have reported the efficacy of using tumor cells in which cytokine genes have been transfected as vaccines for systemic tumors. Dranoff *et al.* (1993) reported such an approach using a variety of cytokines, including IL-5, IL-6, IFN-γ, TNF or GM-CSF. These studies showed that GM-CSF-producing tumor cells were the most effective potentiators of *in vivo* immunogenicity, possibly by virtue of activation of antigen-presenting cells. More recently, Sampson *et al.* (1996a) demonstrated that similar protocols were successful within the CNS. Irradiated B16-F10 murine melanoma (B16) cells, genetically engineered to produce GM-CSF, IL-3 or IL-6 and used as a subcutaneous vaccination, stimulated a potent and persistent response to intracerebral B16 tumors, increasing the survival of tumor-bearing mice. The IL-4- or IFN-γ-transfected cells had no effect. The specific anti-B16 response was abrogated by systemic CD8$^+$ lymphocyte depletion. Interestingly, depletion of CD4$^+$ cells, putatively an important effector in subcutaneous tumors, did not have an adverse effect on the survival of immunized animals. Dranoff *et al.* (1993) and Vieweg *et al.* (1994) also reported that transfection with the gene for IL-2 increased immunogenicity of transfected cells. However, Ram *et al.* (1994) found that transfection of 9L gliosarcoma cells with the *IL-2* gene did not reduce the degree of brain tumor outgrowth as compared with nontransfected controls. Similarly, Sampson *et al.* (1996a) found that vaccination with IL-2-producing cells decreased median survival times significantly in the B16 model.

A number of recent studies carried out in humans have demonstrated that tumor-specific T cells are present in patients bearing tumors. Furthermore, a number of tumor-specific antigens recognized by CD8$^+$ T cells have been isolated and cloned, such as MAGE-1 (*MAGEA1*), MAGE-3 (*MAGEA3*), tyrosinase, MART-1 and gp-100. Much work is currently underway in an attempt to generate meaningful cell-mediated immune responses to these tumor-specific antigens (Kawakami and Robbins, 1995). The epidermal growth factor receptor (*EGFR*) gene in malignant gliomas frequently contains amplifications and rearrangements that are significant and potentially detectable by immunological means, and this gene may represent an example of such a tumor-specific antigen (Batra *et al.*, 1994).

Recently, using the most common variant of the EGFR (EGFRvIII) antigen as a model, we developed and evaluated an active immunotherapeutic strategy. In these studies, we presented the EGFR antigen, which is specific to brain tumors, for processing in the milieu of allogeneic cell rejection. Past studies had demonstrated the utility of an allogeneic antigen presentation system in nontumor models for producing class I-restricted immunity. Such an immunization strategy has been termed 'cross-priming' (Bevan, 1976, 1995). In these experiments, an allogeneic cell line was transfected to express EGFRvIII. Allogeneic cell/EGFRvIII-immunized mice developed significant cytotoxicity against syngeneic B16 cells transfected with EGFRvIII. *In vitro* antibody blockade of lymphocyte function demonstrated the CD8 phenotype of the effector cells involved in this cytolytic activity. After the same immunizations with the allogeneic/EGFRvIII vaccine, 50% of animals immunized survived intracranial tumor challenge with syngeneic B16/EGFRvIII cells. Further studies demonstrated that the generation of this immunity by so-called cross-priming is antigen specific, MHC class I-restricted and is mediated by both $CD8^+$ and $CD4^+$ cells *in vivo* (Ashley *et al.*, 1997b).

Attempts to enhance immunogenicity or cytolytic susceptibility of brain tumor targets, both *ex vivo* and *in vivo*, have met with mixed results. Regionally, increased levels of cytokines may have adverse effects, including stimulation of tumor growth. The cytokines IFN-γ, TGF-β and TNF-α have all been found to enhance glioma cell proliferation (Wrann *et al.*, 1987; Black *et al.*, 1992; Kurpad, Wikstrand and Bigner, 1994; Yin *et al.*, 1994; Paulus *et al.*, 1995). Similarly, IL-6 and IL-10 are also considered to be brain tumor-promoting (Huettner, Paulus and Roggendorf, 1995). In addition, introducing cytokine-producing cells that bear antigens present in the CNS raises the potential for inducing experimental autoimmune encephalitis, as demonstrated by Bigner, Pitts and Wikstrand (1981) in macaques that were given injections of normal CNS or brain tumor tissue. Finally, as now well demonstrated by a number of different studies, these potent immunoregulatory molecules may cause CNS damage through vasogenic effects and edema. Therefore, the effects of *in vivo* introduction of cytokine-secreting brain tumor cells must be carefully examined in further studies before proceeding to human trials.

ALTERATION OF EFFECTOR CELLS

Although glioma cells have repeatedly been shown to express highly immunogenic cell surface molecules (Kurpad, Wikstrand and Bigner, 1994; Wikstrand and Bigner, 1996), the efferent immune response may be insufficient to eradicate an existing tumor burden (Sedlacek, 1994). Accordingly, some investigators are exploring means of augmenting the reactivity of various effector cell populations. Providing bispecific targeting antibody chimeras to an ongoing cell-target interaction has been shown to enhance the cytocidal effect of LAK cells (Obukhov *et al.*, 1992). Such 'directed' LAK cells were well tolerated when administered intralesionally, and were claimed to be effective in tumor cell cytolysis (Nitta *et al.*, 1990). Genotypic enhancement of LAK cells has been attempted by the introduction of the human *TNF-α* gene by liposomal transfection into IL-2-activated LAK cells (Tashiro *et al.*, 1993). These cells secreted high levels of TNF-α and exhibited enhanced cytotoxicity of U-251 MG human glioma cells *in vitro*. The increased expression of TNF-α on the surface of LAK cells was claimed to be the crucial component. Whether this approach will be feasible *in vivo*, considering the brain tumor potentiating effects of TNF-α (Adachi *et al.*, 1992; Black *et al.*, 1992), remains unexamined.

Summary

Brain tumors are not unique in their resistance to the host immune response; they share the same mechanisms of escape from immune surveillance with tumors of nonneural origin. The modes of resistance include inhibition of the afferent and efferent pathways of the immune response, release of immunosuppressive molecules, and down regulation or abnormal expression of MHC and other immunoregulatory molecules. The features that are unique to CNS tumors and that make cell-mediated approaches to therapy difficult include the partial immune afferent and efferent immunoprivilege as demonstrated by Saris *et al.* (1992) and Holladay *et al.* (1994), the paucity and comparative inactivity of TILs in gliomas and the confines of the intrathecal compartment itself, which renders even transient edema or robust inflammatory response potentially lethal. Although methods for *in vivo* transfection of brain tumor targets are in development, problems of delivery to target cells are inevitable. Successful immunotherapeutic regimens must seek to counter the immunosuppressive effects of endogenously produced soluble mediators. The exquisite specificity of target recognition that characterizes the mammalian immune response, both humoral and cell-mediated, makes possible the specific delivery of a variety of cytocidal or cytostatic compounds, including drugs, toxins and substrates for systemic activation. The complex of sequential actions of all of the components of that response, however, must also be understood before a meaningful manipulation of the individual pathways can be attempted.

References

Adachi, K., Belser, P., Bender, H., Li, D., Rodeck, U., Benveniste, E.N., Woo, D., Schmiegel, W.H. and Herlyn, D. (1992) Enhancement of epidermal growth factor receptor expression on glioma cells by recombinant tumor necrosis factor-α. *Cancer Immunology, Immunotherapy* **34**, 370–6.

Akbasak, A., Oldfield, E.H. and Saris, S.C. (1991) Expression and modulation of major histoincompatibility antigens on murine primary brain tumors *in vitro*. *Journal of Neurosurgery* **75**, 922–9.

Aoki, T., Tashiro, K., Miyatake, S., Kinashi, T., Nakano, T., Oda, Y., Kikuchi, H. and Honjo, T. (1992) Expression of murine interleukin 7 in murine glioma cell line results in reduced tumorigenicity *in vivo*. *Proceedings of the National Academy of Sciences U.S.A.* **89**, 3850–4.

Ariza, A., Lopez, D., Mate, J.L., Isamet, M., Musulen, E., Pijol, M., Ley, A. and Navas-Palacios, J.J. (1995) Role of CD44 in the invasiveness of glioblastoma multiforme and the noninvasiveness of meningioma: an immunohistochemistry study. *Human Pathology* **26**, 1144–7.

Asher, R. and Bignami, A. (1992) Hyaluronate binding and CD44 expression in human glioblastoma cells and astrocytes. *Experimental Cell Research* **203**, 80–90.

Ashley, D.M., Kong, F.M., Bigner, D.D. and Hale, L.P. (1997a) Endogenous expression of transforming growth factor β1 inhibits growth and tumorigenicity and enhances *Fas*-mediated apoptosis in a murine high grade glioma model. Submitted

Ashley, D.M., Sampson, J.H., Archer, G.E., Batra, S.K., Bigner, D.D. and Hale, L.P. (1997b) A genetically modified allogeneic cellular vaccine generates MHC class I-restricted cytotoxic responses against tumor-associated antigens and protects against CNS tumors *in vivo*. *Journal of Neuroimmunology*, in press.

Barba, D., Saris, S.C., Holder, C., Rosenberg, S.A. and Oldfield, E.H. (1989) Intratumoral LAK cell and interleukin-2 therapy of human gliomas. *Journal of Neurosurgery* **70**, 175–82.

Batra, S.K., Rasheed, B.K.A., Bigner, S.H. and Bigner, D.D. (1994) Oncogenes and anti-oncogenes in human central nervous system tumors. *Laboratory Investigation* **71**, 621–37.

Bevan, M.J. (1976) Cross-priming for a secondary cytotoxic response to minor H antigens with H-2 congenic cells which do not cross-react in the cytotoxic assay. *Journal of Experimental Medicine* **143**, 1283–8.

——(1995) Antigen presentation to cytotoxic T lymphocytes *in vivo*. *Journal of Experimental Medicine* **182**, 639–41.

Bigner, D.D., Fritz, R.B. and Day, E.D. (1969) Cerebral physiology in dogs after brain tumor induction with Schmidt-Ruppin Rous sarcoma virus: experiences with radioiodinated normal and antiviral immunoglobulin G. *Journal of the National Cancer Institute* **43**, 565–73.

Bigner, D.D., Pitts, O.M. and Wikstrand, C.J. (1981) Induction of lethal experimental allergic encephalomyelitis in nonhuman primates and guinea pigs with human glioblastoma multiforme tissue. *Journal of Neurosurgery* **55**, 32–42.

Bigner, D.D., Self, D.J., Frey, J., Ishizaki, R., Langlois, A.J. and Swenberg, J.A. (1975) Refinement of the avian oncornavirus-induced primary rat brain tumor model for therapeutic screening. *Recent Results in Cancer Research* **51**, 20–34.

Black, K.L., Chen, K., Becker, D.P. and Merrill, J.E. (1992) Inflammatory leukocytes associated with increased immunosuppression by glioblastoma. *Journal of Neurosurgery* **77**, 120–6.

Bosnes, V. and Hirschberg, H. (1989) Immunomagnetic separation of infiltrating T lymphocytes from brain tumors. *Journal of Neurosurgery* **71**, 218–23.

Bourdon, M.A., Wikstrand, C.J., Furthmayr, H., Matthews, T.J. and Bigner, D.D. (1983) Human glioma-mesenchymal extracellular matrix antigen defined by monoclonal antibody. *Cancer Research* **43**, 2796–805.

Brooks, W. H., Markesbery, W.R., Gupta, G.D. and Roszman, T.L. (1978) Relationship of lymphocyte invasion and survival of brain tumor patients. *Annals of Neurology* **4**, 219–24.

Bullard, D.E., Thomas, D.G.T., Darling, J.L., Wikstrand, C.J., Diengdoh, J.V., Barnard, R.O., Bodmer, J.G. and Bigner, D.D. (1985) A preliminary study utilizing viable HLA mismatched cultured glioma cells as adjuvant therapy for patients with malignant gliomas. *British Journal of Cancer* **51**, 283–9.

Cinque, S., Willems, J., Depraetere, S., Vermeire, L. and Joniau, M. (1992) '*In vitro*' effect of interleukin-1 β on human glioma cell lines: regulation of cell proliferation and IL-6 production. *Immunology Letters* **34**, 267–71.

Couldwell, W.T., Dore-Duffy, P., Apuzzo, M.L.J. and Antel, J.P. (1991) Malignant glioma modulation of immune function: relative contribution of different soluble factors. *Journal of Neuroimmunology* **33**, 89–96.

Denlinger, R.H., Swenberg, J.A., Koestner, A. and Wechsler, W. (1973) Differential effect of immunosuppression on the induction of nervous system and bladder tumors by *N*-methyl *N*-nitrosourea. *Journal of the National Cancer Institute* **50**, 87–93.

Dranoff, G., Jaffee, E., Lazenby, A., Golumbek, P., Levitsky, H., Brose, K., Jackson, V., Hamada, H., Pardoll, D. and Mulligan, R.C. (1993) Vaccination with irradiated tumor cells engineered to secrete murine granulocyte-macrophage colony-stimulating factor stimulates potent, specific, and long-lasting anti-tumor immunity. *Proceedings of the National Academy of Sciences U.S.A.* **90**, 3539–43.

Ebato, M., Nitta, T., Yagita, H., Sato, K. and Okumura, K. (1993) Skewed distribution of TCR Vα 7-bearing T cells within tumor-infiltrating lymphocytes of HLA-A24(9)-positive patients with malignant glioma. *Immunology Letters* **39**, 53–64.

— (1994) Shared amino acid sequences in the NDβN and Nα regions of the T cell receptors of tumor-infiltrating lymphocytes within malignant glioma. *European Journal of Immunology* **24**, 2987–92.

Eby, N.L., Grufferman, S., Flannelly, C.M., Schold, S.C. Jr, Vogel, F.S. and Burger, P.C. (1988) Increasing incidence of primary brain lymphomas in the U.S. *Cancer* **62**, 2461–5.

Elliott, L.H., Brooks, W.H. and Roszman, T.L. (1990) Inability of mitogen-activated lymphocytes obtained from patients with maligant primary intracranial tumors to express high affinity interleukin 2 receptors. *Journal of Clinical Investigation* **86**, 80–6.

Fidler, I.J. and Schroit, A.J. (1988) Recognition and destruction of neoplastic cells by activated macrophages: discrimination of altered self. *Biochimica Biophysica Acta* **948**, 151–73.

Fishleder, A.J., Finke, J.H., Tubbs, R. and Bukowski, R.M. (1990) Induction by interleukin-2 of oligoclonal expansion of cultured tumor-infiltrating lymphocytes. *Journal of the National Cancer Institute* **82**, 124–8.

Fitch, F.W., McKisic, M.D., Lancki, D.W. and Gajewski, T.F. (1993) Differential regulation of murine T lymphocyte subsets. *Annual Review of Immunology* **11**, 29–48.

Fraser, J.D., Straus, D. and Weiss, A. (1993) Signal transduction events leading to T-cell lymphokine gene expression. *Immunology Today* **14**, 357–62.

Frey, J.L., Bino, T., Kantor, R.R., Segal, D.M., Giardina, S.L., Roder, J., Anderson, S. and Ortaldo, J.R. (1991) Mechanism of target cell recognition by natural killer cells: characterization of a novel triggering molecule restricted to $CD3^-$ large granular lymphocytes. *Journal of Experimental Medicine* **174**, 1527–36.

Glick, R.P., Lichtor, T., Kim, T.S., Ilangovan, S. and Cohen, E.P. (1995) Fibroblasts genetically engineered to secrete cytokines suppress tumor growth and induce antitumor immunity to a murine glioma *in vivo*. *Neurosurgery* **36**, 548–55.

Goodenow, R.S., Vogel, J.M. and Linsk, R.L. (1985) Histocompatibility antigens on murine tumors. *Science* **230**, 777–83.

Groothuis, D.R., Vriesendorp, F.J., Kupfer, B., Warnke, P.C., Lapin, G.D., Kuruvilla, A., Vick, N.A., Mikhael, M.A. and Patlak, C.S. (1991) Quantitative measurements of capillary transport in human brain tumors by computed tomography. *Annals of Neurology* **30**, 581–8.

Hayes, R.L. (1992) The cellular immunotherapy of primary brain tumors. *Revue Neurologique* **148**, 454–66.

Hayes, R.L., Koslow, M., Hiesiger, E.M., Hymes, K.R., Hochster, H.S., Moore, E.J., Pierz, D.M., Chen, D.K., Budzilovich, G.N. and Ransohoff, J. (1995) Improved long term survival after intracavitary interleukin-2 and lymphokine-activated killer cells for adults with recurrent malignant glioma. *Cancer* **76**, 840–52.

Holladay, F.P., Heitz, T. and Wood, G.W. (1992) Antitumor activity against established intracerebral gliomas exhibited by cytotoxic T lymphocytes, but not by lymphokine-activated killer cells. *Journal of Neurosurgery* **77**, 757–62.

Holladay, F.P., Choudhuri, R., Heitz, T. and Wood, G.W. (1994) Generation of cytotoxic immune responses during the progression of a rat glioma. *Journal of Neurosurgery* **80**, 90–6.

Hong, L.L., Johannsen, L. and Krueger, J.M. (1991) Modulation of human leucocyte antigen DR expression in glioblastoma cells by interferon-γ and other cytokines. *Journal of Neuroimmunology* **35**, 139–52.

Huettner, C., Paulus, W. and Roggendorf, W. (1995) Messenger RNA expression of the immunosuppressive cytokine IL-10 in human gliomas. *American Journal of Pathology* **146**, 317–22.

Iwasaki, K., Kikuchi, H., Miyatake, S., Aoki, T., Yamasaki, T. and Oda, Y. (1990) Infiltrative and cytolytic activities of LAK cells against a human glioma spheroid model. *Cancer Research* **50**, 2429–36.

Jääskelainen, J., Lehtonen, E., Heikkila, P., Kalliomaki, P. and Timonen, T. (1990) Damage to multicellular human H-2 glioma spheroids incubated with LAK cells: an ultrastructural study. *Journal of the National Cancer Institute* **82**, 497–501.

Jääskelainen, J., Maenpaa, A., Patarroyo, M., Gahmberg, C.G., Somersalo, K., Tarkkanen, J., Kallio, M. and Timonen, T. (1992) Migration of recombinant IL-2 activated T and natural killer cells in the intercellular space of human H-2 glioma spheroids *in vitro*. A study on adhesion molecules involved. *Journal of Immunology* **149**, 260–8.

Jellinger, K.A. and Paulus, W. (1992) Primary central nervous system lymphomas—an update. *Journal of Cancer Research and Clinical Oncology* **119**, 7–27.

Kasahara, T., Mukaida, N., Yamashita, K., Yagasawa, H., Akahoshi, T. and Matsushima, K. (1991) IL-1 and TNF-α induction of IL-8 and monocyte chemotactic and activating factor (MCAF) mRNA expression in a human astrocytoma cell line. *Immunology* **74**, 60–7.

Kasid, A., Morecki, S., Aebersold, P., Cornetta, K., Culver, K., Freeman, S., Director, E., Lotze, M.T., Blaese, R.M., Anderson, W.F. and Rosenberg, S.A. (1990) Human gene transfer: characterization of human tumor-infiltrating lymphocytes as vehicles for retroviral-mediated gene transfer in man. *Proceedings of the National Academy of Sciences U.S.A.* **87**, 473–7.

Kawakami, Y. and Robbins, P.F. (1995) Biology of tumor antigens. In DeVita, V.T., Hellman, S. and Rosenberg, S.A. (eds), *Biologic therapy of cancer*. Second edition. Philadelphia: J.B. Lippincott, 53–64.

Kida, S., Weller, R.O., Zhang, E.-T., Phillips, M.J. and Iannotti, F. (1995) Anatomical pathways for lymphatic drainage of the brain and their pathological significance. *Neuropathology and Applied Neurobiology* **21**, 181–4.

Kikuchi, T., Watanabe, M. and Ohno, T. (1991) Cytological characteristics of human glioma-infiltrating lymphocytes stimulated with recombinant interleukin 2 and an anti-CD3 antibody. *Japanese Journal of Cancer Research* **82**, 339–45.

Kitahara, T., Watanabe, O., Yamaura, A., Makino, H., Watanabe, T., Suzuki, G. and Okumura, K. (1987) Establishment of interleukin-2 dependent cytotoxic T lymphocyte cell line specific for autologous brain tumor and intracranial administration for therapy of the tumor. *Journal of Neuro-Oncology* **4**, 329–36.

Knopf, P.M., Cserr, H.F., Nolan, S.C., Wu, T.-Y. and Harling-Berg, C.J. (1995) Physiology and immunology of lymphatic drainage of interstitial and cerebrospinal fluid from the brain. *Neuropathology and Applied Neurobiology* **21**, 175–80.

Koberda, J., Grimm, E.A. and Moser, R.P. (1993) Effect of anti-CD3/anti-CD28/interleukin-2 stimulation of mononuclear cells on transforming growth factor β inhibition of lymphokine-activated killer cell generation. *Journal of Cancer Research and Clinical Oncology* **119**, 131–6.

Koberda, J., Przepiorka, D., Moser, R.P. and Grimm, E.E. (1994) Sequential TNF and TGF-beta regulation of expansion and induction of cytotoxicity in long term cultures of lymphokine-activated killer cells. *Lymphokine and Cytokine Research* **13**, 139–45.

Kovacsovics-Bankowski, M. and Rock, K.L. (1995) A phagosome-to-cytosol pathway for exogenous antigens presented on MHC class I molecules. *Science* **267**, 243–6.

Kuppner, M.C., Hamou, M.-F. and de Tribolet, N. (1990) Activation and adhesion molecule expression on lymphoid infiltrates in human glioblastomas. *Journal of Neuroimmunology* **29**, 229–38.

Kuppner, M.C., Hamou, M.F., Sawamura, Y., Bodmer, S. and de Tribolet, N. (1989) Inhibition of lymphocyte function by glioblastoma-derived transforming growth factor-β2. *Journal of Neurosurgery* **71**, 211–17.

Kuppner, M.C., Van Meir, E., Gauthier, T., Hamou, M.F. and de Tribolet, N. (1992) Differential expression of the CD44 molecule in human brain tumours. *International Journal of Cancer* **50**, 572–7.

Kurpad, S.K., Wikstrand, C.J. and Bigner, D.D. (1994) Immunobiology of malignant astrocytomas. *Seminars in Oncology* **21**, 149–61.

Levine, S. (1973) The role of mononuclear cell deficiency in the production of neutrophilic allergic encephalomyelitis. (Abstract) *Journal of Neuropathology and Experimental Neurology* **32**, 168.

Li, H., Hamou, M.-F., de Tribolet, N.B., Jaufeerally, R., Hofmann, M., Diserens, A.-C. and Van Meir, E.G. (1993) Variant CD44 adhesion molecules are expressed in human brain metastases but not in glioblastomas. *Cancer Research* **53**, 5345–9.

Lillehei, K.O., Mitchell, D.H., Johnson, S.D., McCleary, E.L. and Kruse, C.A. (1991) Long-term follow-up of patients with recurrent malignant gliomas treated with adjuvant adoptive immunotherapy. *Neurosurgery* **28**, 16–23.

List, J., Moser, R.P., Steuer, M., Loudon, W.G., Blacklock, J.B. and Grimm, E.A. (1992) Cytokine responses to intraventricular injection of interleukin-2 into patients with leptomeningeal carcinomatosis: rapid induction of tumor necrosis factor-α, interleukin 1-β, interleukin 6, γ-interferon, and soluble interleukin-2 receptor (M_r 55,000 protein). *Cancer Research* **52**, 1123–8.

Long, D.M. (1970) Capillary ultrastructure and the blood-brain barrier in human malignant brain tumors. *Journal of Neurosurgery* **32**, 127–44.

Lotze, M.T., Line, B.R., Mathisen, D.J. and Rosenberg, S.A. (1980) The *in vivo* distribution of autologous human and murine lymphoid cells grown in T cell growth factor (TCGF): implications for the adoptive immunotherapy of tumors. *Journal of Immunology* **125**, 1487–93.

Medawar, P.B. (1948) Immunity to homologous grafted skin. III. The fate of skin homografts transplanted to the brain, to subcutaneous tissue, and to the anterior chamber of the eye. *British Journal of Experimental Pathology* **29**, 58–69.

Merchant, R.E., Ellison, M.D. and Young, H.F. (1990) Immunotherapy for malignant glioma using human recombinant interleukin-2 and activated autologous lymphocytes. A review of pre-clinical and clinical investigations. *Journal of Neuro-Oncology* **8**, 173–88.

Merchant, R.E., Grant, A.J., Merchant, L.H. and Young, H.F. (1988a) Adoptive immunotherapy for recurrent glioblastoma multiforme using lymphokine-activated killer cells and recombinant interleukin-2. *Cancer* **62**, 665–71.

Merchant, R.E., Merchant, L.H., Cook, S.H.S., McVicar, D.W. and Young, H.F. (1988b) Intralesional infusion of lymphokine-activated killer (LAK) cells and recombinant interleukin-2 (rIL-2) for the treatment of patients with malignant brain tumor. *Neurosurgery* **23**, 725–32.

Miescher, S., Whiteside, T.L., de Tribolet, N. and von Fliedner, V. (1988) *In situ* characterization, clonogenic potential, and antitumor cytolytic activity of T lymphocytes infiltrating human brain cancers. *Journal of Neurosurgery* **68**, 438–48.

Miller, D.C., Hochberg, F.H., Harris, N.L., Gruber, M.L., Louis, D.N. and Cohen, H. (1994) Pathology with clinical correlations of primary central nervous system non-Hodgkin's lymphoma. The Massachusetts General Hospital experience 1958–1989. *Cancer* **74**, 1383–97.

Mizuno, M., Yoshida, J., Takaoka, T. and Sugita, K. (1994) Liposomal transfection of human γ-interferon gene into human glioma cells and adoptive immunotherapy using lymphokine-activated killer cells. *Journal of Neurosurgery* **80**, 510–14.

Morantz, R.A., Shain, W. and Cravioto, H. (1978) Immune surveillance and tumors of the nervous system. *Journal of Neurosurgery* **49**, 84–92.

Moretta, L., Ciccone, E., Mingari, M.C., Biassoni, R. and Moretta, A. (1994) Human natural killer cells: origin, clonality, specificity, and receptors. *Advances in Immunology* **55**, 341–80.

Morioka, T., Baba, T., Black, K.L. and Streit, W.J. (1992) Inflammatory cell infiltrates vary in experimental primary and metastatic brain tumors. *Neurosurgery* **30**, 891–6.

Mosmann, T.R. (1995) Cytokines, differentiation and functions of subsets of CD4 and CD8 T cells. *Behring Institute Mitteilungen* (96), 1–6.

Murphy, J.B. and Sturm, E. (1923) Conditions determining the transplantability of tissues in the brain. *Journal of Experimental Medicine* **38**, 183–97.

Nagane, M., Oyama, H., Shibui, S. and Nomura, K. (1993) Recurrence with tumor bleeding in a patient with malignant astrocytoma during the treatment with intracranial injection of lymphokine-activated killer cells—a case report. *No to Shinkei. Brain and Nerve* **45**, 547–51.

Nakagawa, K., Omori, N., Hashimoto, K., Yamamoto, T., Tsunoda, T. and Nose, T. (1992) The combined effect of lymphokine activated killer cell and radiation therapy on rat brain tumor *in vitro*. *Biotherapy* **4**, 109–15.

Nakagawa, K., Kamezaki, T., Shibata, Y., Tsunoda, T., Meguro, K. and Nose, T. (1995) Effect of lymphokine-activated killer cells with or without radiation therapy against malignant brain tumors. *Neurologica Medico-Chirurgica* **35**, 22–7.

Neuwelt, E.A., Clark, K., Kirkpatrick, J.B. and Toben, H. (1978) Clinical studies of intrathecal autologous lymphocyte infusions in patients with malignant glioma: a toxicity study. *Annals of Neurology* **4**, 307–12.

Nitta, T., Sato, K., Yagita, H., Okumura, K. and Ishii, S. (1990) Preliminary trial of specific targeting therapy against malignant glioma. *Lancet* **335**(8686), 368–71.

Obukhov, S.K., Gennie, M.J., Tutt, A.L., Kemshead, J.T., Coakham, H.B. and Beverely, P.C. (1992) The cytotoxic action of lymphokine activated killer cells upon the human glioma cell line U251 is stimulated by bispecific monoclonal antibody (MoAb) constructs. *Journal of Neuro-Oncology* **13**, 203–10.

Ortaldo, J.R., Mason, A.T. and O'Shea, J.J. (1995) Receptor-induced death in human natural killer cells: involvement of CD16. *Journal of Experimental Medicine* **181**, 339–44.

Ortaldo, J.R., Mason, A. and Overton, R. (1986) Lymphokine-activated killer cells. Analysis of progenitors and effectors. *Journal of Experimental Medicine* **164**, 1193–205.

Packer, R.J., Kramer, E.D. and Ryan, J.A. (1991) Biologic and immune modulating agents in the treatment of childhood brain tumors. *Neurologic Clinics* **9**, 405–22.

Paine, J.T., Handa, H., Yamasaki, T., Yamashita, J. and Miyatake, S. (1986) Immunohistochemical analysis of infiltrating lymphocytes in central nervous system tumors. *Neurosurgery* **18**, 766–72.

Paterson, P.Y. (1960) Transfer of allergic encephalomyelitis in rats by means of lymph node cells. *Journal of Experimental Medicine* **111**, 119–36.

Paulus, W., Baaur, I., Huettner, C., Schmausser, B., Roggendorf, W., Schlingensiepen, K.H. and Brysch, W. (1995) Effects of transforming growth factor β-1 on collagen synthesis, integrin expression, adhesion and invasion of glioma cells. *Journal of Neuropathology and Experimental Neurology* **54**, 236–44.

Picker, L.J., Nakache, M. and Butcher, E.C. (1989) Monoclonal antibodies to human lymphocyte homing receptors define a novel class of adhesion molecules on diverse cell types. *Journal of Cell Biology* **109**, 927–37.

Ram, Z., Walbridge, S., Heiss, J.D., Culver, K.W., Blaese, R.M. and Oldfield, E.H. (1994) *In vivo* transfer of the human interleukin-2 gene: negative tumoricidal results in experimental brain tumors. *Journal of Neurosurgery* **80**, 535–40.

Ratner, S. and Heppner, G.H. (1988) Motility and tumoricidal activity of interleukin-2-stimulated lymphocytes. *Cancer Research* **48**, 3374–80.

Restifo, P.R. and Wunderlich, J.R. (1995) Biology of cellular immune responses. In DeVita, V.T. Jr, Hellman, S. and Rosenberg, S.A. (eds), *Biologic therapy of cancer*. Second edition. Philadelphia: J.B. Lippincott, 3–38.

Ridley, A. and Cavanagh, J.B. (1971) Lymphocytic infiltration in gliomas: evidence of possible host resistance. *Brain* **94**, 117–24.

Romagnani, S. (1992) Human TH1 and TH2 subsets: regulation of differentiation and role in protection and immunopathology. *International Archives of Allergy and Immunology* **98**, 279–85.

Rosenberg, S.A., Lotze, M.T., Muul, L.M., Chang, A.E., Avis, F.P., Leitman, S., Linehan, W.M., Robertson, C.N., Lee, R.E., Rubin, J.T., Seipp, C.A., Simpson, C.G. and White, D.E. (1987) A progress report on the treatment of 157 patients with advanced cancer using lymphokine-activated killer cells and interleukin-2 or high-dose interleukin-2 alone. *New England Journal of Medicine* **316**, 889–97.

Ross, H.J., Antoniono, R.J., Buckmeier, J.A. and Redpath, J.L. (1994) Variable expression of IL-1 β has minimal effect on the radiation sensitivity of three human glioma cell lines. *International Journal of Radiation Biology* **66**, 785–91.

Roszman, T., Elliott, L. and Brooks, W. (1991) Modulation of T-cell function by gliomas. *Immunology Today* **12**, 370–4.

— (1992) Proliferative potential of T cell lymphocytes from gliomas. *Journal of Neurosurgery* **77**, 820–1.

Sakai, K., Chang, A.E. and Shu, S. (1990) Effector phenotype and immunologic specificity of T-cell-mediated adoptive therapy for a murine tumor that lacks intrinsic immunogenicity. *Cellular Immunology* **129**, 241–55.

Salcman, M. and Broadwell, R.D. (1991) The blood-brain barrier. In Salcman, M. (ed.), *Neurobiology of brain tumors, Vol. 4. Concepts in neurosurgery*. Baltimore: Williams & Wilkins, 229–49.

Sampson, J.H., Archer, G.E., Ashley, D.M., Fuchs, H.E., Hale, L.P., Dranoff, G. and Bigner, D.D. (1996a) Subcutaneous vaccination with irradiated, cytokine-producing tumor cells stimulates $CD8^+$ cell-mediated immunity against tumors located in the 'immunologically privileged' central nervous system. *Proceedings of the National Academy of Sciences U.S.A.* **93**, 1279–96.

Sampson, J.H., Ashley, D.M., Archer, G.E., Fuchs, H.E., Hale, L.P. and Bigner, D.D. (1996b) Cytokines abrogate tumorgenicity of TGF-β producing spontaneous murine astrocytoma. (Abstract) *Journal of Neuro-Oncology*, in press.

Saris, S.C., Spiess, P., Lieberman, D.M., Lin, S., Walbridge, S. and Oldfield, E.H. (1992) Treatment of murine primary brain tumors with systemic interleukin-2 and tumor-infiltrating lymphocytes. *Journal of Neurosurgery* **76,** 513–19.

Sawamura, Y. and de Tribolet, N. (1995) Immunotherapy of brain tumours. In Thomas, D.G.T. and Graham, D.I. (eds), *Malignant brain tumours*. London: Springer Verlag, 355–70.

Sawamura, Y., Hosokawa, M., Kuppner, M.C., Kobayashi, H., Aida, T., Abe, H. and de Tribolet, N. (1989) Antitumor activity and surface phenotypes of human glioma-infiltrating lymphocytes after *in vitro* expansion in the presence of interleukin 2. *Cancer Research* **49**, 1843–9.

Scheinberg, L.C., Edelman, F.L. and Levy, W.A. (1964) Is the brain 'an immunologically privileged site'? 1. Studies based on intracerebral tumor homotransplantation and isotransplantation to sensitized hosts. *Archives of Neurology* **11**, 248–64.

Scheinberg, L.C., Levy, A. and Edelman, F. (1965) Is the brain an 'immunologically privileged site'? 2. Studies in induced host resistance to transplantable mouse glioma following irradiation of prior implants. *Archives of Neurology* **13**, 283–6.

Scheinberg, L.C., Suzuki, K., Edelman, F. and Davidoff, L.M. (1963) Studies in immunization against a transplantable cerebral mouse glioma. *Journal of Neurosurgery* **20**, 312–17.

Scheinberg, L.C., Kotsilimbas, D.G., Karpf, R. and Mayer, N. (1966) Is the brain an 'immunologically privileged site'? 3. Studies based on homologous skin grafts to the brain and subcutaneous tissues. *Archives of Neurology* **15**, 62–7.

Schiffer, D., Croveri, G. and Pautasso, C. (1974) Frequenza e significatio degli infiltrati linfo-plasmacellulari nei gliomi umani. *Tumori* **60**, 177–84.

Schneider, J., Hofman, F.M., Apuzzo, M.L.J. and Hinton, D.R. (1992) Cytokines and immunoregulatory molecules in malignant glial neoplasms. *Journal of Neurosurgery* **77**, 265–73.

Schwinzer, R. (1989) N7 Cluster report: CD45/CD45R. In Knapp, W. (ed.), *Leucocyte typing IV. White cell differentiation antigens*. Oxford: Oxford University Press, 628–34.

Sedlacek, H.H. (1994) Vaccination for treatment of tumors: a critical comment. *Critical Reviews in Oncogenesis* **5**, 555–87.

Shau, H. and Roberts, R.L. (1992) Tumor necrosis factor stimulation of neutrophils for antitumor activity. *Immunology Series* **57**, 523–33.

Shimizu, Y. and Shaw, S. (1989–90) T lymphocyte adhesion molecules. *Year in Immunology* **6**, 69–94.

Shirai, Y. (1921) Transplantations of rat sarcomas in adult heterogeneous animals. *Japanese Medical World* **1**, 14–15.

Shuttleworth, E.C. Jr (1972) Barrier phenomena in brain tumors. *Progress in Experimental Tumor Research* **17**, 279–90.

Steinbok, P., Thomas, J.P.W., Grossman, L. and Dolman, C.L. (1984) Intratumoral autologous mononuclear cells in the treatment of recurrent glioblastoma multiforme. A phase 1 (toxicity) study. *Journal of Neuro-Oncology* **2**, 147–51.

Stevens, A., Klöter, I. and Roggendorf, W. (1988) Inflammatory infiltrates and natural killer cell presence in human brain tumors. *Cancer* **61**, 738–43.

Tada, M. and de Tribolet, N. (1993) Recent advances in immunobiology of brain tumors. *Journal of Neuro-Oncology* **17**, 261–71.

Takakura, K., Miki, Y. and Kubo, O. (1975) Adjuvant immunotherapy for malignant brain tumors in infants and children. *Child's Brain* **1**, 141–7.

Takakura, K., Miki, Y., Kubo, O., Ogawa, N., Matsutani, M. and Sano, K. (1972) Adjuvant immunotherapy for malignant brain tumors. *Japanese Journal of Clinical Oncology* **2**, 109–20.

Takaoka, T., Yoshida, J., Mizuno, M. and Sugita, K. (1994) Transfection-induced tumor necrosis factor-α increases the susceptibility of human glioma cells to lysis by lymphokine-activated killer cells: continuous expression of intercellular adhesion molecule-1 on the glioma cells. *Japanese Journal of Cancer Research* **85**, 750–5.

Takeuchi, J. and Barnard, R.O. (1976) Perivascular lymphocytic cuffing in astrocytomas. *Acta Neuropathologica* **35**, 265–71.

Tashiro, T., Yoshida, J., Mizuno, M. and Sugita, K. (1993) Reinforced cytotoxicity of lymphokine-activated killer cells toward glioma cells by transfection with the tumor necrosis factor-α gene. *Journal of Neurosurgery* **78**, 252–6.

Tjuvajev, J., Gansbacher, B., Desai, R., Beattie, B., Kaplitt, M., Matei, C., Koutcher, J., Gilboa, E. and Blasberg, R. (1995) RG-2 glioma growth attenuation and severe brain edema caused by local production of interleukin-2 and interferon-gamma. *Cancer Research* **55**, 1902–10.

Townsend, A. and Bodmer, H. (1989) Antigen recognition by class I restricted T lymphocytes. *Annual Review of Immunology* **7**, 601–24.

Tzeng, J.-J., Barth, R.F., Clendenon, N.R. and Gordon,W.A. (1990) Adoptive immunotherapy of a rat glioma using lymphokine-activated killer cells and interleukin 2. *Cancer Research* **50**, 4338–43.

Vick, N.A., Bigner, D.D. and Kvedar, J.P. (1971) The fine structure of canine gliomas and intracranial sarcomas induced by the Schmidt-Ruppin strain of the Rous sarcoma virus. *Journal of Neuropathology and Experimental Neurology* **30**, 354–67.

Vieweg, J., Rosenthal, F.M., Bannerji, R., Heston, W.D.W., Fair, W.R., Gansbacher, B. and Gilboa, E. (1994) Immunotherapy of prostate cancer in the Dunning rat model: use of cytokine gene modified tumor vaccines. *Cancer Research* **54**, 1760–5.

Watanabe, Y., Kuribayashi, K., Miyatake, S., Hishihara, K., Nakayama, E., Taniyama, T. and Sakata, T. (1989) Exogenous expression of mouse interferon γ cDNA in mouse neuroblastoma C1300 cells results in reduced tumorigenicity by augmented anti-tumor immunity. *Proceedings of the National Academy of Sciences U.S.A.* **86**, 9456–60.

Wen, P.Y. (1993) Clinical experience with immunotherapy. In Black, P.McL., Schoene, W.C. and Lampson, L.A. (eds), *Astrocytomas: diagnosis, treatment, and biology*. Boston: Blackwell Scientific, 123–47.

Whelan, H.T., Przybylski, C., Bajic, D.M. and Schmidt, M.H. (1993) Intracellular growth factor metabolism in proliferation of a brain tumor cell line. Intracellular growth factors and brain tumor proliferation. *Journal of Neuro-Oncology* **15**, 243–50.

Wikstrand, C.J. and Bigner, D.D. (1996) Tumors of the central nervous system. In Keane, R.W. and Hickey, W.F. (eds), *Immunology of the nervous system*. New York: Oxford University Press, in press.

Wrann, M., Bodmer, S., de Martin, R., Siepl, C., Hofer-Warbinek, R., Frei, K., Hofer, E. and Fontana, A. (1987) T cell suppressor factor from human glioblastoma cells is a 12.5 kd protein closely related to transforming growth factor-β. *EMBO Journal* **6**, 1633–6.

Yamada, S., DePasquale, M., Patlak, C.S. and Cserr, H.F. (1991) Albumin outflow into deep cervical lymph from different regions of rabbit brain. *American Journal of Physiology* **261**, H1197–204.

Yamanaka, R., Tanaka, R., Saitoh, T. and Okoshi, S. (1994) Cytokine gene expression on glioma cell lines and specimens. *Journal of Neuro-Oncology* **21**, 243–7.

Yang, S.C., Owen-Schaub, L.B., Roth, J.A. and Grimm, E.A. (1990) Characterization of OKT3-initiated lymphokine- activated effectors expanded with interleukin-2 and tumor necrosis factor α. *Cancer Research* **50**, 3526–32.

Yin, D., Kondo, S., Takeuchi J., Morimura, T., Nakatsu, S., Oda, Y. and Kikuchi, H. (1994) Interferon-gamma induces a decrease in the susceptibility of human glioma cells to lysis by lymphokine-activated killer cells. *Neurosurgery* **35**, 113–18.

Yoshida, S., Takai, N. and Tanaka, R. (1987) Functional analysis of interleukin-2 in immune surveillance against brain tumors. *Neurosurgery* **21**, 627–30.

Young, H., Kaplan, A. and Regelson, W. (1977) Immunotherapy with autologous white cell infusions ('lymphocytes') in the treatment of recurrent glioblastoma multiforme: a preliminary report. *Cancer* **40**, 1037–44.

Yu, J.S., Wei, M.X., Chiocca, E.A., Martuza, R.L. and Tepper, R.I. (1993) Treatment of glioma by engineered interleukin 4-secreting cells. *Cancer Research* **53**, 3125–8.

CHAPTER 8

Antibodies and molecular immunology

Immunohistochemistry and antigens of diagnostic significance

CAROL J. WIKSTRAND, KAR-MING FUNG, JOHN Q. TROJANOWSKI, ROGER E. MCLENDON AND DARELL D. BIGNER

Introduction

Diagnostic neuropathology has benefited in the last two decades from the incorporation of immunohistochemically based technology. The continual development of new, defined reagents to identify epitopes associated with stages of cell lineage, cell cycle, oncogene and suppressor gene products, or cell activation, is helping to clarify the nature of cellular maturation, tissue differentiation, tumor progression and metastasis (Bonnin and Rubinstein, 1984; Kleihues, Kiessling and Janzer, 1987). Thus, the development of these marker-defining reagents has resulted not only in improving diagnostic capability, but also in clarifying developmental pathways within and between cell lineages (Molenaar *et al.*, 1989; Rorke, Molenaar and Trojanowski, 1992; Yachnis *et al.*, 1993). The continuing refinement of reagents and techniques is resulting in the revision of historical classifications (Kleihues,

Kiessling and Janzer, 1987). For example, the unambiguous localization of glial fibrillary acidic protein (GFAP) initially clarified the probable glial origin of several tumors, yet the recent demonstrations that GFAP can be coexpressed with other intermediate filament proteins throughout development (Yachnis *et al.*, 1993), and the localization of GFAP and neurofilament protein (NFP) isoforms in human medulloblastomas (Rorke, Molenaar and Trojanowski, 1992), has led to the conclusion that GFAP is not totally synonymous with astrocytic lineage. Therefore, the molecular characterization of cell types will continue not only to drive classification, but also to redefine the 'markers' themselves.

Several excellent reviews of intracellular, membrane-associated, and secreted neural markers are available to the reader (Wikstrand and Bigner, 1980, 1996; McLendon *et al.*, 1986; Kleihues, Kiessling and Janzer, 1987; McKeever, Davenport and Shakui, 1991; Rorke, Molenaar and Trojanowski, 1992; Kurpad *et al.*, 1995), and it is not within the scope of this chapter to recapitulate these comprehensive references. Instead, the markers discussed herein are those currently of use in the immunohistochemical evaluation of lineage or cell cycle status [intermediate filament proteins (IFPs), neuroendocrine-related markers and nuclear proteins involved in cycling]; those associated with the expression or action of oncogenes or tumor suppressor genes (growth factor receptors and p53); and those oncofetal markers that are operationally specific in the adult central nervous system (CNS), allowing discriminatory localization of specific monoclonal antibodies (MAbs) for diagnostic and therapeutic purposes (tenascin, Gp 240 and cell adhesion molecules). Although the specific determination of tumor grade or the ready distinction of reactive glial cells from differentiated neoplastic cells is still not definitively possible by immunohistochemical means, there is an evolving association among the presence of some markers, tumor grade and prognosis [MIB-1, Ki-67, tenascin, Gp 240, epidermal growth factor receptor (EGFR) and its variants, and oncofetal gangliosides]. Problems and pitfalls of interpretation within these defined antigen–antibody systems are noted in the text of this chapter, and the appendix briefly reviews current techniques, their strengths and limitations, and interpretation of data. This review serves the reader both as a background concerning the general characteristics of each antigen and as an overview of the expression of each antigen in neural neoplasia. More specific characterization of each antigen in diagnostic applications is given in the chapters devoted to each tumor type.

Development of the central nervous system; a temporal overview of cellular and molecular events

For more than a century, our knowledge and classification of brain tumors has been based fundamentally on the comparison of the features of these tumors with the embryonic and postnatal CNS. This classical compare-and-contrast approach has been dramatically augmented by recent technical advancements in immunochemistry, immunohistochemistry, cell biology and molecular biology. With these techniques, the molecular phenotypes of the developing CNS and brain tumors are being explored.

During embryonic development, the neuronal and glial components of the CNS evolve from a layer of stratified primitive epithelium composed of multipotential stem cells collectively known as primitive neuroectodermal cells. This layer of multipotential stem cells undergoes a complex but organized developmental process involving cell proliferation, migration, differentiation and death that ultimately leads to the assembly of the mature CNS. By birth, the basic structure of the human CNS is well established, albeit immature, and robust developmental activities continue for a short postnatal period of about 4 years duration. Early postnatal development of the CNS is not a simple continuation of *in utero* developmental activities; in fact, many of these processes are unique to this stage of life. The assembly of the mature retina (Young, 1985) and the internal granular layer of the cerebellum (Jacobson., 1991) are examples of the several developmental activities unique to the early postnatal period. Disturbance of these normal developmental activities may be the etiology of a variety of disorders ranging from developmental abnormalities and neurodegenerative diseases, to tumor formation in the nervous system.

In the past two decades, the study of the expression and function of a panel of well-characterized and developmentally regulated proteins (Table 8.1), such as NFPs and neural cell adhesion molecules (NCAMs), in the embryonic and mature nervous system, has demonstrated that a number of them play important roles in establishing the mature CNS. Many neuron-specific proteins, such as NFPs, are induced in a stepwise manner during the maturation of postmitotic neurons (Carden *et al.*, 1987: Lee *et al.*, 1987). Further, the post-translational modifications of some of these proteins

Table 8.1 Summary of developmentally regulated proteins in the CNS

Proteins expressed by the primitive neuroepithelium, developing neurons and glia
Nestin
Vimentin
Proteins expressed by neuroendocrine cells
Synaptophysin
Chromogranin
Proteins expressed by neurons
Neurofilament proteins (NF)
Low molecular weight (NF-L)
Middle molecular weight (NF-M)
High molecular weight (NF-L)
α-Internexin
Peripherin (peripheral nervous system)
Hu
Neuron-specific enolase (γ-subunit)
GAP 43
Proteins expressed by photoreceptor cells
S-antigen
Rod-opsin
Interphotoreceptor retinoid binding protein (IRBP)
Proteins expressed by astrocytes
Glial fibrillary acidic protein (GFAP)
S-100 (conditional)
Miscellaneous important proteins in the nervous system
Neural cell adhesion molecules (NCAMs)
MAP 5

(e.g., sialylation of NCAMs, phosphorylation of NFPs) occurs in discrete stages during development (Frost *et al.*, 1991; Gennarini *et al.*, 1984). Indeed, the asynchronous but coordinated induction and subsequent post-translational modifications of these proteins define molecular milestones in the progressive maturation of neurons and glial cells (Tohyama *et al.*, 1991). Further, the commitment of CNS progenitor cells to the neuronal or glial lineage and the maturation of neurons and glia are heralded by the coordinated expression and modification of lineage-specific proteins (see below). Based on these findings, as well as on studies of the expression of these developmentally regulated proteins in different brain tumors, a correlation between the biological identity of brain tumors and the developing CNS has been established.

Expression of intermediate filament proteins in the developing, mature and neoplastic nervous systems

Among the diverse proteins expressed by developing and mature CNS cells, the family of IFP subunits are of particular interest for tumor diagnosis. The IFPs (Lazarides, 1982; Weber and Osborn, 1982; Steiner and Roop, 1988) are intracellular filaments measuring about 10 nm in diameter, and they form a major part of the cytoskeleton. The IFPs are divided into six classes (I–VI) (Table 8.2) that share biochemical and structural similarities (Weber and Osborn, 1982; Osborn and Weber, 1986; Steiner and Roop, 1988). Notably, discrete stages in the development of neurons have been defined by using the expression of different IFPs as molecular markers of developmental milestones, as diagrammed in Fig. 8.1 (Carden *et al.*, 1987; Lee *et al.*, 1987; Tohyama *et al.*, 1991, 1992; Yachnis *et al.*, 1993).

INTERMEDIATE FILAMENTS EXPRESSED IN THE EMBRYONIC CENTRAL NERVOUS SYSTEM NEUROEPITHELIUM

The embryonic CNS neuroepithelium forms along the inner surface of the ventricular zone and harbors the earliest group of progenitor cells committed to give rise to cells of the future CNS. Nestin and vimentin are two IFPs that are expressed early in the embryonic CNS neuroepithelium.

Nestin

Nestin (Frederiksen and McKay, 1988; Geschwind and Hockfield, 1989) is the most recently identified member of the IFP family and is widely expressed by many different types of cells during fetal development. It is biochemically and structurally distinctive enough to be classified as a new class (class VI). Nestin has a molecular mass of 210–240 kilodaltons (kDa) and is the largest among all IFPs. The nestin gene exhibits 16–29% identity with other IFPs, predominantly in the 300 amino acid (aa) interspecies conserved α-helical region responsible for filament formation (Dahlstrand, Collins and Lendahl, 1992). Immunochemically, nestin was first defined by rat MAb 401 raised against fixed spinal cord extracts from embryonic day 15 rats; however, as this MAb failed to recognize human nestin in immunohistochemical assays, polyclonal rabbit antihuman nestin

Table 8.2 Characteristics and distribution of the intermediate filament classes

Type	Molecular mass (kDa)	Class	Tissue/cell type distribution
Keratin (acidic and basic)	40–68	I and II	Epithelium
Vimentin	57	III	Mesenchymal Primitive neuroepithelial cells Astrocytes Developing neurons
GFAP	50–52	III	Astrocytes Ependymal cells Nonmyelinating Schwann cells
Peripherin	57	III	Neurons of the central and peripheral nervous system
NFP	68 (NF-L) 150 (NF-M) 200 (NF-H)	IV	Neurons Adrenal medullary cells
α-Internexin	66	IV	Neurons
Lamin	60–70	V	Nuclear membrane
Nestin	210–240	VI	Primitive neuroepithelium Developing astrocytes Developing neurons Schwann cells

GFAP, glial fibrillary acidic protein; NFP, neurofilament protein; NF-L, low molecular weight neurofilament; NF-M middle molecular weight neurofilament; NF-H, high molecular weight neurofilament.

antisera 129 and 130 were produced by immunization with recombinant rat nestin expressed in *E. coli* (Tohyama *et al.*, 1992).

In the developing CNS, nestin is expressed in the primitive neuroepithelial cells. Nestin is almost completely eliminated toward the end of gestation and is expressed only in endothelial cells of the mature human CNS (Tohyama *et al.*, 1991; Yachnis *et al.*, 1993) and by the Schwann cells in the peripheral nervous system (PNS) (Friedman, Zaremba and Hockfield, 1990). As development proceeds, nestin is replaced by NFP in cells committed to the neuronal lineage and by GFAP in cells committed to differentiate into astrocytes (Yachnis *et al.*, 1993). In view of these findings, nestin should be regarded as a protein marker of embryonic CNS neuroectodermal cells and of immature CNS precursor cells not yet committed to a neuronal or an astrocytic

Table 8.3 Expression of nestin, vimentin, synaptophysin, neurofilament proteins and GFAP in central nervous system tumors

Tumor	Nestin	Vimentin	SYN	NFP	GFAP
Medulloblastomas:					
undifferentiated	+	+	+	–	–
with neuronal differentiation	–	+	+	+	–
with glial differentiation	+	+	+	–	+
with neuronal and glial differentiation	+	+	+	+	+
Astrocytic tumors	+/–	+	–	–	+
Ependymomas	+	+/–	–	–	+

+, All cases are positive; –, All cases are negative; +/–, Some cases are positive and some are negative.
SYN, synatophysin; NFP, neurofilament protein; GFAP, glial fibrillary acidic protein.

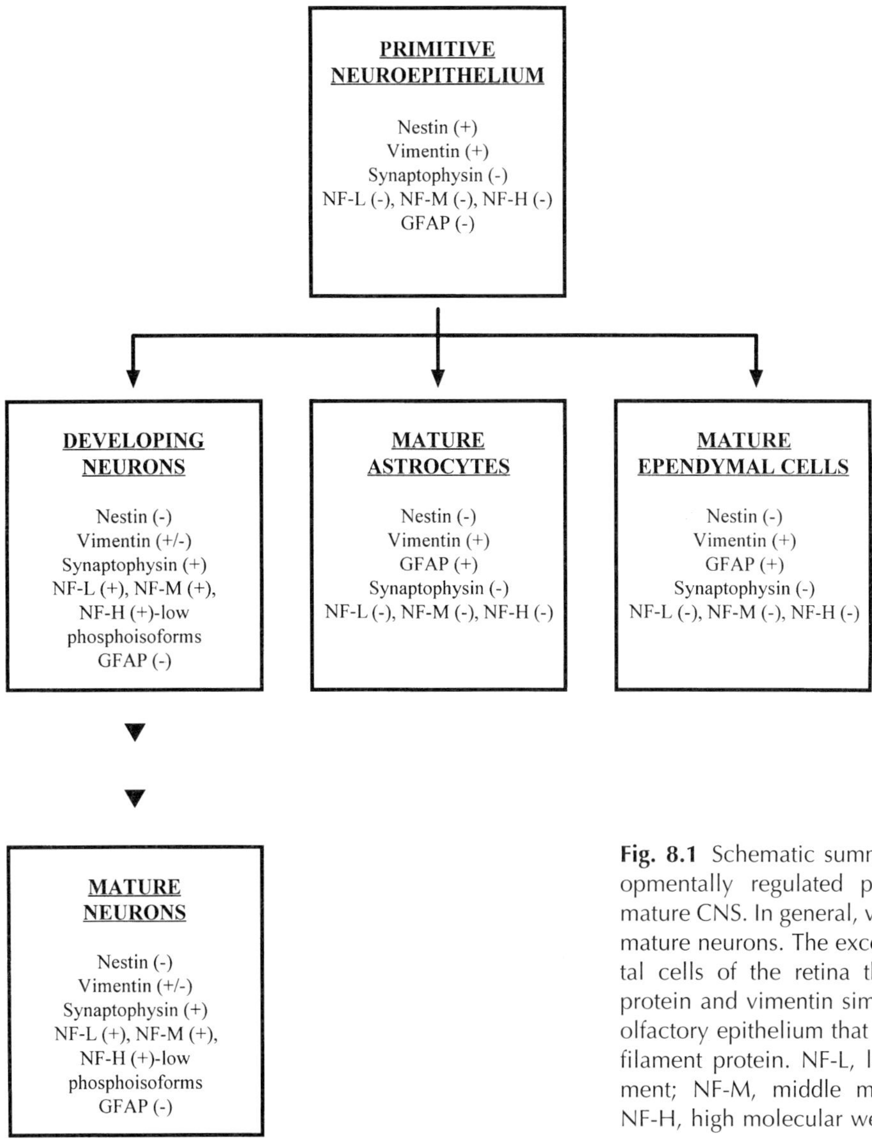

Fig. 8.1 Schematic summary of the expression of developmentally regulated protein in the developing and mature CNS. In general, vimentin is not expressed by most mature neurons. The exceptions to this trend are horizontal cells of the retina that express both neurofilament protein and vimentin simultaneously, and neurons of the olfactory epithelium that express vimentin but not neurofilament protein. NF-L, low molecular weight neurofilament; NF-M, middle molecular weight neurofilament, NF-H, high molecular weight neurofilament.

lineage. However, since nestin also is widely expressed by many types of embryonic tissues (Tohyama *et al.*, 1992), the expression of nestin should not be regarded as an unequivocal phenotypic marker of embryonic CNS neuroepithelial cells. Nestin expression has been demonstrated with antisera 129 and 130 in CNS tumors (Table 8.3); Tohyama *et al.* (1992) reported its coexpression with NFP in medulloblastomas with neuronal or mixed neuronal/glial differentiation, and its expression with GFAP in medulloblastomas with glial differentiation, and with GFAP in glial tumors of all grades [astrocytoma, anaplastic astrocytoma, glioblastoma multiforme (GBM), ependymoma and ganglioglioma]. An example of nestin expression in a GBM is provided in Fig. 8.2(a). Coexpression of nestin and vimentin was observed in two cases of meningioma. Dahlstrand, Collins and Lendahl (1992) reported similar results in a series of 67 primary CNS tumors, with frequency of expression correlated with degree of malignancy in gliomas (1/7 astrocytomas+; 2/5 anaplastic astrocytomas+; 15/15 GBM+). While nestin-positive tumor cells alone were found in 14/36 tumors, nestin positivity was reported in both endothelial cells and tumor cells of the remaining 22 tumors. Notably, no nestin expression was found in nine carcinoma metastases in the CNS (Dahlstrand, Collins and Lendahl, 1992). Recently, Florenes *et al.* (1994) have reported nestin protein expression in 10/15

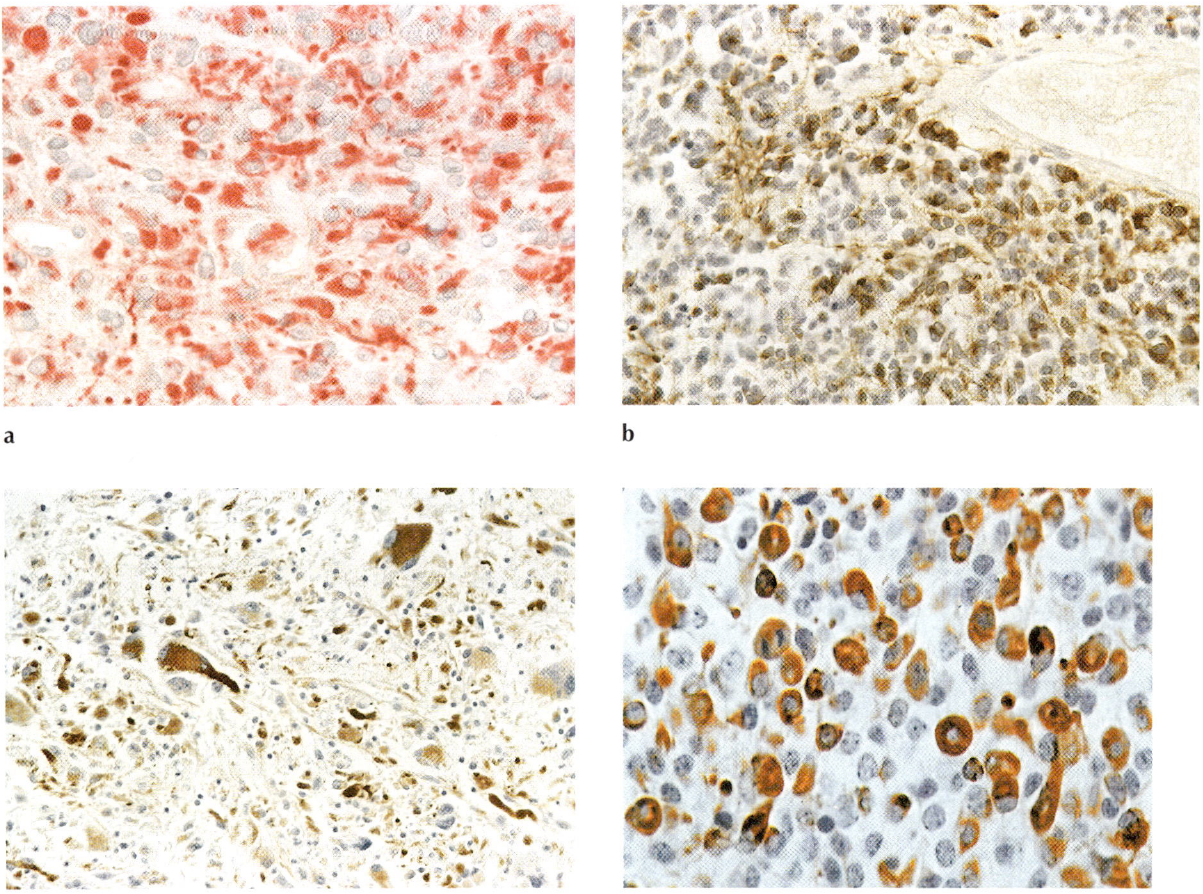

a b c d

Fig. 8.2 Expression of intermediate filament protein (IFP) in primary CNS tumors. (a) Nestin expression in a glioblastoma multiforme (GBM). ×900 (b) NFP expression in a posterior fossa PNET. ×400 (c) GFAP expression in a GBM. ×400 (d) GFAP-positive oligodendroglial tumor. ×400.

primary melanomas and 29/34 metastatic melanomas, with abundant expression in infiltrating tumor cells, suggesting an association of nestin expression and tumor invasion.

Vimentin

Vimentin is a class III IFP with a molecular mass of 57 kDa (Osborn and Weber, 1986). In contrast to nestin, vimentin is widely expressed in a variety of embryonic and mature tissues. During CNS neuronal development, the expression of vimentin closely parallels that of nestin (Tohyama *et al.*, 1992). Vimentin is not expressed in mature neurons, with two exceptions: (1) the horizontal cells of the retina in which neurofilament proteins and vimentin are expressed simultaneously (Shaw and Weber, 1983); and (2) sensory neurons of the olfactory epithelium that express vimentin, but not neurofilament proteins (Vollrath *et al.*, 1985). In addition, vimentin is coexpressed with GFAP in developing and mature astrocytes (Yachnis *et al.*, 1993). Vimentin can almost be considered the default IFP, as it often becomes the predominant IFP in *in vitro* cultures of CNS tumor cells and is coexpressed with the more lineage-distinctive NFP and GFAP in CNS tumors (Tohyama *et al.*, 1992). It has been identified as the major IFP in some cases of undifferentiated medulloblastomas, choroid plexus papillomas and some meningiomas (Tohyama *et al.*, 1992).

NEURON-SPECIFIC INTERMEDIATE FILAMENT PROTEINS

In the CNS, the expression of NFP, α-internexin and peripherin is preceded by the down regulation of nestin and vimentin (Tohyama *et al.*, 1992). Thus, the expression of these neuron-specific proteins signals the commitment of neuroepithelial cells to differentiate into neurons.

Neurofilament proteins

The NFPs are class IV IFPs, and they are expressed exclusively in CNS and PNS neurons, as well as in adrenal chromaffin cells. Notably, the expression of NFP in embryonic CNS cells is a specific indicator of commitment to the neuronal lineage. Neurofilaments are composed of three subunits of different molecular mass: low- (NF-L, 68 kDa), middle- (NF-M, 150 kDa) and high- (NF-H, 200 kDa) NFP subunits. Each NFP subunit is encoded by a separate gene (Nixon, 1993). The NF-M and NF-H undergo a different extent of post-translational phosphorylation during their maturation. The phosphorylation state of NF-M and NF-H may vary from unphosphorylated to highly phosphorylated, leading to the generation of multiple phosphoisoforms of these two neurofilament subunits; NF-L is the least extensively phosphorylated (Lee *et al.*, 1987). Trojanowski and Lee (1983) prepared MAbs to the P 68, P 150 and P 200 subunits of bovine NFP that were applied to the evaluation of CNS and PNS neoplasms; however, it became evident that non- or poorly phosphorylated NFP subunits were not readily detected by these reagents. A complete library of anti-NF-L, anti-NF-M and anti-NF-H reagents were subsequently developed by immunization with enzymatically dephosphorylated NFP. These have been used to demonstrate selective expression of distinct phosphoisoforms of NF-H and NF-M, and expression of NF-L, the epitope of which is phosphorylation independent (Molenaar *et al.*, 1989, 1990) in a variety of CNS and PNS tumors and normal tissues.

In the developing CNS, there is a general trend that the more heavily phosphorylated isoforms of NF-M and NF-H (i.e., isoforms with higher molecular mass and a higher degree of phosphorylation) are expressed in more advanced stages of neuronal development than their less phosphorylated counterparts. In the developing spinal cord, highly phosphorylated NF-H appears much later during development than does highly phosphorylated NF-M (Carden *et al.*, 1987; Foster and Dahl, 1987; Lee *et al.*, 1987, 1988; Nixon, 1993). In a study of archival, paraffin-embedded, Bouin's or formalin-fixed primary CNS tumor tissues, NFPs of all classes were undetectable in 15 astrocytomas, 2 GBMs and 6 ependymomas; GFAP was the detected IFP. In this study 7/7 gangliomas expressed all three NFP isoforms and GFAP (Molenaar *et al.*, 1989). In an analysis of 35 medulloblastomas, 6 expressed all three NFP isoforms, with 5/6 coexpressing GFAP (2 expressed NF-L, NF-M and GFAP, and 3 expressed NF-M only, with or without GFAP expression); 6 expressed only GFAP; and in the remaining, IFP could not be unequivocally identified [Fig. 8.2(b)] (Kivelä, Takkanen and Virtanen, 1989; Molenaar *et al.*, 1989; Maraziotis *et al.*, 1992). Similarly, in a study of snap-frozen material, 9/12 peripheral neuroblastomas expressed all three NFPs, and the remaining 3/12 were negative for NF-H; there was an increase in the amount of NFP immunoreactivity with increasing differentiation (Molenaar *et al.*, 1990). Only highly differentiated tumors (2/2 ganglioneuroblastomas, 4/4 ganglioneuromas; Molenaar *et al.*, 1990) express the heavily phosphorylated isoforms of NF-H; similar patterns of NFP expression have also been described in gangliogliomas, neurocytomas and pineocytomas (Hessler *et al.*, 1992; Hassoun *et al.*, 1993; Kuchelmeister *et al.*, 1994). The distribution of NFP in primary CNS tumors and extracranial tumors is summarized in Table 8.4.

α-Internexin and peripherin

α-Internexin and peripherin are two newly identified neuron-specific IFPs. α-Internexin (Chiu *et al.*, 1989; Fliegner, Ching and Liem, 1990; Ching and Liem, 1991) is a class IV IFP with a molecular mass of 66 kDa that is expressed in the CNS and developing PNS. In the developing cerebellum, α-internexin is expressed from 20 weeks gestational age onward (Yachnis *et al.*, 1993). Peripherin is a class III IFP with a molecular mass of 57 kDa and is detected in neuronal populations originating from different lineages (neural tube, neural crest and placodes) (Baudoin *et al.*, 1993). Since the appearance of α-internexin and peripherin is accompanied by the down regulation of nestin, the expression of α-internexin and peripherin in embryonic nervous system cells signals the commitment of these cells toward a neuronal lineage. Peripherin and, to a lesser extent, α-internexin, have been detected in immature peripheral neuroblastomas, composite peripheral ganglioneuroblastomas and peripheral ganglioneuromas (Foley *et al.*, 1994).

GLIAL FIBRILLARY ACIDIC PROTEIN

Described by Eng *et al.* in 1971, GFAP is a class III IFP of 55 kDa that is conventionally regarded as a useful marker antigen for astroglial cells (Kleihues, Kiessling and Janzer, 1987), although its coexpression in development and CNS neoplasia with other intermediate filaments, primarily vimentin and

Table 8.4 Expression of neurofilament proteins in intracranial and extracranial tumors

Intracranial tumors expressing neurofilament protiens	Intracranial tumors not expressing neurofilament proteins	Extracranial tumors expressing neurofilament proteins
Ganglioneuroblastoma	Astroblastoma	Carcinoid
Ganglioneuroma	Choroid plexus papilloma	Esthesioneuroblastoma
Neurocytoma	Ependymoma	Ewing's sarcoma
Neuronal medulloblastoma (PNET)	Glioblastoma multiforme	Ganglioneuroblastoma
	Gliosarcoma	Ganglioneuroma
Pineoblastoma	Hemangioblastoma	Neuroblastoma
	Mixed glioma	Pheochromocytoma
	Oligodendroglioma	Small-cell lung carcinoma
	Pineocytoma	Teratoma
	Pituitary adenoma	
	Subependymal giant-cell astrocytoma	
	Subependymoma	

NFP, precludes its use as an absolute indicator of astroglial origin (Rorke, Molenaar and Trojanowski, 1992; Yachnis *et al.*, 1993). The distribution of GFAP within normal brain has been extensively described. In general, protoplasmic astrocytes have little GFAP, but they have only GFAP as an intermediate filament protein (Shaw, Osborn and Weber, 1981), whereas reactive fibrous astrocytes demonstrate abundant GFAP in the perikaryon and cytoplasmic processes, with no staining of the nucleus (Smith and Lantos, 1985). Frequently, GFAP is coexpressed with vimentin in a single-cell cytoskeleton (Wang, Cairncross and Liem, 1984). Cutarelli *et al.* (1991), in a study of 10 juvenile pilocytic astrocytomas (JPAs), demonstrated cellular coexpression of GFAP, vimentin and S-100.

As summarized by Kleihues, Kiessling and Janzer (1987), the use of GFAP in the histopathologic diagnosis of gliomas has been extensively reviewed. Decades of experience with this marker have established several major considerations in interpreting GFAP-positive cases. First, the technical aspects of reliable GFAP detection are not straightforward; fixation parameters (type and duration) and the need for permeabilization result in great interlab variability (Dixon and Eng, 1981; Zheng, Ivarsson and Collins, 1986; Kleihues, Kiessling and Janzer, 1987). In addition, the variety of polyclonal anti-GFAP sera available introduces a second source of variability that can be controlled by the use of a cocktail of defined MAbs (McLendon *et al.*, 1986). Second, the distinction between GFAP-positive neoplastic astrocytes and entrapped (or peritumoral) reactive astrocytes, both of which express GFAP, is very difficult (Coffin, Mukai and Dehner, 1983; Nakagawa, Perentes and Rubinstein, 1986). Third, no reliable correlation between GFAP staining and neoplastic progression exists, although there is a general decrease in GFAP expression with increasing anaplasia (Duffy *et al.*, 1980). Examples of GFAP immunoreactive cells are provided in Fig. 8.2(c–d). A summary of the IFP profile of various CNS tumors is presented in Table 8.3.

CYTOKERATINS

The cytokeratins (CKs) comprise the most complex family of IFP, being approximately 20 in number, and are distinguishable by molecular mass, isoelectric point and reactivity spectrum with defined MAbs (Franko *et al.*, 1987; Ng and Lo, 1989). Long considered to be an immunohistochemical marker for epithelial cells and derived neoplasms, cytokeratin reactivity has been used to discriminate poorly differentiated metastatic carcinoma in the CNS from primary neoplasms (Russell and Rubinstein, 1989, p. 32). Although primarily associated with epithelial differentiation, some CK types have been detected in the CNS of several vertebrate species (Bodega *et al.*, 1995). Within the human CNS, cytokeratins have been detected in chordomas and meningiomas (Russell and Rubinstein, 1989, p. 32), and, most notably, in focal areas exhibiting squamous-cell morphology in GBMs and gliosarcomas (Mørk *et al.*, 1988).

These observations have prompted several groups to investigate the expression of various cytokeratins by normal and neoplastic cells in the CNS. Raised against Jakob-Creutzfeldt virus-infected mouse brain cells, a MAb (34C9) that recognizes a 65-kDa protein of rodent brain and multiple cytokeratin proteins isolated from human epidermal cells was used by Franko *et al.* (1987) to demonstrate the existence of cytokeratin in murine and hamster cerebellar granular layer astrocytes, Purkinje cells and ependymal cells. In astrocytes, GFAP and cytokeratin were frequently coexpressed. Cosgrove *et al.* (1989) and Ng and Lo (1989) reported that the anticytokeratin MAbs AE1 (anti-56.5-, 50-, 48- and 40-kDa cytokeratins) and AE3 (anti-65–67-, 64-, 59-, 58-, 56-, 54- and 52-kDa cytokeratins) were reactive with a broad spectrum of human astrocytic neoplasms regardless of histologic grade: 40–66% of well-differentiated astrocytomas, 63–83% of anaplastic astrocytomas and 58–83% of GBMs were immunoreactive with these reagents. In addition, isolated astrocyte-like cells and scattered neoplastic oligodendrocytes were positive in 4/8 cases of oligodendroglioma; ependymomas (4/4) were negative (Ng and Lo, 1989). In an extensive analysis of 24 anticytokeratin MAbs, Franke *et al.* (1991) reported distinct cross-reactivity of eight anticytokeratin MAbs with astrocytic cells in astrocytomas, oligodendrogliomas and GBMs, as well as with reactive glia and normal brain elements. One of these MAbs (KA4) was demonstrated by Western blot to cross-react with GFAP, but the probable specific reactivity of several defined anti-CK reagents with cells in the molecular layer of the cerebellum, glial cells and vascular walls in neoplastic brain tissue (Franke *et al.*, 1991) could lead to the misinterpretation of carcinomatous deposits in malignant gliomas as cautioned by Rubinstein (Russell and Rubinstein, 1989, p. 229). Therefore, the use of anti-CK immunohistochemistry to distinguish between primary CNS neoplasia and metastatic carcinoma must be performed in conjunction with markers for nonepithelial IFP (NFP and GFAP).

Neuroendocrine- and photoreceptor-related proteins and their expression in brain tumors

Neuroendocrine cells comprise a family of cells that share features of both neurons and endocrine cells. Historically, the concept of neuroendocrine cells originated from observations that oxytocin and vasopressin were synthesized by hypothalamic neurons and were stored within neuronal processes in the posterior pituitary prior to their release into the circulation (Sharrer, 1967; for a review of earlier literature, see DeLellis and Dayal, 1992). While these cells have features of neurons, their secretory products are delivered in an endocrine or paracrine fashion rather than by synaptic contacts. The close relationship between neuroendocrine cells and neurons has been most extensively studied in the adrenal medulla, where both chromaffin cells and neurons express NFPs (Bader *et al.*, 1984; Trojanowski and Lee, 1985; Molenaar, Lee and Trojanowski, 1990). The development of a chromaffin or neuronal phenotype in adrenal medullary cells is influenced by local factors, according to Anderson and Axel, 1986; Ogawa, Ishikawa and Ohta, 1986; and Unsicker, 1986. Some tumors that demonstrate neuroendocrine features, such as small-cell carcinoma of the lung, also show features of epithelial cells (e.g., cytokeratin positivity) in addition to their neuroendocrine features (Molenaar, de Leij and Trojanowski, 1991).

Apart from their argentophilic and argyrophilic properties, as well as the demonstration of the characteristic dense-core secretory granules by electron microscopy, many of the neuroendocrine cells also exhibit the 'APUD' phenotype: amine precursor uptake and decarboxylation. In general, neuroendocrine cells share phenotypes characterized by the simultaneous expression of multiple genes encoding a wide variety of neuronal and endocrine traits (DeLellis *et al.*, 1986; Tischler, 1989). Among the many different proteins expressed by neuroendocrine cells (reviewed by DeLellis and Dayal, 1992), synaptophysin and chromogranin represent two conventionally considered markers of the neuroendocrine lineage that have been extensively studied (Wiedenmann and Huttner, 1989).

SYNAPTOPHYSIN

Synaptophysin (SYN) is an acidic, *N*-glycosylated, integral membrane glycoprotein of 38 kDa, first characterized as a major component of synaptic vesicles of bovine brain (Wiedenmann and Franke, 1985); it has since been demonstrated to be a major calcium-binding protein of the synaptic vesicle membrane, with the Ca^{+} binding site residing in the cytoplasmic domain (Rehm, Wiedenmann and Betz, 1986). Shalev *et al.* (1992) have shown that the imperfect repetitive pentapeptide YGP(Q)QG, which recurs 10 times in the synaptophysin cytoplasmic tail, contains the epitope (aa 269–289 of rat synaptophysin) recognized by the antisynaptophysin MAb SY38. This motif has been evolutionarily conserved in various

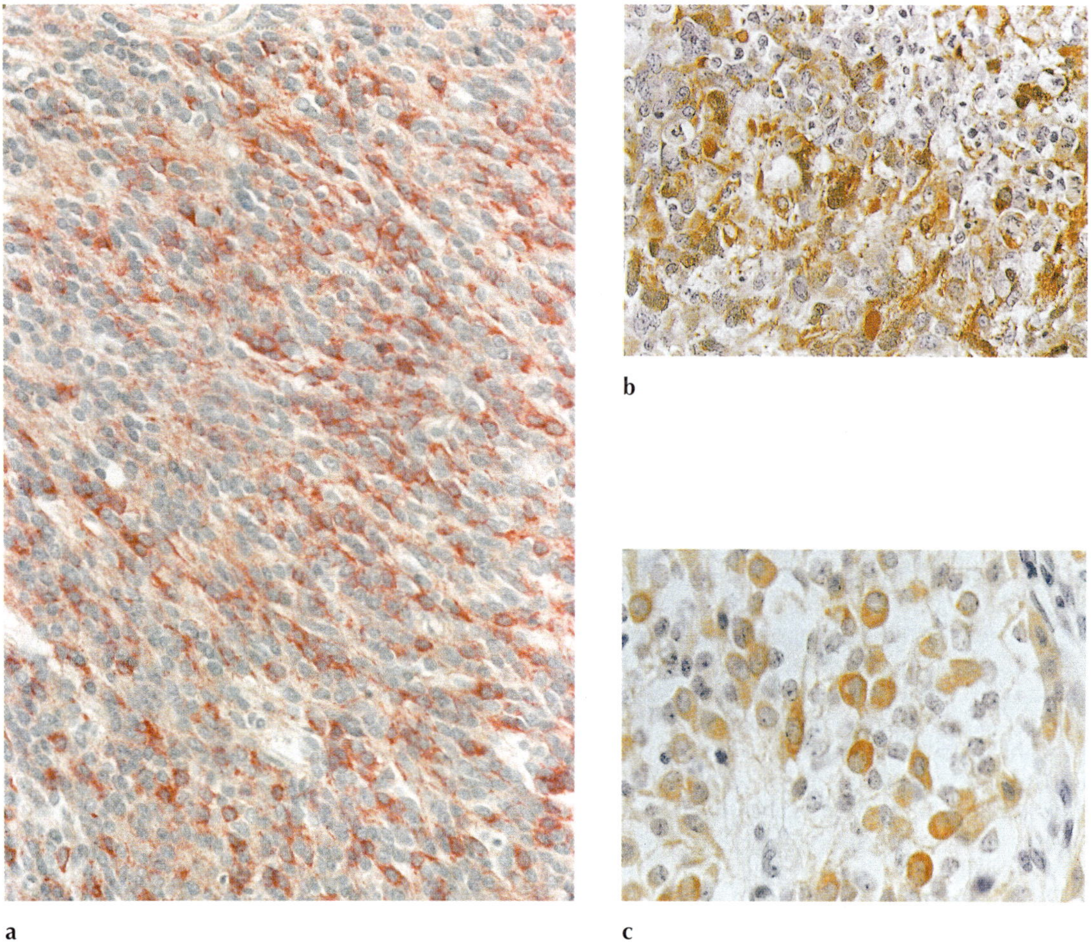

Fig. 8.3 Neuroendocrine-related proteins in primary CNS tumors. (a) Synaptophysin expression in a posterior fossa PNET. ×400 (b) NSE expression in a GBM. ×560. (c) NSE expression in an oligodendroglioma. ×400

granule-associated proteins, including the 40–45-kDa platelet dense-granule membrane glycoprotein granulophysin (Gerrard *et al.*, 1991) and leukophysin (Abdelhaleem *et al.*, 1991), and is now considered an immunodominant construct responsible for the cross-reactivity of conformation-dependent antigranulophysin MAbs for synaptophysin and that of conformation-independent antisynaptophysin MAb SY38 for granulophysin and leukophysin (Shalev *et al.*, 1992). Based on the different patterns of granulophysin and synaptophysin in Western blot analysis, these authors have been able to show a variable distribution of the two. Synaptophysin is dominantly expressed in the brain, and to a far lesser extent in the pituitary, whereas the reverse is true for granulophysin. The latter shares a wider tissue distribution as well, having been demonstrated in 'neutrophils, plasma cells, testis, kidney, heart, muscle and exocrine tissues, which apparently lack synaptophysin' (Shalev *et al.*, 1992).

The observed molecular cross-reactivity and differential tissue distribution of these molecules complicates the interpretation of previously published studies using the MAb SY38 to evaluate normal and neoplastic tissue synaptophysin distribution, assuming correlation with neuroendocrine/neuronal lineage (Wiedenmann *et al.*, 1986; Gould *et al.*, 1990: Maraziotis *et al.*, 1992). In the absence of the determination of the molecular weight of the detected epitope by parallel blot analysis, it can be concluded only that 'granule-associated proteins' may be useful in revealing the neuroendocrine nature of metastatic tumors of unknown origin (Wiedenmann *et al.*, 1988). Granule-associated proteins have been demonstrated in a subset of CNS tumors, including medulloblastomas [Fig. 8.3(a)] (Gould *et al.*, 1987,

1990; Coffin *et al.*, 1990; Molenaar, de Leij and Trojanowski, 1991; Tohyama *et al.*, 1992; Molenaar and Trojanowski, 1994), neurocytomas (Hessler *et al.*, 1992; Hassoun *et al.*, 1993), pineocytomas (Coca *et al.*, 1992; Kuchelmeister *et al.*, 1994), gangliogliomas (Miller, Lang and Epstein, 1993) and ganglioneuromas (Molenaar *et al.*, 1990), but not in astrocytic tumors, ependymomas, choroid plexus papillomas or meningiomas (Tohyama *et al.*, 1992). The localization by these antibodies to oligodendroglial elements is not understood and may represent a cross-reactive epitope or fixation artifact. This family of granule-associated proteins is expressed by many different peripheral neuroendocrine tumors, including pheochromocytomas, carcinoid tumors, small-cell carcinomas of the lung and gastrointestinal tract, and pituitary adenomas (Wiedenmann and Huttner, 1989). Although granule-associated proteins can be detected in formalin-fixed, paraffin-embedded sections, the sensitivity of detection is greatly enhanced by using alcohol-fixed, paraffin-embedded specimens or frozen sections (Hoog *et al.*, 1988). Potential discrimination between members of the granule-associated protein family may be possible with antinonconserved NH_2 terminus-descriptive polyvalent antisera (Shalev *et al.*, 1992) or with MAbs such as EP10 (Honer, Kaufmann and Davies, 1992), which defines an epitope on human synaptophysin not conserved in rat or bovine synaptophysin; whether this epitope is characteristic of other human granule-associate proteins has not been reported.

CHROMOGRANIN A

Chromogranin A is expressed in the intravesicular matrix of the ultrastructurally evident dense-core vesicles of neuroendocrine cells; it is the major constituent of the proteins isolated from vesicles in adrenal chromaffin cells and has a molecular mass of 70–80 kDa (Cohn *et al.*, 1982). The expression of chromogranin A has not been well described in primary brain tumors except gangliogliomas (Diepholder *et al.*, 1991). In contrast, chromogranins are widely expressed in neuroendocrine tumors outside the CNS (reviewed by Wiedenmann and Huttner, 1989).

NEURON-SPECIFIC ENOLASE

The γ-subunit of neuron-specific enolase (NSE) was one of the first marker proteins that was used to identify neuroendocrine cells and neurons and has been used in immunohistochemical analysis of brain tumors [Fig. 8.3(b) and (c)] with striking results. However, it has been shown that most antibodies that recognize the γ-subunit of NSE cross-react with the β-subunit of enolase, an enzyme abundantly expressed in a wide variety of nonneuroendocrine cells (Haimoto *et al.*, 1985; Pählman, Esscher and Nilsson, 1986). Duncan *et al.* (1992) have recently reported the production of γ-NSE MAbs P1 and P2 following immunization protocols using synthetic peptides representing unique hydrophilic loop regions of γ-NSE; however, several nonneuroendocrine cells also express the γ-subunit of NSE, and the γ-subunit of NSE is readily induced in a variety of cells in diverse pathological conditions (Vinores and Rubinstein, 1985). For these reasons, the use of NSE as a lineage-specific marker for neurons and neuroendocrine cells is rather limited.

PROTEINS EXPRESSED BY PHOTORECEPTOR CELLS

Retinal S-antigen (arrestin), rod-opsin and interphotoreceptor retinoid-binding protein (IRBP) are three highly characterized markers of retinal photoreceptors and pinealocytes (Korf *et al.*, 1992). Retinal S-antigen (48 kDa) is a cytosolic protein that regulates phototransduction in retinal rods, and is also found in normal pinealocytes, although its function there is unknown (Perentes *et al.*, 1986; Korf *et al.*, 1992; Mirshahi *et al.*, 1992). Monoclonal antibodies have been produced to the N-terminal region (aa residues 1–74) of the protein, and the immunodominant epitope has been localized to aa 40–50 (epitope S2) (Stiemer *et al.*, 1992). These authors have shown that anti-S2 MAbs, which specifically recognize retinal S-antigen (arrestin), also recognize human TNF-α through the common sequence motif GV*x*L*x*D, and 48-kDa proteins isolated from human kidney proximal tubule cells as well (Mirshahi *et al.*, 1992). The restricted expression of retinal S-antigen within the CNS, however, as defined by MAb A9-C6 and S-series MAbs (Stiemer *et al.*, 1992) has resulted in the attribution of photoreceptor lineage to subsets of retinoblastomas (Perentes *et al.*, 1987; Gonzalez-Fernandez *et al.*, 1992) and medulloblastomas (Bonnin and Perentes, 1988; Czerwionka *et al.*, 1989; Maraziotis *et al.*, 1992).

Similarly, rod-opsin, a rod outer-segment protein, also expressed in pinealocytes (Korf *et al.*, 1992), is defined by specific MAbs (Jaffey *et al.*, 1995); it frequently colocalizes with retinal S-antigen, but is conventionally found in fewer cases of retinoblastoma (Russell and Rubinstein, 1989, p. 361) and medulloblastoma (Jaffey *et al.*, 1995). The IRBP, a 140-kDa glycoprotein, is the major soluble protein present in the interphotoreceptor matrix (produced in retinal photoreceptors) and binds retinol in a light-dependent manner (reviewed in Korf *et al.*, 1992); its role in pinealocytes is undefined, as is the role of retinal S-antigen and rod-opsin. It is reported to be the earliest photoreceptor-associated protein expressed during retinal development (Lopes *et al.*, 1993) and is expressed only in tumors exhibiting rod-opsin and retinal S-antigen: pineal parenchymal tumors (Lopes *et al.*, 1993) and subsets of retinoblastomas and medulloblastomas (Korf *et al.*, 1992). The concomitant expression of these three photoreceptor proteins suggests that subsets of these tumors (but not neuroblastomas, ganglioneuroblastomas, glioblastomas, oligodendrogliomas or astrocytomas) exhibit phenotypic features of the photoreceptor lineage (Korf *et al.*, 1992).

Detection of tumor suppressor genes, oncogenes and related gene products in central nervous system tumors

The frequency of tumor suppressor gene alteration or loss, and of oncogene amplification and/or rearrangement, is thoroughly discussed in Chapter 2 of this book, and in Fuller and Bigner (1992). The following reviews the immunohistochemical detection of the expressed, overexpressed and/or variant proteins resulting from the altered transcription of these genes and the problems inherent in this approach.

Altered suppressor gene p53 protein localization

The p53 protein is a 53-kDa nuclear phosphoprotein that controls elements of the cell cycle; it is encoded by a tumor suppressor gene localized to human chromosome 17p, which is frequently mutated in glioblastomas and is thought to be one of the earliest alterations in human astrocytoma progression (Sidransky *et al.*, 1992; Newcomb *et al.*, 1993; Louis, 1994;Van Meir *et al.*, 1994). As illustrated in Fig. 8.4, the normal p53 protein is conceptually divided into three regions: (1) the NH_2 terminus, which is proline rich, highly acidic and of predicted α-helical conformation, containing the transcriptional activation domain and a heat-shock protein-binding domain; (2) the central region, containing the highly conserved domains II–IV, that is hydrophobic and of predicted β-pleated sheet conformation; and (3) the carboxy terminal region, containing multiple functional sites (nuclear localization signals, DNA binding domains and phosphorylation sites). This portion of the molecule is basic and of predicted α-helical conformation (Vogelstein and Kinzler, 1992; Louis, 1994). The wild-type p53 protein is localized in the nucleus in homo-dimeric or -tetrameric complexes (Louis, 1994), which have a short half-life, rapid turnover and negligible accumulation usually undetectable by immunohistochemistry (Iggo *et al.*, 1990; Louis *et al.*, 1993). Conversely, mutated gene products generally have a slower turnover rate, resulting in nuclear and, occasionally, cytoplasmic accumulation, which is sufficiently stable to allow immunohistochemical localization (Iggo *et al.*, 1990; Ellison *et al.*, 1992; Bruner, Connelly and Saya, 1993; Louis *et al.*, 1993).

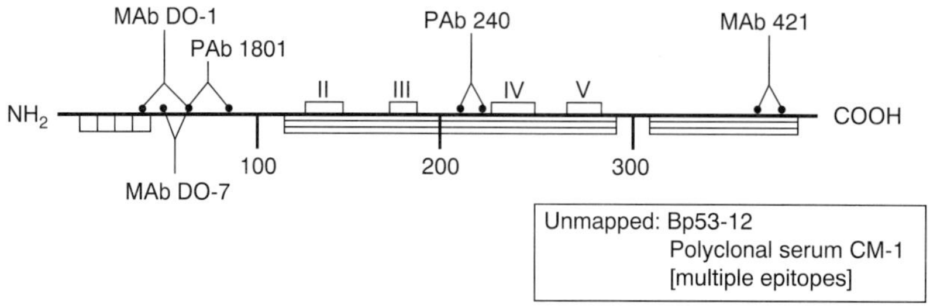

Fig. 8.4 Schematic diagram of the organization of the p53 protein with approximate MAb–epitope locations: ⊢⊢⊢, transcriptional activation domain; ☰, ascribed DNA binding regions; II, III, IV, V, highly conserved domains (Louis, 1994); NH_2, amino terminus; COOH, carboxy terminus; codon numbers lie below the linear structure; Y, mapped epitopic regions of defined anti-p53 MAbs. (Compiled from Vogelstein and Kinzler, 1992; Vojtesek *et al.*, 1992; Louis, 1994; Drach *et al.*, 1996)

The early assumption of a correlation between detectable p53 protein and *TP53* gene mutation led to the development of many MAbs and defined anti-p53 polyclonal antisera for ready immunohistochemical localization of cells presumably expressing a mutant p53 protein. As summarized in Table 8.5, the most widely analyzed and extensively defined reagents all react with wild-type and mutant proteins, with one exception, MAb PAb 240, which reacts with a conformational determinant exposed by denaturation and activating mutations (Drach *et al.*, 1996). The epitopes of the conventionally used reagents have been readily defined using a series of exonuclease-III-generated unidirectional deletions from the 3' end of the coding sequence of plasmid pT7-7 Hup 53 *TP53* DNA, and expression of truncated proteins in bacterial cells (Vojtesek *et al.*, 1992). Figure 8.4 provides the relative localization of epitopes defined by these MAbs, which are precisely described in Table 8.5.

Prior to the development and characterization of MAbs DO-1, DO-7 (Vojtesek *et al.*, 1992) and Bp53-12 (Lang *et al.*, 1994a), polyclonal antibody CM-1 was the most reliable reagent for analysis of archival (routinely formalin-fixed and paraffin-embedded) material (Midgley *et al.*, 1992). Although multiple analyses of anti-p53 antibody panels have established the general reliability of CM-1, Fisher *et al.* (1994) have recently demonstrated that even with this extensively analyzed reagent, the nature of fixative, time of fixation and avoidance of heat during processing and reaction were all crucial to the optimal interaction between CM-1 and p53 protein, especially in cases with a lower frequency of positive nuclei. As the antigen–antibody interaction of each MAb and epitope is unique, similar analyses of optimal conditions for DO-1, DO-7 and Bp53-12 need to be performed; for example, Ellison *et al.* (1995) described the analysis of p53 with MAb DO-7 following two cycles of boiling the tissue via the microwave antigen retrieval technique, whereas Drach *et al.* (1996) reported that MAb DO-7 was the only one of a panel including PAb 1801, Bp53-12 and DO-1 that did *not* require antigen retrieval. In addition, although PAb 1801 has been reported as the sole reagent in analyses of p53 in archival

Table 8.5 Characteristics of defined anti-p53 antibody reagents

Antibody	Defined epitope: Location[b]	Defined epitope: Restriction	Reactivity with[a]: Frozen sections[c]	Reactivity with[a]: Paraffin-embedded sections[d]	Reactivity with[a]: Denatured protein[e§]	Reference(s)[f]
MAb DO-1	Amino terminus; aa 37–45	Wild type and mutants	+	+	+	A, B
MAb DO-7	Amino terminus; aa 35–45	Wild type and mutants	+	+	+	A, B
MAb PAb 1801	Amino terminus; aa 45–79	Wild type and mutants	+	+	+	A, B, C
MAb PAb 240	Central portion; conformational epitope; aa 161–220; 208–220	Mutants only	+	–	+	A, B, C
MAb 421	Carboxy terminus; aa 370–378	Wild type and mutants	+	–	+/–	B, C
MAb Bp53–12	Unknown	Wild type and mutants	+	+	Unknown	A
Polyclonal antiserum CM-1	Multiple	Wild type and mutants	+	+	+	A, C

[a] Observed reactivity (+) or lack thereof (–) under condition listed; no indication of staining intensity given; see Vojtesek *et al.* (1992).
[b] It should be noted that some discrepancies do exist in amino acid sequences mapped (Ellison *et al.*, 1992); the consensus sequences listed here are from the most recent descriptions (Louis, 1994; Drach *et al.*, 1996).
[c] Frozen sections: brief prefixation in acetone:methanol, 1:1.
[d] Paraffin-embedded sections fixed in Methacarn or 10% formalin-saline.
[e] Denatured protein: reactivity with target in Western blot.
[f] References cited: A: Drach *et al.* , 1996; B: Vojtesek *et al.*, 1992; C: Louis, 1994.
MAb, monoclonal antibody.

material (Bruner, Connelly and Saya, 1993; Louis *et al.*, 1993), Vojtesek *et al.* (1992) found it to be a weakly staining antibody under these conditions. These discrepancies highlight the need for both definition of epitope stability for each reagent and the incorporation of antibody panels, as has been performed with frozen-tissue immunohistochemistry.

As summarized by Drach *et al.* (1996), the necessity for anti-p53 antibody panels is established by the inability of any single immunohistochemical reagent to identify all p53 proteins, both mutant and wild type (Ellison *et al.*, 1992; Vojtesek *et al.*, 1992; Louis *et al.*, 1993; Rasheed *et al.*, 1994). This was clearly illustrated in an early study by Ellison *et al.* (1992). Although CM-1 was most effective in identifying the largest proportion of p53+ cases as defined by the entire panel of three MAbs (PAb 1801, PAb 240 and PAb 421) and polyclonal antisera CM-1 and CM-19 (20/34 CM-1+, as opposed to 24/34, total panel), it did not react with four cases identified by the mutant p53-specific MAb PAb 240. Significantly, in this series, 8/34 glioblastoma multiforme cases were positive with all five reagents, 2/34 with 4/5 reagents, 10/34 with 3/5 reagents (not the same three) and 4/34 with one reagent. Similar results were reported by Drach *et al.* (1996) with a six-antibody panel (PAb 1801, PAb 240, DO-1, DO-7, Bp53-12 and CM-1) in childhood astrocytomas. Although CM-1 was the best consensus reagent, it was unreactive with cases readily detectable by Bp53-12, DO-1, DO-7 and PAb 240. Therefore, the reliability of a single anti-p53 reagent analysis is highly questionable in frozen tissue.

In addition to unique MAb–epitope sensitivities, other observations bear on this highly variable demonstration of p53 reactivity. As detailed by Louis *et al.* (1993), the results of MAb PAb 1801 immunohistochemistry of formalin-fixed, paraffin-embedded sections and mutation analyses agreed in only 19/34 cases. In the 15 discrepant cases, five exhibited *TP53* gene alterations but were nonreactive with PAb 1801, and 10 expressed detectable protein, but no detectable gene alterations in exons 5–8. The altered-gene, protein-negative cases can be attributed to truncated proteins either lacking or cloaking the epitopic region, or preventing its binding to proteins that prolong half-life (Louis *et al.*, 1993), thus suggesting that PAb 1801 immunohistochemistry may lead to an underestimate of *TP53* mutations (Louis *et al.*, 1993; Rubio *et al.*, 1993; Louis, 1994). The 10 cases with p53 protein positivity and no evidence of *TP53* gene alteration most likely represent cases in which wild-type p53 protein accumulation occurs (Davidoff *et al.*, 1992; Newcomb *et al.*, 1993; Louis, 1994), either through binding to altered cellular or viral proteins, or

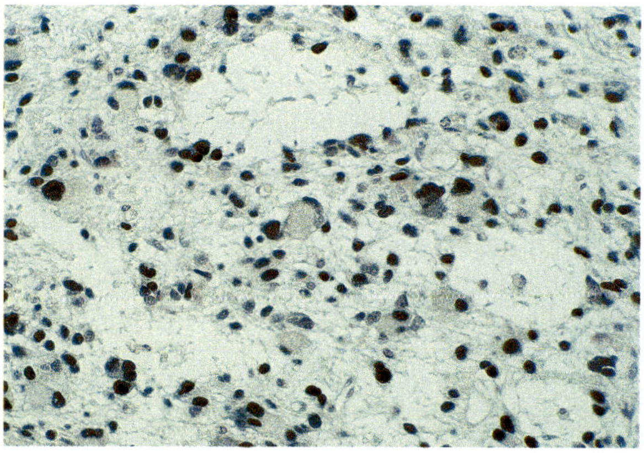

Fig. 8.5 Immunohistochemistry for p53 protein in an anaplastic astrocytoma. The darker nuclei express the stabilized p53 protein, while the lighter ones do not. The labeling is heterogeneous. Immunohistochemistry for p53 (PAb 1801)-BCIP with nuclear fast red. × 250

simply accumulation in rapidly dividing tumor cells independent of *TP53* mutation (Louis *et al.*, 1993). Thus, as summarized by Louis (1994), p53 immunopositivity, when present, may reflect several different underlying biologic conditions, and, where absent, may not be conclusive for the absence of *TP53* gene alteration.

Despite these limitations, several studies of p53 protein expression as determined on panels of both frozen and fixed tumor tissue of neuroectodermal origin have been reported; regrettably, the majority have been performed with one or two reagents and are subject to the caveats listed above. In general, p53 protein accumulation is primarily nuclear and cytoplasmic positivity, when found, is always associated with nuclear positivity (Ellison *et al.*, 1992; Soini *et al.*, 1994), with a wide variation in the percentage of positive cells. Immunoreactivity for p53 protein is primarily associated with astrocytic cells, even in biopsies exhibiting a mixed morphology such as mixed anaplastic oligoastrocytomas (Bruner, Saya and Moser, 1991; Ng *et al.*, 1994) (Fig. 8.5). However, in a study of eight gliosarcomas, Albrecht, Connelly and Bruner (1993) and Biernat *et al.* (1995) demonstrated p53-immunoreactive nuclei in both the glial and sarcomatous components. Within adult tumors of glial origin, there is a general trend for increasing incidence of p53 protein immunoreactivity with increasing malignancy, with well-differentiated astrocytomas being reported to have a lower incidence (18–46%); as compared with anaplastic astrocytomas (29–57%) and glioblastomas (GBMs, 49–70%) (Bruner, Sayer and Moser, 1991; Ellison *et al.*, 1992, 1995; Haapasalo *et al.*, 1993; Newcomb *et al.*, 1993; Iuzzolino *et al.*, 1994; Soini *et al.*, 1994). Although the number of cases examined is too small for statistical significance, the same trend of increasing p53 protein immunoreactivity with increasing malignancy is seen in oligodendrogliomas, with p53 protein incidence projected as 33–75% (Kros *et al.*, 1993; Pavelic *et al.*, 1994; Soini *et al.*, 1994).

Because the more malignant histological features of anaplastic astrocytomas and GBMs appear to be associated with the accumulation of detectable p53 protein, Soini *et al.* (1994) have suggested that it might be a prognostic marker in high-grade astrocytomas or oligodendrogliomas. Kyritsis *et al.* (1995) analyzed the relationship of p53 immunostaining and survival in 182 adult patients (12 astrocytomas, 48 anaplastic astrocytomas and 122 GBMs). Kaplan-Meier survival plots indicated that the 6 astrocytoma and 35 anaplastic astrocytoma p53+ patients had longer survival times than their p53– counterparts. No difference in survival was noted for the 73 p53+ GBM patients. In their series of 123 astrocytic tumors (24 astrocytomas, 31 anaplastic astrocytomas and 68 GBMs), however, Ellison *et al.* (1995) could find no relation between survival and three categories of p53 protein expression: (p53–, p53 labeling index <40% and p53 labeling index >60%). Although the percentage of cells exhibiting p53 protein positivity in low-grade astrocytomas is relatively low, Iuzzolino *et al.* (1994) have reported that in a long-term follow-up study of 52 such patients, the median survival times for p53+ versus p53– cases were not significantly different, although a more aggressive course was seen in patients with p53 immunoreactive tumors 3–4 years after surgery, as indicated by Kaplan-Meier survival estimates at 5 years (21.2% for p53+ tumor patients versus 45.9% for p53– tumor patients). Similarly, in a study of 25 cases of recurrent oligodendroglioma, Kros *et al.* (1993) concluded that tumors exhibiting a high percentage (>75%) of p53 immunolabeled cells predicted an unfavorable clinical course. This association does not appear to hold true for pediatric gliomas. Lang *et al.* (1994b) have reported that as the percentage of tumors exhibiting *TP53* protein immunoreactivity in grade I (juvenile pilocytic astrocytoma, JPA, 5/7, 71%), grade II (juvenile astrocytoma, JA, 5/8, 63%) and grade III (juvenile anaplastic astrocytoma, JAA, 10/16, 63%) was far higher than the percentage of tumors exhibiting *TP53* gene mutation in exons 2–11 as determined by single-strand conformation polymorphism analysis (SSCP) (14%, 25% and 19%, respectively), mechanisms other than *TP53* gene inactivation by mutation or *MDM2* complex formation is operative in pediatric astrocytomas. This conclusion was shared by Drach *et al.* (1996), whose study of JAs and JAAs revealed no significant difference in mean survival time between p53-protein-positive and p53-protein-negative tumors. Although, as concluded by Ellison *et al.* (1995) and Louis (1994), immunohistochemistry for the p53 protein to date appears to have little or no value in the prognostic assessment of these tumors, its biological significance remains to be determined. Given the relative ease of the methodology versus standard molecular techniques, p53 immunohistochemistry will continue to play a significant role in characterizing the biology of this protein in disease and neoplastic conditions; additional efforts need to be made to improve the specificity and sensitivity of detection.

ONCOGENES AND RELATED GENE PRODUCTS

'Cellular proto-oncogenes are a group of conserved nucleotide sequences homologous to transforming genes of oncogenic retroviruses' (Sauceda *et al.*, 1988); and tumors of neuroectodermal origin demonstrate a relatively high incidence of proto-oncogene amplification (Debiec-Rychter *et al.*, 1994). As summarized in this book (Chapter 2) and by Fuller and Bigner (1992), gene amplification, related to increasing grade of glioma malignancy, occurs in approximately 40–50% of all GBM cases, and although amplification of *MYCN* (2–4% overall; 2/47, Wong *et al.*, 1987; 1/57, Fuller *et al.*, 1990) and *GLI* (2–4% overall; 2/45, Kinzler *et al.*, 1987; 1/47, Wong *et al.*, 1987) have been demonstrated, amplification of *MYC* or *KRAS2* or other as yet unidentified oncogenes are merely sporadic. The most commonly amplified proto-oncogene is *EGFR*, or the epidermal growth factor receptor gene, which has been found to be amplified in approximately 50% of cases of GBM (Libermann *et al.*, 1985; Wong *et al.*, 1987; Ekstrand *et al.*, 1992; Schlegel *et al.*, 1994b). The following discussion will briefly summarize the experience with *MYC* and *MYCN* and concentrate on oncogene products that have been evaluated immunohistochemically with reference to incidence, grade discrimination or prognosis.

c-myc and N-myc proteins

Amplification of the gene *MYC* is a rare occurrence in tumors of astrocytic origin (Helseth *et al.*, 1988; Lang *et al.*, 1994b). Although the overall incidence is low, *MYC* is the most common oncogene amplified in medulloblastomas (Wasson *et al.*, 1990). The most widely used antibodies to the *MYC* gene product, a 439 amino acid nuclear phosphoprotein, are MAbs generated to synthethic peptides representing one of two hydrophilic portions of the molecule: aa 171–188 or aa 408–432 (Evan *et al.*, 1985). Engelhard, Butler and Bauer (1989), using these MAbs, detected c-myc protein in 4/4 GBM studied; similarly, Orian *et al.* (1992) found c-myc protein in 1/20 (5%) JPAs, 7/21 (33%) anaplastic astrocytomas and 16/21 (76%) GBMs. The authors reported that this trend of c-myc protein expression increasing with degree of malignancy was highly significant ($P<0.001$), suggesting that it might be an indicator of progression. Two studies have been reported that compare levels of *MYC* gene amplification as determined by Northern and Southern blot, respectively, and protein expression by anti-c-myc protein MAb (NCL-c-myc and 1F7, respectively) immunoperoxidase immunohistochemistry. Both have concluded that detection of the c-myc protein in CNS tumors is not a consequence of gene amplification or rearrangement, but rather of nuclear accumulation of the protein, which has a long half-life (Shindo *et al.*, 1993; Debiec-Rychter *et al.*, 1994). Most notably, Shindo *et al.* (1993) also reported increasing numbers of positive nuclei with increasing degree of malignancy, but in addition noted heterogeneous staining of the nuclei of reactive astrocytes in optic nerves involved by optic sheath meningioma, and in the proliferating endothelial cells of GBM, as well as in the nuclei of the neoplastic cells themselves. The authors were unable to conclude whether the accumulation of c-myc protein in reactive astrocytes and endothelial cells was due to the same mechanism as in glioma cells.

As noted above, amplification of *MYCN* is more frequent than that of *MYC* in CNS tumors (Fuller and Bigner, 1992), but is still a negligible percentage of astrocytic tumors in terms of the contribution of immunohistochemical analysis (Lang *et al.*, 1994a). As was the case with *MYC*, however, Garson *et al.* (1989) readily detected the 63–66 kDa N-myc product protein in a nuclear staining pattern in 6/10 frozen medulloblastoma tissues using a sheep polyvalent anti-*MYCN* exon 3 peptide serum. *MYCN* was not amplified in any of the nine medulloblastoma samples as determined by Southern blot analysis. Considerable heterogeneity in nuclear staining was observed, with no detectable protein in the cytoplasm or nucleoli; binding of the antiserum in the six positive samples could be blocked by preincubation of antibody with the immunizing synthetic peptide. Assay of archival formalin-fixed, paraffin-embedded tissue was uniformly negative. There was no correlation between duration of relapse-free survival and absence or presence of N-myc protein in this small series. Whether N-myc protein expression will be of prognostic utility in CNS tumor evaluation remains to be determined.

Nerve growth factor receptor

Nerve growth factor (NGF) was the first growth factor to be associated with neuroectodermal tumor cells (Fabricant, De Larco and Todaro, 1977), and it is the most extensively studied member of the neurotrophins family. Nerve growth factor receptors (NGFRs) (Pusztai *et al.*, 1993; Chao and Hempstead, 1995) exist in high- and low-affinity forms; the low-affinity NGFR (p75-NGFR) is a protein with a molecular mass of 75 kDa, while the high-affinity receptors are a family of protein tyrosinase receptors with a molecular mass of 140 kDa and known as Trk A, B and C. These high-affinity Trk receptors appear to mediate most of the biological effects of NGF and other neurotrophins (Cordon-Cardo *et al.*, 1991; Pusztai *et al.*, 1993; Chao and Hempstead, 1995) and are widely distributed in the embryonic and adult CNS (Buck *et al.*, 1988; Muragaki *et al.*, 1994) as well as in human medulloblastomas and other pediatric CNS tumors (Segal *et al.*, 1994; Washiyama *et al.*, 1996).

Strong p75-NGFR immunoreactivity has been demonstrated in both formalin-fixed and frozen tissues with the anti-p75-NGFR MAb Me20.4 on the processes of differentiated tumor cells in peripheral neuroblastoma (6/11), ganglioneuroblastoma (2/2) and ganglioneuroma (4/4) (Baker *et al.*, 1991). The expression in adrenal neuroblastomas, however, (Molenaar, Rorke and Trojanowski, 1995) was limited to stromal septae separating nodules of tumor cells and occasional tumor cells. As summarized in the latter report, neuroblastomas were more frequently NGFR positive than negative (6 versus 5), as were astrocytomas (11 versus 3); the staining in these astrocytomas was frequently characterized by a fine fibrillar pattern, corresponding to the fibrillary processes of the tumor cells (Baker *et al.*, 1991). In contrast, medulloblastomas were more frequently p75-NGFR negative than positive (22 versus 13); however, in three of the cases exhibiting NGFR positivity, staining of confluent fields of tumor cells centered around blood vessels was observed; two of these cases exhibited astrocytic differentiation (Molenaar *et al.* 1989; Baker *et al.*, 1991). In summary, NGFR expression was documented in the majority of CNS gliomas and in over a third of medulloblastomas, most strikingly, those with astrocytic features.

The high-affinity nerve growth factor receptors Trk A, B and C bind specifically to the neurotrophin NGF, brain-derived neurotrophic factor (BDNF) and neurotrophin 3 (NT3), respectively. During development, individual receptor-positive cells sequentially respond to those factors in autocrine and paracrine fashion (Washiyama *et al.*, 1996). The role of the various neurotrophins in the induction of differentiation, and the regulation of cell death and apoptosis in tumors has recently been postulated (Barbacid, 1994; Chao and Hempstead, 1995). Washiyama *et al.* (1996) have reported an extensive immunohistochemical analysis of Trk A, B and C receptors and their respective neurotrophins on frozen and paraffin-embedded specimens of 27 medulloblastomas and 15 pediatric brain tumors other than medulloblastomas using a panel of defined MAbs to both extra- and intracytoplasmic domains of the receptors. The Trk A receptors were identified in 8/27 (30%) medulloblastomas, Trk B in 16/27 (59%) and Trk C in 14/27 (52%), suggesting that Trk expression may correlate with neuronal differentiation in medulloblastomas as defined by parallel analysis with MAbs to NFPs. That aberrant expression of these receptors may occur in tumors is suggested by the positive results with Trk A, which is not detectable in the normal developing or adult cerebellum where medulloblastomas arise (Barbacid, 1994). Although the number of cases per tumor category was small (15 pediatric brain tumors: 4 gangliomas and 11 glial tumors), Trk A was found in 2/4 gangliogliomas and 3/11 gliomas, Trk B in 4/4 gangliogliomas and 8/11 gliomas, and Trk C in 2/4 and 9/11, respectively (Washiyama *et al.*, 1996), reflecting the same predominance of Trk B and C as seen in medulloblastomas.

Platelet-derived growth factor and its receptor

The platelet-derived growth factor (PDGF)-β chain, encoded by the *PDGFB* proto-oncogene, was the first cellular growth factor shown to correspond to a known viral oncogene (*PDGF-β*/v-*sis*) (Fujimoto *et al.*, 1988). Following the demonstration by Nister *et al.* (1988, 1991) that long-term cultured glioma cells express both PDGF-α and PDGF-β, it was demonstrated that glioma tissue expressed PDGF-α (42/42 cases) (Mauro *et al.*, 1991) at higher levels than normal nervous tissue. In addition, Potapova *et al.* (1996) have shown that transfection of human glioma cultured cells with the gene for PDGF-β confers a tumorigenic and metastatic potential to these cells. Of interest in terms of autocrine and paracrine stimulation loops is the demonstration by *in situ* hybridization that the receptor for PDGF-α, PDGFR-α, is also expressed by glioma cells (Maxwell *et al.*, 1990). Hermanson *et al.* (1992) combined *in situ* hybridization analysis and immunohistochemistry on a panel of 14 tumors of glial origin (2 JPA, 5 astrocytomas, 2 anaplastic astrocytomas and 5 GBMs) to investigate coexpression of PDGF-α and -β chains and their cognate receptors. Affinity-purified polyvalent serum PDGFR.7 (anti-PDGFR-α COOH-terminal amino acid residues 1066–1084) and MAb PDGFR-β2, directed against the extracellular domain of the receptor (Claesson-Welsh *et al.*, 1988) revealed the same reactivity pattern as did *in situ* hybridization with cRNA probes for the same targets. Glioma cells expressing PDGFR-α were found in tumors of all grades, whereas expression of PDGFR-β was very low or absent in glioma cells. Expression of PDGF-α and -β chains was a consistent finding in high-grade gliomas, lower grade tumors usually being negative. Both PDGF-β and PDGFR-β were found in the endothelial cells of hyperplastic capillaries. The authors concluded that both autocrine and paracrine loops existed in gliomas, related to tumor progression: autocrine stimulation via PDGFR-α in glioma cells, and paracrine, and perhaps autocrine, activation of PDGFR-β in endothelial cells (Hermanson *et al.*, 1988, 1992, 1996). The very limited expression of these molecules in normal brain parenchyma suggests that PDGFR-α and PDGFR-β could serve as targets for immunotherapeutic intervention, even though their ubiquitous expression is not helpful in diagnostic interpretation.

Epidermal growth factor receptor and its variants

The epidermal growth factor receptor (EGFR) is encoded by the *EGFR* cellular oncogene located on human chromosome 7 at region 7p12–p14 (Merlino *et al.* 1985). Overexpression by the *EGFR* gene has been observed in a variety of spontaneous human tumors and studied extensively in human gliomas (Libermann *et al.*, 1985; Wong *et al.*, 1987; Humphrey *et al.*, 1988). The majority of studies implicate gene amplification as the underlying mechanism of EGFR 'overexpression', and estimates of the frequency of *EGFR* gene amplification by genetic analyses in human tumors of astrocytic origin range from 37 to 58% (Libermann *et al.*, 1985; Agosti *et al.*, 1992; Chaffanet *et al.*, 1992; Ekstrand *et al.*, 1992; Schlegel *et al.*, 1994a; Hoi *et al.*, 1995; Schwechheimer, Huang and Cavanee, 1995). Amplification is primarily associated with GBMs and not with astrocytomas of grades II/III or pilocytic astrocytomas (Torp *et al.*, 1991; Agosti *et al.*, 1992; Ekstrand *et al.*, 1992; Schlegel *et al.*, 1994a, 1994b). Although *EGFR* gene amplification has been invariably associated with high levels of protein expression, such protein 'overexpression' without gene amplification has been found in 38% (Schlegel *et al.*, 1994b) and 12% (Chaffanet *et al.*, 1992) of GBMs, suggesting that multiple systems of deregulation in *EGFR* expression may exist at translational and post-translational levels.

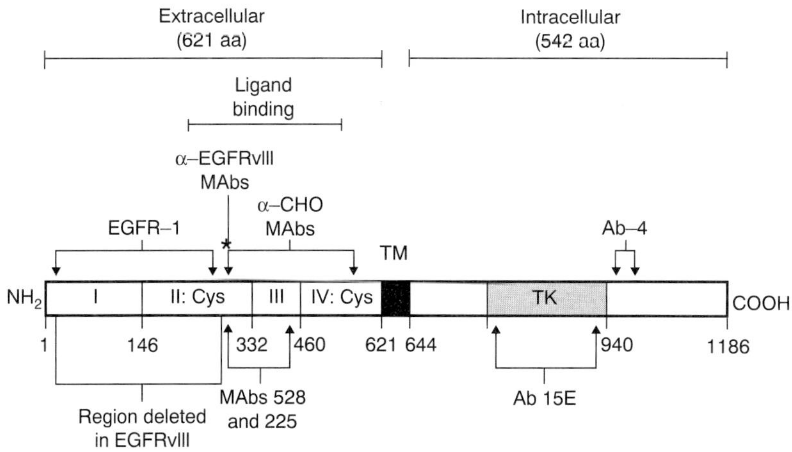

Fig. 8.6 Schematic diagram of the organization of the wild-type EGFR protein with approximate MAb–epitope locations: NH_2, amino terminus; COOH, carboxy terminus; TM: transmembrane segment; TK: tyrosine kinase domain; aa residue numbers lie below the linear structure; ↑⌊⌋↑, mapped epitopic regions of defined anti-EGFR and anti-EGFRvIII MAbs. (Compiled from Humphrey *et al.*, 1988; Ekstrand *et al.*, 1992)

The wild-type EGFR is a transmembrane glycoprotein with an M_r of 170 kDa (1186 aa residues) and comprises three functional domains (Fig. 8.6): (1) the intracellular domain with tyrosine-specific protein kinase activity, (2) a transmembrane segment and (3) an extracellular region divided into four functional regions. Domains I and III are cysteine poor, the latter being the site for ligand (EGF and TGF-α) binding. Cysteine-rich domains II and IV contain sites for *N*-linked glycosylation and disulfide bonds determining the tertiary conformation of the molecule. The original use of affinity-purified polyvalent anti-EGFR sera (Schechter *et al.*, 1979) has been replaced by a series of characterized MAbs against different sites on the receptor (Waterfield *et al.*, 1982). Although polyvalent sera and MAbs are most readily induced to the apparently more immunogenic cytoplasmic domain (Gullick *et al.*, 1985), antibodies specific for the external domain are most relevant in terms of histochemical detection of positive cells, antibody–antigen internalization and potential manipulation of the functional mitogenic properties of the receptor (Table 8.6). Listed are those reagents that have been most extensively used in immunodetection systems, including classical immunohistochemistry and probing Western blots of reduced and nonreduced protein. Not included in this list, because of obvious problems with cross-reactivity, are those anti-EGFR MAbs originally described (Carpentier *et al.*, 1986) which were subsequently found to react with blood group-associated carbohydrate epitopes also expressed in carbohydrate side chains of the EGFR (Herlyn *et al.*, 1993). In addition to the epitopically defined reagents that span the EGFR molecule (Fig. 8.6), three reagents are listed with somewhat unique properties. Reagent AbP2 is a conformation-specific polyvalent serum generated against PDGFR-β cytoplasmic domain aa 964–979 that has been found to react with the acidic tripeptide Asp–Glu–Glu, which is decrypted following tyrosine phosphorylation in both PDGFR-β and EGFR cytoplasmic domains (Panneerselvam *et al.*, 1995). The MAbs L8A4 and Y10 are listed as they specifically react with the most commonly detected EGFR variant form, EGFRvIII, which is described below (Wikstrand *et al.*, 1995).

Wild-type EGFR has been detected in CNS tumors by immunohistochemical methods and this has been reported by several groups. As might be expected with the variety of reagents available (Table 8.6) and their application with lightly methanol- or acetone-fixed, frozen tissue, or in variously fixed, paraffin-embedded tissue, the results reported have been quite variable. Agosti *et al.* (1992) examined 103 formalin-fixed glioma samples (21 pilocytic astrocytomas, 10 astrocytomas, 26 anaplastic astrocytomas and 46 GBMs) with the MAb F4 directed against aa sequence 985–996 of the EGFR cytoplasmic domain, and found positive membrane and cytoplasmic staining of tumor cells in only 17/46 (37%) GBMs. Subsequently, using affinity-purified rabbit polyvalent antiserum AB-4 and MAb 2E9, respectively, with formalin-fixed tissue, Dietzmann and von Bossanyi (1994) reported a higher incidence of EGFR positivity: 0–2/9

Table 8.6 Antibodies used in immunohistochemical evaluation of the epidermal growth factor receptor and its variants

Antibody	Source (class)	Mass (kDa) reactivity (+, –)	Domain or epitopic specificity	Inhibition of EGF-binding	Conformation dependent?	Reference
Ab-4	Rabbit polyvalent serum	170 (+) 145 (+)	aa 1005–1016 of the cytoplasmic domain	No	No	Dietzmann and von Bossanyi, 1994
Ab-15E	Rabbit polyvalent serum	170 (+) 145 (+)	ATP binding site of EGFR TK domain	No	No	Gullick *et al.*, 1986
MAb EGFR-1	IgG_{2b}	170 (+) 145 (–)	Between external domain aa 6–274; protein core	No	No	Waterfield *et al.*, 1982
MAb 225	IgG_1	170 (+) 145 (unknown)	External domain	Yes	Unknown	Sato *et al.*, 1983
MAb 528	IgG_{2a}	170 (+) 145 (+)	External domain; protein core	Yes	No	Kawamoto *et al.*, 1983
MAb 425	IgG_{2a}	170 (+) 145 (+)	External domain; protein core	Yes	No	Murthy *et al.*, 1987
MAb 2E9	IgG_1	170 (+) 145 (unknown)	External domain	Yes	Unknown	Defize *et al.*, 1986
AbP2	Rabbit polyvalent serum	170 (+) 145 (unknown)	aa 964–979 of the cytoplasmic domain PDGFR-β	No	Yes	Panneerselvam *et al.*, 1995
L8A4	IgG_1	170 (–) 145 (+)	aa surrounding fusion junction (6–274)	No	No	Wikstrand *et al.*, 1995
H10	IgG_1	170 (–) 145 (+)	aa surrounding fusion junction (6–274)	No	No	Wikstrand *et al.*, 1995
Y10	IgG_{2a}	170 (–) 145 (+)	aa surrounding fusion junction (6–274)	No	No	Wikstrand *et al.*, 1995

aa, amino acid; EGF, epidermal growth factor; kDa, kilodaltons; EGFR, epidermal growth factor receptor; MAb, monoclonal antibody; PDGFR, platelet-derived growth factor receptor.

(0–22%) pilocytic astrocytomas+; 5–6/18 (27–33%) astrocytomas +; [16–12]/17 [94–71%] anaplastic astrocytomas +; and [17–13]/19 [90–68%] GBMs+. In general, the higher proportion of EGFR+ cases found in this latter series is more consistent with results reported with various reagents applied to acetone-fixed, frozen tissue. Schwechheimer, Huang and Cavanee (1995) reported positive immunoreactivity for EGFR in 14/18 (78%) glioblastomas using an uncharacterized polyvalent rabbit-anti-EGFR external domain antiserum. Schlegel *et al.* (1994a), using the polyvalent antiserum 15E, reported that 34/37 (92%) GBM and 7/10 (70%) (5 astrocytomas and 5 anaplastic astrocytomas) exhibited strong but heterogeneous immunoreactivity for the EGFR with the strongest signals being detectable in large gemistocytic cells. Torp *et al.* (1991) found that anti-EGFR extracellular domain MAbs 528 and EGFR-1 were highly reproducible in identifying EGFR+ cases with the frequency increasing with malignancy in frozen tissue. In 2/6 (33%) astrocytomas, 5/7 (71%) anaplastic astrocytomas and 14/22 (64%) GBM cases studied, weak-to-strong staining intensity was exhibited in at least 25% of tumor cells. In a similar analysis of frozen glioma specimens with MAb 528, Wikstrand *et al.* (1995) reported 4/7 (57%) AA and 18/21 (86%) GBM cases exhibiting ≥25% positive tumor cells. The consistent observation of increasing frequency of EGFR+ cases with tumor grade, however, does not contribute an independent prognostic parameter beyond the grade itself but has provided the rationale for immunolocalization studies with anti-EGFR MAbs in glioma patients. Kalofonos *et al.* (1989) reported selective uptake of the anti-EGFR extracellular domain MAb EGFR-1 in 9/12 patients. Recently, Dadparvar *et al.* (1994) localized 111-indium-labeled anti-EGFR MAb 425 in 23 patients with gliomas, thus demonstrating the potential of glioma-expressed EGFR for immunotherapeutic approaches.

In malignant gliomas, *EGFR* gene amplification is frequently associated with structural gene rearrangement that leads to deletion mutations most frequently described in segments of the gene corresponding to the extracellular domain of the EGFR (Humphrey *et al.*, 1990; Sugawa *et al.*, 1990; Yamazaki *et al.*, 1990), although mutations in the intracellular kinase portion of the molecule have been described (Ekstrand *et al.*, 1992). The most frequently detected variant, EGFRvIII, is characterized by a consistent 801-base-pair in-frame gene deletion resulting in a 267-amino-acid deletion in domains I and II of the extracellular portion of the molecule, with the generation of a glycine residue at the fusion point of the variant 145-kDa molecule (Fig. 8.6) (Humphrey *et al.*, 1990; Yamazaki *et al.*, 1990). As reported by several groups (Humphrey *et al.*, 1988; Yamazaki *et al.*, 1990; Ekstrand *et al.*, 1992; Schlegel *et al.*, 1994a; Schwechheimer *et al.*, 1995), *EGFR* gene amplification is estimated to occur in 40–50% of cases, of which approximately 50% express the EGFRvIII deletion, with or without an additional intracytoplasmic region deletion (Ekstrand *et al.*, 1992). High-affinity MAbs L8A4, H10 and Y10 have been produced to EGFRvIII (Wikstrand *et al.*, 1995) that specifically precipitate the 145-kDa variant molecule, are unreactive with 170-kDa wild-type EGFR in both reduced and nonreduced forms, and are internalized beginning within 5 minutes of binding to target receptors on EGFRvIII-expressing cells in *in vitro* assays (Reist *et al.*, 1995). These MAbs have been used in indirect immunoperoxidase-mediated immunohistochemical assays to survey frozen biopsy tissue of human gliomas (7 anaplastic astrocytomas, 3 gliosarcomas, 21 GBMs) (Wikstrand *et al.*, 1995). The EGFRvIII was expressed by only 1/7 (14%) anaplastic astrocytomas, but in 2/3 (67%) gliosarcomas and 13/21 (62%) GBMs, for an overall incidence of 52% in gliomas in this series. As shown in Fig. 8.7(a), anti-EGFRvIII MAb L8A4 localizes the variant protein strongly in this formalin-fixed, paraffin-embedded GBM using a microwave antigen retrieval technique (Shi *et al.*, 1992). In a recent study of freshly disaggregated cells from 20 serial biopsy specimens of human gliomas, Wikstrand *et al.* (1997) demonstrated that 10/20 cases (50%) were positive for EGFRvIII as detected by MAb L8A4. Indirect and direct (quantitative) flow cytometry analyses demonstrated unequivocal cell membrane localization of EGFRvIII, which was confirmed by confocal microscopic analysis. Cell surface EGFRvIII receptor density as estimated by quantitative flow analysis was greater than 2.5×10^5 receptors/cell in 4/5 cases examined (Wikstrand *et al.*, 1997). Transfection of EGFRvIII either into cells coexpressing normal receptor (Nishikawa *et al.*, 1994) or into non-EGFR-expressing murine fibroblasts (Batra *et al.*, 1995) confers tumorigenic potential to these cells, suggesting that in human patients tumor cells that contain the *EGFRvIII* gene and/or express the EGFRvIII protein may enjoy a growth advantage *in vivo*. This association provides a basis for the use of anti-EGFRvIII MAb immunohistochemical evaluation in a prognostic manner. The demonstration of EGFRvIII receptor density levels sufficient for successful *in vivo* immunotargeting and the rapid internalization of anti-EGFRvIII MAbs following binding to the receptors on the cell surface and processing via the lysosomal pathway (Reist *et al.*, 1995) also suggests the potential of anti-EGFRvIII MAbs coupled to isotopes, toxins (Lorimer *et al.*, 1995) or chemotherapeutic agents for immunotherapeutic approaches.

Additional proteins and glycolipids with predominant expression in central nervous system tumors as opposed to normal central nervous system

The majority of immunohistochemically detected markers discussed above (the intermediate filament proteins, the neuroendocrine proteins, and the nuclear-localized proteins p53, c-myc and N-myc) are all intracellular in location and are suitable for diagnostic purposes, but not for therapeutic applications. As introduced in the preceding discussion of growth factor receptors, several transmembrane proteins, glycoproteins and glycolipids on the surface of cells also demonstrate specificity for cell lineage and/or state of differentiation. These antigens are thus good candidates for antibody localization, not only diagnostically, but also therapeutically. This latter characteristic is common to the target molecules discussed in this section.

CELL SURFACE MOIETIES

Although discussed separately as oncogene products, the PDGFR and EGFR (including EGFRvIII) glycoproteins are also examples of transmembrane molecules suitable for immunotargeting. These molecules are different from those described below, however, in that they are rapidly internalized with bound antibody within moments of binding, thereby providing opportunities and presenting challenges regarding delivery of cytostatic or cytocidal agents. The cell surface-expressed targets presented below have not been demonstrated to internalize and, like the extracellular matrix-elaborated molecules discussed in the following section, may be regarded as a geographically more 'fixed' target.

Adhesion molecules: neural cell adhesion molecule and L1

The neural cell adhesion molecule (NCAM) [encoded by *NCAMI* (*CD56, Leu* 19)] and the related neurite-glia cell adhesion molecule (NG-CAM) (Ng-CAM in the chicken and L1 in mouse and man, encoded by *LICAM* in humans) are both members of the immunoglobulin supergene family (IgSF). In the adult human CNS, discrete isoforms of NCAM exist (Frost *et al.*, 1991), probably generated by alternative splicing of mRNA encoded by a single gene as demonstrated for chicken NCAM (Murray *et al.*, 1986). During embryonic development of the CNS, NCAMs are heavily sialylated and migrate in reducing gels with an apparent mass range of 180–250 kDa. With development, the degree of sialylation decreases with a concomitant increase in adhesiveness (Molenaar, de Leij and Trojanowski, 1991; Behrens *et al.*, 1992). Many MAbs specific for NCAM have been produced with defined reactivity for the extracellular protein backbone (Crossin, Edelman and Cunningham, 1984; Aletsee-Ufrecht *et al.*, 1990; ERIC, Phimister *et al.*, 1991), *N*-linked carbohydrate epitopes (UJ13A, Patel *et al.*, 1989a; SEN-7, Waibel *et al.*, 1993) and the α2–8 polysialic acid linkages (15G8, Crossin, Edelman and Cunningham, 1984; 3F8, Patel *et al.*, 1989b; 12F8, Miller, Lang and Epstein, 1993). Using Western blot analysis and immunohistochemistry, Frost *et al.* (1991) and Patel *et al.* (1991a) examined the expression of NCAM isoforms in normal adult and fetal brain and in a panel of CNS tumor biopsies. Norml adult brain, they found, is characterized by four isoforms of 180, 170, 140 and 120 kDa; a fifth 95-kDa isoform is revealed after *N*-linked carbohydrate and sialic acid residues are removed by *N*-glycanase and neuraminidase treatment, respectively. Embryonic NCAM is more heavily polysialylated than the adult form, resulting in a smear on sodium dodecyl sulfate polyacrylamide gel electrophoresis (SDS-PAGE); the 180-, 170-, 140-, 120- and 95-kDa isoforms are apparent after disialylation. Astrocytomas, ependymomas and meningiomas express only the 140-, 120- and 95-kDa isoforms with little or no sialylation, while oligodendrogliomas express the same pattern plus a sialylated form that reduces to 170 kDa (Figarella-Branger, Durbec and Rougon, 1990; Frost *et al.*, 1991; Patel *et al.*, 1991a). While heavily sialylated, NCAMs isolated from schwannomas consist only of the 140-, 120- and 95-kDa forms. Of greatest interest, in the Figarella-Branger, Durbec and Rougon (1990) study, are medulloblastomas and 4/7 neuroblastomas identical to fetal brain in expressing large amounts of heavily sialylated NCAM and the full spectrum of 'embryonic' isoforms: 180, 170, 140, 120 and 95 kDa. Since Carbone *et al.* (1991) have shown that there is a strong correlation between the expression of NCAM isoform 140, lack of substrate adhesion, and spontaneous aggregation of small-cell lung carcinoma cells in culture, it is not surprising, that in a study of six well-characterized medulloblastoma cell lines that grow as aggregates in suspension, all were found to express the 140 kDa isoform with variable expression of the 170 and 120 kDa forms (Wikstrand, Friedman and Bigner, 1991). As reviewed by Molenaar, Rorke and Trojanowski

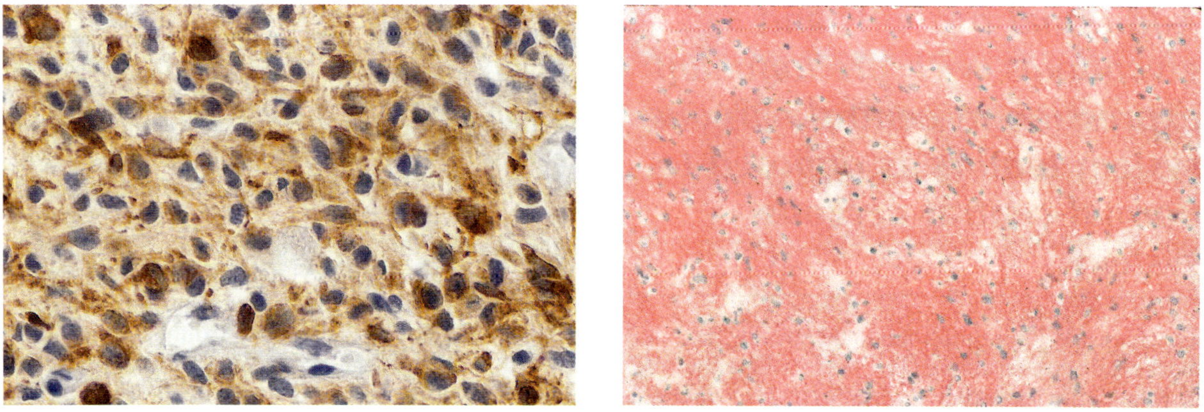

Fig. 8.7 Immunohistochemistry of transmembrane proteins in primary CNS tumors. (a) Anti-EGFRvIII MAb L8A4 strongly reacts with every neoplastic cell in this GBM in a pattern that spares the nuclei of tumor cells and does not react with benign stromal elements such as vascular endothelial cells. Formalin-fixed section, antigen retrieval technique with acidic buffer; ×198. (b). Neural cell adhesion molecule expression in a pilocytic astrocytoma. ×400

(1995), a series of immunohistochemical studies have demonstrated NCAM expression in medulloblastomas, other primitive neuroectodermal tumors, astrocytomas, oligodendrogliomas, ependymomas and meningiomas, in addition to neuroblastomas, ganglioneuroblastomas and ganglioneuromas (Molenaar, de Leij and Trojanowski, 1991; Yamanaka, Tanaka and Saito, 1994), in schwannomas and in retinoblastomas (Frost *et al.*, 1991; Rodrigues *et al.*, 1992), and neuroendocrine tumors (Carbone *et al.*, 1991; Jin, Hemperly and Lloyd, 1991; Patel *et al.*, 1991a). An example of NCAM staining in a pilocytic astrocytoma is presented in Fig. 8.7(b). The anti-NCAM MAb ERIC has been specifically localized to recurrent malignant gliomas successfully in patients receiving either ^{131}I ERIC injection into the resection cavity or glioma cysts, or ^{90}Y ERIC, with minimal toxicity. Early cerebral edema responded readily to dexamethasone, and delayed, mild myelosuppression required no treatment (Papanastassiou *et al.*, 1993; Hopkins *et al.*, 1995).

The related human IgSF L1 adhesion molecule has 92% homology with murine L1 (Hlavin and Lemmon, 1991) and structural similarity to NCAM, which appears to be coexpressed by all L1-positive cells (Kadmon *et al.*, 1990). In normal development, L1 has been predominantly associated with neurite fasciculation and outgrowth (Lagenaur and Lemmon, 1987), and in the CNS it is only present on postmitotic neurons (Patel *et al.*, 1991b). L1 is synthesized as a single transmembrane protein with an estimated mass of 135 kDa and, after modulation, an M_r in SDS-PAGE of approximately 210 kDa (Nybroe and Bock, 1988). L1 is heavily glycosylated, with 22 sites for *N*-linked glycosylation in the extracellular domain. Within this region are six Ig-homology domains and three fibronectin-like repeats (Moos *et al.*, 1988). Monoclonal antibodies specific for L1 and not simply cross-reactive with conserved domains common to many molecules have been difficult to obtain, and early studies were performed with polyvalent antisera to L1 with cross-species reactivity (Figarella-Branger, Durbec and Rougon, 1990). Monoclonal antibodies reactive with human L1 have been isolated following immunization with human fetal brain (UJ127.11 and UJ181.4; Patel *et al.*, 1991b) or neuroblastoma cells (5G3; Wolff *et al.*, 1988). More recently, MAbs with reactivity for defined regions of the L1 extracellular domain (Ig domains 1–4, 5–6) and fibronectin repeats 2–3 have been isolated after fusion proteins, generated in *E. coli* and/or synthetic peptides, were used (Klinz, Schachner and Maness, 1995); however, these latter MAbs have not yet been applied immunohistochemically.

As defined by MAbs 5G3, UJ127.11 and UJ181.4, which identify unique epitopes in the extracellular domain probably not involving carbohydrate (Patel *et al.*, 1991b), L1 immunoprecipitated from human cerebellum comprises several components: a doublet of 190/210 kDa, a band of 140 kDa, and minor components of 65–80 kDa. Following *N*-linked deglycosylation, the 190/210-kDa doublet shifts to 150/165 kDa, and the 140-kDa band to 107 kDa (Wolff *et al.*, 1988). Figarella-Branger, Durbec and Rougon (1990) identified L1 in 7/7 human neuroblastoma biopsies tested by Western blot using a polyclonal anti-L1 serum, but were unable to detect the 190/210-isoform in gliomas, ependymomas or medulloblastomas. In contrast,

Patel *et al.* (1991b), using monoclonal anti-L1 MAbs UJ127.11 and 5G3, readily demonstrated coincident reactivity by Western blot and immunohistochemistry in 21/24 neuroblastomas, 1 each neuroepithelioma and ganglioneuroblastoma, 0/3 medulloblastomas, 1/8 oligodendrogliomas and 0/3 gliomas. Wikstrand, Friedman and Bigner (1991) have reported the detection of both the 140- and 190/210-kDa isoforms of L1 in 6/6 medulloblastoma biopsy-derived cell lines and xenografts tested with MAb UJ127.11. Pilot studies involving the intrathecal administration of anti-L1 MAb UJ181.4 have been reported (Lashford *et al.*, 1988; Moseley *et al.*, 1990). In all, 7 patients (4 medulloblastomas, 1 pineoblastoma, 1 teratoma and 1 ependymoma) have received UJ181.4 with no significant CNS or systemic toxicity. While no localization occurred in the teratoma and ependymoma cases, specific localization was achieved in all others, with long-term disease-free intervals (22–60 months) in the patients with pineoblastoma and medulloblastoma. The absence of CNS toxicity and the range of NCAM and L1 expression within primary CNS tumors is consistent with further therapeutic trials. Even though diagnostically elucidating NCAM and L1 isoforms is probably not of great benefit, their use prognostically, particularly with regard to cell migration and metastasis, has yet to be determined.

Table 8.7 Panel of epitope-defined anti-ganglioside MAbs

MAb	Minimum binding epitope[a]	Defined gangliosides expressing epitope[b]
DMAb-3	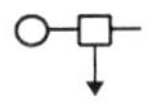	GM2, GalNAc-GD1a
DMAb-20	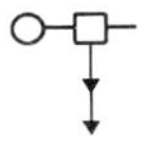	GD2
DMAb-7	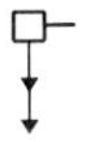	GD3, GT1a, 3',8'-LD1
SL-50	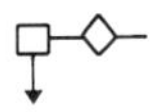	3'-isoLM1
DMAb-22	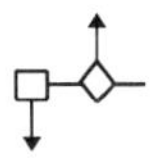	3',6'-isoLD1

[a] As defined by comparative analysis of binding to fast atom bombardment mass spectroscopy analyzed, purified ganglioside standards, ○, *N*-acetylgalactosamine; □, galactose; ◇, *N*-acetylglucosamine; ▼, NeuAc.
[b] Reactivity spectrum of antibody designated.

Oncofetal ganglioside epitopes

Gangliosides are a group of sialic-acid-containing glycosphingolipids that are anchored to the cell membrane by a lipophilic ceramide segment, with the antigenic hydrophilic carbohydrate section extending extracellularly. The sequence of sugar residues that defines classes or 'series' of gangliosides can also be found on glycoproteins. The orderly sequences of glycosylation and sialylation required to produce specific defining linkages are well known, and MAbs specific for the more common 'normal' (GM2, GM3, GD2 and GD3) and 'oncofetal' gangliosides (3'-isoLM1 and 3',6'-isoLD1) have been thoroughly described (Table 8.7) (Wikstrand *et al.*, 1994b). While these reagents are of demonstrably high specificity, they are all of the IgM class, thus requiring the careful use of irrelevant isotype control antibody. The majority of these defined carbohydrate epitopes are sensitive to most fixation methods with the exception of short-duration acetone fixation (Wikstrand *et al.*, 1993).

The appearance of novel or quantitative shifts in ganglioside phenotype following neoplastic transformation has been reported in tumors of diverse origin (Wikstrand *et al.*, 1994a, 1994b). Among tumors of neuroectodermal origin, gliomas have been reported to demonstrate a marked shift from the expression of the more complex oligosialylated gangliosides such as GD1a, GD1b and GT1b found in normal brain, to the simpler, less polar gangliosides (Vick *et al.*, 1992; Sung *et al.*, 1994). Using a panel of MAbs recognizing GM2, GD3 (and 3',8'-LD1) and GD2, and a diverse series of cytologic specimens, Vick *et al.* (1992) found that GD3 was present on a large portion of many tumor types (100% of glial tumors, 69% of non-CNS tumors, 44% of non-small-cell carcinomas and 60% of sarcomas), and is therefore not diagnostically useful alone. While slightly more restricted in expression, GM2 and GD2 were still present in nonglial-CNS tumors (31% and 15%, respectively) and non-small-cell carcinomas (18% and 10%) at levels that were not useful for true differentiation. When a panel of 30 primary CNS tumors (4 astrocytomas, 24 GBMs and 2 gliosarcomas) was examined, the high incidence of expression of GM2 (84%), GD2 (77%) and GD3 (100%) precluded their utility in terms of differential diagnostic application (Wikstrand *et al.*, 1994a, 1994b).

Of greater potential as glioma-distinctive markers are the lactotetraose series gangliosides IV$_3$NeuAc-LcOse4Cer (3'-isoLM1) and IV$_3$NeuAc,III$_6$NeuAc-LcOse4Cer (3',6'-isoLD1) as the major mono- and oligosialogangliosides, respectively, of many human gliomas. Anti-3'-isoLM1 MAb SL-50 and anti-3',6'-isoLD1 MAbs DMAb 21

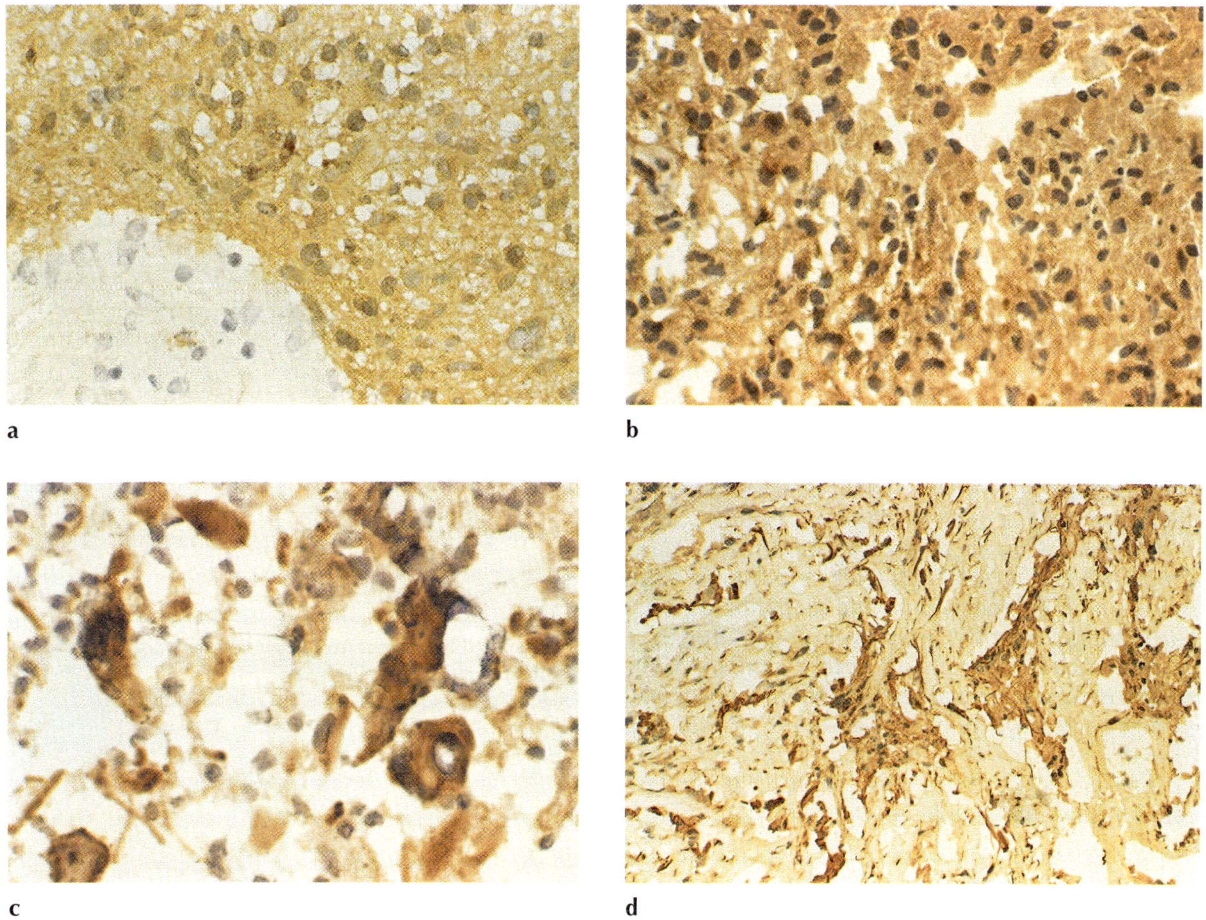

Fig. 8.8 Immunohistchemistry of oncofetal gangliosides in primary CNS tumors. (a) Anti-3'-isoLM1 MAb SL-50 immunostain showing intense reactivity of tumor and absence of blood vessel staining (hematoxylin counterstain) in a GBM. Acetone-fixed, frozen tissue; × 325. (b) Anti-3',6'-isoLD1 DMAb-22 exhibits a diffuse pattern of reactivity with intense staining of nearly all cells in a GBM. Acetone-fixed, frozen tissue; × 520. (c). Anti-3',6'-isoLD1 DMAb-21 intensely stains neoplastic giant cells in this giant-cell GBM. Acetone-fixed, frozen tissue; × 400. (d). Anti-3',6'-isoLD1 DMAb 22 reacts only with the neoplastic glial element and is unreactive with the sarcomatous component of a gliosarcoma. Acetone-fixed, frozen tissue; × 170.

and 22 were generated following immunization with extracted 3'-isoLM1 or the human glioma biopsy-derived xenograft D54 MG, respectively (Table 8.7) (Wikstrand *et al.*, 1991, 1993), and have been used to analyze the distribution of the 3'-isoLM1 and 3',6'-isoLD1 epitopes on a variety of human tumors by immunohistochemistry and high-performance thin-layer chromatography (HPTLC), and immunostaining. Immunohistochemical localization of 3'-isoLM1 was performed on 31 biopsies of human gliomas (2 anaplastic astrocytomas, 2 gliosarcomas and 27 GBMs); 15 (48%) expressed 3'-isoLM1 as defined by >10% of positive neoplastic cells. Staining of small anaplastic cells, giant cells and the glial component of gliosarcomas was observed. Neoplastic gemistocytes, when present, showed particularly intense staining; blood vessels were not appreciably stained (Wikstrand *et al.*, 1991). An example of MAb SL-50 reactivity with a GBM is presented in Fig. 8.8(a). In a similar analysis with the same tumor panel, anti-3',6'-isoLD1 MAbs DMAb-21 and -22 were found specifically to localize to 4/4 anaplastic astrocytomas, 14/23 GBMs and 2/2 gliosarcomas (Wikstrand *et al.*, 1993). Reactivity with the MAbs roughly correlates with glioma cell size; cells with abundant cytoplasm tended to exhibit strong cytoplasmic reactivity, while those with scant cytoplasm tended to be non-reactive. An example of intense staining of a GBM in a diffuse pattern with DMAb-22 is provided in

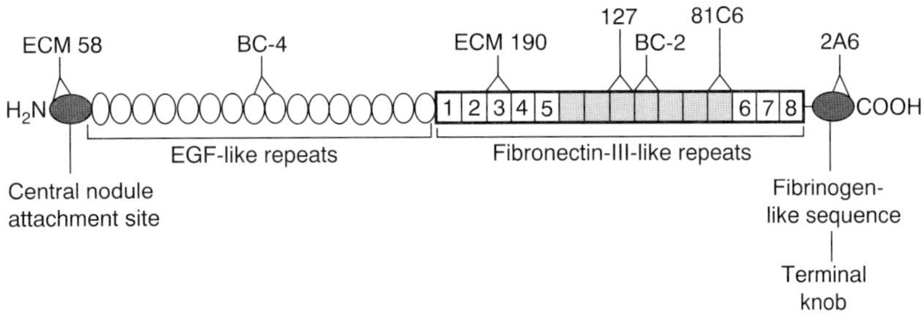

Fig. 8.9 Schematic diagram of a single arm of the tenascin hexabrachion molecule with approximate MAb–epitope locations: NH_2, amino terminus, which joins to five other single arms in the molecule's central nodule; COOH, carboxy terminus, forming each arm's terminal knob; Y, mapped epitopic regions of defined antitenascin MAbs. (Compiled from Murphy-Ullrich *et al.*, 1991; Lightner, 1994; Schenk and Chiquet-Ehrismann, 1994 to indicate MAb–epitope locations; see Lightner, 1994 for current model of tenascin-C structure.)

Fig. 8.8(b); Fig. 8.8(c) illustrates the intense staining of the cells in a gigantocellular GBM. In Fig. 8.8(d), staining of the neoplastic glial element and lack of staining of the sarcomatous component is demonstrated in a gliosarcoma. As these analyses were performed with lightly acetone-fixed, frozen tissue, it is not possible truly to localize the antigen deposition; however, membrane staining is suggested by the observed fibrillar pattern in Figs 8.8(c) and (d). Nuclear staining was rarely noted. Within the CNS, 3'-isoLM1 and 3',6'-isoLD1 appear to serve as operationally specific markers of neoplasia, or in the fetal–newborn period, they seem to mark areas of rapid astroglial proliferation (Svennerholm *et al.*, 1987). The inability to detect 3'-isoLM1 or 3',6'-isoLD1 by either extensive HPTLC analysis (Svennerholm *et al.*, 1987; Fredman *et al.*, 1988) or immunohistochemistry in samples of adult CNS tissue (Wikstrand *et al.*, 1991), and the presence of these epitopes in intense reactive astrocytosis and in gliomas, provides a marker system for hyperplastic/neoplastic or, perhaps, 'nonresting' astrocytes.

EXTRACELLULAR MATRIX MOLECULES

Extracellular matrix (ECM) molecules, elaborated by neoplastic cells within the CNS, have proven to be attractive targets for antibody localization as a result of their distribution throughout the tumor matrix, their absence of expression in normal brain parenchyma and their location in the hyperplastic vessels of gliomas (Wikstrand and Bigner, 1996). The following section summarizes the experience with two such molecules extensively expressed by gliomas: tenascin and GP 240.

Tenascin

Tenascin is a polymorphic ECM glycoprotein which is widely expressed during embryonic development, but is far more restricted in form and distribution in normal adult tissues (Bourdon *et al.*, 1983; Lightner, 1994). Although three members of the tenascin family (tenascin-C, tenascin-R and tenascin-X) have been described, the most extensively studied is tenascin-C, originally described as cytotactin, and being the predominant tenascin molecule expressed during embryogenesis, in the nervous system and in tumors (Schenk and Chiquet-Ehrismann, 1994). Tenascin-C is distinct from other ECM proteins in that it is composed of a radially arranged hexamer joined at the amino-terminal central knob by disulfide bonds. As illustrated in Fig. 8.9, each arm is a single subunit of 220–320 kDa, consisting of a linear array of repeated structural domains including: (1) the amino-terminal triple-helical coil structure stabilized by cysteine residues involved in oligomerization, (2) a linear segment of 14½ epidermal growth-factor-like domains, (3) a region of 8–15 fibronectin type III (FN-III) domains, and (4) a β- and γ-fibrinogen-like region carboxy terminus (Lightner, 1994; Bigner *et al.*, 1995). Different subunits or forms are generated by alternate splicing and variable transcription of up to eight FN-III domains that are inserted between universally conserved FN-III repeat numbers 5 and 6–8; three predominant isoforms of 220, 230 and 320 kDa (considered the complete tenascin-C monomeric arm) have been demonstrated in human glioma cells and normal tissues, including human cerebral cortex (Murphy-Ullrich *et al.*, 1991; Ventimiglia *et al.*, 1992). However, the splicing patterns of human tenascin are quite complex, and it is probable that many other splice variants are routinely produced (Siri *et al.*, 1991). Expression of these variants and their relative proportions are variable in tissues, cell types and tumors (Chiquet-Ehrisman *et al.*, 1991; Ventimiglia *et al.*, 1992). Both polyvalent sera and MAbs specific for various epitopes on tenascin have been produced (Balza *et al.*, 1993; Bourdon *et al.*, 1983; Siri *et al.*, 1991). The mapping of the epitopes recognized by these MAbs was performed by a combination of rotary shadowing immunomicroscopy, Western blotting and analysis of reactivity with β-galactosidase–tenascin fusion proteins expressed in *E. coli* (Murphy-Ullrich *et al.*, 1991; Siri *et al.*, 1991). As shown in Fig. 8.9, MAb BC-4 recognizes an epitope present on all tenascin isoforms, whereas MAb BC-2 defines an epitope the expression of which is controlled by alternative splicing of tenascin pre-mRNA (Siri *et al.*, 1991). Similarly, MAb ECM 58, which binds the central core, MAb 2A6, which localizes to the terminal knob, and MAb 190, which localizes to FN-111 repeat 3, all bind to the predominant 320-, 230- and 220-kDa isoforms; whereas those MAbs recognizing epitopes in alternative splice regions are more discriminatory: MAb 127 binds only to the 320-kDa isoform, and human-specific MAb 81C6 binds to the 320- and 230-kDa isoforms (Murphy-Ullrich *et al.*, 1991).

Polyvalent antitenascin antisera and MAbs 81C6 and 2A6 have been used extensively to determine tenascin distribution immunohistochemically. Tenascin is strongly expressed in mesenchymal tumors and carcinomas, fibrosarcomas, osteosarcomas, melanoma, Wilms' tumor, colon carcinoma, mammary and lung carcinomas, and squamous carcinomas (Bigner *et al.*, 1995; Kurpad and Bigner, 1995; Kurpad *et al.*, 1995). Tenascin has been localized by immunohistochemistry in liver, spleen, kidney, skin and breast (Bourdon *et al.*, 1983; Lightner *et al.*, 1989; Lightner, Marks and McCachren, 1994) and by Western blot in adult human brain cortex (Ventimiglia *et al.*, 1992). In the CNS, extremely low levels are found in cortex, but enhanced levels are found in reactive astrocytes where there is cerebral injury and cerebellar degeneration (McComb and Miller, 1990; Laywell *et al.*, 1992). Tenascin expression has been correlated with increasing degree of malignancy (McComb and Bigner, 1985; Higuchi *et al.*, 1993), it being prominent in the most anaplastic forms of glioma. Bourdon *et al.* (1983, 1985) described intense staining in unfixed, frozen tissue sections of 1/6 (17%) astrocytomas and 14/16 (88%) GBMs. In a larger immunohistochemical study of 54 astrocytomas in paraffin sections, Zagzag *et al.* (1995), using antihuman tenascin murine MAb TN2, found that tenascin was variably expressed in all astrocytomas, but was most pronounced in high-grade tumors. In the majority of low-grade tumors (pilocytic astrocytomas and well-differentiated fibrillar astrocytomas), intercellular matrix or stromal staining was faint, but in GBMs tenascin was frequently expressed around cells in a fibrillar, anastamosing network [Fig. 8.10(a)–(c)]. Intracytoplasmic tenascin immunoreactivity was frequently seen (Zagzag *et al.*, 1995). The predominant localization in all grades, however, was in and around vascular channels in gliomas [Fig. 8.10(c)] and has been postulated to correlate with angiogenesis (Zagzag *et al.*, 1996). This localization and the demonstration that human brain microvessel endothelial cells can synthesize tenascin *in vitro* have led to the hypothesis that tenascin, whether elaborated by tumor cells or endothelial cells, may be associated with endothelial cell activation, playing an active role in neoplastic angiogenesis. As yet, discrimination of tenascin-C isoform expression by various tissues has not been addressed in an extensive manner immunohistochemically.

GP 240

Another ECM molecule similar to tenascin in its distribution is the chondroitin sulfate proteoglycan, characteristic of melanomas and gliomas, and defined by its protein core as GP 240. Further characterization or purification of the molecule has not yet been accomplished (R. Reisfeld, personal communication). The GP 240 molecule is elaborated by gliomas, melanomas and hyperplastic endothelial cells within gliomas (Carrel *et al.*, 1980; Behnke *et al.*, 1988; Colapinto *et al.*, 1990). Two MAbs define separate epitopes on the core protein of this molecule: MAbs 9.2.27 (Bumol and Reisfeld, 1982; Schrappe *et al.*, 1992) and Mel-14, produced by Carrel *et al.* (1980). The GP 240 molecule is not detectable in either white or gray matter from the medulla oblongata, cerebellum or spinal cord (Schrappe *et al.*, 1992) but has been detected immunohistochemically in 5/6 (83%) ependymomas, 4/9 (44%) medulloblastomas, 2/7 (29%) astrocytomas and 28/49 (57%) GBMs (Kurpad *et al.*, 1995) and in colon and breast carcinomas (Carrel *et al.*, 1980). Localization of GP 240 in primary CNS tumors is quite similar to that of tenascin. While diffuse staining is frequently seen, the predominant pattern, characteristic of the more anaplastic tumors, is the blood-vessel-associated and fibrillary staining pattern depicted in Fig. 8.10(d) and reminiscent of the tenascin localization shown in Fig. 8.10(c).

Both antitenascin and anti-GP 240 MAbs have been investigated in phase I studies of compartmental administration of iodinated MAbs to patients with primary CNS tumors or tumors metastatic to the CNS (Bigner *et al.*, 1995). Striking clinical and radiographic responses have been

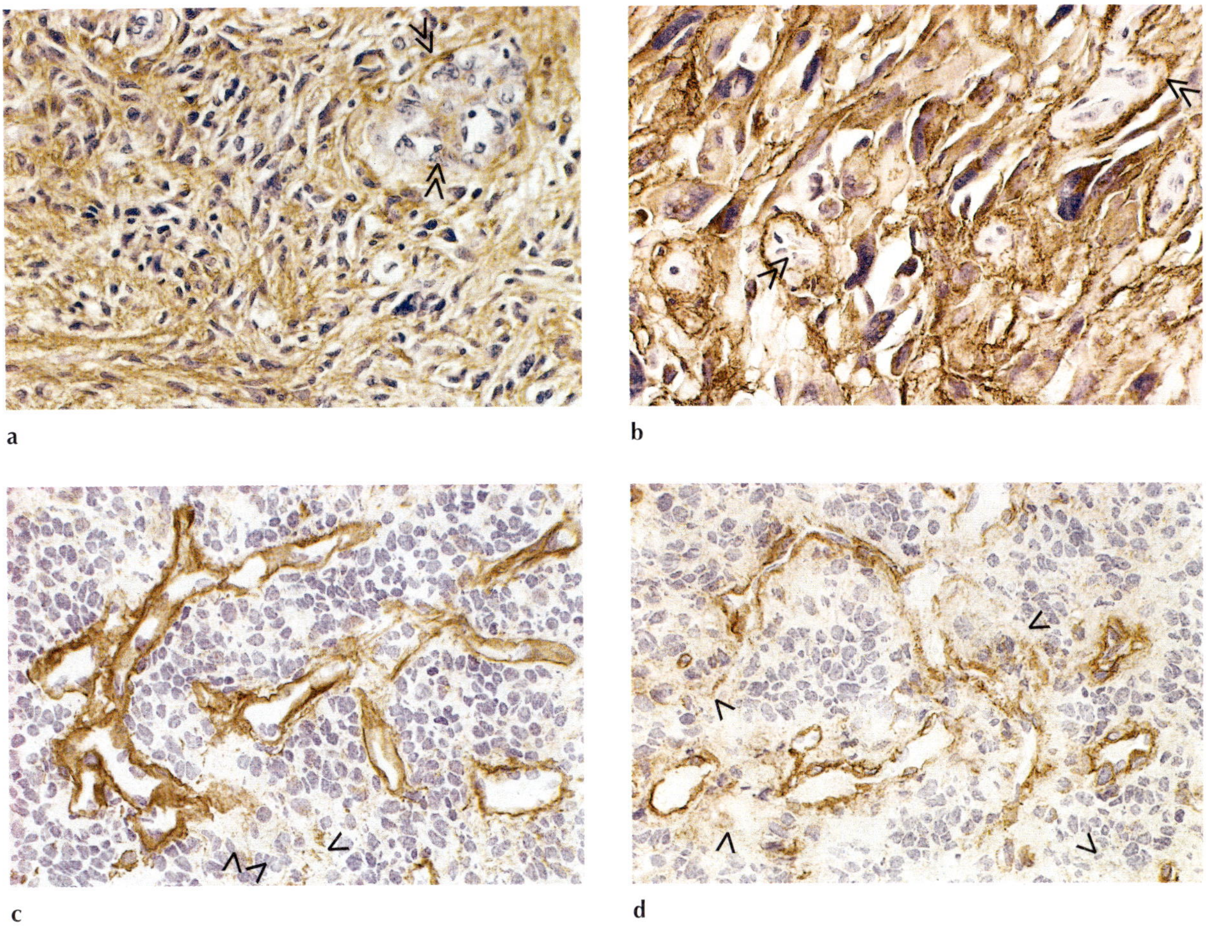

Fig. 8.10 Immunohistochemical localization of ECM proteins in a GBM. (a) Diffuse immunoreactivity is featured by every neoplastic cell in this GBM; in addition, the glomeruloid vascular structure («) is outlined by affinity-purified, polyvalent rabbit antitenascin serum. Formalin-fixed tissue, × 100. (b). This gigantocellular GBM exhibits strong perivascular immunoreactivity («) as well as strong string-like immunoreactivity consistent with localization in the extracellular compartment; or membranous localization. Formalin-fixed tissue, affinity-purified, polyvalent rabbit antitenascin serum; ×100. (c). A strong perivascular localization of tenascin is seen in this GBM; in addition, focal moderate staining is seen in a somewhat string-like pattern (<) which suggests either an extracellular or membranous localization. Acetone-fixed frozen tissue, MAb 81C6; × 100. (d). Same GBM as illustrated in part (c); anti-GP 240 MAb Mel-14 demonstrates an identical localization of the GP 240 antigen to that of tenascin: strong perivascular localization and moderate focal, string-like localization (<) suggesting a pericellular pattern of the GP 240 antigen.

obtained after administration of antitenascin MAb 81C6 into spontaneous cysts of recurrent gliomas or into surgically created cystic resection cavities. In the case of intrathecal administration of MAb 81C6 or Mel-14 $F(ab')_2$ fragments to patients with neoplastic meningitis, clinical responsiveness is more difficult to assess, but, currently, survival prolongation through maintenance of stable disease has been observed in several cases, and clearance of melanoma cells from the CSF and radiographic responses have been seen in several patients.

Markers of historical significance: a redefinition

HNK-1 (LEU 7)

Early studies with anti-Leu 7 (anti-HNK-1) MAb, which was considered as identifying lymphocyte natural killer cells and a subset of activated T cells (Abo and Balch, 1981), revealed that myelin sheath

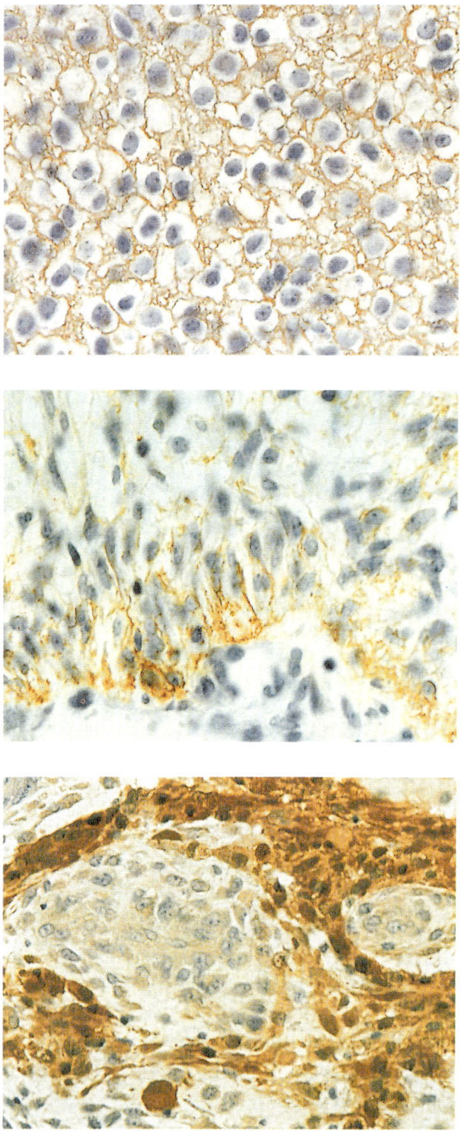

a b c

Fig. 8.11 (a) Anti-HNK-1 immunoreactivity in an oligodendroglioma with anti-Leu 7 antibody. × 400. (b) Anti-HNK-1 immunoreactivity in an astroblastoma with anti-Leu 7 antibody. × 400. (c). Anti-HNK-1 immunoreactivity in a gliosarcoma with anti-Leu 7 antibody; glial tumor cells are immunopositive; perivascular sarcoma cells are negative. × 240

elements in the central and peripheral nervous systems, including oligodendrocytes and Schwann cells, also exhibited cell membrane staining (Russell and Rubinstein, 1989). As summarized by these authors, immunopositivity with anti-Leu 7 in CNS tumors is, in general, found with most types of neoplastic neuroepithelial cells, notably in >90% of oligodendrogliomas, in both GFAP-positive and -negative cells (Perentes and Rubinstein, 1986) [Fig. 8.11(a) and (b)]. Astrocytomas and astroblastomas [Fig. 8.11(b)] are frequently positive, whereas the HNK-1 positivity of central neurocytomas, ependymomas and malignant schwannomas is highly variable (Perentes and Rubinstein, 1986; Russell and Rubinstein, 1989). The authors concluded that less differentiated neuroepithelial tumors tended to be negative, and well-differentiated ones positive, and that although HNK-1 expression was variable within and between classes of CNS tumors, HNK-1 could be used, for example, to differentiate an oligodendroglioma invading the meninges (probably tumor-cell positive) from a meningioma (negative) (Russell and Rubinstein, 1989).

It is now established that HNK-1 is an *N*-linked carbohydrate epitope with a terminal 3-sulfate glucuronic acid residue present on a variety of otherwise nonrelated proteins and some glycolipids prominent on the cell membrane of many normal and neoplastic tissues (Kosaka *et al.*, 1990). The HNK-1 epitope has been found to occur in most neural immunoglobulin superfamily molecules (Yoshihara, Ikeda and Mori, 1991). Proteins so far defined as carrying the HNK-1 epitope include CD57 (Leu 7), high-molecular-weight chondroitin sulfate proteoglycans, integrins, myelin-associated glycoprotein (MAG), NCAM (localized to the 65-kDa NH_2 terminus (Cole and Schachner, 1987; Kleihues, Kiessling and Janzer, 1987), L1 (Kruse *et al.*, 1985) and the ECM adhesion molecules fibronectin and J1 (tenascin-R) (Kruse *et al.*, 1985; Harper *et al.*, 1990). Conventionally used antibodies recognizing the HNK-1 epitope as defined originally on CD57 are the commercially available murine IgM MAbs HNK-1 (anti-Leu 7) and VC1.1, which are mutually inhibitory and are believed to identify identical epitopes (Kosaka *et al.*, 1990). The diverse nature of HNK-1 carrier molecules prompted a re-examination of HNK-1 immunoreactivity as a marker for CNS tumors, especially oligodendrogliomas (Schwechheimer, Gass and Berlet, 1992). In a comparative immunohistochemical and Western blot analysis of 60 CNS and PNS tumors using a panel of MAbs to myelin basic protein (MBP), MAG and HNK-1, the latter authors found that none of the tumors, including oligodendrogliomas, neurinomas and neurofibromas, contained MAG or MBP, although retained myelin sheaths and remnants did. As expected, while anti-HNK-1 MAbs were reactive with the majority of oligodendrogliomas and Schwann-cell tumors, Western blot analysis revealed this activity to be attributable to a wide variety of polypeptides in these samples and in normal brain unrelated to MAG. The authors concluded that the wide distribution of the HNK-1 epitope within different tumor types of the CNS and

PNS cannot support its use as an oligodendroglioma or Schwann-cell tumor marker. In addition, the recognition of a number of carcinomas, adenocarcinomas (Elias, 1990b), rhabdomyosarcomas and Ewing's sarcomas (Wick, Swanson and Manivel, 1988) by anti-Leu 7 reagents limits the use of anti-Leu 7 except in defined cases (see below).

S-100 PROTEIN

The acidic, calcium-binding S-100 protein[s] was first isolated from the CNS by Moore (1965) and was subsequently found to exist as homo- or heterodimers of two highly similar polypeptide chains (α, 93 aa; β, 91 aa) with a total M_r of 20–25 kDa (Kleihues, Kiessling and Janzer, 1987). The S-100 protein has been shown to be a potent inhibitor of phosphorylation via synaptosomal C-kinase and Tau and to modify the activity of adenylate cyclase (Fano *et al.*, 1995). It is routinely localized to the cytoplasm and nucleus of astrocytes, oligodendrocytes and Schwann cells (Matus and Mughal, 1975; Vanstapel *et al.*, 1985), and its presence in some neurons is now established (Vanstapel *et al.*, 1985; Kleihues, Kiessling and Janzer, 1987). As more than 90% of cerebral S-100 contains the β monomer, primarily as a homodimer (Fano *et al.*, 1995), monospecific anti-S-100-β sera yield results similar to those obtained with reagents recognizing both subunits (Kleihues, Kiessling and Janzer, 1987). The highly soluble nature of the protein requires rapid chemical fixation, preferably using aldehyde, to prevent inconsistent localization (Elias, 1990b).

As summarized by Russell and Rubinstein (1989, pp. 34–5), S-100 has been demonstrated in a wide variety of normal cells, 'including stellate cells of the adenohypophysis, chondrocytes, adipose cells, melanocytes, Langerhans cells, T lymphocytes, and the interdigitating reticulum cells of the lymph nodes, as well as in a large number of neoplasms of epithelial and cartilaginous origin'. Within the CNS, S-100 can mirror the distribution of GFAP in recognizing glial neoplasms (astrocytomas, including GBM, oligodendrogliomas and ependymoblastomas), as in the gliosarcoma illustrated in Fig. 8.11(c). The S-100 protein has also been definitively localized to choroid plexus papillomas, central ganglion cell tumors, meningiomas, hemangioblastomas, meningeal melanomas, craniopharyngiomas, chordomas, medulloepitheliomas, schwannomas and peripheral neuroblastomas (Meis, Ordonez and Bruner, 1986; Elias, 1990b). The use of anti-S-100 reagents in neuro-oncology is limited by its presence in poorly differentiated carcinomas, including breast cancers and the vast majority of CNS neoplasms. However, it is an excellent marker for the differential diagnosis of anaplastic schwannomas versus malignant spindle-cell tumors (Elias, 1990b) and, when used in conjunction with anti-Leu 7 MAbs, can differentiate Schwann-cell neoplasms from fibrosarcomas, leiomyosarcomas and undifferentiated spindle-cell sarcomas (Perentes and Rubinstein, 1986).

'A2B5' GANGLIOSIDE

The murine IgM MAb A2B5 (clone 105) was isolated following an immunization protocol using chick retina and was initially reported to react with most neuronal cells therein. The target epitope defined by A2B5 was thought to be distinctive for GQ gangliosides (Eisenbarth, Walsh and Nirenberg, 1979). Subsequently, MAb A2B5 was claimed to differentiate between two types of astrocytes in cultured, developing rat optic nerve cells: A2B5–, tetanus-toxin-binding-negative, GFAP+, fibroblast-like astrocytes (type 1); and A2B5+, tetanus-toxin-binding-positive, GFAP+, neuron-like astrocytes (type 2) (Raff, Miller and Noble, 1983). These latter cells were ultimately designated in mammals, including humans, as oligodendrocyte type 2 astrocyte (O-2A) progenitor cells, defined in studies of cultured cells both by their reactivity with MAb A2B5 and their expression of GD3 (reviewed in Satoh and Kim, 1995). Based on this apparent 'lineage restriction', many histochemical studies examining the distribution of MAb A2B5-reactive cells in CNS tumors have been reported (Bonnin and Rubinstein, 1984; Bishop and de la Monte, 1989; Piepmeier, Fried and Makuch, 1993) with variable results. MAb A2B5+ cells have been demonstrated in several types of tumors, including gliomas (low and high grade), medulloblastomas, schwannomas, meningiomas, neuroblastomas and metastatic carcinomas (review of the above references by McLendon *et al.*, 1988). In addition, conflicting studies of A2B5 expression solely on neurons in fetal human brain cell cultures (Lee *et al.*, 1992), versus A2B5+ astrocytes in similarly cultured cells (Aloisi *et al.*, 1992; Satoh and Kim, 1995) and the demonstration of A2B5 expression in neurofibrillary tangles and dystrophic neurons in Alzheimer's disease brain (Tooyama *et al.*, 1992) have led some to question whether MAb A2B5 can be used to identify specific glial precursors in human cultured cells or tissue.

An explanation for the observed heterogeneity in A2B5+ cells is provided by the redefinition of the epitopic specificity of MAb A2B5. Fredman *et al.* (1984) were the first to determine that MAb A2B5 was reactive with a variety of tri- and polysialoganglioside fractions of chicken retina and brain and with human adult frontal lobe. Subsequently, Dubois *et al.* (1990) established that the minimum binding epitope for MAb A2B5 is the trisialic acid motif of GT3 (NeuAcα2-8NeuAcα2-8NeuAcα2-3Galβ1-4Glc-β1-1 ceramide). The ability of MAb A2B5 to react with the 9-*O*-acetylated derivative of GT3 indicates that the binding site does not include the polyalcohol chain of the terminal sialic acid, the oxidation or acetylation of which does not affect the antibody affinity (Dubois *et al.*, 1990). The reactivity spectrum of MAb A2B5 thus includes the other c-series gangliosides characterized by polysialic acid linkages (Dubois *et al.*, 1990; Freischutz *et al.*, 1994). The diversity of possible glycoprotein and glycolipid A2B5 epitope carrier molecules predicts a heterogeneity of cell types defined as A2B5+. As summarized by Satoh and Kim (1995), 'antigen' A2B5 expression in NSE+ neurons, GFAP+ glial cells and Gal C+ oligodendrocytes in human fetal brain cell cultures abrogates its use as a marker for identifying human glial precursor cells in mixed cell culture populations, and, by extrapolation, in tissue. The original definition of lineage-specific binding in *in vitro* cell cultures was undoubtedly influenced by the concentration of fetal calf serum, the site and developmental stage of the tissue, and the reliability of other cell-specific markers, perhaps creating an artifactually and artificially simple lineage discrimination.

Detection of cell proliferation and cell death in central nervous system tumors

The total number of cells in a population is maintained constant only if cell proliferation is balanced by cell loss. There are several factors that dictate the balance between cell proliferation and cell death. Indeed, one of the most salient features of all malignant neoplasms is uncontrolled cell proliferation that far exceeds cell death. Thus, increasing attention is being given now to both of these aspects in the study of neoplastic growth, since perturbations in the balance between cell proliferation and cell death will influence the growth rate of tumors (Fig. 8.12). Recent studies suggest that programmed cell death, or apoptosis, may play an important role in tumor progression in experimental (Arends, McGregor and Wyllie, 1994; Christofori and Hanahan, 1994; Symonds *et al.*, 1994; Fung, Lee and Trojanowski, 1995) and human tumors (Leoncini *et al.*, 1993; Schiffer *et al.*, 1994). Below, and in Table 8.8, we summarize recently developed methods for monitoring cell proliferation and programmed cell death in tumors.

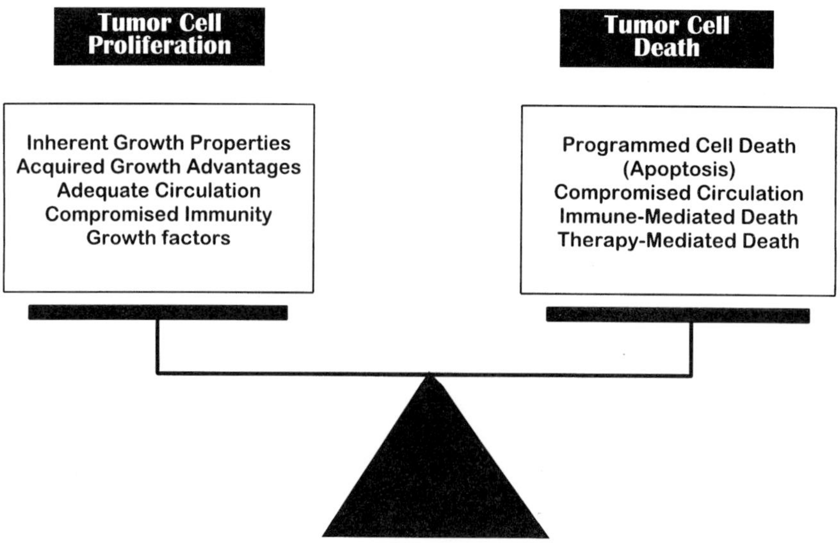

Fig. 8.12 Schematic summary of several important factors regulating the overall balance between cell proliferation and cell death during tumor growth. When tumor cell proliferation exceeds tumor cell death, a gross increase in the total number of tumor cells occurs.

Table 8.8 Summary of techniques for detecting cell proliferation and cell death in tissue sections

Marker	Detection	Principle
Detection of cell proliferation on tissue sections		
Mitotic figures	M phase	Morphologic detection of mitotic figures.
AgNOR staining	Nucleolar organizing region	Silver staining of the nucleolar organizing region.
$[^3H]$-Thymidine	S phase	*In vivo* incorporation of $[^3H]$-thymidine followed by autoradiographic detection on tissue sections.
BrdU/IdU	S phase	*In vivo* or *ex vivo* incorporation of BrdU or IdU followed by immunohistochemical detection of the incorporated thymidine homolog on tissue sections.
Ki-67	G1, S, G2, M phase	Detection of Ki-67 molecules by immunohistochemistry.
PCNA	G1, S, G2, M phase	Detection of PCNA molecules by immunohistochemistry.
Detection of cell death on tissue sections		
Apoptotic bodies	Apoptotic cell death	Conventional nuclear staining (e.g., gallocyanine, hematoxylin, Hoechst, etc.)
TUNEL method	DNA fragmentation	*In situ* labeling of nicked DNA 3'-end by b-dUTP mediated by terminal deoxynucleotidyl transferase. Incorporated b-dUTP visualized by histochemical techniques using avidin.

BrdU, bromodeoxyuridine; IdU, iododeoxyuridine; PCNA, proliferating cell nuclear antigen; TUNEL, terminal deoxynucleotidyl (uracal) nick end labeling.

MARKERS OF CELL PROLIFERATION

Since a high cell proliferation rate is associated with aggressive clinical behavior, determination of mitotic figure incidence has been conventionally used to detect cycling cells in primary CNS tumors. Identifying cells in S phase via autoradiography following *in vivo* or *ex vivo* labeling with $[^3H]$-thymidine, although sensitive, is not practicable in most clinical situations. Various labeling methods that determine indices related to tumor cell proliferation, including the immunohistochemical detection of the incorporation of the thymidine analogs bromodeoxyuridine (BrdU) and iododeoxyuridine (IdU) or of the expression of proliferation-associated nuclear proteins such as Ki-67, PCNA/cyclin or DNA polymerase α have been investigated as adjuncts to classic histologic grading of CNS neoplasms (for review, see Onda *et al.*, 1994). For example, the absorption of the thymidine analogs BrdU and IdU, by biopsy tissue, from buffered solution results in the direct labeling of S-phase cell nuclei. This incorporation is readily detected immunohistochemically (Meyer, Marchosky and Hickey, 1993). The MAb Ki-67 detects two nonhistone proteins of 395 and 345 kDa that are present in all phases of the cell cycle, except G0 and the early G0–G1 transitional phase (Gerdes *et al.*, 1983, 1984, 1991). The proliferating cell nuclear antigen (PCNA) or DNA polymerase subunits α and δ have both been targets of analysis similar to Ki-67 determination.

The most extensive investigations have been reported for both *in vivo* and *in situ* BrdU incorporation and determination of the Ki-67 labeling index (LI), most conveniently expressed as the percentage of positive cells in defined tumor fields. The predominant method is to count in areas of overall high density of labeled cells, a technique conventionally attributed to the principle of considering the most malignant parts of the tumor for diagnostic and prognostic purposes. It must be recognized that determination of BrdU LI, whether following *in vivo* or *in vitro* exposure to BrdU, is hampered by problems of delivery. *In vivo*, high levels of tumor cell proliferation are found perivascularly and in areas where high partial pressure of oxygen exists. These levels decrease with increasing distance from the blood vessels (Morimura, Kita and Budka, 1989). *In vitro* exposure of brain tumor tissues to BrdU labeling results in delivery of label only 0.8 mm from the tissue sample surface, thereby restricting the measurable target population (Morimura *et al.*, 1991). Problems exist with determining Ki-67 LI in frozen tissue; the duration of fixation in acetone and of air drying are crucial factors for the preservation and detection of Ki-67 antigen (Morimura, Kita and Budka, 1989; Raghavan, Steart and

Weller, 1990). These problems have been partially overcome by generation of MIB 1–3 series of anti-Ki-67 MAbs (Gerdes *et al.*, 1992), which can be utilized with paraffin-embedded sections with or without microwave antigen retrieval techniques (Cattoretti *et al.*, 1992; Key *et al.*, 1993). Determining the PCNA LI becomes more difficult owing to the spectrum of protein concentrations produced over the cell cycle. However, protein concentration is not the only variable. In a carefully controlled study of experimental rat gliomas, Nakasu *et al.* (1994a) reported that degrees of staining varied with 10% formalin or periodonate–lysine–paraformaldehyde (PLP) fixation. PCNA and BrdU LI correlated only when 'light' PCNA-staining cells in formalin-fixed tissues were excluded. Further complicating application to archival or multiple-lab-prepared human samples was the observation that overfixation in formalin reduced the number of PCNA-positive cells.

Despite these caveats, there is steadily accumulating evidence that Ki-67 and BrdU LI do correlate fairly well with the prognosis, not only of individual patients with gliomas (Onda *et al.*, 1994), but also with grades of malignancy in general (Burger, Shibata and Kleihues, 1986; Sallinen *et al.*, 1994). Although the numerical value of each index might vary from study to study, intrastudy reliability has been demonstrated in many reports, and the following generalizations can be drawn:

1. Reports of PCNA and anti-DNA polymerase α level determination have been highly variable and infrequent, respectively, and neither enjoys widespread use (Kunishio *et al.*, 1990; Kordek *et al.*, 1994; Sallinen *et al.*, 1994).
2. The BrdU LI appears to correlate directly with conventional histologic grading and with survival of glioma patients (the higher the BrdU LI, the higher the grade and the shorter the survival period) in several series [Fujimaki *et al.*, 1991 (50 cases: 10 astrocytomas, 12 anaplastic astrocytomas and 28 GBMs); Hoshino *et al.*, 1989 (127 cases: 42 astrocytomas, 36 anaplastic astrocytomas and 49 GBMs)]. An example of BrdU labeling in a GBM is provided in Fig. 8.13(a). The BrdU LI did not correlate with the histology (solid or cystic) or clinical outcome in a study of 50 cases of juvenile pilocytic astrocytoma (Ito *et al.*, 1992) nor with survival time of 26 cases of medulloblastoma (Ito *et al.*, 1991).
3. The Ki-67 antigen LI alone has similarly been shown to correlate directly with the histologic grade of gliomas [Raghavan, Steart and Weller, 1990 (90 cases: 26 astrocytomas, 26 anaplastic astrocytomas and 38 GBMs); Schröder *et al.*, 1991 (73 cases: 21 astrocytomas, 20 anaplastic astrocytomas and 32 GBMs)].
4. The introduction of the anti-Ki-67 antigen MIB MAbs, which can be used with paraffin-embedded tissue with good histologic preservation, has increased the reliability of Ki-67 antigen interpretation and its correlation with the conventional parameters of histologic grading: nuclear density, degree of pleomorphism, number of mitoses, necrosis and capillary endothelial proliferation (Karamitopoulou *et al.*, 1994; Onda *et al.*, 1994; Sallinen *et al.*, 1994). An LI correlation with malignancy must be determined for each neoplasm, as relatively low LI is demonstrated in an anaplastic astrocytoma [Fig. 8.13(b) and (c)], whereas a very high LI is demonstrated in a medulloblastoma [Fig. 8.13(c)].
5. When Ki-67 and BrdU LI are determined for the same samples, the higher Ki-67 values are usually attributed to the Ki-67 antigen being detectable from mid–late G1 through S and G2, gradually declining during mitosis, whereas BrdU staining identifies only S-phase cells (Sawhney and Hall, 1992). Comparative studies of Ki-67 and BrdU LI have demonstrated a strong correlation with each other (Morimura, Kita and Budka, 1989; Onda *et al.*, 1994), most especially when *in vitro* BrdU staining was performed (Morimura, 1991).
6. The Ki-67 antigen LIs as defined by MIB-1 have been reported to provide additional help in differentiating between grade II and III astrocytomas (Sallinen *et al.*, 1994). MIB-1-defined LI showed strong prognostic potential with high sensitivity and specificity in placing patients in surviving and nonsurviving categories (50 case retrospective series; $P < 0.0001$) as reported by Sullivan *et al.* (1994). Similarly, Hoshino *et al.* (1988), in a study of 47 cases of low-grade astrocytomas, reported that BrdU LI correctly identified a subset that progressed rapidly among histologically indistinguishable low-grade astrocytomas.

Statin is a 57-kDa nuclear membrane phosphoprotein purported to be a nuclear marker for nonproliferating cells (Tsanaclis *et al.*, 1991; Lee, Sandig and Wang, 1992). Ansari *et al.* (1993) have recently demonstrated however, that statin is expressed by replicating cells as assessed by colocalization with [^{3}H]-thymidine-labeled and Ki-67-labeled cells. Therefore, statin's association with growth arrest is neither absolute nor dependable, and its use as a marker for G0 is not supportable.

It is clear that a single kinetic determinant such as a proliferation index cannot serve as a sole predictor of the complex cellular behaviors involved

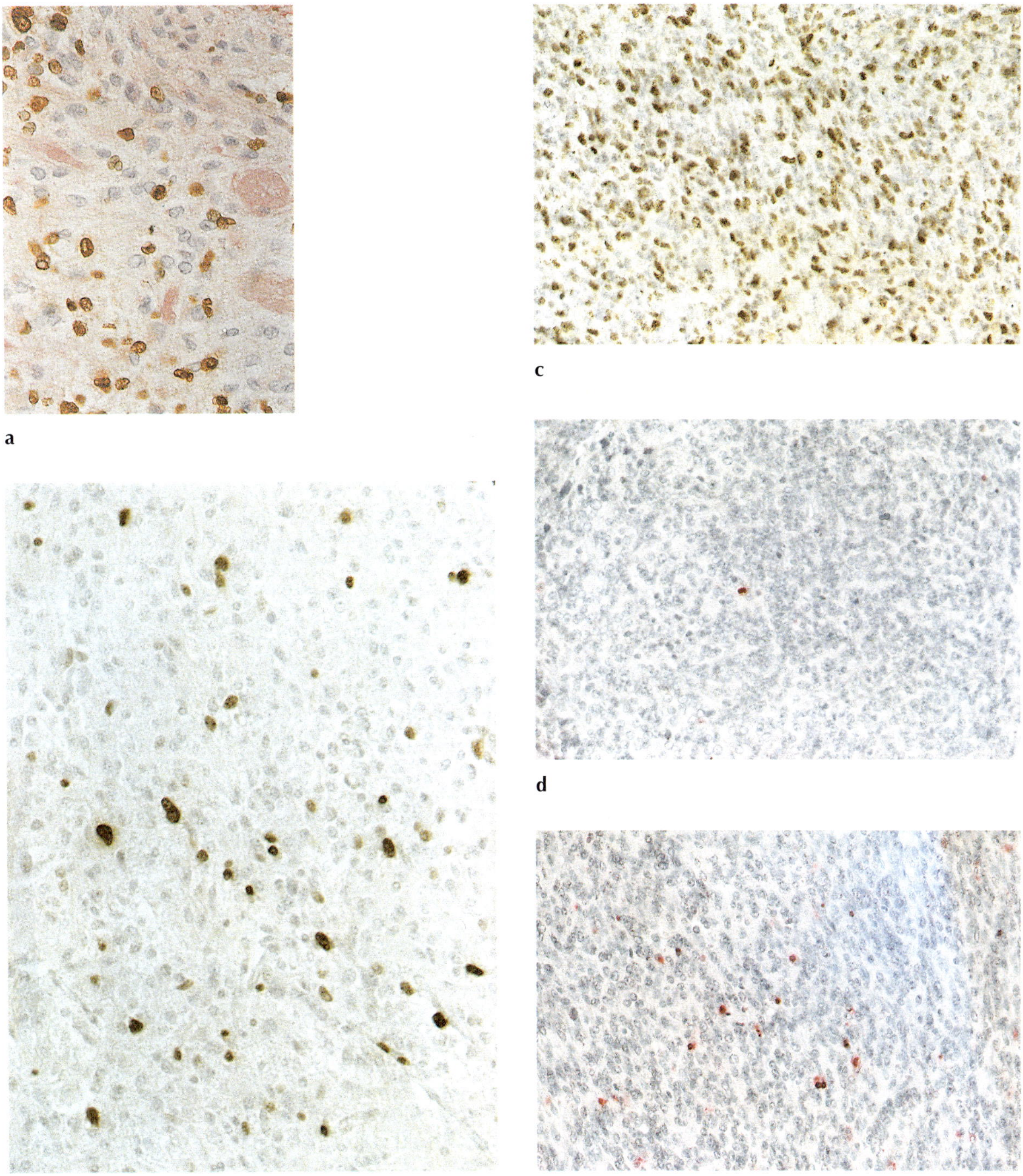

a b c d e

Fig. 8.13 Immunohistochemical demonstration of cell proliferation in primary CNS tumors. (a) Immunopositivity in nuclei of a large number of tumor cells in a GBM stained with an anti-BrdU MAb. × 240. (b) MIB-1 staining of an anaplastic astrocytoma; low index. × 200. (c) MIB-1 staining of a medulloblastoma; high index. × 450. (d) PNET; TUNEL, low index. × 450. (e) PNET; TUNEL, high index, same tumor as in part (d). × 200 in neoplastic progression and therapeutic sensitivity (Morimura, Kita and Budka, 1989). However, these reagents are proving to be useful in initial attempts to characterize these dynamic processes.

DETECTION OF CELL DEATH

Necrosis and apoptosis represent the two major forms of cell death (Farber, 1994). Necrosis is considered to be the end product of irreversible cell injury, and it is thought to be a passive rather than an active pathological process. In contrast, programmed cell death, or apoptosis, represents an active form of cell death initiated as a result of the transcription and/or translation of mediators of the cell death process, and it plays an important role in many physiological (e.g., the development and modeling of the CNS) and pathological processes. Dramatic evidence for the role of cell death in the biology of tumors comes from the well-documented cases of spontaneous regression of some human tumors, including neuroblastomas and infantile mesenchymal tumors (Enzinger and Weiss, 1988; Fukasawa *et al.*, 1994); indeed, apoptosis has been implicated as a critical factor in controlling tumor progression (Arends, McGregor and Wyllie, 1994) and has been observed in human medulloblastomas (Schiffer *et al.*, 1994).

Morphological detection of apoptotic bodies

Fragmentation of the nucleus into smaller, round dense bodies (karyorrhexis) occurs in the latter part of apoptosis; these apoptotic cells are morphologically distinct and contain round, homogeneously stained, condensed (pyknotic) nuclei (Migheli *et al.*, 1994). Gel electrophoretic analysis of apoptotic bodies reveals internucleosomal DNA fragmentation at 185–200 base pair (bp) intervals, identifiable as a DNA 'ladder' (Wyllie *et al.*, 1984). In contrast, coagulative necrosis is characterized by cell swelling, lysis and disrupted membranes at the morphological level, and this is associated with random DNA fragmentation leading to a DNA smear in gel electrophoresis. In general, any good nuclear staining is suitable for morphological detection of apoptotic bodies. However, gallocyanin-chrome alum staining and the bisbenzimide trihydrochloride (Hoechst) dyes are two of the most useful stains for detecting apoptotic bodies with bright field or fluorescent microscopy, respectively (Lasorella, Iavarone and Israel, 1995).

Inhibition of apoptosis in central nervous system tumors by *BCL2*

The *BCL2* mammalian oncogene, located on chromosome 18q21, codes for a 26-kDa protein that localizes to the inner mitochondrial membrane, nuclear envelope and endoplasmic reticulum (Reed *et al.*, 1991; Karp and Broder, 1994). Elevated levels of bcl-2 protein expression have been demonstrated to render the expressing cells resistant to apoptotic induction by various stimuli (Han *et al.*, 1996), including apoptosis induced by overexpression of p53 protein (Alderson *et al.*, 1995). Commercially available affinity-purified rabbit antisera to synthetic peptides representing either conserved mammalian epitopes or unique human sequences have been described (Reed *et al.*, 1991). Use of these reagents in immunoblot analysis revealed Bcl-2 expression by several cell lines of neural origin, including neuroblastomas, ganglioneuromas, neurofibrosarcomas and ganglioneuroblastomas, while in CNS tumor-derived cell lines, 6/6 medulloblastoma lines and 2/5 glial tumor-derived lines were negative for Bcl-2 (Reed *et al.*, 1991). In an immunohistochemical study of tumor specimens derived from 17 pediatric patients with neuroblastomas or ganglioneuromas and using murine anti-Bcl-2 MAb 124 or rabbit antisynthetic Bcl-2 peptide antiserum (Reed *et al.*, 1991), Krajewski *et al.* (1995) reported that Bcl-2 protein was found exclusively in tumor cells of the neuronal lineage that did not express N-myc; Bcl-2 immunoreactivity was pronounced in well-differentiated tumor cells judged to be similar to immature ganglion cells at an intermediate stage of neuronal differentiation. The detection of strong Bcl-2 immunoreactivity in residual tumor cells in 6/7 samples obtained after therapy suggested that the Bcl-2 oncoprotein may be cytoprotective for neuroblastoma cells *in vivo*. Recently, Alderson *et al.* (1995) examined formalin-fixed, paraffin-embedded sections of 28 gliomas (3 astrocytomas, 13 anaplastic astrocytomas and 12 GBMs) immunohistochemically with murine MAbs 124 and PAb 1801 for Bcl-2 and p53 proteins, respectively, and for *TP53* gene mutations by SSCP of exons 5–8. Expression of Bcl-2 was significantly ($P<0.01$) associated with wild-type p53 protein in 16/28 (57%) of the tumors examined and, in cases of p53 protein overexpression, with 7/7 tumors negative for *TP53* gene mutation and with only 1/7 tumors with an exon-7-mutated *TP53* gene. Using MAb 124 and antigen retrieval techniques with formalin-fixed tissue, Nakasu *et al.* (1994b) also observed a higher incidence of Bcl-2 expression in low-grade astrocytomas as opposed to GBMs, suggesting that inhibition of apoptosis by Bcl-2 expression may be a common early event in the development of glial neoplasms.

In situ *end labeling*

Recent advances in molecular biology have led to the development of enzyme-mediated methods for *in situ* labeling of the 'nicked' ends of fragmented DNA (reviewed by Migheli *et al.*, 1994). The *in situ* end labeling (ISEL) family of assays depends upon the use of enzymes such as DNA polymerase or terminal deoxynucleotidyl transferase (Tdt; TUNEL) to insert labeled nucleotides in the 3'-hydroxyl termini of endonuclease-induced DNA breaks (Gorczyca, Gong and Darzynkiewicz, 1993). Labeling is then revealed by colorimetric methods. Using the TUNEL technique, Migheli *et al.* (1994) demonstrated that abundant apoptotic cells were either isolated or grouped in small foci in 5 GBMs, 5 medulloblastomas, 5 cases of cerebral lymphomas and 3 cases of brain metastasis; medulloblastomas had the highest number of labeled cells. An example of the detection of different apoptotic rates in different areas within the same medulloblastoma is provided in Fig. 8.13(d) and (e). In GBM, the highest incidence of apoptotic cells was found in necrotic areas. In a later study, Schiffer *et al.* (1995) analyzed a large panel of formalin-fixed neuroepithelial tumors [30 medulloblastomas, 30 ependymomas, 30 oligodendrogliomas and 90 astrocytic tumors (30 astrocytoma, 30 anaplastic astrocytomas and 30 GBMs)]. An apoptotic index (AI) was determined, and compared with mitotic indices (MIs), MIB-1 (Ki-67) LI and survival. The AI was high in malignant tumors (anaplastic oligodendrogliomas, 0.24) and in tumors of embryonal origin (medulloblastomas, 0.36) and lower in tumors of the glial series (0.05–0.15). The AI:MI ratio was lower in malignant oncotypes than in benign ones, and correlated with very high MIB-1 LI, thereby supporting studies in non-CNS tumors suggesting that apoptosis is linked directly with the ability to proliferate. The authors suggested that AI or AI:MI ratios would be of value in determining the proliferation potential and cell loss in brain tumors.

Summary and future prospects

The histopathologic diagnosis of CNS tumors has been enhanced and refined by the incorporation of immunohistochemical techniques, most notably in the area of cell lineage determination and cell stasis and proliferation. An emerging body of evidence suggests that some markers associated with more aggressive forms of neoplasms do not simply correlate with tumor grade but may indeed identify tumor cell subsets within grades with enhanced growth potential, and thus, a less favorable prognosis. The most promising group of such markers consists of proteins that have been demonstrated to confer drug resistance to the cells expressing them. They can be separated into three general groups: (1) mediators of drug uptake or sequestration (*MDR1* [*PGY1*] gene encoded P-glycoprotein, P-gp; multidrug-resistance protein, MRP); (2) cytoplasmic drug-conjugating agents such as glutathione-*S*-transferases; and (3) nuclear enzymes that effect DNA repair [O^6-methylguanine-DNA methyltransferase (MGMT): O^6-alkylguanine-DNA alkyltransferase and 3-methyladenine DNA glycosylase] (Gerson and Willson, 1995; Walker and Swenberg, Chapter 5, this book). Both P-gp and MRP are large transmembrane glycoproteins (170 kDa and 190 kDa, respectively) of the superfamily of the ATP-binding cassette transporter proteins, the presence of which confer resistance to several lipophilic drugs: taxol (P-gp only), doxorubicin, daunorubicin, etoposide, actinomycin D, vincristine and vinblastine (Breuninger *et al.*, 1995). The P-gp has been demonstrated to function as an energy-dependent efflux pump that transports targeted chemotherapeutic agents across the plasma membrane; MRP may have a similar extrusion capacity, but may also sequester drugs cytoplasmically (Breuninger *et al.*, 1995). The immunohistochemical detection of these proteins by specific MAbs in patient biopsies has been demonstrated to be associated with resistance to pertinent chemotherapy and a poor prognosis in osteosarcoma (P-gp; Chan *et al.*, 1996) and peripheral neuroblastoma (MRP; Norris *et al.*, 1996). Interestingly, P-gp expression was characteristic of a subset of *MYCN* amplification-negative peripheral neuroblastoma patients with a poor outcome (Norris *et al.*, 1996).

The nuclear DNA adduct-repair enzymes have been extensively studied, and MAbs produced to MGMT have already proven useful in correlating levels of alkyltransferase with cancer patient response to alkylating agents (Yarosh, Belanich, and Li, 1996). The MAbs specific for human MGMT have been used in quantitative immunohistochemical image analysis in parallel with biochemical assays of MGMT activity. Results demonstrated that quantitative image analysis correlated strongly with the quantitative estimates of MGMT levels by Western blot and activity by [^{3}H] O^6-methylguanine release in an alkyltransferase assay (Zaidi, Liu and Gerson, 1996). Both conventional and quantitative immunohistochemistry established the heterogeneity of alkyltransferase

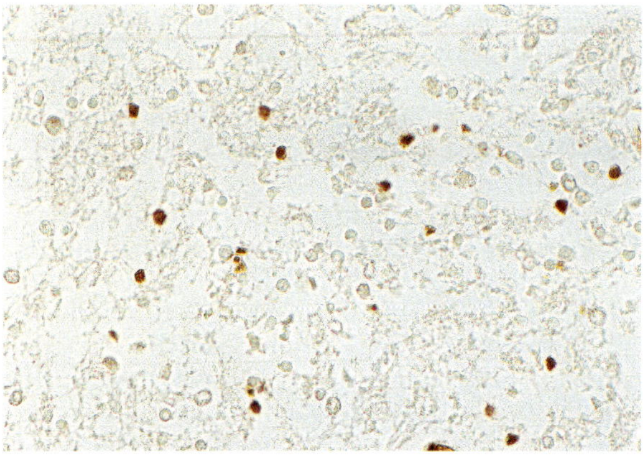

Fig. 8.14 Alkyltransferase gene expression in a glioma stained with the MT3.1 MAb. Note the predominant nuclear staining with some evidence of cytoplasmic staining as well. × 160

expression in both normal and neoplastic colon cells (Zaidi, Liu and Gerson, 1996). Anti-MGMT MAbs have been applied to the immunohistochemical investigation of human gliomas (Citron *et al.*, 1995). Antihuman MGMT MAb MT3.1 (D.D. Bigner, unpublished data) has been used to demonstrate the presence of characteristically predominant nuclear staining, with some isolated cytoplasmic staining on a human GBM (Fig. 8.14) (Gerson *et al.*, unpublished results). MT3.1 has also been demonstrated to react with both active and O^6-benzylguanine-inactivated MGMT in lymphocytes and tumor biopsies of patients receiving O^6-benzylguanine in an attempt to inactivate MGMT. As detected by MT3.1, MGMT, both active and inactive, persisted in lymphocytes up to 24 hours after O^6-benzylguanine administration, whereas MGMT was significantly degraded in tumor tissue within 18 hours (Liu *et al.*, 1996). Although there is some evidence that MAbs to MGMT or P-gp may directly inhibit the action of their targets (Volker *et al.*, 1996), the greatest contribution of MAbs in this area will be in the determination of the incidence of cells within a tumor sample that are capable of escaping specific chemotherapies, thereby predicting therapeutic outcome, or by suggesting strategies to remove the resistant cells by pretreatment with antagonists or specific MAbs.

It is encouraging that several of these potentially prognostic markers may also be functioning as effective targets for immunotherapeutic intervention. Despite the problems—numerous control problems associated with the more demanding technical aspects of immunohistochemical techniques, frequent requirement for libraries of monospecific MAbs for optimal detection of epitopically diverse marker proteins (p53, GFAP and L1), and differing fixation and assay condition requirements for each antigen–antibody pair—the exquisite specificity of the technology and the constantly enlarging library of defined antigen-localizing reagents and candidate markers can only continue to improve our understanding of the biology of nervous system tumors, as well as our understanding of tumor classification and grading. The considerable advances by many investigators over the past decade ensure that the remaining challenges of discriminating reactive cells from infiltrating tumor cells, elucidating those populations with higher growth potential, and improving prognostic accuracy, will be met.

APPENDIX

Technical notes concerning problems and pitfalls associated with interpretation of immunohistochemical results with central nervous system tissue

Several excellent reviews and manuals of immunohistochemical procedures have been published that provide comprehensive overviews of approaches for optimal fixation, permeabilization, selection of enhancing methodologies, and general interpretation (Van Noorden, 1986; Elias, 1990a, 1990b; Leong, 1993; McKeever, Burger and Nelson, 1993). The purpose of this appendix is to highlight those procedures and reagents that are optimal for the sensitive and accurate detection of the marker molecules discussed in this chapter.

GENERAL CONSIDERATIONS

As reviewed by several authors (Van Noorden, 1986; Elias, 1990a, 1990b; Leong, 1993), there are four major sources of potential difficulty in immunohistochemical assays of marker distribution: (1) antigenic target, (2) antibody reagents, (3) experimental design, and (4) correct interpretation.

Table 8A.1 Reported optimal conditions for various markers in CNS immunohistochemistry

Antigen[a]	Optimal fixation methodology	Comments	References
Cell surface antigens			
p75NGFR	Frozen sections; acetone	MAb Me 20.4	Ross *et al.*, 1984
	Formalin	MAb Me 20.4	Baker *et al.*, 1991
EGFR	Frozen sections; acetone	MAb EGFR-1	Torp *et al.*, 1991
EGFRvIII	Frozen sections; acetone	MAb L8A4	Wikstrand *et al.*, 1995
Gangliosides	Frozen sections; acetone	Epitopes sensitive to all other organic solvents	Wikstrand *et al.*, 1993
HNK-1	Frozen sections; EtOH	Sensitive to formalin fixation	McKeever, Burger and Nelson, 1993
		Chloroform delipidization helpful	Elias, 1990a
Cytoplasmic Antigens			
Intermediate filament proteins, general	Frozen sections; EtOH Methacarn; Carnoy's		Elias, 1990b
NFP	Frozen sections; EtOH	Formalin sensitive	McKeever, Burger and Nelson, 1993
	Bouin's fixative	Epitope masking of 68 kD NFP	Elias, 1990b
GFAP	4% NBF; 4% NBF-70% EtOH	May require trypsin digestion	Kleihues, Kiessling and Janzer, 1987
		Some epitopes formalin and paraformaldehyde sensitive	Shi, Kay and Kalra, 1991
		Chloroform delipidization helpful	Elias, 1990a
Vimentin	Frozen sections; EtOH	Protease digestion not recommended	Elias, 1990b
Cytokeratins	Frozen sections; EtOH	Multiple MAb-epitope optima	Elias, 1990b
	Methacarn	MAbs 35BH11, 34BE12	Elias, 1990b
	Formalin Methacarn	MAbs AE1, AE3; trypsin digestion success variable	Elias, 1990b
Synaptophysin (Granulophysin)	Frozen sections; EtOH	Suboptimal detection in formalin-fixed material	Hoog *et al.*, 1988
Nuclear antigens			
p53	Phenol formol saline	Antibody CM-1. No heat treatment for adherence; denatures p53	Fisher *et al.*, 1994
BrdU	Variable	Requires uptake of BrdU *in vivo* or *in vitro*; sensitivity then based on MAb used	Yu, Woods and Levison, 1992
Ki-67	Frozen sections; acetone	Non-MIB series MAbs' epitopes sensitive to most fixatives	Morimura, Kita and Budka, 1989
	Formalin	MIB series MAbs	Yu, Woods and Levison, 1992
PCNA	Periodonate-lysine paraformaldehyde	Formalin sensitive with time	Nakasu *et al.*, 1994a
		Heat sensitive as for p53	Yu, Woods and Levison, 1992
S-100	4% paraformaldehyde	Highly soluble, requires immediate fixation; aldehydes decrease sensitivity	Yang *et al.*, 1995
		Requires trypsin or bromelain digestion	Yang *et al.*, 1995

[a] Antigen localization is based on predominant detected location. Synaptophysin, although an integral synaptic vesicle membrane protein, is conventionally detected by MAbs directed to the cytoplasmic tail. The S-100 protein has been identified both in the cytoplasm, and nucleus; p53 has been found in cytoplasm as well as its predominant localization to the nucleus. NBF, neutral buffered formalin; BrdU, bromodeoxyuridine; PCNA, proliferating cell nuclear antigen; NGFR, nerve growth factor receptor; MAb, monoclonal antibody; EGFR, epidermal growth factor receptor; NFP, neurofilament protein; GFAP, glial fibrillary acidic protein.

Table 8A.2 Antigen–antibody systems of use in CNS immunohistochemistry: effect of µ-wave antigen retrieval procedures[a]

Antigen–antibody pair[b]	Optimal buffer systems	Reference(s)
1. Detection enhanced following µ-wave treatment		
GFAP – GA5	Distilled H_2O Saturated lead thiocyanate	Yachnis and Trojanowski, 1994 Shi, Key and Kalra, 1991
GFAP – 6F2	0.01 M sodium citrate, pH 7.8	McQuaid *et al.*, 1995
NFP – 2F11	Saturated lead thiocyanate	Shi, Key and Kalra, 1991
NF-L – NR4 (p-ind)	Distilled H_2O 0.01 M sodium citrate, pH 7.8	Yachnis and Trojanowski, 1994 McQuaid *et al.*, 1995
NF-M, NF-H – HO14, RM024 (P+)	Distilled H_2O	Yachnis and Trojanowski, 1994
NF-M, NF-H – RMd020, DP1 (P–)	Distilled H_2O	Yachnis and Trojanowski, 1994
NF-M, NF-H – SMI-32 (P–)	4% aluminum chloride	Evers and Uylings, 1994
Vimentin – V9	Saturated lead thiocyanate	Shi, Key and Kalra, 1991
Cytokeratin – AE1	0.05 M citric acid, sodium phosphate pH 2–3, pH 8	Shi *et al.*, 1995
NSE – BBS/NC/VI-H14	0.05 M citric acid, sodium phosphate pH 2–3, pH 8	Shi *et al.*, 1995
Chromagranin – LK3H10	Saturated lead thiocyanate	Shi, Key and Kalra, 1991
Synaptophysin – [polyclonal]	0.01 M sodium citrate, pH 7.8	McQuaid *et al.*, 1995
Retinal S-antigen – C10C10	Distilled H_2O	Yachnis and Trojanowski, 1994
EGFR – H11	0.01 M sodium citrate, pH 5.6	Wikstrand *et al.*, unpublished data
EGFRvIII – L8A4	0.01 M sodium citrate, pH 5.6	Wikstrand *et al.*, 1995
PCNA - PC10	0.05 M citric acid, sodium phosphate pH 2–3, pH 8	Shi *et al.*, 1995
Ki-67 – MIB-1	0.05 M citric acid, sodium phosphate pH 2–3, pH 8	Shi *et al.*, 1995
p53 – KD68/Bp53-121	0.05 M glycine–HCl pH 3.5	Taylor *et al.*, 1994
2. Detection not improved or diminished following µ-wave treatment		
NFP – 2F11	0.01 M sodium citrate, pH 7.8	McQuaid *et al.*, 1995
Synaptophysin – SY-38	Distilled H_2O	Yachnis and Trojanowski, 1994
EGFR – EGFR-1	0.01 M sodium citrate, pH 5.6	Wikstrand *et al.*, unpublished data
3. Detection lost following µ-wave treatment		
p75NGFr – Me20.4	Distilled H_2O	Yachnis and Trojanowski, 1994
NCAM – Moc 1	Distilled H_2O	Yachnis and Trojanowski, 1994

[a] Each reference should be consulted for exact µ-wave treatment parameters and buffer formulations; in general, slides bearing 4–6 µm sections of buffered formalin-, ethanol- or Bouin's solution fixed tissue were heated in a microwave oven for one or two 4–5 minute exposures and allowed to cool for 15–20 minutes before immunohistochemical assay.

[b] The MAbs or polyvalent serum investigated are shown; for anti-NFP MAbs, the designations p-ind, P+ and P– indicate that a MAb recognizes NFP independent of its phosphorylation state, in its heavily phosphorylated state or only in its nonphosphorylated state, respectively (Yachnis and Trojanowski, 1994).

GFAP, glial fibrillary acidic protein; NFP, neurofilament protein; NF-L, low molecular weight neurofilament; NF-M, middle molecular weight neurofilament; NF-H, high molecular weight neurofilament; NSE, neuron-specific enolase; EGFR, epidermal growth factor receptor; PCNA, proliferating cell nuclear antigen; NCAM, neural cell adhesion molecule.

Antigenic target

The two major features of antigen preservation and accessibility that require experimental optimization for each antigen–antibody pair are fixation and permeabilization, either by solvent, enzyme digestion or microwave treatment. Extensive reviews of these topics have been published (Van Noorden, 1986; Elias, 1990a; Ainley and Ironside, 1994), and summaries of relevant marker protocols are provided in Tables 8A.1 and 8A.2. As noted by Van Noorden (1986), the necessity for preserving the structure and 'fixing' the location of soluble markers in fresh tissue using chemical fixatives, primarily aldehydes, also frequently results in the formation of excess aldehyde cross-linkages, leading to insufficient penetration of reactants and potential false-negative results or artifactual false-positive (trapping) staining (Elias, 1990a). As noted in Table 8A.1, some markers are optimally detected in lightly acetone-fixed frozen sections and are only weakly, if at all, detected in conventionally fixed and embedded archival tissue (EGFRvIII, gangliosides, HNK-1, vimentin and synaptophysin), whereas others either require rapid fixation (S-100) or are readily detected following fixation under defined conditions and without further enhancing steps (some NFP epitopes and cytokeratins). Most marker detection, however, is enhanced by either proteolytic digestion (trypsin, pepsin, bromelain and ficin) or lipid solvents (chloroform:methanol) of aldehyde-fixed sections as noted in Table 8A.1; denaturing fixatives such as ethanol or Carnoy's do not require subsequent permeabilization or enhancement (Elias, 1990a). However, the conditions for each of these systems must be experimentally determined to avoid overdigestion and false-negative staining. Vimentin is an example of an antigen quite sensitive to protease digestion (Elias, 1990b).

The most promising recent advance in optimizing antigen availability has been the application, by many groups, of the microwave treatment of tissue sections first extensively described by Shi, Key and Kalra (1991). Since that report, a wide variety of antigen–MAb systems have been investigated with various buffer solutions and microwave treatment protocols. A brief summary of pairs pertinent to this discussion is provided in Table 8A.2. As for conventional immunohistochemistry, the success of the technique is unique for each MAb–epitope pair, as exemplified for the disparate results obtained with detection of EGFR, NFP and GFAP by different MAbs and/or buffers (Table 8A.2). The most extensive analyses pertinent to CNS antigen retrieval by microwave technology are to be found in Ainley and Ironside (1994), Yachnis and Trojanowski (1994) and McQuaid *et al.* (1995).

Antibody reagents

As stressed in this chapter, selection of an epitope-defined primary reagent (either affinity-purified polyvalent sera or similarly purified monoclonal reagents) is crucial to any study attempting unambiguous antigen localization. Most commercially available reagents are provided with defined conditions for optimal sensitivity. Frequently, however, assay parameters must be redefined in each individual laboratory to take into consideration antigen presentation in study material, past tissue-processing fixatives used, etc. As noted in Chapter 8 for several antigens (NFP, GFAP, CK, p53, NGFR, tenascin and HNK-1), a primary antibody panel approach is not only advised, but necessary, to assume even approaching optimal antigen detection.

A frequently overlooked parameter is the selection and optimization of the bridging, or secondary antibody reagent, employed. The secondary reagent must be affinity-purified by the target species immunoglobulin and demonstrated to be noncross-reactive with immunoglobulin of the target tissue species. Crucial also is the selected concentration. The elaborate immunohistochemical sandwich techniques available (Van Noorden, 1986; Elias *et al.*, 1990a; Leong, 1993) are extremely sensitive to deviations from optimal antibody– antigen equivalence zones, with deviation in either direction usually resulting in suboptimal staining.

Experimental design

The most frequently flawed component of an immunohistochemical study is the experimental design, usually by omission of necessary positive and negative controls. After primary and secondary antibody reagents are optimized as discussed above, it is crucial that all steps in the immunohistochemical cascade are demonstrated to be functional in any given assay of an unknown. This requires complete tissue controls for each assay run, including: (1) antigen-expressing tissue as independently established by biochemical or immunohistochemical determination of antigen (antigen, antigen-positive primary antibody and components of the detection system positive control); and (2) nonantigen-expressing tissue (background control for antigen-positive primary antibody and components of the detection system negative control). Complete antibody assays must be run on the positive and negative control tissues and experimental samples. Necessary antibody applications include: (1) use of immunoglobulin isotype control antibodies or normal purified immunoglobulins of the same species to provide the affinity-purified polyvalent primary reagent at identical concentration (not just dilution) as the antigen-positive primary reagents employed; and (2) omission of the secondary reagent in negative control primary slides to ascertain nonspecific tertiary (chromagen system) staining. The following 'controls', frequently encountered in the literature, are not consistent with reliable interpretation.

1. Omitting the primary reagent. This frequent protocol, either using a dilution buffer as primary reagent or omitting the primary incubation and leaving the target in blocking buffer, fails to control for the very possible Fc-mediated binding of primary reagent. This can be subsequently 'specifically' detected by standard protocols and a false positive of experimental MAbs may be incorrectly concluded. Should the irrelevant isotype controls noted above reveal the possibility of nonspecific immunoglobulin binding, additional blocking steps can be attempted or $F(ab)_2$ or F(ab) reagents may be used.
2. Using normal (species) serum at the same dilution as the primary reagent. Primary polyvalent serum reagent should be affinity-purified, or, at least, provided in immunoglobulin fraction form, in which case, the immunoglobulin concentration is known. As hyperimmune serum has an immunoglobulin content several-fold that of preimmune serum, it is obvious that immunoglobulin concentration, not serum dilution, must be equivalent.
3. Using hybridoma supernatants as primary reagents. Since the immunoglobulin concentration of such samples varies hourly, this is unacceptable in that an assay so performed is uncontrollable and unrepeatable.

Interpretation and quantitation

Interpreting and quantifying results require care and skill. Even with optimally performed assays, several factors can complicate interpretation (Yu, Woods and Levison, 1992; Leong, 1993). The most frequently encountered interpretation problems include: (1) diffuse, pale, monotonous background (insufficient blocking; oversufficient developing); (2) atypical localization of positivity (inadequate fixation, overpermeabilization); (3) intrinsic and extrinsic pigments that are confused with applied chromogen (corrected by pretreatment to inactivate endogenous reactivity) (Leong, 1993); and (4) false-positive staining via primary antibody uptake by mitotic cells, necrotic tissue or tissue edges (edge effect) or large cell-bodied neurons (Perentes and Rubinstein, 1987), or via absorption or phagocytosis of antigens by macrophages or histiocytes (Leong, 1993). Appropriate controls, as outlined in the 'Experimental design' section above should help in resolving some of these problems, although antigen 'migration' by diffusion or uptake cannot be readily identified if isotype control slides are appropriately unstained.

Attempts to quantitate immunohistochemical observations, especially for nuclear markers such as Ki-67, PCNA, etc., have historically been time consuming and inaccurate. Manual counting of positive cells per total cells to determine proliferation indices can result in highly variable values per investigator per field (Yu, Woods and Levison, 1992). Problematic also is the functional and kinetic cell heterogeneity within a specimen, rendering interpretation of the proliferation pattern of the biologically and therapeutically relevant cell population within a tumor sample difficult (Yu, Woods and Levison, 1992). Recently, computerized quantitative immunohistochemistry performed by digital image analyzers has been introduced in several settings as a replacement for conventional immunohistochemical assessment (Zaidi, Liu and Gerson, 1996). After blank fields are standardized, randomly selected fields of immunostained samples are assessed for immunostain density on a 'gray' scale ranging from 0 (black) to 255 (white). Parameters that can be measured include: (1) integrated gray (sum of pixel densities), (2) mean gray and (3) percentage area (positive pixels above background/total pixels). While still in the developmental stage, all three digitized parameters have been found to correlate with subjective immunohistochemical assessments in a study of anti-alkyltransferase expression in colonic tumors, and to be more sensitive in describing areas of marked heterogeneity within a tumor (Zaidi, Liu and Gerson, 1996).

SUMMARY

In summary, immunohistochemical evaluation of normal and neoplastic tissue is a constantly evolving and improving technology, not only in terms of the defined specificity of the immune reagents being employed, but also in the variety of options for antigen fixation and detection, the enhanced amplification systems for exquisite sensitivity, and the emerging technologies for objective interpretation and quantitation all now becoming available. When appropriately controlled, immunohistochemical evaluation can serve as a very precise tool in diagnostic assessment and, ultimately, in prognostic assessment as well.

References

Abdelhaleem, M., Hatskelzon, L., Dalal, B.I., Gerrard, J.M. and Greenberg, A.H. (1991) Leukophysin: a 28 kDa granule membrane protein of leukocytes. *Journal of Immunology* **147**, 3053–9.

Abo, T. and Balch, C.M. (1981) A differentiation antigen of human NK and K cells identified by a monoclonal antibody (HNK-1). *Journal of Immunology* **127**, 1024–9.

Agosti, R.M., Leuthold, M., Gullick, W.J., Yasargil, M.G. and Wiestler, O.D. (1992) Expression of the epidermal growth factor receptor in astrocytic tumours is specifically associated with glioblastoma multiforme. *Virchows Archiv A, Pathological Anatomy and Histopathology* **420**, 321–5.

Ainley, C.D. and Ironside, J.W. (1994) Microwave technology in diagnostic neuropathology. *Journal of Neuroscience Methods* **55**, 183–90.

Albrecht, S., Connelly, J.H.H. and Bruner, J.M. (1993) Distribution of p53 protein expression in gliosarcomas: an immunohistochemical study. *Acta Neuropathologica* **85**, 222–6.

Alderson, L.M., Castleberg, R.L., Harsh, G.R.4th, Louis, D.N. and Henson, J.W. (1995) Human gliomas with wild-type p53 express bcl-2. *Cancer Research* **55**, 999–1001.

Aletsee-Ufrecht, M.C., Langley, K., Rotsch, M., Havemann, K. and Gratzl, M. (1990) NCAM: a surface marker for human small cell lung cancer cells. *FEBS Letters* **267**, 295–300.

Aloisi, F., Giampaolo, A., Russo, G., Peschle, C. and Levi, G. (1992) Developmental appearance, antigenic profile, and proliferation of glial cells of the human embryonic spinal cord: an immunocytochemical study using dissociated cultured cells. *Glia* **5**, 171–81.

Anderson, D.J. and Axel, R. (1986) A bipotential neuroendocrine precursor whose choice of cell fate is determined by NGF and glucocorticoids. *Cell* **47**, 1079–90.

Ansari, B., Dover, R., Gillmore, C.P. and Hall, P.A. (1993) Expression of the nuclear membrane protein statin in cycling cells. *Journal of Pathology* **169**, 391–6.

Arends, M.J., McGregor, A.H. and Wyllie, A.H. (1994) Apoptosis is inversely related to necrosis and determines net growth in tumors bearing constitutively expressed *myc, ras*, and HPV oncogenes. *American Journal of Pathology* **144**, 1045–57.

Bader, M.F., Georges, E., Mushynski, W.E. and Trifaro, J.M. (1984) Neurofilament proteins in cultured chromaffin cells. *Journal of Neurochemistry* **43**, 1180–93.

Baker, D.L., Molenaar, W.M., Trojanowski, J.Q., Evans, A.E., Ross, A.H., Rorke, L.B., Packer, R.J., Lee, V.M.-Y. and Pleasure D. (1991) Nerve growth factor receptor expression in peripheral and central neuroectodermal tumors, other pediatric brain tumors, and during development of the adrenal gland. *American Journal of Pathology* **139**, 115–22.

Balza, E., Siri, A., Ponassi, M., Caocci, F., Linnala, A., Virtanen, I. and Zardi, L. (1993) Production and characterization of monoclonal antibodies specific for different epitopes of human tenascin. *FEBS Letters* **332**, 39–43.

Barbacid, M. (1994) The Trk family of neurotrophin receptors. *Journal of Neurobiology* **25**, 1386–403.

Batra, S.K., Castelino-Prabhu, S., Wikstrand, C.J., Zhu, X., Humphrey, P.A., Friedman, H.S. and Bigner, D.D. (1995) Epidermal growth factor ligand-independent, unregulated, cell-transforming potential of a naturally occurring human mutant EGFRvIII gene. *Cell Growth and Differentiation* **6**, 1251–9.

Baudoin, C., Meneguzzi, G., Portier, M.M., Demarchez, M., Bernerd, F., Pisani, A. and Ortonne, J.P. (1993) Peripherin, a neuronal intermediate protein, is stably expressed by neuroendocrine carcinomas of the skin, their xenograft on nude mice, and the corresponding primary cultures. *Cancer Research* **53**, 1175–81.

Behnke, J., Mach, J.-P., Buchegger, F., Carrel, S., Delaloye, B. and de Tribolet, N. (1988) *In vivo* localization of radiolabeled monoclonal antibody in human gliomas. *British Journal of Neurosurgery* **2**, 193–7.

Behrens, J., Frixen, U., Schipper, J., Weidner, M. and Birchmeier, W. (1992) Cell adhesion in invasion and metastasis. *Seminars in Cell Biology* **3**, 169–78.

Biernat, W., Aguzzi, A., Sure, U., Grant, J.W., Kleihues, P. and Hegi, M.E. (1995) Identical mutations of the *p53* tumor suppressor gene in the gliomatous and the sarcomatous components of gliosarcomas suggest a common origin from glial cells. *Journal of Neuropathology and Experimental Neurology* **54**, 651–6.

Bigner, D.D., Brown, M., Coleman, R.E., Friedman, A.H., Friedman, H.S., McLendon, R.E., Bigner, S.H., Zhao, X.-G., Wikstrand, C.J., Pegram, C.N., Kerby, T. and Zalutsky, M.R. (1995) Phase I studies of treatment of malignant gliomas and neoplastic meningitis with ^{131}I-radiolabeled monoclonal antibodies anti-tenascin 81C6 and anti-chondroitin proteoglycan sulfate Mel-14 F(ab')$_2$ – a preliminary report. *Journal of Neuro-Oncology* **24**, 109–22.

Bishop, M. and de la Monte, S.M. (1989) Dual lineage of astrocytomas. *American Journal of Pathology* **135**, 517–27.

Bodega, G., Suárez, I., Rubio, M. and Fernández, B. (1995) Type II cytokeratin expression in adult vertebrate spinal cord. *Tissue and Cell* **27**, 555–9.

Bonnin, J.M. and Perentes, E. (1988) Retinal S-antigen immunoreactivity in medulloblastoma. *Acta Neuropathologica* **76**, 204–7.

Bonnin, J.M. and Rubinstein, L.J. (1984) Immunohistochemistry of central nervous system tumors. Its contributions to neurosurgical diagnosis. *Journal of Neurosurgery* **60**, 1121–33.

Bourdon, M.A., Wikstrand, C.J., Furthmayr, H., Matthews, T.J. and Bigner, D.D. (1983) Human glioma-mesenchymal extracellular matrix antigen defined by monoclonal antibody. *Cancer Research* **43**, 2796–805.

Bourdon, M.A., Matthews, T.J., Pizzo, S.V. and Bigner, D.D. (1985) Immunochemical and biochemical characterization of a glioma-associated extracellular matrix glycoprotein. *Journal of Cellular Biochemistry* **28**, 183–95.

Breuninger, L.M., Paul, S., Gaughan, K., Miki, T., Chan, A., Aaronson, S.A. and Kruh, G.D. (1995) Expression of multidrug resistance-associated protein in NIH/3T3 cells confers multidrug resistance associated with increased drug efflux and altered intracellular drug distribution. *Cancer Research* **55**, 5342–7.

Bruner, J.M., Connelly, J.H. and Saya, H. (1993) p53 protein immunostaining in routinely processed paraffin-embedded sections. *Modern Pathology* **6**, 189–94.

Bruner, J.M., Saya, H. and Moser, R.P. (1991) Immunocytochemical detection of p53 in human gliomas. *Modern Pathology* **4**, 671–4.

Buck, C.R., Martinez, H.J., Chao, M.V. and Black, I.B. (1988) Differential expression of the nerve growth factor receptor gene in multiple brain areas. *Brain Research: Developmental Brain Research* **44,** 259–68.

Bumol, T.F. and Reisfeld, R.A. (1982) Unique glycoprotein-proteoglycan complex defined by monoclonal antibody on human melanoma cells. *Proceedings of the National Academy of Sciences U.S.A.* **79**, 1245–9.

Burger, P.C., Shibata, T. and Kleihues, P. (1986) The use of the monoclonal antibody Ki-67 in the identification of proliferating cells: application to surgical neuropathology. *American Journal of Surgical Pathology* **10**, 611–17.

Carbone, D.P., Koros, A.M.C., Linnoila, R.I., Jewett, P. and Gazdar, A.F. (1991) Neural cell adhesion molecule expression and messenger RNA splicing patterns in lung cancer cell lines are correlated with neuroendocrine phenotype and growth morphology. *Cancer Research* **51**, 6142–9.

Carden, M.J., Trojanowski, J.Q., Schlaepfer, W.W. and Lee, V.M.-Y. (1987) Two-stage expression of neurofilament polypeptides during rat neurogenesis with early establishment of adult phosphorylation patterns. *Journal of Neuroscience* **7**, 3489–504.

Carpentier, J.-L., Rees, A.R., Gregoriou, M., Kris, R., Schlessinger, J. and Orci, L. (1986) Subcellular distribution of the external and internal domains of the EGF receptor in A-431 cells. *Experimental Cell Research* **166**, 312–26.

Carrel, S., Accolla, R.S., Carmagnola, A.L. and Mach, J.-P. (1980) Common human melanoma-associated antigen(s) detected by monoclonal antibodies. *Cancer Research* **40**, 2523–8.

Cattoretti, G., Becker, M.H.G., Key, G., Duchrow, M., Schluter, C., Galle, J. and Gerdes, J. (1992) Monoclonal antibodies against recombinant parts of the Ki-67 antigen (MIB 1 and MIB 3) detect proliferating cells in microwave-processed formalin fixed paraffin sections. *Journal of Pathology* **168**, 357–63.

Chaffanet, M., Chauvin, C., Laine, M., Berger, F., Chedin, M., Rost, N., Nissou, M.F. and Benabid, A.L. (1992) EGF receptor amplification and expression in human brain tumours. *European Journal of Cancer* **28**, 11–17.

Chan, H.S.L., Grogan, T.M., DeBoer, G., Haddad, G. and Ling, V. (1996) Importance of P-glycoprotein as determinant of chemotherapy response in osteosarcoma. (Abstract) *Proceedings of the American Association for Cancer Research* **37**, 326.

Chao, M.V. and Hempstead, B.L. (1995) p75 and Trk: a two-receptor system. *Trends in Neurosciences* **18**, 321–6.

Ching, G.Y. and Liem, R.K. (1991) Structure of the gene for the neuronal intermediate filament protein alpha-internexin and functional analysis of its promoter. *Journal of Biological Chemistry* **266**, 19459–68.

Chiquet-Ehrismann, R., Matsuoka, Y., Hofer, U., Spring, J., Bernasconi, C. and Chiquet, M. (1991) Tenascin variants: differential binding to fibronectin and distinct distribution in cell cultures and tissues. *Cell Regulation* **2**, 927–38.

Chiu, F.C., Barnes, E.A., Das, K., Haley, J., Socolow, P., Macaluso, F.P. and Fant, J. (1989) Characterization of a novel 66 kd subunit of mammalian neurofilaments. *Neuron* **12**, 1435–45.

Christofori, G. and Hanahan, D. (1994) Molecular dissection of multi-stage tumorigenesis in transgenic mice. *Seminars in Cancer Biololgy* **5**, 3–12.

Citron, M., White, A., Decker, R., Wasserman, P., Li, B., Randall, T., Guerra, D., Belanich, M. and Yarosh, D. (1995) O^6-methylguanine-DNA methyltransferase in human brain tumors detected by activity assay and monoclonal antibodies. *Oncology Research* **7**, 49–55.

Claesson-Welsh, L., Eriksson, A., Morén, A., Severinsson, L., Ek, B., Östman, A., Betsholtz, C. and Heldin, C.-H. (1988) cDNA cloning and expression of a human platelet-derived growth factor (PDGF) receptor specific for β-chain-containing PDGF molecules. *Molecular and Cellular Biology* **8**, 3476–86.

Coca, S., Vaquero, J., Escandon, J., Moreno, M., Peralba, J. and Rodriguez, J. (1992) Immunohistochemical characterization of pineocytomas. *Clinical Neuropathology* **11**, 298–303.

Coffin, C.M., Mukai, K. and Dehner, L.P. (1983) Glial differentiation in medulloblastomas. Histogenetic insight, glial reaction, or invasion of brain? *American Journal of Surgical Pathology* **7**, 555–65.

Coffin, C.M., Braun, J.T., Wick, M.R. and Dehner, L.P. (1990) A clinicopathologic and immunohistochemical analysis of 53 cases of medulloblastoma with emphasis on synaptophysin expression. *Modern Pathology* **3**, 164–70.

Cohn, D.V., Zangerle, R., Fischer-Colbrie, R., Chu, L.L., Elting, J.J., Hamilton, J.W. and Winkler, H. (1982) Similarity of secretory protein I from parathyroid gland to chromagranin A from adrenal medulla. *Proceedings of the National Academy of Sciences U.S.A.* **79**, 6056–9.

Colapinto, E.V., Zalutsky, M.R., Archer, G.E., Noska, M.A., Friedman, H.S., Carrel, S. and Bigner, D.D. (1990) Radioimmunotherapy of intracerebral human glioma xenografts with ^{131}I-labeled F(ab')$_2$ fragments of monoclonal antibody Mel-14. *Cancer Research* **50**, 1822–7.

Cole, G.J. and Schachner, M. (1987) Localization of the L2 monoclonal antibody binding site on chicken neural cell adhesion molecule (NCAM) and evidence for its role in NCAM-mediated adhesion. *Neuroscience Letters* **78**, 227–32.

Cordon-Cardo C., Tapley, P., Jing, S.Q., Nanduri, V., O'Rourke, E., Lamballe, F., Kovary, K., Klein, R., Jones, K.R., Reichardt, L.F. and Barbacid, M. (1991) The trk tyrosine protein kinase mediates the mitogenic properties of nerve growth factor and neurotrophin-3. *Cell* **66**, 173–83.

Cosgrove, M., Fitzgibbons, P.L., Sherrod, A., Chandrasoma, P.T. and Martin, S.E. (1989) Intermediate filament expression in astrocytic neoplasms. *American Journal of Surgical Pathology* **13**, 141–5.

Crossin, K.L., Edelman, G.M. and Cunningham, B.A. (1984) Mapping of three carbohydrate attachment sites in embryonic and adult forms of the neural cell adhesion molecule. *Journal of Cell Biology* **99**, 1848–55.

Cutarelli, P.E., Roessmann, U.R., Miller, R.H., Specht, C.S. and Grossniklaus, H.E. (1991) Immunohistochemical properties of human optic nerve glioma. Evidence of type 1 astrocyte origin. Investigative *Ophthalmology and Visual Science* **32**, 2521–4.

Czerwionka, M., Korf, H.W., Hoffmann, O., Busch, H. and Schachenmayr, W. (1989) Differentiation in medulloblastomas: correlation between the immunocytochemical demonstration of photoreceptor markers (S-antigen, rod-opsin) and the survival rate in 66 patients. *Acta Neuropathologica (Berlin)* **78**, 629–36.

Dadparvar, S., Krishna, L., Miyamoto, C., Brady, L.W., Brown, S.J., Bender, H., Slizofski, W.J., Eshleman, J., Chevres, A. and Woo, D.V. (1994) Indium-111-labeled anti-EGFR-425 scintigraphy in the detection of malignant gliomas. *Cancer* **73** (3 Suppl), 884–9.

Dahlstrand, J., Collins, V.P. and Lendahl, U. (1992) Expression of the class VI intermediate filament nestin in human central nervous system tumors. *Cancer Research* **52**, 5334–41.

Davidoff, A.M., Pence, J.C., Shorter, N.A., Iglehart, J.D. and Marks, J.R. (1992) Expression of p53 in human neuroblastoma- and neuroepithelioma-derived cell lines. *Oncogene* **7**, 127–33.

Debiec-Rychter, M., Alwasiak, J., Papierz, W. and Liberski, P.P. (1994) Expression of N-myc, c-myc and c-erbB-1 proto-oncogenes in cerebral primitive neuroectodermal tumors (PNET). *Folia Neuropathologica* **32**, 229–31.

Defize, L.H.K., Molenaar, W.H., van der Saag, P.T. and de Laat, S.W. (1986) Dissociation of cellular responses to epidermal growth factor using anti-receptor monoclonal antibodies. *EMBO Journal* **5**, 1187–92.

DeLellis, R.A. and Dayal, Y. (1992) The neuroendocrine system. In Sternberg, S.S. (ed.), *Histology for pathologists*. New York: Raven Press, 347–62.

DeLellis, R.A., Dayal, Y., Tischler, A.S., Lee, A.K. and Wolfe, H.J. (1986) Multiple endocrine neoplasia syndromes: cellular origins and interrelationship. *International Review of Experimental Pathology* **28**, 163–215.

Diepholder, H.M., Schwechheimer, K., Mohadjer, M., Knoth, R. and Bolk B. (1991) A clinicopathologic and immunomorphologic study of 13 cases of ganglioglioma. *Cancer* **68**, 2192–201.

Dietzmann, K. and von Bossanyi, P. (1994) Coexpression of epidermal growth factor receptor protein and c-erbB-2 oncoprotein in human astrocytic tumors. An immunohistochemical study. *Zentralblatt für Pathologie* **140**, 335–41.

Dixon, R.G. and Eng, L.F. (1981) Glial fibrillary acidic protein in the retina of the developing albino rat: an immunoperoxidase study of paraffin-embedded tissue. *Journal of Comparative Neurology* **195**, 305–21.

Drach, L.M., Kammermeier, M., Neirich, U., Jacobi, G., Kornhuber, B., Lorenz, R. and Schlote, W. (1996) Accumulation of nuclear p53 protein and prognosis of astrocytomas in childhood and adolescence. *Clinical Neuropathology* **15**, 67–73.

Dubois, C., Manuguerra, J.C., Hauttecoeur, B. and Maze, J. (1990) Monoclonal antibody A2B5, which detects cell surface antigens, binds to ganglioside GT3 (II3 (NeuAc)3LacCer) and to its 9-O-acetylated derivative. *Journal of Biological Chemistry* **265**, 2797–803.

Duffy, P.E., Huang, Y.-Y., Rapport, M.M. and Graf, L. (1980) Glial fibrillary acidic protein in giant cell tumors of brain and other gliomas. A possible relationship to malignancy, differentiation, and pleomorphism of glia. *Acta Neuropathologica* **52**, 51–7.

Duncan, M.E., McAleese, S.M., Booth, N.A., Melvin, W.T. and Fothergill, J.E. (1992) A simple enzyme-linked immunosorbent assay (ELISA) for the neuron-specific γ isozyme of human enolase (NSE) using monoclonal antibodies raised against synthetic peptides corresponding to isozyme sequence differences. *Journal of Immunological Methods* **151**, 227–36.

Eisenbarth, G.S., Walsh, F.S. and Nirenberg, M. (1979) Monoclonal antibody to a plasma membrane antigen of neurons. *Proceedings of the National Academy of Sciences U.S.A.* **76**, 4913–17.

Ekstrand, A.J., Sugawa, N., James, C.D. and Collins, V.P. (1992) Amplified and rearranged epidermal growth factor receptor genes in human glioblastomas reveal deletions of sequences encoding portions of the N- and/or C-terminal tails. *Proceedings of the National Academy of Sciences U.S.A.* **89**, 4309–13.

Elias, J.M. (1990a) Immunohistochemical methods. In Elias, J.M. (ed.), *Immunohistopathology: a practical approach to diagnosis*. Chicago: American Society of Clinical Pathologists' Press, 1–90.

— (1990b) Immunohistochemical approach to the diagnosis of malignant disease. In Elias, J.M. (ed.), *Immunohistopathology: a practical approach to diagnosis*. Chicago: American Society of Clinical Pathologists' Press, 91–147.

Ellison, D.W., Gatter, K.C., Steart, P.V., Lane, D.P. and Weller, R.O. (1992) Expression of the p53 protein in a spectrum of astrocytic tumours. *Journal of Pathology* **168**, 383–6.

Ellison, D.W., Steart, P.V., Bateman, A.C., Pickering, R.M., Palmer, J.D. and Weller, R.O. (1995) Prognostic indicators in a range of astrocytic tumours: an immunohistochemical study with Ki-67 and p53 antibodies. *Journal of Neurology, Neurosurgery and Psychiatry* **59**, 413–19.

Eng, L.F., Vanderhaeghen, J.J., Bignami, A. and Gerstl, B. (1971) An acidic protein isolated from fibrous astrocytes. *Brain Research* **28**, 351–4.

Engelhard, H.H.3rd, Butler, A.B.4th and Bauer, K.D. (1989) Quantification of the c-myc oncoprotein in human glioblastoma cells and tumor tissue. *Journal of Neurosurgery* **71**, 224–32.

Enzinger, F.M. and Weiss, S.W. (1988) Tumors of the sympathetic nervous system. In Enzinger, F.M., and Weiss, S.W. (eds), *Soft tissue tumors*. St Louis: C.V. Mosby, 816–35.

Evan, G.I., Lewis, G.K., Ramsay, G. and Bishop, J.M. (1985) Isolation of monoclonal antibodies specific for human c-myc proto-oncogene product. *Molecular and Cellular Biology* **5**, 3610–16.

Evers, P. and Uylings, H.B.M. (1994) Effects of microwave pretreatment on immunocytochemical staining of vibratome sections and tissue blocks of human cerebral cortex stored in formaldehyde fixative for long periods. *Journal of Neuroscience Methods* **55**, 163–72.

Fabricant, R.N, De Larco, J.E. and Todaro, G.J. (1977) Binding and thermal dissociation of nerve growth factor and its receptor on human melanoma cells. *Biochemical and Biophysical Research Communications* **79**, 299–304.

Fano, G., Biocca, S., Fulle, S., Mariggio, M.A., Belia, S. and Calissano, P. (1995) The S-100: a protein family in search of a function. *Progress in Neurobiology* **46**, 71–82.

Farber, E. (1994) Programmed cell death: necrosis versus apoptosis. *Modern Pathology* **7**, 605–9.

Figarella-Branger, D.F., Durbec, P.L. and Rougon, G.N. (1990) Differential spectrum of expression of neural cell adhesion molecule isoforms and L1 adhesion molecules on human neuroectodermal tumors. *Cancer Research* **50**, 6364–70.

Fisher, C.J., Gillett, C.E., Vojtesek, B., Barnes, D.M. and Millis, R.R. (1994) Problems with p53 immunohistochemical staining: the effect of fixation and variation in the methods of evaluation. *British Journal of Cancer* **69**, 26–31.

Fliegner, K.H., Ching, G.Y. and Liem, R.K. (1990) The predicted amino acid sequence of alpha-internexin is that of a novel neuronal intermediate filament protein. *EMBO Journal* **9**, 749–55.

Florenes, V.A., Holm, R., Myklebost, O., Lendahl, U. and Fodstad, O. (1994) Expression of the neuroectodermal intermediate filament nestin in human melanomas. *Cancer Research* **54**, 354–6.

Foley, J., Witte, D., Chiu, F.C. and Parysek, L.M. (1994) Expression of the neural intermediate filament proteins peripherin and neurofilament-66/alpha-internexin in neuroblastoma. *Laboratory Investigation* **71**, 193–9.

Foster, G.A., Dahl, D. and Lee, V.M.-Y. (1987) Temporal and topographic relationships between the phosphorylated and non-phosphorylated epitopes of the 200 kDa neurofilament protein during development *in vitro*. *Journal of Neuroscience* **7**, 2651–63.

Franke, F.E., Schachenmayr, W., Osborn, M. and Altmannsberger, M. (1991) Unexpected immunoreactivities of intermediate filament antibodies in human brain and brain tumors. *American Journal of Pathology* **139**, 67–79.

Franko, M.C., Gibbs, C.J.Jr, Rhoades, D.A. and Gajdusek, D.C. (1987) Monoclonal antibody analysis of keratin expression in the central nervous system. *Proceedings of the National Academy of Sciences U.S.A.* **84**, 3482–5.

Frederiksen, K. and McKay, R.D.G. (1988) Proliferation and differentiation of rat neuroepithelial precursor cells *in vivo*. *Journal of Neuroscience* **8**, 1144–51.

Fredman, P., Magnani, J.L., Nirenberg, M. and Ginsburg, V. (1984) Monoclonal antibody A2B5 reacts with many gangliosides in neuronal tissue. *Archives of Biochemistry and Biophysics* **233**, 661–6.

Fredman, P., von Holst, H., Collins, V.P., Granholm, L. and Svennerholm, L. (1988) Sialyllactotetraosylceramide, a ganglioside marker for human malignant gliomas. *Journal of Neurochemistry* **50**, 912–19.

Freischutz, B., Saito, M., Rahmann, H. and Yu, R.K. (1994) Activities of five different sialyltransferases in fish and rat brains. *Journal of Neurochemistry* **62**, 1965–73.

Friedman, B., Zaremba, S. and Hockfield, S. (1990) Monoclonal antibody rat 401 recognizes Schwann cells in mature and developing peripheral nerve. *Journal of Comparative Neurology* **295**, 43–51.

Frost, G., Patel, K., Bourne, S., Coakham, H.B. and Kemshead, J.T. (1991) Expression of alternative isoforms of the neural cell adhesion molecule (NCAM) on normal brain and a variety of brain tumours. *Neuropathology and Applied Neurobiology* **17**, 207–17.

Fujimaki, T., Matsutani, M., Nakamura, O., Asai, A., Funada, N., Koike, M., Segawa, H., Aritake, K., Fukushima, T., Houjo, S., Tamura, A. and Sano, K. (1991) Correlation between bromodeoxyuridine-labeling indices and patient prognosis in cerebral astrocytic tumors of adults. *Cancer* **67**, 1629–34.

Fujimoto, M., Weaker, F.J., Herbert, D.C., Sharp, Z.D., Sheridan, P.J. and Story, J.L. (1988) Expression of three viral oncogenes (v-sis, v-myc, v-fos) in primary human brain tumors of neuroectodermal origin. *Neurology* **38**, 289–93.

Fukasawa, Y., Ishikura, H., Takada, A., Yokoyama, S., Imamura, M., Yoshiki, T. and Sato, H. (1994) Massive apoptosis in infantile myofibromatosis. A putative mechanism of tumor regression. *American Journal of Pathology* **144**, 480–5.

Fuller, G.N. and Bigner, S.H. (1992) Amplified cellular oncogenes in neoplasms of the human central nervous system. *Mutation Research* **276**, 299–306.

Fuller, G.N., Burger, P.C., Schold, S.C., Preisinger, A., Wong, A.J., Bigner, D.D., Vogelstein, B. and Bigner, S.H. (1990) Gene amplification in human gliomas. (Abstract) *Journal of Neuropathology and Experimental Neurology* **49**, 320.

Fung, K.-M., Lee, V.M.-Y. and Trojanowski, J.Q. (1995) The dynamics of cell proliferation and cell death during the emergence of primitive neuroectodermal tumors of the immature central nervous system in transgenic mice. *American Journal of Pathology* **146**, 1376–87.

Garson, J.A., Pemberton, L.F., Sheppard, P.W., Varndell, I.M., Coakham, H.B. and Kemshead, J.T. (1989) N-myc gene expression and oncoprotein characterisation in medulloblastoma. *British Journal of Cancer* **59**, 889–94.

Gennarini, G., Rougon, G., Deagostini-Bazin, H., Hirn, M. and Goridis, C. (1984) Studies on the transmembrane disposition of the neural cell adhesion molecule N-CAM. A monoclonal antibody recognising a cytoplasmic domain and evidence for the presence of phosphoserine residues. *European Journal of Biochemistry* **142**, 57–64.

Gerdes, J., Schwab, U., Lemke, H. and Stein, H. (1983) Production of a mouse monoclonal antibody reactive with a human nuclear antigen associated with cell proliferation. *International Journal of Cancer* **31**, 13–20.

Gerdes, J., Lemke, H., Baisch, H., Wacker, H.H., Schwab, U. and Stein, H. (1984) Cell cycle analysis of a cell proliferation-associated human nuclear antigen defined by the monoclonal antibody Ki-67. *Journal of Immunology* **133**, 1710–15.

Gerdes, J., Li, L., Schlueter, C., Duchrow, M., Wohlenberg, C., Gerlach, C., Stahmer, I., Kloth, S., Brandt, E. and Flad, H.-D. (1991) Immunobiochemical and molecular biologic characterization of the cell proliferation-associated nuclear antigen that is defined by monoclonal antibody Ki-67. *American Journal of Pathology* **138**, 867–73.

Gerdes, J., Becker, M.H.G., Key, G. and Cattoretti, G. (1992) Immunohistological detection of tumour growth fraction (Ki-67 antigen) in formalin-fixed and routinely processed tissues. *Journal of Pathology* **168**, 85–6.

Gerrard, J.M., Lint, D., Sims, P.J., Wiedmer, T., Fugate, R.D., McMillan, E., Robertson, C. and Israels, S.J. (1991) Identification of a platelet dense granule membrane protein that is deficient in a patient with the Hermansky-Pudlak syndrome. *Blood* **77**, 101–12.

Gerson, S.L. and Willson, J.K. (1995) O^6-alkylguanine-DNA alkyltransferase. A target for the modulation of drug resistance. *Hematology-Oncology Clinics of North America* **9**, 431–50.

Geschwind, D.H. and Hockfield, S. (1989) Identification of proteins that are developmentally regulated during early cerebral corticogenesis in the rat. *Journal of Neuroscience* **9**, 4303–17.

Gonzalez-Fernadez, F., Lopes, M.B.S., Garcia-Fernandez, J.M., Foster, R.G., De Grip, W.J., Rosenberg, S., Newman, S.A. and VandenBerg, S.R. (1992) Expression of developmentally defined retinal phenotypes in the histogenesis of retinoblastoma. *American Journal of Pathology* **141**, 363–75.

Gorczyca, W., Gong, J. and Darzynkiewicz, Z. (1993) Detection of DNA strand breaks in individual apoptotic cells by the *in situ* terminal deoxynucleotidyl transferase and nick translation assays. *Cancer Research* **53**, 1945–51.

Gould, V.E., Wiedenmann, B., Lee, I., Schwechheimer, K., Dockhorn-Dworniczak, B. and Eadosevich, J.A. (1987) Synaptophysin expression in neuroendocrine neoplasms as determined by immunocytochemistry. *American Journal of Pathology* **126**, 243–57.

Gould, V.E., Jansson, D.S., Molenaar, W.M., Rorke, L.B., Trojanowski, J.Q., Lee, V.M.-Y., Packer, R.J. and Franke, W.W. (1990) Primitive neuroectodermal tumors of the central nervous system – patterns of expression of neuroendocrine markers, and all classes of intermediate filament proteins. *Laboratory Investigation* **62**, 498–509.

Gullick, W.J., Downward, J., Parker, P.J., Whittle, N., Kris, R., Schlessinger, J., Ulrich, A. and Waterfield, M.D. (1985) The structure and function of the epidermal growth factor receptor studied by using anti-synthetic peptide antibodies. *Proceedings of the Royal Society of London Series B: Biological Sciences* **226**, 127–34.

Gullick, W.J., Downward, J., Foulkes, J.G. and Waterfield, M.D. (1986) Antibodies to the ATP-binding site of the human epidermal-growth-factor (EGF) receptor as specific inhibitors of EGF-stimulated protein-tyrosine activity. *European Journal of Biochemistry* **158**, 245–53.

Haapasalo, H., Isola, J., Sallinen, P., Kalimo, H., Helin, H. and Rantala, I. (1993) Aberrant p53 expression in astrocytic neoplasms of the brain: association with proliferation. *American Journal of Pathology* **142**, 1347–51.

Haimoto, H., Takahashi, Y., Koshikawa, T., Nagura, H. and Kato, K. (1985) Immunohistochemical localization of gamma-enolase in normal human tissues other than nervous and neuroendocrine tissues. *Laboratory Investigation* **52**, 257–63.

Han, Z., Chatterjee, D., Early, J., Pantazis, P., Hendrickson, E.A. and Wyche, J.H. (1996) Isolation and characterization of an apoptosis-resistant variant of human leukemia HL-60 cells that has switched expression from Bcl-2 to Bcl-x_L. *Cancer Research* **56**, 1621–8.

Harper, J.R., Perry, S.K., Davis, R.M. and Laufer, D.M. (1990) Human neuroectoderm-derived cell line secretes fibronectin that shares the HNK-1/10C5 carbohydrate epitope with neural cell adhesion molecules. *Journal of Neurochemistry* **54**, 395–401.

Hassoun, J., Soylemezoglu, F., Gambarelli, D., Figarella-Branger, D., von Ammon, K. and Kleihues, P. (1993) Central neurocytoma: a synopsis of clinical and histological features. *Brain Pathology* **3**, 297–306.

Helseth, E.G., Unsgaard, A., Dalen, A., Fure, H., Skandsen, A., Ødegaard, A. and Vik, R. (1988) Amplification of the epidermal growth factor receptor gene in biopsy specimens from human intracranial tumours. *British Journal of Neurosurgery* **2**, 217–25.

Herlyn, D., Benderm H., Adachi, K., Takahashi, H., Belser, P. and Rodeck, U. (1993) Monoclonal antibody targeting of epidermal growth factor receptor on human malignant gliomas. In Epentos, A.A. (ed.), *Monoclonal antibodies 2: applications in clinical oncology*. London: Chapman and Hall Medical, 219–26.

Hermanson, M., Nister, M., Betsholtz, C., Heldin, C.H., Westermark, B. and Funa, K. (1988) Endothelial cell hyperplasia in human glioblastomas: coexpression of mRNA for PDGF-β chain and PDGF receptor suggests autocrine growth stimulation. *Proceedings of the National Academy of Sciences U.S.A.* **85**, 7748–52.

Hermanson, M., Funa, K., Hartman, M., Claesson-Welsh, L., Heldin, C.H., Westermark, B. and Nister, M. (1992) Platelet-derived growth factor and its receptors in human glioma tissue: expression of messenger RNA and protein suggests the presence of autocrine and paracrine loops. *Cancer Research* **52**, 3213–19.

Hermanson, M., Funa, K., Koopmann, J., Maintz, D., Waha, A., Westermark, B., Heldin, C.H., Wiestler, O.D., Louis, D.N., von Deimling, A. and Nister, M. (1996) Association of loss of heterozygosity on chromosome 17p with high platelet-derived growth factor α receptor expression in human malignant gliomas. *Cancer Research* **56**, 164–71.

Hessler, R.B., Lopes, M.B.S., Frankfurter, A., Reidy, J. and Vandenberg, S.R. (1992) Cytoskeletal immunohistochemistry of central neurocytomas. *American Journal of Surgical Pathology* **16**, 1031–8.

Higuchi, M., Ohnishi, T., Arita, N., Hiraga, S. and Hayakawa, T. (1993) Expression of tenascin in human gliomas: its relation to histological malignancy, tumor dedifferentiation and angiogenesis. *Acta Neuropathologica* **85**, 481–7.

Hlavin, M.L. and Lemmon, V. (1991) Molecular structure and functional testing of human L1 CAM: an interspecies comparison. *Genomics* **11**, 416–23.

Hoi Sang, U., Espiritu, O.D., Kelley, P.Y., Klauber, M.R. and Hatton, J.D. (1995) The role of the epidermal growth factor receptor in human gliomas: I. The control of cell growth. *Journal of Neurosurgery* **82**, 841–6.

Honer, W.G., Kaufmann, C.A. and Davies, P. (1992) Characterization of a synaptic antigen of interest in neuropsychiatric illness. *Biological Psychiatry* **31**, 147–58.

Hoog, A., Gould, V.E., Grimelius, L., Franke, W.W., Falkmer, S. and Chejfec, G. (1988) Tissue fixation methods alter the immunohistochemical demonstrability of synaptophysin. *Ultrastructural Pathology* **12**, 673–8.

Hopkins, K., Chandler, C., Bullimore J., Sandeman, D., Coakham, H. and Kemshead, J.T. (1995) A pilot study of the treatment of patients with recurrent malignant gliomas with intratumoral yttrium-90 radioimmunoconjugates. *Radiotherapy and Oncology* **34**, 121–31.

Hoshino, T., Rodriguez, L.A., Cho, K.G., Lee, K.S., Wilson, C.B., Edwards, M.S.B., Levin, V.A. and Davis, R.L. (1988) Prognostic implications of the proliferative potential of low-grade astrocytomas. *Journal of Neurosurgery* **69**, 839–42.

Hoshino, T., Prados, M., Wilson, C.B., Cho, K.G., Lee, K.-S. and Davis, R.L. (1989) Prognostic implications of the bromodeoxyuridine labeling index of human gliomas. *Journal of Neurosurgery* **71**, 335–41.

Humphrey, P.A., Wong, A.J., Vogelstein, B., Friedman, H.S., Werner, M.H., Bigner, D.D. and Bigner, S.H. (1988) Amplification and expression of the epidermal growth factor receptor gene in human glioma xenografts. *Cancer Research* **48**, 2231–8.

Humphrey, P.A., Wong, A.J., Vogelstein, B., Zalutsky, M.R., Fuller, G.N., Archer, G.E., Friedman, H.S., Kwatra, M.M., Bigner, S.H. and Bigner, D.D. (1990) Anti-synthetic peptide antibody reacting at the fusion junction of deletion-mutant epidermal growth factor receptors in human glioblastoma. *Proceedings of the National Academy of Sciences U.S.A.* **87**, 4207–11.

Iggo, R., Gatter, K., Bartek, J., Lane, D. and Harris, A.L. (1990) Increased expression of mutant forms of p53 oncogene in primary lung cancer. *Lancet* **335**, 675–9.

Ito, S., Hoshino, T., Prados, M.D. and Edwards, M.S.B. (1992) Cell kinetics of medulloblastomas. *Cancer* **70**, 671–8.

Ito, S., Hoshino, T., Shibuya, M., Prados, M.D., Edwards, M.S.B. and Davis, R.L. (1992) Proliferative characteristics of juvenile pilocytic astrocytomas determined by bromodeoxyuridine labeling. *Neurosurgery* **31**, 413–19.

Iuzzolino, P., Ghimenton, C., Nicolato, A., Giorgiutti, F., Fina, P., Doglioni, C. and Barbareschi, M. (1994) p53 protein in low-grade astrocytomas: a study with long-term follow-up. *British Journal of Cancer* **69**, 586–91.

Jacobson, M. (1991) Histogenesis and morphogenesis of cortical structures. In Jacobson, M. (ed.), *Developmental neurobiology*. New York: Plenum Press, 401–514.

Jaffey, P.B., To, G.T., Xu, H.-J., Hu, S.-X., Benedict, W.F., Donoso, L.A. and Campbell, G.A. (1995) Retinoblastoma-like phenotype expressed in medulloblastomas. *Journal of Neuropathology and Experimental Neurology* **54**, 664–72.

Jie, Z., Ivarsson, B. and Collins, V.P. (1986) Monoclonal antibodies to GFAP epitopes available in formaldehyde-fixed tissue. *Acta Pathologica, Microbiologica, et Immunologica Scandinavica Section A* **94**, 353–61.

Jin, L., Hemperly, J.J. and Lloyd, R.V. (1991) Expression of neural cell adhesion molecule in normal and neoplastic human neuroendocrine tissues. *American Journal of Pathology* **138**, 961–9.

Kadmon, G., Kowitz, A., Altevogt, P. and Schachner, M. (1990) Functional cooperation between the neural adhesion molecules L1 and N-CAM is carbohydrate dependent. *Journal of Cell Biology* **110**, 209–18.

Kalofonos, H.P., Pawlikowska, T.R., Hemingway, A., Courtenay-Luck, N., Dhokia B., Snook, D., Sivolapenko, G.B., Hooker, G.R., McKenzie, C.G., Thomas, D.G.T., Lavender, P.J. and Epenetos, A.A. (1989) Antibody-guided diagnosis and therapy of brain gliomas using radiolabeled monoclonal antibodies against epidermal growth factor receptor and placental alkaline phosphatase. *Journal of Nuclear Medicine* **30**, 1636–45.

Karamitopoulou, E., Perentes, E., Diamantis, I. and Maraziotis, T. (1994) Ki-67 immunoreactivity in human central nervous system tumors: a study with MIB 1 monoclonal antibody on archival material. *Acta Neuropathologica* **87**, 47–54.

Karp, J.E. and Broder, S. (1994) New directions in molecular medicine. *Cancer Research* **54**, 653–65.

Kawamoto, T., Sato, J.D., Le, A., Polikoff, J., Sato, G.H. and Mendelsohn, J. (1983) Growth stimulation of A431 cells by epidermal growth factor: identification of high affinity receptors for epidermal growth factor by an anti-receptor monoclonal antibody. *Proceedings of the National Academy of Sciences U.S.A.* **80**, 1337–41.

Key, G., Becker, M.H.G., Baron, B., Duchrow, M., Schlüter, C., Flad, H.D. and Gerdes, J. (1993) New Ki-67-equivalent murine monoclonal antibodies (MIB 1-3) generated against bacterially-expressed parts of the Ki-67 cDNA containing three 62-base pair repetitive elements encoding for the Ki-67 epitope. *Laboratory Investigation* **68**, 629–36.

Kinzler, K.W., Bigner, S.H., Bigner, D.D., Trent, J.M., Law, M.L., O'Brien, S.J., Wong, A.J. and Vogelstein, B. (1987) Identification of an amplified, highly expressed gene in a human glioma. *Science* **236**, 70–3.

Kivelä, T., Tarkkanen, A. and Virtanen, I. (1989) Synaptophysin in the human retina and retinoblastoma. *Investigative Ophthalmology and Visual Science* **30**, 212–19.

Kleihues, P., Kiessling, M. and Janzer, R.C. (1987) Morphological markers in neuro-oncology. *Current Topics in Pathology* **77**, 307–38.

Klinz, S.G., Schachner, M. and Maness, P.F. (1995) L1 and N-CAM antibodies trigger protein phosphatase activity in growth cone-enriched membranes. *Journal of Neurochemistry* **65**, 84–95.

Kordek, R., Bratosiewicz, J., Biernat, W., Alwasiak, J. and Liberski, P.P. (1994) Expression of p53-protein, epidermal growth factor receptor (EGFR) and proliferating cell antigens in human gliomas. *Folia Neuropathologica* **32**, 227–8.

Korf, H.-W., Korf, B., Schachenmayr, W., Chader, G.J. and Wiggert, B. (1992) Immunocytochemical demonstration of interphotoreceptor retinoid-binding protein in cerebellar medulloblastoma. *Acta Neuropathologica* **83**, 482–7.

Kosaka, T., Isogai, K., Barnstable, C.J. and Heizmann, C.W. (1990) Monoclonal antibody HNK-1 selectively stains a subpopulation of GABAergic neurons containing the calcium-binding protein parvalbumin in the rat cerebral cortex. *Experimental Brain Research* **82**, 566–74.

Krajewski, S., Chatten, J., Hanada, M. and Reed, J.C. (1995) Immunohistochemical analysis of the Bcl-2 oncoprotein in human neuroblastomas. Comparisons with tumor cell differentiation and N-myc protein. *Laboratory Investigation* **72**, 42–54.

Kros, J.M., Godschalk, J.J., Krishnadath, K.K. and Van Eden, C.G. (1993) Expression of p53 in oligodendrogliomas. *Journal of Pathology* **171**, 285–90.

Kruse, J., Keilhauer, G., Faissner, A., Timpl, R. and Schachner, M. (1985) The J1 glycoprotein – a novel nervous system cell adhesion molecule of the L2/HNK-I family. *Nature* **316**, 146–8.

Kuchelmeister, K., von Borcke, I.M., Klein, H., Bergmann, M. and Gullotta, F. (1994) Pleomorphic pineocytoma with extensive neuronal differentiation: report of 2 cases. *Acta Neuropathologica (Berlin)* **88**, 448–53.

Kunishio, K., Miashima, N., Matsuhisa, T., Tsuno, K., Matsumi, N., Satoh, T., Matsumoto, K., Furuta, T., Nishimoto, A. and Shiraishi, T. (1990) Immunohistochemical demonstration of DNA polymerase alpha in human brain-tumor cells. *Journal of Neurosurgery* **72**, 268–72.

Kurpad, S.N. and Bigner, D.D. (1995) Immunotherapy of malignant gliomas. In Black, P. (ed.), *Cancer of the nervous system*. Cambridge, Mass.: Blackwell Science, 264–87.

Kurpad, S.N., Zhao, X.G., Wikstrand, C.J., Batra, S.K., McLendon, R.E. and Bigner, D.D. (1995) Tumor antigens in astrocytic gliomas. *GLIA* **15**, 244–56.

Kyritsis, A.P., Bondy, M.L., Hess, K.R., Cunningham, J.E., Zhu, D., Amos, C.J., Yung, W.K.A., Levin, V.A. and Bruner, J.M. (1995) Prognostic significance of p53 immunoreactivity in patients with glioma. *Clinical Cancer Research* **1**, 1617–22.

Lagenaur, C. and Lemmon, V. (1987) An L1-like molecule, the 8D9 antigen, is a potent substrate for neurite extension. *Proceedings of the National Academy of Sciences U.S.A.* **84**, 7753–7.

Lang, F.F., Miller, D.C., Koslow, M. and Newcomb, E.W. (1994a) Pathways leading to glioblastoma multiforme: a molecular analysis of genetic alterations in 65 astrocytic tumors. *Journal of Neurosurgery* **81**, 427–36.

Lang, F.F., Miller, D.C., Pisharody, S., Koslow, M. and Newcomb, E.W. (1994b) High frequency of p53 protein accumulation without p53 gene mutation in human juvenile pilocytic, low grade and anaplastic astrocytomas. *Oncogene* **9**, 949–54.

Lashford, L.S., Davies, A.G., Richardson, R.B., Bourne, S.P., Bullimore, J.A., Eckert, H., Kemshead, J.T. and Coakham, H.B. (1988) A pilot study of ^{131}I monoclonal antibodies in the therapy of leptomeningeal tumors. *Cancer* **61**, 857–68.

Lasorella, A., Iavarone, A. and Israel, M.A. (1995) Differentiation of neuroblastoma enhances Bcl-2 expression and induces alterations of apoptosis and drug resistance. *Cancer Research* **55**, 4711–16.

Laywell, E.D., Dorries, U., Bartsch, U., Faissner, A., Schachner, M. and Steindler, D.A. (1992) Enhanced expression of the developmentally regulated extracellular matrix molecule tenascin following adult brain injury. *Proceedings of the National Academy of Sciences U.S.A.* **89**, 2634–8.

Lazarides, E. (1982) Intermediate filaments: a chemically heterogeneous, developmentally regulated class of proteins. *Annual Review of Biochemistry* **51**, 219–50.

Lee, M.J., Sandig, M. and Wang, E. (1992) Statin, a protein specifically present in nonproliferating cells, is a phosphoprotein and forms a complex with a 45-kilodalton serine/threonine kinase. *Journal of Biological Chemistry* **267**, 21773–81.

Lee, S.C., Liu, W., Brosnan, C.F. and Dickson, D.W. (1992) Characterization of primary human fetal dissociated central nervous system cultures with an emphasis on microglia. *Laboratory Investigation* **67**, 465–76.

Lee, V.M.-Y., Carden, M.J., Schlaepfer, W.W. and Trojanowski, J.Q. (1987) Monoclonal antibodies distinguish several differentially phosphorylated states of the two largest rat neurofilament subunits (NF-H and NF-M) and demonstrate their existence in the normal nervous system of adult rats. *Journal of Neuroscience* **7**, 3474–88.

Lee, V.M.-Y., Otvos, L.Jr, Carden, M.J., Hollosi, M., Dietzschold, B. and Lazzarini, R.A. (1988) Identification of the major multiphosphorylation site in mammalian neurofilaments. *Proceedings of the National Academy of Sciences U.S.A.* **85**, 1998–2002.

Leoncini, L., Del Vecchio, M.T., Megha, T., Barbini, P., Galieni, P., Pileri, S., Sabattini, E., Gherlinzoni, F., Tosi, P., Kraft, R. and Cottier, H. (1993) Correlations between apoptotic and proliferative indices in malignant non-Hodgkin's lymphomas. *American Journal of Pathology* **142**, 755–63.

Leong, A.S.-Y. (1993) Immunohistochemistry – theoretical and practical aspects. In Leong, A.S.-Y. (ed.), *Applied immunohistochemistry for the surgical pathologist.* London: Edward Arnold, 1–22.

Libermann, T.A., Nusbaum, H.R., Razon, N., Kris, R., Lax, I., Soreq, H., Whittle, N., Waterfield, M.D., Ullrich, A. and Schlessinger, J. (1985) Amplification, enhanced expression and possible rearrangement of EGF receptor gene in primary human brain tumours of glial origin. *Nature* **313**, 144–7.

Lightner, V.A. (1994) Tenascin: does it play a role in epidermal morphogenesis and homeostasis? *Journal of Investigative Dermatology* **102**, 273–7.

Lightner, V.A., Marks, J.R. and McCachren, S.S. (1994) Epithelial cells are an important source of tenascin in normal and malignant human breast tissue. *Experimental Cell Research* **210**, 177–84.

Lightner, V.A., Gumkowski, F., Bigner, D.D. and Erickson, H.P. (1989) Tenascin/hexabrachion in human skin: biochemical identification and localization by light and electron microscopy. *Journal of Cell Biology* **108**, 2483–93.

Liu, L., Zaidi, N.H., Spiro, T.P., Majka, S., Willson, J.K.V. and Gerson, S.L. (1996) Differential degradation rates of inactivated alkyltransferase in lymphocytes and tumors of patients after treatment with O^6-benzylguanine. (Abstract) *Proceedings of the American Association for Cancer Research* **37**, 380.

Lopes, M.B., Gonzalez-Fernandez, F., Scheithauer, B.W. and VandenBerg, S.R. (1993) Differential expression of retinal proteins in a pineal parenchymal tumor. *Journal of Neuropathology and Experimental Neurology* **52**, 516–24.

Lorimer, I.A.J., Wikstrand, C.J., Batra, S.K., Bigner, D.D. and Pastan, I. (1995) Immunotoxins that target an oncogenic mutant epidermal growth factor receptor expressed in human tumors. *Clinical Cancer Research* **1**, 859–64.

Louis, D.N. (1994) The p53 gene and protein in human brain tumors. *Journal of Neuropathology and Experimental Neurology* **53**, 11–21.

Louis, D.N., von Deimling, A., Chung, R.Y., Rubio, M.P., Whaley, J.M., Eibl, R.H., Ohgaki, H., Wiestler, O.D., Thor, A.D. and Seizinger, B.R. (1993) Comparative study of p53 gene and protein alterations in human astrocytic tumors. *Journal of Neuropathology and Experimental Neurology* **52**, 31–8.

Maraziotis, T., Perentes, E. Karamitopoulou, E., Nakagawa, Y., Gessaga, E.C., Probst, A. and Frankfurter, A. (1992) Neuron-associated class III beta-tubulin isotype, retinal S-antigen, synaptophysin, and glial fibrillary acidic protein in human medulloblastomas: a clinicopathological analysis of 36 cases. *Acta Neuropathologica* **84**, 355–63.

Matus, A. and Mughal, S. (1975) Immunohistochemical localization of S-100 protein in brain. *Nature* **258**, 746–8.

Mauro, A., Bulfone, A., Turco, E. and Schiffer, D. (1991) Coexpression of platelet-derived growth factor (PDGF) B and PDGF B-type receptor in human gliomas. *Childs Nervous System* **7**, 432–6.

Maxwell M., Naber, S.P., Wolfe, H.J., Galanopoulos, T., Hedley-Whyte, E.T., Black, P.M. and Antoniades, H.N. (1990) Co-expression of platelet-derived growth factor (PDGF) and PDGF-receptor genes by primary human astrocytomas may contribute to their development and maintenance. *Journal of Clinical Investigation* **86**, 131–40.

McComb, R.D. and Bigner, D.D. (1985) Immunolocalization of monoclonal antibody-defined extracellular matrix antigens in human brain tumors. *Journal of Neuro-Oncology* **3**, 181–6.

McComb, R.D. and Miller, K.A. (1990) Developmental and reactive expression of tenascin (TN) in the human cerebellum. *Journal of Neuropathology and Experimental Neurology* **49**, 344–9.

McKeever, P.E., Burger, P.C. and Nelson, J.A. (1993) Introduction to neurooncology. In Nelson, J.S., Parisi, J.E. and Schochat, S.S. (eds), *Principles and practice of neuropathology*. St Louis: Mosby, 109–122.

McKeever, P.E., Davenport, R.D. and Shakui, P. (1991) Patterns of antigenic expression of human glioma cells. *Critical Reviews in Neurobiology* **6**, 119–47.

McLendon, R.E., Burger, P.C., Pegram, C.N., Eng, L.F. and Bigner, D.D. (1986) The immunohistochemical application of three anti-GFAP monoclonal antibodies to formalin-fixed, paraffin-embedded, normal and neoplastic brain tissue. *Journal of Neuropathology and Experimental Neurology* **45**, 692–703.

McLendon, R.E., Vick, W.W., Bigner, S.H. and Bigner, D.D. (1988) Monoclonal antibodies and diagnosis of brain neoplasms. In Kupchik, H.Z. (ed.), *Cancer diagnosis* in vitro *using monoclonal antibodies*. New York: Marcel Dekker, 31–66.

McQuaid, S., McConnell, R., McMahon, J. and Herron, B. (1995) Microwave antigen retrieval for immunocytochemistry on formalin-fixed, paraffin-embedded post-mortem CNS tissue. *Journal of Pathology* **176**, 207–16.

Meis, J.M., Ordonez, N.G. and Bruner, J.M. (1986) Meningiomas: an immunohistochemical study of 50 cases. *Archives of Pathology and Laboratory Medicine* **110**, 934–7.

Merlino, G.T., Ishii, S., Whang-Peng, J., Knutsen, T., Xu, Y.H., Clark, A.J.L., Stratton, R.H., Wilson, R.K., Ma, D.P., Roe, B.A., Hunts, J.H., Shimizu, N. and Pastan, I. (1985) Structure and localization of genes encoding aberrant and normal epidermal growth factor receptor RNAs from A431 human carcinoma cells. *Molecular and Cellular Biology* **5**, 1722–34.

Meyer, J.S., Marchosky, J.A. and Hickey, W.F. (1993) Cell kinetic classification of tumors of the nervous system by DNA precursor labeling *in vitro. Human Pathology* **24**, 1357–64.

Midgley, C.A., Fisher, C.J., Bartek, J., Vojtesek, B., Lane, D. and Barnes, D.M. (1992) Analysis of p53 expression in human tumours: an antibody raised against human p53 expressed in *Escherichia coli. Journal of Cell Science* **101**, 183–9.

Migheli, A., Cavalla, P., Marino, S. and Schiffer, D. (1994) A study of apoptosis in normal and pathologic nervous tissue after *in situ* end-labeling of DNA strand breaks. *Journal of Neuropathology and Experimental Neurology* **53**, 606–16.

Miller, D.C., Lang, F.F. and Epstein, F.J. (1993) Central-nervous-system gangliogliomas. 1. Pathology. *Journal of Neurosurgery* **79**, 859–66.

Mirshahi, M., Razaghi, A., Vandewalle, A., Cluzeaud, F., Tarraf, M. and Faure, J.P. (1992) Immunodetection and localization of protein(s) related to retinal S-antigen (arrestin) in kidney. *Biology of the Cell* **76**, 175–84.

Molenaar, W.M. and Trojanowski, J.Q. (1994) Primitive neuroectodermal tumors of the central nervous system in childhood: tumor biological aspects. *Critical Reviews in Oncology-Hematology* **17**, 1–25.

Molenaar, W.M., de Leij, L. and Trojanowski, J.Q. (1991) Neuroectodermal tumors of the peripheral and the central nervous system share neuroendocrine, N-CAM-related, antigens with small cell lung carcinomas. *Acta Neuropathologica (Berlin)* **83**, 46–54.

Molenaar, W.M., Baker, D.L., Pleasure, D., Lee, V.M.-Y. and Trojanowski, J.Q. (1990a) The neuroendocrine and neural profiles of neuroblastomas, ganglioneuroblastomas and ganglioneuromas. *American Journal of Pathology* **136**, 375–82.

Molenaar, W.M., Lee, V.M.-Y. and Trojanowski, J.Q. (1990b) Early fetal acquisition of the chromaffin and neuronal immunophenotype by human adrenal medullary cells. An immunohistological study using monoclonal antibodies to chromogranin A, synaptophysin, tyrosine hydroxylase and neuronal cytoskeletal proteins. *Experimental Neurology* **108**, 1–9.

Molenaar, W.M., Rorke, L.B. and Trojanowski, J.Q. (1995) Neural tumors. In Colvin, R.B., Bhan, A.K. and McCluskey, R.T. (eds), *Diagnostic immunopathology*. New York: Raven Press, 651–68.

Molenaar, W.M., Jansson, D.S., Gould, V.E., Rorke, L.B., Franke, W.W., Lee, V.M.-Y., Packer, R.J. and Trojanowski, J.Q. (1989) Molecular markers of primitive neuroectodermal tumors and other pediatric central nervous system tumors. Monoclonal antibodies to neuronal and glial antigens distinguish subsets of primitive neuroectodermal tumors. *Laboratory Investigation* **61**, 635–43.

Moore, B.W. (1965) A soluble protein characteristic of the nervous system. *Biochemical and Biophysical Research Communications* **19**, 739–44.

Moos, M., Tacke, R., Scherer, H., Teplow, D., Früh, K. and Schachner, M. (1988) Neural adhesion molecule L1 as a member of the immunoglobulin superfamily with binding domains similar to fibronectin. *Nature* **334**, 701–3.

Morimura, T., Kitz, K. and Budka, H. (1989) *In situ* analysis of cell kinetics in human brain tumors. A comparative immunocytochemical study of S phase cells by a new *in vitro* bromodeoxyuridine-labeling technique, and of proliferating pool cells by monoclonal antibody Ki-67. *Acta Neuropathologica* **77**, 276–82.

Morimura, T., Kitz, K., Stein, H. and Budka, H. (1991) Determination of proliferative activities in human brain tumor specimens: a comparison of three methods. *Journal of Neuro-Oncology* **10**, 1–11.

Mørk, S.J., Rubinstein, L.J., Kepes, J.J., Perentes, E. and Uphoff, D.F. (1988) Patterns of epithelial metaplasia in malignant gliomas. II. Squamous differentiation of epithelial-like foci in gliosarcomas and glioblastomas. *Journal of Neuropathology and Experimental Neurology* **47**, 101–18.

Moseley, R.P., Davies, A.G., Richardson, R.B., Zalutsky, M.R., Carrell, S., Fabre, J., Slack, N., Bullimore, J., Pizer, B., Papanastassiou, V., Kemshead, J.T., Coakham, H.B. and Lashford, L.S. (1990) Intrathecal administration of ^{131}I-radiolabeled monoclonal antibody as a treatment for neoplastic meningitis. *British Journal of Cancer* **62**, 637–42.

Muragaki, Y., Timothy, N., Leight, S., Hempstead, B.L., Chao, M.V., Trojanowski, J.Q. and Lee, V.M.-Y. (1995) Expression of Trk receptors in the developing and adult human central and peripheral nervous system. *Journal of Comparative Neurology* **356**, 387–97.

Murphy-Ullrich, J.E., Lightner, V.A., Aukhil, I., Yan, Y.Z., Erickson, H.P. and Höök, M. (1991) Focal adhesion integrity is downregulated by the alternatively spliced domain of human tenascin. *Journal of Cell Biology* **115**, 1127–36.

Murray, B.A., Hemperly, J.J., Prediger, E.A., Edelman, G.M. and Cunningham, B.A. (1986) Alternatively spiced mRNAs code for different polypeptide chains of the chicken neural cell adhesion molecule (N-CAM). *Journal of Cell Biology* **102**, 189–93.

Murthy, U., Basu, A., Rodeck, U., Herlyn, M., Ross, A.H. and Das, M. (1987) Binding of an antagonistic monoclonal antibody to an intact and fragmented EGF-receptor polypeptide. *Archives of Biochemistry and Biophysics* **252**, 549–60.

Nakagawa, Y., Perentes, E. and Rubinstein, L.J. (1986) Immunohistochemical characterization of oligodendrogliomas: an analysis of multiple markers. *Acta Neuropathologica* **72**, 15–22.

Nakasu, S., Nakaima, M., Nioka, H., Matsumara, K. and Handa, J. (1994a) Proliferating cell nuclear antigen expression in a rat glioma model: comparison with bromodeoxyuridine labeling index. *Neurologica Medico-Chirurgica* **34**, 269–73.

Nakasu, S., Nakasu, Y., Nioka, H., Nakajima, M. and Handa, J. (1994b) bcl-2 protein expression in tumors of the central nervous system. *Acta Neuropathologica* **88**, 520–6.

Newcomb, E.W., Madonia, W.J., Pisharody, S., Lang, F.F., Koslow, M. and Miller, D.C. (1993) A correlative study of p53 protein alteration and p53 gene mutation in glioblastoma multiforme. *Brain Pathology* **3**, 229–35.

Ng, H.-K. and Lo, S.T.H. (1989) Cytokeratin immunoreactivity in gliomas. *Histopathology* **14**, 359–68.

Ng, H.-K., Lo, S.Y., Huang, D.P. and Poon, W.S. (1994) Paraffin section p53 protein immunohistochemistry in neuroectodermal tumors. *Pathology* **26**, 1–5.

Nishikawa, R., Ji, X.D., Harmon, R.C., Lazar, C.S., Gill, G.N., Cavenee, W.K. and Huang, H.J.S. (1994) A mutant epidermal growth factor receptor common in human glioma confers enhanced tumorigenicity. *Proceedings of the National Academy of Sciences U.S.A.* **91**, 7727–31.

Nister, M., Libermann, T.A., Betsholtz, C., Pettersson, M., Claesson-Welsh, L., Heldin, C.H., Schlessinger, J. and Westermark, B. (1988) Expression of messenger RNAs for platelet-derived growth factor and transforming growth factor α and their receptors in human malignant glioma cell lines. *Cancer Research* **48**, 3910–18.

Nister, M., Claesson-Welsh, L., Eriksson, A., Heldin, C.H. and Westermark, B. (1991) Differential expression of platelet-derived growth factor receptors in human malignant glioma cell lines. *Journal of Biological Chemistry* **266**, 16755–63.

Nixon, R.A. (1993) The regulation of neurofilament protein dynamics by phosphorylation: clues to neurofibrillary pathobiology. *Brain Pathology* **3**, 29–38.

Norris, M.D., Bordow, S.B., Hagber, P.S., Marshall, G.M., Stewart, B.W. and Haber, M. (1996) The MDR1 gene predicts for outcome in subsets of patients with primary neuroblastoma. (Abstract) *Proceedings of the American Association for Cancer Research* **37**, 312.

Nybroe, O. and Bock, E. (1988) Structure and function of the neural cell adhesion molecules NCAM and L1. *Advances in Experimental Medicine and Biology* **265**, 185–96.

Ogawa, M., Ishikawa, T. and Ohta, H. (1986) Transdifferentiation of endocrine chromaffin cells into neuronal cells. *Current Topics in Developmental Biology* **20**, 99–110.

Onda, K., Davis, R.L., Wilson, C.B. and Hoshino, T. (1994) Regional differences in bromodeoxyuridine uptake, expression of Ki-67 protein, and nucleolar organizer region counts in glioblastoma multiforme. *Acta Neuropathologica* **87**, 586–93.

Orian, J.M., Vasilopoulos, K., Yoshida, S., Kaye, A.H., Chow, C.W. and Gonzales, M.F. (1992) Overexpression of multiple oncogenes related to histological grade of astrocytic glioma. *British Journal of Cancer* **66**, 106–12.

Osborn, M. and Weber, K. (1986) Intermediate filament proteins: a multigene family distinguishing major cell lineages. *Trends in Biochemical Sciences* **11**, 469–72.

Påhlman, S., Esscher, T. and Nilsson, K. (1986) Expression of gamma-subunit of enolase, neuron-specific enolase, in human non-neuroendocrine tumors and derived cell lines. *Laboratory Investigation* **54**, 554–60.

Panneerselvam, K., Reitz, H., Khan, S.A. and Bishayee, S. (1995) A conformation-specific anti-peptide antibody to the beta-type platelet-derived growth factor receptor also recognizes the activated epidermal growth factor receptor. *Journal of Biological Chemistry* **270**, 7975–9.

Papanastassiou, V., Pizer, B.L., Coakham, H.B., Bullimore, J., Zananiri, T. and Kemshead, J.T. (1993) Treatment of recurrent and cystic malignant gliomas by a single intracavity injection of ^{131}I monoclonal antibody: feasibility, pharmacokinetics and dosimetry. *British Journal of Cancer* **67**, 144–51.

Patel, K., Rossell, R.J., Bourne, S., Moore, S.E., Walsh, F.S. and Kemshead, J.T. (1989a) Monoclonal antibody UJ13A recognizes the neural cell adhesion molecule (NCAM). *International Journal of Cancer* **44**, 1062–8.

Patel, K., Rossell, R.J., Pemberton, L.F., Cheung, N.K., Walsh, F.S., Moore, S.E., Sugimoto, T. and Kemshead, J.T. (1989b) Monoclonal antibody 3F8 recognises the neural cell adhesion molecule (NCAM) in addition to the ganglioside GD2. *British Journal of Cancer* **60**, 861–6.

Patel, K., Frost, G., Kiely, F., Phimister, E., Coakham, H.B. and Kemshead, J.T. (1991a) Expression of the cluster 1 antigen (neural cell adhesion molecule) in neuroectodermal tumours. *British Journal of Cancer–Supplement* **14**, 20–3.

Patel, K., Kiely, F., Phimister, E., Melino, G., Rathjen, F. and Kemshead, J.T. (1991b) The 200/220 kDa antigen recognized by monoclonal antibody (Mab) UJ127.11 on neural tissues and tumors is the human L1 adhesion molecule. *Hybridoma* **10**, 481–91.

Pavelic, J., Hlavka, V., Poljak, M., Gale, N. and Pavelic, K. (1994) p53 immunoreactivity in oligodendrogliomas. *Journal of Neuro-Oncology* **22**, 1–6.

Perentes, E. and Rubinstein, L.J. (1986) Immunohistochemical recognition of human neuroepithelial tumors by anti-Leu-7 (HNK-1) monoclonal antibody. *Acta Neuropathologica* **69**, 227–33.

——(1987) Recent applications of immunoperoxidase histochemistry in human neuro-oncology. An update. *Archives of Pathology and Laboratory Medicine* **111**, 796–812.

Perentes, E., Rubinstein, L.J., Herman, M.M. and Donoso, L.A. (1986) S-antigen immunoreactivity in human pineal glands and pineal parenchymal tumors. A monoclonal antibody study. *Acta Neuropathologica (Berlin)* **71**, 224–7.

Perentes, E., Herbort, C.P., Rubinstein, L.J., Herman, M.M., Uffer, S., Donoso, L.A. and Collins, V.P. (1987) Immunohistochemical characterization of human retinoblastomas *in situ* with multiple markers. *American Journal of Ophthalmology* **103**, 647–58.

Phimister, E., Kiely, F., Kemshead, J.T. and Patel, K. (1991) Expression of neural cell adhesion molecule (NCAM) isoforms in neuroblastoma. *Journal of Clinical Pathology* **44**, 580–5.

Piepmeier, J.M., Fried, I. and Makuch, R. (1993) Low-grade astrocytomas may arise from different astrocyte lineages. *Neurosurgery* **33**, 627–32.

Potapova, O., Fakhrai, H., Baird, S. and Mercola, D. (1996) Platelet-derived growth factor-β/v-sis confers a tumorigenic and metastatic phenotype to human T98G glioblastoma cells. *Cancer Research* **56**, 280–6.

Pusztai, L., Lewis, C.E., Lorenzen, J. and McGee, J.O'D. (1993) Growth factors: regulation of normal and neoplastic growth. *Journal of Pathology* **169**, 191–201.

Raff, M.C., Miller, R.H. and Noble, M. (1983) A glial progenitor cell that develops *in vitro* into an astrocyte or an oligodendrocyte depending on culture medium. *Nature* **303**, 390–6.

Raghavan, R., Steart, P.V. and Weller, R.O. (1990) Cell proliferation patterns in the diagnosis of astrocytomas, anaplastic astrocytomas and glioblastoma multiforme: a Ki-67 study. *Neuropathology and Applied Neurobiology* **16**, 123–33.

Rasheed, B.K.A., McLendon, R.E., Herndon, J.E., Friedman, H.S., Friedman, A.H., Bigner, D.D. and Bigner, S.H. (1994) Alterations of the TP53 gene in human gliomas. *Cancer Research* **54**, 1324–30.

Reed, J.C., Meister, L., Tanaka, S., Cuddy, M., Yum, S., Geyer, C. and Pleasure, D. (1991) Differential expression of *bcl2* protooncogene in neuroblastoma and other human tumor cell lines of neural origin. *Cancer Research* **51**, 6529–38.

Rehm, H., Wiedenmann, B. and Betz, H. (1986) Molecular characterization of synaptophysin, a major calcium-binding protein of the synaptic vesicle membrane. *EMBO Journal* **5**, 535–41.

Reist, C.J., Archer, G.E., Kurpad, S.N., Wikstrand, C.J., Vaidyanathan, G., Willingham, M.C., Moscatello, D.K., Wong, A.J., Bigner, D.D. and Zalutsky, M.R. (1995) Tumor-specific anti-epidermal growth factor receptor variant III monoclonal antibodies: use of the tyramine-cellobiose radioiodination method enhances cellular retention and uptake in tumor xenografts. *Cancer Research* **55**, 4375–82.

Rodrigues, M.M., Rajagopalan, S., Lee, L., Nair, C.N., Advani, S.H., Donoso, L., Chader, G.J. and Wiggert, B. (1992) Retinoblastoma: messenger RNA for interphotoreceptor retinoid binding protein. *Current Eye Research* **11**, 425–33.

Rorke, L.B., Molenaar, W.M. and Trojanowski, J.Q. (1992) Advances in diagnosis and basic science. The impact of monoclonal antibody studies on changing nosology and biological concepts of brain tumors. In Packer, R.J., Bleyer, W.A. and Pochedly, C. (eds), *Pediatric neuro-oncology. New trends in clinical research*. Philadelphia: Harwood Academic, 8–32.

Ross, A.H., Grob, P., Bothwell, M., Elder, D.E., Ernst, C.S., Marano, N., Ghrist, B.D.F., Slemp, C.C., Herlyn, M., Atkinson, B. and Koprowski, H. (1984) Characterization of nerve growth factor receptor in neural crest tumors using monoclonal antibodies. *Proceedings of the National Academy of Sciences U.S.A.* **81**, 6681–5.

Rubio, M.-P., von Deimling, A., Yandell, D.W., Wiestler, O.D., Gusella, J.F. and Louis, D.N. (1993) Accumulation of wild type p53 protein in human astrocytomas. *Cancer Research* **53**, 3465–7.

Russell, D.S. and Rubinstein, L.G. (1989) *Pathology of tumours of the nervous system*. Fifth edition. London: Edward Arnold.

Sallinen, P.K., Haapasalo, H.K., Visakorpi, T., Helen, P.T., Rantala, I.S., Isola, J.J. and Helin, H.J. (1994) Prognostication of astrocytoma patient survival by Ki-67 (MIB-1), PCNA, and S-phase fraction using archival paraffin-embedded samples. *Journal of Pathology* **174,** 275–82.

Sato, J.D., Kawamoto, T., Le, A.D., Mendelsohn, J., Polikoff, J. and Sato, G.H. (1983) Biological effects *in vitro* of monoclonal antibodies to human epidermal growth factor receptors. *Molecular Biology and Medicine* **1**, 511–29.

Satoh, J. and Kim, S.U. (1995) Ganglioside markers GD3, GD2, and A2B5 in fetal human neurons and glial cells in culture. *Developmental Neuroscience* **17**, 137–48.

Sauceda, R., Ocadiz, R., Gutierrez, A.L., Salcedo, M., Ortega, V., Figureroa, H.H. and Gariglio, P. (1988) Novel combination of c-myc, N-myc, and N-ras oncogene alteration in brain tumors. *Brain Research: Molecular Brain Research* **427**, 123–32.

Sawhney, N. and Hall, P.A. (1992) Editorial: Ki67 – structure, function, and new antibodies. *Journal of Pathology* **168**, 161–2.

Schechter, Y., Hernaez, L., Schlessinger, J. and Cuatrecasas, P. (1979) Local aggregation of hormone-receptor complexes is required for activation by epidermal growth factor. *Nature* **278**, 835–8.

Schenk, S. and Chiquet-Ehrismann, R. (1994) Tenascins. *Methods in Enzymology* **245**, 52–61.

Schiffer, D., Cavalla, P., Chiò, A., Giordana, M.T., Marino, S., Mauro, A. and Migheli, A. (1994) Tumor cell proliferation and apoptosis in medulloblastoma. *Acta Neuropathologica (Berlin)* **87**, 362–70.

Schiffer, D., Cavalla, P., Migheli, A., Chiò, A., Giordana, M.T., Marino, S. and Attanasio, A. (1995) Apoptosis and cell proliferation in human neuroepithelial tumors. *Neuroscience Letters* **195**, 81–4.

Schlegel, J., Merdes, A., Stumm, G., Albert, F.K., Forsting, M., Hynes, N. and Kiessling, M. (1994a) Amplification of the epidermal-growth-factor-receptor gene correlates with different growth behaviour in human glioblastoma. *International Journal of Cancer* **56**, 72–7.

Schlegel, J., Stumm, G., Brandle, K., Merdes, A., Mechtersheimer, G., Hynes, N.E. and Kiessling, M. (1994b) Amplification and differential expression of members of the erbB-gene family in human glioblastoma. *Journal of Neuro-Oncology* **22**, 201–7.

Schrappe, M., Bumol, T.F., Apelgren, L.D., Briggs, S.L., Koppel, G.A., Markowitz, D.D., Mueller, B.M. and Reisfeld, R.A. (1992) Long-term growth suppression of human glioma xenografts by chemoimmunoconjugates of 4-desacetylvinblastine-3-carboxyhydrazide and monoclonal antibody 9.2.27. *Cancer Research* **52**, 3838–44.

Schröder, R., Bien, K., Kott, R., Meyers, I. and Vössing, R. (1991) The relationship between Ki-67 labeling and mitotic index in gliomas and meningiomas: demonstration of the variability of the intermitotic cycle time. *Acta Neuropathologica* **82**, 389–94.

Schwechheimer, K., Gass, P. and Berlet, H.H. (1992) Expression of oligodendroglia and Schwann cell markers in human nervous system tumors. An immunomorphological study and western blot analysis. *Acta Neuropathologica* **83**, 283–91.

Schwechheimer, K., Huang, S., and Cavenee, W.K. (1995) EGFR gene amplification – rearrangement in human glioblastomas. *International Journal of Cancer* **62**, 145–8.

Segal, R.A., Goumnerova, L.C., Kwon, Y.K., Stiles, C.D. and Pomeroy, S.L. (1994) Expression of the neurotrophin receptor and TrkC linked to a favorable outcome in medulloblastoma. *Proceedings of the National Academy of Sciences U.S.A.* **91**, 12867–71.

Shalev, A., Gerrard, J.M., Robertson, C., Greenberg, A.H. and Linial, M. (1992) Sharing of antigenic epitopes between synaptophysin and granulophysin. *Journal of Cellular Biochemistry* **49**, 59–65.

Sharrer, B. (1967) The neurosecretory neuron in neuroendocrine regulatory mechanisms. *American Zoology* **7**, 161–9.

Shaw, G. and Weber, K. (1983) The intermediate filament complement of the retina: a comparison between different mammalian species. *European Journal of Cell Biology* **33**, 95–104.

Shaw, G., Osborn, M. and Weber, K. (1981) An immunofluorescence microscopical study of the neurofilament triplet proteins, vimentin and glial fibrillary acidic protein within the adult rat brain. *European Journal of Cell Biology* **26**, 68–82.

Shi, S.-R., Key, M.E. and Kalra, K.L. (1991) Antigen retrieval in formalin-fixed, paraffin-embedded tissues:

an enhancement method for immunohistochemical staining based on microwave oven heating of tissue sections. *Journal of Histochemistry and Cytochemistry* **39**, 741–8.

Shi, S.-R., Cote, C., Kalra, K.L., Taylor, C.R. and Tandon, A.K. (1992) A technique for retrieving antigens in formalin-fixed, routinely acid-decalcified, celloidin-embedded human temporal bone sections for immunohistochemistry. *Journal of Histochemistry and Cytochemistry* **40**, 787–92.

Shi, S.-R., Imam, S.A., Young, L., Cote, R.J. and Taylor, C.R. (1995) Antigen retrieval immunohistochemistry under the influence of pH using monoclonal antibodies. *Journal of Histochemistry and Cytochemistry* **43**, 193–201.

Shindo, H., Tani, E., Matsumuto, T., Hashimoto, T. and Furuyama, J. (1993) Stabilization of c-myc protein in human glioma cells. *Acta Neuropathologica* **86**, 345–52.

Sidransky, D., Mikkelsen, T., Schwechheimer, K., Rosenblum, M.L., Cavenee, W. and Vogelstein, B. (1992) Clonal expansion of p53 mutant cells is associated with brain tumour progression. *Nature* **355**, 846–7.

Siri, A., Carnemolla, B., Saginati, M., Leprini, A., Casari, G., Baralle, F. and Zardi, L. (1991) Human tenascin: primary structure, pre-mRNA splicing patterns and localization of the epitopes recognized by two monoclonal antibodies. *Nucleic Acids Research* **19**, 525–31.

Smith, D.A. and Lantos, P.L. (1985) Immunocytochemistry of cerebellar astrocytomas: with a special note on Rosenthal fibers. *Acta Neuropathologica* **66**, 155–9.

Soini, Y., Niemela, A., Kamel, D., Herva, R., Bloigu, R., Paakko, P. and Vahakangas, K. (1994) p53 immunohistochemical positivity as a prognostic marker in intracranial tumours. *Acta Pathologica, Microbiologica, et Immunologica Scandinavica* **102**, 786–92.

Steiner, P.M. and Roop, D.R. (1988) Molecular and cellular biology of intermediate filaments. *Annual Review of Biochemistry* **57**, 593–625.

Stiemer, R.H., Gausepohl, H., Mirshahi, M., de Kozak, Y., Kraft, M., Faure, J.-P. and Frank, R.W. (1992) Immunological characterization of an immunomodulatory epitope in S-antigen/arrestin with a sequence motif common to tumor necrosis factor α. *Immunology Letters* **32**, 233–40.

Sugawa, W., Ekstrand, A.J., James, C.D. and Collins, V.P. (1990) Identical splicing of aberrant epidermal growth factor receptor transcripts from amplified rearranged genes in human glioblastomas. *Proceedings of the National Academy of Sciences U.S.A.* **87**, 8602–6.

Sung, C.C., Pearl, D.K., Coons, S.W., Scheithauer, B.W., Johnson, P.C. and Yates, A.J. (1994) Gangliosides as diagnostic markers of human astrocytomas and primitive neuroectodermal tumors. *Cancer* **74**, 3010–22.

Svennerholm, L., Fredman, P., Jungbjer, B., Mänsson, J.-E., Rynmark, B.-M., Bostrom, K., Hagberg, B., Noren, L. and Santavauori, P. (1987) Large alterations in ganglioside and neutral glycolipid patterns in brains from cases with infantile neuronal ceroid lipofuscinosis/polyunsaturated fatty acid lipidosis. *Journal of Neurochemistry* **49**, 1772–83.

Symonds, H., Krall, L., Remington, L., Saenz-Robles, M., Lowe, S., Jacks, T. and Van Dyke, T. (1994) p53-dependent apoptosis suppresses tumor growth and progression *in vivo*. *Cell* **78**, 703–11.

Taylor, C.R., Shi, S.-R., Chaiwun, B., Young, L., Imam, S.A. and Cote, R.J. (1994) Strategies for improving the immunohistochemical staining of various intranuclear prognostic markers in formalin-paraffin sections: androgen receptor, estrogen receptor, progesterone receptor, p53 protein, proliferating cell nuclear antigen, and Ki-67 antigen revealed by antigen retrieval techniques. *Human Pathology* **25**, 263–70.

Tischler, A.S. (1989) The dispersed neuroendocrine cells: the structure, function, regulation and effects of xenobiotics on this system. *Toxicologic Pathology* **17**, 307–16.

Tohyama, T., Lee, V.M.-Y., Rorke, L.B. and Trojanowski, J.Q. (1991) Molecular milestones that signal axonal maturation and the commitment of human spinal cord precursor cells to the neuronal or glial phenotype in development. *Journal of Comparative Neurology* **310**, 285–99.

Tohyama, T., Lee, V.M.-Y., Rorke, L.B., Marvin, M., McKay, R.D.G. and Trojanowski, J.Q. (1992) Nestin expression in embryonic human neuroepithelium and in human neuroepithelial tumor cells. *Laboratory Investigation* **66**, 301–13.

Tooyama, I., Yamada, T., Kim, S.U. and McGeer, P.L. (1992) Immunohistochemical study of A2B5-positive ganglioside in postmortem human brain tissue of Alzheimer disease, amyotrophic lateral sclerosis, progressive supranuclear palsy and control cases. *Neuroscience Letters* **136**, 91–4.

Torp, S.H., Helseth, E., Dalen, A. and Unsgaard, G. (1991) Epidermal growth factor receptor expression in human gliomas. *Cancer Immunology, Immunotherapy* **33**, 61–4.

Trojanowski, J.Q. and Lee, V.M.-Y. (1983) Anti-neurofilament monoclonal antibodies: reagents for the evaluation of human neoplasms. *Acta Neuropathologica* **59**, 155–8.

——(1985) Expression of neurofilament antigens by normal and neoplastic human adrenal chromaffin cells. *New England Journal of Medicine* **313**, 101–4.

Tsanaclis, A.M., Brem, S.S., Gately, S., Schipper, H.M. and Wang, E. (1991) Statin immunolocalization in human brain tumors. Detection of noncycling cells using a novel marker of cell quiescence. *Cancer* **68**, 786–92.

Unsicker, K. (1986) Differentiation and phenotypical conversion of adrenal medullary cells: the effects of neuronotrophic, neurite-promoting, hormonal, and neuronal signals. In Panula, P., Päivăriuta, H. and Soinila, S. (eds), *Neurochemistry: modern methods and applications*. New York: Alan R. Liss, 181–206.

Van Meir, E.G., Polverini, P.J., Chazin, V.R., Su-Huang, H.J., de Tribolet, N. and Cavenee, W.K. (1994) Release of an inhibitor of angiogenesis upon induction of wild type *p53* expression in glioblastoma cells. *Nature Genetics* **8**, 171–6.

Van Noorden, S. (1986) Tissue preparation and immunostaining techniques for light microscopy. In

Polak, J.M. and Van Noorden, S. (eds), *Immunocytochemistry: modern methods and applications*. Second edition. Bristol: John Wright, 26–53.

Vanstapel, M.J., Peeters, B., Cordell, J., Heyns, W., De Wolf-Peeters C., Desmet, V. and Mason, D. (1985) Production of monoclonal antibodies directed against antigenic determinants common to the α- and β-chain of bovine brain S-100 protein. *Laboratory Investigation* **52**, 232–8.

Ventimiglia, J.B., Wikstrand, C.J., Ostrowski, L.E., Bourdon, M.A., Lightner, V.A and Bigner, D.D. (1992) Tenascin expression in human glioma cell lines and normal tissues. *Journal of Neuroimmunology* **36**, 41–55.

Vick, W.W., Tello, J.W., Wikstrand, C.J., He, X., Longee, D., Fredman, P., Svennerholm, L., Bigner, D.D., Johnston, W.W. and Bigner, S.H. (1992) Application of a panel of antiganglioside monoclonal antibodies to cytologic specimens. *Acta Cytologica* **36**, 697–705.

Vinores, S.A. and Rubinstein, L.J. (1985) Simultaneous expression of glial fibrillary acidic (GFA) protein and neuron-specific enolase (NSE) by the same reactive or neoplastic astrocytes. *Neuropathology and Applied Neurobiology* **11**, 349–59.

Vogelstein, B. and Kinzler, K.W. (1993) The multistep nature of cancer. *Trends in Genetics* **9**, 138–41.

Vojtesek, B., Bartek, J., Midgley, C.A. and Lane, D.P. (1992) An immunochemical analysis of the human nuclear phosphoprotein p53. New monoclonal antibodies and epitope mapping using recombinant p53. *Journal of Immunological Methods* **151**, 237–44.

Volker, K., Pearson, J.W., Wiltrout, R.H., Longo, D.L. and Fogler, W.E. (1996) MRK-16 $(Fab')_2$ and Fab mediates the *in vivo* reversal of multidrug resistance. (Abstract) *Proceedings of the American Association for Cancer Research* **37**, 332.

Vollrath, M., Altmannsberger, M., Weber, K. and Osborn, M. (1985) An ultrastructural and immunohistological study of the rat olfactory epithelium: unique properties of olfactory sensory cells. *Differentiation* **29**, 243–53.

Waibel, R., Mannhart, M., O'Hara, C.J., Brocklehurst, C., Zangemeister-Wittke, U., Schenker, T., Lehmann, H.-P., Weber, E. and Stahel, R.A. (1993) Monoclonal antibody SEN7 recognizes a new epitope on the neural cell adhesion molecule present on small cell lung cancer but not on lymphocytes. *Cancer Research* **53**, 2840–5.

Wang, E., Cairncross, J.G. and Liem, R.K.H. (1984) Identification of glial filament protein and vimentin in the same intermediate filament system in human glioma cells. *Proceedings of the National Academy of Sciences U.S.A.* **81**, 2102–6.

Washiyama, K., Muragaki, Y., Rorke, L.B., Lee, V.M.-Y., Feinstein, S.C., Radeke, M.J., Blumberg, D., Kaplan, D.R. and Trojanowski, J.Q. (1996) Neurotrophin and neurotrophin receptor proteins in medulloblastomas and other primitive neuroectodermal tumors of the pediatric central nervous system. *American Journal of Pathology* **148**, 929–40.

Wasson, J.C., Saylors, R.L.3rd, Zeltzer, P., Friedman, H.S., Bigner, S.H., Burger, P.C., Bigner, D.D., Look, A.T., Douglass, E.C. and Brodeur, G.M. (1990) Oncogene amplification in pediatric brain tumors. *Cancer Research* **50**, 2987–90.

Waterfield, M.D., Mayes, E.L.V., Stroobant, P., Bennet, P.L.P., Young, S., Goodfellow, P.N., Banting, G.S. and Ozanne, B. (1982) A monoclonal antibody to the human epidermal growth factor receptor. *Journal of Cellular Biochemistry* **20**, 149–61.

Weber, K. and Osborn, M. (1982) Cytoskeleton: definition, structure and gene regulation. *Pathology Research and Practice* **175**, 128–45.

Wick, M.R., Swanson, P.E. and Manivel, J.C. (1988) Immunohistochemical analysis of soft tissue sarcomas. Comparisons with electron microscopy. *Applied Pathology* **6**, 169–79.

Wiedenmann, B. and Franke, W.W. (1985) Identification and localization of synaptophysin, an integral membrane glycoprotein of Mr 38000 characteristic of presynaptic vesicles. *Cell* **41**, 1017–28.

Wiedenmann, B. and Huttner, W.B. (1989) Synaptophysin and chromogranins/secretogranins – widespread constituents of distinct types of neuroendocrine vesicles and new tools in tumor diagnosis. *Virchows Archiv B, Cell Pathology including Molecular Pathology* **58**, 95–121.

Wiedenmann, B., Franke, W.W., Kuhn, C., Moll, R. and Gould, V.E. (1986) Synaptophysin: a marker protein for neuroendocrine cells and neoplasms. *Proceedings of the National Academy of Sciences U.S.A.* **83**, 3500–4.

Wiedenmann, B., Kuhn, C., Schwechheimer, K., Waldherr, R., Raue, F., Brandeis, W.E., Kommerell, B. and Franke, W.W. (1988) Synaptophysin identified in metastases of neuroendocrine tumors by immunocytochemistry and immunoblotting. *American Journal of Clinical Pathology* **88**, 560–9.

Wikstrand, C.J. and Bigner, D.D. (1980) Immunobiological aspects of the brain and human gliomas. A review. *American Journal of Pathology* **98**, 515–67.

——(1997) Tumors of the central nervous system. In Keane, R.W. and Hickey, W.F. (eds), *Immunology of the nervous system*. New York: Oxford University Press, 760–84.

Wikstrand, C.J., Friedman, H.S. and Bigner, D.D. (1991) Medulloblastoma cell-substrate interaction *in vitro*. *Invasion and Metastasis* **11**, 310–24.

Wikstrand, C.J., He, X., Fuller, G.N., Bigner, S.H., Fredman, P., Svennerholm, L. and Bigner, D.D. (1991) Occurrence of lacto series gangliosides 3'-isoLM1 and 3',6'-isoLD1 in human gliomas *in vitro* and *in vivo*. *Journal of Neuropathology and Experimental Neurology* **50**, 756–69.

Wikstrand, C.J., Longee, D.C., McLendon, R.E., Fuller, G.N., Friedman, H.S., Fredman, P., Svennerholm, L. and Bigner, D.D. (1993) Lactotetraose series ganglioside 3',6'-isoLD1 in tumors of central nervous and other systems *in vitro* and *in vivo*. *Cancer Research* **53**, 120–6.

Wikstrand, C.J., Fredman, P., McLendon, R.E., Svennerholm, L. and Bigner, D.D. (1994a) Altered expression of ganglioside phenotypes of human gliomas *in vivo* and *in vitro*. *Molecular and Chemical Neuropathology* **21**, 129–38.

Wikstrand, C.J., Fredman, P., Svennerholm, L. and Bigner, D.D. (1994b) Detection of glioma-associated gangliosides GM2, GD2, GD3, 3'-isoLM1, and 3',6'-isoLD1 in central nervous system tumors *in vitro* and *in vivo* using epitope-defined monoclonal antibodies. *Progress in Brain Research* **101**, 213–23.

Wikstrand, C.J., Hale, L.P., Batra, S.K., Hill, M.L., Humphrey, P.A., Kurpad, S.N., McLendon, R.E., Moscatello, D., Pegram, C.N., Reist, C.J., Traweek, S.T., Wong, A.J., Zalutsky, M.R. and Bigner, D.D. (1995) Monoclonal antibodies against EGFRvIII are tumor specific and react with breast and lung carcinomas and malignant gliomas. *Cancer Research* **55**, 3140–8.

Wikstrand, C.J., McLendon, R.E., Friedman, A.H. and Bigner, D.D. (1997) Cell surface localization and density of the tumor-associated variant of the epidermal growth factor receptor, EGFRvIII. *Cancer Research* **57**, 4130–40.

Wolff, J.M., Frank, R., Mujoo, K., Spiro, R.C., Reisfeld, R.A. and Rathjen, F.G. (1988) A human brain glycoprotein related to the mouse cell adhesion molecule L1. *Journal of Biological Chemistry* **263**, 11943–7.

Wong, A.J., Bigner, S.H., Bigner, D.D., Kinzler, K.W., Hamilton, S.R. and Vogelstein, B. (1987) Increased expression of the epidermal growth factor receptor gene in malignant gliomas is invariably associated with gene amplification. *Proceedings of the National Academy of Sciences U.S.A.* **84**, 6899–903.

Wyllie, A.H., Morris, R.G., Smith, A.L. and Dunlop, D. (1984) Chromatin cleavage in apoptosis: association with condensed chromatin morphology and dependence on macromolecular synthesis. *Journal of Pathology* **142**, 67–77.

Yachnis, A.T. and Trojanowski, J.Q. (1994) Studies of childhood brain tumors using immunohistochemistry and microwave technology: methodological considerations. *Journal of Neuroscience Methods* **55**, 191–200.

Yachnis, A.T., Rorke, L.B., Lee, V.M.-Y. and Trojanowski, J.Q. (1993) Expression of neuronal and glial polypeptides during histogenesis of the human cerebellar cortex including observations on the dentate nucleus. *Journal of Comparative Neurology* **334**, 356–69.

Yamanaka, R., Tanaka, R. and Saito, T. (1994) Immunohistochemical analysis of tumor-infiltrating lymphocytes and adhesion molecules (ICAM-1, NCAM) in human gliomas. *Neurologica Medica Chirurgica (Tokyo)* **34**, 583–7.

Yamazaki, H., Ohba, Y., Tamaoki, N. and Shibuya, M. (1990) A deletion mutation within the ligand binding domain is responsible for activation of epidermal growth factor receptor gene in human brain tumors. *Japanese Journal of Cancer Research* **81**, 773–9.

Yang, Q., Hamberger, A., Hyden, H., Wang, S., Stigbrand, T. and Haglid, K.G. (1995) S-100β has a neuronal localisation in the rat hindbrain revealed by an antigen retrieval method. *Brain Research* **696**, 49–61.

Yarosh, D., Belanich, M. and Li, B. (1996) Monoclonal antibodies to O^6-alkylguanine-DNA alkyltransferase: cellular localization, protein conformation and resistance to nitrosourea chemotherapy. (Abstract) *Proceedings of the American Association for Cancer Research* **37**, 364.

Yoshihara, Y., Oka, S., Ikeda, J. and Mori, K. (1991) Immunoglobulin superfamily molecules in the nervous system. *Neuroscience Research* **10**, 83–105.

Young, R.W. (1985) Cell differentiation in the retina of the mouse. *Anatomical Record* **212**, 199–205.

Yu, C.C.-W., Woods, A.L. and Levison, D.A. (1992) The assessment of cellular proliferation by immunohistochemistry: a review of currently available methods and their applications. *Histochemical Journal* **24**, 121–31.

Zagzag, D., Friedlander, D.R., Miller, D.C., Dosik, J., Cangiarella, J., Kostianovsky, M., Cohen, H., Grumet, M. and Greco, M.A. (1995) Tenascin expression in astrocytomas correlates with angiogenesis. *Cancer Research* **55**, 907–14.

Zagzag, D., Friedlander, D.R., Dosik, J., Chikramane, S., Chan, W., Greco, M.A., Allen, J.C., Dorovini-Zis, K. and Grumet, M. (1996) Tenascin-C expression by angiogenic vessels in human astrocytomas and by human brain endothelial cells *in vitro*. *Cancer Research* **56**, 182–9.

Zaidi, N.H., Liu, L. and Gerson, S.L. (1996) Quantitative immunohistochemical estimates of O^6-alkylguanine-DNA alkyltransferase expression in normal and malignant human colon. *Clinical Cancer Research* **2**, 577–84.

PART II

Pathologic anatomy

CHAPTER 9

Tumors of central neuroepithelial origin

ROGER E. MCLENDON, DAVID S. ENTERLINE, ROBERT D. TIEN, WADE L. THORSTAD AND JANET M. BRUNER

Classification and grading

The tumors considered in this chapter arise from cells derived from the primitive neuroepithelium. By far the greatest number are composed of neuroglial cells and are collectively known as *gliomas*, in the strict sense of the term. Historically, however, the name 'glioma' has been used as a generic term that encompasses all the tumors of central neuroepithelial origin, including those composed exclusively or predominantly of undifferentiated precursor cells, of neuroblastic cells in various stages of differentiation and of mixed populations exhibiting different directions of cellular maturation.

Numerically, the gliomas, taken in either sense, constitute the most important group of intracranial tumors. Their complexity is due to the considerable number of cell types involved in neoplasia; to the histologic heterogeneity found within the major classes of glioma and often in different parts of one individual tumor; and, in some cases, to interpretative difficulties raised by cytogenetic assumptions and by the role frequently played by malignant progression in the constitution of many of these neoplasms. The problems entailed in their classification have long provoked a good deal of controversy. By and large, however, most classifications have reflected a general acceptance of histologic tumor types that are based on the identification of reasonably precise cytologic features linking neoplastic elements to normal cell types found in the mature and developing central nervous system (CNS). It is not our intent to review all the classifications that have been proposed, and what follows is a summary of the major historic and more recent schemes.

CLASSIFICATION

Most modern classifications are based upon that of Bailey and Cushing (1926). These authors studied the embryogenesis of the various cellular components of the CNS in light of the work of the Spanish school. They then attempted to classify the tumors observed in terms of the different morphologic stages through which these cells pass in ontogenesis, using metallic techniques to supplement routine staining methods. Having enumerated 20 cell types, they proposed a classification based on a pyramidal scheme of *cytogenesis*, including 14 main groups, as follows:

1. Medulloepithelioma
2. Medulloblastoma
3. Pineoblastoma
4. Pinealoma
5. Ependymoblastoma
6. Ependymoma
7. Neuroepithelioma
8. Spongioblastoma:
   (a) multiforme, (b) unipolare
9. Astroblastoma
10. Astrocytoma:
    (a) protoplasmaticum, (b) fibrillare
11. Oligodendroglioma
12. Neuroblastoma
13. Ganglioneuroma
14. Papilloma choroideum

While most CNS tumors recognized today can be identified in that list, current terminologies reflect a number of significant modifications in the definition of some. Thus, the term 'glioblastoma' has now widely replaced that of 'spongioblastoma multiforme'. The name 'ependymoblastoma' – employed by Bailey and Cushing to describe a variant of well-differentiated ependymoma, and subsequently discarded – has been revived to designate a recognizable form of embryonal neoplasm with ependymal differentiation. The 'unipolar (or polar) spongioblastoma', applied by them to a fairly characteristic variant of astrocytoma with pilocytic elements, now more generally refers to a distinctive histologic growth pattern within several types of neuroglial tumors. The 'neuroepithelioma' has been deleted as a separate entity from the tumors originating in the central neuraxis and is reserved for a variant of the common retinoblastoma. The term 'pinealoma', used to signify a tumor of the pineal parenchyma composed of mature pineocytes, has today been replaced by that of 'pineocytoma'.

Bailey and Cushing were well aware of the range of morphologic variations that may normally be expected in malignant neoplasms in general and of the phenomena of anaplasia that accompany rapid increases in tumor growth. They did not claim that their scheme of classification indicated an embryogenic derivation. However, the weight and wealth of their cytologic observations seemed to overshadow the role played by malignant progression in the composition and evolution of many gliomas. Subsequent to the publication of the classification of Bailey and Cushing, increasing attention was directed to the frequency with which *anaplasia* determines the morphologic characteristics of tumor cell populations and their diversity in malignant gliomas. This invited a reappraisal of those constituent cells that are structurally reminiscent of primitive embryonal types. The problem was especially applicable in the case of the common glioblastoma and its multifold variants. The association of 'polar spongioblast'-like or 'astroblast'-like cells with others showing extremes of polymorphism, including various types of giant cells, with foci of increased cellular density and with

Table 9.1 Glioma classification according to degree of malignancy

New	Old (with new in parentheses)	
Astrocytoma, grades 1–4	Astrocytoma (astrocytoma, grade 1) Astrocytoma (astrocytoma, grade 2) Polar spongioblastoma (obsolete) Glioblastoma multiforme (astrocytoma, grades 3 and 4)	
Ependymoma, grades 1–4	Ependymoma (ependymoma, grade 1) Ependymoma (ependymoma, grades 2–4) Neuroepithelioma (obsolete) Medulloepithelioma (ependymoma, grade 4)	
Oligodendroglioma, grades 1–4	Oligodendroglioma (oligodendroglioma, grade 1) Oligodendroglioma (oligodendroglioma, grades 2–4)	
Neuroastrocytoma, grades 1–4	Neurocytoma Ganglioneuroma Gangliocytoma Ganglioglioma	(neuroastrocytoma, grade 1)
	Neuroblastoma Spongioneuroblastoma Glioneuroblastoma Others	(neuroastrocytoma, grades 2–4)
Medulloblastoma	Medulloblastoma	

the development of more embryonal small-cell forms represents the cacophony induced by malignant progression.

Influenced by such considerations, Kernohan and his coworkers (Kernohan *et al.*, 1949; Kernohan and Sayre, 1952) swung the pendulum hard in the direction of simplification and, by introducing a system of grading from 1 to 4 in ascending order of malignancy, reduced the glioma types to five main groups (Table 9.1). This resulted in the elimination of several tumor entities, including the glioblastoma multiforme.

This radical bid for simplicity was certainly of value in its insistence upon the importance of anaplasia and, as a result, has often been welcomed by general pathologists and clinicians. Through succeeding years, the existence of a number of rare gliomas, previously proposed as embryonal, has been called into question by virtue of modern ultrastructural, immunohistologic, and molecular genetic investigations. For these reasons, in this text, the astroblastoma has been located with the ependymomas, due to the former's ultrastructural features in common with the tanycyte. The 'polar spongioblastoma' will be considered as an unusual, but distinctive, histologic growth pattern that may be recognized in both gliomas and neuronal tumors, but without a clearly defined independent prognostic or cytogenetic implication (Schiffer *et al.*, 1993). As to the glioblastoma multiforme, many examples are certainly derived from the anaplastic progression of a more differentiated astrocytoma, but such a derivation cannot be clearly demonstrated in all instances; the term therefore remains convenient to designate a highly characteristic, highly malignant and common type of neoplasm that may have histologic features suggesting an origin from other forms of malignant glioma.

The 'International classification of central nervous system tumors' drafted under the auspices of the World Health Organization (WHO) (Zülch, 1979) represented the first consensus achieved after many years of study and discussion by proponents of different schools. It is, in its essential lines, derived from the classification of Bailey and Cushing. While, as with any other classification scheme, criticisms of detail were leveled against it, its main contribution was to reconcile the terminologies and concepts of sometimes widely differing viewpoints and thus achieve, by compromise, a reasonable measure of uniformity on the most commonly recognized tumor entities and their most frequent variants. This first WHO classification of tumors derived from neuroepithelial tissues was detailed in the previous edition of this book (Russell and Rubinstein, 1989, pp. 83–161).

The classification adopted in this edition follows, with some modifications, the scheme proposed by the WHO revision of 1993 (Kleihues, Burger and Scheithauer, 1993). In regard to the gliomas in the restricted sense of the term, the various types seen in practice will be described according to their derivation from the main classes of [illegible]oglia, including some of their more primiti[illegible]ages. Those composed of neoplastic neurogli[illegible]umed to be derived from the more [illegible]d cell types form the largest group and [illegible]umors prone to malignant progression and to development of features of glioblastoma. It is well known, however, that examples of glioblastoma are found in which cytologic evidence of evolution from one of the more differentiated forms of glioma is lacking (Louis and Gusella, 1995). Indeed, many such tumors, appear to arise *de novo*, and their clinical evolution, combined with their typical gross and microscopic features, makes them distinctive as a level of ultimate glial transformation. Nevertheless, we feel that the characterization of glioblastoma as a separate category of anaplastic glioma no longer deserves to be maintained.

In the scheme we have elected, we have separated (as is generally done today) the tumors of neuroglial cells from those composed of neuronal elements or of primitive bipotential precursors. We have retained the distinction between the common tumors of embryonal neuroectodermal origin found in the cerebellum, grouping them under the term 'medulloblastoma' and distinguishing them from the histologically similar neuroblastic growths arising, albeit much less frequently, in the supratentorial compartment. The disparity of incidence between these various forms of primitive neoplasia and the ontogenetic differences that characterize the cellular development, migration and maturation of the neuroepithelial elements in the forebrain from those in the cerebellum continue to justify such a separation. The bipotential capacity of the cerebellar medulloblastoma to express divergent glial and neuronal phenotypes, and the frequency with which glial elements, participating in the proliferation of mature ganglion cell tumors, result in the development of gangliogliomas are further reasons why it is convenient to continue to group together the tumors of neuronal cells with those of their primitive bipotential precursors. In this group is included, also, the rare medulloepithelioma, which, by virtue of its multipotential capacity to express all the stages of central neurogenic maturation from the most embryonal to the most differentiated, constitutes the prototype of embryonal central neuroepithelial tumors.

Finally, it will be convenient to consider separately those neoplasms related to the other specialized tissues to which the central neuroepithelium may give rise. These include the neuroepithelial tumors of the retina, those of the optic nerve and chiasm, those of the neurohypophysis, those of the pineal body and those that arise from the epithelium of the choroid plexus.

The complete scheme of classification adopted here is given in full below, following the general outline of the WHO classification (Kleihues, Burger and Scheithauer, 1993):

I. Tumors of neuroglial cells
  A. Astrocytic tumors
    1. Astrocytoma (including protoplasmic and fibrillary variants)
    2. Anaplastic astrocytoma (including gemistocytic variant)
    3. Gliomatosis cerebri
    4. Glioblastoma multiforme
    5. Pilocytic astrocytoma (including adult and juvenile variants)
    6. Pleomorphic xanthoastrocytoma
    7. Desmoplastic infantile astrocytoma
    8. Subependymal giant-cell astrocytoma (tuberous sclerosis)
  B. Oligodendroglial tumors
    1. Oligodendroglioma
    2. Mixed oligoastrocytoma
    3. Anaplastic oligodendroglioma
  C. Ependymal tumors
    1. Ependymoma
    2. Anaplastic ependymoma
    3. Astroblastoma
    4. Subependymoma
    5. Ependymoblastoma

II. Tumors of neuronal cells and of primitive bipotential precursors
  A. Medulloepithelioma
  B. Medulloblastoma and cerebellar neuroblastoma
  C. Neuronal tumors and mixed neuronal–glial tumors
    1. Cerebral neuroblastoma
    2. Central neurocytoma
    3. Gangliocytoma
    4. Ganglioglioma
    5. Desmoplastic infantile ganglioglioma
    6. Dysembryoplastic neuroepithelial tumor

III. Tumors of specialized tissues of central neuroepithelial origin
  A. Tumors of the neurohypophysis
    1. Astrocytoma
    2. Granular-cell tumor
  B. Tumors of the parenchymal and glial cells of the pineal body
    1. Pineoblastoma
    2. Pineocytoma
    3. Mixed or transitional forms
    4. Glioma
  C. Tumors of the choroid plexus epithelium
    1. Papilloma
    2. Carcinoma

Grading astrocytomas

Any scheme of histologic grading has two main goals: (1) the tumor grade must predict clinical behavior and (2) the grading criteria must be sufficiently objective and defined to minimize variation among observers and to maximize reproducibility (Fulling and Nelson, 1984). Of the numerous grading systems in use for astrocytomas, most utilize three or four grades of malignancy. In addition, a key assumption of any valid grading scheme of malignancy is that representative histologic material has been obtained and evaluated.

Histologic grading of diffuse infiltrating gliomas may present important technical problems. Since anaplastic features may be focal, the prognostic value attached to the grading of small or stereotactic needle biopsies is totally dependent on adequate and representative sampling of the neoplasm. Not infrequently, the peripheral portion of a glioma has the classic appearance of a well-differentiated or low-grade astrocytoma, but the deep parts less accessible to resection or biopsy may already have developed the histologic character of a glioblastoma.

Even when the restriction of the sample is taken into account, the problem of correlating a particular histologic picture with subsequent clinical behavior is a significant hurdle. The first category of glioma for which a prognostically significant scale of malignancy grades was accepted was the diffuse cerebral astrocytoma. More recently, several histologic features of oligodendrogliomas have been recognized that permit classification of these tumors into prognostically significant grades of malignancy. For the ependymomas, attempts at grading have, to date, not been generally accepted to be of clinical significance. Even in the astrocytomas, grading carries limitations with respect to predicting prognosis because it does not take into account the anatomic location of the tumor, an aspect that determines surgical accessibility and the likelihood of complete resection. Further consideration must be given to the defined population of tumors being graded by these methods, as they are generally validated only for diffusely infiltrating gliomas of the adult cerebrum. Thus, the clinical course of certain examples of specific types of astrocytoma, such as the pilocytic form of juvenile type or the pleomorphic xanthoastrocytoma, is that of a distinct histopathologic entity completely different from that of the diffusely infiltrating forms of astrocytoma.

Though, for most tumors, it is recognized that higher grades of malignancy are associated with a poorer patient prognosis, the grading criteria for astrocytomas–and for all gliomas–are somewhat inexact. Increasingly more malignant examples show a continuum of histologic features that permits classification into grades. The individual histologic criteria used to define these grades vary somewhat for different schemes. Some histologic features used to grade astrocytomas are the presence of increasing cellularity, microcysts (which suggest an improved prognosis) and nuclear and cellular pleomorphism, and the identification of vascular mural cell proliferation, mitotic activity and coagulative tumor necrosis. These features are illustrated in Figs 9.1–9.4. Within a single grade, the prognosis for individual patients may be difficult to predict on the basis of grade; i.e., astrocytomas with similar histologic features may behave in a widely disparate clinical fashion. There is, however, a general correlation of decreasing postoperative patient survival with increasing grade of malignancy.

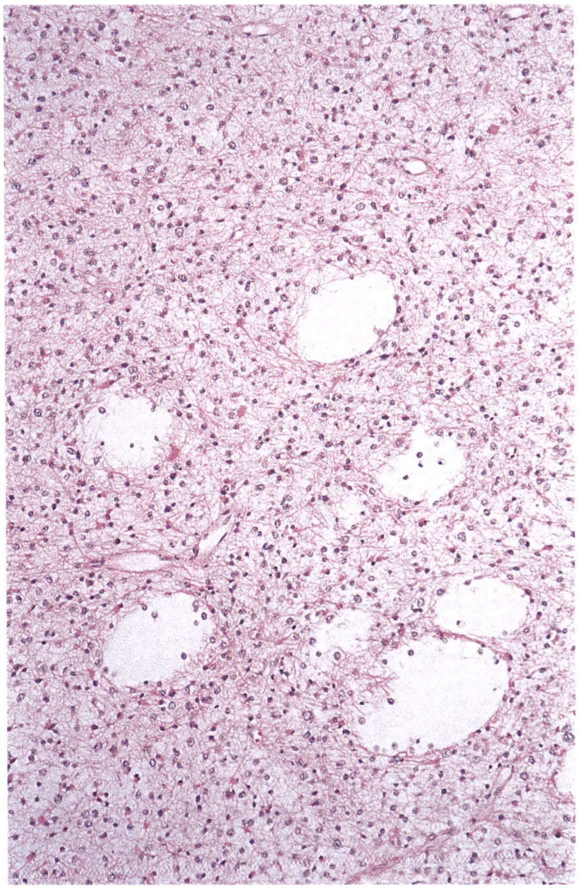

Fig. 9.1 Well-differentiated or low-grade astrocytoma showing increased cellularity, beyond that of normal brain, and the presence of microcysts. Hematoxylin and eosin (H&E), × 125

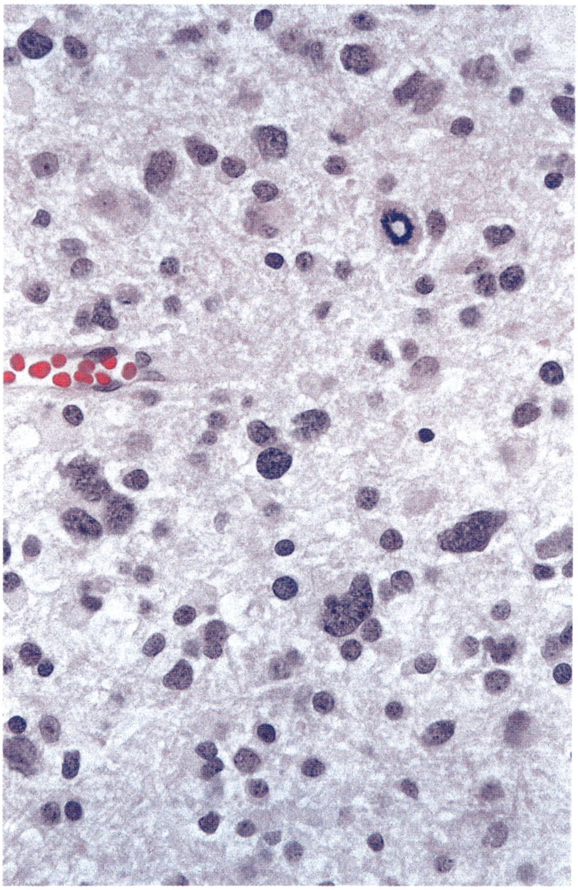

Fig. 9.2 Anaplastic astrocytoma showing nuclear pleomorphism and mitotic figures. H&E, × 500

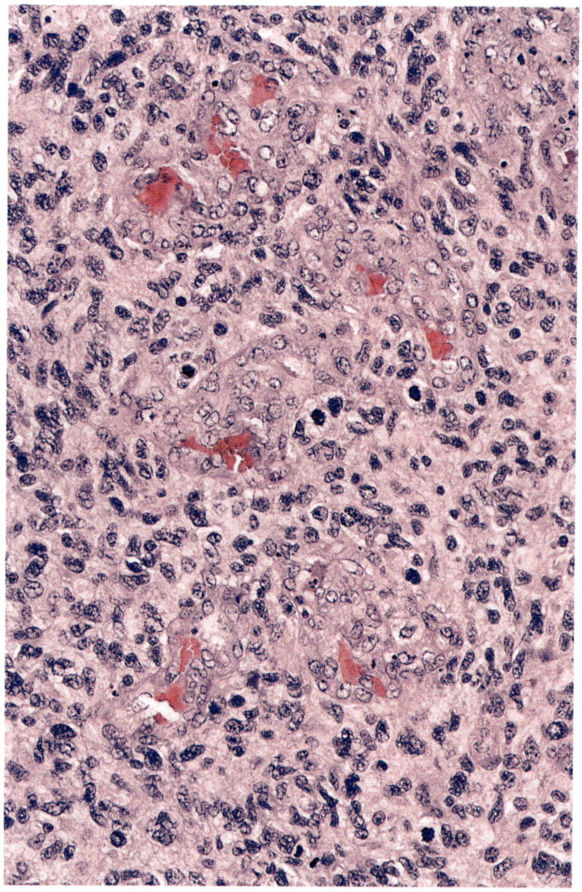

Fig. 9.3 Additional histologic features of anaplastic astrocytoma include dense cellularity with mitotic figures and glomeruloid microvascular proliferation. H&E, × 250

Historically, the first systems for grading gliomas were presented at about the same time (Kernohan *et al.*, 1949; Svien *et al.*, 1949; Ringertz, 1950). Svien *et al.* and Kernohan *et al.* used a four-grade system (designated as grades 1 through 4) that was patterned after the histologic grading system for epithelial neoplasms used at the Mayo Clinic. Ringertz's system had three grades of astrocytoma malignancy: astrocytoma, intermediate-type astrocytoma, and glioblastoma multiforme. Necrosis was the single histologic feature used by Ringertz to divide the intermediate-type astrocytoma from the glioblastoma. Both systems (four-grade system, Svien *et al.*, 1949, and Kernohan *et al.*, 1949; three-grade system, Ringertz, 1950) based the histologic grade on the recognition of cellular anaplasia. However, the system of Svien *et al.* and Kernohan *et al.* was largely based on the proportion of normal tissue remaining mixed with the invading tumor and the morphologic configuration of the invading edge of tumor into the surrounding normal brain tissue. Because of the usual infiltrative growth pattern of gliomas, these features are notoriously difficult to distinguish, especially in well-differentiated tumors. Also, it has subsequently been considered that the presence of even a single highly malignant focus of glioblastoma in an otherwise lower-grade astrocytoma portends a grave prognosis. These two difficulties with the original system of Kernohan *et al.* – the invading edge and the proportion of cellular anaplasia – may have contributed to the lack of clinical relevance in separating the individual tumor grades. From the original publications, there was no clinical distinction in survival at 3 years between grades 2 and 3 astrocytomas of Svien *et al.* and Kernohan *et al.*, whereas there was a clear survival difference among the three groups of patients in Ringertz's study. The more recent study of Fulling and Nelson (1984), using the Kernohan grading system to classify 503 patients with malignant astrocytoma, found no survival difference between grades 3 and 4 of Kernohan *et al.*(respectively, 10

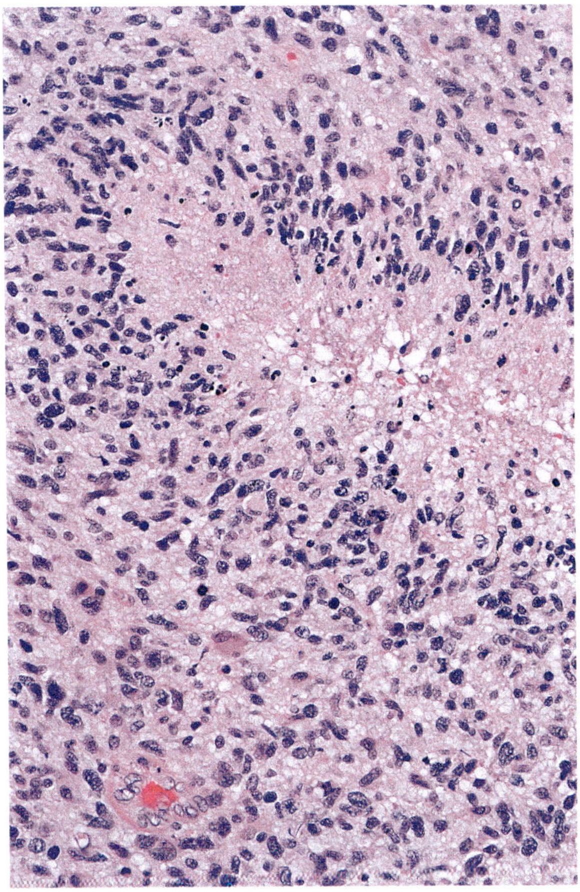

Fig. 9.4 Histologic features of glioblastoma multiforme include foci of coagulative necrosis and peripheral pseudopalisades of neoplastic cells. H&E, × 250

months median survival time versus 9 months), while there was a significant difference in survival among the patients when these same tumors were reclassified using necrosis as the factor distinguishing anaplastic astrocytoma from glioblastoma (28 months median survival for anaplastic astrocytoma versus 8 months for glioblastoma), a similar system to that proposed by Ringertz. Thus, the three-tiered grading schemes were popularized.

Three-tiered grading systems have been shown to be more closely correlated with clinical survival for diffuse infiltrating astrocytomas, and are more widely used today in diagnostic neuropathology. These grading systems include those of Ringertz (1950), as modified by Nelson *et al.* (1983), Fulling and Nelson (1984), Burger *et al.* (1985) and Burger and Green (1987); a scheme proposed by Daumas-Duport *et al.* (1988b) (widely called the 'St Anne-Mayo system'); and the current system advocated by the WHO in its 1993 revision (Kleihues, Burger and Scheithauer, 1993).

The three-tiered system of Ringertz (1950) proposed necrosis as the distinguishing feature of the glioblastoma from the intermediate-grade astrocytoma. It used features of cytologic pleomorphism, mitotic activity and microvascular proliferation changes to distinguish the intermediate-grade astrocytoma from the lower-grade astrocytoma. The three-tiered systems used by Nelson (Nelson *et al.*, 1983; Fulling and Nelson, 1984) and by Burger (Burger *et al.*, 1985; Burger and Green, 1987) have similar criteria and changed the designation of the intermediate-grade tumor to anaplastic (or malignant) astrocytoma and that of the lowest-grade tumor to well-differentiated astrocytoma. Studies by these two authors and their colleagues have shown a clinical correlation with postoperative survival, and a reproducibility of the three-tiered systems in distinguishing three significantly different survival curves. The mean survival times (MSTs) are somewhat variable among the studies, but can be summarized as about 24–30 months for anaplastic astrocytoma and about 8–12 months for glioblastoma, depending somewhat on the types of postoperative therapy. These figures are comparable to those first published by Ringertz in 1950. No large studies by these authors discussed the well-differentiated astrocytoma, but the MST in the original Ringertz group was 63 months. Though the position of gemistocytic astrocytoma has been variably placed with respect to grade, Krouwer *et al.* (1991), in a study of 51 astrocytomas with gemistocytic features, concluded that those astrocytomas with 20% or more gemistocytes had a median survival time of 35 months, placing them more in the range of anaplastic astrocytomas than well-differentiated astrocytomas. For this reason, we have included the discussion of this tumor in the section about anaplastic astrocytomas.

The St Anne-Mayo scheme detailed by Daumas-Duport *et al.* (1988b) names four histologic features to be used in grading and nominally has four grades of astrocytoma (1–4). This system uses a simple tabulation of the four features as present or absent in a standardized and objective numeric scale: cellular pleomorphism, mitotic activity, microvascular proliferation and necrosis. Each feature present receives one scoring point, and the grade for an individual tumor is based solely on the cumulative numeric score. Thus, astrocytomas with none of the four features are grade 1, those with one feature are grade 2, those with two features are grade 3, and those with three or four features present are grade 4. In the most recent publication of the WHO classification (Kleihues, Burger and Scheithauer, 1993), the criteria used for grading of astrocytomas (I–IV) are similar to those used in this system. The diagnosis of glioblastoma requires microvascular proliferation *and/or* necrosis. The essential variance of this system from the other three-tiered systems discussed above is that an astrocytoma can be classified as a grade IV tumor (or WHO glioblastoma) based on the presence of vascular changes and without the feature of necrosis. In most cases of glioblastoma (using necrosis as the criterion for diagnosis), both of these features are present. The apparent discordance between the presence of microvascular proliferation and tumor necrosis occurred in only 14/181 (7.7%) tumors in the series published by Kim *et al.* (1991) and in 32/275 (11.6%) tumors in the series of Barker *et al.* (1996). Thus, although this represents a major discrepancy in criteria, it may not affect the practicality of grading in the vast majority of tumors. The concordance among individual pathologists who use the St Anne-Mayo system is reported to be as high as 94% (Kim *et al.*, 1991). Their grade 1 tumor, however, is exceedingly rare (<0.25% in one series), and the other three grades produce three distinct survival curves; thus, this scheme may also be considered practically as a three-tiered scale. One study undertaken by Kim *et al.* (1991) to validate this system, soon after its inception, examined 251 cases of astrocytomas and also suggested, because of survival data, that the presence of necrosis should cause a tumor to be immediately classified as grade 4, even using this system. In the original study of the St Anne-Mayo system published by Daumas-Duport *et al.* (1988b), and in the validation study of Kim *et al.* (1991), the MST for grade 2 astrocytomas was about 45+ months, for grade 3 astrocytomas about 16+ months and for grade 4 astrocytomas about 8+ months. In a multivariate analysis, however, Kim *et al.* found no significant difference in survival between grades 2 and 3 of the St Anne-Mayo grading scale. There was a significant survival difference between grades 3 and 4.

The MSTs for glioblastomas and grade 4 astrocytomas are generally about the same for all grading schemes in use today. However, the MSTs for the lower-grade astrocytomas, those well-differentiated and anaplastic tumors, are more disparate, depending on the system in use. In general, the currently used three-tiered grading schemes for the diffuse fibrillary astrocytomas in adults show significantly differing MSTs among grades and may be considered as clinically relevant in separating the grades of tumors. It is essential that the pathologist, surgeon and oncologist jointly determine the grading system for common use at each institution and that criteria for grading be applied consistently so that survival information can be predicted for the patient population. Survival times will also vary according to the effectiveness of any current or future treatment administered for these tumors.

It should be remembered that increasing grades of malignancy within the astrocytoma group are associated directly with patient age. Well-differentiated astrocytomas (grade II) are most common in patients in the third or fourth decade, anaplastic astrocytomas (grade III) in the fourth or fifth decade and glioblastomas (grade IV), or the most malignant astrocytomas, in the sixth decade and beyond (Burger, Scheithauer and Vogel, 1991, pp. 107–12). A low-grade astrocytoma (grades I and II) rarely occurs in a person over age 50 years; the reverse is not necessarily true. Glioblastomas occur with some frequency in young children (Dohrmann, Farwell and Flannery, 1976; Georges, Notermann and Flament-Durand, 1983). Most notable are the brainstem glioblastomas. A distinct trough in incidence, however, appears between the ages of 18 and 23 years, when the age-specific incidence approaches one per million population (McLendon *et al.*, 1985).

For this discussion, the terms 'well-differentiated astrocytoma', 'anaplastic astrocytoma' and 'glioblastoma' will be used to describe fibrillary astrocytomas. That the glioblastoma is primarily derived from astrocytes in most cases can be assumed, even though its morphology may be so bizarre as to obscure such recognition.

Classification of embryonal tumors of the central nervous system

Special diagnostic and conceptual problems exist in the identification and classification of CNS neoplasms because, in the central neuraxis, the cells of renewal that are the presumed target for neoplastic transformation are at their most abundant during development, and, consequently, the distinction between adult-type and embryonal tumors may be blurred. The problem is further complicated by the frequency and multifocality of neoplastic progression, presenting the difficulty of distinguishing anaplastic from embryonal-cell forms. Despite these difficulties, the distinction needs to be maintained as precisely as possible, and the application of some kind of cytogenetic scheme for the definition of those embryonal tumors that can be recognized as having distinct morphologic features is necessary. While the classic, historical scheme of normal neurocytogenesis is likely to undergo modifications in the light of the immunomorphologic markers currently used for the recognition and identification of different neuroepithelial cell types, many embryonal CNS tumors can still be classified according to such a scheme, each demonstrating a range and a restriction in its differentiating capabilities that generally conform to the neurocytogenetic lineage to which it can be related. This historic classification

Table 9.2 Cytogenetic classification of embryonal tumors of the central neuroepithelium

Stages of neurocytogenesis		Normal cell type	Equivalent embryonal CNS tumor	Differentiating potential of the tumor
Forebrain	First	Primitive ventricular (matrix, neuroepithelial) cell	Medulloepithelioma	Divergent (neuronal, glial and/or ependymal)
Forebrain	Second	Neuroblast	Cerebral neuroblastoma	Neuronal
Forebrain	Third	Glioblast (spongioblast) (? radial glia)	Polar spongioblastoma	Astrocytic and/or oligodendroglial
	Third	Ependymoblast (? ependymoglioblast)	Ependymoblastoma	Ependymal and primitive glial
Cerebellum	Neuroepithelial roof of 4th ventricle ↓	Undifferentiated neuroepithelial cell ('medulloblast') ↓	Cerebellar medulloblastoma	Divergent (glial and/or neuronal)
Cerebellum	External granular layer	Undifferentiated neuroepithelial cell		
Pineal anlage		Pineoblast	Pineoblastoma	Pineocytic, astrocytic, neuronal and/or photosensory
Neuroepithelium of primitive optic cup		Retinoblast	Retinoblastoma	Neuroblastic and photosensory

scheme, with its corresponding proposed correlations to the normal stages of cytogenesis, is shown in Table 9.2.

In 1973, Hart and Earle proposed that certain supratentorial tumors of infancy should be classified as primitive neuroectodermal tumors (PNETs); these tumors were characterized microscopically by a high nuclear-to-cytoplasmic ratio and had greater than 95% of the tumor cells lacking differentiation by light microscopy. The advent of immunologic reagents has subsequently aided in the characterization of many of these neoplasms, several of which are now recognized as small-cell gliomas of infancy (Friede, Janzer and Roessmann, 1982). Nevertheless, cases still exist that either lack phenotypic markers for accurate characterization or require ultrastructural analysis for classification. The vast majority of these remaining cases can be shown to express markers of a neuronal phenotype. Histologically, the similarities to the classical medulloblastomas were recognized by Rorke (1983) and Becker and Hinton (1983) who proposed that the term 'primitive neuroectodermal tumor' should be used to characterize all CNS neoplasms of embryonal neuroectodermal origin, including those tumors also known as *medulloepithelioma, neuroblastoma, polar spongioblastoma, pineoblastoma, ependymoblastoma, retinoblastoma* and *olfactory neuroblastoma*. The rationale for this recharacterization was explained by Becker and Hinton (1983) as follows: '[F]rom a practical, histologic point of view, these tumors are often indistinguishable from one another and are best thought of as PNETs with or without differentiating features.' Indeed, the objectivity, reproducibility and ease of application inherent to the system led to an acceptance of the system among some pathologists who were no longer dependent on the site of origin to place a label on an otherwise undifferentiated neuroectodermal neoplasm. Furthermore, supporters of the system note that it also encompasses the plasticity of the transformed embryonal neuroectodermal cell to express divergent neuroectodermal phenotypes.

It is obvious from multiple viewpoints that acceptance of this system is not universal. The most obvious defect with this classification is clinical. Up to 75% of medulloblastomas may be cured with a combined surgical, radiotherapeutic and chemotherapeutic approach, and over 50% 5-year survival has been documented in patients with this tumor. In contrast, only 30% 5-year survival is usual for the tumors known as cerebral neuroblastomas (Bennett and Rubinstein, 1984) despite similarly aggressive therapy. Radiographically, cerebral neuroblastomas are prone to calcification, a feature they have in common with retinoblastomas but that is rare in medulloblastomas. Also, cerebral neuroblastomas are prone to cyst formation, a feature noted by Berger *et al.* (1983) to signify a better prognosis.

Histologically, a number of factors distinguish these tumors at a light microscopic level. Flexner-Wintersteiner rosettes are common in retinoblastomas, infrequent in pineoblastomas, rare in medulloblastomas and absent in cerebral neuroblastomas. Calcification is common in retinoblastomas and cerebral neuroblastomas but absent in medulloblastomas. 'Pale islands' of tumor cells are present in up to two thirds of childhood medulloblastomas and some medulloepitheliomas but are lacking in cerebral neuroblastomas, retinoblastomas and pineoblastomas. Finally, true ependymal rosettes define the ependymoblastoma (Mørk and Rubinstein, 1985; Rubinstein, 1970) but are absent in the other neoplasms.

In this text, we have maintained the cytogenetic approach used in previous editions to characterize these malignant embryonal tumors of neuroectodermal origin. The considerations that prompted the genesis of this approach have been reviewed (Rubinstein, 1985).

Applications of the classification: divergent differentiation, mixed gliomas and heterogeneous cell populations

The classification of embryonal CNS tumors outlined above therefore allows a place for the original concept of Bailey and Cushing tumor types in which the component cells recapitulate a stage of neuroepithelial cytogenesis. Examples of such entities can, however, be accepted only when the morphology of the individual neoplastic cells and the architectural pattern of the tumor are compatible with such an interpretation. In other words, this system is acceptable when the range of variation in cell forms, and in differentiation features expressed, and the essential cytologic and nuclear characteristics of the tumor cells do not warrant the alternative interpretation of malignant progression. Because the latter is a frequent development in tumors of the glioma group, especially in astrocytomas, careful scanning of all parts of a tumor for variations in appearance, texture and morphologic features, as well as multiple samplings for histologic examination, are essential.

Many tumors, however, display an impressive heterogeneity that cannot simply be explained by malignant progression. In the case of the embryonal tumors listed above, the diversity of cell populations is usually due to the maturation of primitive cells along a single determined path of cell lineage or according to a range of differentiating capabilities imprinted at the particular stage of ontogenesis at which transformation is presumed to have taken place. It should be recognized that divergent differentiation is a feature of embryonal tumors in general (Willis, 1958, p. 410). The exceptional expression of aberrant elements, such as striated muscle cells in medulloblastoma ('medullomyoblastoma') and medulloepithelioma, may possibly be viewed in that context. Advances in our understanding of the mechanisms involved in phenotypic regulation will undoubtedly contribute to our understanding of this phenomenon.

In the central neuroepithelial tumors that are not part of the embryonal group, cellular heterogeneity, when not attributable to the selective advantage gained by more actively proliferating cell populations and culminating in the picture of anaplasia, usually results in two forms of *mixed glioma*: a more or less diffuse blend of differing glial cell types or, less often, examples in which large areas of tumor, of distinct microscopic structure and even dissimilar macroscopic appearance, are found in close juxtaposition.

The former is common enough to be almost the general rule in certain types of glioma, e.g., the oligodendrogliomas and the optic nerve gliomas. But, insofar as distinct glioma types can be recognized in the face of such a cellular heterogeneity, the distinction must, in practice, be based upon the common habit of naming the tumor by the prevalent kind of cell identified after a comprehensive survey of many histologic fields. Thus, even in the presence of quantitatively minor tumor cell populations that are clearly nonoligodendroglial, the overall architectural pattern, the outline of the supporting vasculature and the cellular characteristics of the preponderant cell type justify the histologic identity of the oligodendroglioma. In the presence of marked anaplasia, however, the typical phenotype of oligodendroglioma may be retained, or may be so masked by cellular atypia and heterogeneity that no distinction from glioblastoma is possible. On the other hand, different adult types of glia may be found intermingled in varying proportions throughout a single tumor, as in many astrocytomas, and it cannot be argued that any one type is derived from another. In extreme instances, such varieties may defy classification. Portmanteau names such as, 'oligoastrocytoma', may be devised for these tumors. In other cases, a distinctive label (e.g., 'subependymoma') will be appropriate in denoting a specific histologic entity. The mechanism by means of which such different cell populations enter into the composition of mixed gliomas is unclear. In some examples, such as the subependymoma just mentioned and in some instances of mixed astrocytoma and oligodendroglioma, the simultaneous participation of different glial cell types in the initial transformation process is a possibility. In some other cases, however, diversity of mature cell populations may result from a process of divergent differentiation from within a monoclonal population. This could be explained by a neoplastic initiation transforming a cell that is in the process of selecting (imprinting) different effective genomes for the expression of different phenotypes. The character and extent to which different glial cell forms are mingled in the astrocytomas, oligodendrogliomas and ependymomas are examined in the appropriate sections of this chapter.

The *gangliogliomas* constitute a type of mixed neoplasm in which advanced differentiation is displayed by cells of two separate neuroepithelial lineages. These tumors pose two problems that are, respectively, of a diagnostic and a biologic order. The first is concerned with the need for discrimination between tumoral elements that are, although numerically inferior, nevertheless neoplastic, and those similar cell types that represent normal entrapped elements of the invaded tissues of the host. The second problem has to do with the distinction to be drawn between the different anaplastic potential of the tumor cells in each lineage: this is recognized to be almost always restricted to the glial elements and almost unknown in differentiated gangliocytes. But, here again, a further distinction has to be made between the gangliogliomas, taken as representing a mixture of cell populations with mature characteristics, and those more primitive tumors in which the development of adult gangliocytes more specifically defines the end stage of a maturing cerebral neuroblastoma.

Finally, a mixture of populations implicating tumor cells of even more disparate character is exemplified by the mixed gliomas and sarcomas. Most instances appear to fall within one of two classes. In the type known as 'gliosarcoma'–by far the more common–the sarcomatous change is surmised to be the malignant transformation of mesenchymal elements belonging to the proliferating vascular stroma of a glioblastoma. In the second type, or 'sarcoglioma', the gliomatous element is a secondary development proposed as originating from the hyperplastic gliosis encountered at the edges of an infiltrating malignant meningioma or sarcoma (Pettinato *et al.*, 1989). Exceptional examples of 'angiogliomas', representing mixed capillary hemangioblastomas and gliomas, may possibly represent a third class. The occurrence of these different forms of mixed neuroepithelial and mesenchymal neoplasms provides the most convincing evidence, so far, for at least biclonal transformation of cells of different lineage in the CNS. The inference is that the initial neoplastic cell populations could have induced malignancy into putatively normal, supportive or reactive and hyperplastic stromal cells by means of an as yet unexplained molecular mechanism. An alternative explanation is that of cellular metaplasia in a glial or mesenchymal neoplasm. Some molecular genetic studies of gliosarcomas support this hypothesis (Biernat *et al.*, 1995).

Diversity of cytologic composition is strongly reflected also in the experimental production of animal gliomas by various agents. Biologically, and therefore clinically, the importance of these mixed types lies in the recognition that histologic variation is not necessarily an expression of anaplasia. Furthermore, the prognostic implications of cellular heterogeneity are made considerably more complex by the problem of determining which of the different cell populations should be accorded the most decisive predictive significance. Thus, in an oligoastrocytoma, it is usually impossible to foretell, in the individual case, whether its subsequent clinical behavior will be more akin to that of an astrocytoma or an oligodendroglioma, or it may be difficult to assess which of the two cell populations displays the potentially more malignant, and therefore more premonitory, cytologic characteristics. These general implications are considered in greater detail in the sections that follow.

Tumors of neuroglial cells

ASTROCYTIC GROUP

This group comprises the many varieties of astrocytoma and the glioblastoma multiforme. We also include gliomatosis cerebri, although this currently is considered by WHO to be a tumor of uncertain histologic origin. The *astroblastoma*, also considered to be of uncertain origin but showing ultrastructural features of tanycytes, is discussed with the ependymoma group. The remaining tumor considered to be of uncertain origin is the polar spongioblastoma, which we consider to be a distinctive growth pattern that may occur in either gliomas or tumors of neuronal origin (Schiffer *et al.*, 1993) (see Fig. 9.97).

Astrocytomas

Astrocytomas constitute a large and rather heterogeneous group of tumors, with wide differences in their clinical incidence, gross and microscopic features and biologic behavior. Their morphologic diversity is attributed partly to the various structural forms displayed by developing, mature and reactive astrocytes, and partly, in diffusely infiltrating examples, to the propensity of neoplastic cells to accommodate their shape to the persistence of pre-existing structures in the neural parenchyma. A brief review of the principal structural features of normal, reactive and developing astrocytic cells is, therefore, desirable as a preliminary to a discussion of their neoplastic proliferations.

Normal, reactive and developing astrocytic cells

Fully developed stellate astrocytes are conventionally divided into *protoplasmic* and *fibrillary* (or *fibrous*) types. In the normal brain, protoplasmic astrocytes are largely confined to the middle layers of the cortex and to the basal ganglia, while the fibrous astrocytes are found in the white matter and in the narrow zones of central neural parenchyma that interface with the supporting vasculature. In some areas of the CNS, mature astrocytes are normally polar, or fusiform. These polar astrocytes include the fibrous astrocytes that are attached to the pia or are situated beneath the ependyma. They also include the distinctive astrocytes that occupy the molecular layer of the cerebellar cortex that have a single major process directed outward toward the pia and have their cell bodies lying in or near the Purkinje cell layer: i.e., the feathered cells of Fañanás, which are protoplasmic, and the Bergmann astrocytes, which are fibrillary.

The morphologic distinction between protoplasmic and fibrillary astrocytes is based on the shape of their arborizing cell processes and on the presence of intracytoplasmic fibrils, as demonstrated in light microscopy by traditional neurohistologic methods. That distinction is maintained by most electron microscopists (Peters, Palay and Webster, 1976, pp. 105–31). By electron microscopy, both cell types are characterized by the presence of intracellular cytoskeletal intermediate filaments measuring 7–11 nm in diameter, forming compact bundles in the fibrillary astrocytes and scantier arrays in protoplasmic astrocytes. These filaments are structural polymers in which the major polypeptide is represented by a biochemically and antigenically distinct class of protein, the glial fibrillary acidic protein (GFAP). This protein, estimated to have a molecular mass of about 49 kilodaltons (kDa) in the human, contains relatively large amounts of aspartic and glutamic acid, alanine, leucine and arginine. Following its original isolation from old multiple sclerosis plaques and its purification by ammonium sulfate precipitation, isoelectric precipitation and preparative polyacrylamide gel electrophoresis (Eng *et al.*, 1971), it was localized by specific immunofluorescence to fibrillary astrocytes (Bignami *et al.*, 1972; Bignami and Dahl, 1974). It has since become one of the most valuable markers for the study of normal, developing and pathologically altered glia (see comprehensive reviews by Dahl and Bignami, 1983; Eng and DeArmond, 1983; McLendon and Bigner, 1994). Its molecular sequence has now been revealed, and the gene has been cloned (Reeves *et al.*, 1989; Kumanishi *et al.*, 1992). Further studies of the structure and regulation of the gene will help to elucidate its role in astrocyte function and are being facilitated by the creation of transgenic mice (Brenner, 1994; Brenner *et al.*, 1994; Galou *et al.*, 1994; Galea, Dupouey and Feinstein, 1995; W.B. Johnson *et al.*, 1995).

Another intermediate filament protein, vimentin, which is found in various cells of mesenchymal origin and has a molecular mass of 57 kDa, has been shown to coexist with GFAP in mature astrocytes (Bjørklund *et al.*, 1984), but only as a minor cytoskeletal component. On the other hand, in some mammalian species it constitutes the major cytoskeletal protein of the developing neuroglia (Bignami, Raju and Dahl, 1982).

Under pathologic stimuli of varying duration, protoplasmic astrocytes are rapidly and permanently converted into fibrous astrocytes. This process of fibrillary gliosis, probably the most frequent and the least specific of the cellular reactions demonstrable in neuropathology, is characterized by a speedy synthesis of GFAP. It has also been shown that the intensity of GFAP immunostaining in reactive or neoplastic processes does not always correlate with GFAP content, but may be more defined by the dissociation of glial filament bundles to expose more epitopes to the antibody (Eng, D'Amelio and Smith, 1989). Studies using a GFAP-*lacZ* transgene in mice have shown that up regulation of GFAP transgene expression occurs within 1 hour after focal mechanical injury (Mücke *et al.*, 1991). The architectural pattern of the protein expression is influenced partly by the original shape of the reacting astrocytes, partly by the degree of local neural tissue destruction and partly by the extent to which preserved nerve fiber tracts will determine the alignment of the glial cell processes. Thus, in the molecular layer of the cerebellum, gliosis involving the Bergmann glia and the Fañanás cells is characteristically vertical, or radial. The laying down of long, parallel glial fibers, or 'isomorphic' gliosis, along the major white matter tracts, such as the corpus callosum, the internal capsule and the pyramids, results in the development of astrocytes that are thinned and elongated and that have been termed 'piloid' or 'pilocytic' due to their hair-like appearance.

Reactive gliosis is also characterized by the manifestations of astrocytic hyperplasia, hypertrophy and degeneration. A common form of reactive astrocyte is one in which the cell body becomes greatly swollen, rounded and hyaline, with an enlarged eccentric nucleus and short stubby cell processes. These cells are the gemistocytic astrocytes of classic neuropathology. By electron microscopy, the bundles of intermediate-size filaments are largely to be found only at the periphery of the perikaryon and in the cell processes, whereas the distended perinuclear cytoplasm is rich in mitochondria, stacks of granular endoplasmic reticulum and ribosomal rosettes. The cytoplasm of these cells stains intensely for GFAP.

In the normal course of development, the embryonal glia go through a transient stage during which they are radial and thereby able to span the entire width of the primitive neural tube. The radial glia are strongly positive for GFAP in both the nonhuman (Levitt and Rakic, 1980) and human (Antanitus, Choi and Lapham, 1976; Choi and Lapham, 1978; Veronina and Preobrazhensky, 1994) primate brain. In the rhesus monkey, they enter a period of amitosis in midgestation, during which they persist between the proliferative ventricular zone and the expanding, developing cerebral cortex (Schmechel and Rakic, 1979a). In late fetal development they re-enter the mitotic cycle and become converted into mature protoplasmic and fibrillary astrocytes (Choi, 1981). They are the source of Bergmann glia relatively early in ontogenesis, i.e., in the first half of pregnancy (Choi and Lapham, 1980). In addition, at the time of myelinogenesis, some of the radial glial cells transform into myelin-forming oligodendroglia (Choi, Kim and Lapham, 1983). It is noteworthy that, in the human, immature spinal oligodendrocytes have been shown transiently to express GFAP immediately before myelinogenesis (Choi and Kim, 1985). In the rat brain, the radial glia do not express GFAP, but instead express vimentin: conversion of glia into mature astrocytes is associated with a decrease of vimentin and the appearance of GFAP as the dominant chemical constituent of the intermediate filaments (Dahl, 1981; Pixley and de Vellis, 1984; Landry, Ivy and Brown, 1990; Zerlin, Levison and Goldman, 1995).

Classification and histologic type

Various classifications of astrocytomas have been proposed at different times in an attempt to relate them to the diverse structural aspects adopted by the normal and reactive astrocytes in the circumstances outlined above. None can be said to satisfy entirely the requirements of consistency, logic or comprehensiveness. Bailey and Cushing (1926) separated astrocytomas into two groups: protoplasmic and fibrillary. Elvidge, Penfield and Cone (1937) classified them as diffuse, pilocytic and gemistocytic. Increasing recognition of the tendency of astrocytomas to show anaplastic changes then led to the system of grading instituted at the Mayo Clinic (Kernohan and Sayre, 1952) and discussed on pp. 308 and 312 herein. Zülch (1957) divided astrocytomas into protoplasmic, fibrillary, gigantocellular, astroblastoma and malignant astrocytoma. The 'polar spongioblastoma', which, in his classification, included the cerebellar astrocytoma and was separately considered as a distinct form of relatively benign, usually circumscribed, glioma, then came to be regarded as representing a common form of pilocytic astrocytoma. Davis (1971) separated the astrocytomas into three main groups: those with prominent cytoplasm, which he subdivided into protoplasmic, gemistocytic and the subependymal giant-cell type; those with prominent fibrils, which were divided into fibrillary and piloid; and a mixed group, labeled juvenile or cerebellar. The international classification proposed by the WHO (Zülch, 1979) divided the astrocytic tumors into astrocytoma (fibrillary, protoplasmic or gemistocytic), pilocytic astrocytoma, subependymal giant-cell astrocytoma, astroblastoma and anaplastic (or malignant) astrocytoma. Burger and Vogel (1982) broadly classified astrocytic neoplasms according to their primary location: i.e., cerebral hemispheric, third-ventricle region, cerebellum, brainstem and optic nerve, with the separate consideration of different subgroups that included fibrillary, protoplasmic, pilocytic and anaplastic variants, subependymal giant-cell astrocytoma and subependymoma.

The general histologic classification used in the revised WHO scheme (Kleihues, Burger and

Scheithauer, 1993) will be generally followed here, with modifications, as follows:

1. Well-differentiated astrocytoma, diffusely infiltrating (including protoplasmic and fibrillary variants)
2. Anaplastic astrocytoma, diffusely infiltrating (including gemistocytic variant)
3. Gliomatosis cerebri
4. Pilocytic astrocytoma (including juvenile and diffuse types)
5. Subependymal giant-cell astrocytoma
6. Pleomorphic xanthoastrocytoma
7. Desmoplastic cerebral astrocytoma of infancy

Such a classification scheme, because of diagnostic needs, should remain based upon both the various cell types encountered in these tumors and the grade of histologic anaplasia. These categories, sanctioned by usage, deserve retention because of their descriptive value. This classification scheme obviates the problem of classifying astrocytomas into mixed histologic types, as the diffusely infiltrating varieties are instead grouped by histologic grade. Fibrillary, protoplasmic and gemistocytic astrocytes are often intermixed, a phenomenon that is further reflected in their fine structural aspects in which intermediate forms between different astrocytes are commonly found (Duffell *et al.*, 1963; Hossmann and Wechsler, 1965; Raimondi, 1966). The special variants of astrocytoma that are not generally subjected to grading have their own characteristic clinical behavior and may be more accurately considered as 'noninfiltrating' or 'circumscribed' tumors: pilocytic, pleomorphic xanthoastrocytoma, subependymal giant-cell astrocytoma and desmoplastic cerebral astrocytoma of infancy.

Any mixture of neoplastic cell populations may include glial elements that are not astrocytic–in particular, oligodendroglia–a feature that will be considered in greater detail in the section on oligodendrogliomas (p. 370).

The histologic classification adopted here takes into consideration the predominance of different types of astrocytes normally present in different parts of the central neuraxis. Among the 'noninfiltrating' astrocytoma variants, most are associated with distinctive localizations within the CNS. The subependymal giant-cell astrocytoma has, as recalled on pp. 353 and 354, a definite morphologic kinship with the 'candle gutterings' of tuberous sclerosis and with the dysgenic type of glial cell characteristic of the disease. The tumor cells of the pleomorphic xanthoastrocytoma and of the superficial desmoplastic cerebral astrocytoma of infancy may, by virtue of their distinctive pericytoplasmic basal lamina, be related to a recognized feature of the normal subpial cerebral astrocyte.

A close relationship exists between the sites of astrocytomas, their age incidence and their biologic behavior. Numerous studies have been published in which these important correlations are examined in detail. Some of these will be referred to in subsequent sections of this chapter. Those concerned with the astrocytomas in general are exemplified by the reports of Elvidge and Martinez-Coll (1956), Levy and Elvidge (1956), Elvidge (1968), Marsa *et al.* (1975), Burger and Fuller (1991) and VandenBerg (1993). Those dealing more specifically with various forms of astrocytoma in the cerebral hemispheres include the follow-up studies by Laws *et al.* (1984), Clark, Henry and McKeever (1985), Garcia, Fulling and Marks (1985), Palma and Guidetti (1985), Afra *et al.* (1986), Krouwer *et al.* (1991), Louis *et al.* (1992), Forsyth *et al.* (1993), Kepes (1993) and Shaw, Scheithauer and O'Fallon (1993). Those reviewing the clinical evolution of childhood astrocytomas include the series published by Marsa *et al.* (1973), Mercuri, Russo and Palma (1981), Duffner *et al.* (1986), Marchese and Chang (1990), Hayostek *et al.* (1993), VandenBerg (1993), Sinson *et al.* (1994) and Pollack *et al.* (1995). Follow-up data on the diencephalic astrocytomas have been contributed by Bernstein *et al.* (1984), Albright, Price and Guthkelch (1985) and Krouwer and Prados (1995); on the childhood chiasmal gliomas by Imes and Hoyt (1986) and Listernick *et al.* (1994); on the brainstem astrocytomas by Albright, Price and Guthkelch (1983), Alvisi, Cerisoli and Maccheroni (1985), Albright *et al.* (1986), Cohen *et al.* (1986), Epstein and McCleary (1986), Stroink *et al.* (1986), Jenkin *et al.* (1987, US Children's Cancer Study Group), Epstein and Wisoff (1990), Epstein and Farmer (1993) and Pollack *et al.* (1993); and on spinal cord astrocytomas in children by Reimer and Onofrio (1985) and Rossitch *et al.* (1990). The reader is also referred to a comprehensive account of the clinical features of a large series of cerebral gliomas investigated and treated at the National Hospital for Nervous Diseases over a period of 20 years (McKeran and Thomas, 1980, pp. 94–5).

General incidence

In most series, astrocytomas account for 25–30% of the gliomas in the cerebral hemispheres. In the cerebellum, they make up about 30% of the gliomas in children. In general, males are more commonly affected than females.

Certain types of astrocytoma may be associated with malformative or dysgenetic conditions: i.e., pilocytic astrocytomas of the third ventricle and of the anterior optic structures with neurofibromatosis (NF) type 1, subependymal giant-cell astrocytomas with tuberous sclerosis, and spinal cord astrocytomas with syringomyelia. In addition, certain of the specific varieties may be associated with certain more characteristic locations within the CNS. These will be indicated as each type is discussed.

Well-differentiated (protoplasmic and fibrillary) astrocytomas

Protoplasmic astrocytomas

This variety, in its pure form, constitutes one of the rare histologic types and, in the intracranial compartment, is largely restricted to the cerebrum. In cerebellar astrocytomas and in the pilocytic astrocytomas of juvenile type in other locations, protoplasmic astrocytes may be numerous, but they do not dominate the histologic picture. Foci of protoplasmic astrocytoma may also occasionally be seen in diffuse cerebral astrocytomas that are largely fibrillary. Scherer (1940a) found that, in many cerebral astrocytomas, the cortical parts were nonfibrillary, whereas fibrils were plentiful in the deeper tissues.

Incidence

According to Zülch (1957) and to Prayson and Estes (1995), the temporal and frontal lobes are the most frequent sites. Examples may also originate in the spinal cord (Russell and Rubinstein, 1989, p. 100). They are most often found in children and young adults (Prayson and Estes, 1995). In this same series, covering a 23-year period, protoplasmic astrocytomas constituted just 5.2% of all low-grade astrocytomas. In most cases, a protracted clinical history with years of epileptic seizures is documented and suggests that the tumor is slowly growing.

Macroscopic appearance

In the cerebrum, protoplasmic astrocytomas are superficial, producing a soft gray expansion of the affected cortex. The cut surfaces reveal variable degrees of involvement of the subjacent white matter by tissue of soft semitranslucent homogeneous appearance and rather gelatinous texture. The borders are poorly defined. Degenerative changes are prone to occur as well as cyst formation. The cysts may be numerous and very small, producing a honeycombed appearance; occasionally, a large cyst replaces much of the tumor.

Microscopic appearance

The better preserved parts of the tumor are composed of evenly distributed cells separated by a considerable amount of eosinophilic matrix that resembles a fine cobweb (Fig. 9.5) but is devoid of glial fibrils. The individual tumor cells correspond

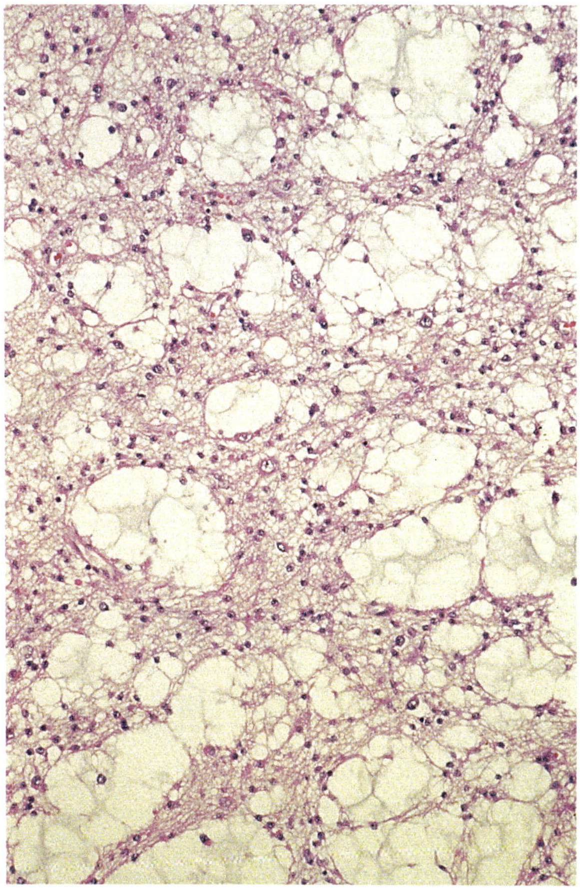

Fig. 9.5 Protoplasmic astrocytoma showing microcystic degeneration. H&E, × 125

to protoplasmic astrocytes (Fig. 9.6), but their processes may be fewer, shorter and sometimes less extensively branched than those of normal cells. In some examples, areas show trapped normal neurons or a mild degree of vascular proliferation. Immunoreactivity for GFAP is sparse and weak in most of the tumors. Microcyst formation is characteristic, especially in the cortical parts of the tumor. In general, the clinical behavior is that of a low-grade astrocytoma (Prayson and Estes, 1995). If features of anaplasia, such as nuclear pleomorphism, mitotic activity or coagulative tumor necrosis, are found, the tumor should be classified as an anaplastic astrocytoma or glioblastoma.

The superficial leptomeninges may rarely be invaded by tumor growth. The tumor seldom disseminates, but Rubinstein (Russell and Rubinstein, 1989, p. 101) noted three examples that developed extensive cerebrospinal spread.

Observations on the fine structure of this tumor are rare. Duffell *et al.* (1963) illustrate an example

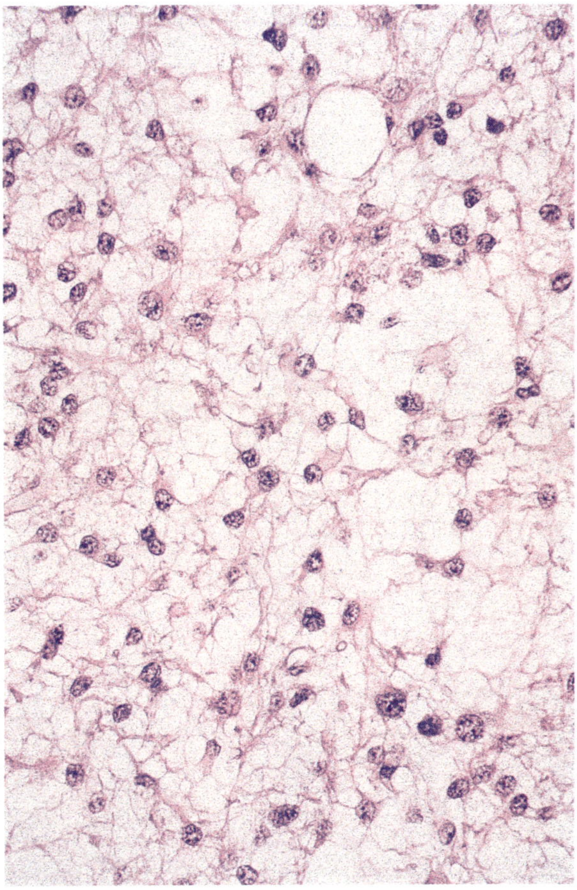

Fig. 9.6 Higher magnification from another case of protoplasmic astrocytoma to show details of tumor cells. H&E, × 500

in which the plasma membrane is disposed into broad processes and from which intracytoplasmic filaments are absent. They stress, however, the frequency of transitional forms between protoplasmic and fibrillary tumor astrocytes.

Fibrillary astrocytomas

The diffuse forms of fibrillary astrocytoma are most often encountered in the cerebral hemispheres of adults and in the brainstem in children and adolescents; in the cerebellum, diffuse fibrillary astrocytomas are more commonly seen in young and middle-aged adults. By contrast, the circumscribed or noninfiltrative forms of astrocytoma are characteristically found in the cerebellum and in the diencephalic region of young subjects, with only relatively occasional involvement of one of the cerebral lobes.

Macroscopic appearance

The tumor may arise in any part of either hemisphere, but the occipital lobes are relatively spared, as confirmed by the figures of McKeran and Thomas (1980, pp. 94–5). The growth may be deeply seated (Fig. 9.7), involving such structures as the corpus callosum, septum pellucidum and basal ganglia. In these examples, there is often neoplastic spread into both hemispheres. These differ from the protoplasmic astrocytomas in their more extensive production of glial fibrils by the tumor cells. In proportion to this character the tumor acquires firmness; it may even be tough and rubbery. In conjunction with this, the appearance

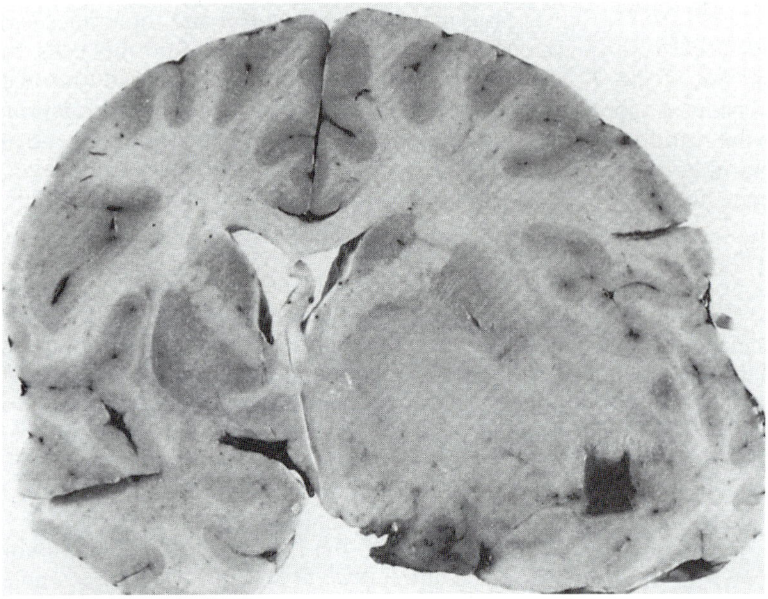

Fig. 9.7 Diffuse cerebral astrocytoma infiltrating the basal ganglia and temporal lobe. Note the herniation and pressure necrosis of the uncinate region. (Courtesy of Dr P.C. Blumbergs)

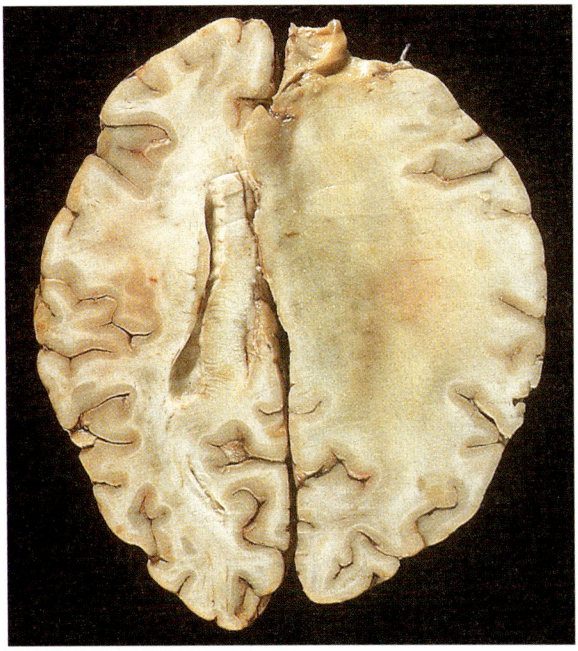

Fig. 9.8 Diffuse fibrillary astrocytoma infiltrating the right cerebral hemisphere and the corpus callosum. Note the segmental loss of distinction of the boundary between the gray and the white matter in the right frontal region.

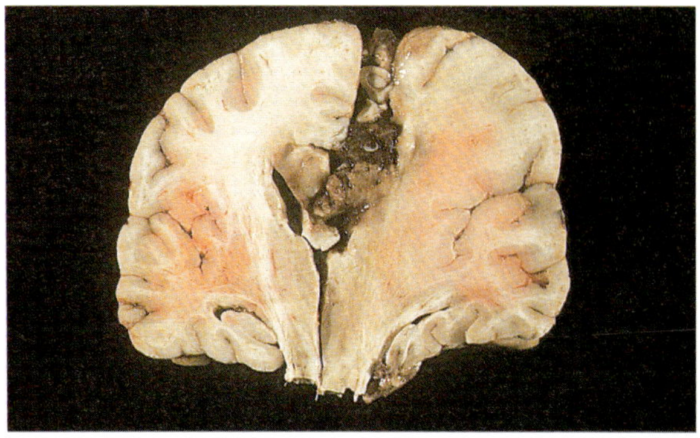

Fig. 9.9 Anaplastic astrocytoma involving the corpus callosum. An area of recent hemorrhage is shown superior to the tumor.

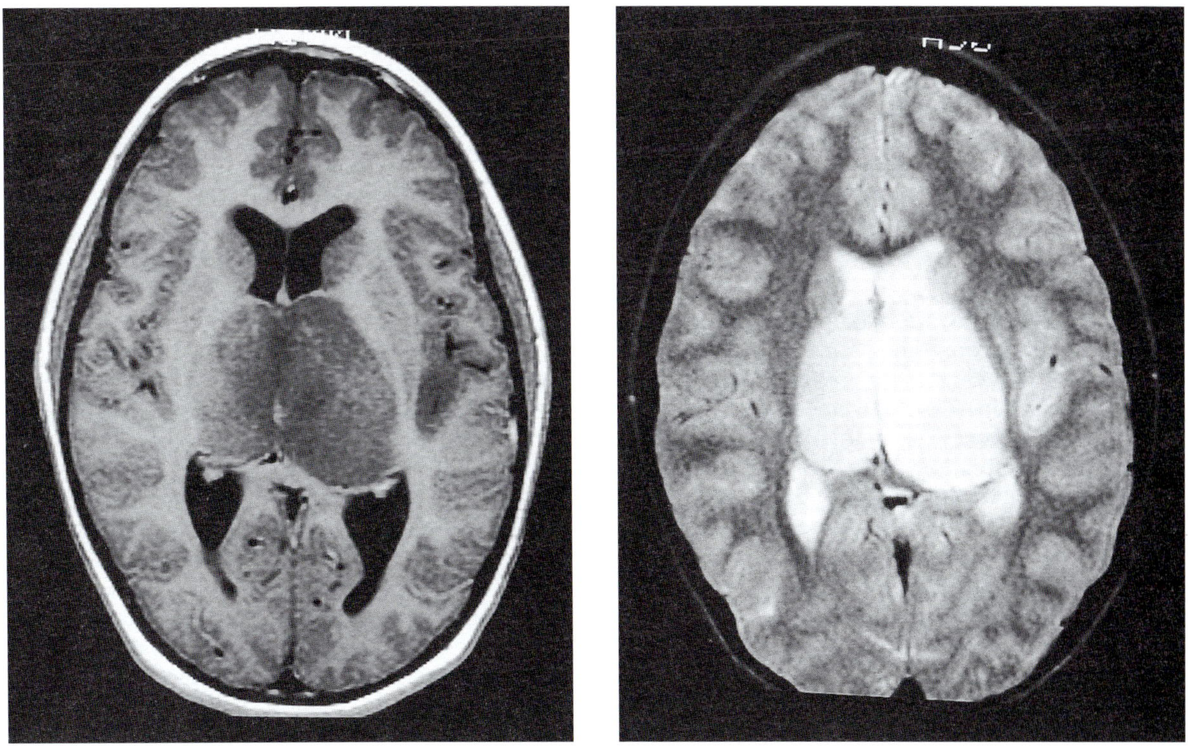

a b

Fig. 9.10 Two MRIs of an 8-year-old girl. (a) Axial T1-weighted postcontrast MRI demonstrates abnormal T1 signal intensity involving the thalami, more so on the left side. There is enlargement and mass effect with marked decrease in signal intensity. No abnormal enhancement is noted. (b) Axial T2-weighted image demonstrates marked abnormal T2 signal intensity of the bithalamic mass. This case represents a well-differentiated astrocytoma. The more well-defined margins, lack of adjacent edema and lack of contrast enhancement favor a lower-grade astrocytoma.

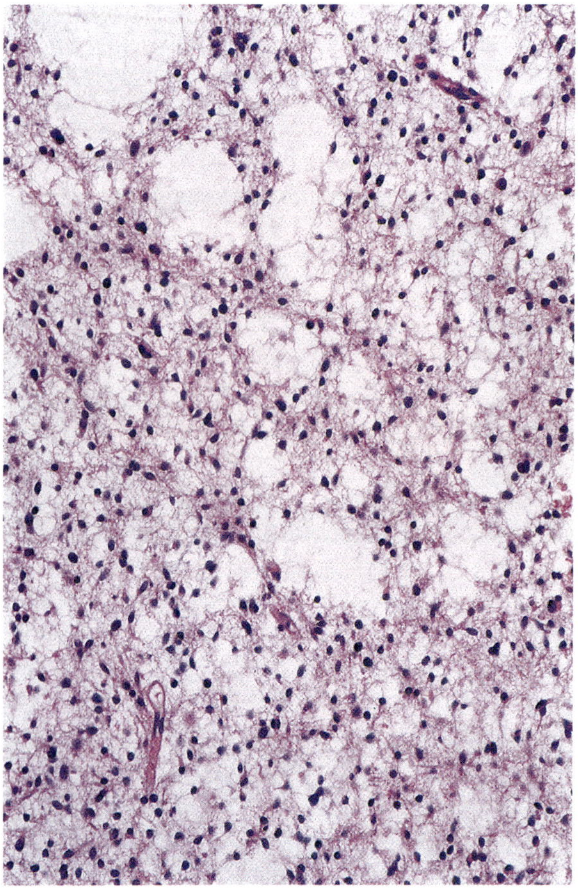

Fig. 9.11 Fibrillary astrocytoma showing early microcystic degeneration. H&E, × 250

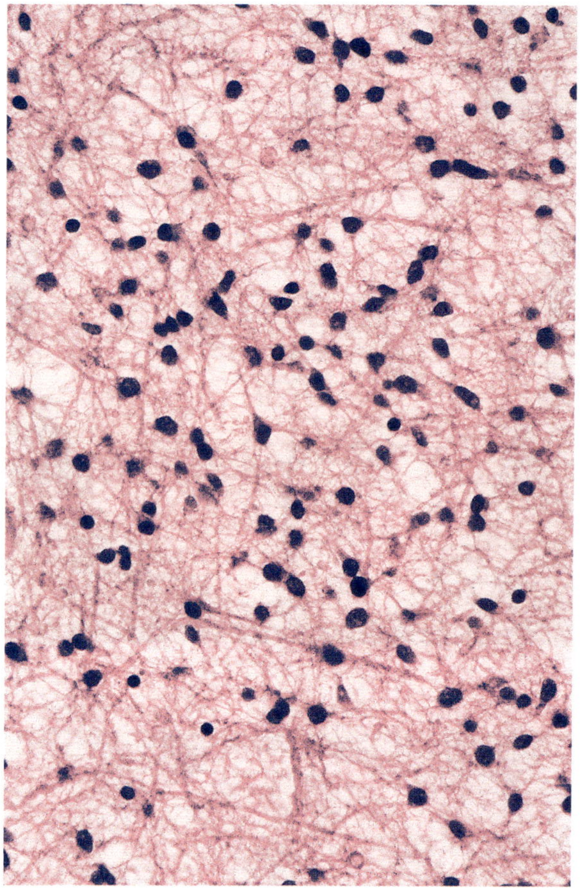

Fig. 9.12 Well-differentiated fibrillary astrocytoma without microcystic change. H&E, × 500

of the cut surfaces is whiter, and it is difficult to distinguish tumor from the adjacent white matter (Fig. 9.8). However, the appearance of expansion combined with increased firmness is diagnostic. The adjacent cortex, where infiltrated, is paler and thicker; its demarcation from the subjacent white matter is characteristically blurred (Figs 9.8 and 9.9). Cysts of variable size may be encountered in the central parts, but are inconstant. The tumor is usually solid, but macroscopic cysts are sometimes present. Because the fibrillary variety is the most common form, the texture is generally uniformly firm or tough, and the appearances of the cut surfaces are very like those of the white matter as a whole (Figs 9.8 and 9.9). Grayer and more granular areas, possibly accompanied by necrosis and hemorrhage, are not uncommon due to the frequency with which anaplasia occurs.

Radiographic appearance

Low-grade astrocytomas have features that tend to be more homogeneous than glioblastomas. Often there is no enhancement; if enhancement is present, it tends to be mild or more homogeneous.

Fibrillary astrocytomas typically represent most of the low-grade astrocytomas that are imaged. These tumors may infiltrate the brain and have ill-defined margins, or they may be relatively focal masses (Fig. 9.10). The more infiltrating lesions are hypodense on computed tomography (CT) scans and typically do not enhance. Calcifications may be seen in up to 20% of cases. There is frequently very little edema around the mass. These tumors may extend across the corpus callosum. Upon magnetic resonance imaging (MRI), the more infiltrating type of fibrillary tumor demonstrates mildly decreased T1 signal intensity and more prominent abnormal T2 signal intensity.

Fibrillary astrocytomas that are more focal have more well-defined low T1 signal and high T2 signal intensity on MRI. At CT scanning, they frequently are hypodense; though these masses most commonly do not enhance. Mild enhancement may be seen in up to 40% of cases.

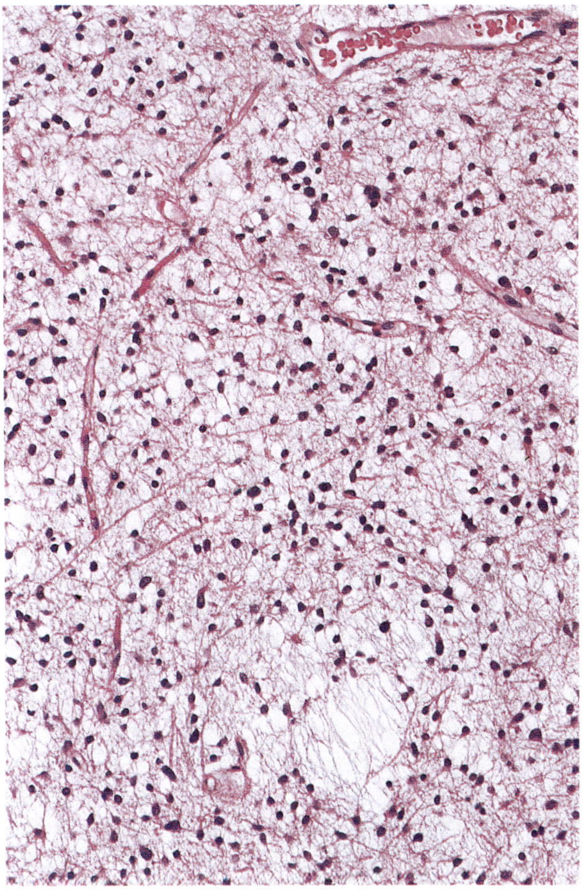

Fig. 9.13 Well-differentiated astrocytoma with delicate capillary vasculature and no endothelial cell proliferation. H&E, × 250

Microscopic appearance

Microscopically, the picture is that of diffuse replacement of the cerebral tissue by neoplastic cells in which there is variable participation of small and large astrocytic types, stellate or pilocytic, either randomly dispersed or arranged in small or larger groups. This morphologic diversity reflects the cellular heterogeneity that, even in the absence of anaplasia, is a common feature in astrocytomas in general. Fine and coarse neuroglial fibrils occupy the matrix and form a criss-cross arrangement between the cells from which they are derived (Fig. 9.11). They are of considerable length and can sometimes be traced over a number of low-power fields. The cell bodies are dispersed unevenly and may vary considerably in shape and size.

In some tumors, the cellular distribution is more uniform, without microcysts, and this type of diffuse cerebral astrocytoma is well recognized (Fig. 9.12). Here, the cells are of simple form, rounded, triangular or fusiform, and their fibrils are of relatively fine caliber. When the cortex is infiltrated, it is common to find a subpial zone in which the cell bodies are more densely collected than elsewhere.

The tougher and therefore more densely fibrillary examples usually have cell bodies of larger size, and these are more characteristically stellate, although simpler variants are also found. Mitoses are absent, and the nuclei, although variable in size, are otherwise consistent in their round or oval shape and in their chromatin content.

The infiltrated tissues are usually well preserved: the pre-existing neurons are evenly separated where the astrocytoma occupies the cortex, and the myelinated nerve fiber tracts are forced apart when the tumor is situated in the white matter. The blood vessels share in this process; they usually exhibit little or no proliferative activity (Fig. 9.13).

Degenerative changes, with the formation of microcysts, are frequent (Fig. 9.10): this entails a corkscrew-like deformation of the fibrils in the tumor matrix, following which they ultimately break up. Calcification may occasionally be present, its early stages being sometimes demonstrable in the walls of the capillary blood vessels.

When fibrillary astrocytomas infiltrate the nerve tracts, there is a tendency for the tumor cells to adapt themselves to their environment. They become elongated bipolar cells with oval nuclei, and the fibrils likewise lie in parallel rows (e.g., see Fig. 9.290). This pilocytic appearance is, therefore, a secondary change imposed upon the tumor elements and is well seen in astrocytomas infiltrating the corpus callosum, the internal capsule, the cerebral peduncles and the pontine tracts.

Electron microscopy

Numerous observations on this type of tumor (Luse, 1960; Raimondi, Mullan and Evans, 1962; Duffell *et al.*, 1963; Raimondi, 1967; Hossmann and Wechsler, 1971; Scheithauer and Bruner, 1987) have stressed the variations in cell outline, but agree on the characteristic presence of conspicuous bundles of intermediate filaments ranging from 7 to 11 nm in diameter, which occupy the perikaryon and especially the cell processes (Fig. 9.14). Free ribosomes, rough and smooth endoplasmic reticulum, lamellar mitochondria and dense bodies are all observed. Some examples may exhibit a greater volume of extracellular space variably filled with flocculent material, the ultrastructural correlate of the frequent microcysts observed by light microscopy (Fig. 9.15) (Scheithauer and Bruner, 1987). The architectural complexity of the tumor resulting from the network of numerous long, radiating and branching cell processes is evocatively brought to light by scanning electron microscopy (Fig. 9.16).

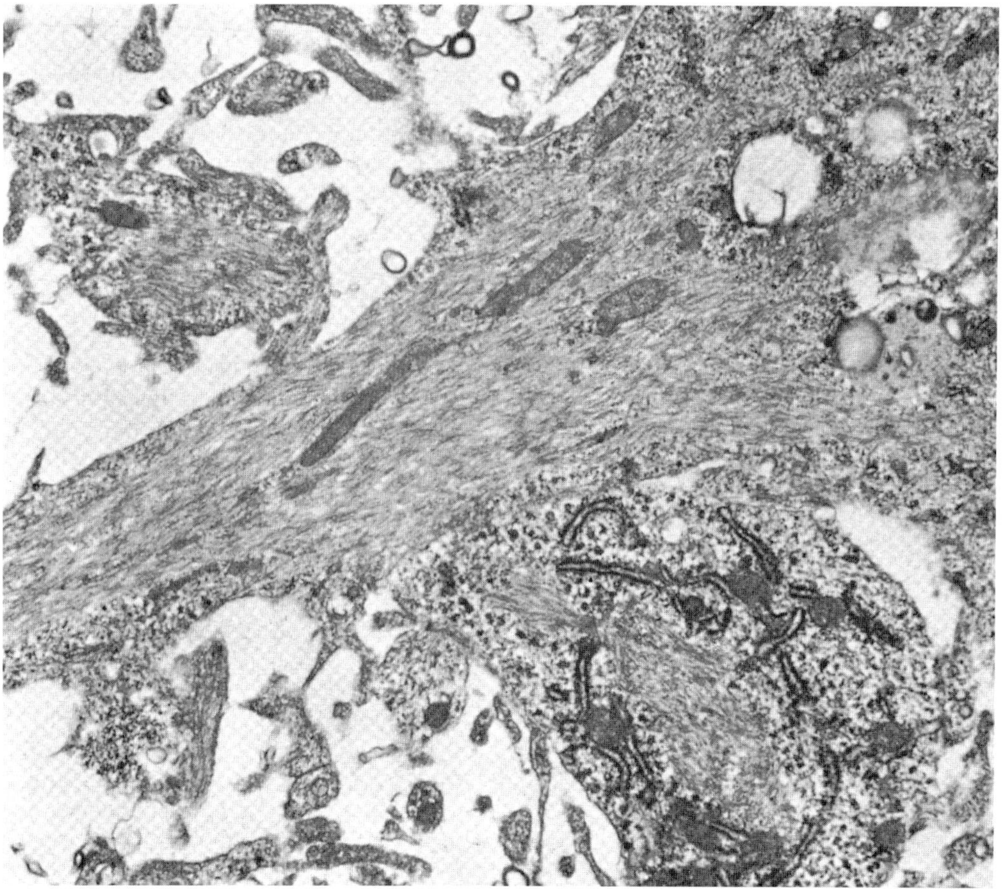

Fig. 9.14 Cerebellar astrocytoma maintained in organ culture for 29 days. Glial filaments form compact bundles in tumor cell processes and are associated with increased granular endoplasmic reticulum and free ribosomes (lower right). × 15 000 (In collaboration with Dr J.C. Sipe and Dr Mary M. Herman and reprinted from the *American Journal of Pathology*, 1973, figure 8, pp. 588–606, with kind permission of the American Society for Investigative Pathology.)

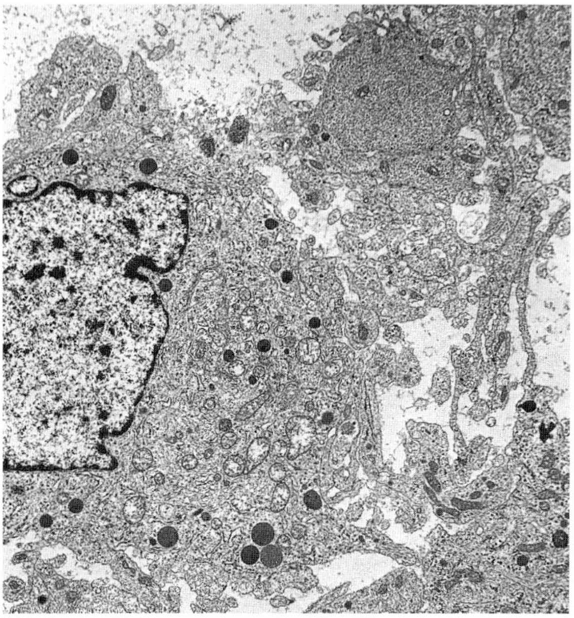

Fig. 9.15 Microcystic astrocytoma with flocculent material surrounding a neoplastic astrocyte that formed part of the lining of a microcyst. × 1500 (mag. to negative)

Immunohistochemistry

The immunopositivity of neoplastic astrocytes for GFAP has been extensively documented, with the agreed observation that it is roughly commensurate with the state of differentiation of the tumor cells (Eng and Rubinstein, 1978; van der Meulen, Houthoff and Ebels, 1978; Velasco *et al.*, 1980) (Fig. 9.17). It has been shown that the amount of GFAP mRNA expression and immunoreactivity in the SF-126 astrocytoma cell line stably transfected with GFAP cDNA correlates inversely with astrocytoma proliferation and growth in soft agar, two properties indicating increased malignancy (Rutka and Smith, 1993). Astrocytomas have also been shown

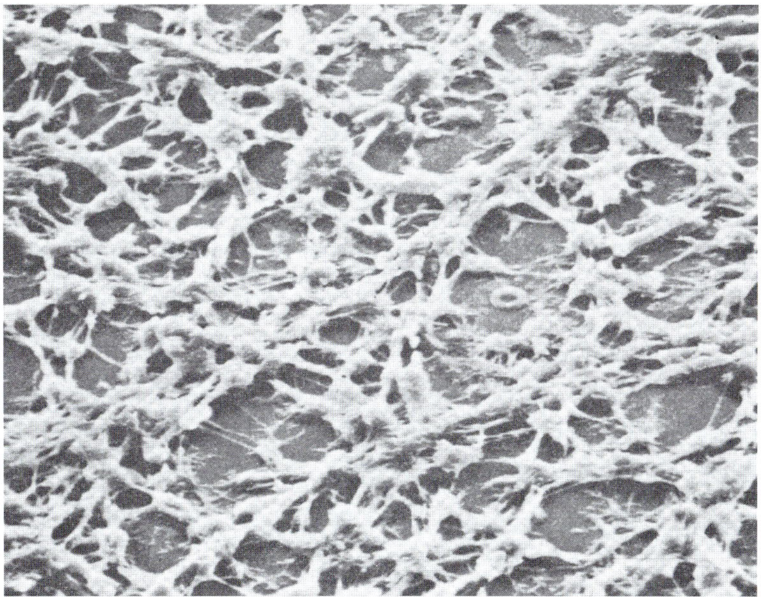

Fig. 9.16 Low-power scanning electron micrograph of astrocytic tumor cells demonstrating the network formed by innumerable radiating and branching cell processes. × 600 (Courtesy of Dr A. Arnold)

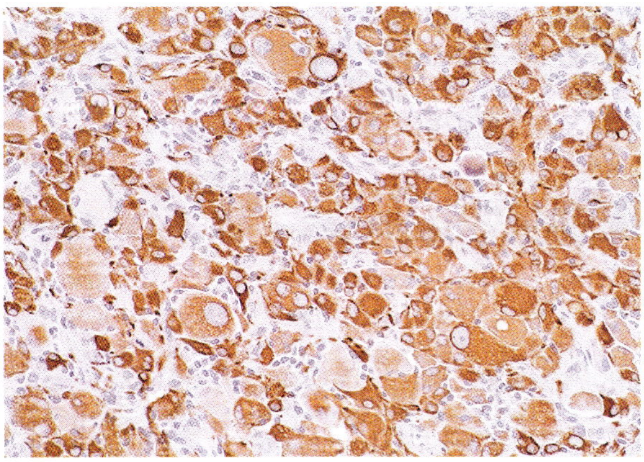

Fig. 9.17 Immunoperoxidase stain for GFAP showing strong reactivity in the cytoplasm of neoplastic astrocytes in this glioblastoma multiforme. GFAP immunoperoxidase and hematoxylin, × 250

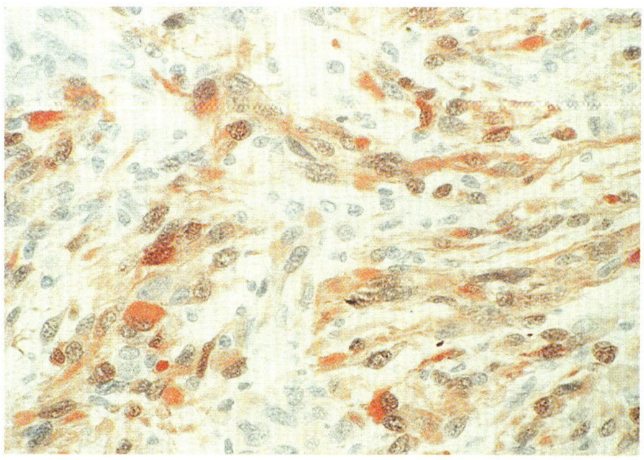

Fig. 9.18 Immunoperoxidase for S-100 protein showing both nuclear and cytoplasmic reactivity in neoplastic astrocytes of this cerebellar astrocytoma. S-100 immunoperoxidase and hematoxylin, × 325

to be immunopositive for glutamine synthetase (Pilkington and Lantos, 1982), with the enzyme better demonstrated in the poorly fibrillated cells and less clearly in the cell processes. The aldolase C isoenzyme, which normally is found chiefly in the brain, has also been localized in the better differentiated astrocytomas (Kumanishi, Watabe and Washiyama, 1985). Other proteins that have been demonstrated by immunoperoxidase in a large proportion of astrocytomas include the S-100 protein (Fig. 9.18) (Tabuchi *et al.*, 1982; Nakamura, Becker and Marks, 1983; Kimura, Budka and Soler-Federsppiel, 1986) and vimentin (Yung, Luna and Borit, 1985; Herpers *et al.*, 1986; Schiffer *et al.*, 1986), but their diagnostic specificity cannot be compared to that of GFAP. Most astrocytomas show a similar pattern of reactivity for S-100 protein and GFAP (Nakapoulou *et al.*, 1990). The expression of vimentin does not seem to correlate with either immaturity or anaplasia of the astrocytic

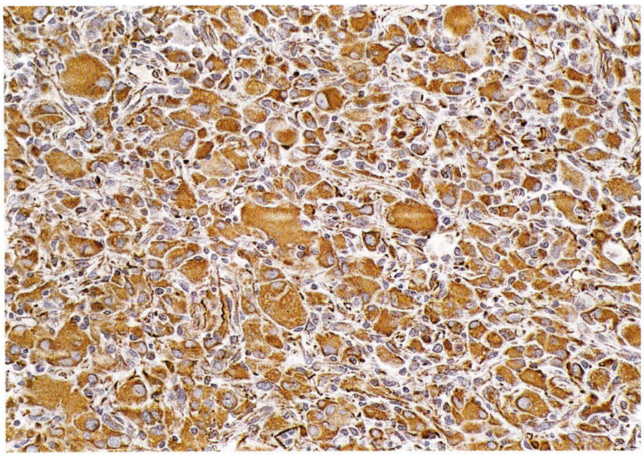

Fig. 9.19 Same case as Fig 9.17. Immunoperoxidase for vimentin, which is strongly reactive in the cytoplasm of the neoplastic astrocytes of a glioblastoma multiforme. Vimentin immunoperoxidase and hematoxylin, × 250

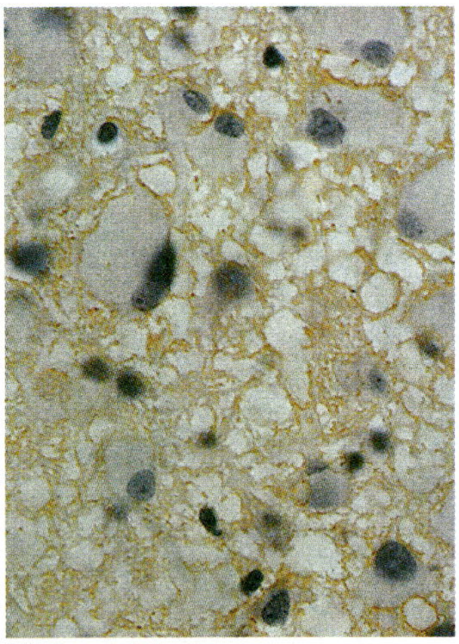

Fig. 9.20 Immunoperoxidase for Leu 7 showing labeling of the cytoplasmic membranes of the astrocytes of this gemistocytic astrocytoma. Leu 7 immunoperoxidase, × 400

cells (Fig. 9.19) (Nakapoulou *et al.*, 1990). According to Herpers *et al.* (1986), it is localized in a more juxtanuclear position, in contrast to GFAP, which is characteristically more intense in the cell processes. Astrocytic tumor cells are often immunopositive with the anti-Leu 7 monoclonal antibody (MAb), which typically stains the outer cytoplasmic membranes (Perentes and Rubinstein, 1986) (Fig. 9.20). This antigen, too, is neither specifically nor exclusively expressed by astrocytes or astrocytoma cells.

Kinetic aspects

The kinetic data on low-grade astrocytomas obtained from ^{3}H-thymidine labeling *in vitro* and *in vivo* have been collated by Steel (1980) and indicate a spread of labeling indices (LIs) ranging from 0.44% to 2%, with a mean of 1.27%. Flow cytometry studies designed to measure the DNA contents in single cells (Hoshino *et al.*, 1978; Lehmann and Krug, 1980; Fitzgibbons *et al.*, 1988; Salmon and Kiss, 1993; Salmon *et al.*, 1993) have not so far provided information on cellular malignancy that supersedes the information from histologic analyses. On the other hand, the labeling of the S phase by immunohistochemistry using a MAb against bromodeoxyuridine (BrdU), discussed more fully in the section on glioblastomas (p. 446), carries the notable advantage of permitting the proliferation potential of a tumor *in situ* to be estimated within 1 or 2 days after its resection. As detailed in the reports from Hoshino's group (Nagashima *et al.*, 1985; Hoshino *et al.*, 1986; Murovic *et al.*, 1986; Hoshino *et al.*, 1993; Ito *et al.*, 1994), the LI obtained in this manner correlates well with the data available from ^{3}H-thymidine autoradiography, with the more benign astrocytomas having an LI of less than 1%. Few studies are yet available for correlation of MIB-1 LIs with survival in low-grade astrocytomas and the significance of the LIs is conflicting (Coons and Johnson, 1996; Giannini *et al.*, 1996).

Anaplastic astrocytomas

It has been shown that most variants of astrocytoma are capable of histologic and biologic progression to a malignant phase, but this capacity is not uniform. Thus, the anaplastic propensities of the diffuse cerebral astrocytomas of adults and of the diffuse brainstem astrocytomas of young patients are well known, but the majority of the cerebellar astrocytomas in children and of the pilocytic astrocytomas of juvenile type in various other locations seldom exhibit this tendency.

The age-related incidence of anaplastic astrocytomas differs from that of glioblastomas. In the large series reviewed by McKeran and Thomas (1980, pp. 94–5), of almost exclusively supratentorial gliomas from the National Hospitals for Nervous Diseases, the mean age of patients when first seen ranged from 37 years for the well-differentiated astrocytomas to 52 years for the least differentiated. Likewise, in their review of 1440 patients with cerebral glioblastomas and anaplastic astrocytomas, Burger *et al.* (1985) found that the mean age incidence in anaplastic astrocytoma was 10 years younger than for glioblastoma.

Incidence of anaplastic change in astrocytomas

The systematic anatomic studies of Scherer, who emphasized the necessity of examining the whole extent of the cerebral astrocytomas, have been paramount in recognizing the anaplastic proclivities of these tumors. He found evidence of anaplasia in 13/18 examples investigated by making complete sections of the hemispheres (Scherer, 1940a). As repeatedly confirmed since, it was often the deeper parts of the tumor that showed malignant features. This may be obvious to the naked eye or may be demonstrable only by microscopy.

With the objective of independently assessing the histologic incidence of anaplasia, Rubinstein (Russell and Rubinstein, 1989, p. 126) reviewed a series of 55 gliomas that arose in various parts of the brain, were obtained at necropsy over a period of 10 years (1946–55) and had already been diagnosed as astrocytoma. In 29 cases (53%), anaplastic changes were found. This analysis can be compared with that of 129 cases originally diagnosed as glioblastomas (Russell and Rubinstein, 1989, p. 225). In the first series, 6 cases had proceeded to focal glioblastoma, whereas in the second, at least 28 were identified as astrocytomas progressing to glioblastoma, while an additional 15 were recognized as anaplastic astrocytomas.

When both series were pooled and analyzed together, it was found that, of a total of 98 astrocytomas, 72 cases (73%) had features of anaplasia, while nearly half (34 cases) of the latter had progressed to frank glioblastoma. If the cerebral group alone was assessed, the number of diffuse cerebral astrocytomas in which microscopic evidence of anaplasia was lacking was only 10 cases out of a total of 243 intracranial gliomas. This figure agrees remarkably closely with Scherer's estimate of five microscopically benign astrocytomas in his series of 125 gliomas.

A discriminating analysis of the different histologic types is important when evaluating the incidence of anaplasia in astrocytomas. A simple numeric grading of their general cytologic features carries limitations because, as is detailed elsewhere, there are distinct differences in the biologic behavior of different types of cerebral astrocytoma; it is particularly in the diffusely infiltrating fibrillary astrocytoma that anaplasia is to be anticipated. The data reported by Laws *et al.* (1984) on the incidence and postoperative patient survival lengths for low-grade astrocytomas of the cerebral hemispheres, while informative within the limited context of a cellular grading system, do not provide the information that permits an analysis of their cases according to their histologic pattern. Where this criterion has been observed, the high frequency of malignant change in the diffuse forms of cerebral astrocytomas has been confirmed. In a study of cerebral astrocytomas in adults treated at the Washington University School of Medicine, Garcia, Fulling and Marks (1985) found only eight well-differentiated examples as compared with 78 anaplastic astrocytomas. Of these eight cases, six were of the juvenile pilocytic type. Thus, only two of their patients had well-differentiated diffuse astrocytomas, and autopsy examination in one patient disclosed a large tumor with foci of marked anaplasia 8 months after diagnosis. In a series of 35 adult patients with low-grade cerebral astrocytomas of nonpilocytic type, all treated with external beam radiotherapy, six cases (17%) developed tumor progression and died. Median survival in this series was 9.8 years (Lunsford *et al.*, 1995).

Time factors in the evolution of anaplasia

The incidence and timing of the conversion of a diffuse cerebral astrocytoma with a low degree of malignancy into an anaplastic astrocytoma or a glioblastoma, while to be anticipated, are impossible to predict in the individual case. Information of a general nature can, however, be gained from neurosurgical series dealing with the incidence and histologic features of recurrences in cerebral astrocytomas. Of the 79 recurrent low-grade tumors reviewed by Laws *et al.* (1984), about half had converted to a higher grade of malignancy (grades 3 or 4), but this development, as already noted, was not correlated with the histologic tumor type. In their survey of 137 examples, Müller, Afra and Schröder (1977a) concluded that an increase of malignancy was to be expected in approximately two thirds of the patients. Since their series was based largely on biopsy material, it is possible that their estimate minimizes the frequency of such an occurrence. Moreover, as brought to light by the clinicopathologic analysis of Müller, Afra and Schröder, already referred to, there was no statistically significant relationship between the time interval preceding clinical recurrence and the demonstration of increased malignancy on subsequent histologic examination. Rather, the incidence and the speed of clinical recurrence remained primarily dependent on the original nature of the astrocytoma at the time of its initial surgical sampling. In the study of Soffietti *et al.* (1989), recurrences were histologically proved in 24/85 adults (28%) with cerebral well-differentiated astrocytomas. Of these, 19 had progressed to anaplastic astrocytoma or glioblastoma, usually from 1 to 5 years after the initial diagnosis. A similar 5-year interval was seen by Vertosick, Selker and Arena (1991), with 7/25

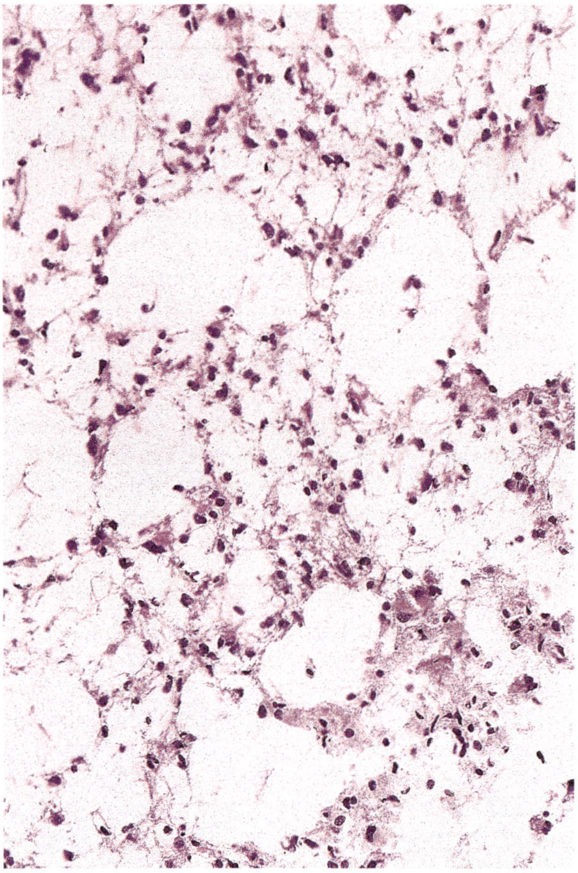

a

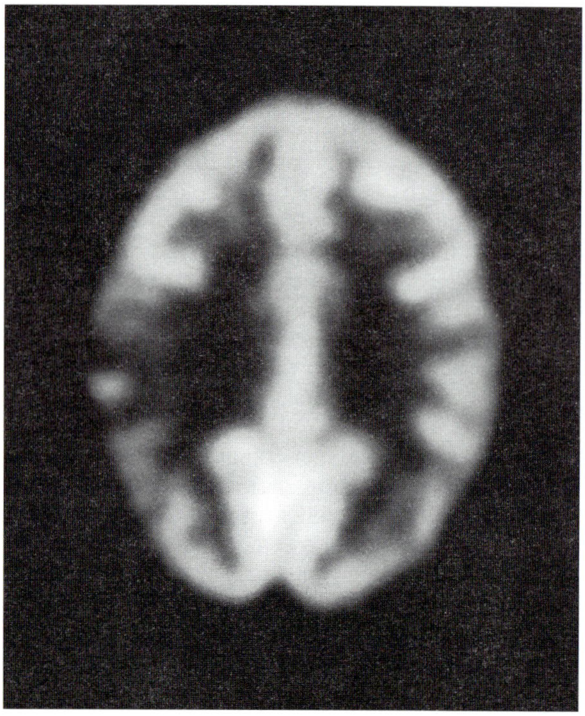

c

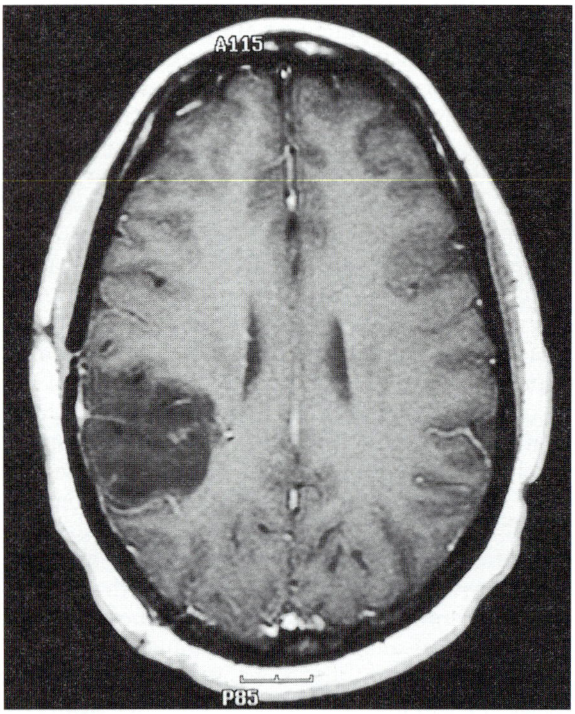

b

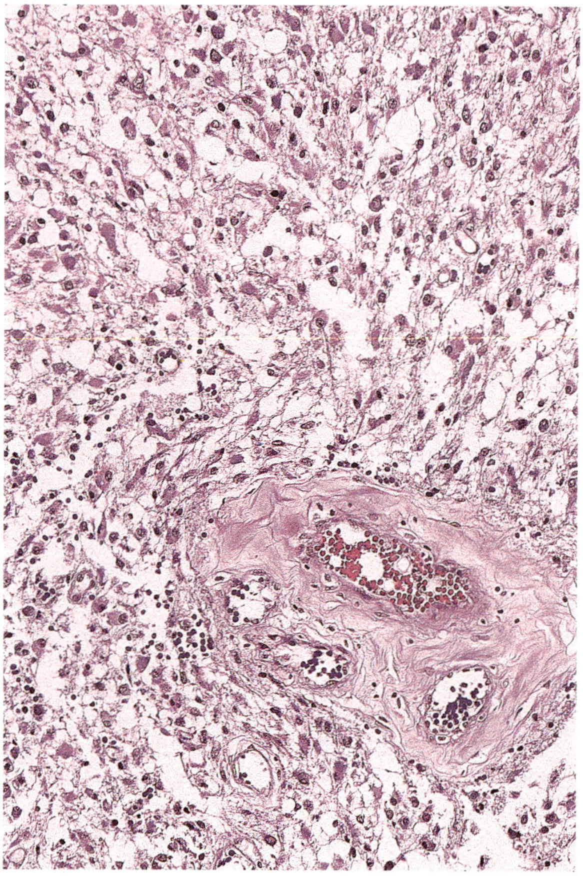

d

patients (28%) showing malignant progression, and by McCormack *et al.* (1992). In McCormack's series, there was radiologic evidence of recurrence with features of higher-grade astrocytoma in 24/41 patients (58.5%) who had an initial surgical resection. In the series of Philippon *et al.* (1993), 18/25 patients (72%) who were biopsied after recurrence of a low-grade astrocytoma showed malignant histologic features. The total number of patients in this last series was 179. This points to unpredictable variations in the incidence and chronologic evolution of anaplasia in cerebral astrocytomas.

Macroscopic appearance

Evidence of anaplasia is manifest where the smooth, homogeneous texture and color of an astrocytoma is replaced by more friable, granular, gray tumor tissue with areas of necrosis and hemorrhage (Figs 9.8 and 9.9). The regional blood vessels may be visibly increased in both number and size. In some cerebral tumors, more than one large area of anaplasia may arise; an initial impression of multifocal glioblastomas may be created, especially when the intervening tissue is macroscopically indistinguishable from normal brain. Microscopic examination may prove that the apparently distinct foci are linked by infiltrating tumor cells. An example of anaplastic change over time is demonstrated in Fig. 9.21.

Finally, the anaplastic foci may be very small and disseminated. These are apt to be perivascular and are sometimes recognizable by their softer and more granular texture and by a pinker color than that of the surrounding tumor.

Fig. 9.21 An example of anaplastic change over time. (a) This patient was diagnosed with a biopsy-proven, low-grade astrocytoma and was followed, without treatment, for 4.5 years before a subtle increase in her symptoms was noticed. H&E, × 66 (b) A follow-up MRI was unchanged from prior scans. (c) An 18-fluoro-deoxyglucose-positron emission tomography (FDG-PET) scan showed a small hypermetabolic focus within a larger region of hypometabolism in the right parietal lobe, suggesting a small region of anaplasia in the larger low-grade tumor. (d) A subsequent biopsy in the region of the FDG-PET 'hot spot' showed anaplastic astrocytoma. H&E, × 100

Radiographic appearance

The radiologic findings of this tumor lie between the more benign-appearing, well-differentiated astrocytoma and the more aggressive glioblastoma multiforme. At CT scanning, the mass is frequently of mixed density, most commonly hypodense. There is usually irregular enhancement, which may be ring-like with a thick rim. Cystic areas or hemorrhage may occur, although less frequently than in patients with glioblastoma. On MRI, the masses are most commonly centered in the white matter with low T1 signal intensity and heterogeneous T2 signal intensity (Fig. 9.22). Enhancement is most often seen and is frequently heterogeneous and irregular. Calcification is uncommon. At angiography, the tumors have a variable vascularity.

Microscopic appearance

The histologic features of the anaplastic astrocytoma include increased cellularity, nuclear and cytoplasmic pleomorphism of the tumor cells, the

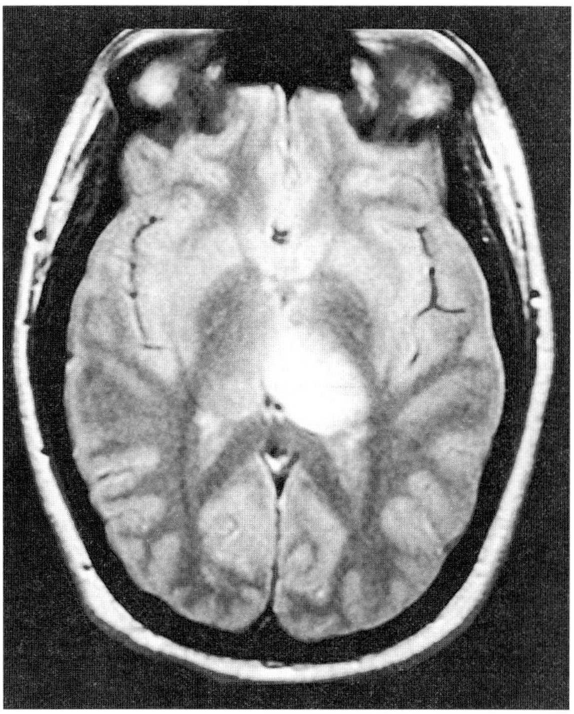

Fig. 9.22 Axial proton density-weighted imaging of a 38-year-old woman with anaplastic astrocytoma. There is abnormal increased T2 signal intensity of the left thalamus. While mass effect is noticed with compression on the third ventricle and internal cerebellar veins, there was no abnormal contrast enhancement in this area. No enhancement was present in this case.

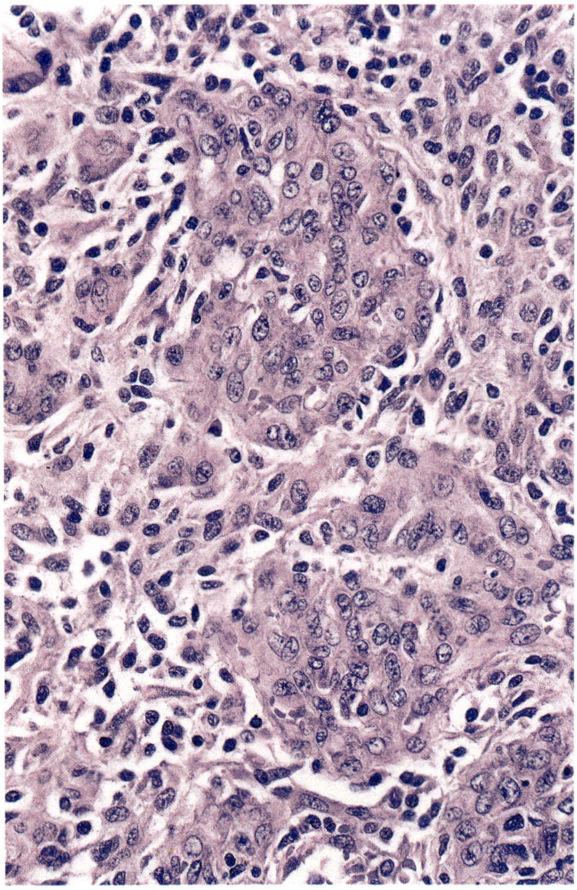

Fig. 9.23 Anaplastic astrocytoma showing glomeruloid vascular proliferation. H&E, × 500

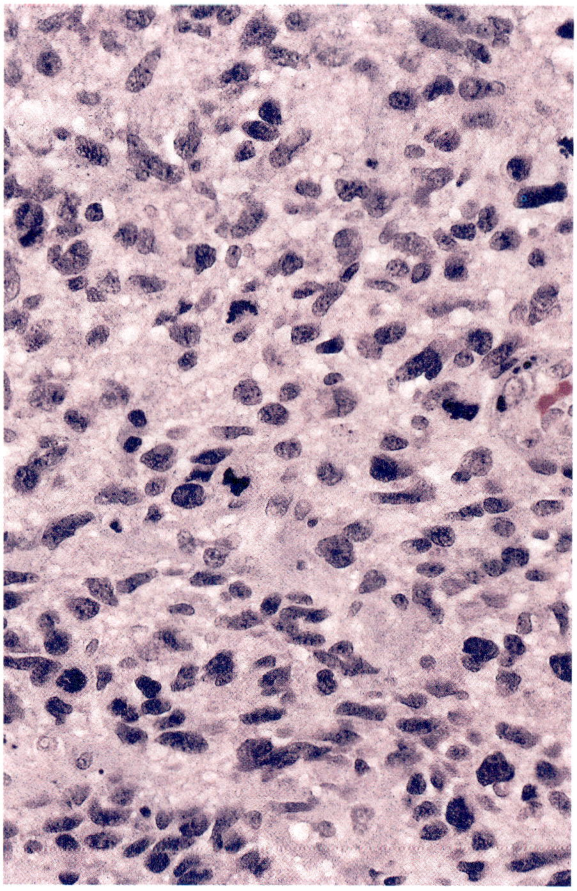

Fig. 9.24 Anaplastic features of dense cellularity, nuclear pleomorphism and abundant mitotic activity in an astrocytoma. H&E. × 500

presence of mitotic figures (some of which may be abnormal) and alterations in the architectural arrangements of the cells (Figs 9.2 and 9.3). These features, as well as the electron microscopic characteristics of anaplastic astrocytoma cells, are dealt with in greater detail in the section on glioblastomas and therefore are not further elaborated here. In fact, the heterogeneity of anaplastic astrocytomas and glioblastomas is a well-known histologic characteristic, and a continuum exists from one to the other in many cases.

It is, however, apparent that some features are of greater prognostic significance than others in the correlations with postoperative survival of the patient. Thus, the presence of microscopic necroses in an astrocytoma with anaplastic foci renders it a glioblastoma (Nelson *et al.*, 1983, 1985). Fulling and Garcia (1985), in an analysis of 78 anaplastic astrocytomas removed from adults, found that no correlation could be established between postoperative patient survival times and cellular density or nuclear pleomorphism. On the other hand, the presence of mitotic figures and of microvascular proliferation was highly significant. Likewise, Burger *et al.* (1985), in their independent review of 175 anaplastic astrocytomas, reported a significant inverse relation between microvascular proliferation and the length of patient survival. It has indeed long been recognized that, in the diffuse astrocytomas, proliferation of the smaller blood vessels (Fig. 9.23) represents an early stage in malignant evolution, commonly associated with other evidence of cytologic anaplasia (Fig. 9.24). Not only are the capillary blood vessels increased in number, but also multiplication of the lining endothelial cells is obvious, and mitosis may be seen. Similar correlates have been reported by Schiffer *et al.* (1988). More recently, the importance of microvascular proliferation and its usual coexistence with foci of necrosis has been re-emphasized (Barker *et al.*, 1996).

In other areas of the tumor, the astrocytic character of the growth is typical. In many examples,

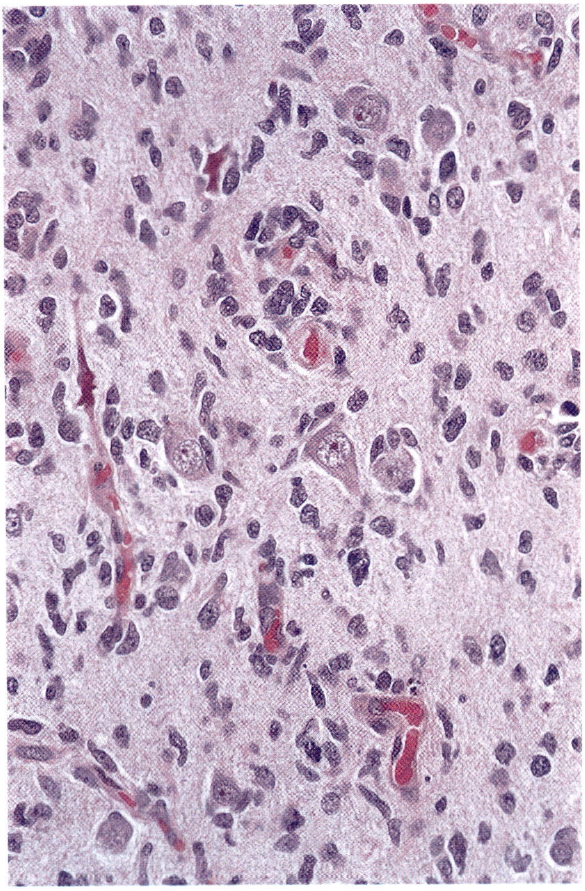

Fig. 9.25 Evidence of tumor invasion of the cerebral cortex, noted as neoplastic satellitosis around cortical neurons. H&E, × 500

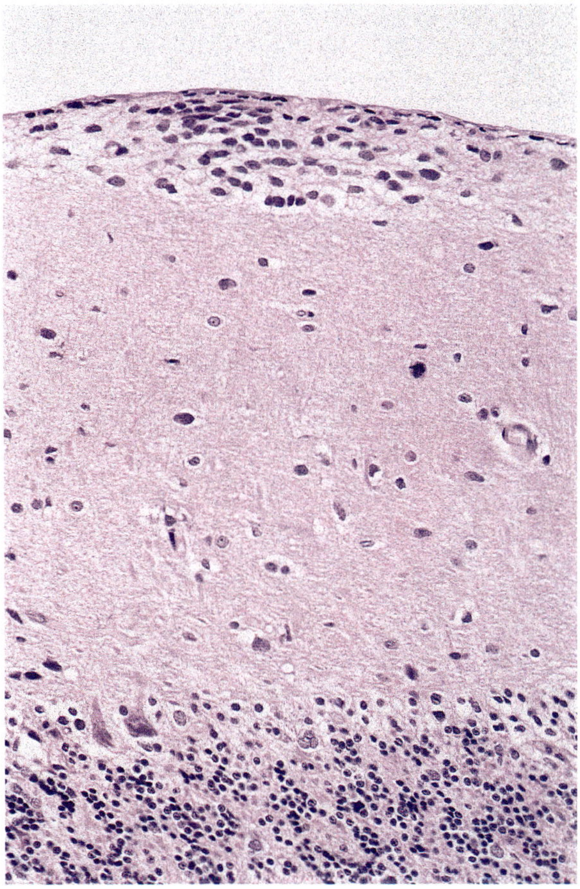

Fig. 9.26 Anaplastic astrocytoma of the cerebellum showing subpial infiltration with neoplastic astrocytes. H&E, × 250

there is evidence of the 'secondary structures' described by Scherer (1938). Details of the latter are given later in this chapter, where the histologic aspects of infiltrating gliomas are described. Although Scherer originally defined his 'secondary structures' as cell patterns determined by the host's tissues, he later (1940a) was clearly of the opinion that 'secondary structures' were confined to malignant astrocytomas. These 'structures' certainly seem to indicate proliferative and infiltrative processes that are manifest beyond the immediate confines of the tumor and are then recognized as foci or zones of increased cellularity. In these diffuse astrocytomas, the focal tumor cell aggregates seen at the interfaces of the neural parenchyma may or may not be positive for GFAP. Scherer's interpretation of these aggregates as evidence of anaplasia has since been repeatedly confirmed, especially the significance to be attached to the subpial zone of the molecular layer, which, in a limited biopsy, may provide a valuable diagnostic clue to the malignant nature of the neoplastic process (see Figs 9.25 and 9.26). On the other hand, within the group of cerebral astrocytomas with anaplastic foci, the presence, by itself, of these 'secondary structures' could not be correlated with shorter survival times of patients (Fulling and Garcia, 1985). These secondary structures are not entirely characteristic of astrocytomas with anaplasia, however, as they are also commonly recognized in infiltrating oligodendrogliomas (see Figs 9.101 and 9.102) (Bruner, 1987).

Focal increases in the density of the cells within the tumor itself, accompanied perhaps by mitotic figures and increased pleomorphism, are certainly indicative of anaplasia. When carefully sought, these distinctive masses of increased cellular density are more often multiple than single. It may be argued that they are the expression of a multicentric progression of anaplasia within the limits of a given neoplastic field, presumably related to the propagation of clonogenic subpopulations. The development of an *in vitro* clonogenic cell assay based on the colony-forming efficiency of astrocytic gliomas was proposed as a first step in the laboratory testing of newly developed cytotoxic and cytostatic agents (Rosenblum *et al.*, 1978); preliminary results suggested that a relatively limited measure of correlation was achieved between sensitivity in culture and patient response (Rosenblum and Gerosa, 1984). In general, this type of *in vitro* test predicts clinical resistance more consistently than clinical sensitivity (Yung, 1989). Because of the small percentage of total tumor cells that grow in culture, such assays may not be predictive of the behavior of tumors. Direct measurement of resistance mechanisms, such as DNA repair enzymes, discussed in Chapter 5, pp. 130–3, may provide more reliable data on susceptibility and resistance to treatment.

Gemistocytic astrocytomas

Gemistocytic astrocytomas are restricted to the cerebral hemispheres (Krouwer *et al.*, 1991) and, as a pure form, are rare. Scherer (1940a) stated that he had seen only one in 18 examples of cerebral astrocytoma. Elvidge and Martinez-Coll (1956) listed 24 gemistocytic astrocytomas in their series of 106 cases of astrocytoma. They were all found in the cerebrum. Since their study was based on biopsy material, it cannot be concluded that their 24 examples were of purely gemistocytic type, for it is commonly found that foci of this character form considerable areas within the diffuse fibrillary cerebral astrocytomas. The series of Krouwer *et al.* (1991) summarized 28 cases in which the diagnosis was confirmed, and concluded that those examples with 20% or more gemistocytes should be considered to be anaplastic astrocytomas, as judged by the characteristically limited patient survival times.

Macroscopic appearance

The typical growth has a gray, almost granular, homogeneous appearance and a soft texture. Its borders are usually relatively circumscribed. Small- or medium-sized cysts may be encountered.

Microscopic appearance

The component cells are exceptionally large and may be fairly closely packed, but the latter feature may vary from field to field. The outlines of the cell bodies are angulated, with relatively short, coarse, fibrillated processes (Fig. 9.27). Often the distension of the cell bodies may be such as to give them an almost globoid appearance. Their cytoplasm is filled with homogeneous hyaline and strongly eosinophilic material, whereas glial fibrils are typically confined to the periphery of the cell bodies and to the cell processes. The cell bodies are intensely positive for GFAP (Fig. 9.28). The tumor cell nuclei are usually eccentric, of variable size, with coarse chromatin nodes and, frequently, relatively conspicuous nucleoli. The amount of intercellular matrix is relatively scanty, but is traversed by coarse glial fibrils. As already noted, there are transitions between this distinctive form and the fibrillary astrocytomas. In these transitional areas, the cells are less bulky, and there is a more abundant fibrillary matrix, which separates the cells rather evenly.

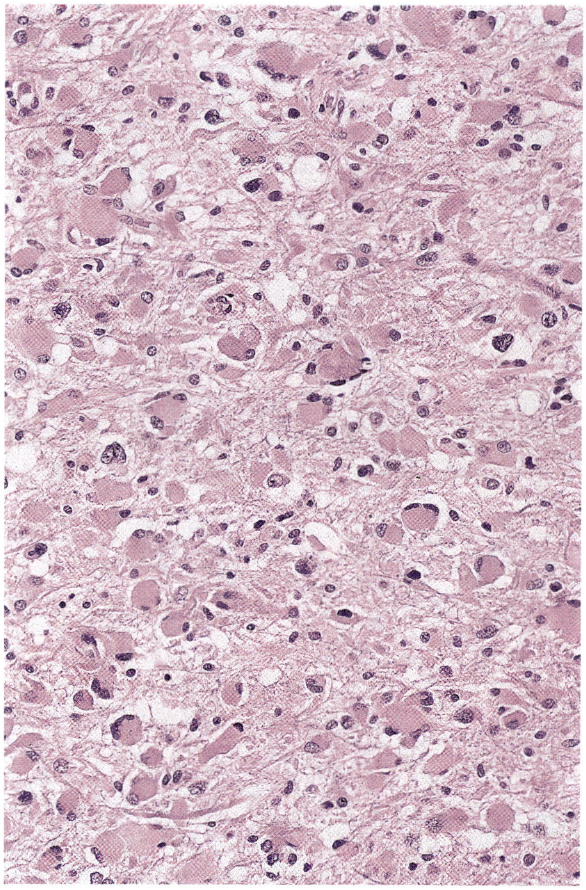

Fig. 9.27 Gemistocytic astrocytoma. H&E, × 250

The significance of this type of neoplastic astrocyte in terms of human glioma kinetics has been provocatively discussed in an autoradiographic study by Hoshino, Wilson and Ellis (1975) on seven patients who were given a single pulse of tritiated thymidine at operation and of whom three had also subsequent autoradiography after death. Surprisingly, despite the biologic malignancy of

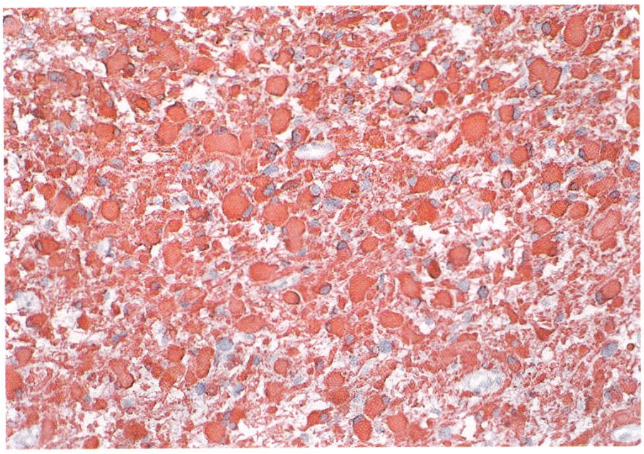

Fig. 9.28 Gemistocytic astrocytoma showing strong positive cytoplasmic reactivity for GFAP. GFAP immunoperoxidase and hematoxylin, × 500

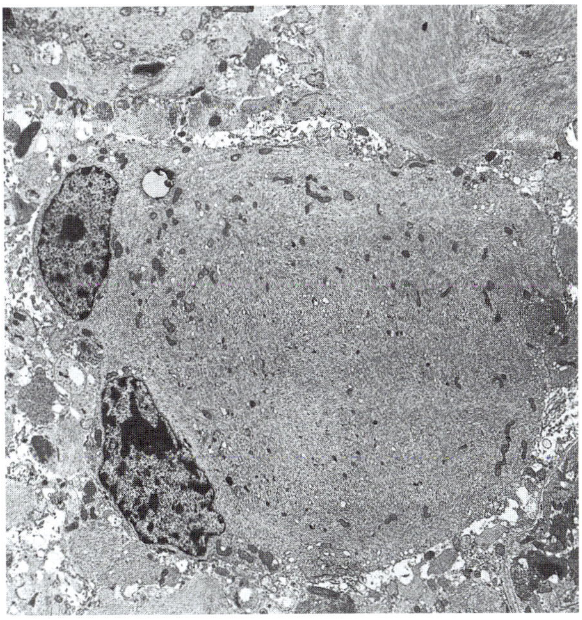

Fig. 9.29 Electron micrograph of a gemistocytic tumor astrocyte. The distended cytoplasm is filled with ribosomal rosettes, stacks of rough endoplasmic reticulum, mitochondria, a few dense autophagic vacuoles and numerous fine glial filaments. Note the numerous small pseudopodial projections of the plasma cell membrane. × 1000 (mag. to negative)

gemistocytic astrocytomas, these cell forms, while associated with considerable proliferative activity on the part of adjacent neoplastic cells, show little evidence of proliferation themselves.

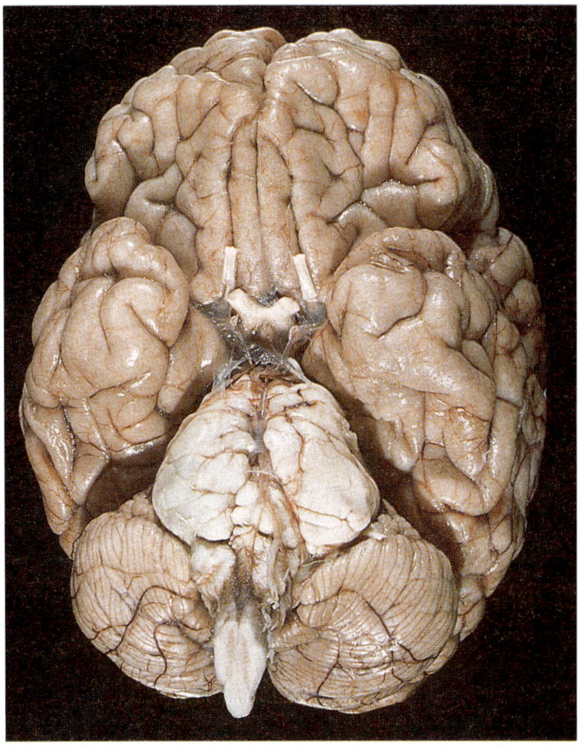

Fig. 9.30 Pontine astrocytoma in a 10-year-old female.

Electron microscopy

Fine structural study of this type of astrocytoma (Luse, 1960; Duffell *et al.*, 1963; Scheithauer and Bruner, 1987) has shown that its cytoplasm is filled with various amounts of endoplasmic reticulum, mitochondria (occasionally of giant size), a few dense lysosome-like bodies and bundles of compact glial filaments. The last, however, predominantly occupy the periphery of the cell, which has short blunt processes. These features are demonstrated in the electron micrograph shown in Fig. 9.29. Exceptionally, the perikaryon is almost completely filled by intertwining cables of filaments that may largely displace the other organelles to the periphery (see illustration of a glioblastoma cell in Fig. 9.199).

Astrocytomas of the brainstem

These gliomas form a fairly common group of which the pontine examples are the best known. The gross and often symmetric enlargement created by the tumor gave rise to the term 'diffuse hypertrophy' that was sometimes applied to this condition. The external surface, as viewed from the base, is seldom regular, but tends to be either slightly or massively, often unevenly, nodular (Fig. 9.30).

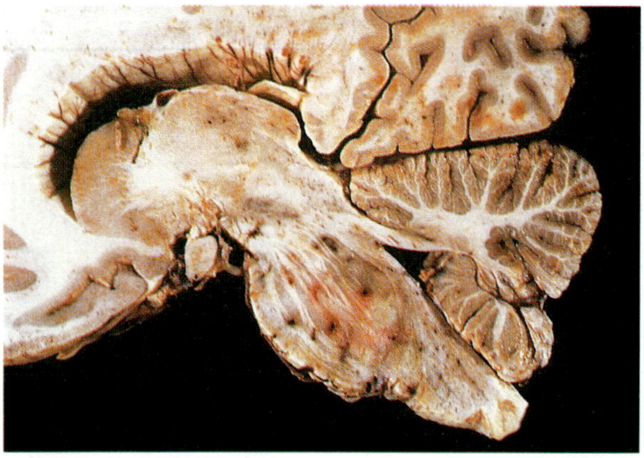

Fig. 9.31 Sagittal view of a different case of pontine astrocytoma confirming the diffuse pontine enlargement and absence of a discrete tumor mass.

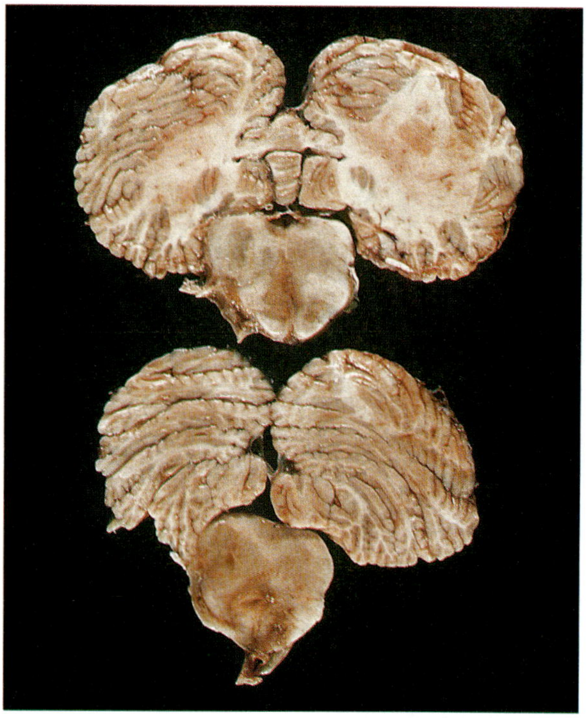

Fig. 9.32 Brainstem glioma that originated in the medulla of a 30-year-old woman who survived for 3 years after diagnosis and radiation therapy.

Characteristically, it is deeply grooved by the basilar artery, and the nodules are then often prominent along the borders of the groove. The cut surface of the involved brainstem is firm and white, with confirmation of the diffuse enlargement and absence of a discrete tumor mass (Fig. 9.31). The medulla is often spared; occasionally, however, the tumor spreads to this region, or it originates in the medulla (Fig. 9.32) and may then extend caudally into the upper cervical segments.

An uncommon variant is seen in the pontine and medullary growths in the restriction to one half of the brainstem. In these cases, it is remarkable how sharply the median raphe defines the border of the tumor upon sectioning. On the other hand, the tumor may spread along the cerebellar peduncles, and in some instances the central white matter of the cerebellum is heavily involved.

Epstein and Farmer (1993) have proposed an anatomic hypothesis to identify brainstem glioma growth patterns and those tumors with a more favorable patient prognosis. In general, those brainstem tumors that can be identified, using MRI, as cervicomedullary or focally medullary and dorsally exophytic have this favorable prognosis. These data are in agreement with those cases presented by May *et al.* (1991) and Pollack *et al.* (1993). It can be emphasized that this favorable prognosis includes lesions arising in the tectal plate and those that are incompletely resected. When a biopsy or resection of these tumors is performed, histologic examination shows a low-grade astrocytoma of either the diffuse fibrillary or the juvenile pilocytic type. Even if additional surgery is performed in the event of recurrence, a tendency for histologic stability rather than anaplastic progression is usual (Pollack *et al.*, 1993).

It is generally accepted that brainstem gliomas tend to occur in childhood and adolescence, accounting for 10–25% of intracranial childhood neoplasms (Epstein and Farmer, 1993). Rubinstein's autopsy figures (Russell and Rubinstein, 1989, p. 150), relating to a total of 46 cases, show that death occurred before the age of 20 years in 36 cases. In the remaining 10 cases, the age at death showed a wide variation, the oldest patient being 64 years of age. The sex ratio was in the proportion of 25 males to 21 females.

Radiographic appearance

Brainstem gliomas represent a diversity of mixed glial tumors unified by their site of occurrence in the brainstem. At MRI, the brainstem is optimally imaged and this reveals enlargement, usually of the pons. Morphologically, the tumor usually deviates the fourth ventricle posteriorly and has exophytic expansion to encase the basilar artery. The mass has low T1 signal intensity and high T2 signal intensity. This may be well defined or diffusely infiltrative. The mass may cause obstructive hydrocephalus and frequently extends to include cranial nerves adjacent to the pons. A more infiltrative appearance

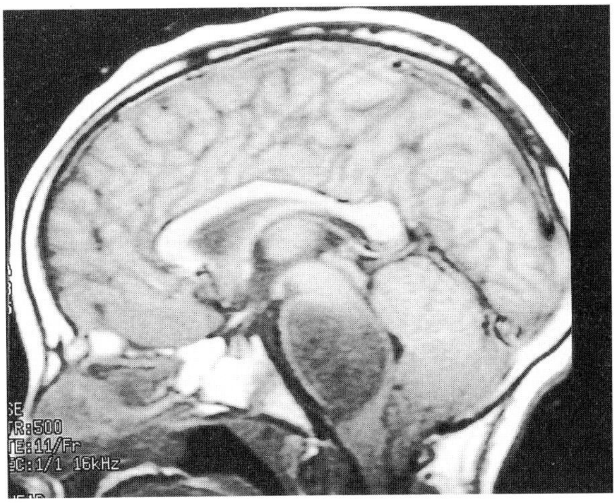

Fig. 9.33 Sagittal T1-weighted noncontrasted MRI image demonstrating marked enlargement of the pons in a 5-year-old girl. This causes compression of the fourth ventricle. There was no enhancement with contrast. This appearance represents brainstem glioma.

favors a predominantly fibrillary histopathology (Fig. 9.33), while cystic or enhancing nodular components are more typically seen with pilocytic tumors (Fig. 9.34). Areas of ring enhancement with irregular margins and cystic necrosis are typically seen when glioblastoma multiforme predominates. The enhancement pattern is variable in brainstem gliomas. This ranges from no enhancement, often seen in early detection, to large areas of irregular ring enhancement.

At CT scanning, detection of small brainstem gliomas may be difficult. The brainstem may be suboptimally visualized by CT due to streak artifacts. Enlargement of the pons with exophytic expansion around the basilar artery may be the only indication of neoplasm. Larger tumors may show hypodensity or heterogeneous hypodensity. The enhancement pattern by CT is also variable, ranging from none to areas of ring enhancement.

Microscopic appearance

With respect to their histology, it is largely accepted that many brainstem gliomas are composed of elongated bipolar cells and are, therefore, pilocytic astrocytomas (Fig. 9.35). However, some have many features in common with the diffuse fibrillary astrocytomas of the cerebral hemispheres. Their manner of growth is similar, involving the infiltration of the tumor cells into pre-existing structures to separate them widely, but without destruction. Because of this relative preservation of normal structures, signs and symptoms may be evoked only at a late clinical stage, when pressure is exerted upon the regional nerve roots and increased intracranial pressure has become evident.

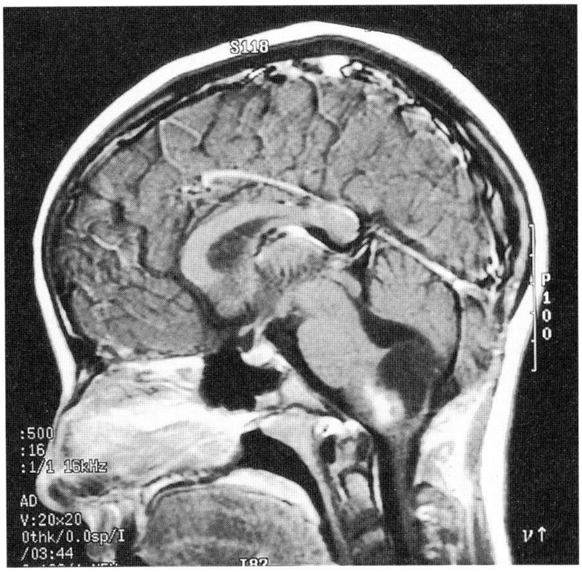

Fig. 9.34 Sagittal T1-weighted postcontrast MRI demonstrating an enhancing mass of the medulla, which is relatively well defined, in a 12-year-old girl. Posterior to the enhancement is an area of rounded low T1 signal indicating an adjacent cyst. This deviates the fourth ventricle posteriorly and superiorily. This tumor represents juvenile pilocytic astrocytoma of the medulla. The cystic area and nodular enhancing mass is a typical finding with this histopathology.

In most of these diffusely infiltrating gliomas, perhaps as many as 80%, the microscopic appearance is similar to that of the diffuse cerebral astrocytomas, with small, but usually well-fibrillated, cells. When the nerve fiber tracts of the basis pontis are infiltrated, the tumor cells become pilocytic; this is clearly a 'secondary structure' within the scope of Scherer's definition (1938), in parallel with what is sometimes seen in diffuse cerebral astrocytomas.

Furthermore, a substantial number of these intrinsic pontine gliomas are glioblastomas. These areas are seldom seen externally in autopsy specimens, but are obvious as the cut surfaces of the tumor are examined. They include soft foci of gray granular tissue, often associated with necrosis and hemorrhage. These appearances have been well correlated with those seen by neuroradiologic imaging (Tsuchida *et al.*, 1985). Evidence of anaplasia was identified in as many as 29 of Rubinstein's 46 necropsied cases (63%, Russell and Rubinstein, 1989); in 20 of these, the age of the subject was under 20 years, the youngest two patients being 3

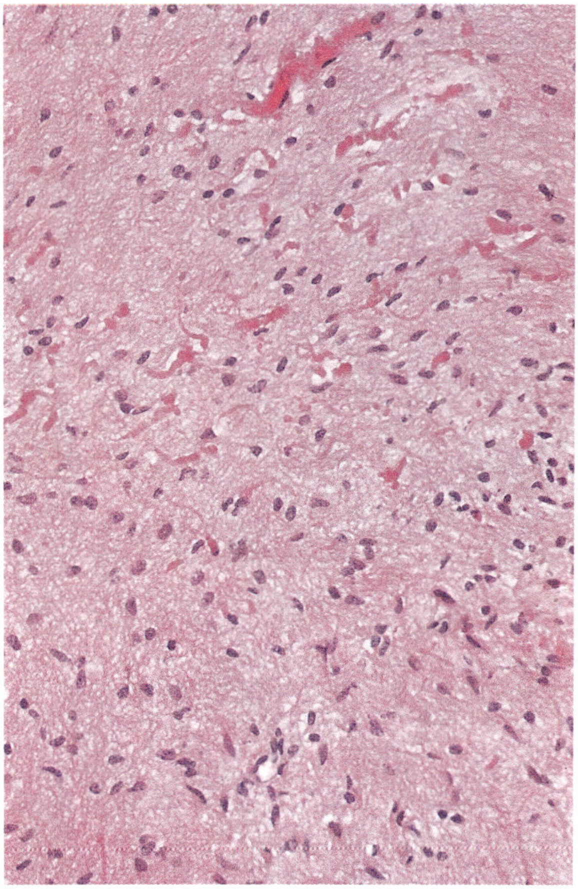

Fig. 9.35 Low-grade pilocytic astrocytoma of the brainstem showing scattered Rosenthal fibers. H&E, × 250.

years old. Therefore, it cannot be argued that age is directly related to this anaplastic histology. This point is important because, as documented by Tomita, McLone and Naidich (1984), there may be a significant discrepancy between the histologic picture presented in a necessarily restricted surgical biopsy and the pathologic picture revealed at postmortem.

A minority of these tumors (in the region of 20%), however, resemble those cerebellar astrocytomas of juvenile pilocytic type that are made up of small, delicate, bipolar and stellate cells with scanty processes. They have a finely reticulated neuroglial matrix and show no focal increase in the density of the cells, no mitotic activity and no evidence of anaplasia. But they are apt to be highly vascular, and endothelial proliferation may be prominent in the capillary blood vessel walls. Small foci of necrosis, with or without hemorrhage, can be sometimes seen in the center of the tumor. The tumors in three of Rubinstein's cases were circumscribed, a contrasting feature when compared with the much more common diffuse variety. Three also contained Rosenthal fibers, one example being in a 64-year-old man. Therefore, the biologic behavior of this subset of brainstem gliomas may be expected to parallel the evolution of pilocytic astrocytomas at other sites, i.e., to display a slower growth and a more prolonged course, including an unusually long period of patient survival following clinical diagnosis.

According to Epstein and McCleary (1986) and Epstein and Farmer (1993), the more benign forms of astrocytoma occur mostly at the cervicomedullary junction and do not extend into the pons. They also include the focal and/or the cystic tumors in this group (Epstein and Wisoff, 1990; Epstein and Farmer, 1993).

The actuarial 5-year survival of patients with brainstem gliomas varies widely in different series (Albright, Price and Guthkelch, 1983; Tomita, McLone and Naidich, 1984; Alvisi, Cerisoli and Maccheroni, 1985; Albright *et al.*, 1986; Cohen *et al.*, 1986; Epstein and McCleary, 1986; Stroink *et al.*, 1986; Jenkin *et al.*, 1987) and is dependent on tumor location within the brainstem, as well as histology. Nevertheless, there does seem to be some predictable association of the focal medullary, cervicomedullary and dorsally exophytic tumors with a lower-grade histology (May *et al.*, 1991; Epstein and Farmer, 1993; Pollack *et al.*, 1993). The differential aspect in the histology of brainstem gliomas was not considered by Albright *et al.* (1986) in their series of 27 children with biopsied brainstem gliomas, but it is of interest that they found a clear correlation between the absence of mitotic activity in the biopsy specimens and a longer survival period. The follow-up studies of Alvisi, Cerisoli and Maccheroni (1985), Epstein and McCleary (1986), Stroink *et al.* (1986) and Albright *et al.* (1986) have further confirmed the existence of a significant correlation between surgical results and the histologic type of the tumor. The histologic features (Rosenthal fibers and microcysts), mentioned by the latter workers as characteristic of the tumors with a better prognosis, contrasted with the features of mitotic activity, hyperchromatism, pleomorphism and necrosis associated with an unfavorable prognosis are, again, consistent with the view that we are dealing with two biologically different types of astrocytoma: one low-grade and the other anaplastic.

The patterns of growth and spread of brainstem astrocytomas have already been indicated and are well described by Epstein and Farmer (1993). Malignant changes are usually restricted to the deeper parts of the tumor, so invasion of the meninges and metastasis by way of the cerebrospinal fluid (CSF) are relatively unusual.

Nevertheless, several examples have been reported (Packer *et al.*, 1983) in which either the basal leptomeninges or the fourth ventricle were transgressed, leading to metastases in the floor of the third ventricle or heavy infiltration of the spinal meninges by anaplastic growth.

Astrocytomas of the spinal cord

Although the spinal intramedullary astrocytomas form about 25% of the gliomas in this location, they must be still regarded as rare. Because they more often affect the upper segments of the cord, they may be more frequent than the ependymomas in that region, the latter of which collectively are far more numerous but predominate in the caudal segments. Thus, in their analysis of intraspinal neoplasms of the cervical region, Webb, Craig and Kernohan (1953) found that, of 41 gliomas, 19 were astrocytomas while only 17 were ependymomas. Occasionally, the upper cervical segments may be involved in a spreading growth that arose primarily in the brainstem. In the series of Slooff, Kernohan and MacCarty (1964), 35/66 astrocytomas (grades 1 and 2) arose in the thoracic segments, 11 in the cervical segments and 10 in the cervicothoracic region. A recent series of cases showed an equal distribution of astrocytomas between the cervical and thoracic cord, with only 1/79 tumors confined to the lumbar region (Minehan *et al.*, 1995). In children and adolescents, the cervical segments seem to be the most frequently involved (Reimer and Onofrio, 1985; Rossitch *et al.*, 1990).

Most spinal cord astrocytomas are relatively circumscribed and produce a limited fusiform swelling of the cord. Most extend over fewer than four spinal cord segments (Minehan *et al.*, 1995). Occasionally, they may be extensive and may then infiltrate the leptomeninges, both locally and further afield. The cut surfaces are moderately firm, homogeneous and grayish white after fixation. A few are partly, or largely, cystic.

The radiologic findings of spinal cord astrocytoma indicate an elongated intramedullary mass that expands the cord. The imaging study of choice is MRI. While T1-weighted images demonstrate a hypointense to isointense mass, T2-weighted images show a hyperintense mass. Contrast enhancement is usually intense, with some areas of cystic necrosis or intratumor cysts frequently being seen (Fig. 9.36). Intramedullary cysts extending far from the tumor most likely represent areas of syringomyelia (Fig. 9.37).

Myelography and CT show enlargement of the cord secondary to the intramedullary mass, but do not identify the extent of the tumor. There may be enlargement of the spinal canal due to bone remodeling.

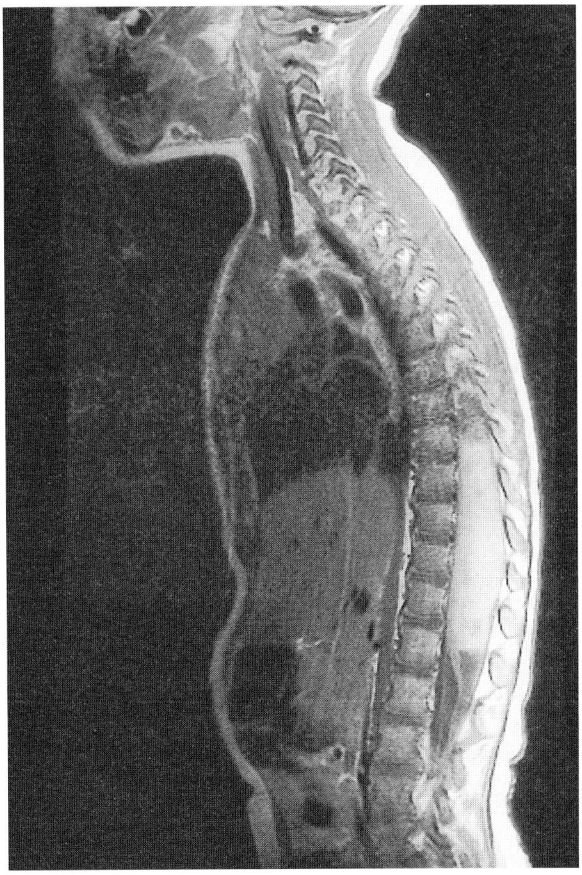

Fig. 9.36 Sagittal T1-weighted postcontrast MRI of the spine demonstrating a large enhancing intramedullary mass extending over approximately six vertebral body segments at the thoracolumbar junction. There are small cystic areas within the mass, as well as a cystic area more anteriorly and expansion of the spinal canal indicating long-standing mass effect. This tumor is an anaplastic astrocytoma.

Microscopically, the astrocytomas of the spinal cord may resemble either the juvenile pilocytic astrocytomas or the diffuse fibrillary astrocytomas of the cerebrum. These histologic types seem to be about equally common (Minehan *et al.*, 1995). In the lower-grade examples, their relatively poor cellularity may raise the differential diagnosis of spinal cord gliosis; this is particularly likely to occur when only a limited biopsy is available. As in other astrocytomas, those of the spinal cord may display various degrees of cytologic anaplasia, and the histologic grade is predictive of patient survival (Cohen *et al.*, 1989; Rossitch *et al.*, 1990; Epstein,

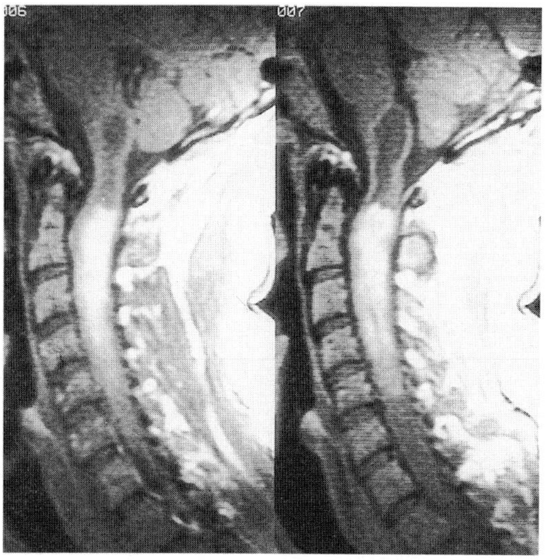

Fig. 9.37 Two sagittal T1-weighted postcontrast MRIs of a 29-year-old man. There is an intramedullary enhancing mass of the upper cervical spine present from C2 to C5 More superiorly, there is a cyst that extends into the medulla. Tumors may have cystic component; however, extension beyond the tumor without enhancement or at a distant site suggest syringomyelia. This tumor is an anaplastic astrocytoma with syringomyelia and syringobulbia.

Farmer and Freed, 1992; O'Sullivan *et al.*, 1994; Minehan *et al.*, 1995).

Although usually solitary, multiple tumors may be found in association with NF type 2 (al-Wahhabi *et al.*, 1992). Syringomyelia may further complicate the pathologic picture, whether the tumors are multiple or solitary. The precise nature of the latter association is obscure, for syringomyelia accompanies a wide variety of intramedullary tumors, and the cavitation is not always in anatomic continuity with the neoplasm. This problem was analyzed in detail by Poser (1956; see also Ferry, Hardman and Earle, 1969; Samii and Klekamp, 1994).

Gliomatosis cerebri

This extreme form of diffusely infiltrating tumor, termed gliomatosis by Nevin (1938) but also described under several other names, is one in which invasion by neoplastic glia has involved more than one lobe and sometimes the major part of the brain. The condition is rare (Couch and Weiss, 1974; Artigas *et al.*, 1985). Most of the reported cases have been of patients in their first or second decade. However, there are a few case reports of older patients presenting with symptoms of dementia (Gottesman, Laufer and Patel, 1991; Ross *et al.*, 1991; Koslow *et al.*, 1992; Vassallo and Allen, 1995). Grossly (Fig. 9.38) and microscopically, these cases closely resemble the diffuse cerebral astrocytomas. Considerable emphasis has sometimes been placed on the concentrations of small glial cells in the molecular layer of the cortex (Fig. 9.39) and also on the elongated–or 'spongioblastic'–form of many of the tumor cells. These features can hardly be regarded as sufficiently distinctive to separate this type of growth from the general group of astrocytomas. The term 'central diffuse schwannosis', which has sometimes been suggested, is a misnomer because astrocytes are clearly an important, and usually predominant, element. The remarkable diffuseness of the process, which in some cases implicates not only the cerebrum but also the cerebellum, brainstem

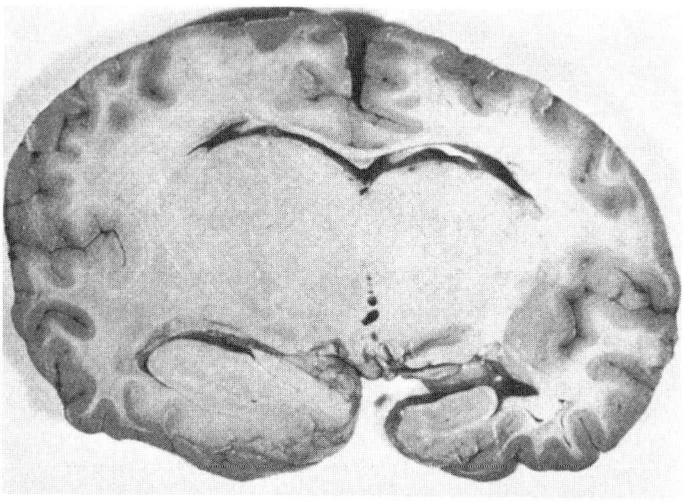

Fig. 9.38 Diffuse glioma (gliomatosis cerebri).

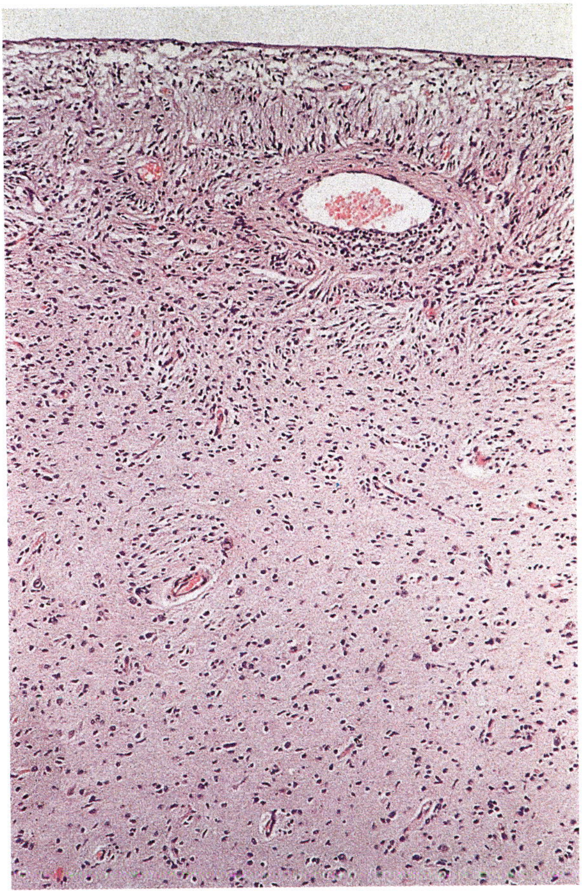

Fig. 9.39 Tumor cells in gliomatosis cerebri infiltrating the cerebral cortex and accumulating in the molecular layer, sometimes invading the pia and surrounding pial vessels (top). H&E, × 125

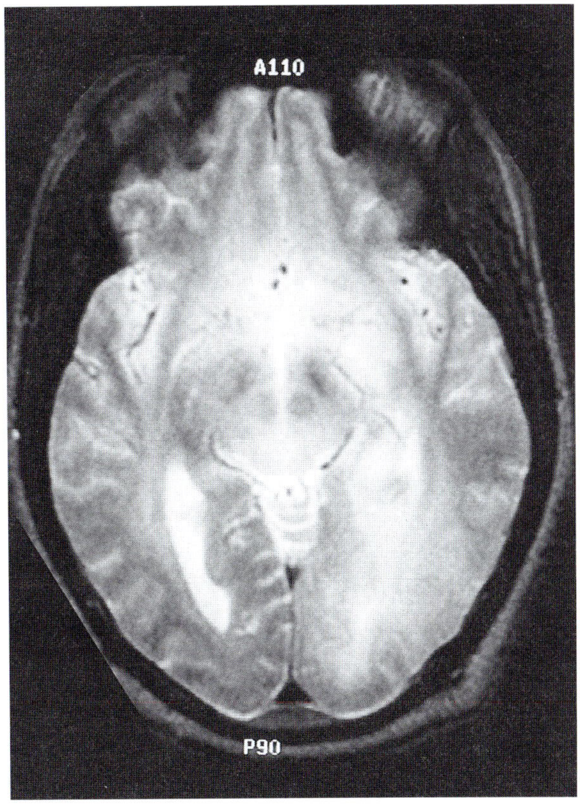

Fig. 9.40 Axial T2-weighted MRI of a 34-year-old man. There is ill-defined, abnormal, increased T2 signal intensity involving both frontal lobes inferiorly, the left temporal lobe and the left occipital lobe. The ill-defined and diffuse infiltrative appearance of this tumor, with multilobe involvement, is compatible with gliomatosis cerebri. No contrast enhancement was present.

and even the spinal cord, tends to support Scherer's contention (1940a) that neoplasia has arisen over a wide field and that the appearances cannot reasonably be interpreted as the result of cellular infiltration from a solitary focus. It also argues against the premise that, in this type of glioma, at least, the sequence of somatic mutations responsible for neoplastic transformation must necessarily be restricted to a very small number of cells, let alone a single cell. An alternative explanation for the diffuseness of the process is that the transformed neoplastic cells are extraordinarily motile (Jennings *et al.*, 1995). Future molecular genetic analysis of widely separated regions within the neoplasm may be useful to resolve the issue. Investigation of cell surface characteristics and comparison with ordinary diffuse astrocytomas may be of value.

The radiologic findings of gliomatosis cerebri reflect the diffuse infiltrative nature of this tumor. The imaging study of choice is MRI. The T2-weighted images demonstrate the tumor involvement through the white matter in multiple lobes of the brain (Fig. 9.40). The T1-weighted sequences may show mild decrease in signal intensity. Contrast enhancement is not usually evident. If a focal area of enhancement is seen, degeneration into a more malignant glioma should be suspected. At CT scanning, gliomatosis cerebri may be difficult to detect. There may be alteration of gray–white distinction, mild mass effect and mild hypodensity in areas of tumor.

In one of Nevin's (1938) cases, an area of glioblastoma was identified, and Rubinstein confirmed a similar change in several of the examples he examined (Russell and Rubinstein, 1989, pp. 146–7). These, as well as other instances in the literature, lend additional support to our inclusion of these cases with the diffuse cerebral astrocytomas

(Fig. 9.41), although a case of oligodendroglial gliomatosis has been reported (Balko, Blisard and Samaha, 1992).

Gliomatosis cerebri should not be confused with the diffuse involvement of the leptomeninges by astrocytoma, the process called 'leptomeningeal gliomatosis'. This latter condition arises from an intra-axial astrocytoma that breaches the pia and spreads secondarily through the leptomeninges. Rare cases have arisen from extra-axial heterotopic glial rests in the meninges. This type of dissemination from parenchymal astrocytomas will be covered more fully under the discussion of growth and dissemination of gliomas later in this chapter on p. 511. Cervós-Navarro *et al.* (1987) have described the electron microscopic features of five examples of gliomatosis cerebri.

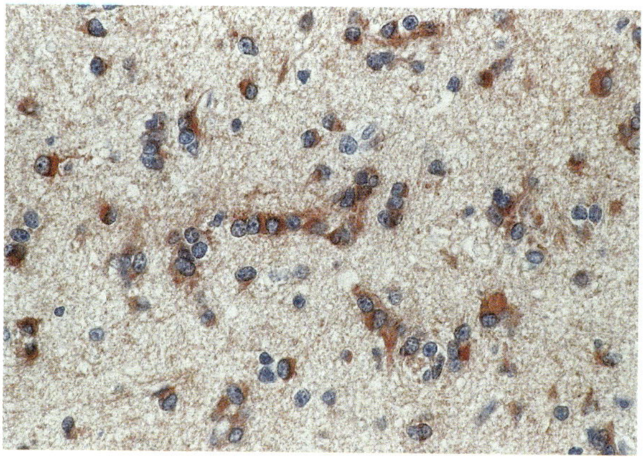

Fig. 9.41 Same case as Fig. 9.39. Positive cytoplasmic reactivity for GFAP confirming the astrocytic derivation of the neoplastic cells in this patient with gliomatosis cerebri. GFAP immunoperoxidase and hematoxylin, × 500

Special variants of astrocytoma (circumscribed forms)

Pilocytic astrocytomas

Many low-grade astrocytomas, especially the cerebellum and the hypothalamic region, exhibit a largely pilocytic character that is independent of the restraints imposed by their environment. In these examples, the cell of origin may have a polar configuration, as exemplified by the Bergmann astrocyte of the cerebellar cortex, the subependymal glia of the central neuraxis or the radial glia seen in normal fetal development.

In the adult type of pilocytic astrocytoma, the tumor is composed of closely packed interwoven bundles of relatively broad, bipolar, fibrillated cells that form an intersecting pattern, have no distinct relationship to the blood vessels and demonstrate little or no tendency to undergo microcystic degeneration (Fig. 9.42). This variant, in which the uniform histologic picture contrasts with the diversified appearances of the juvenile type, tends to occur in older patients and is likely to have attributes of anaplastic astrocytoma, two features that further contribute to its separation. It is not further discussed here, since it cannot be considered a 'circumscribed' variant of astrocytoma.

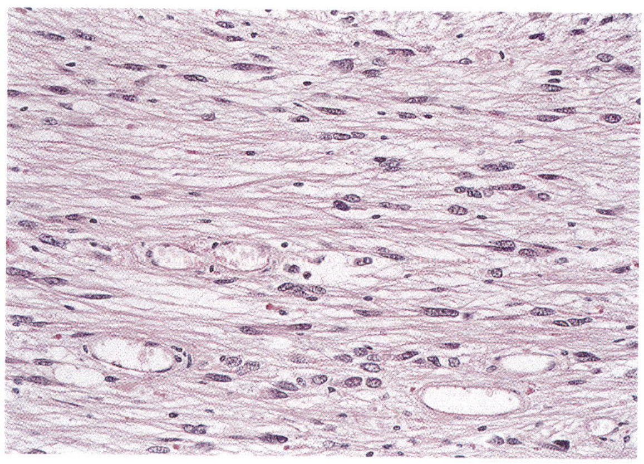

Fig. 9.42 Diffuse pilocytic astrocytoma. H&E, × 250

The tumor cells of the juvenile type of pilocytic astrocytoma may represent a morphologically simple type of fiber-forming glia, hence the term 'polar spongioblastoma', which was originally used for their designation (Bailey and Eisenhardt, 1932).

Astrocytomas with this distinctive histology occur most commonly in the cerebellum. Any part of the cerebellum may be the site of origin. According to Elvidge, Penfield and Cone (1937), the juvenile examples occur in the midline, whereas the hemispheres are involved in adults. But, neither Bucy and Gustafson (1939) nor Ringertz and Nordenstam (1951) confirmed this in their larger series. Rubinstein (Russell and Rubinstein, 1989, pp. 83–161) indicated a slight predominance of tumors in the lateral lobe in subjects under 20 years of age; in subjects over 20 years, all tumors were lateral; but, in some cases of both groups, the vermis as well as one or both lobes were involved.

Other classic locations include the optic apparatus and the region of the third ventricle. An uncommon location is the cerebral hemisphere. These tumors will be considered together, with the exception of the optic pathway gliomas that are discussed separately in this chapter.

Cerebellar astrocytomas have long been known to differ in several points from the majority of astrocytomas arising in the cerebral hemispheres. First, they are predominantly tumors of early life, most

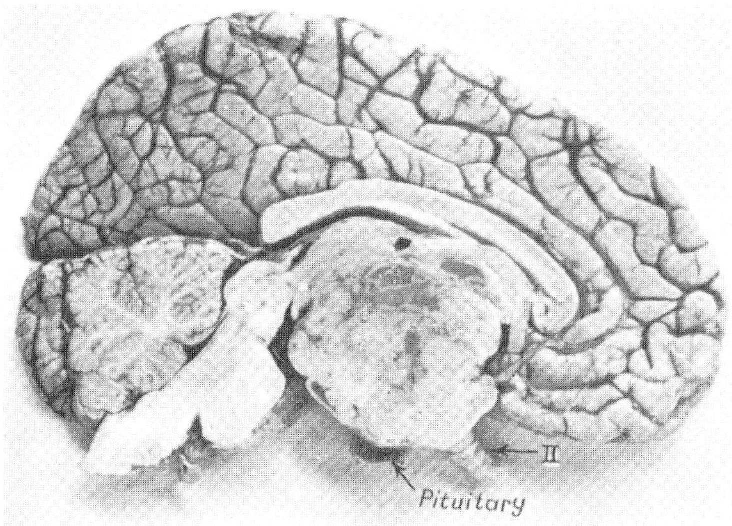

Fig. 9.43 Pilocytic astrocytoma of the third ventricle (juvenile type) infiltrating optic nerve (II) in a case of NF type 1.

being recognized in the first two decades (Bucy and Gustafson, 1939; Ilgren and Stiller, 1987, literature review; Schneider, Raffel and McComb, 1992). Second, they are often circumscribed and have a characteristic tendency to be grossly cystic. They are, therefore, more amenable to surgical treatment than the diffuse cerebral astrocytomas. Third, cellular anaplasia is an uncommon development. The following points should, however, be added: some cerebellar astrocytomas are solid throughout; many, microscopically, display diffusely infiltrative edges; and anaplastic changes have been described only rarely (Tomlinson *et al.*, 1994; Coakley *et al.*, 1995).

The astrocytomas of the region of the third ventricle are also tumors of childhood and adolescence, and, less often, of young adults in their third decade. Although they are, for the most part, macroscopically well defined in relation to the dorsal contiguous structures, they usually infiltrate the optic tracts and chiasm as well as the hypothalamus (Fig. 9.43). Because of this, they are prone to create various hypothalamic disturbances as well as visual disorders. Surprisingly, however, the hypothalamus may be extensively involved in some instances without giving rise to any such manifestations. Diabetes insipidus, Fröhlich's disease, precocious puberty and the syndrome of extreme emaciation with bulimia (diencephalic syndrome) have all been observed in association with these tumors. Those in which the main bulk of the tumor occupies the cavity of the ventricle produce internal hydrocephalus, which may often be considerable. Occasionally, the tumor protrudes caudally through the tentorial opening to compress the brainstem or, when laterality is pronounced, into the temporal lobe.

In recent years, there has been increasing awareness of the existence of cerebral hemispheric pilocytic astrocytomas of juvenile type and of the importance of separating these from the diffuse cerebral astrocytomas, not only because of their pathologic features, but also in the light of their considerably more favorable clinical behavior (Katsetos and Krishna, 1994).

This form of cerebral astrocytoma, by no means new (see Palma and Guidetti, 1985, for references), has many features in common with the growths originating in the hypothalamic region and in the cerebellar hemispheres of young subjects, and, like them, is found mostly in patients in younger age groups. Most of the patients are in their first or second decade; the series from the Armed Forces Institute of Pathology reviewed by Clark, Henry and McKeever (1985) indicates a somewhat higher mean age of onset, i.e., at 22 years. Garcia and Fulling (1985) reported seven patients in their second and third decade. Both sexes are about equally affected. Compared with the diffuse cerebral astrocytomas, there is a distinctly higher tendency for the temporal and parieto-occipital lobes to be involved. Cyst formation is characteristic and conspicuous, the tumor often presenting, as in the cerebellar examples, as a large cyst containing a small mural nodule. The follow-up studies of Palma and Guidetti (1985), Clark, Henry and McKeever

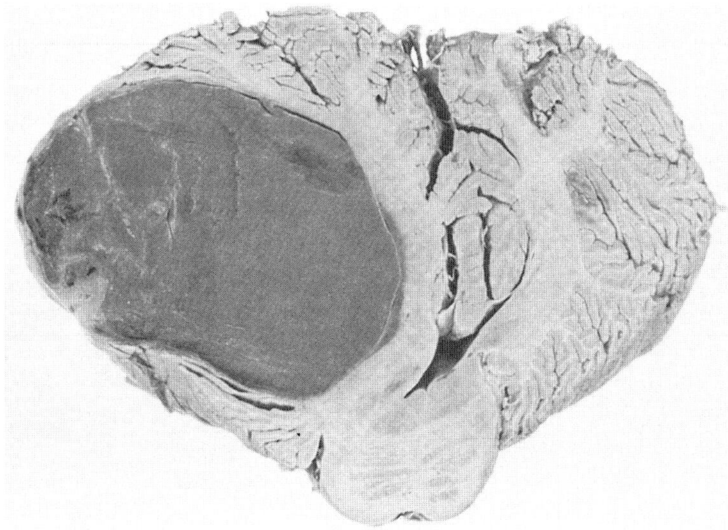

Fig. 9.44 Largely cystic cerebellar astrocytoma. (Courtesy of Dr H. Budka)

(1985), Garcia and Fulling (1985), Garcia, Fulling and Marks (1985), Afra *et al.* (1986), Forsyth *et al.* (1993) and Pollack *et al.* (1995) confirm the favorable outcome of this type of hemispheric astrocytoma, the infrequency of recurrence after surgical excision and the virtual absence of anaplastic change.

Macroscopic appearance

Grossly, the pilocytic astrocytomas of juvenile type, whether situated in the region of the third ventricle or in the cerebellum, and those less commonly involving a cerebral hemisphere, the brainstem or the walls of the fourth ventricle, are often relatively circumscribed, except that those in the neighborhood of the third ventricle are apt to infiltrate the optic chiasm and tracts. In any situation, these tumors often penetrate the regional leptomeninges without spreading further afield, but examples of distant dissemination in the cerebrospinal pathways have been seen and reported (Obana *et al.*, 1991; Mishima *et al.*, 1992; Hayostek *et al.*, 1993; Versari *et al.*, 1994).

In the large cystic tumors, the neoplasm may present as a mural nodule; the cyst, which contains clear limpid yellow or brownish fluid, is then virtually outside the growth (Fig. 9.44). In other instances, the cyst is fringed by a zone of tumor that is either soft, gray and gelatinous or of tough consistency (Ilgren and Stiller, 1987). Tumors of the vermis are apt to encroach on the cavity of the fourth ventricle and may even gain an attachment to the floor. In some of the lateral lobe examples, the tonsil is also implicated, and a few are found to extend into the restiform body.

Radiographic appearance

Pilocytic astrocytomas are usually well defined and contain a solid enhancing nodule and a cystic component. Solid pilocytic astrocytomas occur infrequently. The solid nodule tends to be hypointense to gray matter on T1-weighted sequences and hyperintense on T2-weighted sequences, often with a mildly lobulated contour. With contrast administration, the solid component of the tumor usually enhances intensely (Figs 9.45 and 9.46), although the pattern may be inhomogeneous (Fig. 9.47). The cystic components have very low T1 and high T2 signal intensity. The rim of the cyst usually does not enhance. The tumor causes localized mass effect but usually has little, if any, edema associated with it.

At CT scanning, pilocytic astrocytomas tend to be hypodense. Associated cysts are of near water density. With contrast enhancement, there usually is intense enhancement. Occasionally, this is heterogeneous. Approximately 10% of pilocytic astrocytomas will have calcification.

Microscopic appearance

With the proviso that transitional aspects can sometimes be demonstrated, two fairly distinct histologic patterns can usually be recognized.

First, in a minority of cerebellar astrocytomas, usually reported as about 15% of cases (Hayostek *et al.*, 1993), the tumor as a whole is similar to the diffuse cerebral astrocytomas; the constituent elements are fibrillated stellate or piloid cells (Fig. 9.48). The latter, as in the cerebral examples, are closely packed in intersecting bundles and tend to be stouter than the slender cells characteristic of the typical form. Microcysts are rare. These diffuse

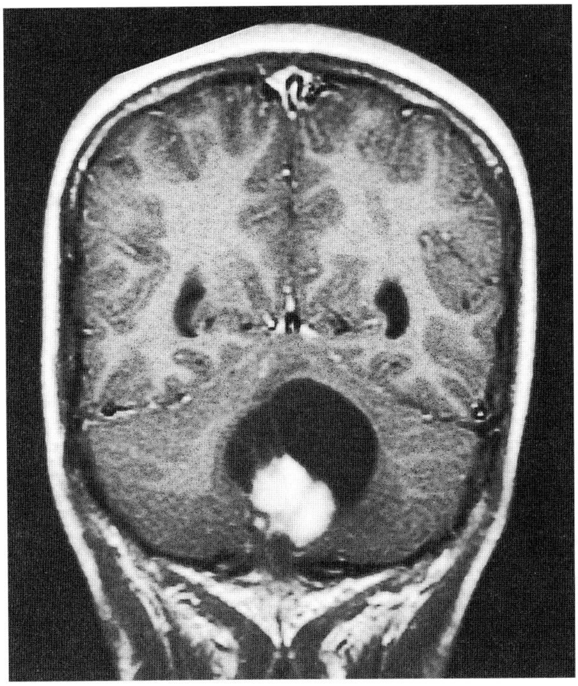

Fig. 9.45 Coronal T1-weighted postcontrast MRI demonstrating a well-defined, nodular, intensely enhancing mass in the midline of the cerebellum in a 14-year-old boy. Well-defined cyst is noted without enhancement. The pathology was that of juvenile pilocytic astrocytoma.

astrocytomas tend to arise more often in adolescence and, especially, in early adult life. Some are grossly cystic on macroscopic examination; more often, they are solid and toughly fibrillated. They are more widely infiltrative than the cerebellar astrocytomas with the more typical histologic pattern. They usually do not contain protoplasmic astrocytes, and the fibrillary character of the tumor cells suggests that the neoplastic process primarily involved the stellate and pilocytic astrocytes of the cerebellar white matter. Long-term follow-up in an older series showed that the 25-year cumulative survival rate for patients with this diffuse form of cerebellar astrocytoma was less than half as favorable as for the other form (Gjerris and Klinken, 1978). Diffusely infiltrating adult fibrillary astrocytomas may have been included in this series, however, since more recent data suggests no significant prognostic difference between this low-grade diffuse type and the juvenile type of pilocytic astrocytoma (Hayostek *et al.*, 1993). These two variants of pilocytic astrocytoma must be distinguished from the diffusely infiltrative cerebellar fibrillary astrocytomas – those with a significantly decreased patient survival rate (Hayostek *et al.*, 1993).

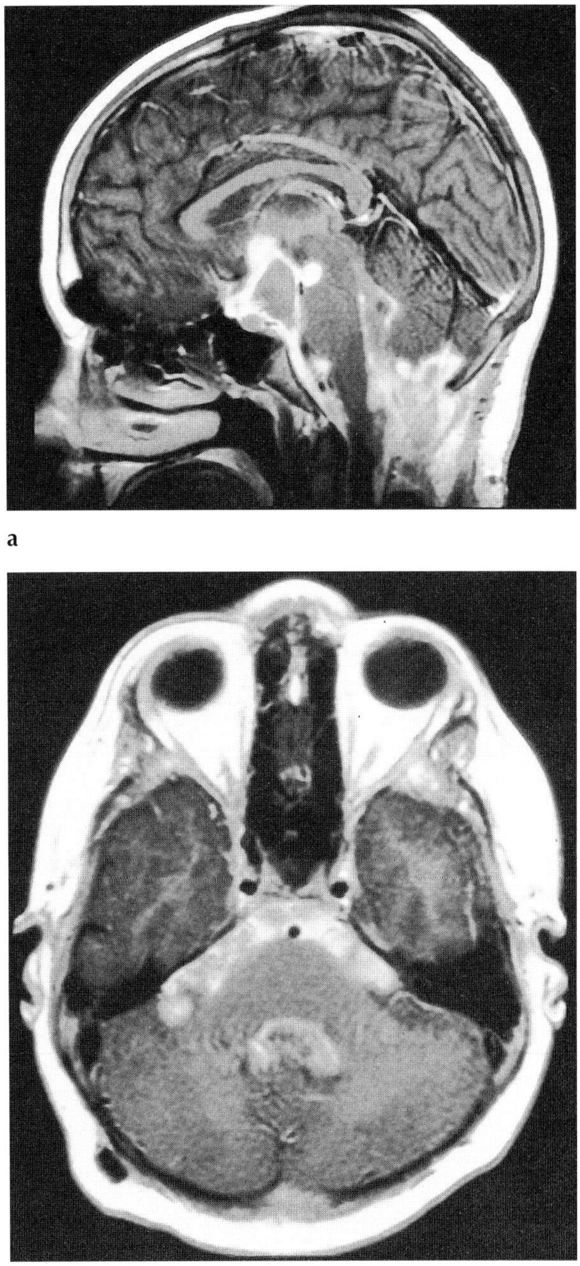

a

b

Fig. 9.46 Postcontrast MRIs of a 16-year-old boy. (a) Sagittal T1-weighted image demonstrates enhancing mass surrounding the brainstem and extending into the fourth ventricle, along the prepontine cistern and into the suprasellar cistern and hypothalamic region. Note the tumor extending to the suboccipital craniotomy surgical site. (b) Axial T1-weighted image demonstrates enhancing tumor along the anterior brainstem surrounding the cranial nerves and encasing the basilar artery. Abnormal enhancing tumor also extends through the fourth ventricle. This appearance represents CSF seeding of pilocytic astrocytoma.

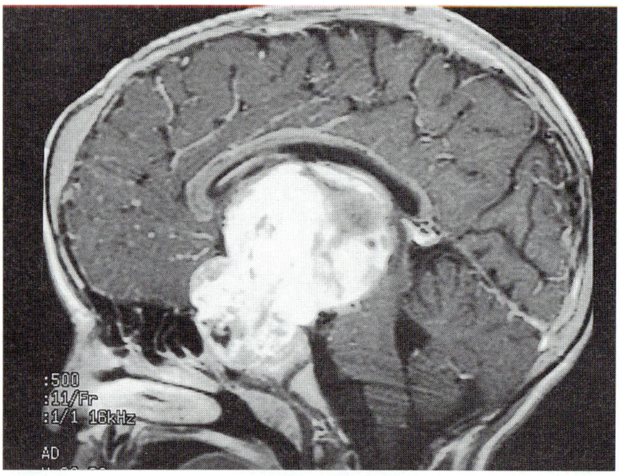

a

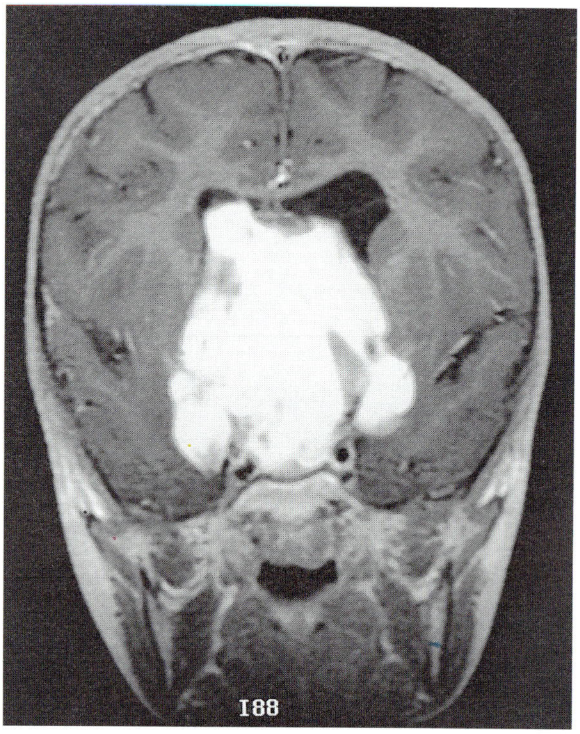

b

Fig. 9.47 Postcontrast MRIs of a 4-year-old 'happy' child with polyphagia. (a) Sagittal T1-weighted image demonstrates a very large hypothalamic mass with marked enhancement and areas of heterogeneous low T1 signal intensity. (b) Coronal T1-weighted image demonstrates intense contrast enhancement of the large, lobulated mass. Superior extension deviating the lateral ventricles is identified. This represents juvenile pilocytic astrocytoma of the hypothalamus.

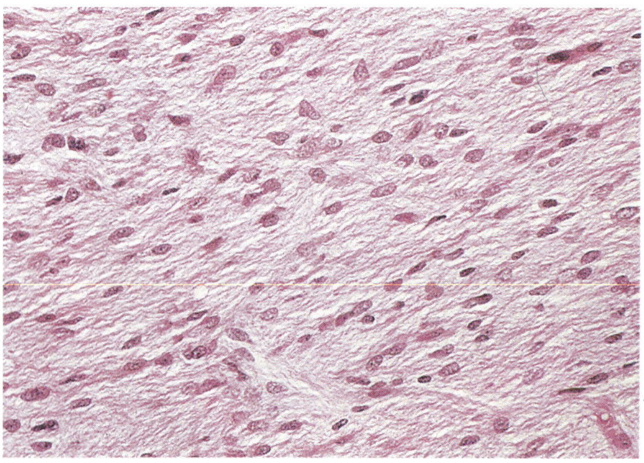

Fig. 9.48 Diffuse component of an otherwise biphasic juvenile type of cerebellar astrocytoma. H&E, × 325

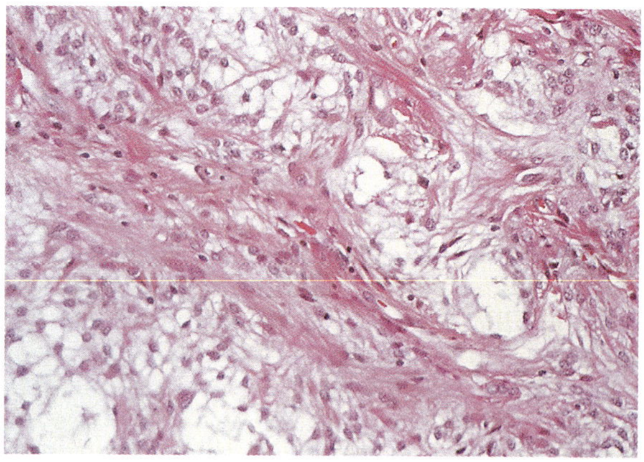

Fig. 9.49 Biphasic pattern of solid and microcystic regions in a typical juvenile pilocytic astrocytoma. H&E, × 250

Second, in the great majority of cases, the picture is characteristically that of an intimate and contiguous association of areas of compact pilocytic growth with other areas of loose-textured spongy character (Fig. 9.49), the classic biphasic pattern. In this typical juvenile form, the compact areas are composed mainly of closely interwoven, elongated and slender hair-like cells containing stout glial fibrils (Fig. 9.50). Variable numbers of stellate astrocytes are included. Rosenthal fibers are usually abundant (Fig. 9.51). These areas vary in size and shape and have irregular borders; they are devoid of microcystic degeneration.

The tumor cells are mostly elongated, thin and tapering. In parallel formations, they often and characteristically sheathe the blood vessels longitudinally (Fig. 9.52). Their astrocytic nature is quite evident in immunoperoxidase staining for the

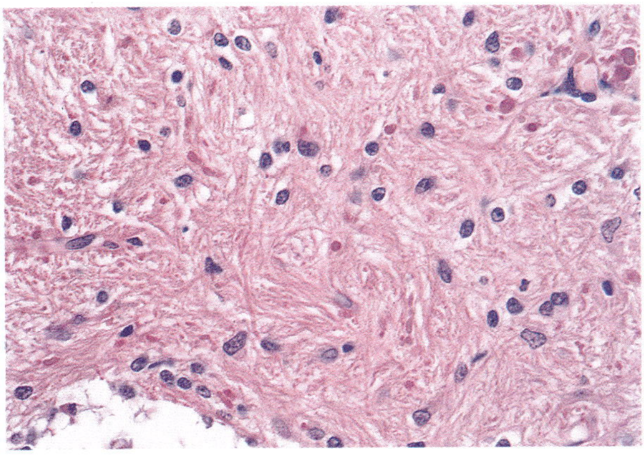

Fig. 9.50 Densely fibrillar character of compact regions of juvenile pilocytic astrocytoma. H&E, × 500

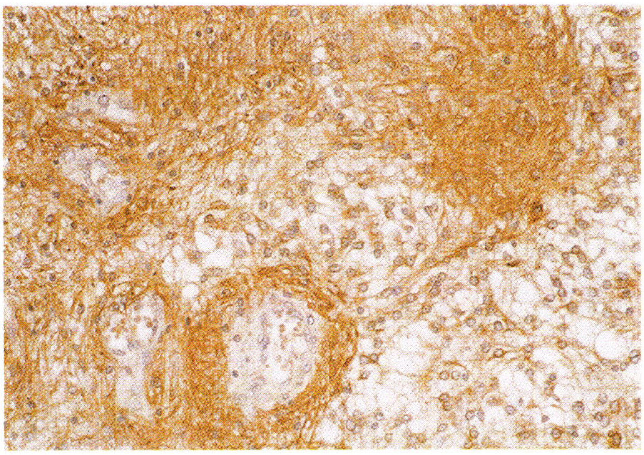

Fig. 9.52 Compact fibrillar areas of juvenile pilocytic astrocytoma, showing a tendency to ensheathe the blood vessels, with the spongy areas in between. GFAP immunoperoxidase and hematoxylin, × 250

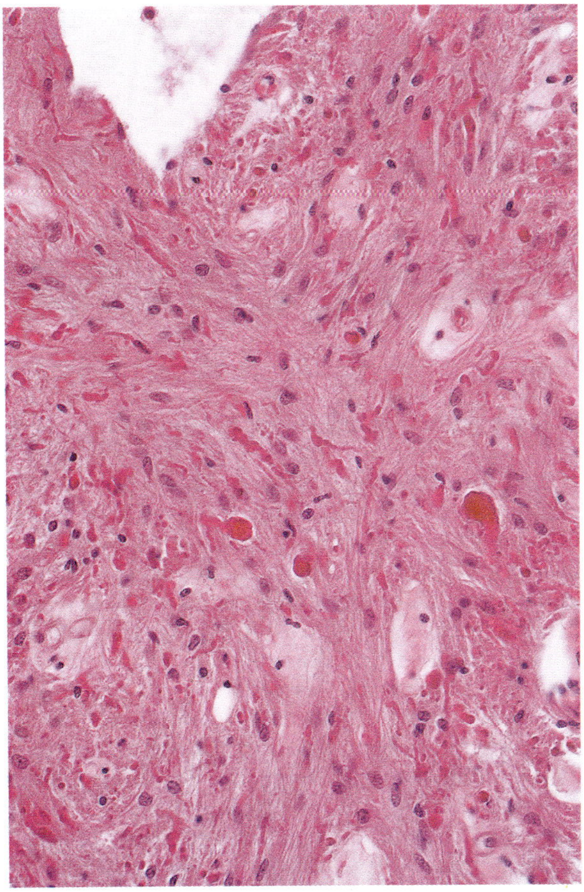

Fig. 9.51 Compact area of juvenile pilocytic astrocytoma from the lateral ventricle showing abundant eosinophilic Rosenthal fibers. H&E, × 250

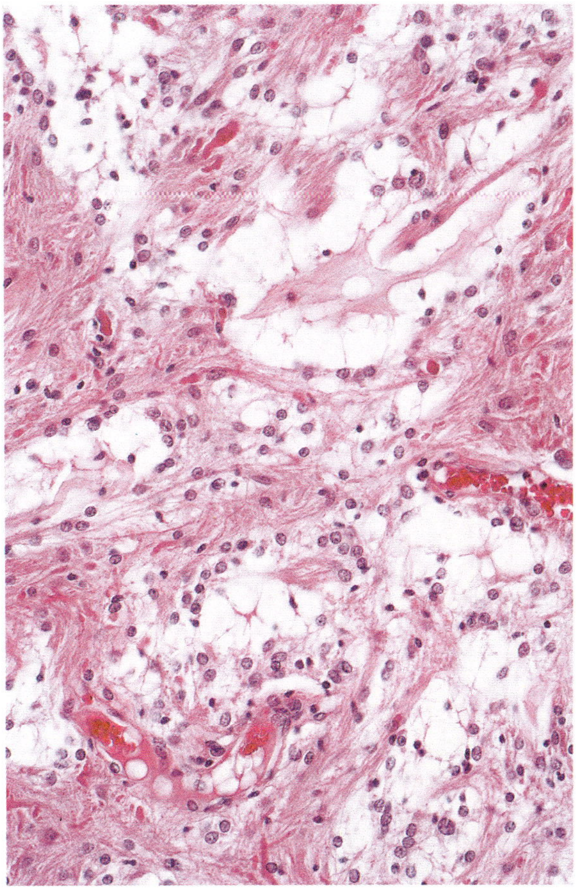

Fig. 9.53 Microcystic area in a juvenile pilocytic astrocytoma. H&E, × 250

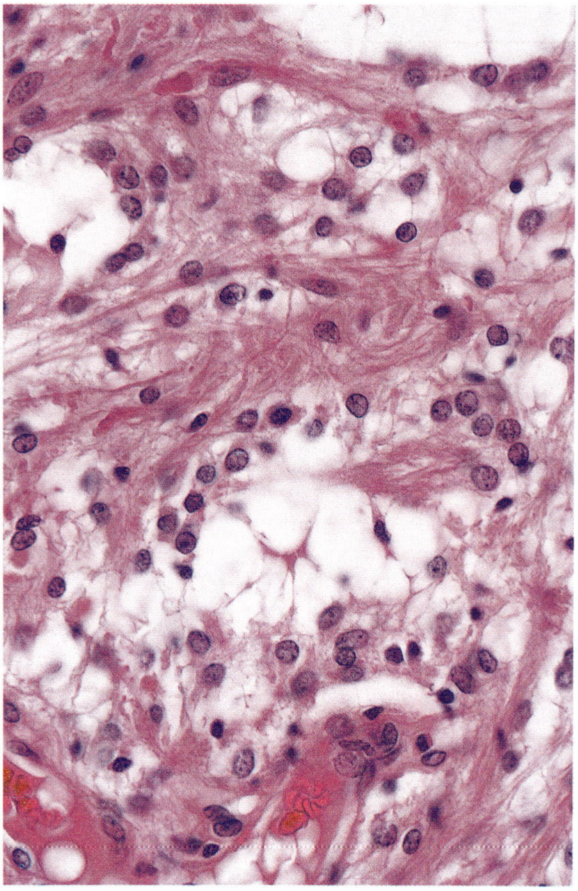

Fig. 9.54 Juvenile pilocytic astroctyoma: individual cells in the microcystic areas, with a tendency to be more protoplasmic than pilocytic. H&E, × 500

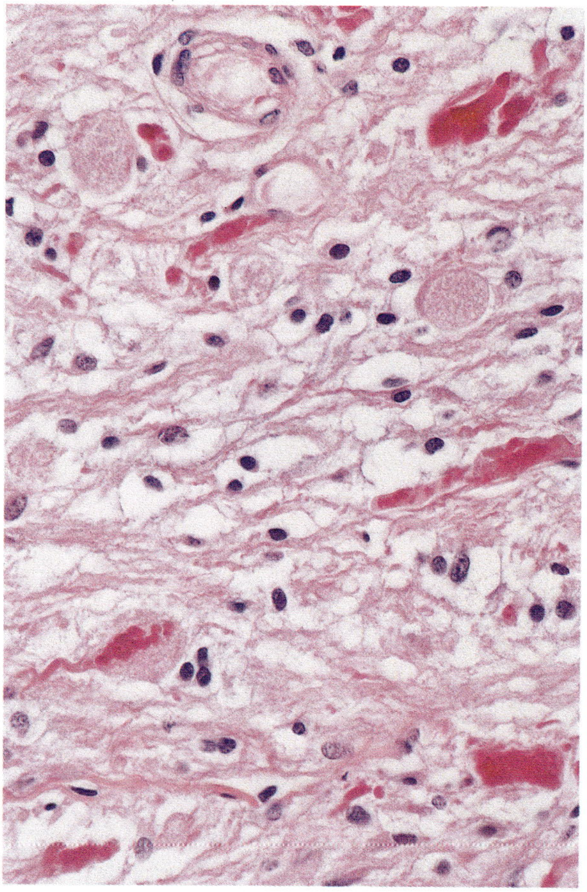

Fig. 9.55 Eosinophilic granular bodies and Rosenthal fibers in a juvenile pilocytic astrocytoma. H&E, × 500

presence of GFAP; the cell bodies and cell processes are intensely positive (Fig. 9.52). Although fibrils are easily demonstrable in their cytoplasm, there is little or no tendency for the formation of an intercellular fibrillary matrix: on the contrary, areas remote from the blood vessels have a rarefied and sparsely cellular appearance, and it is these areas that are prone to undergo microcystic degeneration (Fig. 9.53). Where such areas are well preserved, the cells are not piloid but feebly stellate (Fig. 9.54): many appear to be protoplasmic astrocytes. Occasionally, rows of tumor cells are orientated vertically towards the blood vessel walls, and here, too, their form is stellate, with rather short fibrillated feet.

Cyst formation is a feature common to the three histologic forms of astrocytoma considered above. This evolution ranges from microcyst formation (Figs 9.49, 9.53 and 9.54) to their coalescence into larger cysts, which may culminate in the development of a largely cystic tumor, as exemplified in the cerebellum in Fig. 9.44.

Cyst formation may be associated with the formation of *eosinophilic granular bodies* (Fig. 9.55). Using electron microscopy, these correspond to the incorporation of many small autophagic vacuoles into larger membrane-bound bodies as the result of the progressive pinocytosis of protein material by tumor astrocytes, as illustrated in Fig. 9.56 (for further discussion of this cellular mechanism, see Rubinstein and Herman, 1972; Caine *et al.*, 1980). The protein has been identified by immunoperoxidase staining as originating from the serum (Brett and Weller, 1978), an interpretation that has been supported by *in vitro* experiments on primary explants from various astrocytic gliomas (Caine *et al.*, 1980). However, some of the material has also been demonstrated to be GFAP (Barnard and Scott, 1980), thus suggesting an alternative, perhaps secretory or degenerative mechanism, as well.

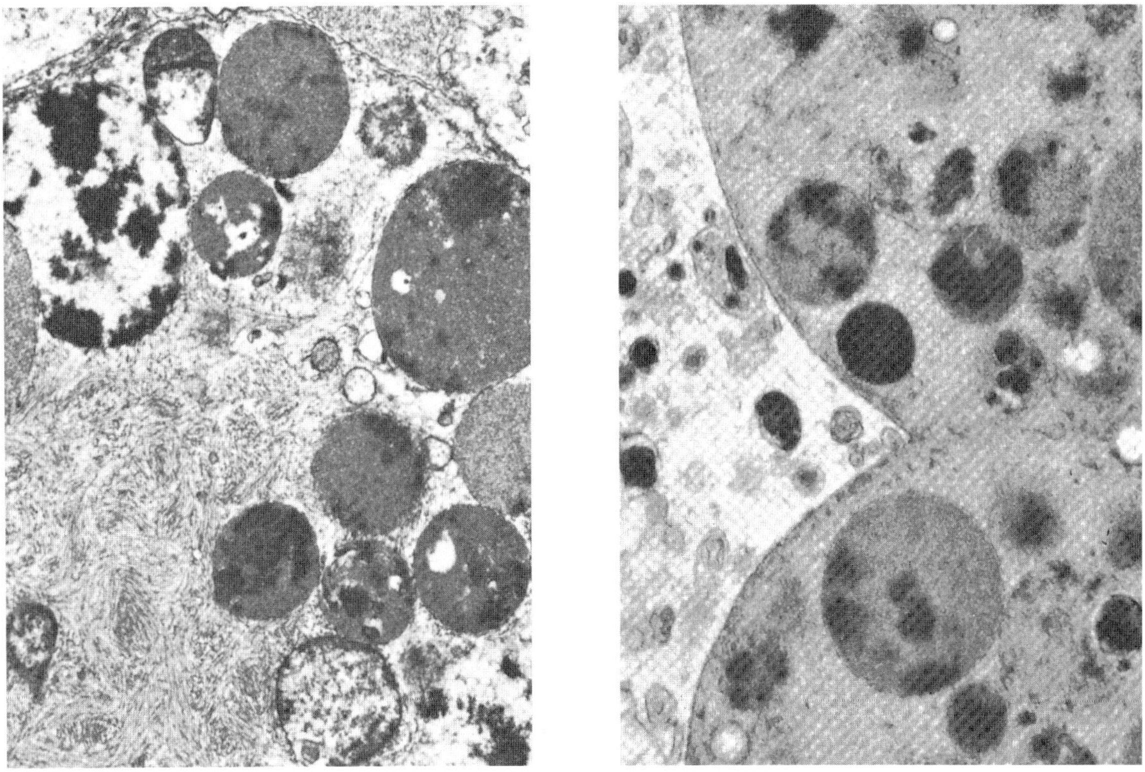

a b

Fig. 9.56 Glial tumor cell from a ganglioglioma. (a) Cytoplasm shows round membrane-bound autophagic vacuoles and numerous filaments. Cell nucleus is in the upper left. × 15 300. (b) Several autophagic vacuoles are enclosed within a much larger membrane-bound profile, only part of which is included in the figure. × 17 300 (In collaboration with Dr Mary M. Herman)

Recently, reactivity of these structures with antibodies to serum protease inhibitors, ubiquitin-protein conjugates and β-amyloid precursor protein has been reported (Katsetos *et al.*, 1994).

Rosenthal fibers are a characteristic degenerative change found in juvenile-type pilocytic astrocytomas, whether the tumors are present in the region of the third ventricle or in the cerebellum. These so-called 'cytoid bodies' form in the cytoplasm of the tumor cells (Figs 9.51 and 9.57). They are opaque, homogeneous, strongly eosinophilic carrot-shaped or beaded masses that assume a dense purple color with phosphotungstic acid–hematoxylin (PTAH) and stain positively with various other histochemical dyes that have an affinity for protein (Herndon *et al.*, 1970).

A considerable body of literature has accumulated on the incidence, morphologic features and functional nature of these Rosenthal fibers (reviews by Grcevic and Yates, 1957; Hallervorden, 1961; Herndon *et al.*, 1970; Horoupian *et al.*, 1982). It has long been known that they are not peculiar to the pilocytic astrocytomas and that they may be found in various situations where a reactive gliosis has long been in progress, e.g., in the regions adjacent to craniopharyngiomas (Fig. 9.58) and capillary hemangioblastomas and about syringomyelic cavities; they may also be found in the pineal body, in the walls of small central cysts. While it is likely, as suggested by Grcevic and Yates (1957), that the neuroglia of some parts of the neuraxis may be more prone to this kind of degeneration than others, Rosenthal fibers, when seen in a glial tumor, are not exclusively associated with pilocytic astrocytomas of the juvenile type or with cerebellar astrocytomas, but may occasionally be found in other variants, even in glioblastomas. Their connection with gliofibrillogenesis or with the degradation of glial filaments remains enigmatic. The central portion is usually not reactive with antibodies against GFAP, but the periphery of the fiber stains intensely (Smith and Lantos, 1985; Kobayashi *et al.*, 1990). The implication is that their development is associated with a profound change

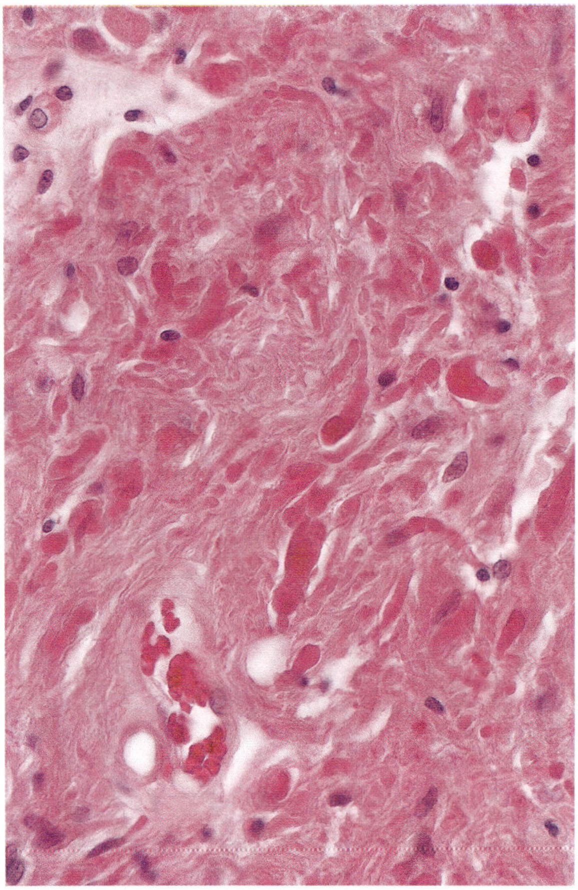

Fig. 9.57 Rosenthal fibers in a juvenile pilocytic astrocytoma. H&E, × 500

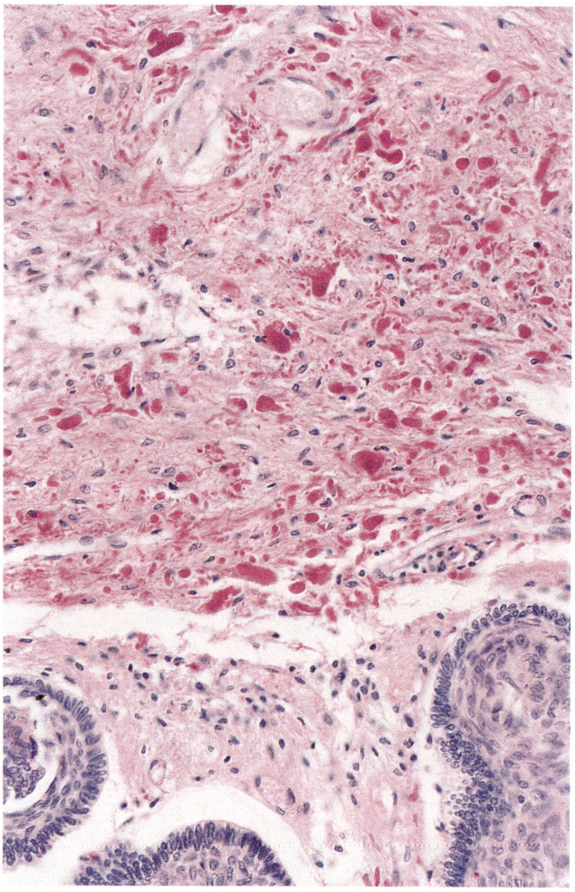

Fig. 9.58 Abundant Rosenthal fibers in the neuropil adjacent to a craniopharyngioma (bottom). H&E, × 250

in the chemical and antigenic constituents of glial fibers.

In *tissue culture*, the presence of Rosenthal fibers in astrocytic tumors has been documented using both light and electron microscopy (Gullotta, 1965; Gullotta and Fliedner, 1972; Escalona-Zapata and Diez-Nau, 1981) and Rubinstein illustrated (Russell and Rubinstein, 1989, pp. 83–161), in Fig. 9.59, their appearance in a tumor cell process of a cerebellar astrocytoma maintained in an organ culture system for 15 days (Sipe, Herman and Rubinstein, 1973). *Experimentally*, Rosenthal fibers have been produced by the intracerebral implantation of nickel wires (Horoupian *et al.*, 1982), and electron immunocytochemical labeling has shown that, in this experimental model, at least, the fibers may largely be made up of plasma protein rather than of proteins derived from fibrillated glia. The suggestion by these workers that gliofibrillogenesis and Rosenthal fiber production might be independent developments, resulting when astrocytes are subjected to prolonged periods of saturation with protein-rich fluid, is of some relevance because the glial tumors most commonly associated with the formation of Rosenthal fibers are often abnormally vascularized and cystic, and they frequently show the concomitant presence of the granular, membrane-bound protein-positive bodies, thus indicating either protein intake or abnormal protein secretion by the tumor cells.

These membrane-bound granules should be differentiated from the non-membrane-bound electron-dense bodies that constitute an early stage in the development of Rosenthal fibers and that are not part of the autophagic system. By light microscopy, the latter may present as multiple eosinophilic cytoplasmic inclusions with the staining reactions of protein, as illustrated by Herndon *et al.* (1970) and others. Both types of granular bodies, which may therefore not be distinguishable by light microscopy, can be encountered, in variable proportions, in glial tumors rich in Rosenthal fibers.

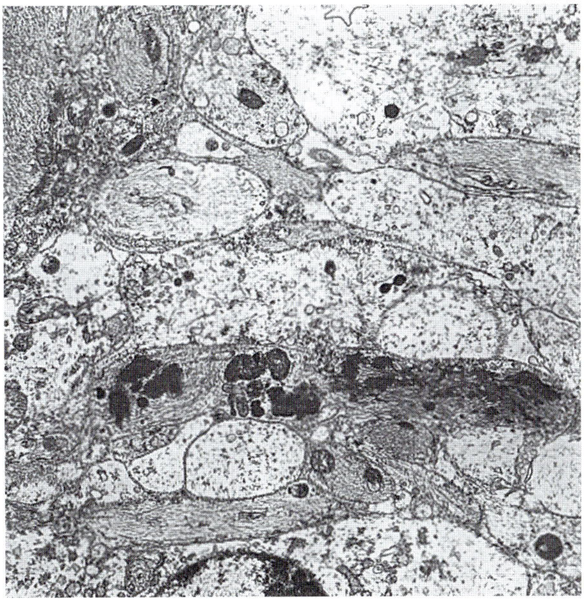

Fig. 9.59 Ultrastructure of a cerebellar astrocytoma shows intensely osmiophilic bodies, corresponding to Rosenthal fibers, with glial filaments. × 1250 (mag. to negative)

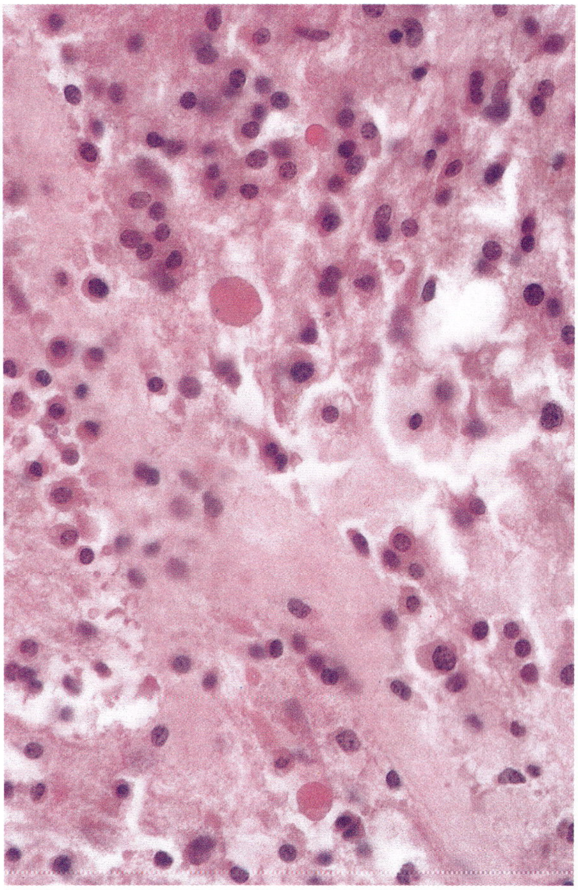

Fig. 9.60 Eosinophilic hyaline globules representing protein droplets in a juvenile pilocytic astrocytoma. H&E, × 500

Foci of oligodendroglial-like cells are occasionally found in juvenile pilocytic astrocytomas. These have the ballooned aspect of 'acute swelling', as is usual in tumors of these cells. This appearance, noted also by others in the cerebellar astrocytomas, was interpreted by Ringertz and Nordenstam (1951) as the result of degeneration in tumor astrocytes.

In addition to the Rosenthal fibers already mentioned (Figs 9.51 and 9.57), the densely pilocytic areas often contain variable numbers of intra- and extracellular eosinophilic hyaline droplets (Fig. 9.60).

Calcospherites, usually discrete, are found in about 25% of the cases.

Leptomeningeal invasion is common in both the juvenile and the diffuse forms and may sometimes be conspicuous. It is demonstrable in up to 30% of cases and carries no adverse prognostic significance in relation to long-term survival (Hayostek *et al.*, 1993). The cells that invade the leptomeninges are predominantly pilocytic, perhaps because of their presumptive origin from the polar cells of the superficial cerebellar cortex.

Microvascular proliferation, without accompanying anaplasia or increased cellularity of the tumor, is common, and is found in at least 15% of the cases. In contrast to its prognostic significance in the diffuse cerebral astrocytomas, its presence in the typical form of cerebellar astrocytoma does not connote a malignant change and, even in patients in whom the tumor has been incompletely removed, it has been associated with long postoperative survival.

Atypical cellular features, such as hyperchromatic nuclei and multinucleated giant cells, have been noted in juvenile pilocytic astrocytomas, sometimes accompanied by microvascular proliferation (Hayostek *et al.*, 1993). However, in the absence of other criteria of malignant change, such as increased mitotic activity, these features are more likely to be due to cellular degeneration, as argued by Bucy and Gustafson (1939), Zülch (1957) and others. It is notable that these examples were found mostly in patients in the higher age groups and that they were accompanied by other evidence of degeneration, such as hyaline thickening of the blood vessels, the presence of large numbers of sizable eosinophilic bodies and smaller hyaline droplets (Fig. 9.60), and variable degrees of cyst formation.

Electron microscopy

Electron microscopic study of pilocytic astrocytomas confirms the presence of compact bundles of intracellular filaments in the cell processes (Hossmann and Wechsler, 1965). Ultrastructural examination (Duffell *et al.*, 1963; Schlote, 1966; Herndon *et al.*, 1970; Horoupian *et al.*, 1982) has corroborated the intracellular localization of Rosenthal fibers and their close topographic relationship to glial filament formation in the astrocytes. As illustrated in Fig. 9.59, they are identifiable as distinct, irregular, densely osmiophilic bodies, separate from – but in places merging into – thickened glial filaments.

Evolution, recurrence and anaplastic change

It has long been known that the circumscribed astrocytoma of childhood, with the typical histologic pattern described above, carries an excellent postoperative prognosis. The figures of Gjerris and Klinken (1978), ranging over a 25-year period, give a 94% survival rate in patients operated on for this form of cerebellar astrocytoma. A more recent study (Hayostek *et al.*, 1993) indicates survival rates of 85%, 81% and 79% at 5, 10 and 20 years, respectively. A similar survival rate of about 80% was seen in a series of 99 patients who were treated before 1980, as summarized by Kehler, Arnold and Muller (1990).

An interesting, presumably spontaneous, evolution of some of the large cystic tumors should also be mentioned. It is likely that some of the large intracerebellar cysts lined by degenerated glia, including numerous Rosenthal fibers, and occasionally reported as 'simple glial cysts', represent the end stage of a slow-growing, burnt-out astrocytoma. The problem is discussed by Silverberg (1971) in his report of four cases. All these cases, as well as the few from the literature that were documented at autopsy, occurred in older adults, usually in their fifth to seventh decade.

It is clear from various follow-up series (Marsa *et al.*, 1973; Leibel *et al.*, 1975; Bernstein *et al.*, 1984; Imes and Hoyt, 1986) that, despite their deep-seated localization in the brain, many cases of hypothalamic pilocytic astrocytomas may pursue a relatively favorable postoperative course, characterized by many years' survival, even after only exploratory biopsy (Sutton *et al.*, 1995). Many patients are given adjuvant local radiotherapy or chemotherapy for these tumors, but indications are controversial, and the criteria are not well defined. Earlier studies (Bernstein *et al.*, 1984) suggested that no statistically significant improvement in patient survival rate could be detected as a result of cranial irradiation. More recent treatment trials, however, advocate this adjuvant therapy (Sutton *et al.*, 1995).

Recurrences are rare. They may be considerably delayed, as recorded by Bernell, Kepes and Seitz (1972), who described two cases of childhood cerebellar astrocytoma that recurred, one 20 years and the other 23 years after surgical excision. An additional late recurrence of a benign pilocytic cerebellar astrocytoma was recorded by Pagni, Giordana and Canavero (1991), 36 years after initial radical resection. In some cases, recurrence is not accompanied by malignant change but, as shown in case 2 of Bernell, Kepes and Seitz (1972), and as apparent from other reports (Budka, 1975; Kleinman *et al.*, 1978; Alpers, Davis and Wilson, 1982; Steinberg *et al.*, 1985; Schwartz and Ghatak, 1990), late recurrence may be associated with the development of anaplasia and the appearance of a malignant astrocytoma or a glioblastoma. In a reported series of 107 patients with cerebellar pilocytic astrocytomas, anaplastic histologic features were noted in only 0.9%, all at recurrence. A notable finding was brisk mitotic activity. Clinical behavior was still benign in some of these cases with anaplastic histology (Tomlinson *et al.*, 1994).

Remarkable among those reported are the case of Kleinman *et al.* (1978) concerning a 51-year-old man who died from a malignant cerebellar astrocytoma 48 years after partial removal of a previously benign astrocytoma at the same site; the case of Budka and Wöber (1974) that involved both cerebellar hemispheres in a 60-year-old male and may have been an early example of diffuse cerebral gliomatosis; and case 3 of Steinberg *et al.* (1985) regarding a 6-year-old female diagnosed with a juvenile-type cerebellar astrocytoma, the patient having succumbed 21 years later to a glioblastoma located at the same site but extending into the brainstem, diencephalon and thalamus.

A notable feature of some of the cerebellar astrocytomas with histologic evidence of malignancy is their apparent association with NF type 1. Attention was drawn to this association by Ilgren, Kinnier-Wilson and Stiller (1985). It has indeed long been known (Russell and Rubinstein, 1989, p. 774) that the cerebellar astrocytoma, like optic nerve gliomas, may be one of the gliomas that is found with an unusual frequency in NF type 1. The pattern of the astrocytoma in these cases is often one of diffuse infiltration of the cerebellar cortex, associated with massive permeation of the cerebellar leptomeninges and the formation of numerous glial bridges transgressing the pia. It is noteworthy that the case of cerebellar glioblastoma in a 14-year-old girl, as reported by Chin *et al.* (1984), was also an example of NF type 1. More examples of this association were collected by Blatt *et al.* (1986), two of them being low grade and the other two malignant.

Subependymal giant-cell astrocytomas

This distinctive tumor is characteristically associated with tuberous sclerosis. Earlier reported examples of this tumor were not uncommonly encountered in the apparent absence of tuberous sclerosis (Bonnin *et al.*, 1984b), but the advent of modern radiologic imaging has more recently documented the occurrence of tuberous sclerosis in nearly all cases of subependymal giant-cell astrocytoma (Shepherd *et al.*, 1991). This tumor has a number of unique morphologic features that, highlighted in some of their fine structural and immunohistochemical aspects, suggest that its cell of origin may have been the target of a dysgenetic event in early development.

Discrepancies in cellular differentiation are evident in the tumor. Despite these qualifications, it is best regarded as a variant of astrocytoma.

Age and sex incidence

These neoplasms are found mostly in subjects in the first and second decades, the patients with tuberous sclerosis being generally younger than those in whom the tumor is an isolated event. Both sexes are about equally affected. Congenital examples, which tend to be of large size, are recognized (Hahn, Bejar and Gladson, 1991; Oikawa, Sakamoto and Kobayashi, 1994).

Sites and macroscopic appearance

Subependymal giant-cell astrocytomas classically occupy the walls of one of the lateral ventricles over the basal ganglia (Fig. 9.61) and, when large, are apt to cause obstruction following blockage of the foramen of Monro. Occasionally, they occlude the third ventricle. They are sharply defined and usually well vascularized. In places, the blood vessels may be greatly dilated, resulting in an angiomatous appearance. Some of the tumors may be coarsely nodular, and cysts of various sizes are often present (Fig. 9.61). Focal calcifications are common.

Radiographic appearance

The radiologic findings of subependymal giant-cell astrocytoma show a slow-growing mass arising from a calcified subependymal 'candle dripping' at the foramen of Monro in a patient with tuberous sclerosis.

At CT scanning, the calcified subependymal nodule is seen at the foramen of Monro, and has an associated soft tissue mass within the frontal horn of the lateral ventricle. The nodule is frequently of mixed density or is isodense to brain; but, with contrast, there is intense enhancement. Cysts or heterogeneous enhancement may also be found in these nodules.

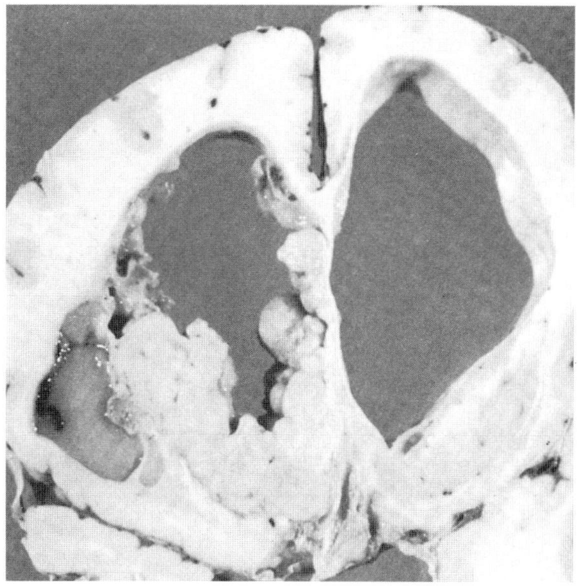

Fig. 9.61 Tumor of the lateral ventricle in a case of tuberous sclerosis. (Courtesy of Dr J. Michaud)

At MRI, the calcified subependymal tuber is usually of low T1 and T2 signal intensity. If this nodule enhances, giant-cell astrocytoma should be suspected. This slow-growing mass frequently is of heterogeneous, increased T2 signal intensity and is heterogeneous to isointense on T1-weighted images. Enhancement is usually intense, although somewhat heterogeneous (Fig. 9.62).

Other findings of tuberous sclerosis are identified in these cases. These include cortical and subcortical tubers, best seen on T2-weighted images as areas of increased T2 signal intensity. Subependymal tubers are commonly seen elsewhere in the lateral ventricles as focal rounded areas of low signal intensity on MRI and as calcified nodules by CT.

Microscopic appearance

These tumors are remarkable. The cells, although variable in size, are mainly very large and often fusiform or pyramidal (Fig. 9.63). They have a bulky homogeneous hyaline cytoplasm (Fig. 9.64), usually elongated into processes that are either coarse and nonfibrillated or fine and fibrillated; the latter form a matrix that often separates the cells rather widely. Many of the cells are indistinguishable from gemistocytic astrocytes, whereas others are extremely elongated with a strap-like appearance, and yet others are more suggestive of large astroblasts. Perivascular pseudorosettes are fairly common. Giant, bizarre forms may be found, but are inconstant. In any event, the nuclei of these

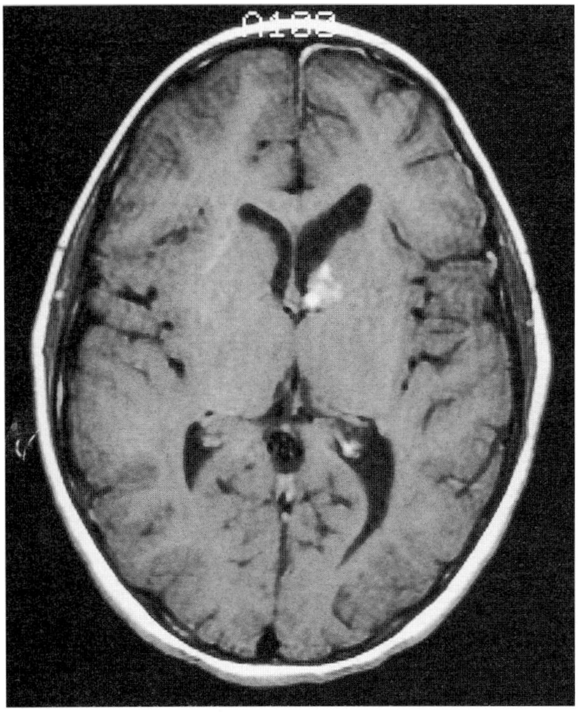

a

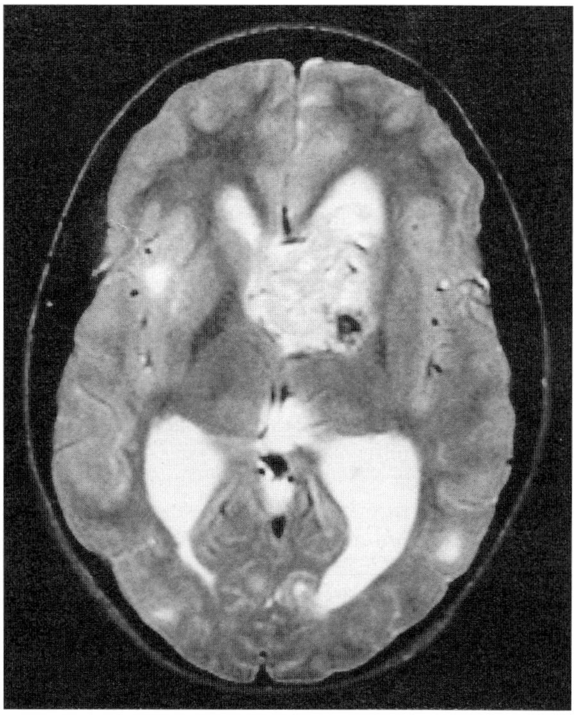

b

Fig. 9.62 Two MRIs of a young girl with tuberous sclerosis. (a) Axial T1-weighted postcontrast image demonstrates an area of abnormal enhancement in the basal ganglion adjacent to the left foramen of Monro. The subependymal enhancement is heterogeneous. Note the subependymal nodule adjacent to the left occipital pole. (b) Axial T2 weighted image 2 years later demonstrates that the subependymal left frontal mass has significantly increased in size. There is heterogeneous T2 signal intensity with an area of lower T2 signal indicating calcification. Enlargement of the ventricular system is present due to obstruction at the foramen of Monro. Also note, on this image, the cortical and subcortical tubers characteristic of tuberous sclerosis. A subependymal tuber near the foramen of Monro is suspicious and should be closely followed. Subependymal giant-cell astrocytoma of tuberous sclerosis is suspected if enhancement is identified in this location.

bizarre cells are remarkably uniform and do not suggest a malignant neoplasm. They are usually eccentric, of variable size, and have a finely granulated nucleoplasm and distinct nucleoli (Fig. 9.64). Mitotic figures are recognized with variable frequency, and their presence does not indicate a worse prognosis (Shepherd *et al.*, 1991). Foci of necrosis similarly have no adverse prognostic implication. Bi- and multinucleated forms occur, and, occasionally, the nuclei are so large and vesiculated as to closely mimic those of neurons (Fig. 9.64). Demonstrable ganglionic participation seems exceptional (Ferraro and Doolittle, 1936). The supporting blood vessels have thin walls and are usually devoid of endothelial proliferation.

Cytogenesis

The interpretation of this glioma has been debated, and some of the more recent electron microscopic and immunohistochemical studies, referred to below, suggest that the cytogenetic points at issue are not clear cut. Its incidence, widely recognized, in cases of tuberous sclerosis suggests an origin in the nests of atypical astrocytes that are so characteristic of the cerebrum in the disease. Thus, examples of tuberous sclerosis may demonstrate, at the periphery of the centrum ovale, foci, of variable size, composed of these swollen glial cells dispersed among intersecting bundles and whorls of glial fibrils, and associated with numerous small calcospherites: these foci might be interpreted as an intermediate stage between the well-defined tumors and the smaller heterotopias of tuberous sclerosis. In the older literature (see Jervis, 1954, for references to previously reported cases), the tumors have mostly been regarded as a variety of astrocytoma or spongioblastoma, but have not always been distinguished from some giant-cell forms of

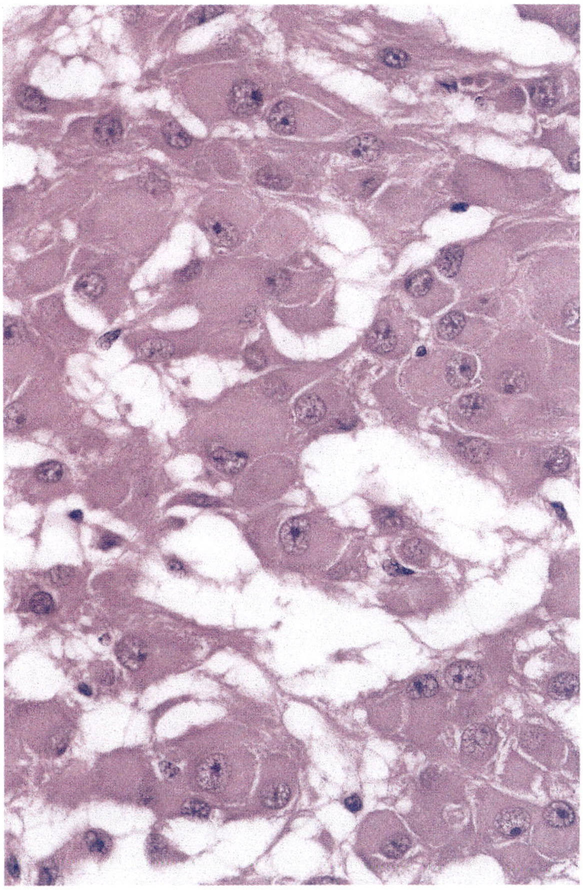

Fig. 9.63 Large fusiform cells with abundant eosinophilic cytoplasm in a subependymal giant-cell astrocytoma. H&E, × 500

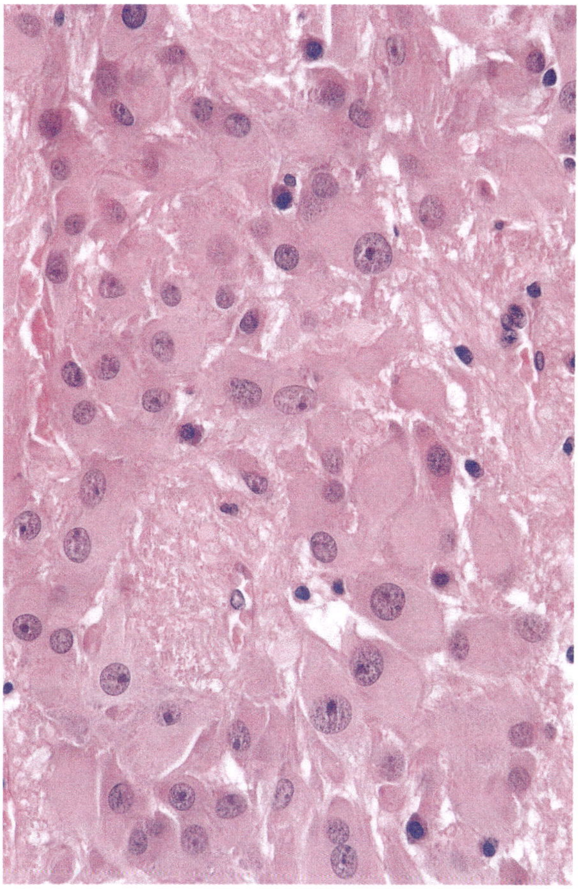

Fig. 9.64 Same case as Fig. 9.63. Some areas of subependymal giant-cell astrocytoma showing epithelioid or pyramidal cells and resembling both neurons and gemistocytic astrocytes. H&E, × 500

glioblastoma (p. 000) and from ganglion cell neoplasms (as discussed on p. 000).

Electron microscopy

Several fine structural studies (Ribadeau-Dumas, Poirier and Escourolle, 1973; Sima and Robertson, 1979; Trombley and Mirra, 1981; Nakamura and Becker, 1983, case 4) have confirmed the astrocytic nature of some of the tumor cells and their identity with the monster astrocytes that are one of the features of tuberous sclerosis. Rosenthal fibers were observed by Sima and Robertson (1979) in some of the cell processes. The same workers, however, also reported the presence of numerous membrane-bound dense bodies measuring 350–900 nm in diameter and of occasional dense-core vesicles measuring 100–200 nm. These findings were subsequently confirmed by de Chadarévian and Hollenberg (1979) and, in one example, by Nakamura and Becker (1983, case 7), who also observed synaptic structures in their case.

Immunohistochemistry

Doubt was cast on the astrocytic nature of the tumor cells by the immunohistochemical findings of Stefansson and Wollmann (1980, 1981), who reported GFAP negativity in the cells of three tumors associated with tuberous sclerosis and their positivity for neuron-specific enolase (NSE), thus reviving an older suggestion that the tumors might be neuronal rather than astrocytic. However, the demonstration of NSE in CNS neoplasms is not indicative of neuronal derivation, and divergent observations on the presence of GFAP in the cells of subependymal giant-cell astrocytomas (see discussion in Bonnin *et al.*, 1984b) tended to suggest a good deal of heterogeneity in the cellular composition of these tumors, despite their relatively uniform histologic appearance by conventional microscopy. The subsequent studies by Nakamura and Becker (1983) on seven examples associated with tuberous sclerosis and by Bonnin *et al.* (1984b) on another 22 cases, of which five were definitely associated with the disease, have independently shown that GFAP positivity is often, but by no means invariably, absent in the subependymal astrocytomas accompanying tuberous sclerosis (Fig. 9.65). Occasional cells containing the 68-kDa neurofilament protein (NFP) were found in 6/22 tumors in the series of Bonnin *et al.*, usually in association with GFAP-positive cells. Some cases show immunohistochemical labeling for synaptophysin, another indication of neuronal derivation (Fig. 9.66). The presence of NSE was confirmed in the cells of 13/18 tumors tested (Bonnin *et al.*, 1984b). According to Nakamura and Becker, S-100 protein-positive cells are also found in the majority of cases (Fig. 9.67).

The difficulty of morphologically relating this tumor to a recognized normal mature or immature glial cell type renders its derivation a matter of conjecture, but the collective evidence suggests that it probably originates from a dysplastic cell with a potential for astrocytic and neuronal differentiation that may be either incompletely or aberrantly expressed.

Clinical behavior

Subependymal giant-cell astrocytomas are characteristically slow growing, and long survival is generally achieved after surgical resection. A case described by Rubinstein (Russell and Rubinstein, 1989, pp. 83–161), of a 22-year-old male with classic tuberous sclerosis admitted for shunting treatment of his hydrocephalus, was known to have had a tumor subtotally removed from the region of the foramen of Monro 17 years previously. Long-delayed recurrences have been reported (Halmagyi, Bignold and Allsop, 1979). Ploidy and kinetic studies have revealed a diploid DNA content in 13/14 examples and a low proliferative rate (Nishizaki *et al.*, 1990; Shepherd *et al.*, 1991).

Pleomorphic xanthoastrocytomas

The recognition of this entity, first defined in 1979 (Kepes, Rubinstein and Eng, 1979), is important on two counts: first, because of the striking disparity between its ominous-looking histologic features and its usually favorable postoperative course; and, second, because of its pleomorphic microscopic appearance, which led to its designation under several different diagnostic labels. Thus, examples of this tumor associated either with a successful clinical cure or with an unusually protracted length

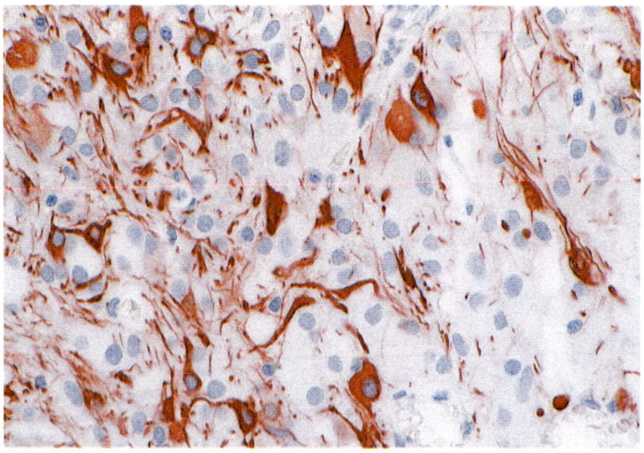

Fig. 9.65 Neoplastic cells of subependymal giant-cell astrocytoma can show cytoplasmic reactivity for GFAP. GFAP immunoperoxidase and hematoxylin, × 500

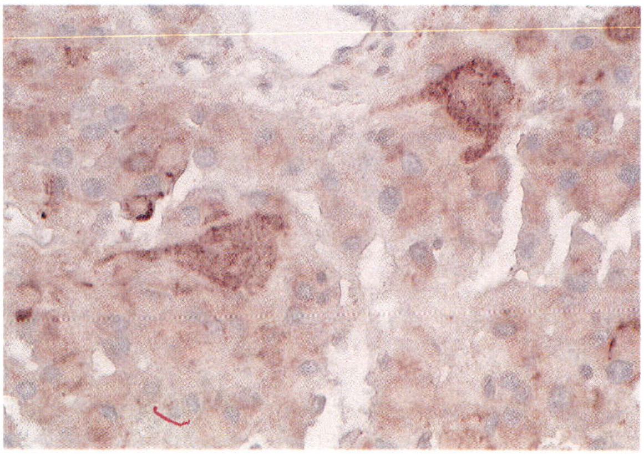

Fig. 9.66 Synaptophysin immunoreactivity seen in the cytoplasm of some cells of subependymal giant-cell astrocytoma. Synaptophysin immunoperoxidase and hematoxylin, × 500

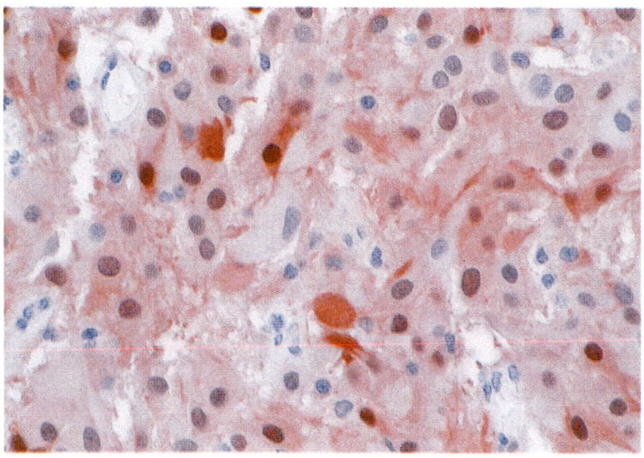

Fig. 9.67 Many cells of subependymal giant-cell astrocytoma showing both nuclear and cytoplasmic reactivity for S-100 protein. S-100 immunoperoxidase and hematoxylin, × 500

of postoperative survival were formerly interpreted in previous editions of this text as superficially situated anaplastic pilocytic astrocytomas (Russell and Rubinstein, 1977, p. 7 and Figs 169 and 170), as recurrent giant-cell glioblastomas (Russell and Rubinstein, 1977, p. 243), or as atypical fibroxanthomas or xanthosarcomas (Russell and Rubinstein, 1977, p. 111). Similar tumors were first labeled 'fibroxanthomatous' by Kepes, Kepes and Slowik (1973), and one was reported by Garcia-Bengochea and Collins (1969) as a monstrocellular sarcoma with long postoperative survival. The application of the immunoperoxidase technique for GFAP has been crucial in identifying all such cases as a distinctive form of superficial cortical astrocytoma, given the name 'pleomorphic xanthoastrocytoma', thereby underscoring some of its histologic features. Since the publication of the original series of 12 cases (Kepes, Rubinstein and Eng, 1979), subsequent reports (Kuhajda *et al.*, 1981; Strøm and Skullerud, 1983; Weldon-Linne *et al.*, 1983; Gomez, Garcia and Colon, 1985; Palma *et al.*, 1985; Pasquier *et al.*, 1985; Grant and Gallagher, 1986) have corroborated the existence of this tumor as an entity *sui generis*. It has now been defined as a specific nosologic category in the most recent revision of the WHO classification (Kleihues, Burger and Scheithauer, 1993). A delightful historic account of its description has been summarized by Kepes (1993).

Age incidence

Pleomorphic xanthoastrocytomas characteristically are tumors of young patients, most frequently in their second decade, less often in the first or third. A history of epileptic seizures, sometimes dating back several years, is usually elicited. There is no obvious preponderance of either sex.

Sites

Although all of the earlier reports were of supratentorial examples, several pleomorphic xanthoastrocytomas originating in the cerebellum have now been reported, although many of these posterior fossa examples have been mixed with apparent neuronal elements (Lindboe, Cappelen and Kepes, 1992; Glasser *et al.*, 1995; Powell *et al.*, 1996). One tumor arising in the thoracic spinal cord has also been reported (Herpers, Freling and Beuls, 1994). Pleomorphic xanthoastrocytomas are typically superficial, often occupying the cerebral cortex over a relatively restricted field only and extending massively in the overlying leptomeninges, but not into the dura. The temporal lobe is preferentially involved, but the tumor may also arise in the parietal or frontal lobes, with or without concomitant temporal involvement.

Macroscopic appearance

Pleomorphic xanthoastrocytomas are often large, part-solid/part-cystic growths in which the cystic component may be extensive. The tumors present as a mural nodule of yellow or reddish tissue, with the cysts containing amber proteinaceous fluid. While the mass often seems to blend with the underlying brain, it is almost always relatively circumscribed, making its gross total resection frequently possible.

Radiographic appearance

The radiologic findings of this well-differentiated astrocytoma demonstrate a cystic neoplasm with a well-defined enhancing mural nodule. The nodule is hypointense on T1-weighted images and of increased T2 signal on T2-weighted images. Intense homogeneous enhancement of the nodule is noted. The associated cyst has low T1 signal and high T2 signal intensity. This mass is classically located in a cortical site.

At CT scanning, the cystic portion of the tumor is of low density. The mural nodule is hypodense and enhances strongly with contrast. A more infiltrative appearance or absence of a cyst is an unusual presentation.

Microscopic appearance

These tumors are distinctive, but are apt to cause considerable diagnostic uncertainties when viewed outside the context of previous experience. As indicated by its name, the cellular features of the tumor are quite variable, ranging from large plump eosinophilic cells with rounded outlines and eccentric nuclei (Figs 9.68 and 9.69) to intersecting bundles of elongated cells in a densely fibrillated matrix (Fig. 9.70). In fact, this extreme cellular pleomorphism is a unifying histologic feature. Cellular atypia, nuclear irregularity and hyperchromatism, multinucleation with giant-cell formation, and mitotic activity may all be present, but necrosis is notably absent and should, when observed, raise the suspicion that the lesion belongs to a more malignant form of glioma that shares with the pleomorphic xanthoastrocytoma the tendency to develop large amounts of intracellular lipid, i.e., the lipidized glioblastoma (Kepes and Rubinstein, 1981). This propensity for cellular lipidization, which may be marked (Fig. 9.71) and which initially led to its interpretation as an atypical fibroxanthoma, is not, however, invariable and may be inconspicuous or even absent. Another feature that originally invited the diagnosis of xanthosarcoma is the demonstration of an abundant reticulin network that often surrounds individual tumor cells (Fig. 9.72) or is aligned along the intersecting spindle-shaped bundles. This abundance of young

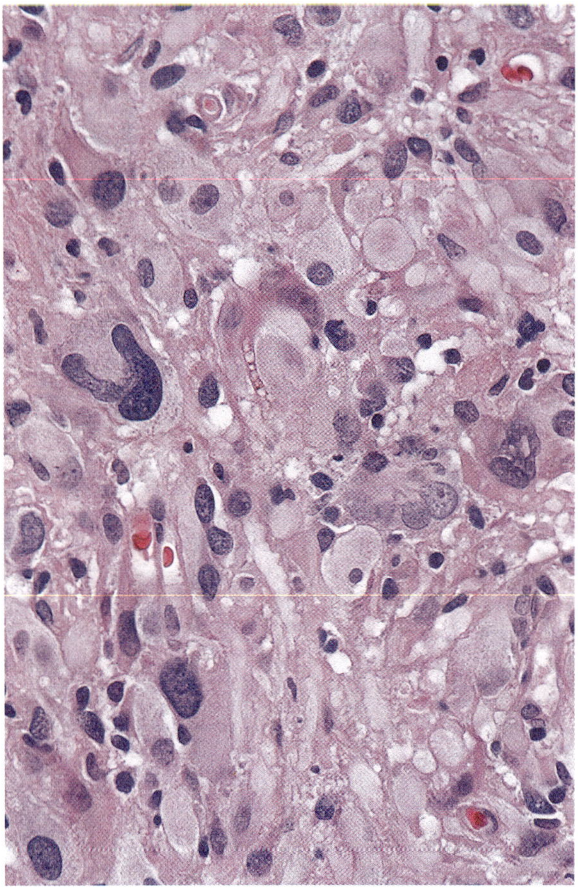

Fig. 9.68 Marked pleomorphism of both nuclei and cytoplasm in neoplastic cells of pleomorphic xanthoastrocytoma. H&E, × 500

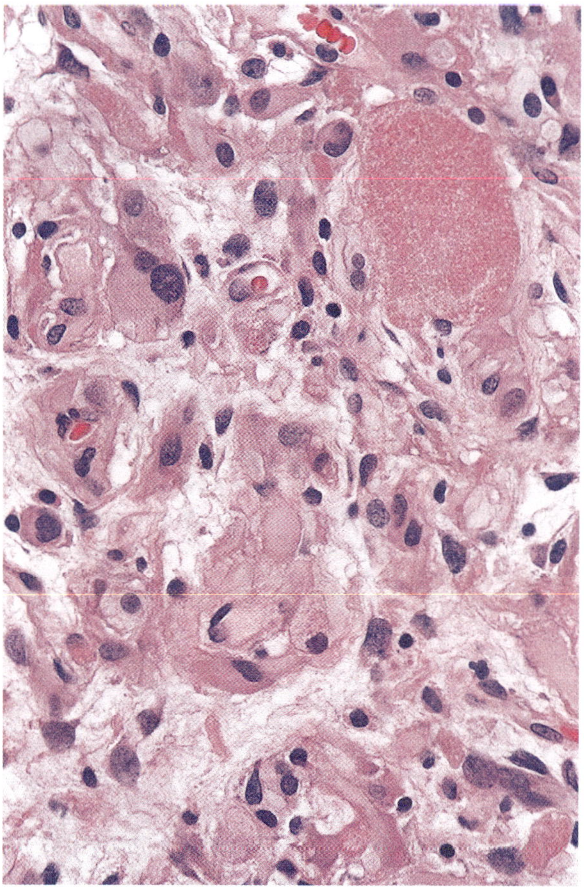

Fig. 9.69 Eosinophilic granular bodies and lipidized cells in pleomorphic xanthoastrocytoma. H&E, × 500

connective tissue seems to be due partly to the predominant involvement of the leptomeninges by the growth and partly to the investment of tumor cells by a basal lamina, as shown by electron microscopy. Additional histologic patterns have been subsequently documented, including an epithelioid variant and an angiomatous form rich in blood vessels (Iwaki *et al.*, 1987; Sugita *et al.*, 1990).

Immunohistochemically, the tumor cells, including those infiltrating the leptomeninges, are positive for GFAP (Fig. 9.73), a finding that establishes their astrocytic nature. Several recent reports have commented on the demonstration of immunoreactivity for neuronal antigens, either synaptophysin or NFPs, in the cytoplasm of individual, large atypical cells, an immunoreactivity rarely coexpressed in cells also demonstrating GFAP (Kros, Vecht and Stefanko, 1991; Furuta *et al.*, 1992; Lindboe, Cappelen and Kepes, 1992; Hirato, Nagayata and Ogawa, 1994; Glasser *et al.*, 1995; Kordek *et al.*, 1995; Powell *et al.*, 1996). These reports have broadened the diagnostic spectrum of pleomorphic xanthoastrocytomas and suggested that the cell of origin might retain a capability for expression of a neuronal phenotype. The relationship of this tumor to other slow-growing glioneuronal neoplasms, such as ganglioglioma, is as yet undefined.

Electron microscopy

As originally reported (Kepes, Rubinstein and Eng, 1979) and later confirmed (Kuhajda *et al.*, 1981; Weldon-Linne *et al.*, 1983), the tumor cells are covered by a well-defined basal lamina, as illustrated in the example obtained from a cystic left temporal tumor in an 18-year-old boy (Fig. 9.74). The subpial cerebral astrocyte, the free surface of which is known to possess that feature, was first suggested as the cell of origin.

Clinical behavior and anaplastic change

Most of the examples have, even in the absence of postoperative irradiation, run a relatively favorable

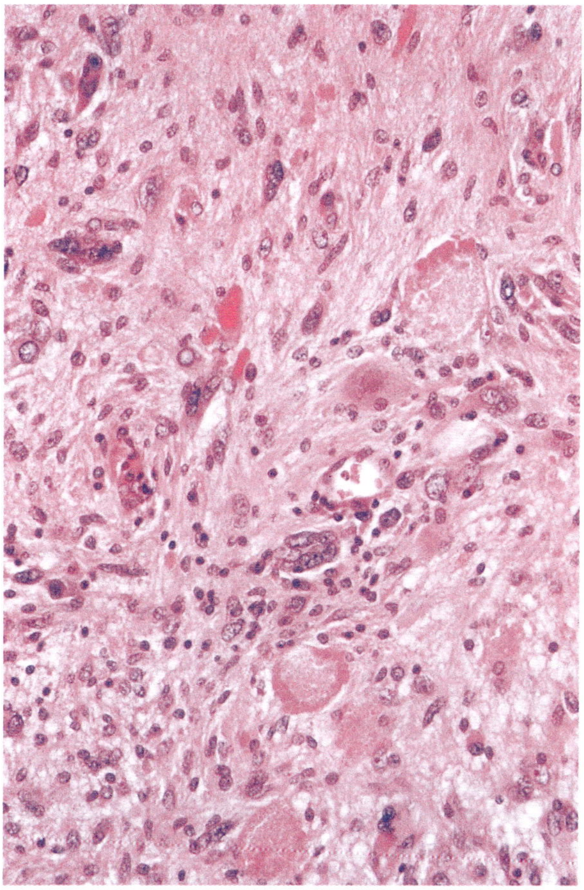

Fig. 9.70 Elongated cells in a fibrillary matrix, with Rosenthal fibers and eosinophilic granular bodies in pleomorphic xanthoastrocytoma. H&E, × 250

course, characterized by apparent clinical cure or long periods of postoperative survival. Recurrences have, however, been documented, sometimes without any demonstrable increase of histologic malignancy. Several examples of recurrence with malignant histologic features have now been reported (Weldon-Linne *et al.*, 1983; Kepes *et al.*, 1989; Allegranza *et al.*, 1991a; Macaulay *et al.*, 1993). Malignant evolution is still exceptional, but its recognition raises caution about regarding this tumor as benign.

Desmoplastic cerebral astrocytomas of infancy

Another rare form of superficial cerebral astrocytoma, characterized by intense desmoplasia and restricted to infants, has been described by Taratuto *et al.* (1984) and reviewed by VandenBerg (1993). As with the pleomorphic xanthoastrocytoma, its recognition was largely made possible by the immunoperoxidase stain for GFAP (Fig. 9.75),

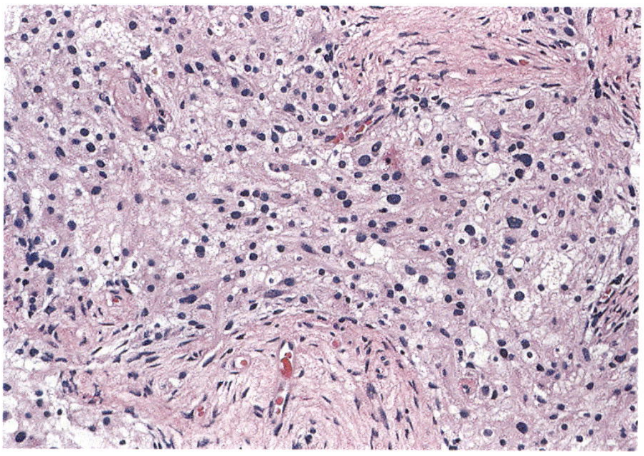

Fig. 9.71 Focal area of lipidized cells in pleomorphic xanthoastrocytoma. H&E, × 250

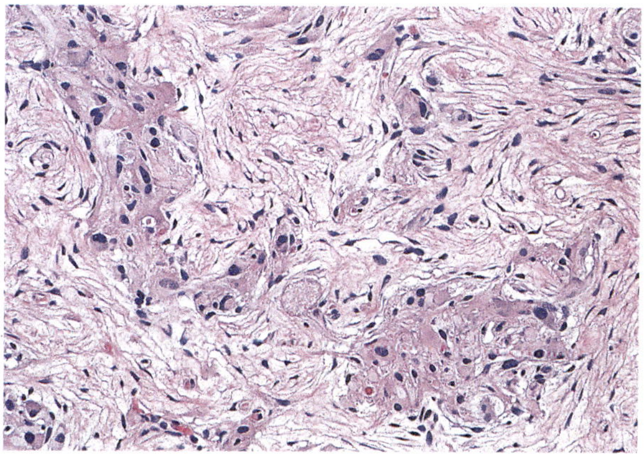

Fig. 9.72 Dense fibrous stroma surrounding groups of neoplastic cells in pleomorphic xanthoastrocytoma. H&E, × 250

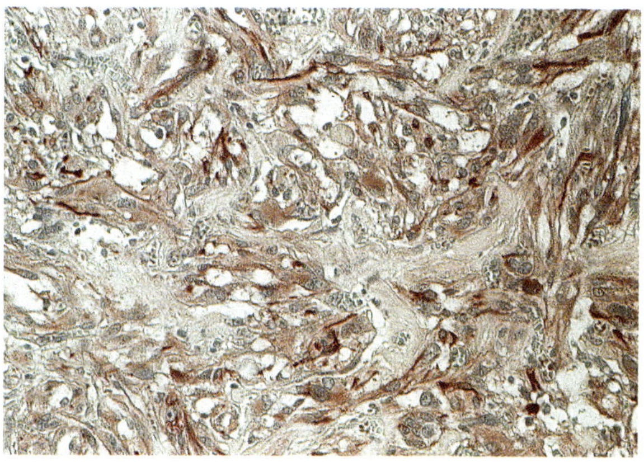

Fig. 9.73 Cells of pleomorphic xanthoastrocytoma showing variable cytoplasmic reactivity for GFAP. GFAP immunoperoxidase and hematoxylin, × 250

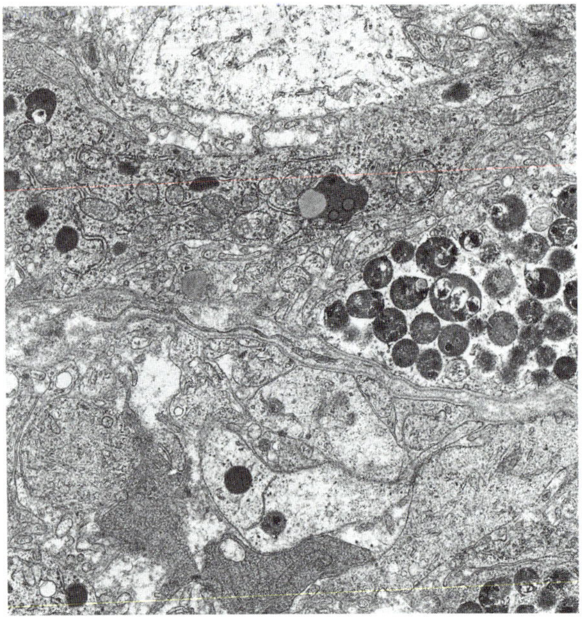

Fig. 9.74 Electron micrograph of a pleomorphic xanthoastrocytoma showing lipidized cells (right side) and investment of tumor cells and their processes by a well-defined basal lamina. × 1250 (mag. to negative)

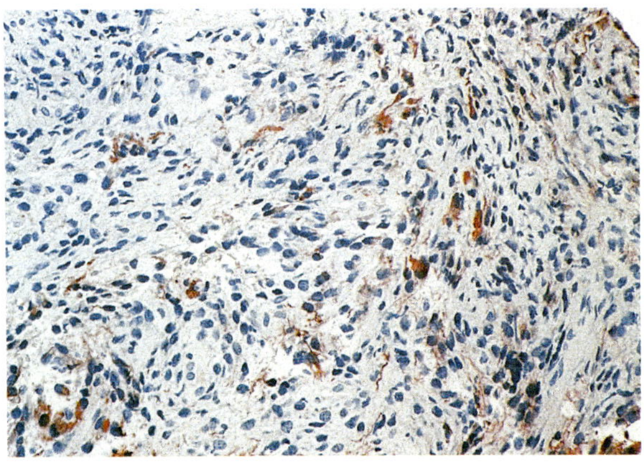

Fig. 9.75 Cytoplasmic reactivity for GFAP in tumor cells of a desmoplastic cerebral astrocytoma of infancy. GFAP immunoperoxidase and hematoxylin, × 250

and here, too, the tumor cells may, in the light of their electron microscopic features, be derived, at least in part, from subpial astrocytes (de Chadarévian, Pattisapu and Faerber, 1990; Louis *et al.*, 1992). The growths, which typically involve the frontal and parietal lobes, are usually massive and grossly cystic. Like the pleomorphic xanthoastrocytomas, they have an apparently favorable prognosis when completely or even partially resected. This neoplasm seems similar to the desmoplastic tumors identified in the same age group and which, with appropriate neurohistologic and immunohistochemical methods, have been shown to express divergent glial and neuronal differentiation (VandenBerg *et al.*, 1987). They have therefore been termed 'desmoplastic infantile gangliogliomas'. Their features are discussed later in this chapter (p. 507). In these superficial desmoplastic tumors, restriction of differentiation to astrocytic cells only is exceptional, but its occurrence justifies the inclusion of some of these examples among the purely astrocytic tumors.

Other astrocytomas with special desmoplastic features

Increasing attention is currently being paid to the presence, in some astrocytic and other neuroglial neoplasms, of extracellular products that may be derived either from the glial cells themselves or from other elements participating in the neoplastic process. This problem has long been familiar in some glioblastomas and is discussed on p. 442 under the heading 'Gliosarcomas'.

Gliofibromas

This term was coined to designate a tumor in which neoplastic astrocytes in a young subject seemed to form basal lamina and collagen directly, without a mesenchymal cell component, as reported by Friede (1978). A case of a mixed glial–mesenchymal tumor in an adult was described by Budka and Sunder-Plassmann (1980). The question as to whether these tumors represent a tumor analogous to what has now been termed 'desmoplastic astrocytoma' is still controversial. Most authors would retain the terminology of 'gliosarcoma' or 'sarcoglioma' for a mixed glial–mesenchymal neoplasm in which both components are malignant. For mixtures in which the mesenchymal tissue is benign, the argument hinges on the presence of mesenchymal cells producing collagen versus astrocytes directly producing basal lamina and collagen. An excellent review and discussion has been published by Cerda-Nicolas and Kepes (1993), who advocate maintaining the distinction of gliosarcomas, but accede to the use of the term 'desmoplastic astrocytoma' for tumors with a benign mesenchymal component. This terminology has also been advocated by Rushing, Rorke and Sutton (1993). The observation by Iglesias *et al.* (1984) that both types of cells can be invested by a common basal lamina raises the possibility of aberrant metaplasia in glial cells. This suspicion is strengthened by the occasional development, also in young subjects, of cartilage in astrocytomas.

The incorporation of mesenchymal elements in the better-differentiated astrocytomas is of more recent interest. Cell lines derived from human gliomas have been shown to display evidence of mesenchymal or epithelial-like features when the cells are transplanted into the brains of nude mice (Mørk *et al.*, 1988; Jacobsen and Papadimitriou, 1989). Unfortunately, as with many glioma cell lines, some of these failed to express GFAP, thus leaving their actual origin open to conjecture. While, as illustrated in Fig. 9.295, a considerable degree of connective tissue proliferation about the tumor cells may result simply from a predominant infiltration of the leptomeninges by an astrocytoma, its demonstration in the two entities described in the preceding paragraphs seems attributable, at least in part, to a neoproliferation of astrocytes whose cytoplasmic membranes are known to be normally invested by a basal lamina on their free surfaces facing the mesenchymal pia. The development of periglial basement membranes has also been shown to take place *in vitro*, namely in organotypic cultures of mouse spinal cord (Kusaka *et al.*, 1985), in experimental rat astrocytomas maintained in an organ culture system (Sipe *et al.*, 1974) and, as recalled on p. 000, in human ependymomas similarly maintained. Also, the transient intracellular expression of laminin has been reported in mature rat astrocytes after injury (Liesi *et al.*, 1984) and in early rat astrocyte cultures (Liesi, Dahl and Vaheri, 1983), followed in the latter circumstances by the appearance of pericellular matrix deposits. The finding, by Alitalo *et al.* (1983), that the widely used human astrocytic glioma cell line U-251 MG, known to express GFAP, is able to synthesize laminin, type IV procollagen and two other collagen polypeptides *in vitro* may also be significant. The rare reports on the development of gliofibromas and the occasional occurrence of cartilage apparently produced by astrocytoma cells *in situ* can, therefore, be viewed in the light of those experimental observations.

Cartilage in astrocytomas

The presence of cartilage nodules in gliomas, originally noted in fourth-ventricle ependymomas where they have usually been ascribed to chondroid metaplasia in the mesenchymal stroma (see Russell and Rubinstein, 1989, p. 200), may in some instances be attributable to the production, by the neoplastic astrocytes, of an intercellular chondroid matrix that stains positively for acid mucopolysaccharides. As a result, the astrocytes gradually develop morphologic features that make them indistinguishable from chondrocytes. Kepes, Rubinstein and Chiang (1984) reported four such cases. These examples suggest that metaplastic transformation of neoplastic glial cells into cells capable of synthesizing native mesenchymal cell products, although an exceptional event, can no longer be disregarded. However, the distinction between a mesenchymal origin and an astrocytic origin of the cartilage cannot be made on the basis of GFAP production since both benign and malignant cartilage produce GFAP (Kepes and Perentes, 1988; Dolman, 1989).

Angiogliomas

A number of tumors, especially those arising in the cerebellum, have been described under this term (see Henschen, 1955, pp. 528 and 735 for discussion and literature; see also Fischer, Sotrel and Welch, 1982). The designation of these tumors as a distinct clinicopathologic entity has been questioned (Lombardi *et al.*, 1991b). Most cases can be interpreted as examples of intensely vascularized gliomas in which the range of the vascular support extends from a pattern of hyalinized telangiectases and cavernous spaces to the development of large arteriovenous and venous fistulae (Russell and Rubinstein, 1989, p. 160; Lombardi *et al.*, 1991b). Most of the gliomas are low grade, whether oligodendrogliomas or pilocytic astrocytomas (Lombardi *et al.*, 1991b). Other examples seem to represent vascular anomalies, especially arteriovenous malformations and, to a lesser extent, cavernous or venous angiomas, all associated with a pronounced astrocytic gliosis. These cases do not represent examples of composite tumors in which both the glial and the vascular elements are intrinsically neoplastic.

Some examples have, however, been interpreted as true mixed tumors (Henschen, 1955, p. 648), and Bonnin, Peña and Rubinstein (1983) described the features of four cases of mixed capillary hemangioblastoma and glioma for which the term 'angioglioma' might be appropriate.

Gliomas of the optic nerve and chiasm

The optic nerve shares with the retina its derivation from the primary cerebral vesicle, but its fibers differ from those of the retinal optic nerve in being supported by oligodendroglia and fibrillary astrocytes, as in the white matter elsewhere. In contrast to either white matter or retina, the optic nerve is partitioned by vascularized connective tissue septa derived from the sheath of Schwalbe, a continuation of the dura mater, which is itself separated from the nerve proper by an extension of the pia–arachnoid. Nests of meningeal cells resembling arachnoid villi are readily found in normal material derived from the optic nerve.

Because of the close relationship of meningeal sheath elements to the parenchyma of the optic nerve, consideration of the tumors arising from these elements might perhaps be warranted either in this chapter or along with the orbital tumors described in Chapter 10. However, it will be more convenient to take up the description of orbital meningiomas in Chapter 11 because of the need to examine, in some detail, their relationship to those meningiomas that have arisen primarily in the anterior fossa and have spread secondarily into the orbit. Also, the histologic and biologic characteristics of meningiomas originating from the optic nerve sheath are the same as those of meningiomas in general. Likewise, the tumors of the optic nerve and chiasm share histologic and biologic identity with hypothalamic gliomas. Thus, in this edition, we have chosen to discuss these tumors along with gliomas rather than in Chapter 10.

As their cytologic features make clear, the cells participating in these neoplasms are predominantly, or maybe exclusively, astrocytic. Historically, however, the group as a whole has been referred to as 'optic nerve gliomas'.

Clinically and biologically, *two subgroups* of anterior optic nerve gliomas have been recognized (e.g., J.Y.C. Wong *et al.*, 1987; Wright, McNab and McDonald, 1989). The largest group by far (1) involves young subjects, (2) may or may not remain localized to the optic nerve and chiasm and (3) most often pursues a favorable clinical course, even in patients in whom the tumor has been either incompletely excised or subjected to a diagnostic biopsy only. Ten-year disease-free survivals approach 95% in this group. The relatively large series of optic nerve gliomas reviewed in the last several years from the standpoint of their clinicopathologic features and long-term follow-up have been of this category and include those of Hoyt and Baghdassarian (1969, 36 cases of which 21 were histologically verified), with follow-up series subsequently updated by Yanoff, Davis and Zimmerman (1978, 63 cases), Borit and Richardson (1982, 30 cases), Horwich and Bloom (1985, 30 cases), Imes and Hoyt (1986), Cutarelli *et al.* (1991, 10 cases) and Burnstine *et al.* (1993, 31 cases). In addition, more recent studies have emphasized the clinical aspects of these tumors as represented in the studies by the North American Study Group for Optic Glioma (NASGOG, 1989, 106 cases), Hoffman *et al.* (1993, 62 children), Jenkin *et al.* (1993, 87 cases), Janss *et al.*(1995, 46 children, <5 years old) and Deliganis, Geyer and Berger (1996), or have emphasized the link with NF type 1 (Hurst, Newman and Cail, 1988; Wright McNab and McDonald, 1989; Dunn and Purvin, 1990; Imes and Hoyt, 1991; Kuenzle *et al.*, 1994; Rossi *et al.*, 1994). Smaller series include those of Kanamori *et al.* (1985, 11 cases) and Weiss *et al.* (1987, 16 cases). The data of 623 examples from the literature were also extensively analyzed by Alvord and Lofton (1988). The consensus is that the vast majority of these neoplasms have a distinctive histologic and cytologic pattern that closely aligns them with the pilocytic astrocytomas of juvenile type.

The other, much less common, form of optic glioma characteristically (1) occurs in middle age, (2) often shows massive hypothalamic and even temporal lobe infiltration and (3) behaves in a much more malignant manner (Hoyt *et al.*, 1973; Harper and Stewart-Wynne, 1978; Spoor *et al.*, 1980; J.Y.C. Wong *et al.*, 1987; Wulc *et al.*, 1989, 7 cases in adults). Microscopically, these latter tumors show the cytologic features of anaplastic astrocytoma or glioblastoma and may result in the gross and radiographic appearance of gliomatosis cerebri.

Incidence

Optic nerve gliomas are either a solitary manifestation or a component of NF type 1. As pointed out in the review by Dutton (1991), optic nerve gliomas are rare, comprising about 1% of intracranial tumors (3.6% of pediatric brain tumors) and, according to Reese (1956), about 6% of the orbital tumors. In clinical ophthalmologic practice, only one such tumor may be encountered among 100 000 patients (Garner and Klintworth, 1994a). The overwhelming majority occur in childhood; according to Dutton (1991), 71% occur in children less than 10 years of age and 90% are diagnosed within the first two decades, with a median age of 7 years (age range: birth to 74 years). The sex incidence among patients with optic nerve gliomas shows a female:male preponderance of 3:2, while the data from patients with chiasmatic gliomas approach an equal sex incidence.

The association of optic nerve lesions with NF type 1 has long been well documented. In many instances, these gliomas, as with sporadic gliomas, are part of a more diffuse neoplasia involving the optic chiasm and the hypothalamus (Davis, 1940; Ortiz de Zarate, 1954).

Usually, there are no significant cytologic differences between the gliomas that accompany NF type 1 and those that are deemed to be sporadic. Davis (1940), although recognizing an oligodendroglial component microscopically in the tumors that he reviewed, found that here, too, astrocytes predominated. Possible differences between NF type-1-associated gliomas and sporadic gliomas include an apparently more common association of the former with extensive arachnoidal hyperplasia and with a more florid local gliomatous infiltration of the leptomeninges, as suggested by Stern, Jakobiec and Housepian (1980) and by Borit and Richardson (1982).

From their review of the literature, Garner and Klintworth (1994a) estimated that a link with NF type 1 may be found in up to one third of the cases of optic nerve glioma, a rate upheld by the recent studies of Janss *et al.* (1995), Deliganis, Geyer and Berger (1996) and by the review of Dutton (1991). Since most optic nerve gliomas occur in young children in whom the other features of peripheral neurofibromatosis have not as yet developed, previous estimates, such as those by Reese (1976), are unduly low. As Stern, Jakobiec and Housepian (1980), Kuenzle *et al.* (1994) and Janss *et al.* (1995) point out, the mean age of patients presenting with an optic nerve glioma is lower in cases associated with NF type 1 than in those without the disease. Thus, the association of the two conditions may be judged only by the existence of familial disease or by such minor manifestations as café-au-lait pigmentation of the skin.

Macroscopic appearance

When primarily intraorbital, the optic nerve glioma produces a fusiform expansion of the nerve (Fig. 9.76). However, spread through the optic foramen results in a dumbbell, or hourglass, expansion, which is partly within and partly outside the skull, constricted by the bony foramen. Enlargement of the foramen is radiologically demonstrable in about two thirds of the cases (Rubinstein, 1988). Alternatively, the nerve may be diffusely infiltrated by a glioma originating in the optic chiasm, in the floor of the third ventricle or in the walls of the hypothalamus (see Fig. 9.47). The reported origin of the tumor, limited either to the intraorbital portion of the nerve or to the optic chiasm, varies with different series, with chiasmatic involvement being found in 25–80% of patients (Hoyt and Baghdassarian, 1969; Yanoff, Davis and Zimmerman, 1978; Borit and Richardson, 1982; Jenkin *et al.*, 1993; Janss *et al.*, 1995). Deliganis, Geyer and Berger (1996) noted that expression of the NF type 1 phenotype strongly influences the location of the tumor. Patients exhibiting the disease predominantly have lesions confined to the anterior optic pathway (16/16 NF type 1 patients), while those lacking the disease are more likely also to exhibit involvement of the hypothalamus (7/28 non-NF type 1 patients). This observation, though, is far from a rule (see Fig. 16.2 p. 379). Intracranial involvement, as will be seen, carries important, and poor, prognostic implications.

On sectioning (Fig. 9.77), the nerve is found to be expanded by growth, but the major part of the

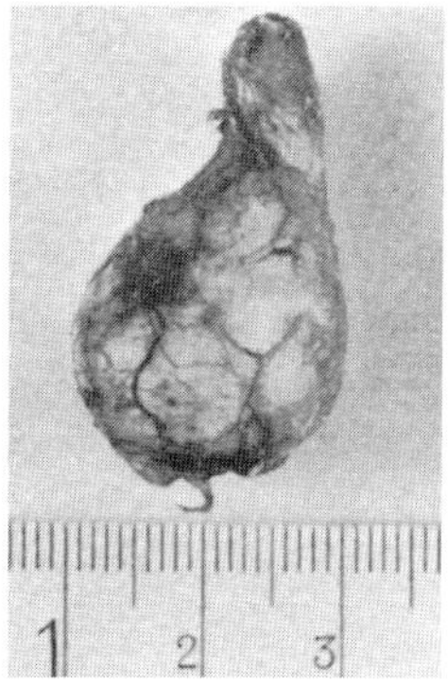

Fig. 9.76 Extracranial, intraorbital optic nerve glioma in a girl aged 6 years.

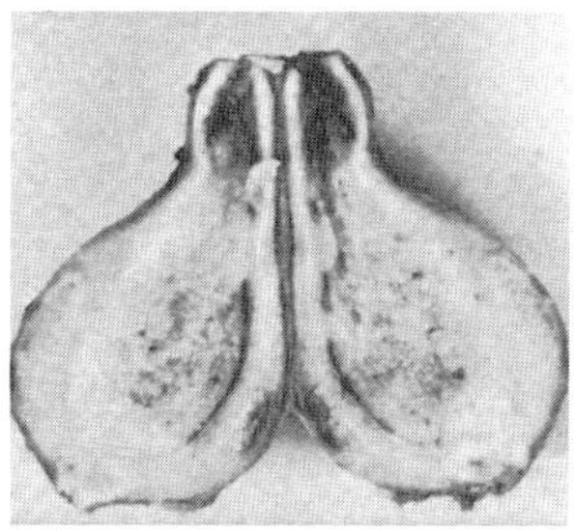

Fig. 9.77 Same case as Fig. 9.76. Bisected nerve reveals fusiform enlargement of the optic nerve with irregular central mucoid change and hemorrhage.

swelling is often due to extension of the tumor into the subarachnoid space, resulting in distension of the enveloping sheath. This is beautifully illustrated by Verhoeff's (1965) Fig. 2, which also demonstrates a remarkable infiltration of the optic disk by tumor. Small cystic areas may be apparent to the naked eye.

Radiographic appearance

The imaging modality of choice in detecting optic nerve gliomas is MRI. The location of the tumor and its extent are well delineated by the multiplanar approach. Optic nerve gliomas may involve the optic nerve alone and cause a fusiform expansion and redundancy of the nerve, or they may extend posteriorly (Fig. 9.78). Alternatively, the glioma may involve primarily the chiasm, demonstrated by enlargement with or without abnormal signal and enhancement. Gliomas of the optic tracts and radiations can also be seen, but frequently have chiasmatic involvement.

The imaging of optic nerve gliomas is variable. The tumor may have normal signal intensity on

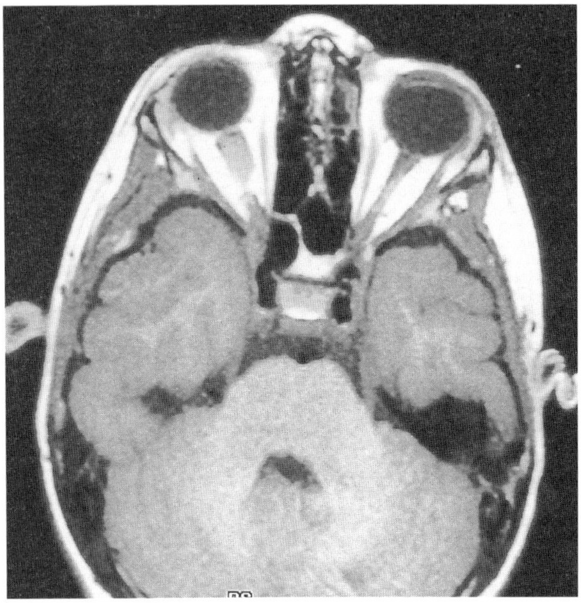

a

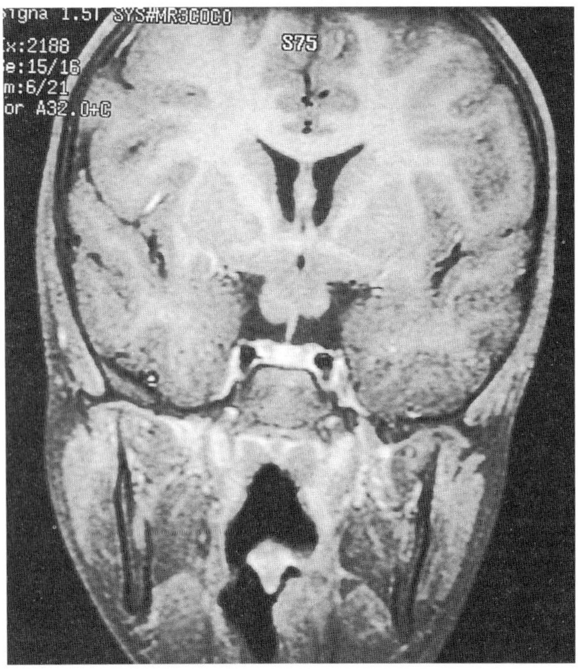

b

Fig. 9.78 Two MRIs of 5-year-old child having NF type 1 with photophobia. (a) Axial T1-weighted MRI at the level of the orbits demonstrates asymmetric enlargement of the right optic nerve, which is redundant. There is no abnormal enhancement. Appearances indicate optic nerve glioma along the intraorbital segment. (b) Coronal T1-weighted postcontrast MRI demonstrates that the optic nerve glioma causes marked enlargement of the optic chiasm, worse on the right side than on the left. There is no abnormal enhancement or signal intensity abnormality.

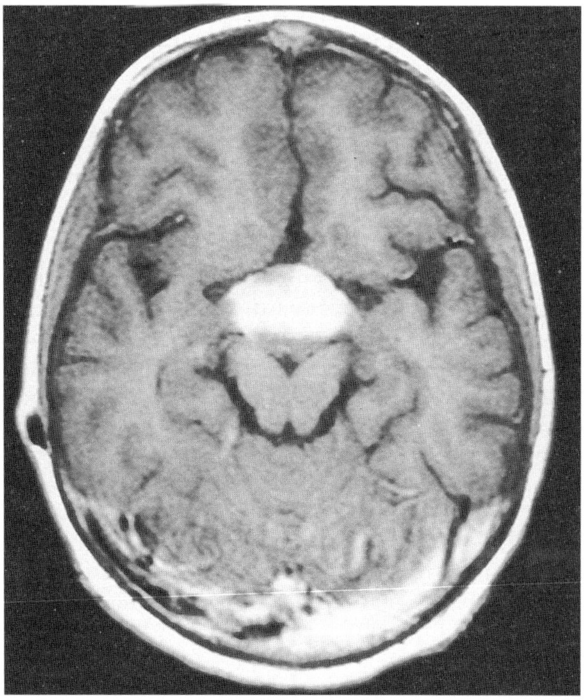

Fig. 9.79 Axial T1-weighted postcontrast MRI of an 8-year-old girl with a history of severe headaches, decreased vision and precocious puberty. Marked enhancement of the optic chiasm is seen, with intense enhancement of the soft tissue mass. This causes mild displacement of the midbrain posteriorly. The mass did not extend into the prechiasmatic optic nerves or optic radiations. These findings indicate chiasmatic optic nerve glioma.

both T1- and T2-weighted sequences and may lack enhancement. In these cases, diagnosis is made by enlargement of the nerve or chiasm alone. Other tumors have mildly hypointense T1 signal of the affected optic nerve, with increased T2 signal intensity. The enhancement may be intense or patchy (Figs 9.79 and 9.80). If there is extension of the tumor posteriorly into the optic radiations and the region of the lateral geniculate body, enhancement is often present. The pattern of enhancement usually involves a cross section of the nerve rather than a 'tram track' appearance that is more commonly seen in optic nerve meningioma and orbital pseudotumor. In more benign cases, the nerve remains well defined and is solely involved. More aggressive cases may extend into the hypothalamus.

Fat saturation techniques with contrast administration are particularly helpful in detection since the high signal intensity of intraorbital fat is removed, allowing better visualization of the optic nerve. In patients with optic nerve gliomas, it is

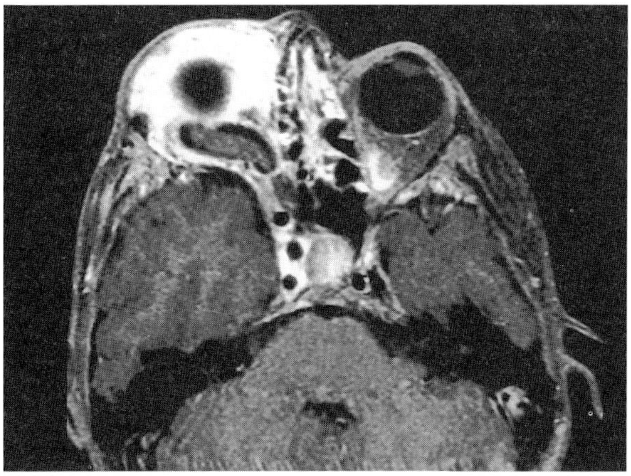

Fig. 9.80 Axial T1-weighted postcontrast MRI with fat saturation in a 13-year-old girl with visual difficulty and a disfigured right eye. The right optic nerve is enlarged, but has normal T1 signal intensity and no abnormal enhancement. This finding indicates optic nerve glioma. There is dilatation of the surrounding dural sheath and elongation of the optic nerve. Also present is a striking, enhancing mass within the right orbit representing a plexiform neurofibroma and dysplasia of the greater sphenoid wing. These findings are typical in a patient with developed NF type 1.

important to look for signs of NF type 1. Approximately 25% of patients with optic nerve gliomas have NF type 1, while 5–15% of patients who have NF type 1 develop optic nerve gliomas. Frequently, in these cases, the tumor is bilateral. Other findings, such as hamartomas, gliomas, plexiform neurofibromas or sphenoid wing dysplasias, can be well demonstrated by MRI. There may be dural ectasia associated with the intraocular component, seen most commonly in patients with NF type 1 (Fig. 9.80).

Enlargement of the optic nerve is also the major finding of optic nerve glioma on CT evaluation. The tumor may be low density and there may be enlargement of the orbital apex due to bone remodeling. Enhancement pattern is variable, ranging from no abnormal enhancement to prominent enhancement along the course of the glioma.

Microscopic appearance

The optic nerve gliomas are almost all pilocytic astrocytomas; therefore, the histologic patterns described reflect the morphologies of this tumor. In his original report, Verhoeff (1965) described the three patterns that Rubinstein (1988) and others (Yanoff, Davis and Zimmerman, 1978) have confirmed as the basic patterns found in optic nerve glioma, noting that all might be found in any one specimen. The first pattern noted by Verhoeff (1965) is finely reticulated, suggesting an exaggeration of the normal neuroglia (Figs 9.81 and 9.82). The second pattern is coarsely reticulated, with microcystic foci. In the third pattern, the cells are spindle shaped, forming bundles, and are coarsely fibrillated; this pattern predominates in areas where the sheath is invaded. Sometimes, the cells are oriented towards blood vessels to form pseudorosettes. The blood vessels vary in number and are often hyalinized. In the overwhelming majority of cases, mitotic figures are not found; when present, their significance in children is controversial, although the same finding in adults is considered ominous. Rosenthal fibers are often conspicuous. Verhoeff's analysis has been recapitulated in some detail because it has set the pattern for many subsequent published descriptions.

By equating certain of the spindle-shaped tumor cells with the elongated schwannoid oligodendroglia demonstrable in the normal white matter of the brain, some workers—particularly del Rio-Hortega (1944), Christensen and Andersen (1952) and Liss (1961)—interpreted the optic nerve gliomas as being chiefly oligodendrogliomas. However, these cells, which are indeed characteristic of the tumors under discussion, can usually, be shown, with the appropriate stains, to contain stout neuroglial fibrils and thus are bipolar astrocytes. The histologic similarity between the optic nerve tumors and the cerebellar astrocytomas of the pilocytic variant is, therefore, quite evident, and current classifications generally include the optic nerve gliomas among the pilocytic astrocytomas (Rubinstein, 1988; Burger, Scheithauer, and Vogel, 1991; Kleihues, Burger, and Scheithauer, 1993; Garner and Klintworth, 1994b).

Russell and Rubinstein (1959) were convinced that oligodendroglial cells participated in at least some of these tumors (as subsequently reiterated by Rubinstein, 1988). While they doubted that pure oligodendrogliomas were found in the anterior optic pathways, they recognized the theoretical possibility of such a group. They stated that, in their experience, oligodendroglial cells were largely confined to the retro-orbital segments; however, other authors have failed to support these differences. The primarily chiasmatic cases were found by Borit and Richardson (1982) to be microscopically identical with those of the primarily orbital cases, except for the absence of partitioning connective tissue septa, which are, of course, lacking in the normal optic chiasm. Furthermore, the cells with oligodendroglial appearances most often accompany myxomatous change and appear to represent a morphologic variant of the astrocyte.

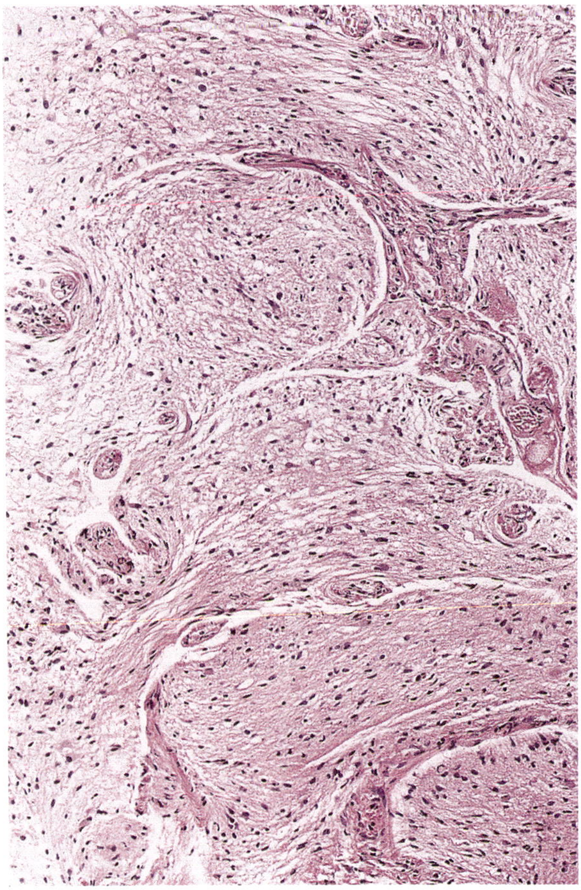

Fig. 9.81 Optic nerve glioma. The normal lobulated appearance of the optic nerve may be disrupted by this glioma.

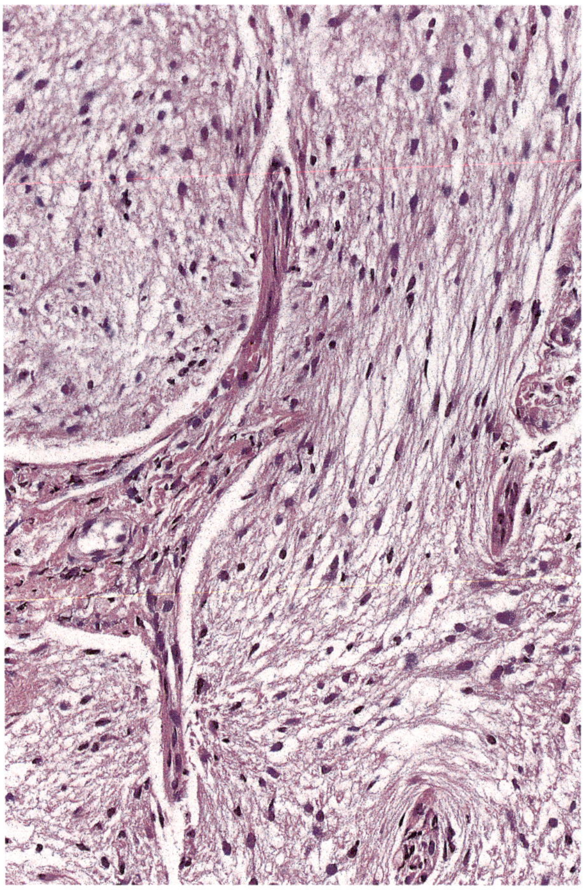

Fig. 9.82 Same case as Fig. 9.81. The lobular architecture of the optic nerve is disrupted by a growth that suggests an exaggeration of the normal neural glia occupying the optic nerve. H&E, × 66

Electron microscopy

Observations on these tumors have confirmed the affinity of the neoplastic cells with astrocytes, since they contain abundant cytoplasmic filaments, often arranged in bundles (Raimondi, 1966; Walter, 1978; Borit and Richardson, 1982). In addition, according to Raimondi, parts of the plasma membrane of these cells appear to fold and invaginate themselves to form rudimentary spirals around axonal structures, a phenomenon that recalls the role of the oligodendrocyte in myelinogenesis and is, apparently, also characteristic of the normal pituicyte (see below). Thus, electron microscopy adds further support to a role of oligodendroglial cells in these tumors.

Immunohistochemistry

The astrocytic nature of most optic nerve gliomas has been well supported by most immunohistochemical assays of these gliomas. Reactions for GFAP have shown the tumor cells to be strongly immunoreactive, highlighting the prominent fibrillary processes of the tumor cells. The only study (Cutarelli *et al.*, 1991) to investigate myelin basic protein (MBP) immunoreactivity in optic nerve gliomas has shown reactivity confined to native oligodendroglia, with no apparent staining of tumor cells. Thus, the presence of human natural killer-1 (HNK-1) reactivity in optic nerve gliomas, and the absence of A2B5 reactivity, has been interpreted as reflecting an origin of these tumors from so-called type 2 astrocytes (Cutarelli *et al.*, 1991). Given the glial nature of these tumor cells, it is not surprising to note that vimentin and S-100 immunoreactivity are also constant findings in these tumors (Cutarelli *et al.*, 1991).

The characterization of DNA synthesis as an indicator of proliferation potential has not been extensively applied to optic nerve gliomas. The

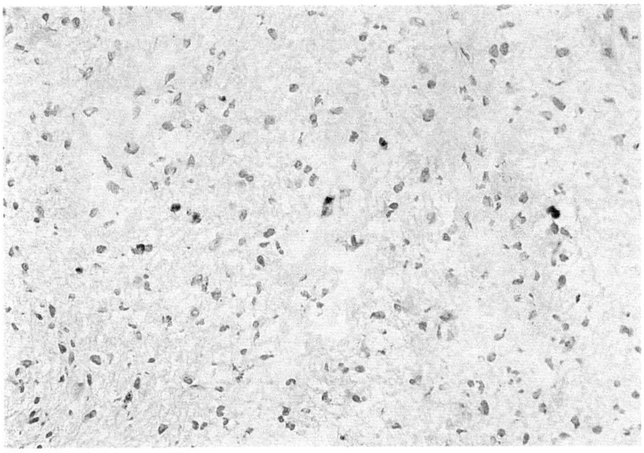

Fig. 9.83 Optic nerve glioma. Proliferation activity may be detected by the MIB-1 MAb against the Ki-67 antigen. Here, the LI approaches 3% and reflects the presence of rare mitoses in this tumor. MIB-1, × 66

study of Louis *et al.* (1991) noted that one optic nerve glioma had an LI of 6%. The significance of this observation is unknown, but may reflect the general tendency of pilocytic astrocytomas occurring in young children to have high BrdU incorporation indices (Ito *et al.*, 1992b) and to exhibit mitoses (Fig. 9.83).

Growth and spread: biologic behavior

It has already been noted that, from the standpoint of their infiltrative extensions, the boundary that separates the gliomas originating in the retro-orbital portion of the optic nerve pathways from those arising chiefly in the neurohypophysis (chapter 21, p. 642) and from those described on p. 342 as pilocytic astrocytomas of the third ventricle of the juvenile type is so tenuous as to be practically nonexistent. This lack of distinction in their gross features is evident from all the reported series. For example, in the series of Borit and Richardson (1982), 4/14 cases that presented primarily as orbital optic nerve gliomas also involved the chiasm, and 2/14 the hypothalamus; whereas 14/16 chiasmatic tumors implicated one and usually more often both optic nerves, and 13/16 involved also the hypothalamus. It is also well recognized that whatever primary designation is the presumed starting point, the histologic features of all these astrocytomas, including nucleolar organizer region (AgNOR) counts (Burnstine *et al.*, 1993), are virtually interchangeable, an identity that is perhaps to be expected from the common derivation of their respective sites of origin from the diencephalon.

As already noted the optic nerve gliomas are prone to infiltrate and expand the adjacent sheath, but do not penetrate the dura. In common with gliomatous infiltrations of the meninges in the CNS proper, the invasive tumor cells excite an obvious proliferation of connective tissue elements: there is an increase of spindle fibroblasts, and an excess of reticulin and collagen fibrils is formed throughout the zone (Fig. 9.84). A striking feature, in some examples, is the concomitant associated *hyperplasia of arachnoidal cells*, a development already noted by Verhoeff (1932) and subsequently emphasized by Davis (1940) in his study of optic nerve gliomas accompanying NF type 1. Arachnoidal cell hyperplasia can also accompany optic nerve gliomas, and may be severe enough to expand the optic canal and even to cause confusion with an orbital meningioma (Cooling and Wright, 1979). As a general incidence, Yanoff, Davis and Zimmerman (1978) found arachnoidal hyperplasia to be present in over half of their cases.

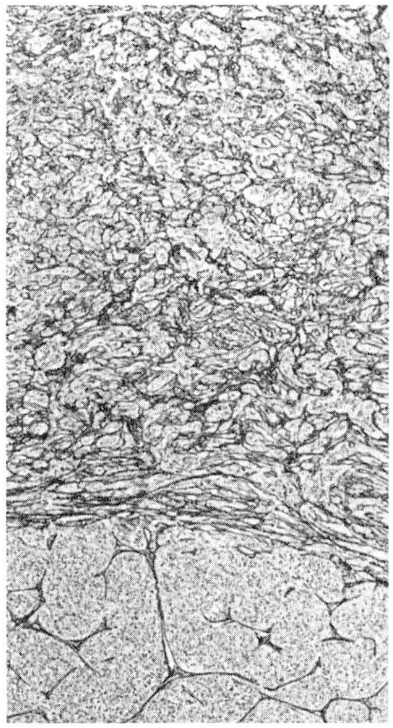

Fig. 9.84 Optic nerve glioma showing invasion of the sheath of Schwalbe with production of reticulin. Reticulin, × 28

The reports quoted above have repeatedly confirmed Verhoeff's (1965) view that the optic nerve gliomas carry, in general, a good prognosis, and an excellent one if the tumor is intraorbital and can be completely excised. The early reports on survival rates of patients with primarily intraorbital growths exceeded 90% in the series of Yanoff, Davis and Zimmerman (1978) and Borit and Richardson (1982). These reports also suggested that in several instances incomplete removal was not followed by progression, thus indicating arrest of tumor growth.

In contrast to these earlier reports, however, it is now apparent that there is some growth potential retained in these gliomas even after 12 years of relative quiescence (Aarabi, Long and Miller, 1978; McDonnell and Miller, 1983). In particular, reference is made to the study of J.Y.C. Wong *et al.* (1987), who noted that 50–85% of optic nerve gliomas involving the chiasm have a more aggressive clinical course and a poorer prognosis than did those confined to a single optic nerve. However, even gliomas confined to one optic nerve can progress; Wright, McDonald and Call (1980) noted that 8/17 gliomas confined to one optic nerve progressed without further treatment. Analysis of these cases has usually suggested that there is no correlation among the extent of the surgical resection or radiation, the demonstration of residual tumor, and the length of survival or degree of postoperative disability. However, it is not entirely clear that there is no role for megavoltage radiation therapy, particularly with regard to recurrent lesions. The original study of Hoyt and Baghdassarian (1969) employed patients treated with orthovoltage irradiation and was the basis of these investigators' original recommendation against radiotherapy. The subsequent study of patients treated more contemporaneously by J.Y.C. Wong *et al.* (1987), and including several of the patients also studied by Hoyt and Baghdassarian (1969), seems to suggest a role for radiation therapy. Similarly, Jenkin *et al.* (1993) have recommended megavoltage irradiation in the therapy of recurrent lesions from incompletely resected lesions. In the case of chiasmatic tumors, the survival rates are less favorable, with estimates ranging from 50% in the series of Borit and Richardson (1982) to 64% according to Yanoff, Davis and Zimmerman (1978). Even in those instances, the less favorable course appears to be due not to any intrinsic differences in the biologic or histologic features of the neoplasm, but rather to its location, which usually precludes extensive surgical resection. The fact that these gliomas, including those with demonstrable hypothalamic involvement, may display long periods of arrest in their growth after mere diagnostic biopsy is an enigmatic observation that has already been commented upon in our account of the juvenile-type pilocytic astrocytomas of the third ventricle. To what extent postoperative radiation treatment influences the further behavior of these tumors is quite unclear, but the overall weight of evidence suggests that mortality is not significantly altered by radiotherapy (Jenkin *et al.*, 1993). More recently, chemotherapy has been found to play a role in the treatment of hypothalamic gliomas (Petronio *et al.*, 1991) and has also been recommended for both progressive and metastatic chiasmatic gliomas (Bruggers *et al.*, 1991; Moghrabi *et al.*, 1993; McCowage *et al.*, 1996). In particular, the effects of radiation on the brains of young children are not insignificant and must be considered in any therapeutic plan. The postoperative management of these patients remains, therefore, a controversial issue (see Weiss *et al.*, 1987; J.Y.C. Wong *et al.*, 1987; and Dutton, 1991, for discussion).

While these neoplasms seem, therefore, to be characterized by protracted delay in their progression and even, in many cases, by apparently complete cessation of growth, we think it erroneous simply to regard them as developmental malformations rather than true new growths. The life-table analysis of 623 examples of optic glioma by Alvord and Lofton (1988) clearly confirms their proliferative capability. Moreover, from the histologic point of view, penetration and expansion of the sheath of Schwalbe can be explained only in terms of invasion, and the occasional development of anaplastic change, to be described, indicates that, although rare, this potential exists.

In the study of Deliganis, Geyer and Berger (1996), the influence of NF type 1 on survival was analyzed in a comparison of 44 patients diagnosed with optic nerve gliomas at the National Institutes of Health. Among their 16 patients with NF type 1, the 5- and 10-year survival rates were 93% and 81%, respectively, versus 83% and 76% among 28 patients without NF type 1 (not significant). In contrast, recurrences were significantly delayed in patients with NF type 1 (8.3 years to first relapse) versus those with sporadic tumors (2.39 years, $P<0.01$), a point also identified by Janss *et al.* (1995).

From a different angle, Lewis *et al.* (1984), in their prospective study of a large population of patients with NF type 1, have estimated the frequency of gliomas involving either the optic nerve or chiasm, or both, to be about 15% of the patients, with most of the cases having been detected by CT. This incidence is surprisingly high when compared with that recorded in previously compiled series, which give a frequency ranging only from 1% to 5%. In the series of Lewis *et al.* (1984), however, only 5% of the cases surveyed had a clinically symptomatic optic nerve or chiasmatic lesion, which would agree with the lower range reported by others. Of the 33 patients suspected radiologically to have a glioma of the anterior visual pathways, seven were operated on and six had histologic confirmation of the neoplasm. All of these patients were also those with clinical symptoms. The main uncertainty lies, therefore, in the nature of the lesion demonstrated by CT in the 10% of patients with NF type 1 without any symptoms or signs pointing to an optic nerve lesion and on whom, consequently, no histologic data are available. Whether such lesions have any growth potential, or could represent preneoplastic changes, or could be hamartomatous, remains entirely speculative.

In this regard, however, it should be noted that the optic nerve lesions accompanying NF type 1, whether glial or meningeal, are not always frankly neoplastic. A *diffuse hyperplastic gliosis* of the optic nerve can be associated with the disease. In one such case noted by Rubinstein (1963, case 13), in a 24-year-old woman without cutaneous manifestations or a familial history but who harbored multiple neurofibromas of the cervical nerve roots and right vagus nerve, the left optic nerve and adjacent chiasm were thickened by a dense cellular and pilocytic fibrillary gliosis that widely separated the individual nerve fibers. Another such case was reported by Spencer and Borit (1967), who briefly referred to a few previously recorded examples. While it is difficult to distinguish such a lesion from an early stage of neoplasia, the question may be raised whether it might not provide the histologic basis for some of the asymptomatic cases observed by Lewis *et al.* (1984).

Malignant forms

The development of a malignant change in the optic nerve glioma of childhood is quite exceptional. In their series of 30 cases, Borit and Richardson (1982) quote one example (their case 23), in a 2-year-old male with NF type 1, in which increased cellular anaplasia was associated with tumor cell dissemination in the cerebrospinal pathways. Rubinstein has noted a focal malignant transformation in a pilocytic astrocytoma of the third ventricle and optic nerves arising in a 14-year-old boy with a family history of NF type 1 (Rubinstein, 1963, case 12). Another unusual example was reported by Wilson *et al.* (1976), in a 9-year-old female diagnosed with a pilocytic astrocytoma of the chiasm, in which anaplastic change took place 18 years after the original biopsy. In all of these cases, the histologic features of a pilocytic astrocytoma of juvenile type were retained in most of the tumor, except for the local development of cytologic anaplasia.

By contrast, middle-aged and older adults may develop optic nerve gliomas that display aggressive growth characteristics, extensive infiltration of the hypothalamus and adjacent cerebral structures, rapid clinical evolution and histologic features that are classic for anaplastic astrocytoma or glioblastoma. This group of cases was first recognized by Hoyt *et al.* (1973), who described five examples and reviewed 10 previously recorded cases; several subsequent examples have been reported by Harper and Stewart-Wynne (1978) and by Spoor *et al.* (1980). Three of the cases reviewed by J.Y.C. Wong *et al.* (1987) appear to belong to this category. These tumors are, despite their location, clearly different histologically and biologically from the optic nerve gliomas of childhood.

Differential diagnosis

In addition to the optic nerve gliomas described above, two other entities deserve mention in this discussion of anterior pathway tumors of glial origin: choristomas and gangliogliomas. Benign optic nerve choristomas involve smooth muscle cells and dense fibrous connective tissue intertwined within atrophic optic nerve parenchyma. Instances of these have been described by Zimmerman *et al.* (1983) and Kazim *et al.* (1992). In the latter case, chiasmatic involvement was noted by an MRI scan.

Gangliogliomas are also exceedingly rare tumors that have been described both in optic nerve and optic chiasm. The examples described by Cohen (1919); Gritzman, Snyckers and Proctor (1983) and Bergin *et al.* (1988) were restricted to the optic nerve, while the examples described by Cogan, Poppen and Hicks (1961), Lowes *et al.* (1978), Chilton, Caughron and Kepes (1990), Rodriguez, Edwards and Levin (1990), Lu *et al.* (1993), Hoffman *et al.* (1993), and Sadun, Hinton and Sadun (1996) involved variably the optic chiasm and hypothalamus. The ages of all these patients ranged from 2 years to 38 years old, reflecting the general age range of gangliogliomas of the cerebrum. The embryogenesis presumably reflects the tissue's origin as a cerebral vesicle; however, an origin from perivascular sympathetic neurons has been suggested (Cogan, Poppen and Hicks, 1961). The cases of Bergin *et al.* (1988) and Sadun, Hinton and Sadun (1996) occurred in the setting of NF type 1. Obviously, care must be taken to accurately characterize the source of the tissue, particularly near the hypothalamus, as local involvement of hypothalamic neurons along the edge of a pilocytic astrocytoma may also present a confusing picture. The prognosis is not known but is presumably good in most cases. An apparent exception is the case of Sadun, Hinton and Sadun (1996) in which rapid growth and visual decline prompted excision, and was apparently related to a high mitotic rate, although 2-year follow-up did not reveal further growth of the tumor.

Controversial or unresolved issues and future directions

Data are beginning to emerge that challenge our concepts of the optic nerve glioma as a low-grade, nonrecurring neoplasm of astrocytes. The fact that recurrence rate increases with postoperative follow-up is established; however, the fact that some neoplasms will exhibit prolonged quiescence, and even regression, following minimal resections is also evident. Similarly, at what point therapeutic intervention is indicated in these children is not clear. The concept of the adult optic nerve glioma as a biologic entity distinct from the pediatric tumor with a tendency to infiltrate and exhibit neoplastic progression is also beginning to be recognized. These unresolved issues necessarily engender controversies with regard to prognostication, monitoring and therapy. More information on the proliferative potential and molecular aspects involved in oncogenesis and progression are obviously needed. The influence of NF type 1 and the *NF1* gene in the biology of optic nerve gliomas will certainly provide a starting point. Information on therapeutic sensitivity and mechanisms of resistance also seem to be fruitful areas of investigation.

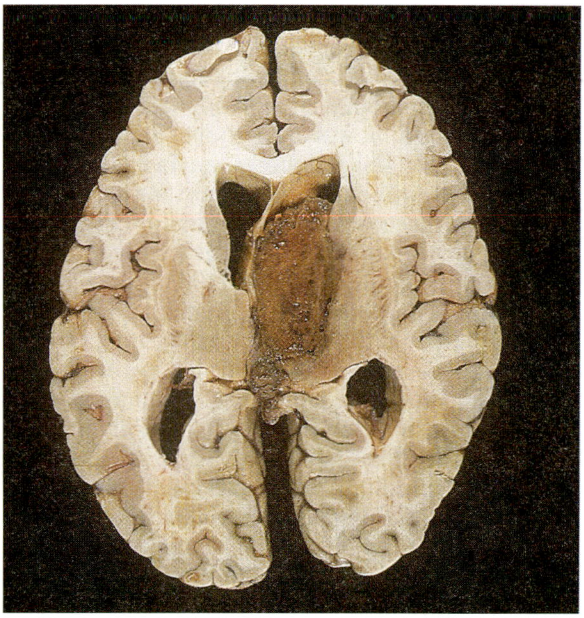

Fig. 9.85 Hemorrhagic oligodendroglioma invading the right lateral ventricle in a 35-year-old man.

OLIGODENDROGLIOMAS

The historic approach to the characterization of gliomas of this type is outlined by Bailey and Bucy (1929) in a classic paper that should be regarded as the formal introduction of this important group of tumors to neuropathology. In that excellent account, the authors noted the predilection of oligodendrogliomas for cerebral hemisphere involvement, incidence in adult life, calcification and slow clinical evolution. The last-mentioned feature, however, calls for considerable modification, especially in regard to the postoperative behavior of these tumors. In addition to the clear demonstration, by silver impregnation, of oligodendroglia as the principal tumor element, Bailey and Bucy described other constituent glial forms that, morphologically, appeared to be transitional between oligodendroglia and astrocytes. The latter are an important component in most neoplasms of this type. Moreover, a growing awareness of the cellular heterogeneity displayed by so many gliomas has increased the amount of attention paid in recent years to the different glial cell types represented in oligodendrogliomas. This is reflected by the greater frequency with which we have come to label such tumors as mixed oligodendrogliomas and astrocytomas and to recognize their phenotypic variability *in vitro*. The visualization of the astrocytic component in oligodendrogliomas has also been considerably facilitated by the introduction of immunohistochemical staining techniques, thus drawing further attention to the role that astrocytic cell elements may play in the subsequent biologic evolution of this group of neoplasms.

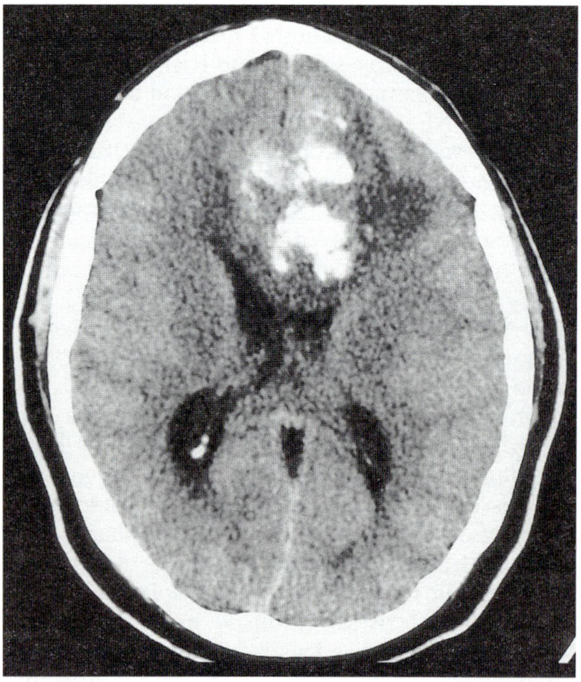

Fig. 9.86 Axial CT scan without contrast in a patient with increasing headaches. This is the classic location and appearance for oligodendroglioma. Dense irregular calcification is identified in both frontal lobes, with significant mass effect. There may be varying amounts of contrast enhancement.

Incidence

Most observers agree that these tumors constitute about 5% of intracranial gliomas (see McKeran and Thomas, 1980), with the exception of Zülch (1986, p. 241), who recorded an appreciably higher incidence of 18.8%. The various figures on sex distribution tabulated by Mørk *et al.* (1985) indicate a male:female ratio ranging from 3:2 to 2:1.

Although not uncommon in childhood and adolescence (Favier, Pizzolato and Berney, 1985, literature), oligodendrogliomas are mostly identified in adults (Fig. 9.85): Zülch's curve (1986, p. 89) shows a peak at the age of 45 years; the series of Mørk *et al.* (1985), as well as the studies of others, agree on the highest incidence in the fifth and sixth decades (Shaw *et al.*, 1992). A more recent series of 111 patients, published by Kros *et al.* (1990), reported a greater number of cases with first diagnosis in the fourth decade, rather than in the fifth or sixth decade. In a smaller series of 54 patients, Chin *et al.* (1980) noted a biphasic age distribution, with a small peak between the ages of 6 and 12 years, and a larger peak between the ages of 25 and 50 years.

Sites

The cerebral hemispheres are the location of the great majority of these tumors, most often in the frontotemporal region. Rarer sites are the cerebellum and the spinal cord (see Fortuna, Celli and Palma, 1980, for a review of 35 published spinal intramedullary examples). A small number of tumors with the typical light microscopic features of oligodendroglioma arise from the ventricular wall (Markwalder *et al.*, 1979), but immunohistochemistry and electron microscopy have confirmed that most or all of them are of neuronal origin (see 'Central neurocytomas', p. 000).

Macroscopic appearance

The cerebral cortex and subcortical white matter are most often affected. Local infiltration of the leptomeninges is not unusual. Some oligodendrogliomas are situated more deeply in the white matter and may abut on, or secondarily invade, the ventricular system (Fig. 9.85). The tumors are a solid mass, grayish pink, often well defined and

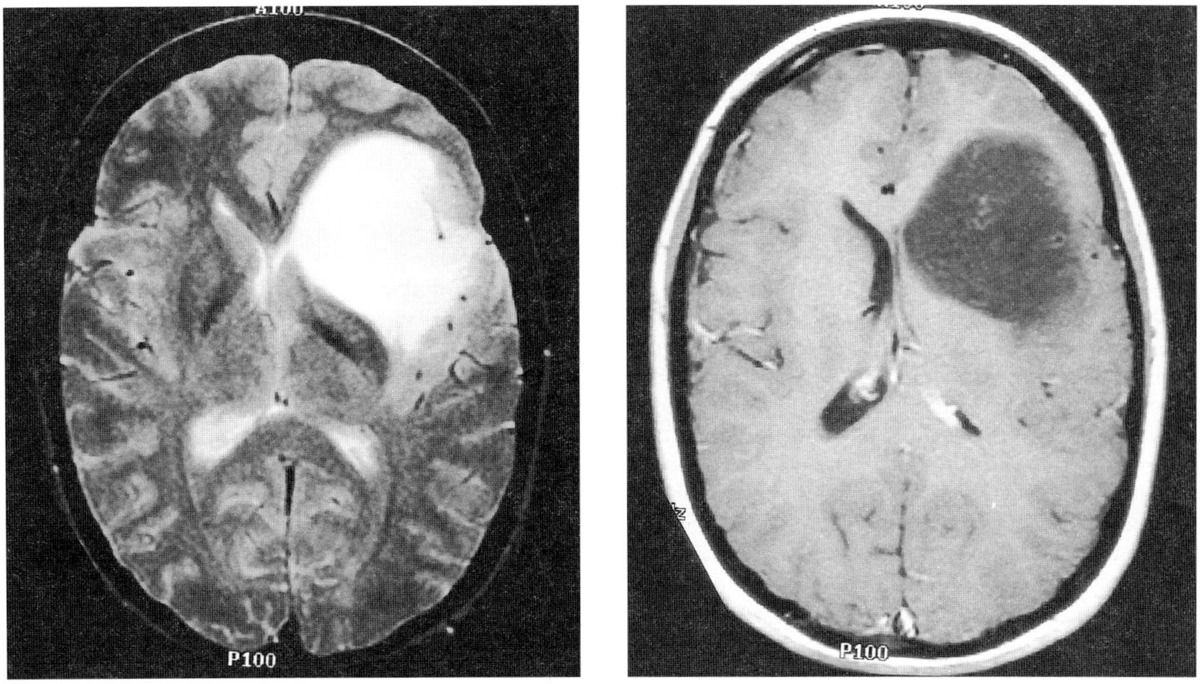

a b

Fig. 9.87 Two MRIs of a 36-year-old woman with headaches. (a) Axial T2-weighted image demonstrates a well-defined area of abnormal T2 signal involving the left frontal and anterior temporal lobe. There is mass effect noted. (b) Axial T1-weighted postcontrast image demonstrates marked decreased T1 signal corresponding to the area of high T2 signal. No abnormal enhancement is identified. This imaging appearance is nonspecific, and low-grade glioma would be favored. Oligodendroglioma was diagnosed at biopsy.

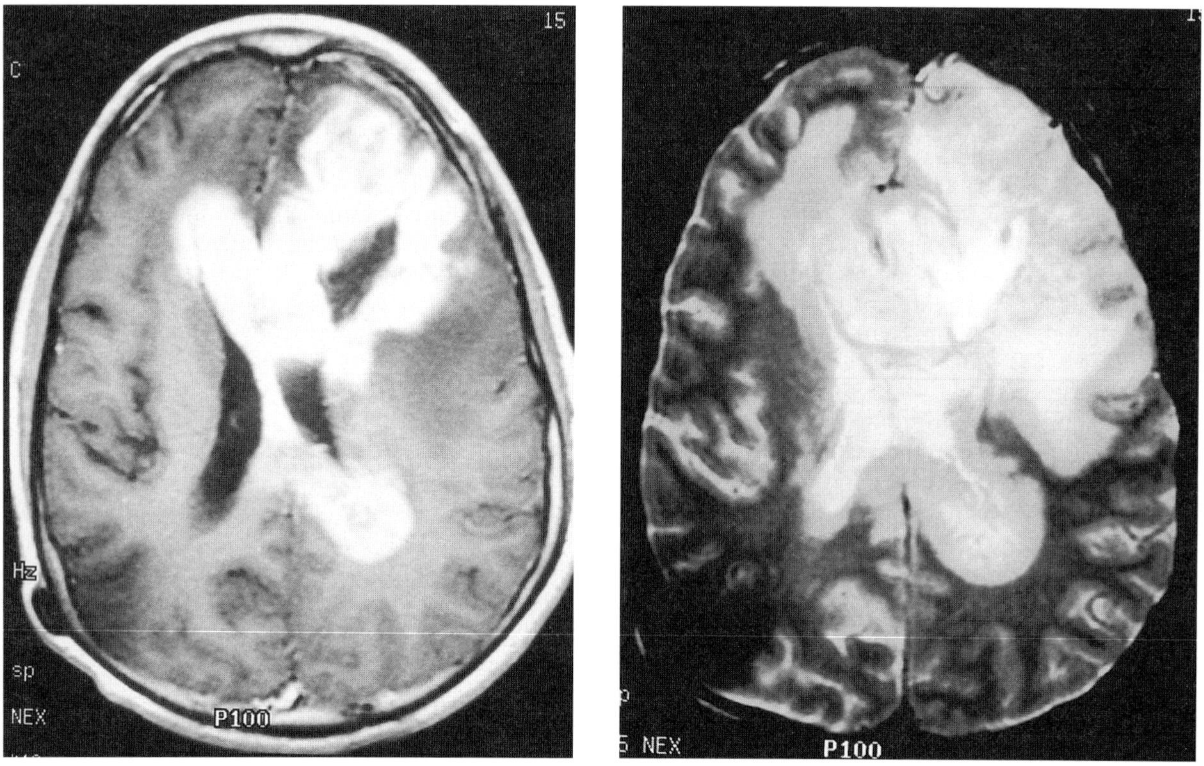

a b

Fig. 9.88 Two MRIs of a 15-year-old boy. (a) Axial T1-weighted postcontrast image demonstrates marked enhancement in both frontal lobes with extension across the corpus callosum and prominent subependymal abnormal enhancement. There is significant mass effect, subfalcine herniation and adjacent edema shown as decreased T1 signal. A central area of cystic necrosis is present. (b) Axial T2-weighted image demonstrates the mass to be of increased T2 signal. Surrounding vasogenic edema is also noted. The more aggressive appearance in this case represents anaplastic oligodendroglioma.

rather soft. Those in which mucinous change is extensive are likely to be gelatinous. Central foci of necrosis and cystic degeneration occur in the larger specimens. Many examples, ranging from 28% (Mørk *et al.*, 1985) to almost 40% of the cases (Earnest, Kernohan and Craig, 1950), demonstrate calcification on routine skull x-ray, the deposits being particularly apt to occur near the periphery. Spontaneous hemorrhage seems a special liability and may occur on a considerable scale and be responsible for sudden coma and death. The possible relationship of this event to the structure of the neoplastic capillary blood vessels has been discussed by Liwnicz, Wu and Tew (1987).

Radiographic appearance

The radiologic findings of oligodendroglioma demonstrate a heterogeneous mass that is frequently calcified and has variable enhancement. Low-grade oligodendrogliomas demonstrate chunky, irregular calcification in 70–90% of cases and usually do not enhance with contrast. On CT scanning, the calcification is well defined. The soft tissue components of the tumor are iso- to hypodense as compared with normal brain, and mass effect is usually found. The frontal lobes are a frequent site, and the lesion may be bilateral. Cortical extension is common. With contrast, the soft tissue component of the tumor may show variable enhancement, usually mild to moderate in degree, if any (Fig. 9.86).

By MRI, calcifications are more difficult to discern. The mass usually has low T1 signal and high T2 signal intensities and is heterogeneous (Fig. 9.87). Involvement of the cortex is common, and inhomogeneous contrast enhancement is most frequently present. Cysts and cystic necrosis are frequently identified.

The frequency of mixed oligodendroglial–astrocytic histology makes the imaging characteristics of low-grade gliomas nonspecific. More malignant

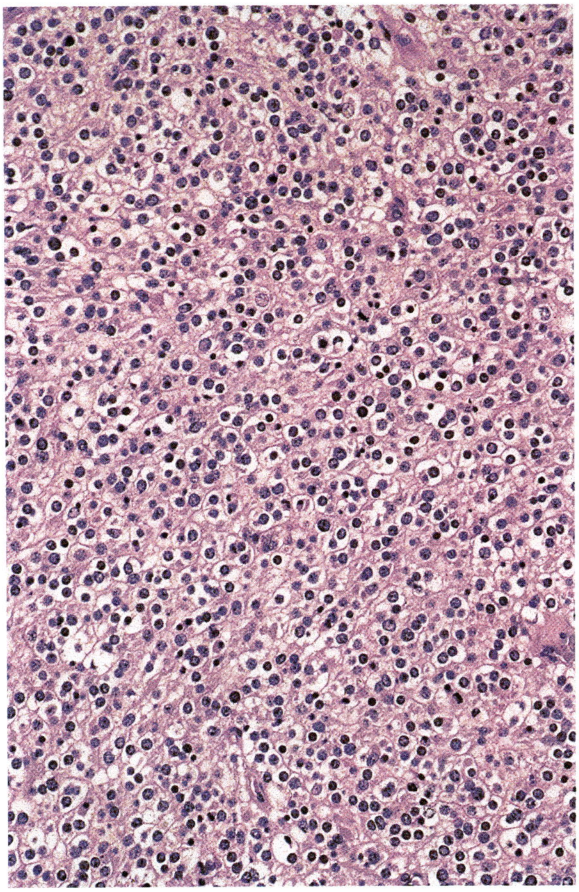

Fig. 9.89 Low-power micrograph of the typical pattern of oligodendroglioma. H&E, × 250

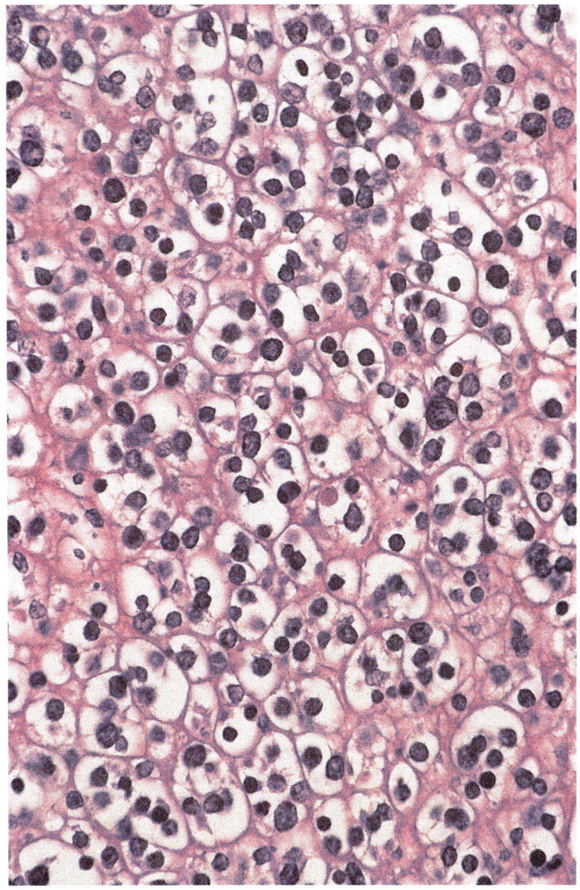

Fig. 9.90 Typical cytologic features of oligodendroglioma. H&E, × 500

forms of oligodendroglioma are demonstrated by more intense, irregular enhancement and/or profound areas of vasogenic edema and mass effect. Subependymal spread is also a characteristic of high-grade gliomas (Fig. 9.88).

Microscopic appearances

To interpret oligodendrogliomas microscopically, it is necessary to recall the normal morphology of the oligodendroglia and the pronounced liability of these cells to undergo degeneration and 'acute swelling'. As this change progresses, the perikaryon undergoes expansion and vacuolation, with a concomitant retraction and ultimate loss of the cell processes that are normally present. The final picture is that of an enlarged rounded cell with a well-defined cytoplasmic membrane and an empty-looking cytoplasm, in the center of which the small spherical nucleus appears to float. Varying degrees of acute swelling are found in the white matter of the brain in all postmortem material; the cortical oligodendroglia are better preserved, but fresh biopsy tissue is essential for the demonstration of the normal morphologic features, a problem that is considerably magnified when these cells are studied with the electron microscope.

This 'acute swelling' determines the characteristic microscopic appearance of the classic oligodendroglioma (Figs 9.89–9.91). The tumor is composed of sheets of swollen cells intersected by a prominent and rather delicate supporting stroma of blood vessels and scant collagen, well-demonstrated in reticulin silver or periodic acid–Schiff (PAS) preparations (Fig. 9.92). This characteristic capillary network is not sufficiently emphasized in some descriptions, but is a helpful diagnostic clue, best appreciated in areas of white matter, since it is similar to the normal vascular pattern of the cerebral cortex. Mitotic figures are variable. Although these tumors are invasive of the adjacent brain, their borders may occasionally seem deceptively

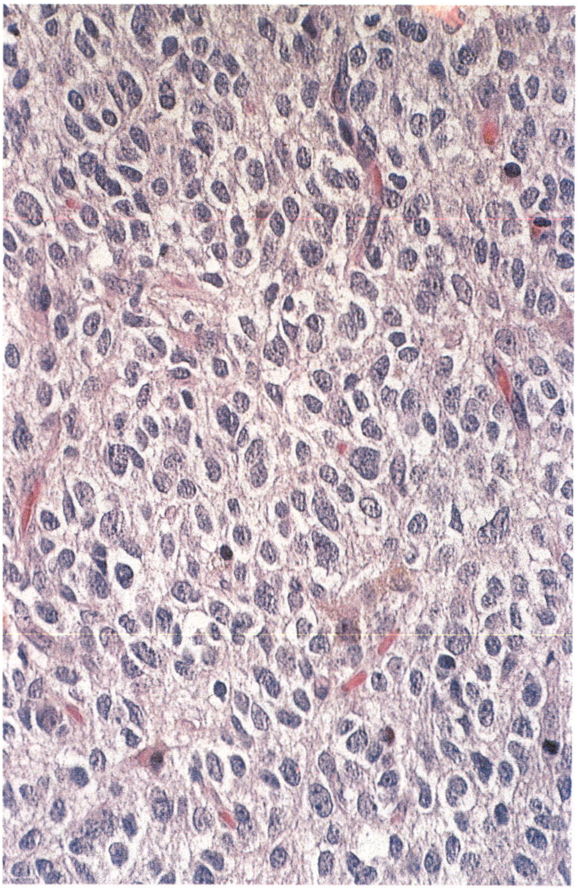

Fig. 9.91 Increased nuclear pleomorphism and nuclear enlargement of oligodendroglioma. Cytoplasmic clearing and branching vascular stroma are maintained, however. H&E, × 315

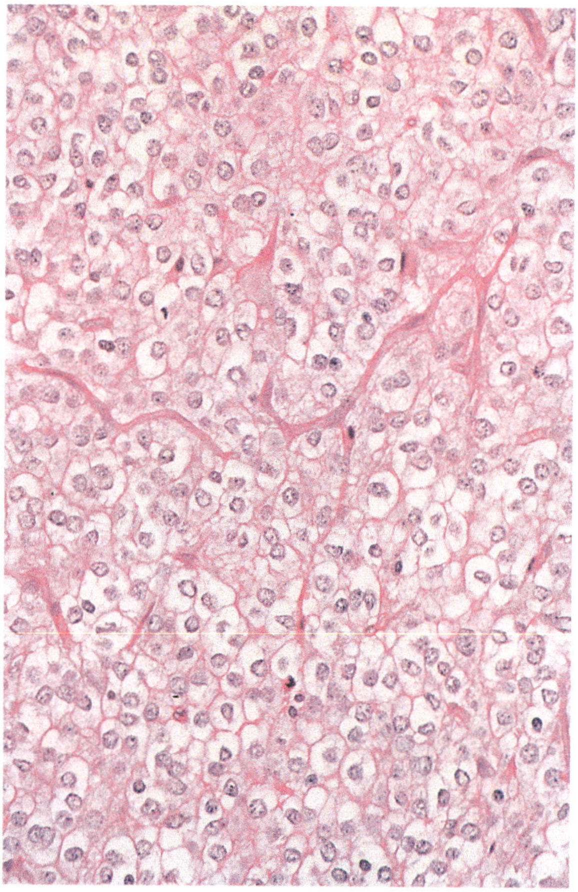

Fig. 9.92 Delicate thin-walled vascular pattern of oligodendroglioma emphasized by a periodic acid–Schiff stain (PAS). PAS with diastase, × 250

well defined (Fig. 9.93). Because of their often well-defined cytoplasmic borders, this tendency for demarcation can lead to misidentification as a metastatic carcinoma, especially in frozen sections. The distinction generally becomes clear when paraffin sections are examined.

In surgical specimens, especially frozen sections or promptly fixed paraffin-embedded tissue, considerable areas of tumor may be devoid of the acute swelling (Fig. 9.94). The cells then lie in small clusters, recalling the picture of satellitosis of cortical neurons in nonneoplastic conditions. The spaces between the clumps may be bridged by fine cobwebs of delicate branching processes (Fig. 9.95). The picture may resemble that seen in small-cell astrocytomas, and the use of the immunoperoxidase stain for GFAP may be helpful in confirming the absence of significant astrocytic fibrillarity. An

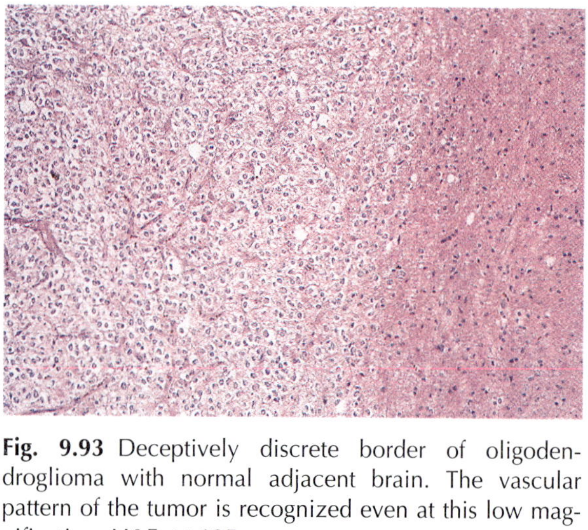

Fig. 9.93 Deceptively discrete border of oligodendroglioma with normal adjacent brain. The vascular pattern of the tumor is recognized even at this low magnification. H&E, × 125

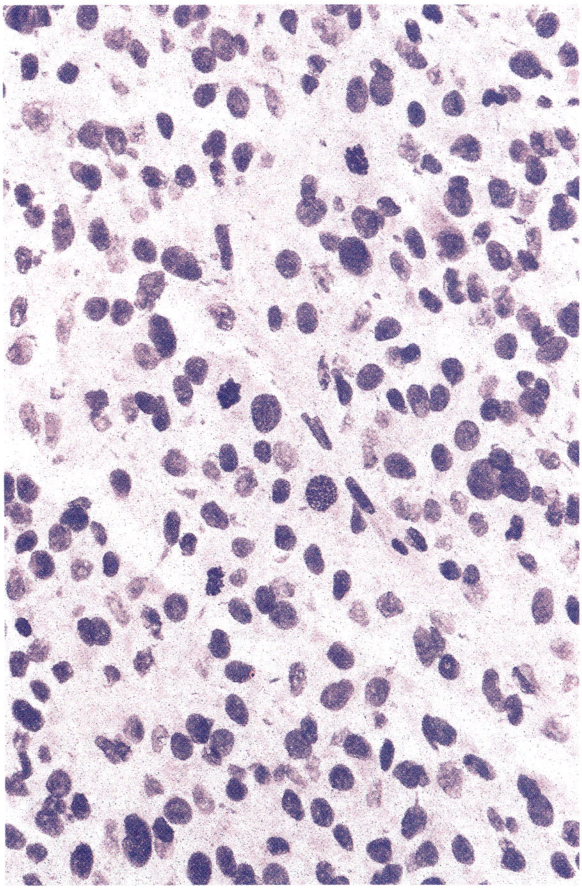

Fig. 9.94 Frozen section of oligodendroglioma showing relatively uniform nuclei. Cytoplasmic clearing, however, is not seen. H&E, × 500

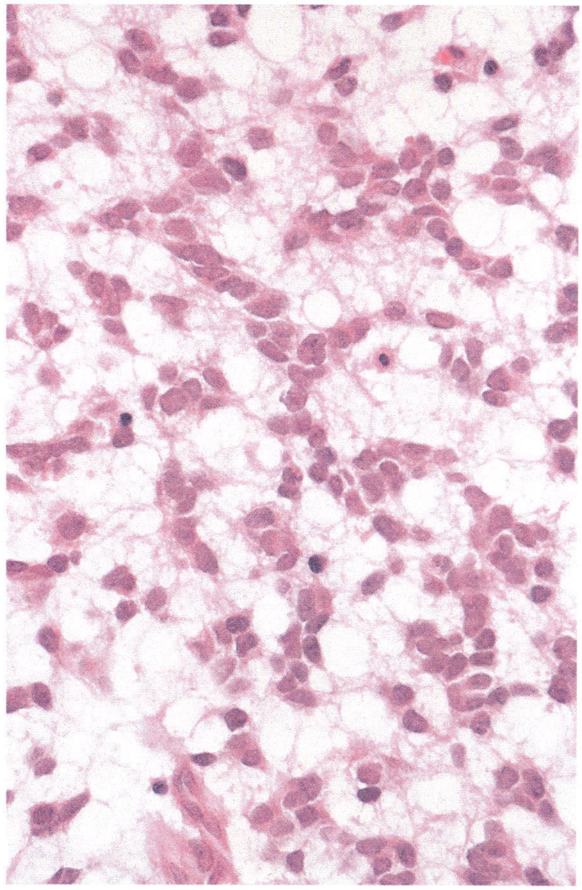

Fig. 9.95 Clustering cytologic pattern of oligodendroglioma. H&E, × 500

additional helpful technique for rapid diagnosis is the examination of alcohol-fixed imprint or smear preparations stained with hematoxylin and eosin (H&E) (Fig. 9.96). The characteristic roundness of the nuclei and lack of fibrillary cytoplasm is easily appreciated and should suggest the diagnosis of oligodendroglioma (Bruner, 1987).

Although the microscopic picture in the typical case is highly distinctive, oligodendrogliomas may demonstrate a fairly wide variety of tissue patterns and cell forms. Some nuclear variability may be present. In places, the tumor cells are no longer round, but may be elongated and display fusiform nuclei (Fig. 9.91). A further, although rare, variation is a cellular arrangement in which the nuclei form distinct palisades, leaving extensive clear zones between them (Fig. 9.97). Such an alignment may also be found in the white matter when the

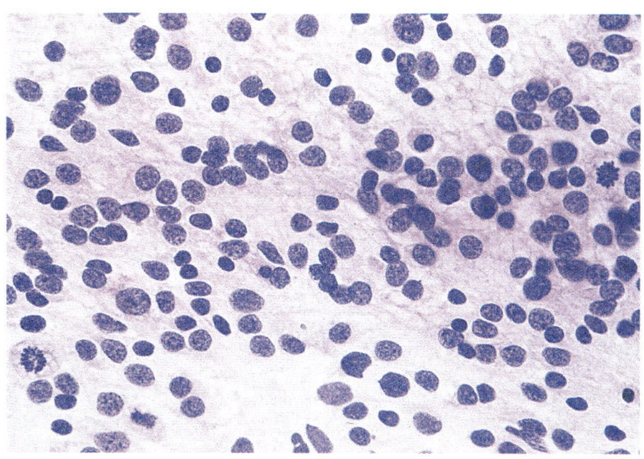

Fig. 9.96 Smear preparation of oligodendroglioma showing rounded regular nuclei without fibrillary cytoplasm. H&E, × 500

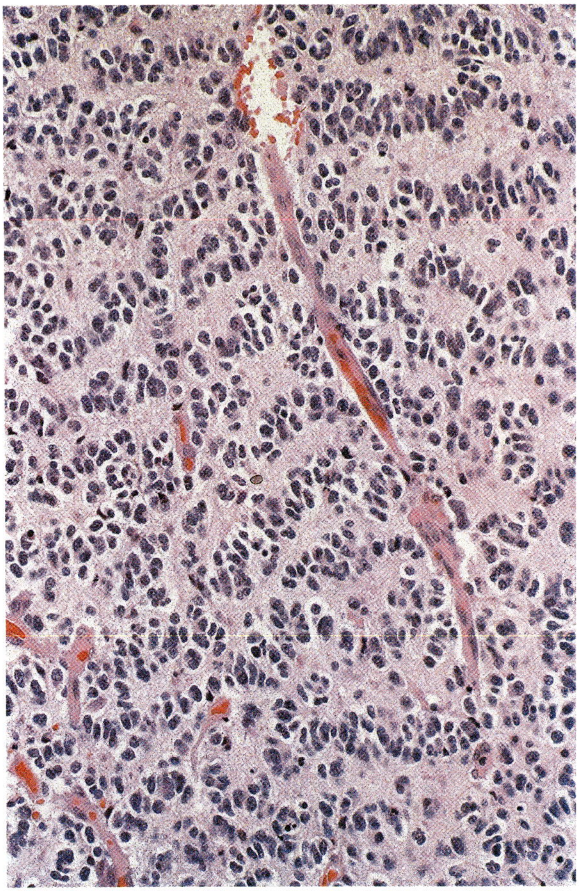

Fig. 9.97 Rhythmic palisading in an oligodendroglioma. H&E, × 250

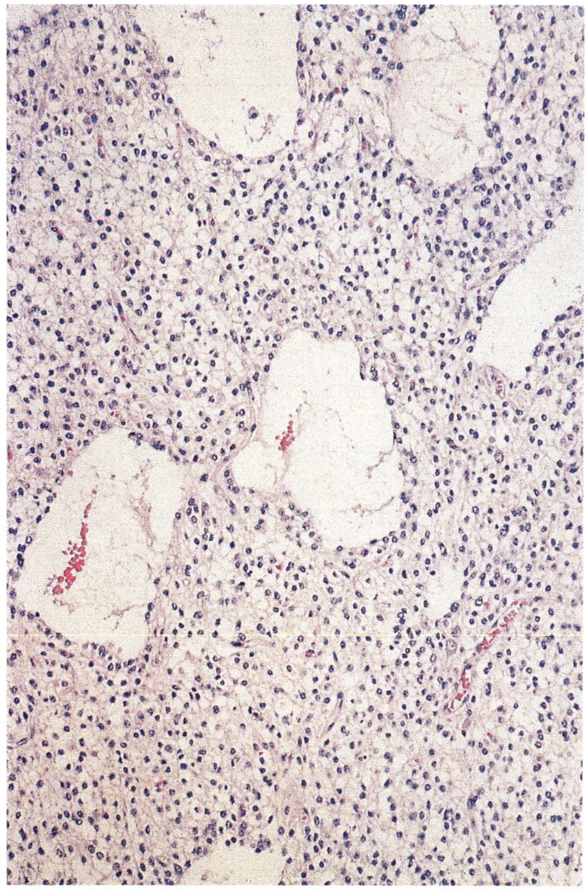

Fig. 9.98 Microcysts in a low-grade oligodendroglioma. H&E, × 125

tumor cells penetrate along bundles of myelinated nerve fibers. The effect produced is well illustrated in Fig. 101 of Zülch and Christensen's large monograph (1956, pp. 90–6). Another common pattern includes the presence of microcysts, which may contain a mucopolysaccharide substance, possibly chondroitin sulfate (Smith and Butler, 1973), that stains with Alcian blue or mucicarmine (Figs 9.98 and 9.99). Other areas may show an arrangement of cells around blood vessels, with the formation of perivascular pseudorosettes (Fig. 9.100).

Occasionally, the tumor cells present an unusual ballooned signet-ring appearance, with a pale eosinophilic or granular cytoplasm. This may be a degenerative phenomenon; by electron microscopy (Takei, Mirra and Miles, 1976), the granules are found to be formed by membrane-bound autophagic vacuoles that are identical with those found in some astrocytomas (see Fig. 9.56).

Calcification, when present, is related to the intrinsic blood vessels. Salts are laid down in their walls as calcospherites, which later become confluent to form masses of considerable size. Occasionally, calcification may progress to lamellar bone formation.

Oligodendrogliomas have an exceptional tendency to invade cerebral cortex, not only forming cell clusters surrounding neurons and blood vessels (satellitosis), but also invading up to the pial surface and growing along it (subpial spread) (Figs 9.101 and 9.102). The tendency is more pronounced than in astrocytomas and can be a suggestive feature in frozen-section material when the cytoplasmic clearing is not well developed and the classification of a glioma is uncertain.

Like other gliomas, these tumors may, on occasion, be superficially situated in the cerebral hemispheres, and then show marked focal infiltration of the leptomeninges and even of the inner layer of the dura. This process may induce a vigorous desmoplastic reaction of the infiltrated meninges and result in the acquisition, by the tumor, of a lobular

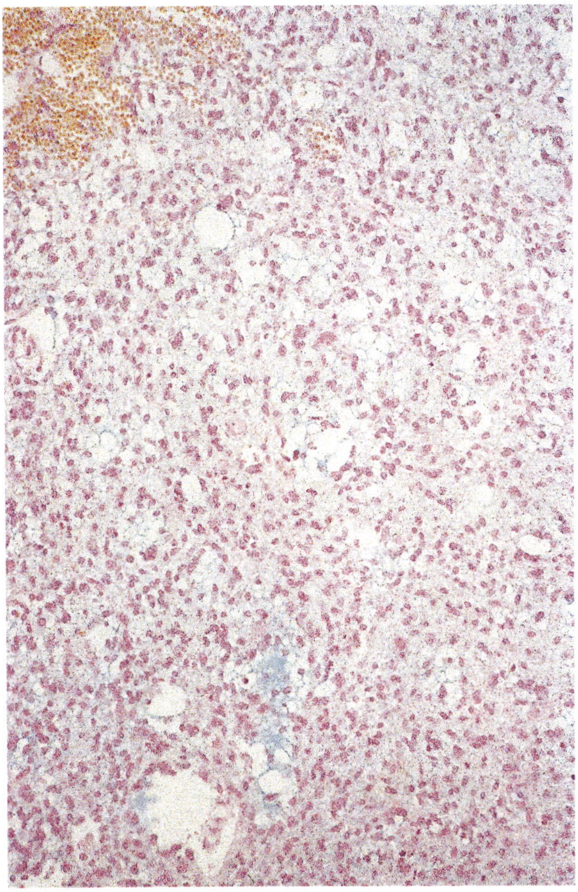

Fig. 9.99 Same case as Fig. 9.98 Mucopolysaccharide material is seen in some of the microcysts. Alcian blue, × 125

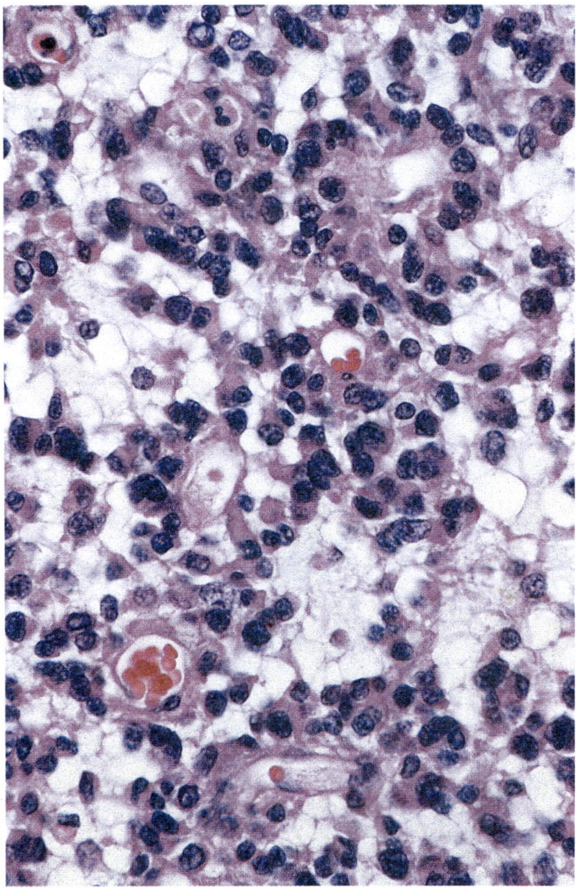

Fig. 9.100 Oligodendroglioma with a perivascular papillary pattern. H&E, × 500

pattern that, both grossly and microscopically, may mimic the pattern of a syncytial meningioma. In our experience, such a growth may rarely spread to the bone. Figure 9.103, from a large superficial oligodendroglioma (Figs 9.104 and 9.105) that presented in a 28-year-old man as a soft scalp nodule in the left frontal region and had eroded the skull through its complete thickness, illustrates that transgression of the dura has stimulated an intense proliferative fibrous connective tissue reaction that encompasses the tumor cells, either singly or in small nests.

The thin-walled capillary blood vessels may show endothelial proliferation in the more anaplastic examples (see below). Malignant change in the vascular stroma has, exceptionally, been observed (see below).

Immunohistochemistry

Normal oligodendrocytes do not possess cytoplasmic intermediate filaments arranged in bundles and do not contain GFAP. Nevertheless, immunoreactivity for GFAP may be found in classic oligodendrocytic tumor cells, in which it has been estimated to occur in approximately 50% of pure oligodendrogliomas. The presence, therefore, of GFAP-positive tumor cells in oligodendrogliomas has presented a diagnostic dilemma, especially in cases where an unexpected number of cells have been positive in sections of the tumor that, in routine stains, have the classic features of neoplastic oligodendrocytes. The problem in earlier years generated a good deal of uncertainty (see De Armond, Eng and Rubinstein, 1980), but now seems to have been largely resolved (Herpers and Budka, 1984; Nakagawa, Perentes and Rubinstein, 1986; Kros *et al.*, 1990) after more comprehensive scrutiny. Both the pure forms of oligodendroglioma and the mixed oligodendrogliomas and astrocytomas (or oligoastrocytomas) have been studied.

The GFAP-reactivity in the tumor may be due to different factors. Well-differentiated reactive

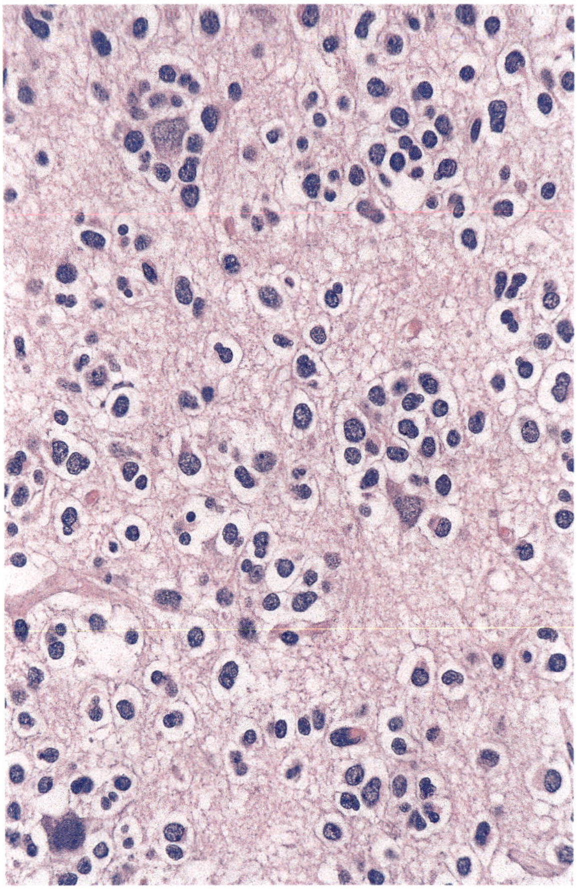

Fig. 9.101 Perineuronal satellitosis in the cerebral cortex with oligodendroglioma invasion. H&E, × 500

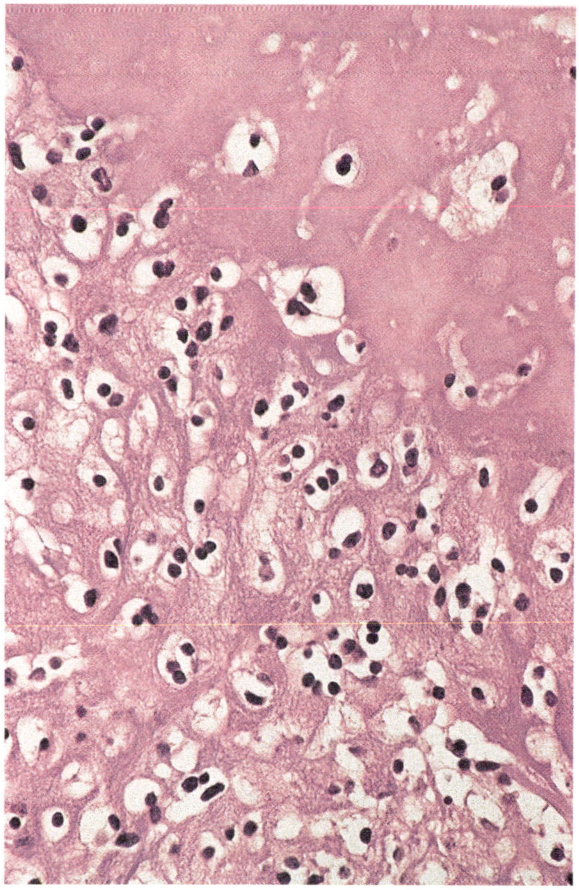

Fig. 9.103 Pronounced desmoplastic reaction in an oligodendroglioma resulting from invasion of the dura and bone by tumor. H&E, × 315

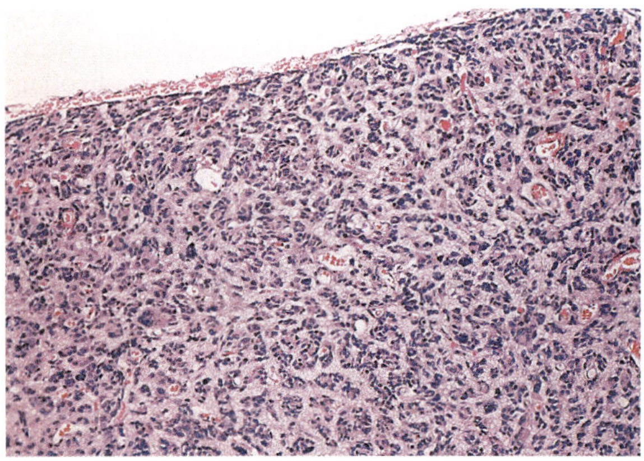

Fig. 9.102 Cortical invasion by oligodendroglioma with subpial accumulation of neoplastic cells. H&E, × 125

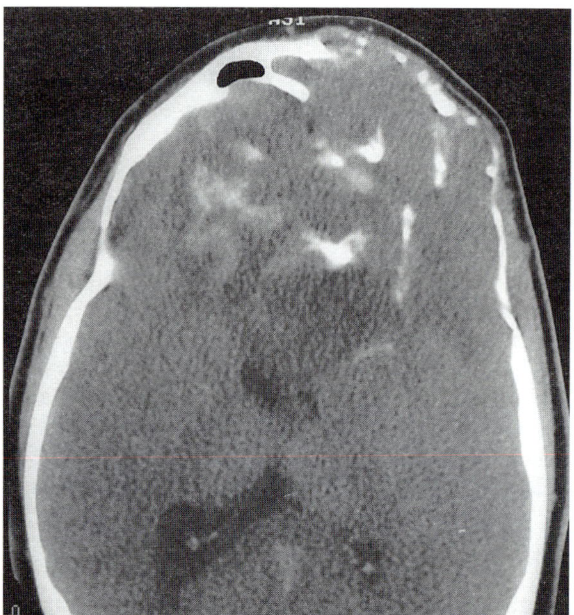

Fig. 9.104 A CT scan of a left frontal oligodendroglioma destroying the bone of the calvarium. The tumor is heterogeneously enhancing.

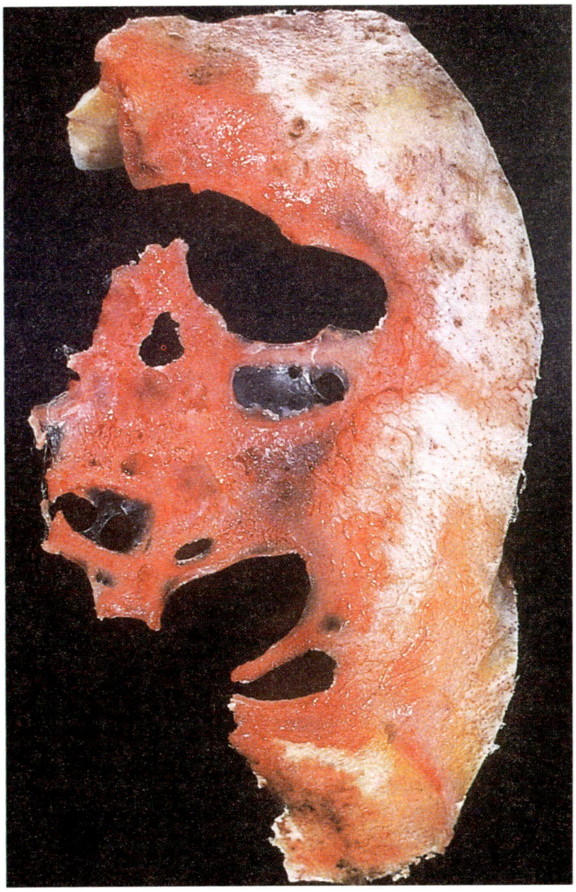

Fig. 9.105 Same case as Fig. 9.104. Calvarial bone eroded by tumor. (Courtesy of Dr Lauren A. Langford)

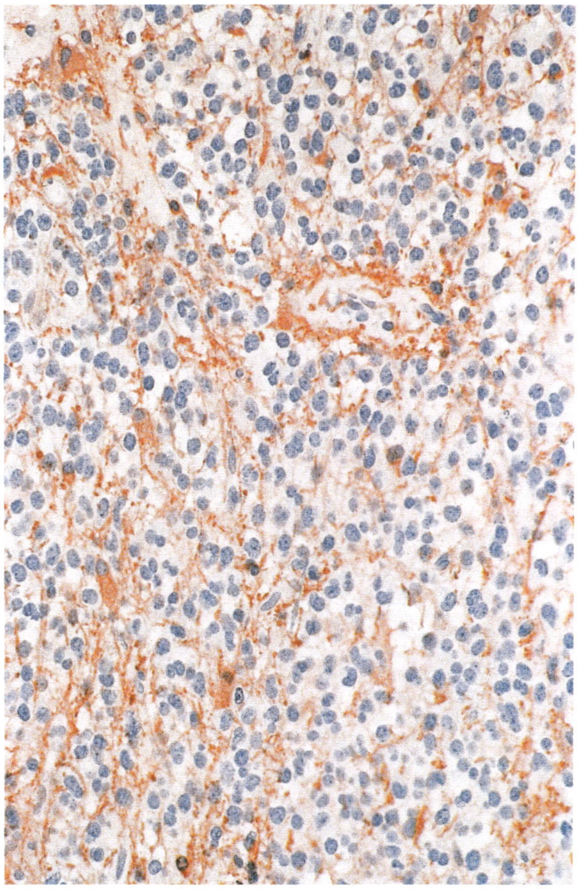

Fig. 9.106 Typical pattern of GFAP immunoreactivity in an oligodendroglioma showing absence of diffuse cytoplasmic staining and some positivity between the neoplastic cells and around blood vessels. GFAP immunoperoxidase, × 250

astrocytes, estimated to be demonstrable in about 60% of the cases, may be scattered throughout the oligodendroglioma (Figs 9.106 and 9.107). Alternatively, the tumor may consist of a mixture of neoplastic astrocytes and oligodendrocytes. In up to 60% of the tumors, as quantitated by Kros *et al.* (1990), neoplastic oligodendrocytes and astrocytes may be bridged by transitional forms, called 'minigemistocytes' and 'gliofibrillary oligodendrocytes' (GFOCs). Both forms have previously been held to exist on the basis of silver carbonate impregnations (Ravens, Adamkiewicz and Groff, 1955). These forms have been determined to represent two cell types that seem to be transitional between astrocytes and oligodendrocytes. The minigemistocytes have a small balloon of eosinophilic cytoplasm that can be easily recognized with routine H&E

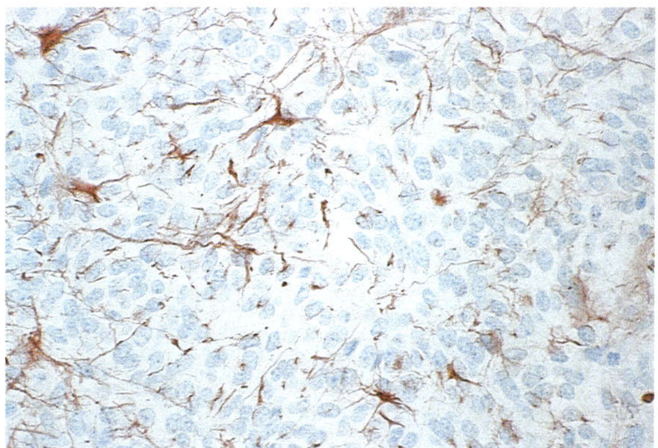

Fig. 9.107 Reactive astrocytes scattered in an oligodendroglioma. GFAP immunoperoxidase, × 315

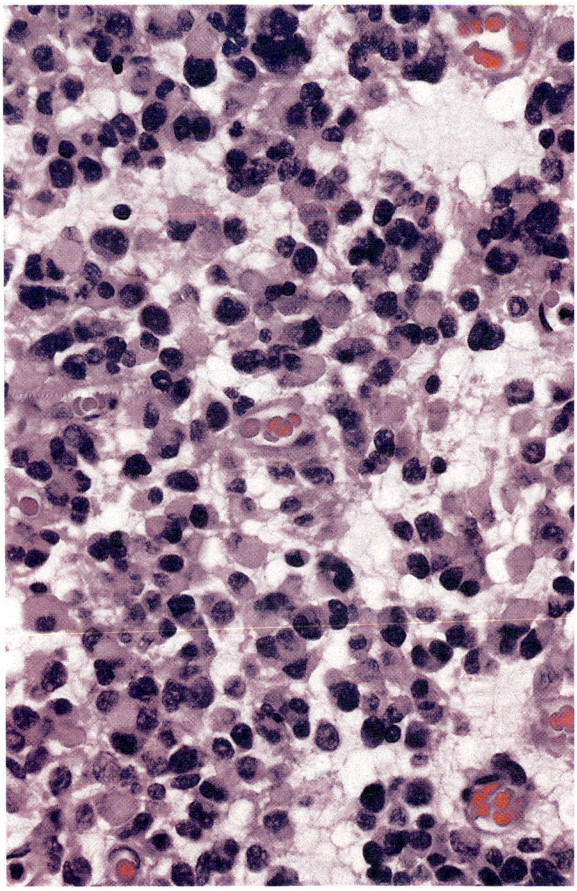

Fig. 9.108 Minigemistocytes in an oligodendroglioma. H&E, × 500.

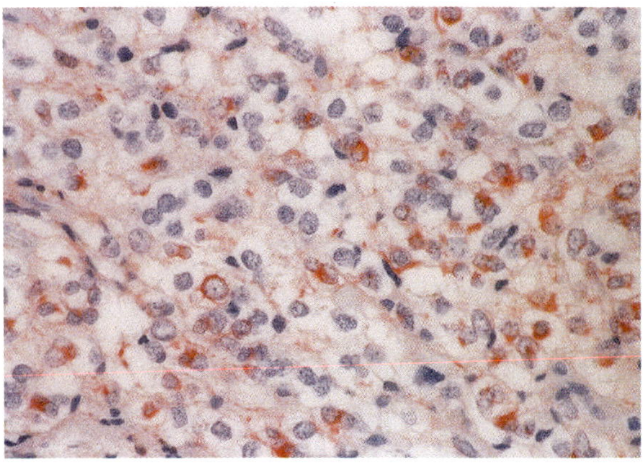

Fig. 9.109 Tumor cells immunopositive for GFAP as a narrow zone around the nucleus in a pattern typical of GFOCs. GFAP immunoperoxidase, × 500

staining (Fig. 9.108). With the same staining, the GFOCs have an appearance identical to the usual oligodendroglia, with vacant cytoplasm; only with GFAP immunohistochemistry do GFOCs exhibit a thin perinuclear rim of positive cytoplasmic reactivity (Fig. 9.109). Both of the transitional forms have been evaluated for their influence on prognosis, and recognition of them in 68% of oligodendrogliomas in this study (Kros *et al.*, 1990) did not adversely affect clinical prognosis.

Collectively, some of these conclusions about GFAP reactivity are explained by relating them to the observations of Choi and Kim (1984, 1985), according to whom the fetal radial glia give rise to cells of both astroglial and oligodendroglial lineage (Choi, Kim and Lapham, 1983), and immature human oligodendrocytes, in normal ontogeny, may transiently express GFAP immediately before myelinogenesis. This view has received support from other workers based on *in vitro* studies on immature mouse oligodendrocytes (Ogawa *et al.*, 1985), although it has been questioned by some (Bullon *et al.*, 1984; Muñoz-Garcia and Ludwin, 1985). In any event, the positivity of many typical neoplastic oligodendrocytes for GFAP and the frequency with which mixed oligodendrogliomas and astrocytomas occur suggest the possibility that the cell type targeted for neoplastic transformation, prior to its phenotypic expression, might be a glial precursor cell capable of either astrocytic or oligodendroglial differentiation. The examination of oligodendrogliomas by de la Monte (1989) for expression of MAb A2B5, galactocerebroside and GFAP lends credence to the existence of a transitional form of oligoastrocyte and suggests a possible explanation for the preponderance of mixed oligoastrocytomas over pure oligodendrogliomas as a phenotype. The MAb A2B5-positive progenitor cells normally differentiate into both type 2 astrocytes and galactocerebroside-positive oligodendrocytes (Raff, Abney and Fok-Seang, 1985). Given the wide distribution of epitopes recognized by MAb A2B5, alternative hypotheses should not be excluded. Mature oligodendrocytes in mice have been shown to be capable of proliferation after trauma (Ludwin, 1984) or demyelination (Arenella and Herndon, 1984). In the normal primate brain, however, it seems that the proliferating capacity of oligodendrocytes is largely restricted to prepubertal animals and found predominantly in the white matter of the forebrain and the pyramidal tracts, i.e., at sites of active myelination (Rakic, 1985). Labeling experiments in postpubertal rhesus monkeys have shown that astrocytes are virtually the only neuroepithelial cells that remain in the mitotic cycle.

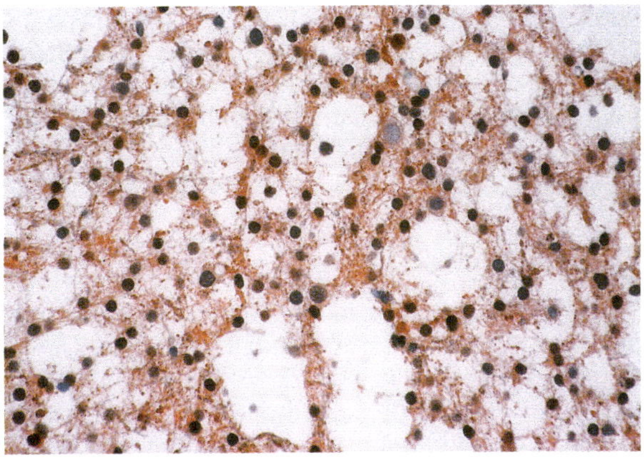

Fig. 9.110 Diffuse nuclear and faint cytoplasmic reactivity for S-100 protein in an oligodendroglioma. Absence of cytoplasmic cellular processes is emphasized by this technique. S-100 protein immunoperoxidase, × 500

Immunoreactivity for the S-100 protein has also been reported in oligodendrogliomas (Nakamura, Becker and Marks, 1983; Kimura, Budka and Soler-Federsppiel, 1986; Nakopoulou, *et al.*, 1990), irrespective of their positivity for GFAP (Fig. 9.110).

The anti-Leu 7 (HNK-1) MAb has been proposed as a marker for these tumors (Motoi *et al.*, 1985; Nakagawa, Perentes and Rubinstein, 1986; Perentes and Rubinstein, 1986), although it is far from specific. Over 90% of oligodendrogliomas demonstrate Leu 7 immunopositivity, which may be found in both GFAP-positive and GFAP-negative oligodendrocytic tumor cells, and characteristically delineates the outer cytoplasmic membranes (Fig. 9.111). However, Leu 7 also labels many astrocytomas. So far, a specific marker exclusive for oligodendrogliomas has yet to be identified. Immunostaining for MBP has been successfully obtained in normal oligodendrocytes of human infants (Itoyama *et al.*, 1980) and adult rats (Sternberger *et al.*, 1985), and has been claimed to be positive in oligodendrogliomas by Figols, Iglesias-Rozas and Kazner (1985). This could not be confirmed, however, by Nakagawa, Perentes and Rubinstein (1986); immunopositivity of the material in that study was found only in the myelin sheaths and myelin fragments (Fig. 9.112). Positivity for the myelin-associated glycoprotein (MAG) has been noted in 3/11 canine oligodendrogliomas by Vandevelde, Fankhauser and Luginbühl (1985), but in only 1/30 tumors in the material of Russell and Rubinstein (1989, pp. 172–87); the immunopositive cells were few (Fig. 9.113).

Carbonic anhydrase C, which has been demonstrated immunohistochemically in normal rodents and, occasionally, in human oligodendrocytes, may show a variable degree of positivity in a minority of oligodendrogliomas (Nakagawa, Perentes and Rubinstein, 1986), where it is usually discrete. However, further study on a variety of neoplasms, both within and outside the CNS, has shown that it cannot serve as a specific marker for any tumor type (Nakagawa, Perentes and Rubinstein, 1987).

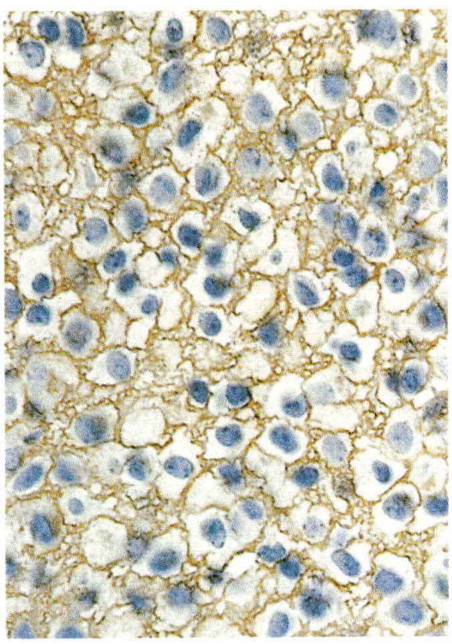

Fig. 9.111 Peripheral cytoplasmic reactivity in an oligodendroglioma. Leu 7 immunoperoxidase, × 400

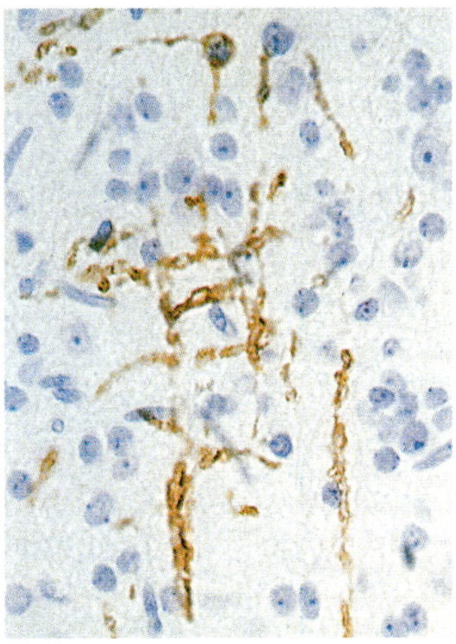

Fig. 9.112 Immunopositive fragments of myelin sheaths scattered among the immunonegative tumor cells in an oligodendroglioma. MBP immunoperoxidase, × 400 (Reprinted from *Acta Neuropathologica*, 1986, pp. 15–22, figure J.)

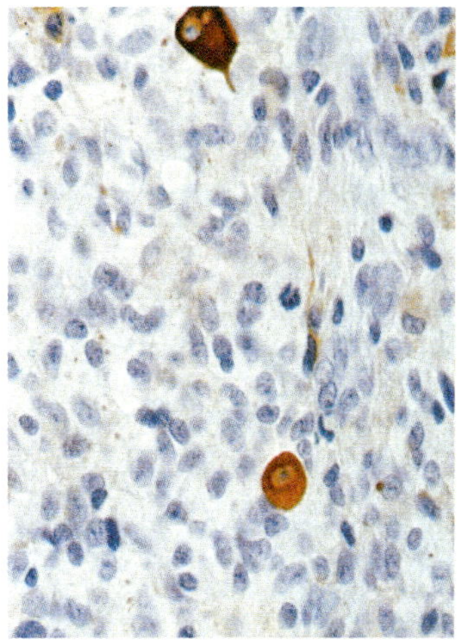

Fig. 9.113 Reaction for MAG in an oligodendroglioma. MAG immunoperoxidase, × 400

The differential immunohistochemical demonstration of soluble lectins has been claimed to help in distinguishing differentiated from anaplastic oligodendrogliomas (Bardosi, Dimitri and Gabius, 1988; Cruz-Sanchez *et al.*, 1991).

Electron microscopy

Earlier electron microscopic observations of oligodendrogliomas included those of Luse (1960), who noted the presence of numerous mitochondria, abnormally enlarged in some examples, and the discontinuity of the vascular basement membrane, which partly incorporated tumor cells into the adventitia. Raimondi (1966) mentioned the presence of discrete cytoplasmic filaments in these tumors. As expected, the oligodendroglioma tumor cells lacked the large numbers of glial filaments, arranged in compact bundles, that are characteristic of astrocytes. Subsequent electron microscopic observations have been made by Garcia and Lemmi (1970), Hossmann and Wechsler (1971), Baloyannis (1981) and Min and Scheithauer (1994). Typically, when adequately fixed and well preserved, the tumor cells may show either a scanty or an abundant cytoplasm that may be rich in organelles, including numerous microtubules and free ribosomes, as well as the large numbers of mitochondria already noted by Luse (1960). The presence of abundant microtubules in the perikarya may be associated with fusiform membrane-bound bodies and a prominent Golgi apparatus (Garcia and Lemmi, 1970). Polygonal intracytoplasmic crystalline inclusions have been described (Tani *et al.*, 1969), but are not specific. Of particular interest is the observation by Robertson and Vogel (1962) of the highly laminar organization, in some cases, of overlapping or concentrically arranged glial cell processes, suggesting their capacity to form sheath-like structures. Such a feature appears to be quite exceptional, but has been confirmed by Hossmann and Wechsler (1971). It is, however, not specific to the oligodendroglioma and has been noted in other forms of glioma, including astrocytomas (Kamitani *et al.*, 1986) and gliomatosis cerebri (Cervós-Navarro *et al.*, 1987). Narrow, laminated cell processes overlying the cell body are more commonly present, and are typical of oligodendroglioma (Min and Scheithauer, 1994). The ultrastructure of the transitional cells in oligodendrogliomas has been extensively detailed by Kros, de Jong and van der Kwast (1992). These miniature gemistocytes or GFOCs have features of both astrocytes and oligodendrocytes, and GFAP is detected in the cytoplasm of both. Using immunoelectron microscopy, Kros and colleagues described bundles of GFAP-positive filaments with a parallel arrangement filling the perinuclear cytoplasm of GFOCs. No other features separated them from GFAP-negative oligodendrocytes. This is in contrast to the finding in astrocytes, which have abundant intermediate filaments filling their cell processes.

Tissue culture

Tissue culture studies of oligodendrogliomas, first detailed by Russell and Bland (1933) and Canti, Bland and Russell (1937), have demonstrated the unique properties of these tumors with respect to cell motility and phenotypic modulation. Details of these studies may be found in the previous edition of this text (Russell and Rubinstein, 1989, pp. 172–87).

Oligodendroglioma cell lines have so far been very difficult to establish from either animal or human tissue cultures. However, such a line, obtained from a mixed human glioma negative for the expression of GFAP but able to synthesize S-100 protein, has been reported (Miyake, 1979) with its response to dibutyryl cyclic adenosine monophosphate (cAMP), which resulted in marked narrowing and elongation of the cell processes. Two additional human oligodendroglioma cell lines have been examined by Kashima *et al.* (1993): HOG (described by Post and Dawson, 1992) and TC620 (described by Manuelidis, Yu and Manuelidis, 1977). Neither line was found, by molecular hybridization techniques, to express GFAP messenger RNA (mRNA), but both expressed mRNA for a specific cytokeratin, K7, a class II intermediate filament protein with a significant homology to GFAP. This unexpected finding raises a question regarding the GFAP immunopositivity seen in the transitional cells of oligodendrogliomas and prompts the speculation by these authors that it may be due to cross-immunoreactivity between these two intermediate filament antigens, GFAP and cytokeratin K7.

Significance of histologic variations

Quite aside from the apparent capacity on the part of neoplastic oligodendrocytes to modulate *in vitro*, and from the additional information provided on their heterogeneous character by their immunopositivity for GFAP, morphologic variation has long been known to be a feature in tissue sections. Although the histologic appearances in the typical case are so characteristic as to be immediately recognizable, the heterogeneity of the microscopic picture may be considerable, as demonstrated in the photomicrographs illustrating this chapter. These variations have been shown more extensively elsewhere (Rubinstein, 1972b) and have been recalled by Escalona-Zapata (1981). They were already emphasized in the early publications on oligodendrogliomas, when silver impregnation techniques were employed to reveal the presence of glial elements other than oligodendrocytic ones (Bailey and Bucy, 1929); these aspects were further developed, at length, by del Rio-Hortega (1944) and Ravens, Adamkiewicz and Groff (1955).

In many examples, such additional glial forms, especially the astrocytic kind, are distributed widely throughout the tumor, sometimes with a tendency to be concentrated in the immediate neighborhood of the blood vessels. The intimate mixture of cell types may be evident in routinely stained sections (Fig. 9.114), but is heightened in immunoperoxidase preparations for GFAP, in which the participation by neoplastic astrocytes and GFAP-positive oligodendrocytes is easily demonstrable. As mentioned above and quantified by Kros *et al.* (1990), the presence of these GFAP-positive oligodendrocytes, either minigemistocytes or GFOCs, does not confer an adverse prognosis over those oligodendrogliomas without GFAP expression. On the other hand, some examples display an apparent juxtaposition of two distinct types of glioma, rather than this intimate cellular mixture (Figs 9.115 and 9.116).

Evolution and malignancy

In the earlier publications on oligodendrogliomas, the view was generally held that these tumors are relatively benign, and undoubtedly many of them are. The clinical presentation, often characterized by focal symptoms, such as Jacksonian or temporal lobe epilepsy, may precede the diagnosis by 5–15 years (Elvidge, Penfield and Cone, 1937): Examples with an evolution spanning two or three decades continue to be reported, either as isolated cases (Freeman and Feigin, 1963; Pelc *et al.*, 1977; Aebi and Kraus-Ruppert, 1978) or in large clinical series (Chin *et al.*, 1980). In the context of such an evolution, postoperative survival of patients for more than 30 years has also been reported (Roberts and German, 1966).

It has long been noted that the postoperative survival of patients from whom oligodendrogliomas had been removed may be disproportionately short in comparison with the preoperative duration of symptoms (Elvidge, Penfield and Cone, 1937). There is, however, no evidence that surgical intervention accelerated growth of the tumor (Weir and Elvidge, 1968). While recurrence is a frequent sequel, estimated to occur in about 50% of cases (Roberts and German, 1966; Chin *et al.*, 1980), some of the more recent clinical follow-up figures

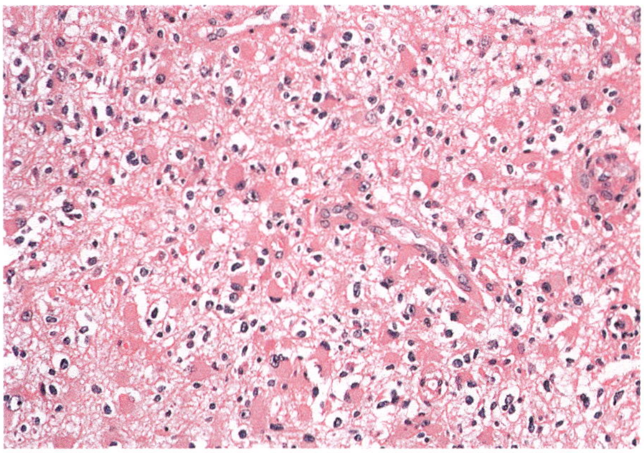

Fig. 9.114 Mixed oligodendroglioma and astrocytoma. H&E, × 250

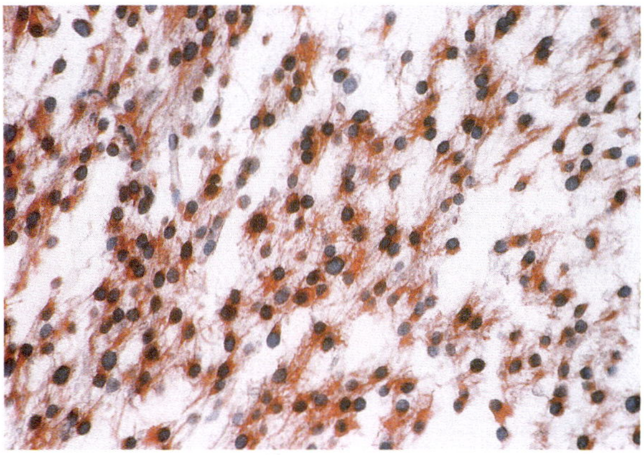

Fig. 9.115 Immunostaining for GFAP of oligodendroglioma and astrocytoma in separate areas. This area shows the rounded cytoplasm and stubby cytoplasmic processes of minigemistocytes in the oligodendroglioma component. GFAP immunoperoxidase, × 500

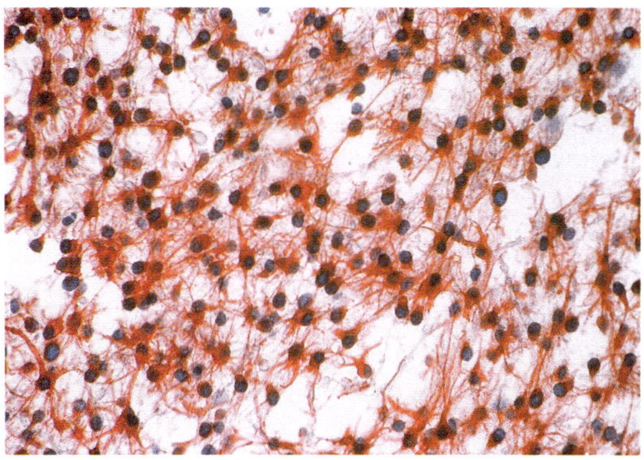

Fig. 9.116 Same case as Fig. 9.115. Immunostaining for GFAP of oligodendroglioma and astrocytoma in separate areas. This area shows the luxuriant cytoplasmic processes of the astrocytoma component. GFAP immunoperoxidase, × 500

on patients who have undergone radical surgery followed by radiotherapy indicate a modest improvement in survival figures compared with the older series. Thus, in the series of Roberts and German of 38 patients, the average postoperative survival was 5–6 years. In the Montreal series (Weir and Elvidge, 1968), 41% of the patients had survived for 5 years. In the series of 29 oligodendrogliomas reported by Wallner, Gonzales and Sheline (1988), postoperative radiation appears to have increased the 5-year survival from about 55% without radiotherapy to 80% with it. The 10-year survival rate was 56% with radiation therapy, but only 18% without. In the series reported by Chin *et al.* (1980), all 24 patients who underwent radical surgery and postoperative radiation survived for at least 5 years. Other recent, larger series of the comparative survival advantage of radiotherapy in totally resected oligodendrogliomas fail to distinguish a difference between the irradiated and nonirradiated groups in Norway (Lindegaard *et al.*, 1987), with 170 patients, or at the Mayo Clinic (Shaw *et al.*, 1992), with 81 patients. Even for those patients with subtotal resections, radiation therapy increased the median survival time, but seemed to offer no improvement in long-term survival. Two other recent series, at Duke University (Bullard *et al.*, 1987) and Princess Margaret Hospital in Toronto (Nijjar *et al.*, 1993), failed to show any improved survival with postoperative radiation therapy. To date, all of these clinical studies involve retrospective analysis. No prospective trials of radiation therapy in patients with oligodendroglioma have been published.

Combination chemotherapy has shown promise by improving survival for patients with oligodendrogliomas or mixed oligoastrocytomas. These regimens can be especially useful in palliation treatment of patients with recurrent disease. The combination of procarbazine, lomustine (*N*-2(chlorethyl)-*N*'-cyclohexyl-*N*-nitrosourea: CCNU) and vincristine, commonly referred to as 'PCV', has produced a significant clinical response rate, ranging up to 100% (Cairncross and Macdonald, 1988; Glass *et al.*, 1992; Kyritsis *et al.*, 1993b). The rationale for applying the same chemotherapy in oligodendrogliomas and mixed oligoastrocytomas hinges on the assumption that all may arise through transformation of the single O2A progenitor lineage, the primitive cell type that developmentally expresses the antigen A2B5 (see 'Immunohistochemistry' above).

Another perspective on the apparent disproportion between length of postoperative patient survival and duration of preoperative symptoms is that many cases of oligodendroglioma present with a relatively short history of a lesion of rapidly increasing size, analogous to that of a glioblastoma, although often preceded by a relatively protracted history of focal, irritative symptoms. In the light of such an evolution, the apparent disproportion becomes understandable. Relevant in this context are the histologic criteria that might predict the prognosis of the tumor, the grading of oligodendrogliomas and the frequency of more differentiated and cytologically benign tumors to undergo subsequent malignant change, with conversion into glioblastomas.

Several studies have addressed themselves to those problems, including the older series of Shenkin, Grant and Drew (1947), Roberts and German (1966) and Weir and Elvidge (1968), and more recent studies, including those of Smith *et al.* (1983), Mørk *et al.* (1986a), Burger *et al.* (1987), Kros *et al.* (1990) and Shaw *et al.* (1992). Most workers have concluded that there is no single reliable histologic criterion by which the malignant examples can be confidently separated from those that are relatively benign. There is general agreement, however, regarding the significance of some combinations of histologic features. Thus, Mørk *et al.* (1986a) found that, alone, neither mitotic activity, nor vascular endothelial proliferation, nor necrosis, nor the age of the patient had any prognostic value, but that when some of these parameters were grouped (such as increased cellular density, the presence of necrosis and the absence of microcyst formation), these features together became associated with a statistically significant reduction in the length of postoperative survival. In contrast, Burger *et al.* (1987) found that 5/15 histologic features evaluated were significant by univariate analysis and suggested that oligodendrogliomas with many of these features (including atypia, mitotic activity, vascular proliferation, vascular hypertrophy, and necrosis) be classified as 'anaplastic'. Histologic features with which to grade anaplasia have been investigated by other authors using large series (Smith *et al.*, 1983, with 323 patients; Kros *et al.*, 1990, with 72 patients; Shaw *et al.*, 1992, with 81 patients), and include nuclear/cytoplasmic ratio or pleomorphism, cell density, mitotic activity, vascular proliferative abnormalities and necrosis (Figs 9.117–9.121). Although median survival intervals vary among patient groups, the general conclusion is that tumors which possess many or all of these histologic features tend to behave in an aggressive fashion. Necrosis, as a feature, seems to distinguish the highest clinical grade of oligodendroglioma from those with other features of anaplasia but without necrosis (Fig. 9.121). Based on several of these histologic features, a prognostically significant justification seems to exist for separating these tumors into at least two malignancy grades: oligodendrogliomas and anaplastic oligodendrogliomas.

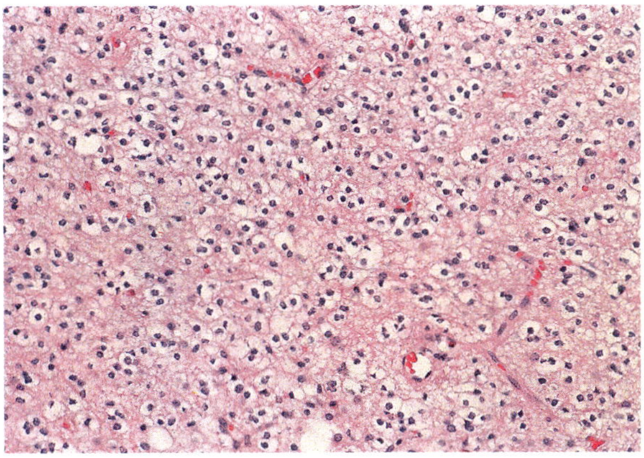

Fig. 9.117 Low-grade oligodendroglioma showing delicate vascular pattern and intervening neuropil between tumor cells. H&E, × 250

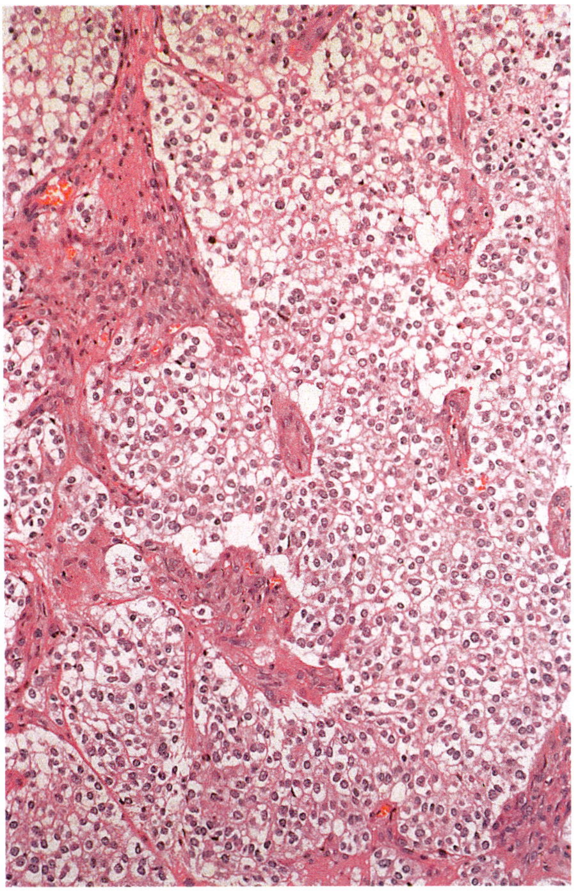

Fig. 9.118 Marked vascular endothelial proliferation in an oligodendroglioma. H&E, × 125

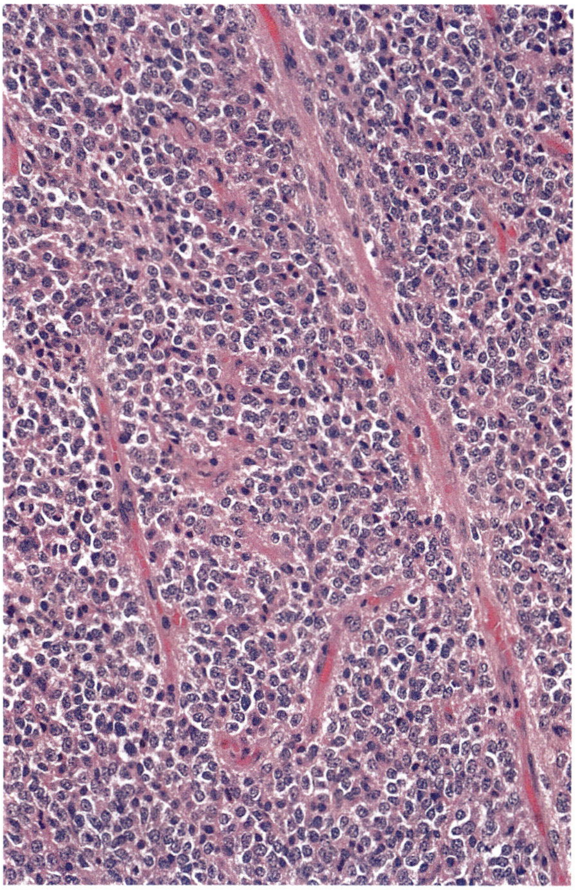

Fig. 9.119 Anaplastic oligodendroglioma with high cellularity and nuclear enlargement. The cytoplasmic clearing is maintained, however. Branching vessels show proliferative changes. H&E, × 250

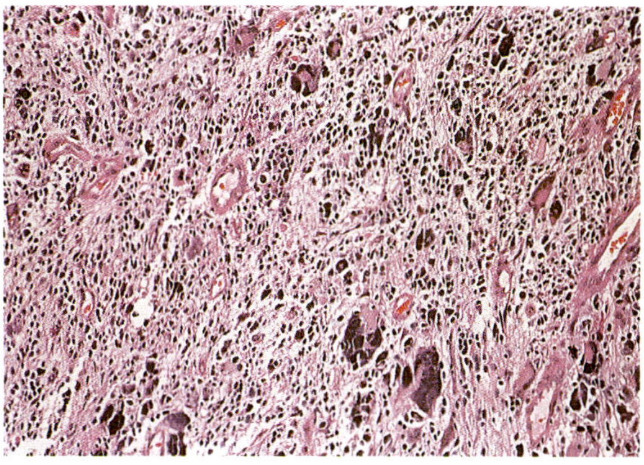

Fig. 9.120 Anaplastic oligodendroglioma showing marked nuclear pleomorphism, but some cytoplasmic clearing. H&E, × 100

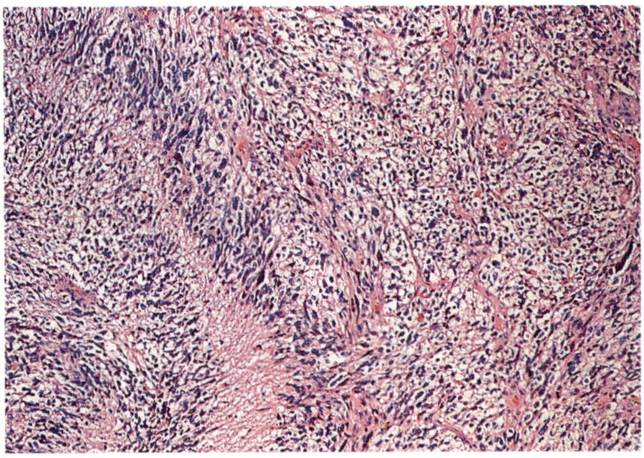

Fig. 9.121 Glioblastoma with focal coagulative necrosis and pseudopalisading of neoplastic cells. The vascular pattern and cytoplasmic clearing suggest that it may have developed from an oligodendroglioma. H&E, × 125

In the case of well-differentiated oligodendrogliomas, quantitative analysis by nuclear morphometry has been claimed to be of value as a reliable predictor of postoperative patient survival (Scarpelli *et al.*, 1987), but the problem is complicated by the fact that a number of oligodendrogliomas undergo malignant change and convert into glioblastomas. In the case of a highly cellular and poorly differentiated round-cell glioblastoma, an oligodendroglial origin may be hard to establish; but when, in such a tumor, many microscopic fields are present that closely resemble those of an oligodendroglioma, it becomes entirely reasonable to assume that the glioblastoma has arisen in a preexisting oligodendroglioma. More precisely, one may assume that the resulting picture of cellular density and anaplasia represents the development of rapidly proliferating clonogenic subpopulations within an oligodendroglioma. This can be inferred not only from an analysis of the final histologic appearance at necropsy, but also by the observation of repeated biopsies. Thus, many reports have documented a general trend towards increasing malignancy in a fair number of cases, as detailed, for example, in the articles by Davis *et al.* (1949), Barnard (1968), Schuier (1976) and Schmitt (1983a, case 2).

We would restrict the term 'anaplastic oligodendroglioma', then, to a relatively pure type of rapidly growing, highly cellular and poorly differentiated oligodendroglioma with the microscopic features illustrated in Figs 9.118–9.120. High cellularity, increased mitotic activity, nuclear or cellular pleomorphism, vascular changes and the presence of necroses without pseudopalisading are characteristically associated with such an anaplastic change. A large proportion of malignant gliomas that present difficulty in precise classification display a microscopic picture of combined oligodendroglioma and astrocytoma in various progressive stages of anaplasia, an appearance that may better justify a diagnosis of glioblastoma. Although precise quantitative data are not available, the experience of Russell and Rubinstein (1989, pp. 172–87) suggests that, in a mixed glioma, it is the astrocytic element that is particularly liable to show anaplastic change to a glioblastoma. Such a view is also held by Müller, Afra and Schröder (1977b) in their correlative clinical and histologic study. Therefore, of the six patients with oligodendroglioma studied by Burger *et al.* (1987), none whose tumors exhibited necrosis with pseudopalisading of tumor cells lived more than 3½ years, a survival equivalent to that of patients with glioblastoma.

In these examples, the resemblance to glioblastoma multiforme is completed by the development of extensive necroses with pseudopalisading of tumor cells (Fig. 9.121), endothelial and vascular proliferation being conspicuous elements in the viable areas of the tumor. The progression to sarcomatous transformation of the proliferating blood vessels—an example of which Rubinstein observed in a 30-year-old man with a temporal lobe oligodendroglioma having extensive mucinous degeneration (Rubinstein, 1972b, Figs 100 and 101)—has been confirmed in more recent reports, such as those by Feigin, Ransohoff and Lieberman (1976) and by Pasquier *et al.* (1978), the latter example being one in which the mesenchymal component was both fibrosarcomatous and angiosarcomatous.

Metastases

The curious behavior of oligodendrogliomas is further exemplified when their spread along the cerebrospinal pathway is considered: this may be massive, highly cellular and rapidly fatal, analogous to the behavior of medulloblastomas, or it may be a chronic process leading to meningeal fibrosis and sustained over many years (Beck and Russell, 1942; Blumenfeld and Gardner, 1945). Furthermore, it seems, from these and other reports, that this form of spread is not associated with the anaplastic oligodendrogliomas described in the foregoing section, but with primary growths that retain their typical appearances. Moreover, the disseminated cells preserve this cytologic uniformity. Some examples may be characterized by extensive formation of mucin (Voldby, 1974).

The growths concerned usually impinge on some part of the cerebral ventricles, but meningeal spread resulting in cerebral oligodendrogliomatosis has also been reported in a significant proportion of oligodendrogliomas originating in the spinal cord (Fortuna, Celli and Palma, 1980). A case in which meningeal metastases were derived from an oligodendroglioma of the olfactory bulb was described by del Rio-Hortega (1944).

Microscopic study provides no clue as to why the clinical evolution in some cases should be rapid, in others protracted. This absence of correlation between the length of preoperative symptoms and the development of subsequent spinal or cerebral meningeal oligodendrogliomatosis is evident from the literature review by Fortuna, Celli and Palma (1980) of 35 examples of spinal intramedullary oligodendroglioma: the interval between diagnosis or surgical removal of the spinal tumor and the evidence of cerebrospinal spread was usually relatively short, but individual cases suggest that there are remarkable exceptions in both the spinal and the cerebral examples. Thus, the total length of history attributable to the metastases was 7 years in case 1 of Beck and Russell (1942) and 14 years in the case reported by Blumenfeld and Gardner (1945). The primary tumor abutting on the ventricle in these cases remained small, whereas the leptomeninges assumed the appearances of a chronic inflammation with resulting hydrocephalus. A similar diagnostic problem was presented in the second of Best's (1963) two reported examples of intracranial oligodendrogliomatosis. Indeed, care is required to form the correct interpretation because the tumor cells in the interstices of the meninges may be mistaken for desquamated arachnoid cells. Ventricular deposits, if present, will correct this impression even if the primary tumor is not, at first, obvious; a more constant clue is found in the diffuse thickening of the nerve roots of the cauda equina from neoplastic infiltration.

Extracranial metastases

Remote metastasis was first studied, in an unequivocal case, by James and Pagel (1951). Here, as in many other intracranial gliomas with a similar sequel, the way seemed to have been paved by previous craniotomy and spread of the tumor to the extracranial soft tissues (see p. 523). Further acceptable cases are those reported by Spataro and Sacks (1968), in which extracranial metastases developed after four craniotomies and massive local infiltration of the calvarium and scalp in the operation area; by Jellinger, Minauf and Salzer-Kuntschik (1969), in which the lower vertebral bodies were the only site of extraneural metastases in a 58-year-old woman previously operated on for a frontal oligodendroglioma; by Kernohan (1971), in which an extensive tumor in a 3½ year-old child demonstrated, after the third craniotomy, metastases in the skull, lungs, hilar lymph nodes and adrenal gland; and by Kummer, Volk and Dorndorf (1977), in which a recurrent parietal oligodendroglioma in a 40-year-old man was found to invade the falx cerebri 4 years after the original tumor had been removed and in whom, 3 years later, necropsy disclosed permeation of the sagittal sinus, as well as remote metastases in the lung, lymph nodes, vertebrae and femur. The material of Rubinstein (Russell and Rubinstein, 1989, pp. 172–87) included one example in which spread to the extracranial soft tissues was conspicuous, but remote metastasis had not occurred.

TUMORS OF THE EPENDYMOMA GROUP

Under this heading are included the *ependymomas*, the *subependymomas* and the *ependymoblastomas*. For an understanding of these neoplasms, it is necessary to recall some of the current views on the origin and development of the ependymal cell and of the subependymal glia, and to appreciate the potential of these cell types to undergo morphologic change in non-neoplastic conditions.

World Health Organization classification

Inclusion of neoplasms in this section is based on their morphologic similarities to the benign ependymal cell and the subependymal neuroglia. The ability of these neoplasms to produce phenotypic features at the light microscopic, ultrastructural, and biochemical levels of ependymal cells results in the cytogenetic grouping of these tumors. The recently revised World Health Organization's *Histological Typing of Tumours of the Central Nervous System* (Kleihues, Burger and Scheithauer, 1993) classifies the neoplasms discussed here as follows:

1. Tumors of neuroepithelial tissue
   - 1.3. Ependymal tumors
     - 1.3.1. Ependymoma
       - Variants
         - 1.3.1.1. Cellular
         - 1.3.1.2. Papillary
         - 1.3.1.3. Clear-cell
     - 1.3.2. Anaplastic (malignant) ependymoma
     - 1.3.3. Myxopapillary ependymoma
     - 1.3.4. Subependymoma
   - 1.6. Neuroepithelial tumors of uncertain origin
     - 1.6.1. Astroblastomas
   - 1.9. Embryonal tumors
     - 1.9.3. Ependymoblastoma

Although astroblastomas were described in the astrocytoma section of earlier editions of this book, additional analyses, performed by Rubinstein and Herman (1989) using tissue culture and electron microscopy, suggested a tanycytic origin of at least some of these tumors. Tanycytes are developmental precursors of ependymal cells. For this reason, and because their cytologic appearance resembles ependymal cells, astroblastomas are discussed here with the ependymal neoplasms. It should be realized, however, that the definitive cell of origin for astroblastomas remains in doubt and that astroblastoma as a discrete clinicopathologic entity is not universally accepted. In the current WHO classification, astroblastomas are considered as neuroepithelial tumors of uncertain origin.

Cytogenesis

Broadly speaking, two cytogenetic concepts have been proposed. One view is that, during the migration and maturation of cells originating from the primitive neural tube, the residual undifferentiated elements lining its lumen progressively acquire the differentiating features of adult ependymal cells. These consist of an increase in granular endoplasmic reticulum, the development of microvilli on the luminal cell surfaces, the appearance of basal bodies and the formation of cilia with the 9 + 2 configuration of an axial filament complex. This concept gains support from observations of primitive neuroepithelial cells in the experimental transplantable mouse testicular teratoma, OTT-6050. Gradual cellular transitions are found in this xenograft from the primitive cells present in the medullary rosettes to more differentiated cells forming ependymoblastic rosettes containing mitotic figures and cell surface specializations that are, however, less well developed than those cells found in mature ependymal rosettes (Herman *et al.*, 1975). Similarly, the findings in the ependymoblastoma, a primitive embryonal tumor that focally exhibits the differentiating features of ependymal cells, lend support to this theory.

A different cytogenetic concept assumes the existence of a primitive 'polar ependymoglioblast', or tanycyte, intermediary between primitive glioblasts and mature ependymal cells, through which maturation of ependymal cell precursors from either glioblasts (Wechsler, 1966), or an unknown undifferentiated ventricular zone cell (Schaper, 1897a), is effected. Since Levitt, Cooper and Rakic (1981) demonstrated that cellular differentiation in the CNS could be detected immunohistochemically in the ventricular zone of 12-week rhesus monkey fetuses, efforts have been directed towards the cellular dissection of the individual components of the developing CNS. In thc human, the tanycyte has come to represent either an immature phase of the developing ependymal cell (Gould, Howard and Papadaki, 1990) or a cell whose function is largely enigmatic (Russell and Rubinstein, 1989), though capable of chemical transportation and/or secretion (Flament-Durand and Brion, 1985; Gould, Howard and Papadaki, 1990).

The term 'polar ependymoglioblast' has been abandoned, but the concept of the tanycyte has not. Resurrected by electron microscopists (Wechsler, 1966) and immunohistochemists (Roessmann *et al.*, 1980), the concept of the human tanycyte has undergone considerable revisions since its conception. Silver impregnation, immunohistochemical and electron microscopic studies (Ramón y Cajal, 1952; Choi and Lapham, 1978; Roessmann *et al.*, 1980; Hajos and Basco, 1984; Gould, Howard and Papadaki, 1990) have confirmed the existence of a primitive cell, along the ventricular lining in human fetal brains, that exhibits a short simple basilar cytoplasmic process superficially and that extends into the subventricular (terminology according to Angevine *et al.*, 1970), but not the intermediate, zone. At the 19/20 week stage in most areas of the CNS, the ventricular zone has thinned, allowing light microscopic distinction between these cells and the radial glia in the subventricular and intermediate zones (Roessmann *et al.*, 1980). Both Roessmann (Roessmann *et al.*, 1980) and Gould (Gould, Howard and Papadaki, 1990) agree that stages of the maturing brain are encountered where these GFAP-positive tanycytes are found amidst mature cuboidal, or epithelial, ependymal cells. However, while Roessmann states that the two cells are distinct and unrelated, Gould presents strong evidence that, through shortening of the basal process, production of cilia, loss of GFAP and the production of microvilli, most tanycytes mature into ependymal cells.

The origin(s) of tanycytes remain unknown. Although hypothesized to arise from radial glia (Schmechel and Rakic, 1979b), there is evidence to suggest otherwise (Roessmann *et al.*, 1980; reviewed in Gould, Howard and Papadaki, 1990). As pointed out by Gould (Gould, Howard and Papadaki, 1990), tanycytes are visible over the ganglionic eminence on the lateral ventricular wall, a region in which radial glia cannot be demonstrated. The assumption is that tanycytes arise directly from undifferentiated cells in the ventricular zone. Furthermore, the possibility remains that a population of mature ependymal cells arise without a transient tanycytic phase.

A second question left unanswered, to date, concerns the fate of the bipolar tanycytes. While recognized in the immediate subependymal regions up to birth by Gould, he did not find these cells in 1 month postterm infants. While he did note that bipolar tanycytes undergo an embryonal phase of active ciliogenesis, he found no evidence that they became mature ependymal cells, suggesting that the subependymal, GFAP-positive cell identified by Deck *et al.* (1978) may be the fate of these cells.

Evidence from ependymomas neither supports nor refutes the hypotheses concerning the fate of the tanycyte. Historically, Bailey and Cushing (1926) invoked the tanycyte to explain the morphology of certain ependymomas exhibiting elongated fibrillated tails attached to a central blood vessel, a tumor originally called 'ependymoblastoma'. This name was later abandoned (see Rubinstein, 1970, for further details). Similarly, Rubinstein invoked the tanycyte to explain the morphology of a tumor called 'astroblastoma' (Rubinstein and Herman, 1989), but it is clear that he considered the tanycyte as an embryonal intermediary. The finding of the embryonal intermediate filament nestin in ependymomas (Tohyama *et al.*, 1992; McLendon *et al.*, 1995b) has been stated to represent evidence of an uncommitted embryonal cell (Tohyama *et al.*, 1992). And Roessmann *et al.* (1980) argue that most ependymomas exhibit GFAP immunoreactivity, cilia production and elongated cell processes because they arose from persistent tanycytes. The concept of the tanycyte as an immature, GFAP-producing phase in the development of the epithelial ependymal cell (Gould and Howard, 1987) can similarly be invoked to explain the morphologies identified in the ependymoma. Thus, Deck *et al.* (1978) hypothesize that GFAP production in most ependymomas reflects this immature, but regulated, expression of this protein.

The capacity of both the adult ependymal cell and the underlying subependymal neuroglia to undergo reactive changes is relevant to the histomorphology of ependymomas. When the ependymal cells are dislocated so that they no longer form surface epithelium, they form either 'rosettes', in which the cells are grouped about a small central lumen, or solid clusters of irregular outline. These formations are commonly found on microscopic examination of any brain in sections taken from parts where the ventricles are sharply angulated, or at the rear end of the occipital horn. In these regions, the subependymal neuroglia continues as a streak or band in the adjacent white matter and incorporates nests of polygonal ependymal cells (see Fig. 9.122). Similar nests are frequently seen in the ventral spur of the aqueduct, in the thin sheet of neuroglial tissue that extends outwards about the foramen of Luschka, and in the commonly obliterated central canal of the spinal cord. The

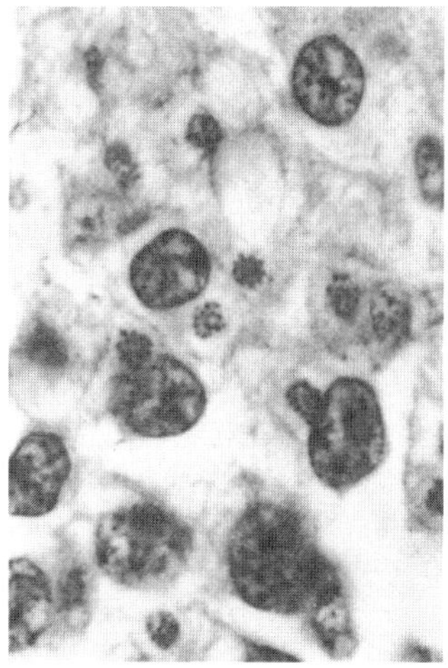

Fig. 9.122 Groups of juxtanuclear blepharoplasts in ectopic periventricular ependymal cells. Mallory's phosphotungstic acid–hematoxylin (PTAH), × 1280

exceptional development of ependymomas or ependymoblastomas apparently unrelated to either a ventricular cavity or the spinal canal presumably results from the neoplastic transformation of such ectopic ependymal elements. The filum terminale also contains scattered groups of these cells but, as detailed below (p. 406), possesses some unique additional features that explain the peculiar histologic characteristics of the ependymomas originating from that structure.

In chronic low-grade inflammations of the ependyma, there is often a reactive proliferation of the subependymal neuroglia resulting in the protrusion of knobs, or 'granulations', of fibrillary glia into the ventricular lumen, and in the disruption of the surface epithelium. The granulations may then enlarge and ultimately form a confluent layer upon the surface. The submerged ependymal cells respond by the formation of *rosettes*. In general, they give the impression of being remarkably inert, with little or no regenerative capacity when their continuity has been breached. Yet, not infrequently, the stimulus of an adjacent tumor (e.g., a glioblastoma) will evoke the production of tapering fibrillated processes that stream from the cell bodies into the neighboring tissues. This appearance, not normally seen in the adult lateral ventricle, closely resembles that of the ependymal tanycytes demonstrable in late fetal life (Roessmann *et al.*, 1980). The importance of this reactive, nonneoplastic phenomenon lies in the fact that cells of this character often form an important component in tumors of the ependymoma group and should not, therefore, be regarded as an embryonal feature.

Intermediate filament production

The capacity of nonneoplastic reactive and neoplastic ependymal cells for intracytoplasmic fibrillogenesis has been repeatedly confirmed and refined by both immunochemistry and electron microscopy (Brightman and Palay, 1963; Zülch and Wechsler, 1968; Wolff, Santiago and Duby, 1972; Rawlinson, Herman and Rubinstein, 1973; Choi and Lapham, 1978; McLendon *et al.*, 1986; Migheli and Mocellini, 1990; Figarella-Branger *et al.*, 1991; Kasper, Perry and Stosiek 1991; Tohyama *et al.*, 1992). The spectrum of intermediate filament production in immature ependymal cells includes nestin (Tohyama *et al.*, 1992), vimentin (Schnitzer, Franke and Schachner, 1981; Bignami, Raju and Dahl, 1982; Miettinen, Clark and Virtanen, 1986; Kasper, Perry and Stosiek, 1991), and cytokeratin (Kasper, Perry and Stosiek, 1991) and GFAP (Roessmann *et al.*, 1980; Choi, 1986; Miettinen, Clark and Virtanen, 1986; Gould and Howard, 1988; Gould, Howard and Papadaki, 1990; Tohyama *et al.*, 1991). Although scanty intermediate filaments (see Fig. 9.123) are identifiable by electron microscopy in the mature ependymal cell, the identity of these filaments is largely unknown as few cells react in immunohistochemical assays for vimentin (Deck *et al.*, 1978; Figarella-Branger *et al.*, 1991) and none react against cytokeratin, GFAP (Tohyama *et al.*, 1991; Sarnat, 1995) or nestin (Tohyama *et al.*, 1992). Possibly, by analogy with the protoplasmic astrocyte, the mature ependymal cell contains too few intermediate filaments to be histologically detectable. Only with the development of conspicuous numbers of intracytoplasmic filaments arranged in bundles, such as occurs in pathologically altered ependymal cells, can the synthesis of large amounts of the protein become immunomorphologically demonstrable. This contrasts with GFAP positivity of the tanycytes in the mouse hypothalamus that retain GFAP once it has been acquired, endowing them early in postnatal life with a feature characteristic of fully differentiated astrocytes (de Vitry *et al.*, 1981).

Cilia and blepharoplasts

The development of 9 + 2 cilia with their basal blepharoplasts should be regarded as the most important hallmark of the mature, fully differentiated ependymal cell. The primitive medullary epithelium is nonciliated. In well-preserved adult material, cilia and blepharoplasts can always be found in the ependyma lining the ventricles. In these cells, the blepharoplasts are usually easily seen along the abluminal border of the cytoplasm. However, ependymal cells found embedded in parenchyma do not have cilia, and the blepharoplasts are clustered near the nucleus (Fig. 9.122), often grouped within a halo of more lightly staining cytoplasm. By electron microscopy, they are seen to represent the basal bodies in which shafts of cilia terminate in the cytoplasm, as beautifully illustrated by Brightman and Palay (1963) in their classic paper on the fine structure of the rat ependyma (cf. Fig. 9.123). The PTAH stain may be useful to experienced eyes in recognizing the basal bodies, but only a tentative diagnosis may be possible without electron microscopy or other architectural evidence for confirmation. To date, no studies report the application of a MAb that recognizes cilia on ependymoma tissues, an antibody that, parenthetically, is one of the few immunoreagents capable of binding mature ependymal cells in humans (Klotz *et al.*, 1986).

Other developmentally regulated ependymal antigens

The application of immunologic techniques has proven to be a powerful tool in the dissection of molecular constituents of the cell. Thus, Hockfield and McKay (1985) generated the MAb Rat 401 against an antigen that was developmentally regulated in glial cells. Subsequent studies by Lendahl, Zimmerman and McKay (1990) proved the antigen recognized by Rat 401 to be nestin, the intermediate filament reviewed previously.

Similarly, MAbs generated against membranes of human milk fat globules resulted in the characterization of an antibody specific for epithelial membranes, the epithelial membrane antigen (EMA) antibody (Ceriani *et al.*, 1977; Heyderman, Steele, and Ormerod, 1979). This antibody has been found by Uematsu *et al.* (1989) to bind fetal ependymal cells between 27 and 40 weeks gestational age, as well as all postnatal ependymal cells, including those from the brains of five children and eight adults studied. No immunoreactivity was noted in a 10-week gestational age fetus. The immunoreactivity patterns were described as 'similar to those of epithelial cells' and included membrane reactivity, irregular punctate cytoplasmic reactivity and smooth ring-like intracytoplasmic reactivity. Similarly, Perentes and Rubinstein (1986) reported epithelial membrane antigen reactivity in normal ependymal cells.

Immunohistochemical studies for neurofilaments, microtubule-associated protein (MAP), clathrin, MBP, synaptophysin and nerve growth factor receptor have not found these antigens in ependymomas (Tohyama *et al.*, 1991).

Subependymal neuroglia

The ependymal cells invariably rest upon a layer of rather dense fibrillary neuroglia, which, as already mentioned, is capable of considerable proliferative

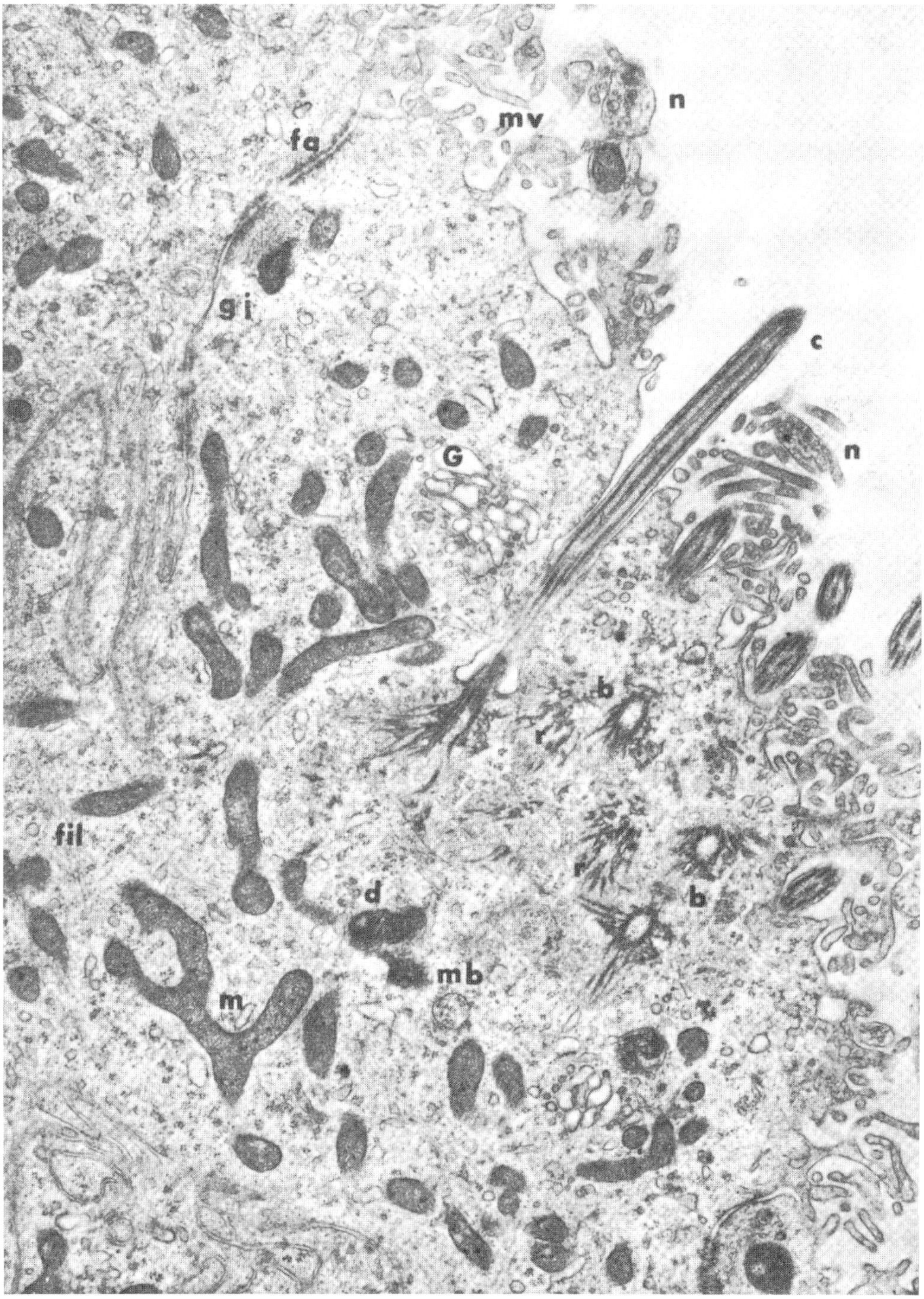

Fig. 9.123 Normal ependymal cell of an adult hamster. The apical cytoplasm of one cell is mainly seen, and part of another. The free surface is thrown into irregular folds, or microvilli (mv), that partially or completely surround the ciliary shafts (c), seen in both longitudinal and transverse sections. The apical cytoplasm contains three basal bodies, or blepharoplasts (b), and three ciliary rootlets (r). The other cytoplasmic components include pleomorphic mitochondria (m), occasionally membrane-bound multivesicular bodies (mb), dense bodies (d), cisterns of the Golgi apparatus (G) and delicate filaments (fil). Note the interdigitations of the plasmalemma of the adjacent cells, with surface specializations consisting of fasciae adherentes (fa) joined by gap junctions (gj). Two neuronal processes (n) lie free in the ventricle. × 20 000. (Courtesy of Dr Milton W. Brightman)

activity. Whether this layer is derived from bipolar tanycytes (Gould, Howard and Papadaki, 1990) or, alternatively, from local immature glial cell precursors that later differentiate into mature astrocytes is of relatively little practical importance. Either hypothesis would readily account for the fact that the subependymal glia often appears to contribute a large and sometimes preponderant element to some of the tumors of this group. The first hypothesis suggests a re-expression of GFAP produced transitionally during development; the second hypothesis indicates cellular heterogeneity, i.e., to both ependymal cells and the subependymal neuroglia participating in the neoplastic process. Recognition of this latter morphology has led to the coining of the name 'subependymoma' (Scheinker, 1945), which, as detailed on p. 410, constitutes a fairly distinct variant of ependymoma.

In the simple scheme of classification proposed for the tumors of the ependymoma group, there seems no need to invoke the existence or the role of a primitive cell. The speculation that neoplastic change involving ependymal structures recapitulates the features of common primitive ancestor cells adds little to the discussion of the growth characteristic of the ependymoma or its clinical prognosis. Unlike primitive neuroepithelial tumors in which the malignant cells may or may not bear a superficial resemblance to embryonal cell forms, the tumors under discussion are well differentiated with characteristic ependymal nuclear features and do not present the cytologic features of either anaplastic or embryonal neoplasms. Embryonal characteristics are confined to the ependymoblastoma (p. 417) and the astroblastoma (p. 419) features for which the hypothesis of an intermediate ependymoglial precursor cell might possibly account for some of the cellular appearances (see p. 417).

The epithelium of the choroid plexus, like the ependyma, takes its origin from the differentiation of primitive neuroepithelial ventricular cells or their progeny. However, both its structure and function are different from those of the ependyma, and these differences are reflected in the neoplasms arising from that organ. As recounted below (Volume 2, p. 35), the epithelial elements of choroid plexus papillomas may occasionally show evidence of focal neuroglial differentiation consistent with the neuroepithelial origin of the parent structure. Accordingly, we have included the choroid plexus neoplasms in Chapter 10 with other tumors derived from primitive ventricular neuroepithelium, but which have developed highly specialized structures and functions. In a similar vein, 'colloid cysts' of the third ventricle, in view of their maldevelopmental nature and the current controversies on their histogenesis, are separately described in the chapter on tumors and tumor-like lesions of maldevelopmental origin (Chapter 15).

Ependymomas

Although most ependymomas are slow growing, their intracranial location may constitute a poor operative risk, resulting in an incomplete resection and increasing the likelihood of recurrence (Goldwein *et al.*, 1990; Sutton *et al.*, 1990–91; Ernestus, Wilcke and Schröder, 1991; Lyons and Kelly, 1991; Ferrante *et al.*, 1994). In particular, the microanatomic location of fourth-ventricular ependymomas has been shown to influence the degree of resection obtainable (Ikezaki *et al.*, 1993). Although controversial (Ross and Rubinstein, 1989), histologic grading of ependymomas also appears to impact upon prognosis, especially of those ependymomas arising in the supratentorial compartment (Rawlings *et al.*, 1988; Papadopoulos, Giri and Evans, 1990; Figarella-Branger *et al.*, 1991; Schiffer *et al.*, 1991b; Chiu *et al.*, 1992). In contrast, the prognosis in spinal examples appears to be significantly better in those with low-grade histology (Waldron *et al.*, 1993) and is also related to the completeness of resection (Wen *et al.*, 1991; Ferrante *et al.*, 1992; Cervoni *et al.*, 1994a).

Incidence

The epidemiology and incidence of ependymomas is covered more completely by Davis and Preston-Martin in Chapter 1. Briefly reviewed here, the incidence of ependymomas in different series range from 2% to 6% of all gliomas. Zülch and Christensen (1956, pp. 295–335) estimated their incidence to be 4.6%. These are predominantly tumors of children and adolescents, in whom they account for up to 10% of all brain tumors (Jellinger and Seitelberger, 1970), but examples in adults are not rare. Among inherited brain tumor syndromes, multiple spinal cord ependymomas are found in association with NF type 2 (central).

Sites

The primary site of ependymomas is heavily age dependent. The fourth ventricle is the most common site and accounts for up to 60% of these tumors in most series (Kernohan and Sayre, 1952; Mørk and Løken, 1977; Cruz-Sanchez *et al.*, 1988b; Rawlings *et al.*, 1988; Schiffer *et al.*, 1991b). Among children (<20 years), approximately 60% of ependymomas arise in the posterior fossa, or, more precisely, in the fourth ventricle (Goldwein *et al.*, 1990; Chiu *et al.*, 1992). Among adults, the location of intracranial ependymomas has not been clearly

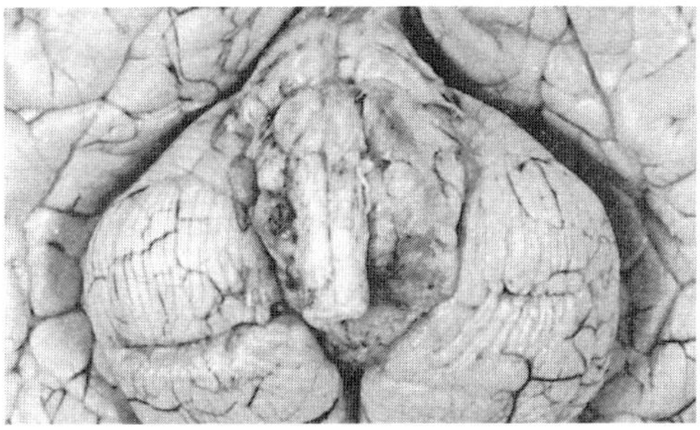

Fig. 9.124 Ependymoma originating from the fourth ventricle in a 10-month-old male infant and partly surrounding the brainstem.

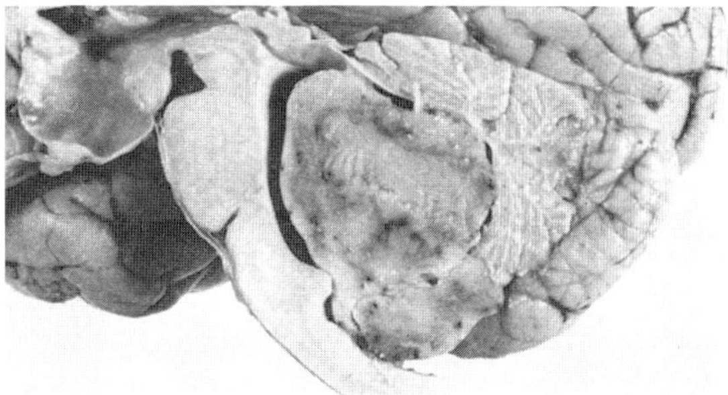

Fig. 9.125 Same case as Fig. 9.124. Tumor filling the fourth ventricle and causing marked dilatation of the third ventricle.

reported, but appears to be approximately evenly divided among infratentorial and supratentorial locations. In contrast, the vast majority of spinal cord ependymomas occur in adults (Ferrante *et al.*, 1992; Waldron *et al.*, 1993; Cervoni *et al.*, 1994a) and comprise the preponderant glioma of the spinal cord and filum terminale (over 60%, according to Slooff, Kernohan, and MacCarty, 1964). The lumbosacral segments are the most frequently involved: this topographic selectivity is largely due to the fact that spinal ependymomas appear to be almost equally divided between the intramedullary cellular ependymomas and the myxopapillary variants, which arise in the region of the conus medullaris, the filum terminale and the cauda equina. When the myxopapillary variants are excluded, the cervical and thoracic regions appear to bear the burden of ependymomas (Mørk and Løken 1977; Cervoni *et al.*, 1994a).

Ectopic locations of ependymomas have been described, and include the broad ligament (Bell, Woodruff and Scully, 1984), the uterosacral ligament (Duggan *et al.*, 1989), the lung (Crotty *et al.*, 1992), the ovary (Selvaggi, 1992; Guerrieri and Jarlsfelt, 1993) and the subcutaneous tissues of the sacrococcygeal region (Gupta and Pratap, 1992; King, Cooper and Malcolm 1993; Bourlond, Bourlond and Rousseau, 1994). These non-CNS locations are discussed more fully in the chapter on tumors of maldevelopmental origin (Chapter 15).

Macroscopic appearance

The macroscopic appearance of the ependymoma varies considerably. Tumors that project into the cavity of a ventricle or from the foramen of Luschka into the cerebellopontine angle may be rather soft and papillary, mimicking a choroid plexus papilloma (Figs 9.124 and 9.125). Those arising within the substance of the brain or cord are usually well defined, homogeneous, gray and granular, but the larger examples in the cerebrum are often partially or extensively cystic (Fig. 9.126).

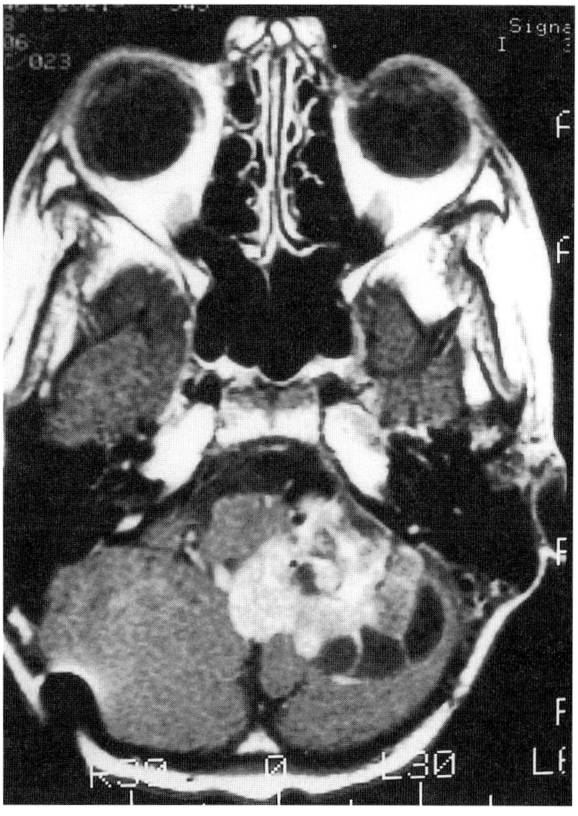

Fig. 9.126 Ependymoma from a 9-year-old male. This axial T1-weighted postcontrast MRI shows an inhomogeneously enhanced mass with multiple cystic components that occupy the fourth ventricle and extend from the foramen of Luschka to the cerebellopontine angle region.

The classic appearance of a posterior fossa ependymoma is a somewhat lobulated soft tissue mass that appears to form a cast or mold of the

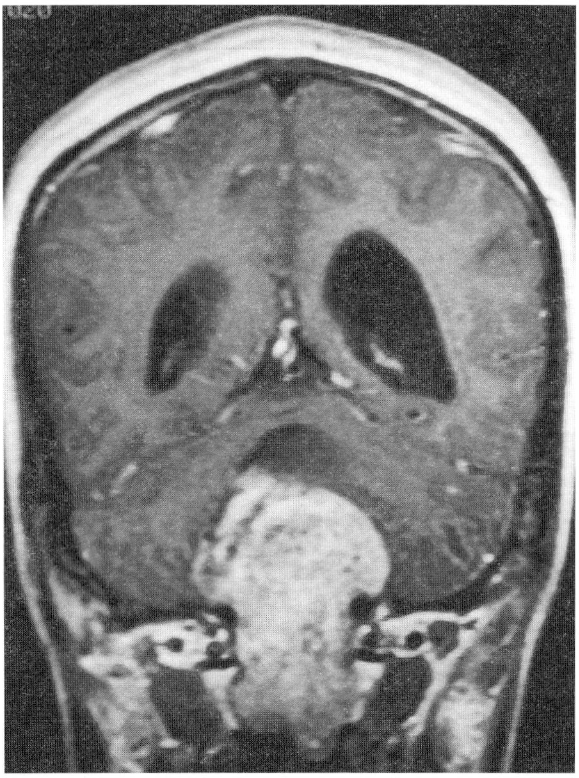

Fig. 9.127 Ependymoma from a 15-year-old female. This coronal T1-weighted postcontrast MRI demonstrates an inhomogeneously enhanced large mass occupying the middle and inferior portion of the fourth ventricle, with hydrocephalus.

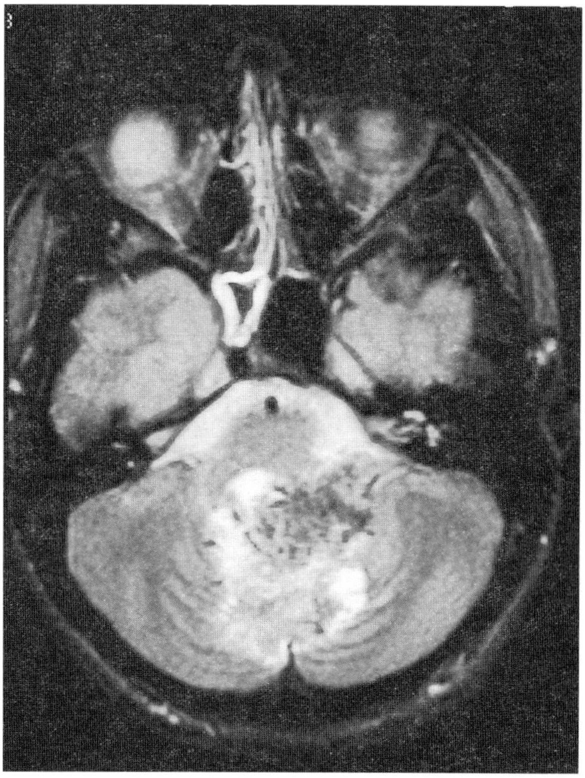

Fig. 9.128 Same case as Fig. 9.127. This axial T2-weighted MRI shows a mass originating in the fourth ventricle and extending to the foramen of Luschka. The mass has inhomogeneously low-signal intensity that, most likely, represents parenchymal calcification.

fourth ventricle. It extrudes through the foramina of Luschka, then Magendie, and then downward through the foramen magnum, resulting in caudal tongue-like projections of tumor that compress dorsal and lateral aspects of the upper cervical cord. This characteristic morphology has been termed the 'plastic ependymoma' by Courville and Broussalian 1961) (Fig. 9.124).

Radiographic appearance

Examination by MRI (Figs 9.126-129) often shows marked heterogeneity within these neoplasms, as a reflection of cystic regions; areas of necrosis; acute, subacute, and chronic hemorrhage; and calcification (Spoto *et al.*, 1990). These tumors are often situated within the ventricle and consequently are frequently associated with hydrocephalus. They have the highest frequency of calcification of all posterior fossa tumors (45%) (Armington *et al.*, 1985). Calcification within these masses can be seen as marked hypointensity on gradient-echo MRIs or as high density by CT. The solid components of ependymomas are typically hypo- or isointense as compared with brain on T1-weighted images and hyperintense on proton density- and T2-weighted scans. The cystic portions of ependymomas are slightly hyperintense to CSF on T1-weighted images and hyperintense to brain on T2-weighted images. Contrast enhancement occurs in virtually all ependymomas, but it is often heterogeneous and irregular. Seeding of the CSF pathways with metastases occurs not infrequently, with estimates varying with the location of the primary neoplasm. Infratentorial ependymomas reportedly produce radiographically demonstrated metastases in up to 6% of cases in contrast with supratentorial tumors in which this phenomenon is exceedingly rare.

Supratentorial ependymomas are often indistinguishable from other gliomas. Because they are primarily extraventricular lesions, supratentorial ependymomas can mimic astrocytoma. Homogeneous solid or ring-enhancing patterns are commonly seen (Courville and Broussalian, 1961).

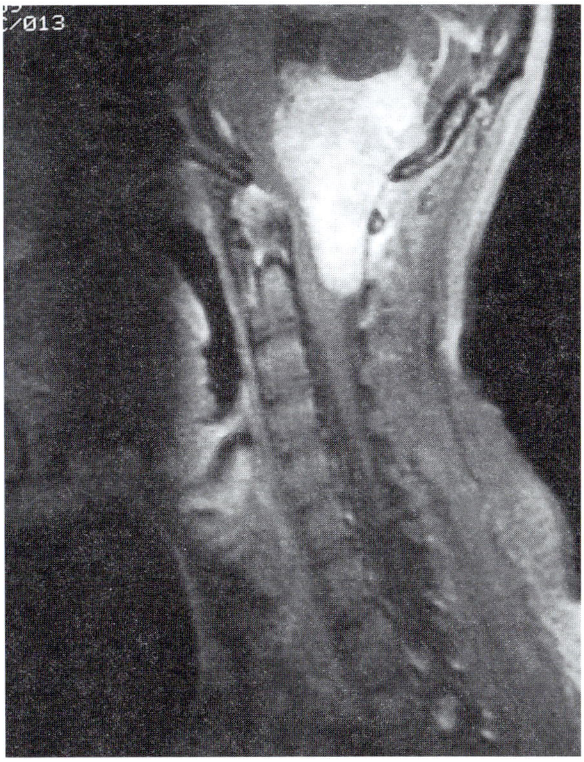

Fig. 9.129 Same case as Fig. 9.127. A sagittal T1-weighted postcontrast MRI shows the mass occupying the middle and interior portions of the fourth ventricle with inferior extension through the foramen magnum to the level of C2, with compression of the medulla and upper cervical cord. There is also a small cystic component on the upper portion of the tumor.

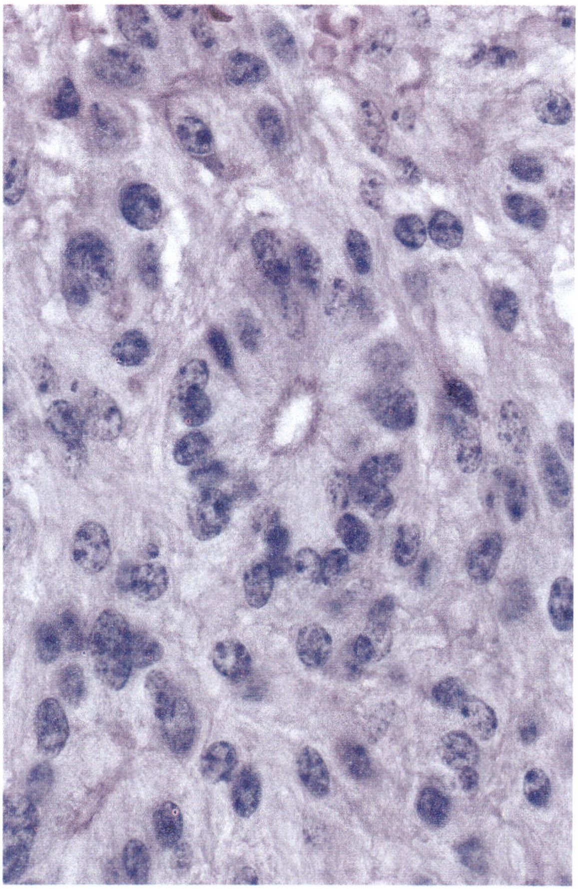

Fig. 9.130 Ependymoma with rosettes. Occasionally, an otherwise typical ependymoma may reveal diminutive spaces lined by ependymal cells, evidencing true ependymal rosette formation. H&E, × 400

Calcification may also be found in the cerebral examples.

Microscopic appearance

The cellularity and architecture of ependymomas may vary, not only from case to case, but also in different locations within the same tumor. A diagnostic feature, the *ependymal rosette* (Fig. 9.130), is found in only a minority of examples and typically in the infratentorial location (Rawlings *et al.*, 1988). Ependymal differentiation may also be inferred by the presence of elongated clefts, or spaces of irregular shape, bordered by typical ependymal epithelium. An epithelial appearance may be manifest in some tumors that exhibit uniform masses of polygonal cells with well-defined borders, the epithelial appearance of which is characteristic of normal ependymal cells. They may be relatively cellular, with little supporting stroma aside from the intrinsic blood vessels. In many examples, the tumor cells appear separated by fibrillary neuroglia (Fig. 9.131). Sometimes neighboring cells are encountered. These are separated by a minute circular space bordered by blepharoplasts or traversed by a small brush of cilia, representing either diminutive ependymal rosettes or an abortive attempt at rosette formation.

Most ependymomas contain areas in which *perivascular pseudorosettes* are conspicuous. In these formations, the blood vessel is the central focus of an eosinophilic halo formed by the radiating, tapering processes of the neoplastic cells with the nucleus of the cell and its perikaryon remote from the blood vessel. The arrangement is, therefore, similar to that seen in astroblastomas, but the neoplastic ependymomal cells have no footplates on the vessel walls; the perikaryon does not extend

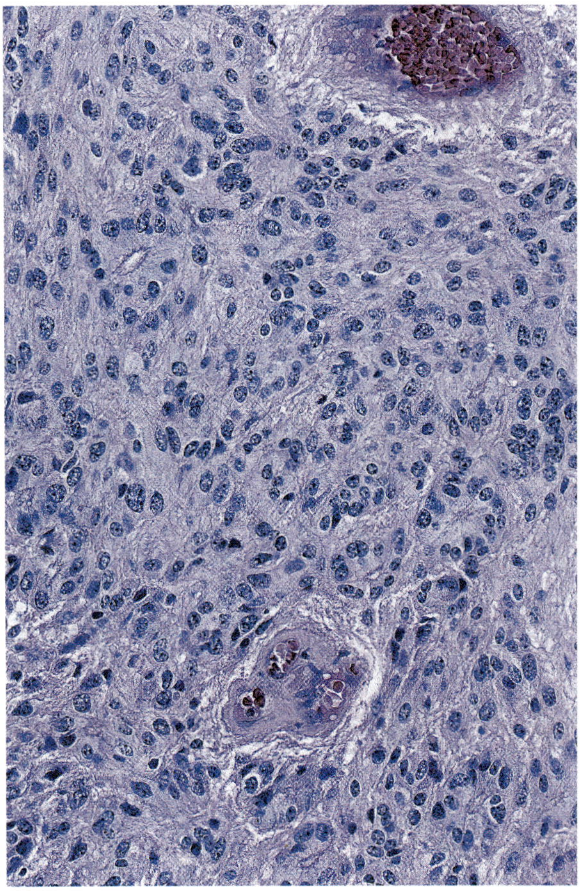

Fig. 9.131 Same case as Fig. 9.130. Typical fibrillar appearance of a cellular ependymoma interrupted by occasional rosettes. H&E, × 200

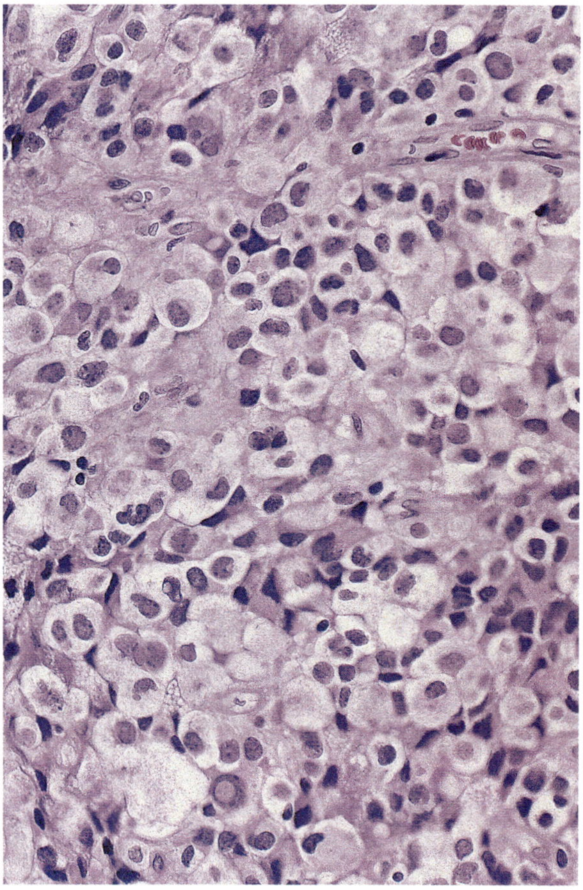

Fig. 9.133 Ependymoma with clear cells. These cells may compose the entire neoplasm. H&E, × 200

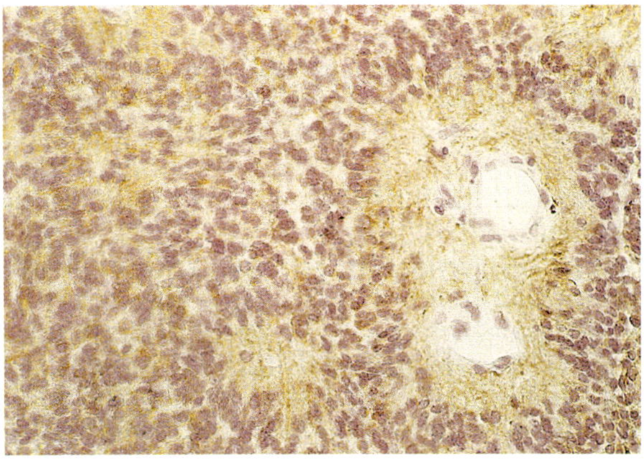

Fig. 9.132 Perivascular pseudorosettes in an ependymoma. GFAP, × 400

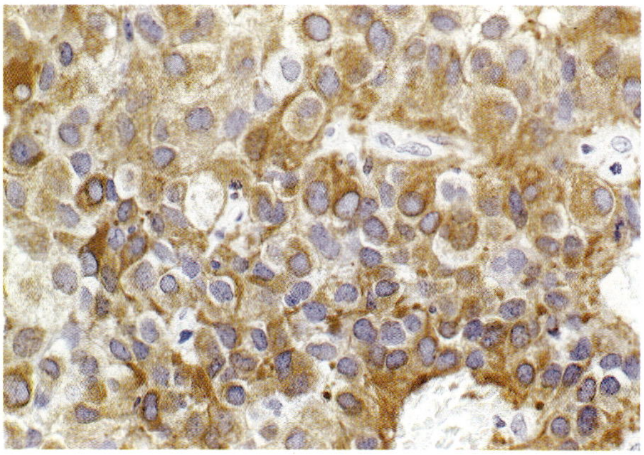

Fig. 9.134 Ependymoma: the glial nature of these clear cells is identified by the strong cytoplasmic expression of GFAP. GFAP immunostaining, × 200

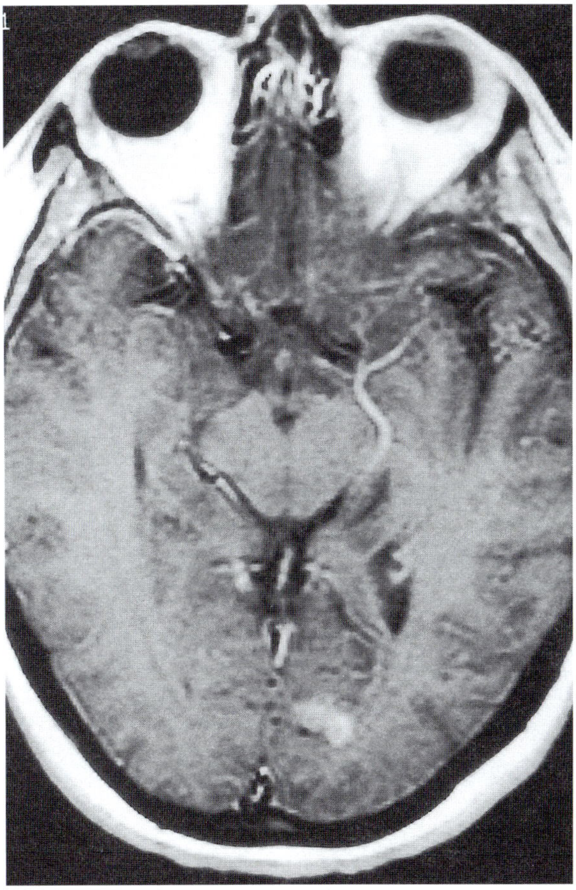

Fig. 9.135 An MRI of a clear-cell ependymoma.

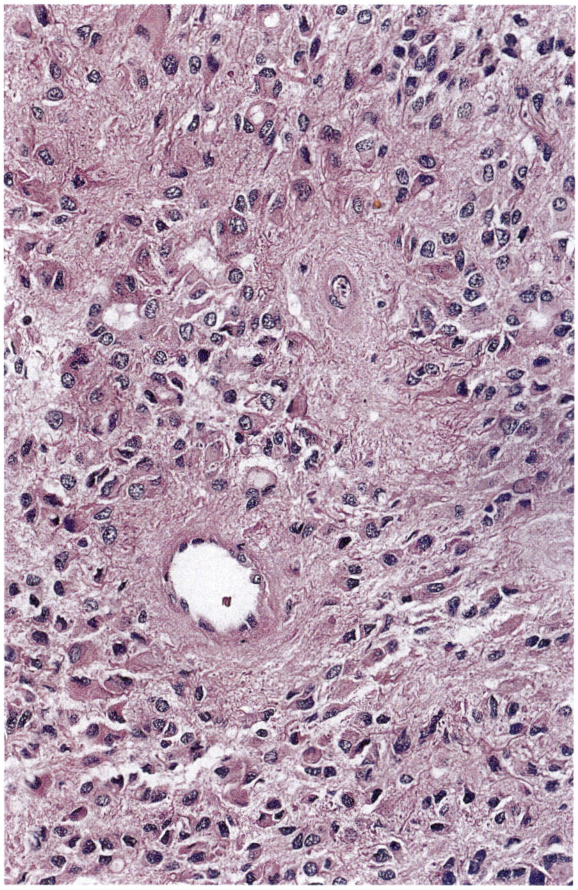

Fig. 9.136 Pseudogemistocytic-type cells found in a posterior fossa ependymoma. H&E, × 200

as a cytoplasmic process to become attached to the blood vessel; and the cellular intervascular architecture of the tumor is usually compact. The tapering perivascular end of the ependymoma tumor cell is strongly fibrillated, as can readily be confirmed with immunohistochemical stains for GFAP (Fig. 9.132).

Clear cells may be found in ependymomas and were identified by Kernohan and Fletcher-Kernohan (1937) as oligodendroglial by silver impregnation in two specimens. Disagreement exists on their interpretation: recent examples have been reported to display the fine structural features of neoplastic ependymal cells (Kawano *et al.*, 1983; Kawano, Yada and Yagishita, 1989). Occasionally, an entire neoplasm may be composed of large clear cells, whereby the diagnosis requires the ultrastructural recognition of cilia and the immunohistochemical determination of GFAP immunoreactivity. We have had the opportunity to examine such a so-called 'clear-cell' variant of ependymoma, which had strenuous mitotic activity and bizarre mitotic figures that arose in the occipital lobe of a 30-year-old female (Figs 9.133–9.135). Ultrastructural examination not only confirmed the presence of cilia but also demonstrated an abundance of cytoplasmic projections.

Pseudogemistocytic cells with eccentric globular GFAP-positive eosinophilic inclusions in the cytoplasm have also been reported in ependymomas (Figs 9.136–9.138) (Twiss, Anderson and Horoupian, 1993). A so-called 'anemone' variant of ependymomal cell was described by Deck, Ramjohn and Dardick (1990) and represents a cell exhibiting extensive membranous projections and resembling an ultrastructural cell type previously also described in lymphomas and carcinomas.

A relatively rare variant, the papillary ependymoma (Fig. 9.139), may be confused with a choroid plexus papilloma. The papillary ependymoma is more characteristic of the forms originating in the region of the cauda equina, but it may also be found in other locations. This variant is distinguished from

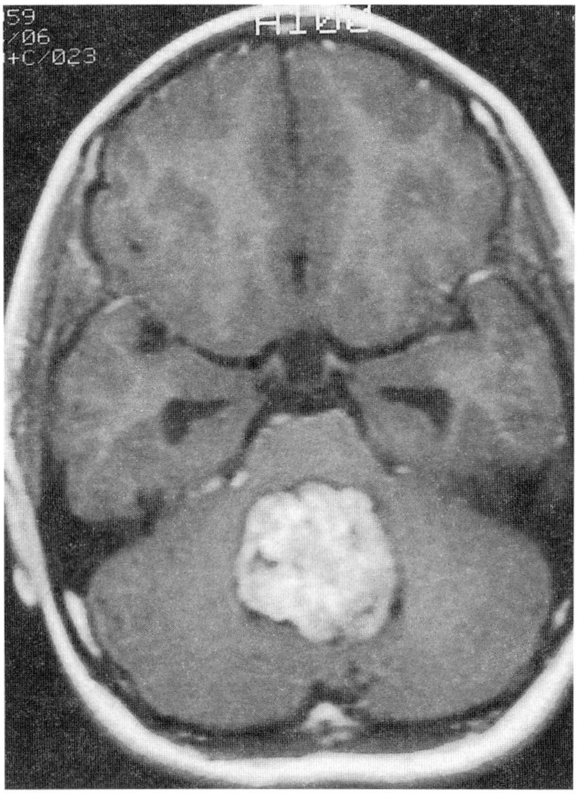

Fig. 9.137 Same case as Fig. 9.136. An MRI of the posterior fossa ependymoma.

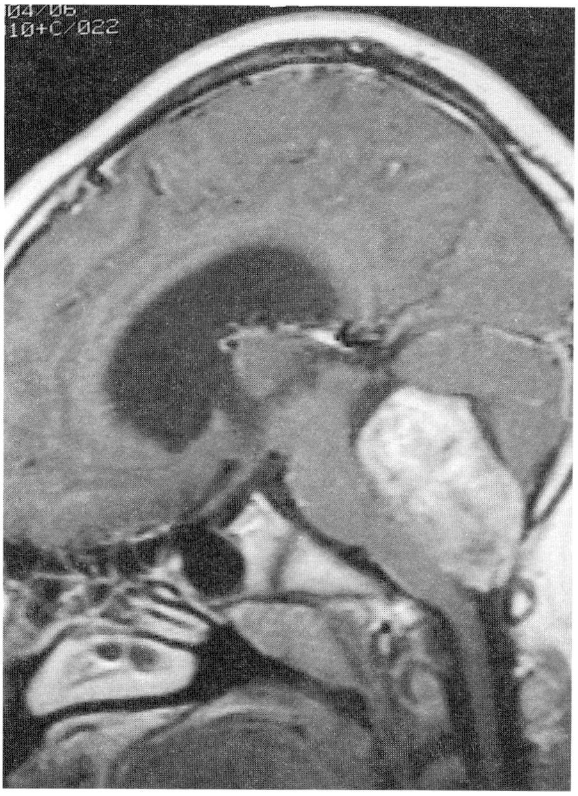

Fig. 9.138 Same case as Fig. 9.136. An MRI of the posterior fossa ependymoma.

the choroid plexus papilloma by the frequent arrangement of cells in multiple layers, the formation of epithelial-like surfaces, occasionally forming tubules, and the presence of a neuroglial stroma. These features contrast with the delicate vascular stroma and 'hobnail' surface characteristic of the choroid plexus tumors. However, as noted in Volume 2, p. 43, focal ependymal features, with the development of elongated fibrillated cells showing positivity for GFAP, may also be occasionally expressed in choroid plexus papillomas.

Cartilage and other mesenchymal cell products in ependymomas

The intriguing inclusion of nodules of cartilage in fourth-ventricle ependymomas, described by several observers (Mackay, 1935; Willis, 1962a: two cases; Siqueira and Bucy, 1966; Mathews and Moossy, 1974, cases 1 and 2), merits discussion. Rubinstein (Russell and Rubinstein, 1989) personally reviewed four such cases, all of which were well differentiated, including two recurrent examples in children. The first arose in a 5-year-old boy, in whom the recurrent tumor at autopsy contained large foci of cartilage, although the growth resected 3 years earlier at the same site showed no hint of this feature (courtesy of Dr Ricardo Ceballos). The second was in a 19-month-old boy from whom a fourth-ventricle tumor had been incompletely resected at the age of 7 months and in whom the recurrence at necropsy included small nodules of cartilage and bone. In this tumor, the chondrocytes were arranged in an orderly pattern that recalled the progressive calcification of cartilage in the mature epiphysis (courtesy of Dr E.L. Shiau). Rubinstein also reviewed an example of chondroid metaplasia in a well-differentiated ependymoma that arose in the cerebellopontine angle of a 54-year-old woman, which case was illustrated in Kepes, Rubinstein and Chiang (1984, Figs 12 and 13). In these cases, as in most of those reported by others, the cartilage and bony nodules were surrounded by a variable layer of mesenchymal connective tissue stroma of nonuniform cellular density. No other tissue elements were present to suggest atypical teratoma.

When these various cases are confronted, an association of this phenomenon with midline posterior-fossa ependymomatous tumors emerges, most often affecting male children in the first

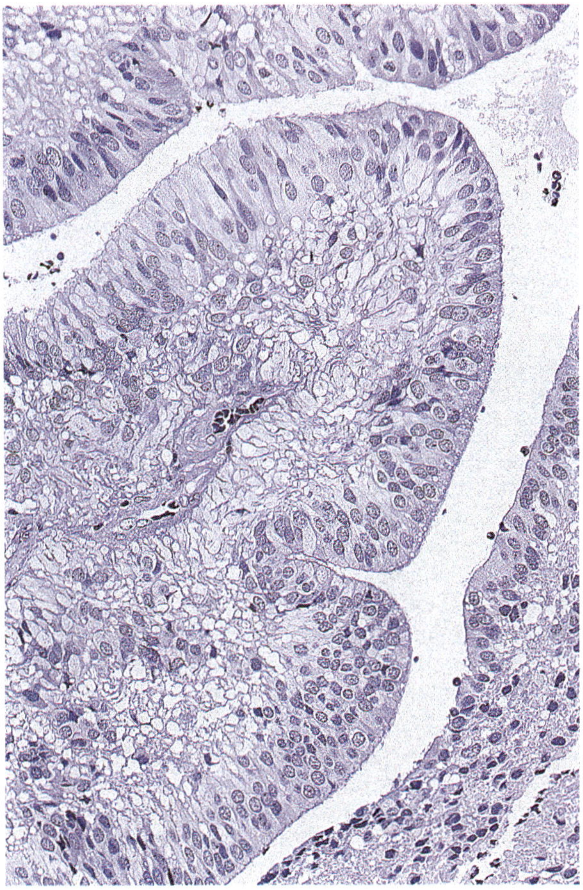

Fig. 9.139 Papillary ependymoma. These tumors may be recognized by the formation of uniform epithelial surfaces. H&E, × 300. (Courtesy of Dr Ashraf Ali, Riyadh, Saudi Arabia)

decade, and with a tendency, on the part of the cartilage and bone, to occur most frequently in the recurrent growths. A tempting explanation of this development could be a deviant inductive interaction between neoplastic neuroepithelial cells and included mesenchymal tissue elements, by analogy with the induction of cartilage in specific somites by the adjacent primitive neuroepithelium of the spinal cord, a known stage of normal development in the chick embryo (Willis, 1962b, p. 12; Lash, 1968, references). In a neoplastic context, it might be recalled that Reese (1956) emphasized the occurrence of cartilage in medulloepitheliomas of the ciliary epithelium, an embryonal type of growth observed usually in children and young subjects, and in which, as mentioned in Volume 2, p. 17, other teratoid features may also be present.

Observations suggest that neoplastic ependymal cells, like astrocytes, are capable, in certain circumstances, of manufacturing collagen precursor products. An example illustrating this potential is the myxopapillary ependymoma. Basement membrane material has likewise been identified in a fourth-ventricle subependymoma in tissue culture (Fu *et al.*, 1974), and its conspicuous increase has been noted when a fourth-ventricle ependymoma and a myxopapillary ependymoma of the cauda equina were separately maintained in an organ culture system (Rawlinson, Rubinstein and Herman, 1974; Vraa-Jensen *et al.*, 1976). The massive production of thick collagen fibers in a well-differentiated intramedullary ependymoma has been documented in one case (Soeur *et al.*, 1979).

Melanin pigment in ependymomas

The occurrence of melanin pigment in an otherwise typical cystic temporal lobe ependymoma in a 30-year-old woman, clinically suspected to harbor a brain tumor over the preceding 8 years, has been reported by McCloskey *et al.* (1976). The presence of melanosomes was confirmed by electron microscopy. Rubinstein examined this tumor, as well as another example arising in the fourth ventricle of a 36-year-old male (Russell and Rubinstein, 1989). Two additional cases examined by light and electron microscopy have recently been reported (Rosenblum, *et al.*, 1990). These exceptional cases raise the problem of melanin production in neuroepithelial tumors, a feature noted elsewhere as occurring in a variant of cerebellar medulloblastoma (see p. 470), in equally exceptional instances of malignant choroid plexus tumors (see Volume 2, p. 49) and, again exceptionally, in olfactory neuroblastoma. Also, as noted in Volume 2, p. 29, melanin, which is a transient feature in the human fetal pineal gland, may occasionally be expressed in pineoblastomas. Collectively, and recalling in this context the existence of the curious melanotic neuroectodermal tumor of infancy referred to in Volume 2, p. 349, these intriguing occurrences suggest that melanin formation may represent yet another expression of cellular differentiation in neuroectodermal neoplasms, similar to what may occasionally take place in meningiomas (Volume 2, p. 95) and in nerve sheath tumors (Volume 2, p. 174). The significance of the increasingly documented relationship between melanogenesis and neurogenic tumors needs further elucidation: the reader is referred to the paper by VandenBerg *et al.* (1981) and to the parallel biochemical and immunomorphologic findings by Erdelyi *et al.* (1981) for further discussion. What emerges at this time is that, while the structure and the chemical composition of the melanotic pigment in these tumors may be heterogeneous, there is little doubt that central neuroepithelial cells are capable of melanosomal melanin formation and that the presence of this pigment need not be attributed, as is often the case, to a neural crest derivation of the pigment-forming cells.

Immunohistochemistry

A positive reaction for GFAP is a frequent but inconstant finding in ependymomas (Vraa-Jensen *et al.*, 1976; Deck *et al.*, 1978; Duffy *et al.*, 1979; Furness, Lowe and Tarrant, 1990; Kaneko *et al.*, 1990; Figarella-Branger *et al.*, 1991). The presence of this protein, which may be expressed in the different variants of ependymoma, including the epithelial, the papillary, the myxopapillary, the clear-cell (Fig. 9.132 and Fig. 9.134) and the subependymomatous variants, is predictable and is consistent with the capability of neoplastic and other pathologically altered ependymal cells for gliofibrillogenesis.

Along with the reported finding of GFAP, other intermediate filaments have also been found in ependymomas. Although not carrying the positive diagnostic import of GFAP, vimentin, cytokeratin and nestin have all been found in ependymomas. Not unexpectedly, vimentin immunoreactivity has been reported in virtually all cases of ependymomas reported in the literature (Schiffer *et al.*, 1986; Cruz-Sanchez *et al.*, 1988b; Tohyama *et al.*, 1992). Cytokeratin expression, on the other hand, is restricted to a very few ependymomas (Mannoji and Becker, 1988; Kaneko *et al.*, 1990), generally of the papillary type (Mannoji and Becker, 1988). The class VI intermediate filament nestin has also been reported in ependymomas (Tohyama *et al.*, 1992; McLendon *et al.*, 1995b).

Immunopositivity for the S-100 protein has been reported (Tabuchi *et al.*, 1982; Nakamura, Becker and Marks, 1983; Kimura, Budka and Soler-Federsppiel, 1986; Coffin *et al.*, 1993), parallel to the expression of GFAP, and is also an inconstant finding. A reaction to the anti-Leu 7 (HNK-1) MAb has also been reported in occasional neoplasms (Perentes and Rubinstein, 1986). In the study by Kaneko *et al.* (1990), 3/13 'anaplastic' ependymomas were found to be reactive with a MAb against cytokeratin, while none of their low-grade ependymomas were immunoreactive. Using a MAb against the EMA, two studies have demonstrated occasional low-grade ependymomas and 'anaplastic' ependymomas to be immunoreactive (Kaneko *et al.*, 1990; Figarella-Branger *et al.*, 1991).

Electron microscopy

The electron microscopic features have been described by several workers (Luse, 1960; Raimondi, 1966; Goebel and Cravioto, 1972; Vraa-Jensen *et al.*, 1976; Friede and Pollak, 1978; Haustein, Cruz-Sanchez and Cervós-Navarro, 1988; Sara, Bruner and Mackay, 1994). The overall appearances of ependymomas are those of a complex mosaic of cell bodies and processes characteristically arranged in a pavement-like manner, but often exhibiting polarity, with the plasma membranes of two or more adjacent cells contributing to the development of one, and sometimes several, complex intercellular *microrosettes*. The latter display variable numbers of surface microvilli that, in extreme cases, may be enormously increased so as to fill entirely the lumen of the microrosette (Figs 9.140 and 9.141). In addition, various numbers of cilia are demonstrable within the microrosettes and in the cytoplasm of the lining cells (Fig. 9.140). The cilia may either display the normal 9 + 2 configuration of the axial filament complex or various abnormal internal configurations (Figs 9.142 and 9.143) (Sara, Bruner and Mackay, 1994). These have been extensively described, respectively, by K.L. Ho (1986) and Kubota *et al.* (1986). Another feature characteristic of microrosette formation is the presence of conspicuous *junctional complexes* (zonulae or fasciae adherentes) (Figs 9.140 and 9.141), irregularly linked by zonulae occludentes (more accurately interpreted as gap junctions) (Fig. 9.144), and connecting at their apices the plasma membranes of the cells participating in the microrosettes (Fig. 9.141). The structure of these junctions and their possible significance in terms of intercellular coupling, as well as their possible relationship to cell malignancy, have been discussed by Tani and Higashi (1972). The cell specializations typical of the normal ependymal cells lining the ventricular cavity are, therefore, not only recapitulated, but also often exaggerated in the microrosettes that constitute one of the diagnostic electron microscopic features of the ependymoma (Guccion and Saini, 1991). These ultrastructural features, in unusual variants such as clear-cell ependymoma or signet-ring-cell ependymomas, are often the first clue that a tumor is ependymal (Zuppan, Mierau and Weeks, 1994). K.L. Ho suggests that microtubular aggregates (1990a) and intercellular septate-like junctions (1990b) may characterize the myxopapillary ependymoma of the tumors located in the region of the filum terminale.

As described in Volume 2, p. 43, electron microscopic studies on choroid plexus papillomas have shown significant fine structural differences between these tumors and ependymomas; these differences essentially confirm the distinction already evident by light microscopy.

Intermediate filaments have been repeatedly demonstrated in neoplastic ependymal cells in the electron microscopic studies mentioned above, as might have been expected from their presence, usually much less conspicuous, in normal ependymal cells (Brightman and Palay, 1963). Their

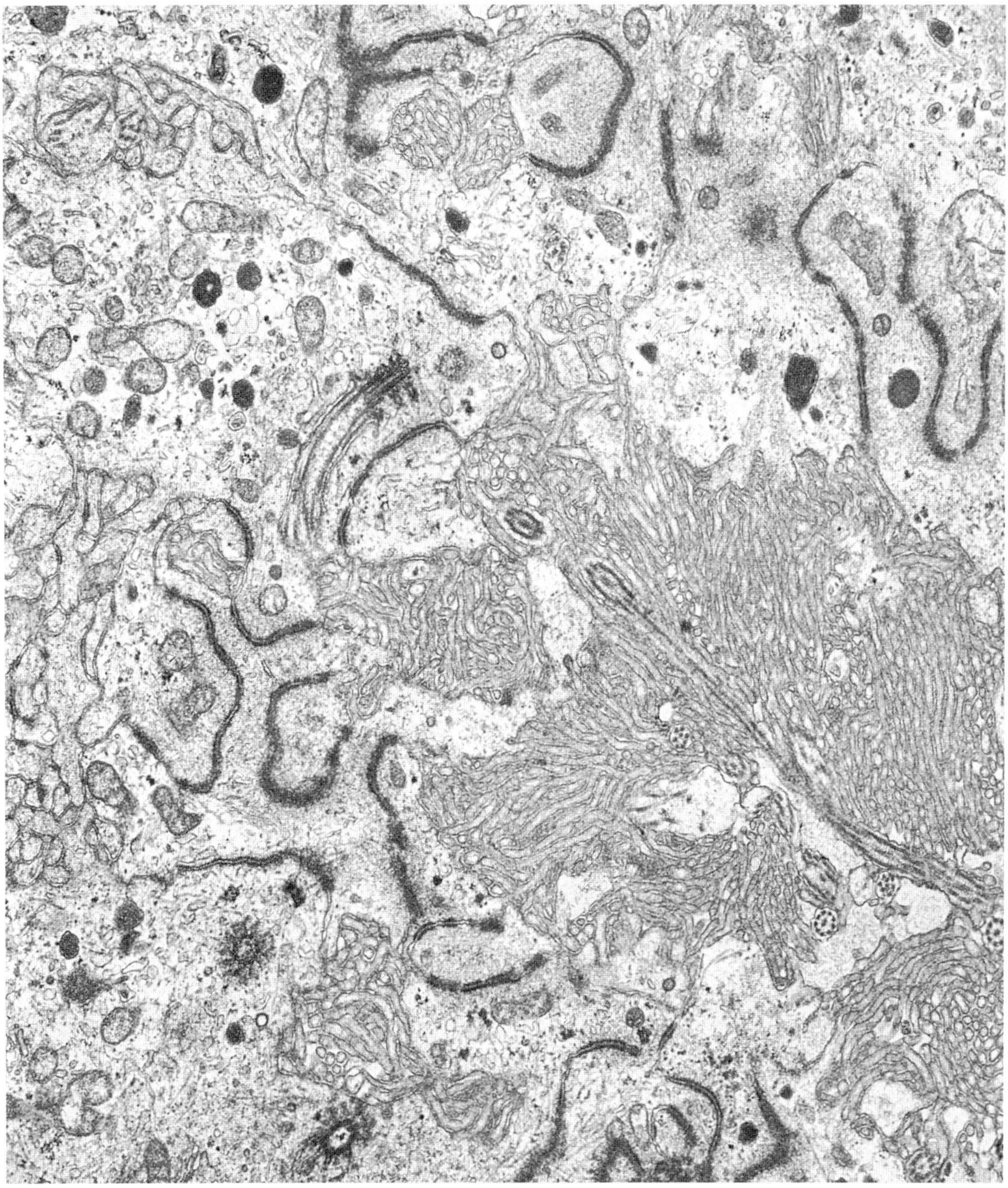

Fig. 9.140 Electron micrograph (montage) of a complex microrosette in a fourth-ventricle ependymoma maintained in organ culture for 30 days. The microrosette is packed with large numbers of surface microvilli. Several profiles of cilia are seen both within the microrosette and, occasionally, in the cytoplasm (left upper middle) of the lining cells. Numerous interrupted zonulae adherentes in series link the apices of the cells contributing to the microrosette. × 9000 (Courtesy of Dr Mary M. Herman and Dr J. Vraa-Jensen)

biochemical identity with either vimentin or GFAP may be inferred from the immunomorphologic demonstration of these proteins in these tumors. Their development in a fourth-ventricle ependymoma is demonstrated in Figs 9.145 and 9.146 and has also been seen in a myxopapillary ependymoma of the filum terminale (see Fig. 9.159). Twiss, Anderson and Horoupian (1993) have demonstrated GFAP immunoreactivity in an unusual globular inclusion by ultrastructural immunohistochemistry of an otherwise typical ependymoma, but, to date, we are not aware of any other ultrastructural immunohistochemical studies on the intermediate filaments of ependymomas.

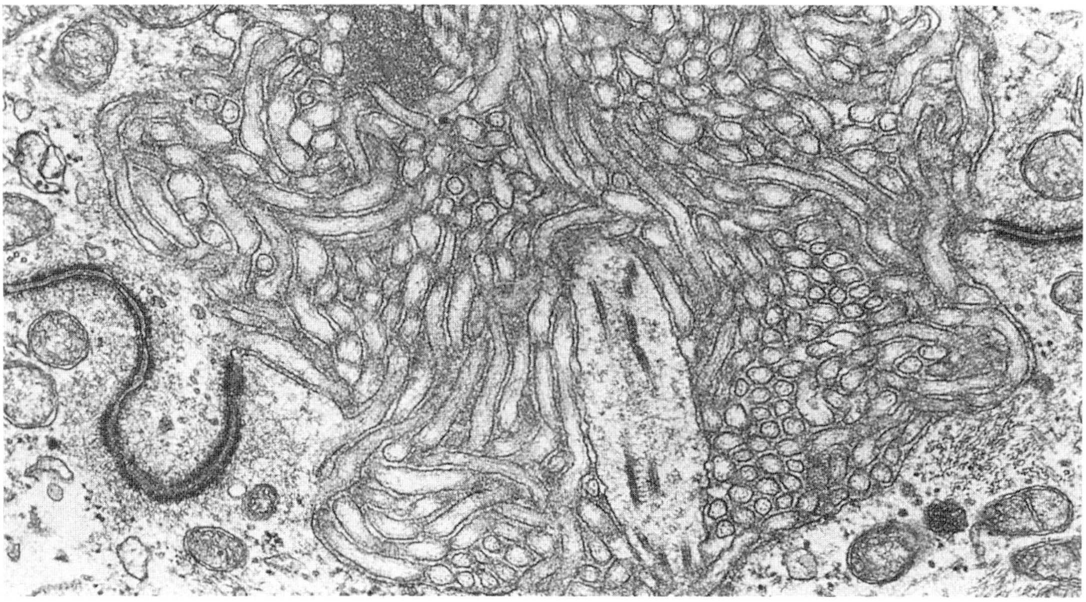

Fig. 9.141 Same case as Fig. 9.140. Original tumor from the fourth ventricle. Part of a microrosette is filled by numerous interdigitating surface microvilli at the apical ends of two cells linked by convoluted zonulae adherentes. × 28 000 (Courtesy of Dr Mary M. Herman and Dr J. Vraa-Jensen and reprinted from *Neuropathology and Applied Neurobiology*, 1976, pp. 349–364, figure 6, with kind permission of Blackwell Science Ltd.)

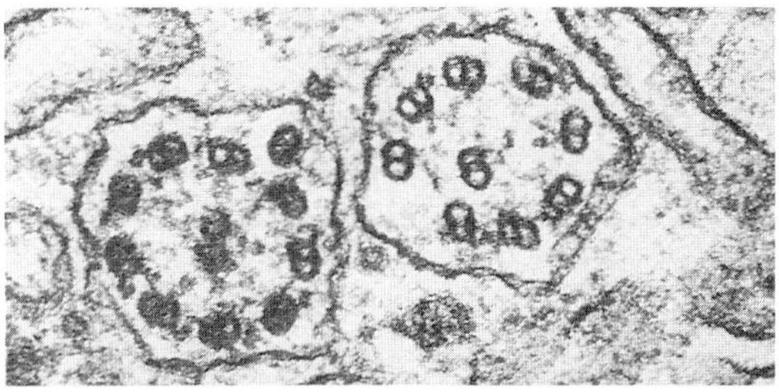

Fig. 9.142 Profile of abnormal cilia showing atypical axial filament complexes of 10 + 2 and 8 + 1 configurations. Note the eccentric outer doublets in the left cilium. × 27 500 (Courtesy of Dr Mary M. Herman and Dr J. Vraa-Jense and reprinted from *Neuropathology and Applied Neurobiology*, 1976, pp. 349–364, figure 6 inset, with kind permission of Blackwell Science Ltd.)

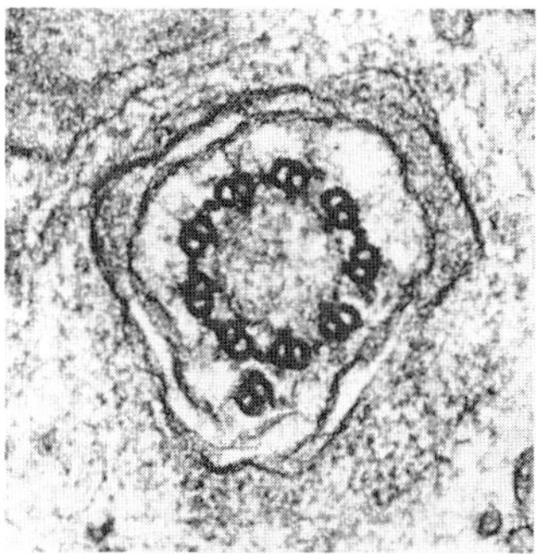

Fig. 9.143 Same case as Fig. 9.142. Profile of abnormal cilia showing atypical axial filament complex of 10 + 0 configuration. Note the eccentric outer doublets in the cilium. × 72 500 (Courtesy of Dr Mary M. Herman and Dr J. Vraa-Jense and reprinted from *Neuropathology and Applied Neurobiology*, 1976, pp. 349–364, figure 7 upper inset, with kind permission of Blackwell Science Ltd.)

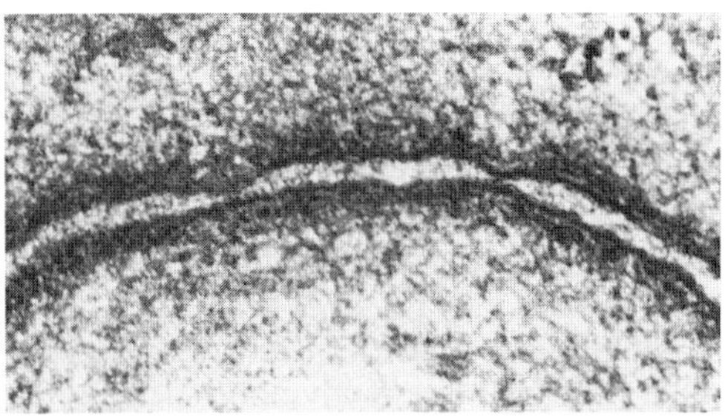

Fig. 9.144 Higher magnification of a zonula adhererens, showing two focal constrictions of the intercellular space. This explant of the same tumor shown in Fig. 9.140 had been maintained in organ culture for 44 days. × 96 000 (Courtesy of Dr Mary M. Herman and Dr J. Vraa-Jensen and reprinted from *Neuropathology and Applied Neurobiology*, 1976, pp. 349–364, figure 7 lower inset, with kind permission of Blackwell Science Ltd.)

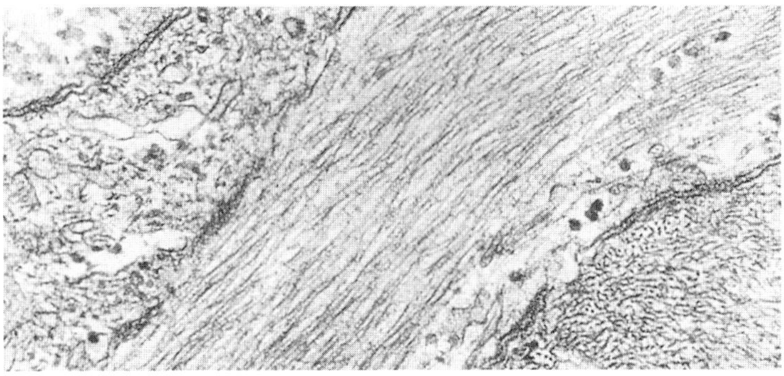

Fig. 9.145 Same tumor as Figs. 9.142 and 9.143, after 36 days in culture, showing arrays of cytoplasmic filaments almost completely filling the cell processes. × 36 500 (Courtesy of Dr Mary M. Herman and Dr J. Vraa-Jensen and reprinted from *Neuropathology and Applied Neurobiology*, 1976, pp. 349–364, figure 9, with kind permission of Blackwell Science Ltd.)

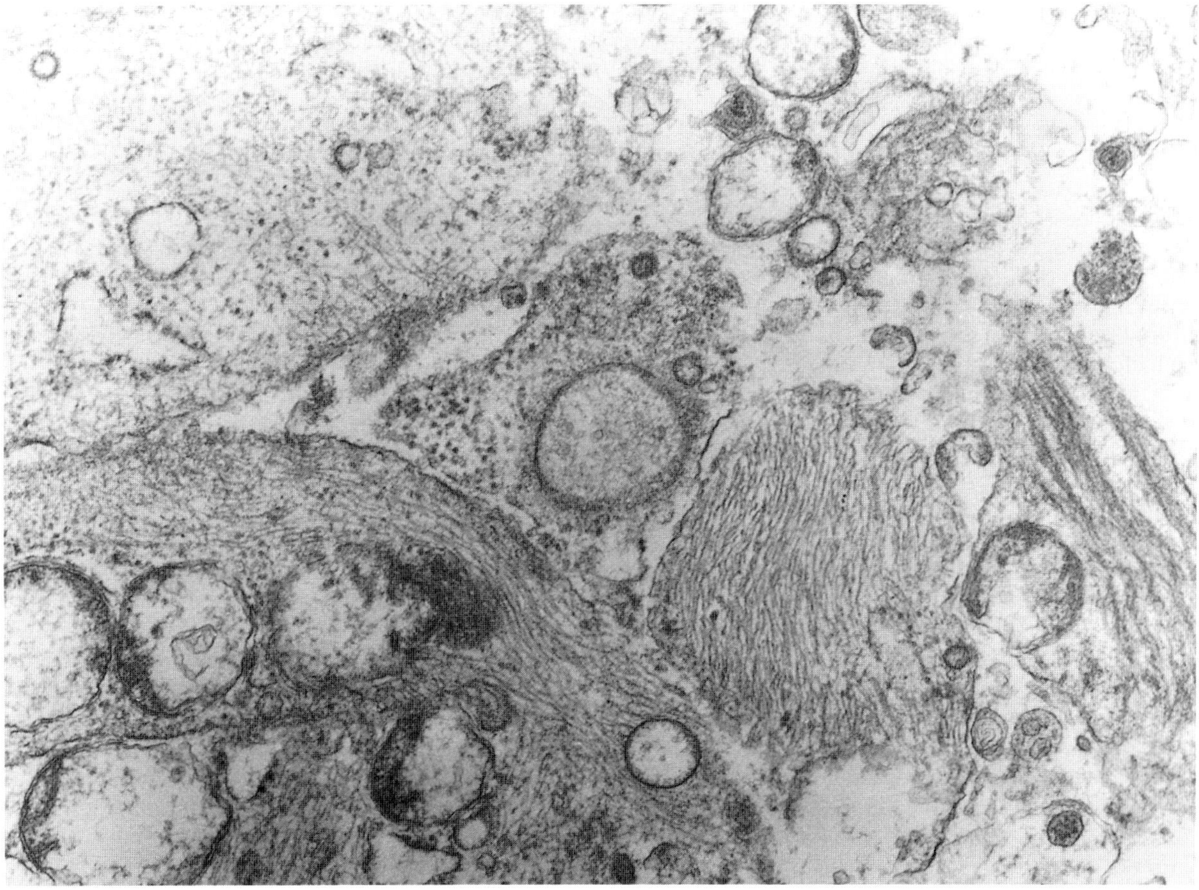

Fig. 9.146 Intermediate filament production. Ultrastructurally, abundant skeins of intermediate filaments are demonstrable, correlating with the immunohistochemical demonstration of both GFAP and vimentin. (Courtesy of Dr Rex Bentley, Durham, NC)

Kinetics

Proliferation-related studies have grown in number in the past several years; however, inroads into the kinetics of ependymomas are only beginning. A study by Spaar, Blech and Ahyai (1986) on the flow cytometry of 10 surgically removed ependymomas from various sites in the neuraxis showed usually diploid histograms, with four of the tumors showing an aneuploid or polyploid pattern. The percentage of cells in the S phase varied greatly, from about 3% up to 27%, whereas subsequent tissue culture of three of the surgical specimens yielded ratios of cells in the S phase ranging from 15% to 25%.

Preliminary data on proliferation indices obtained by immunohistochemical means have been reported. These studies predominately focus on assessing the prognostic utility of these methods in determining recurrence, and they do not focus on cell cycle times. Techniques that use BrdU incorporation and its immunohistochemical identification suggest that tumors with 1% of the cells labeled have a stronger tendency to recur than those with less than 1% labeled (Asai *et al.*, 1992). Using the Ki-67 MAb, Schröder, Ploner and Ernestus (1993) suggest that LI correlates well with mitotic counts. They further suggest that an increased LI may correlate with an increased tendency of a tumor to recur; however, their material was limited with respect to long-term follow-up. The study of Reyes-Mugica, Chou and Myint (1994) fails to show any correlation among DNA ploidy, histologic variables and patient survival.

These data, however, do indicate considerable heterogeneity within the tumors, and the clinicopathologic correlations to be derived are limited, with the obvious generalization that ependymomas of low malignancy show a low LI with either flow or histologic assessment methods.

A recent report on the identification of the polyomavirus SV40 large-T-antigen gene in both choroid plexus papillomas and ependymomas, by polymerase chain reaction (PCR) amplification, appears to have significance in relation to the oncogenesis of at least a certain proportion of these neoplasms (Bergsagel *et al.*, 1992). These factors and others are discussed in Chapters 2, 3 and 6.

Cytogenetics and molecular genetics

Cytogenetic studies of ependymomas, which are also reviewed in Chapter 2, have indicated that these tumors may show considerable variation among patients, variations that do not necessarily correlate with histologic grade (Stratton *et al.*, 1989; Thiel *et al.*, 1992). Although consistent rearrangements and breakpoints have not been identified within ependymomas by using these methods, abnormalities affecting chromosomes 2, 4, 9, 10, 11, 13, 16, 17 and 22 have been identified more commonly than is suggested by random occurrence (Savard and Gilchrist, 1989; Metzger *et al.*, 1991; Griffin *et al.*, 1992; Ransom *et al.*, 1992; Sainati *et al.*, 1992; Weremowicz *et al.*, 1992; Neumann *et al.*, 1993; Rogatto *et al.*, 1993; Sawyer *et al.*, 1994; Wernicke *et al.*, 1995). Among these changes, losses of chromosome 22 have been most prevalent in these various series. A high incidence of loss of chromosome 22 was confirmed by molecular studies in a restriction fragment length polymorphism (RFLP) analysis reported by James *et al.* (1990). A mutation of the *NF2* gene, which is located on chromosomal arm 22q, was demonstrated in 1/8 ependymomas by Rubio *et al.* (1994). These findings suggest that the *NF2* gene may be the target of chromosome 22 loss in a subset of ependymomas.

Xenogeneic transplantation

A well-differentiated fourth-ventricle ependymoma from an 11-year-old girl was successfully passaged in immunologically conditioned mice (Horowitz *et al.*, 1987). The transplants were karyotypically characterized, and the kinetics parameters were estimated *in vivo* using the fraction of labeled mitoses after a single pulse of ^{3}H-thymidine. The considerable dampening of the second peak was presumably due to the kinetic heterogeneity of the tumor cell population: the total cell cycle time was estimated to be about 80 hours, the S phase being approximately 12 hours and the LI being about 10%. The calculated growth fraction was in the region of 70%, with a cell loss of about 90%. The transplants showed very little necrosis, and their estimated doubling time was long (approximately 40 days), suggesting that most of the estimated cell loss may be due to a large number of cells leaving the mitotic cycle as they become well differentiated. Unfortunately, this xenograft has since died.

More recent examples of ependymoma xenografts include the D528 EP (Figs 9.147–9.150) and D612 EP derived from the Duke University material. These xenografts, which have been grown in both intracranial and subcutaneous systems, exhibit immunoreactivity for GFAP, vimentin and nestin, while D612 EP is also immunoreactive for neural cell adhesion molecule (NCAM). There was no immunoreactivity with any of the neurofilament subunit antibodies or against synaptophysin. The D528 EP xenograft grows intracranially with a median postimplantation survival of 85 days; D612 EP produces a median postimplantation survival of 72.5 days (n = 10). Both xenografts grow as well-formed masses with no evidence of infiltration into either brain or subcutaneous tissues. Histologically, perivascular pseudopalisading is found in both xenografts, although true rosette formation is not found. Ultrastructurally, neither xenograft exhibits cilia, but both exhibit abundant intermediate filaments that are immunoreactive for GFAP. Karyotypically, D528 EP exhibits 46,XX,del(6)(q22q26), while D612 EP exhibits 50,XX,+X,t(1;8)(p11;q11), t(1;8)(p11;q11),+1,–4,der(5)t(4;5)(q12;q35),+der(5) t(4;5)(q12;q35),–6,+9,+9,–16,+i(17q),+mar.

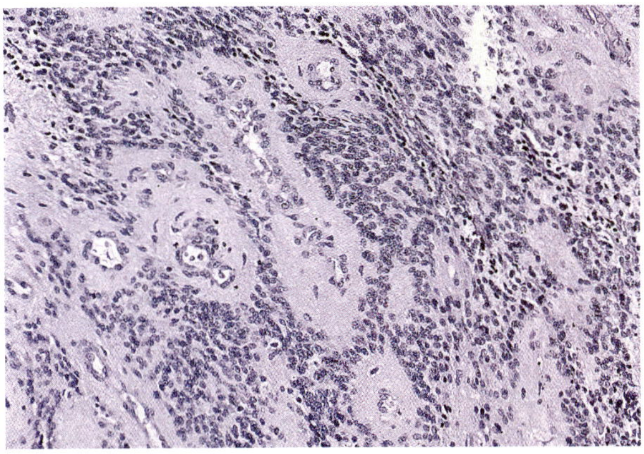

Fig. 9.147 Ependymoma arising in the posterior fossa from which the D528 EP xenograft, shown in Fig. 9.149, was derived. H&E, × 200

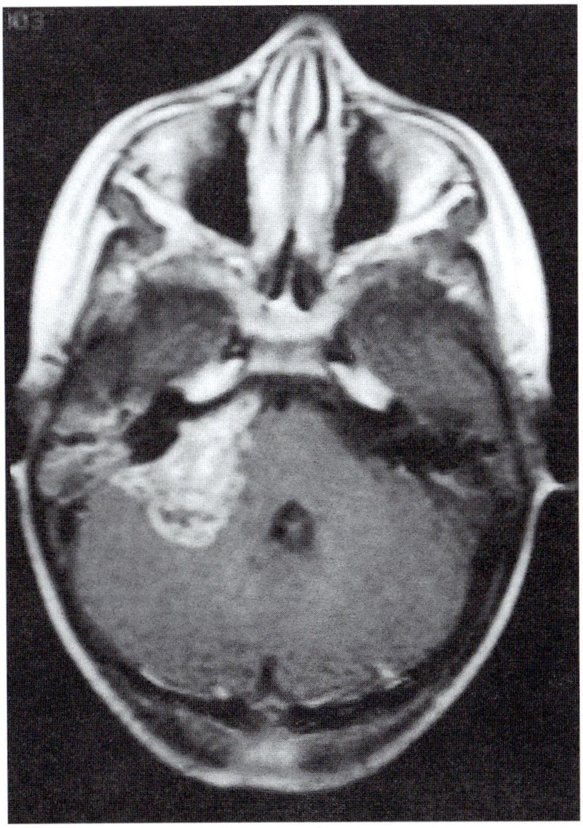

Fig. 9.148 An MRI of a posterior fossa ependymoma from which the xenograft D528 EP, shown in Fig. 9.149, was derived. H&E, × 200

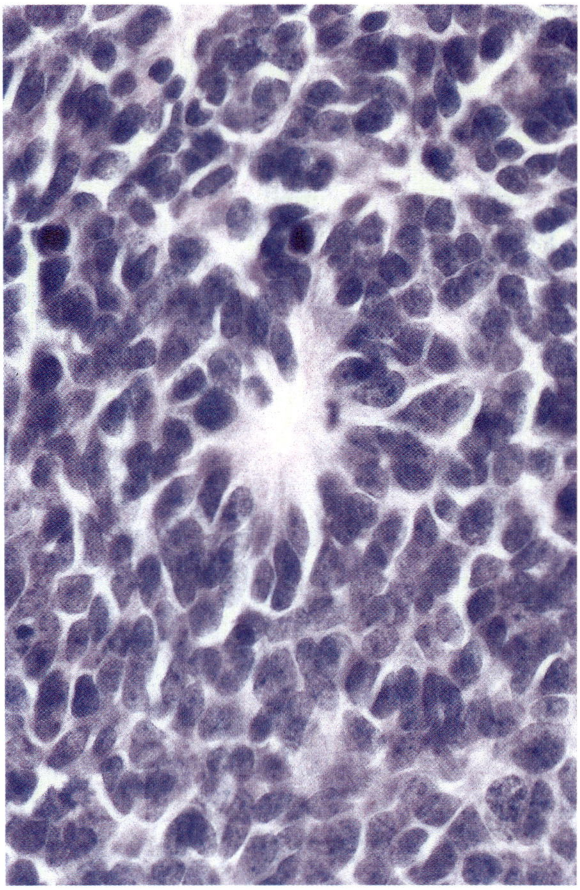

Fig. 9.149 The D528 EP xenograft showing a high nuclear-to-cytoplasmic ratio and small tubular spaces formed by the ependymal cells. No cilia are identifiable by light or electron microscopy. H&E, × 400

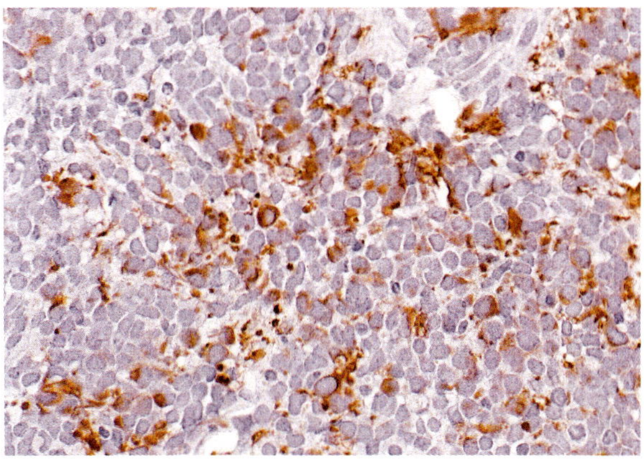

Fig. 9.150 Immunohistochemical demonstration of GFAP intracytoplasmically in the cells of D528 EP. GFAP, × 400

The RFLP studies comparing the primary brain tumor tissue from each patient against multiple passages of the resulting xenografts confirmed the origin of both xenografts (McLendon *et al.*, 1995b).

Myxopapillary ependymomas

This variant of ependymoma, originally defined by Kernohan (1932), represents a distinctive subentity of ependymoma that is virtually restricted to the region of the cauda equina and originates from the conus medullaris or the filum terminale. It must, however, be emphasized that ependymomas from all areas may also display the more classic epithelial, cellular or papillary patterns as noted by Slooff, Kernohan and MacCarty (1964) in their large series of 96 tumors in the lumbosacral region. Moreover, although the distinctive histologic features of the myxopapillary form may be attributable to the mucinous change undergone by the collagenous stroma of the papillary formations and by the development of mucin secretion by the tumor cells themselves, it should be recognized that mucinous change is not universally found in the papillary tumors of the cauda equina. Indeed, a not uncommon histologic presentation is that of densely hyalinized cords of connective tissue, only occasionally lined by epithelial-type ependymal cells.

The unusual character of the supporting stroma of myxopapillary ependymomas is evidently determined by the special features of the filum terminale. The latter is a unique structure composed of connective tissue derived from the pia mater, nerve fibers, neurons and various neuroglial elements, amongst which ependymal cells are conspicuous (Tarlov, 1938; Miller, 1968). The ubiquity of the fibrous tissue may account for the fact that the tumors arising from the filum are often characterized by the presence of an abundant supportive connective tissue stroma that is absent from other histologic types of ependymoma, as well as from other papillary variants. However, exceptional examples originating in spinal nerve roots (Sharma, 1991; Moser *et al.*, 1992), as well as supratentorially, both in the lateral ventricles and intraparenchymally, have been recorded (Sato *et al.*, 1983; Maruyama *et al.*, 1992; Warnick *et al*, 1993).

Myxopapillary tumors of the sacral cord are most frequently harbored by patients in the third or fourth decade of life, although they may also present in childhood (Chan *et al.*, 1984; Ross *et al.*, 1993). They vary in size, but symptomatic patients usually have tumors that are massive, well-defined, sausage-shaped growths with smooth or irregularly nodular surfaces that may be multifocal. They compress, or may even envelop, the roots of the cauda equina, and a determination of their origin from the filum terminale or the conus medullaris may not always be evident at surgery. Occasionally, the tumor may infiltrate the roots of the cauda equina so diffusely that complete surgical removal is impossible, an event that is, fortunately, exceptional. With the more massive growths, especially on recurrence, the adjacent bone may be deformed and even eroded. As discussed below (p. 416), several examples have been reported in which the protracted clinical history over a period of many years ultimately led to the development of remote metastases (Fig. 9.151). Further clinicopathologic correlations have been presented by Sonneland, Scheithauer and Onofrio (1985) in their review of 77 such tumors from the Mayo Clinic, by Celli, Cervoni and Cantore (1993) and by Ross *et al.* (1993).

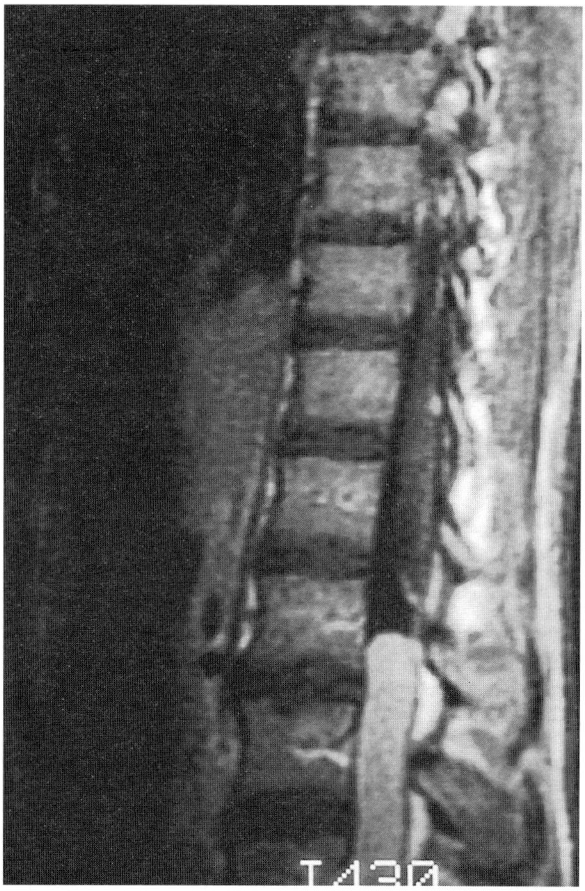

Fig. 9.151 An MRI demonstrating extensive leptomeningeal spreading of a myxopapillary ependymoma.

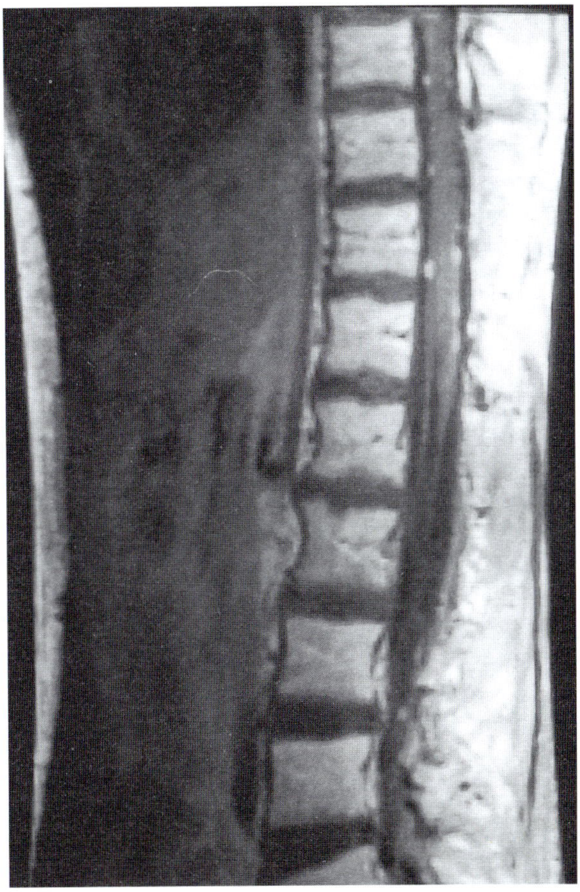

Fig. 9.152 An MRI of a myxopapillary ependymoma.

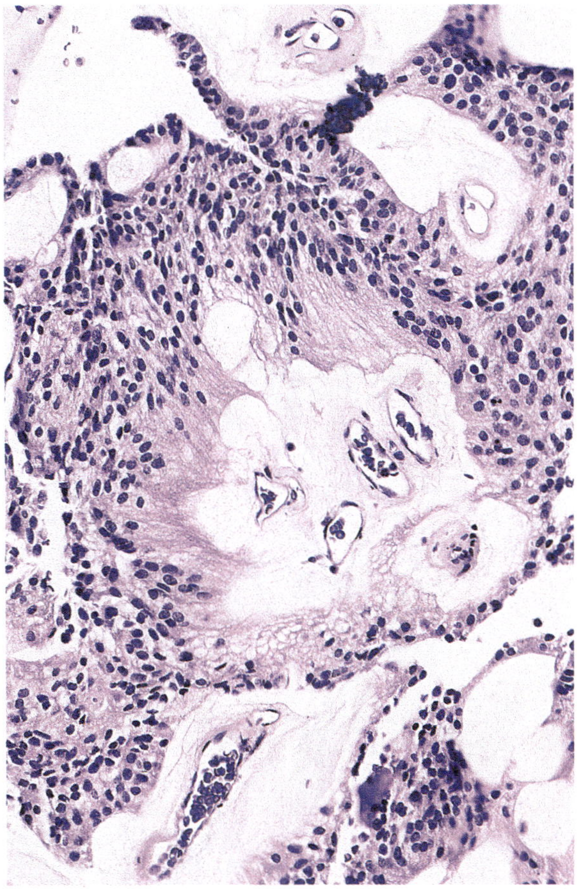

Fig. 9.153 Same tumor as Fig. 9.152. Origin is in the filum terminale. H&E, × 100

Radiographic appearance

Small conus medullaris and filum terminale ependymomas are seen as well-delineated intradural masses with a contracted 'meniscus' around the tumor (Fig. 9.152). Large myxopapillary ependymomas can fill the entire canal. Examination by MRI shows a widened cord or filum terminale mass. Most ependymomas are isointense as compared with cord on T1-weighted images. Mixed signal lesions are seen if cyst formation, tumor necrosis or hemorrhage has occurred. Ependymomas typically become hyperintense on T2-weighted sequences. Virtually all ependymomas enhance strongly following contrast administration. Contrast-enhanced scans clearly delineate tumor extent and are helpful in distinguishing neoplastic cyst from benign syrinx. The major differential diagnosis for intramedullary ependymoma is cord astrocytoma. Ependymomas often hemorrhage and are typically more sharply delineated than astrocytomas, but there is no specific pattern that permits reliable differentiation between these two common intramedullary tumors. The differential diagnosis of small conus and filum ependymomas is schwannoma. Imaging findings of these two entities are often indistinguishable. Other tumors, such as ganglioglioma and paraganglioma, occur in the filum terminale but are rare. Large myxopapillary ependymomas that cause sacral destruction can be confused with aneurysmal bone cyst, chordoma, and giant-cell tumor.

Microscopic appearance

The myxopapillary ependymoma is made up of well-defined cuboidal to low columnar cells surrounding central vascular cores containing abundant hyaline acellular connective tissue (Fig. 9.153). A positive reaction for mucin is usually obtainable in these clear areas (Fig. 9.154). In other areas, the central cores surrounded by the ependymal cells appear empty. Solid sheets of compact, polygonal

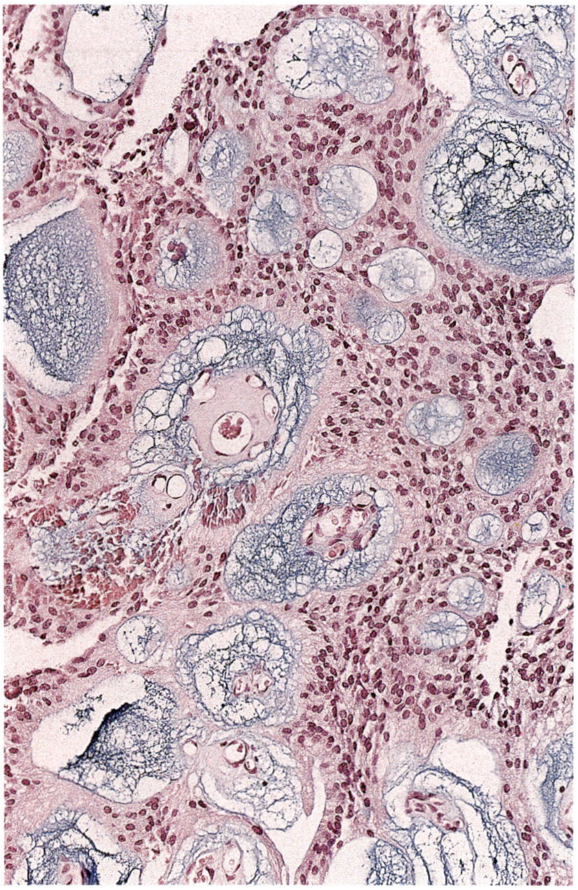

Fig. 9.154 Mucin can be demonstrated in the myxopapillary ependymoma. Alcian blue, × 100

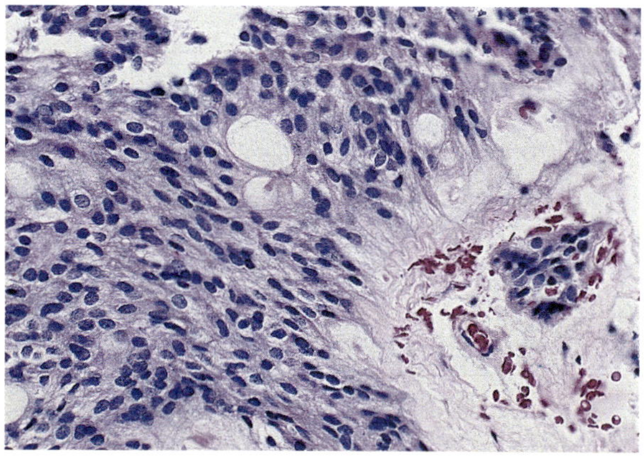

Fig. 9.155 Myxopapillary ependymoma arising in the filum terminale. H&E, × 200

cells may also be encountered apart from the papillae. More rarely, tubules or elongated channels lined with low columnar cells resting on a collagen basement membrane can be detected. Microcystic change is frequent (Fig. 9.153) and serves to highlight the strongly fibrillated, elongated cells attached by their finely pointed umbilicated processes to the supporting blood vessels (Figs 9.153, 9.155 and 9.156) or to the capsule of the tumor. The glial nature of the fibrils can be easily confirmed by the demonstration of GFAP in the cytoplasm of these cells. The demonstration of blepharoplasts is usually not possible. The tumors are often highly vascular and hemosiderin is commonly found. Although subtotal resection has been most commonly associated with recurrence, Ross *et al.* (1993) have suggested that staining for AgNOR in the nuclei may also be helpful in identifying lesions likely to recur.

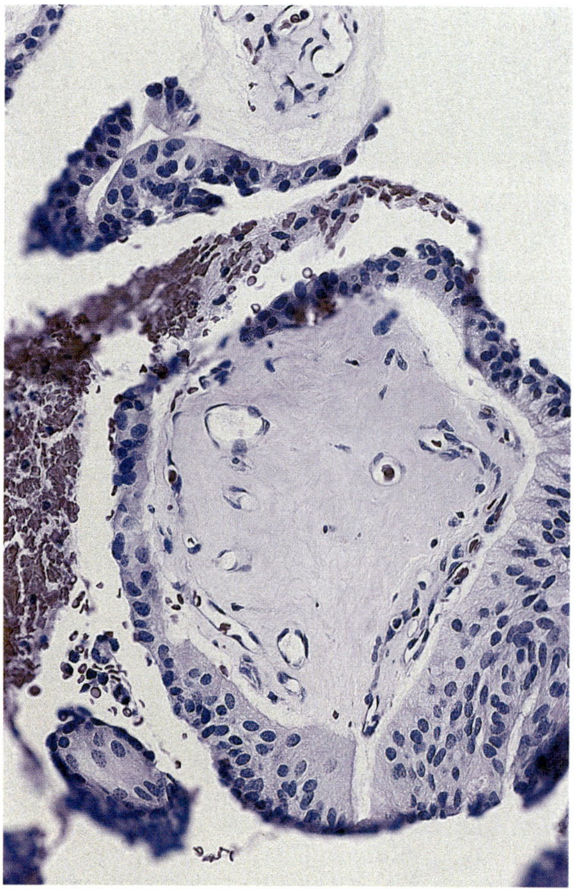

Fig. 9.156 Myxopapillary ependymoma arising in the filum terminale. H&E, × 200

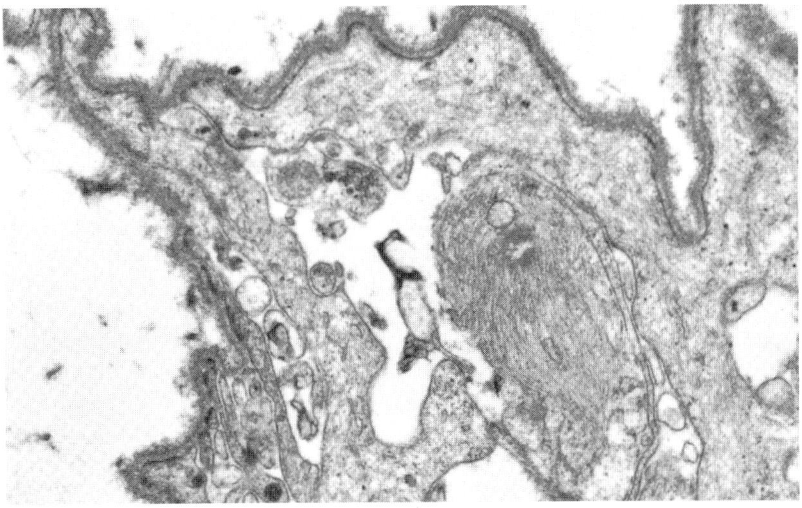

Fig. 9.157 Electron micrograph of a myxopapillary ependymoma. The free surfaces of three adjacent tumor cells are covered by a single continuous basement membrane. × 15 000 (Courtesy of Dr Mary M. Herman and Dr D.G. Rawlinson and reprinted from *Acta Neuropathologica*, 1973, pp. 1–13, figure 4b with kind permission of Springer-Verlag GmbH & Co. KG.)

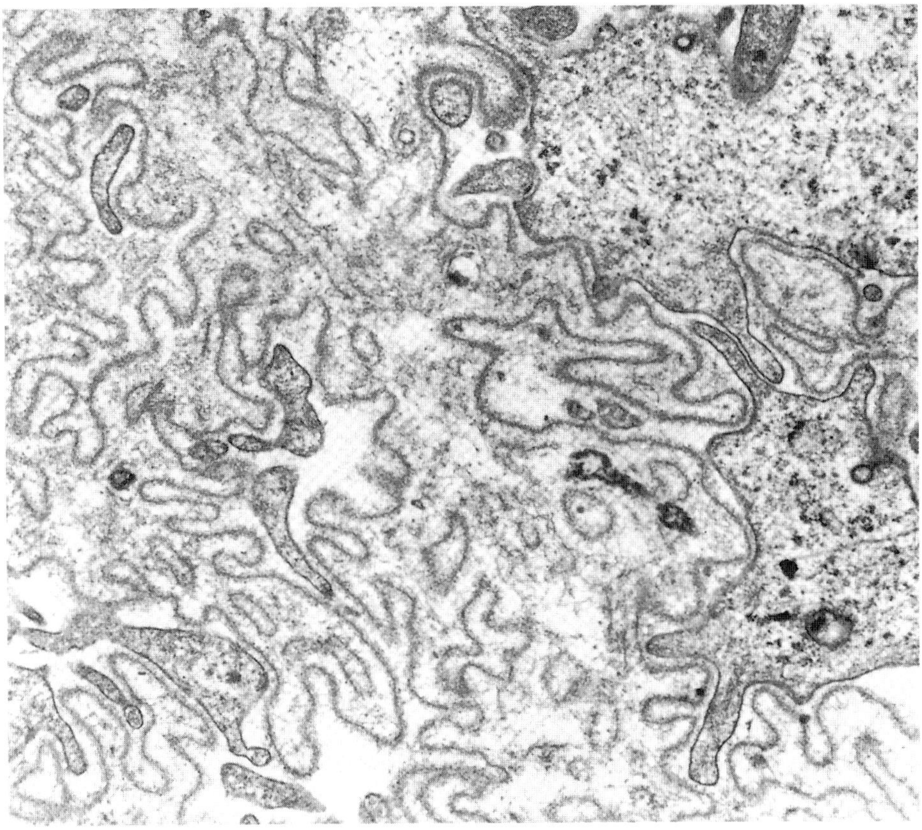

Fig. 9.158 Electron micrograph of a myxopapillary ependymoma of the filum terminale, maintained in organ culture for 20 days and showing extracellular space filled with elaborate convolutions of basement membrane material, with separation of the tumor cell processes. × 19 000 (Courtesy of Dr Mary M. Herman and Dr D.G. Rawlinson and reprinted from *Acta Neuropathologica*, 1973, pp. 1–13, figure 6 with kind permission of Springer-Verlag GmbH & Co. KG.)

Electron microscopy

The fine structural features of this tumor have been repeatedly studied by, among others, Wolff, Santiago and Duby (1972), Rubinstein (Rawlinson, Herman and Rubinstein, 1973; Rawlinson, Rubinstein and Herman, 1974), Specht *et al.* (1986) and Sara, Bruner and McKay (1994). Essentially, they have confirmed its ependymomatous nature, with, however, a number of additional features that appear restricted to the myxopapillary type, features that suggest similarities to choroid plexus epithelium rather than to ependyma. These include the presence of relatively few cilia, complex cellular interdigitations and abundant basement membrane material, often topographically related to collagen fibrils; the last feature is obviously linked to the normal structure, noted above, of the filum terminale and conus medullaris, where ependymal cells may be directly apposed to connective tissue derived from the leptomeninges instead of resting on the neuropil. As shown in Figs 9.157 and 9.158, the free surface of the tumor cells may be covered by a continuous basement membrane. In agreement with the light microscopy and immunohistochemical findings, the tumor cells may contain abundant numbers of glial filaments (Fig. 9.159). Specht *et al.* (1986) have drawn attention to the presence of large numbers of abnormal microtubular aggregates enclosed by a limiting membrane.

Subependymomas

The recognition of this variant of ependymoma as a distinct tumor entity dates back to the report by Scheinker (1945), although it had been previously observed and reported (see Chason, 1956, for review). Subsequent descriptions and designations as 'subependymal astrocytoma' (French and Bucy, 1948) and 'subependymal glomerate astrocytoma' (Boykin *et al.*, 1954) emphasized the participation of astrocytes in the tumor: indeed, a characteristic feature of this neoplasm is the extent to which the proliferation of fibrillary subependymal astrocytes dominates the histologic picture.

The tumors are distinctive: intraventricular location, frequent multiplicity, sharp demarcation with a lobulated appearance, slow growth and usually noninvasive behavior characterize this neoplasm. By far the most frequent examples arise in the cavity or lateral recesses of the *fourth ventricle* (accounting for over 70% of the cases, according to the review by Scheithauer, 1978); however, the lateral ventricles (Iqbal and Sutcliffe, 1994), the spinal cord (Matsumura, Hori and Spoerri, 1988; Guha, Resch and Tator, 1989; Pagni *et al.*, 1991;

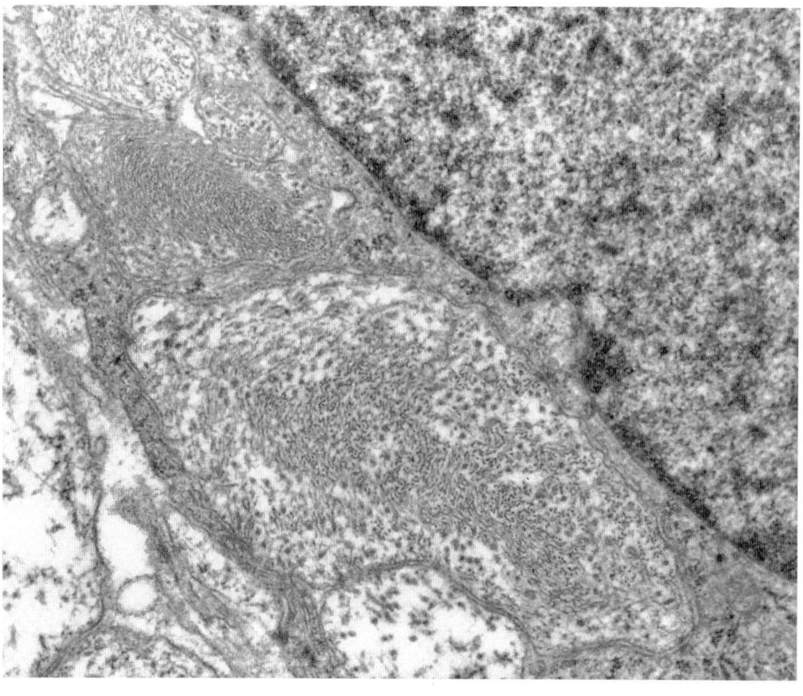

Fig. 9.159 Same case as Fig. 9.157. Tumor cell processes contain tightly packed filaments and discrete microtubules. × 21 500 (Courtesy of Dr Mary M. Herman and Dr D.G. Rawlinson)

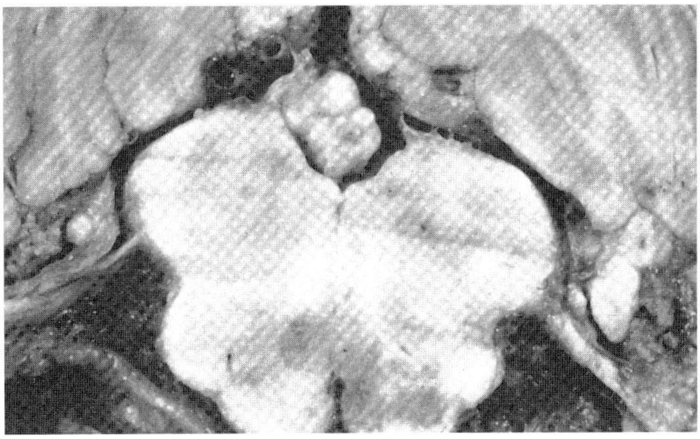

Fig. 9.160 Multiple subependymomas occupying the cavity and lateral recesses of the fourth ventricle in a patient with granular ependymitis due to chronic meningeal cryptococcosis.

Salvati *et al.*, 1992), the cerebral aqueduct (K.L. Ho, 1982), the third ventricle (K.C. Ho *et al.*, 1987) or the filum terminale (Roeder, Jinkins and Bazan, 1994) may play host. In a considerable proportion of cases, a small tumor or tumors, measuring less than 1 cm in diameter, may be found incidentally at necropsy (Fig. 9.160), almost filling the cavity of the fourth ventricle without associated obstructive hydrocephalus. As confirmed in Scheithauer's (1978) review, these *asymptomatic* tumors are most frequently found in male patients whose ages range from the fifth to the eighth decade, with a mean of about 60 years. Similar observations have been made by Chason (1956) in a well-documented and illustrated article.

The consensus that the tumor represents a variant of ependymoma is based on the almost invariable recognition of ependymal cellular features, despite the conspicuous involvement of the subependymal neuroglia in its histologic make-up. Electron microscopy and tissue culture confirm these observations and are further supported by the not infrequent existence of transitional or mixed forms in which the histologic picture of typical ependymoma and subependymoma is juxtaposed within the same example (Scheithauer, 1978). As already noted in regard to ependymomas in general, the astroglial component of subependymomas varies greatly from one specimen to another, and sometimes in different parts of the same tumor. It is maximal in the small and symptomless growths encountered incidentally in later life.

However, an appreciable number of subependymomas will grow to a size large enough to become

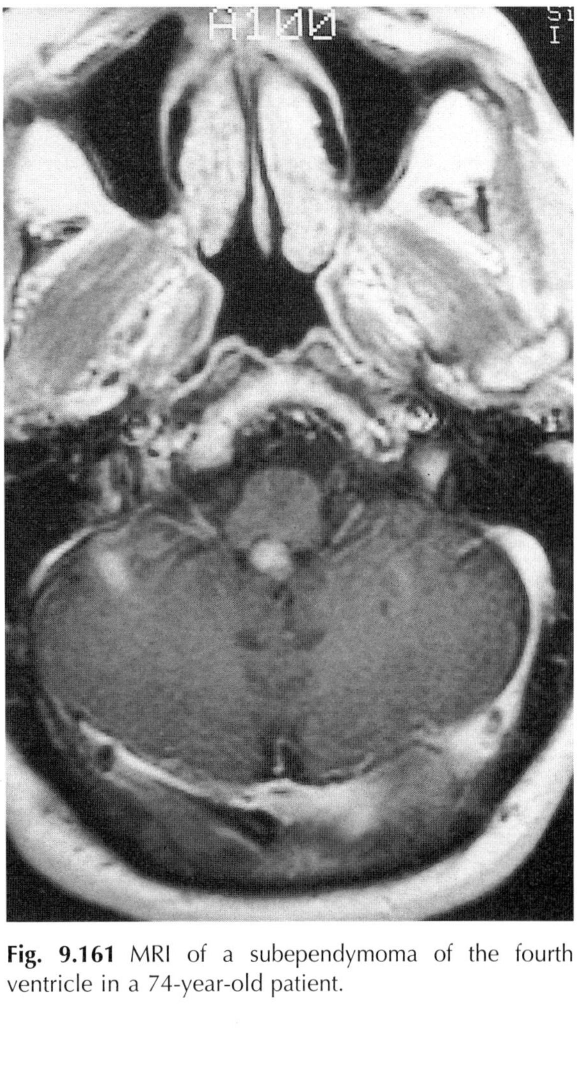

Fig. 9.161 MRI of a subependymoma of the fourth ventricle in a 74-year-old patient.

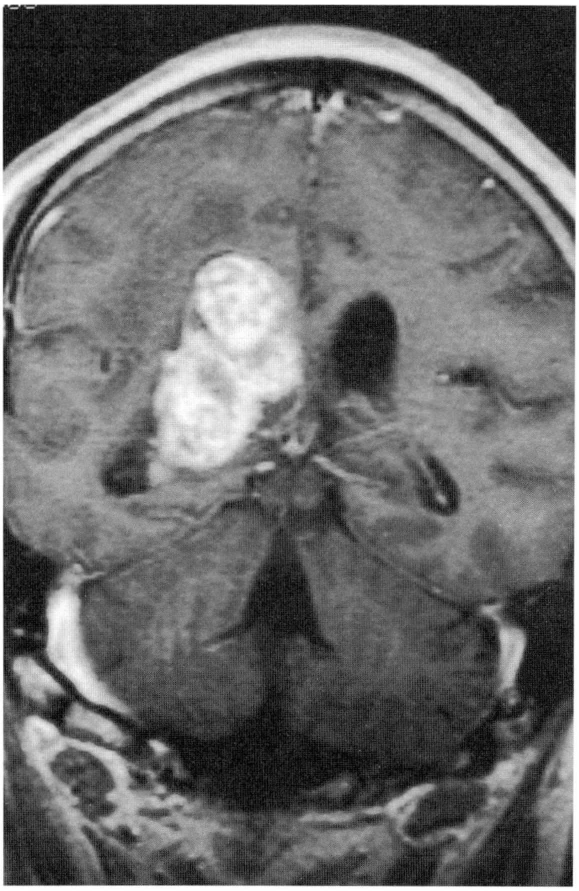

Fig. 9.162 MRI of the subependymoma shown in Fig. 9.164.

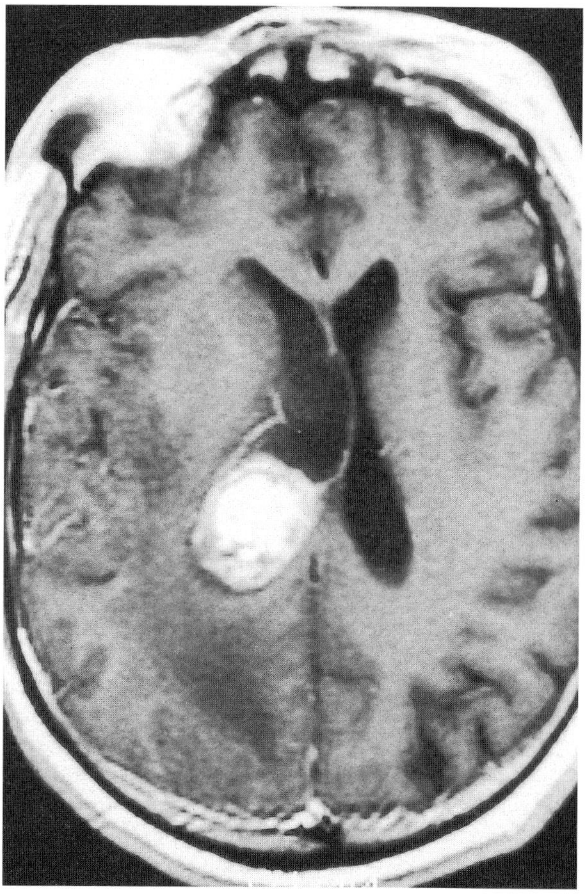

Fig. 9.163 MRI of the subependymoma shown in Fig. 9.164.

symptomatic (Scheithauer, 1978; Lombardi *et al.*, 1991a). Those that seem peculiarly liable to do so have involved the septum lucidum, the foramen of Monro, the aqueduct (Lee *et al.*, 1987; Lombardi *et al.*, 1991a) and the spinal cord (Guha, Resch and Tator, 1989), but subependymomas arising in the fourth ventricle (Fig. 9.161), particularly from its floor, may also become symptomatic. Occasionally, those originating in a lateral ventricle are pedunculated (Vaquero *et al.*, 1980). These larger examples, most of which measure about 5 cm in their greatest dimension, frequently demonstrate cyst formation, focal calcifications and hemorrhage (Figs 9.162–9.164). Unlike the small asymptomatic growths of elderly patients, the symptomatic tumors span a much wider range in their age incidence, with a number presenting in the first decade of life. As expected, it is in the symptomatic examples that transitional features combining those of ependymoma and of subependymoma are most likely to occur. Of the symptomatic subependymomas, Lombardi *et al.* (1991a) reported flow cytometry for ploidy analysis on 15 symptomatic neoplasms, identifying tetraploid peaks in two, hyperdiploid aneuploidy in one, and diploid peaks in 12.

An unusual variant of subependymoma that recurred in a 60-year-old man revealed sarcomatous transformation of the vasculature and was reported by Louis, Hedley-Whyte and Martuza (1989). Similarly, Tomlinson *et al.* (1991) reported a subependymoma, arising in the brainstem of a 52-year-old man, that exhibited rhabdomyosarcomatous elements.

Radiographic appearance

Nonenhanced CT scans show a well-delineated mass that is hypo- or isodense to brain parenchyma. Calcification is sometimes identified. Minimal or no enhancement is seen on postcontrast studies.

The MRI diagnosis of subependymoma relies on the intraventricular location, with the most common site being the fourth ventricle (Figs 9.161–9.163), typically in an asymptomatic middle-

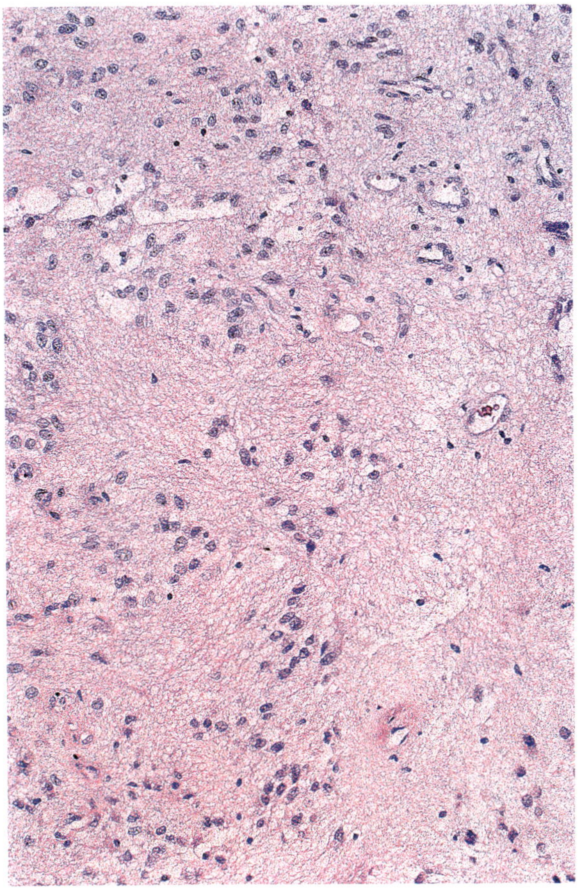

Fig. 9.164 Low-power view of a poorly cellular, delicately fibrillar subependymoma of the medial wall of the lateral ventricle. H&E, × 150

aged or elderly male. Lesions related to the lateral ventricle are usually in contact with the septum pellucidum. Most small subependymomas are homogeneously hypo- to isointense masses on T1-weighted images. Subependymomas may appear mildly hyperintense on T2-weighted scans. Large lesions reveal intensities that reflect their pathologic heterogeneity. Contrast enhancement is usually absent (Kim *et al.*, 1993). The differential diagnosis includes other gliomas (i.e., ependymoma, astrocytoma, oligodendroglioma and central neurocytoma), intraventricular meningioma, choroid plexus tumor, and subependymal hamartoma/subependymal giant-cell astrocytoma (e.g., in a patient with tuberous sclerosis) (Jelenik *et al.*, 1990) or gray matter heterotopia (which would be isointense to normal gray matter on all sequences).

Cytogenesis

Various hypotheses can be suggested to account for the development of this variant of ependymoma. The frequency with which large, symptom-producing examples exhibit transitional features bridging subependymoma and classic ependymoma, and the frequency with which rare cells immunoreactive against the Ki-67 (proliferation-related) antigen are found, point to an actively proliferating role on the part of the more cellular ependymomatous subpopulations in these tumors. As a corollary, the smaller, more fibrillar masses, which appear devoid of active growth because of an absence of mitotic figures and an absence of immunoreactivity with Ki-67, may conceivably represent an arrested stage in a benign neoplasm. Another hypothesis is that it represents a dysgenic event. This possibility is raised by the finding of K.L. Ho (1983) of an association between subependymomas and the presence of heterotopic leptomeningeal neuroglial tissue, combined with the occasional occurrence of this tumor in identical twins (Clarenbach *et al.*, 1979) or with the unusual case of father–son subependymomas (Ryken, Robinson and VanGilder, 1994). In one of Rubinstein's cases, there was an associated syringomyelia, in another, a cavernous angioma of the putamen, but these may have been fortuitous. In a few cases, quoted by Scheithauer (1978), a subependymoma may accompany other primary neoplasms of the CNS, but again the association could be accidental or related to the development of secondary hydrocephalus induced by the other tumor.

The possibility that these lesions are, in some cases, the result of a reactive process involving the ependyma and the subependymal glia, such as long-standing hydrocephalus or chronic ependymitis, cannot be dismissed, especially in view of their frequent multiplicity in those circumstances.

Thus, Russell and Rubinstein (1989) have previously noted the association of small multiple subependymomas occupying the lateral recess in combination with a choroid plexus papilloma of the cerebellopontine angle in an 18-year-old girl; of multiple subependymomas occupying the cavity and lateral recesses of the fourth ventricle, with a chronic granular ependymitis due to a protracted cryptococcal meningitis of several years' duration in a 59-year-old male (Fig. 9.160); and of similar multiple subependymomas in the fourth ventricle, with long-standing hydrocephalus secondary to a diffuse primary leptomeningeal melanomatosis in a 41-year-old man. Fenstermaker, Ganz and Roessmann (1989) reported a subependymoma-like reaction to a dermoid cyst in a 43-year-old woman. The suggestion of a reactive etiology in these cases is further reinforced by the report by K.C. Ho *et al.* (1987) of the remarkable association of a subependymoma of the third ventricle with a suprasellar craniopharyngioma known to have been present in a 42-year-old woman for at least 18 years and resulting in obstructive hydrocephalus. In this case, the patient had received multiple doses of radiation directed to the suprasellar neoplasm over a period of 15 years, so the alternative possibility of a radiation-induced second tumor originating in a region of intense reactive gliosis may also have to be entertained. In any event, the resemblance that exists between the microscopic picture of subependymomas and the ependymal granulations that typically accompany chronic low-grade ventricular inflammation is undeniable.

Microscopic appearance

Microscopically, the pattern is that of a densely fibrillar but rather sparsely nucleated glioma throughout which ependymal cells are unevenly scattered (Fig. 9.164). These well-differentiated cells may form hollow rosettes or perivascular pseudorosettes, but usually only small clumps of fibrillar cells with no special orientation are found. Blepharoplasts may be demonstrable. This was further clearly established by the electron microscopic observations on such an example by Fu *et al.* (1974), and subsequently confirmed by other electron microscopic studies by Azzarelli, Rekate and Roessmann (1977) and Friede and Pollak (1978).

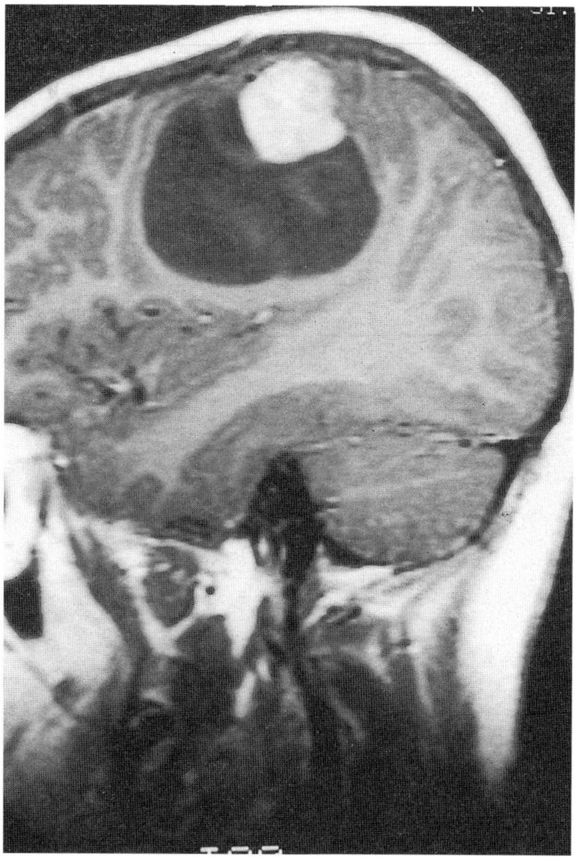

Fig. 9.165 An MRI of the supratentorial ependymoma shown in Fig. 9.167, associated with a large parenchymal cyst.

Malignant forms of ependymoma

Anaplastic (malignant) ependymomas

Although ependymomas are notably benign in their circumscription and cytologic features, there is evidence, on rare occasions, of rapid growth accompanied by anaplasia. This development may occur in patients of any age and may involve cerebral examples (Figs 9.165 and 9.166), as well as those arising in the posterior fossa and even, exceptionally, myxopapillary ependymomas of the cauda equina.

There is, at this time, relatively little detailed information on these malignant examples except for the consensus that they form a small minority of the ependymomas and that histologic grading plays an limited role in identifying these lesions prospectively. Craig and Kernohan (1938), in a study of tumors of the fourth ventricle, found that fewer than 5% of ependymomas were highly malignant with a tendency to rapid recurrence after removal. Ringertz and Reymond (1949) also found six malignant cases in their survey of 72 ependymomas. In their series of 133 ependymomas, Fokes and Earle (1969) mention only one example in the frontoparietal lobe of a 34-year-old man in whom a grade 3 cellular ependymoma converted into a glioblastoma 6 months later. In their series of 75 ependymomas in children, Shuman, Alvord and Leech (1975) reported three malignant examples. Seven anaplastic ependymomas were recorded by Mørk and Løken (1977) in their series of 101 tumors; five of them were supratentorial, three of which were in adults.

In spinal ependymomas, malignant change appears to be quite exceptional. Only five malignant examples were reported by Slooff, Kernohan and MacCarty (1964) in their series of 169 cases. Mørk, Risberg and Krogness (1980) reported an unusual example in the spinal cord of a 12-year-old boy who later developed extensive spinal and intracranial dissemination.

Ignoring the group of embryonal neoplasms best categorized as ependymoblastomas, the concept of features of prognostic significance among ependymomas continues to be an area of controversy. While the vast majority of studies indicate that some histologic factors portend a poor prognosis, there remains little consensus on which factors are

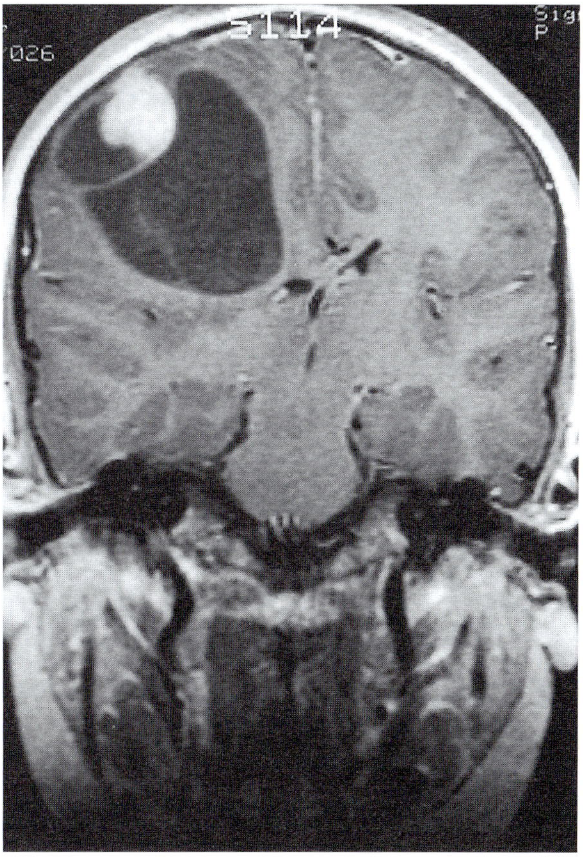

Fig. 9.166 An MRI of the ependymoma shown in Fig. 9.167, associated with a large parenchymal cyst.

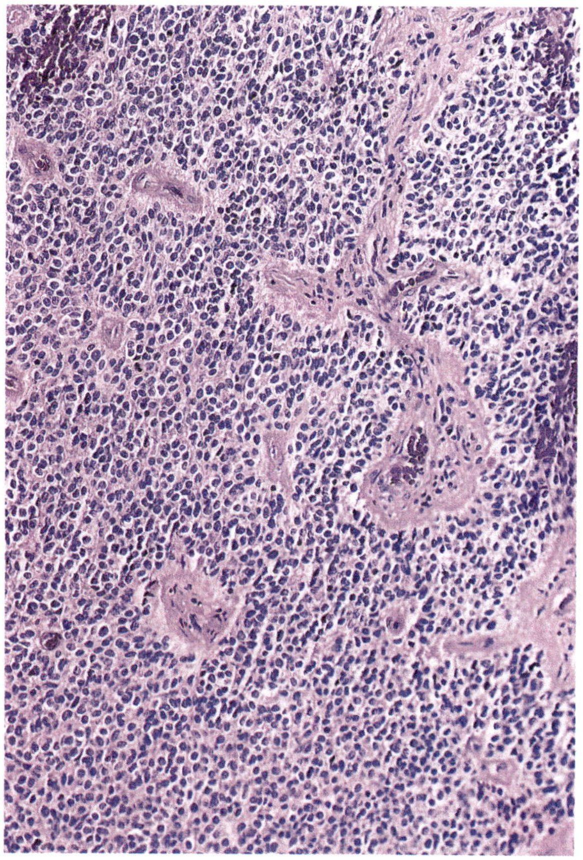

Fig. 9.167 Ependymoma arising in the cerebral hemispheres showing high cellularity and vascular proliferation, a feature associated with poor survival rate for the patient when the tumor is in this location. H&E, × 200

useful. These tumors reflect the well-recognized problem of location *versus* histology, such that a lesion in an eloquent area can be clinically devastating despite a mature phenotype. Thus, studies that do not indicate the location of the tumors or the age of the patients at diagnosis are usually unsuccessful in identifying factors of prognostic significance. Studies such as these are further complicated by their retrospective nature, the lack of uniform staging and examination, and inconsistent therapy. Even such a relatively simple concept as total *versus* partial resection is complicated by the location of a tumor and its proximity to eloquent regions (Ikezaki *et al.*, 1993) and to CSF pathways. Thus, one study found that infants with 'flagrant' signs of hydrocephalus were poor candidates to benefit from any therapy (Rawlings *et al.*, 1988). Anatomic location of primary tumor occurrence is also age dependent, with one study indicating that the mean age of a patient with a posterior fossa tumor was 7 years, that of a patient with a supratentorial tumor was 17 years and that of a patient with a spinal cord tumor was 41 years (Rawlings *et al.*, 1988).

Clearly, few, if any, histologic features will be useful independently in evaluating the posterior fossa ependymomas. For example, Schiffer *et al.* (1991a, 1991b) found that, among patients with infratentorial ependymomas, an age of less than 4 years connotes a poor prognosis, while the presence of subependymomatous regions indicates a good prognosis. Furthermore, the same studies found that the presence of mitoses and necroses in supratentorial tumors is a reliable indicator of a poor prognosis, though not if they are present in infratentorial tumors. In contrast, Figarella-Branger *et al.* (1991), in their study of childhood infratentorial tumors, suggest that mitotic activity and necroses are indicative of a poor prognosis, while abundant GFAP production by the tumor cells is indicative of a prolonged survival of the patient. Rawlings *et al.* (1988) further confound issues by finding that the presence of 'epithelial features', defined as clefts or tubules lined by columnar cells, indicate a good survival rate for the patient, while the presence of subependymomatous regions foretells a poor survival rate. Rawlings *et al.* (1988) denied the utility of mitoses, necroses and vascular proliferation in infratentorial tumors. In context, supratentorial tumors with mitoses, nuclear pleomorphism and vascular proliferation tended toward a poor survival rate (Fig. 9.167) as opposed to the presence of microcysts, which foretold a good prognosis.

Clinicopathologic correlation

All studies confirm the fact that local recurrence is the major factor involved in morbidity and mortality in ependymomas. The intimate relationship of cranial ependymomas to the ventricular system, however, might be expected to promote the dispersal of tumor cells in the CSF, with the growth of seedlings at remote points. Earlier studies were largely drawn from autopsy data and thus were subject to clinical bias of selection. These studies, including the reports of Cairns and Russell (1931), Tarlov and Davidoff (1946), Svien *et al.* (1953) and Fokes and Earle (1969), suggest metastatic rates of up to 25%, but the clinical significance of these findings is not known. More recent studies have suggested that clinical staging appears to be a useful area for exploitation of prognostic information. Rawlings *et al.*, (1988) noted that, from their review of the literature, the rate of metastasis in patients with ependymomas ranged from 3% to 10%, with an average rate of clinically evident metastasis of 1% to 3%. Their study confirmed that the presence of positive CSF cytologic studies for tumor cells was, independently, a poor prognostic finding, regardless of the presence of clinically evident metastasis. In this study, 10% of patients with supratentorial tumors and 15% of patients with infratentorial tumors were found to have positive CSF cytology for tumor cells. (One patient had a symptomatic compressive metastasis; the remaining patients had positive cytologic findings associated with recurrence at the primary site.) All of these patients died within 36 months of original diagnosis, a mortality rate that is supported by the literature. The presence of histologic anaplasia also apparently raises the likelihood of spinal and cerebral seeding as indicated by Renaudin, DiTullio and Brown (1979) in a series of 19 intracranial ependymomas in children. The issue of spinal irradiation is controversial and requires further study. Goldwein *et al.* (1991) noted that age (greater than 4 years) and treatment by total spinal irradiation were the only factors independently predictive of a prolonged survival among 17 children with 'histologically' malignant ependymomas. Nevertheless, treatment with total spinal irradiation did not increase survival in patients with histologically low-grade ependymomas (Goldwein *et al.*, 1990). The cautions of Rubinstein (Ross and Rubinstein, 1989) must be remembered: the prognosis of patients with ependymomas exhibiting malignant histology must still be considered unpredictable, with up to two thirds of the cases considered to have anaplastic features histologically being expected to pursue a favorable course.

Extraneural metastasis

Spread of *cerebral* ependymomas in continuity with the extracranial soft tissues, without histologic evidence of enhanced malignancy, has been observed as a postoperative development in several examples (Feigin and Volk, 1951; Maass, 1954; Sherbaniuk and Shnitka, 1956; Wen and Barrows, 1957; Newton, Henson and Walker, 1992). In four of these reports, this spread led ultimately to remote metastasis. A similar complication was reported by Perry (1957), Nigogosyan, De La Pava and Pickren (1962, case 2) and Glasauer and Yuan (1963). No nodules were found in the scalp in these cases, but the regional cervical lymph nodes were involved in the case of Glasauer and Yuan (1963): repeated craniotomy was invariably featured in all three instances. The microscopic description and illustrations suggest, in the last-mentioned case, a highly malignant form of ependymoma probably similar to the ependymoblastoma as defined below. The lungs were the site of metastases in most examples. In that of Perry (1957), the microscopic description leaves some doubt as to whether it was an ependymoma, as claimed, or an oligodendroglioma; metastases were confined to the liver and bone marrow. The total length of the clinical history was greatest (13 years) in the case of Sherbaniuk and Shnitka (1956). Paradoxically, one report indicated prolonged survival in a factor predisposing to extraneural spread (Newton, Henson and Walker, 1992).

In *spinal* ependymomas, spread to the extravertebral soft tissues has similarly been reported prior to distant metastases. The tumors described by Weiss (1955) and by Patterson, Campbell and Parsons (1961) were, respectively, myxopapillary and papillary ependymomas of the cauda equina. Both recurred after the initial operation and were re-explored twice when the growth had spread into the adjacent soft tissues. At necropsy, 10 and 17 years, respectively, from the start of the illness, metastases were found in the liver, lungs and mediastinal lymph nodes. The papillary character of the tumor was reflected in the metastases in both cases. A similar case in which the total length of the clinical history was almost 30 years has been reported by Rubinstein (Rubinstein and Logan, 1970). In this latter case, the metastatic foci were reported to be well differentiated at necropsy, although some areas at the primary site reportedly showed cellular anaplasia. Further examples of sacral cord ependymomas characterized by a similar protracted clinical evolution ultimately followed by distant body metastases, but without anaplastic change in the original growth, have since been reported by Barone and Elvidge (1970), Wight, Holley and Finbow (1973) and Newton, Henson and Walker (1992). Of particular interest in this context is the case reported by Wolff, Santiago and Duby (1972) in which an ectopic myxopapillary ependymoma of the sacrococcygeal region, in a 4-year-old child, resulted in metastases in an inguinal lymph node 2½ years later and in the right lung at the age of 23 years. There was no evidence of tumor recurrence 13 months after lobectomy, i.e., 20 years after removal of the original sacral growth. Mavroudis, Townsend and Wilson (1977) reported a similar course demonstrated by the patient who had an ependymoma of the cauda equina that was followed by multiple local recurrences over a period of 29 years and multiple pulmonary metastases (with numerous mitotic figures). This patient was alive at the time of reporting having received two courses of radiotherapy and eight of chemotherapy.

Experience with these neoplasms indicates that long postoperative survival of the patient with ultimate recurrence of the tumor is often unattended by any cytologic features of malignancy: earlier editions of this book record an example of this kind following 16 years after removal of a fourth-ventricle ependymoma in a man aged 21 years. Thus, ependymomas share with other differentiated gliomas the same uncertainties as to whether, when, and how often anaplastic features may later manifest themselves in a residual or recurrent growth. The prognostic significance of such delayed recurrences has been further discussed by Shuman, Alvord and Leech (1975) in the context of their experience of three such examples in children. Similarly, an earlier edition (1989, p. 213) records an instance of delayed recurrence in a histologically malignant ependymoma in which the recurrent tumor appeared to be benign. The patient was a 16-year-old boy, in whom the recurrence presented 11 years after the excision and postoperative radiation of a fourth-ventricle tumor.

Ependymoblastomas

The name 'ependymoblastoma' was originally applied by Bailey and Cushing (1926) to a purely histologic variant of benign ependymoma composed of fibrillar cells termed 'ependymal spongioblasts'. This separation from the other forms of ependymoma was subsequently rejected as insignificant and discarded (Bailey, 1927; Cox, 1933). While, therefore, the ependymoblast has long remained enigmatic as a tumor cell type, the studies of Herman *et al.* (1975) on the progressive differentiation of primitive neuroepithelial elements in the mouse testicular teratoma, the investigations by others on the normal developing avian and mammalian CNS and the electron microscopic observations on such a tumor by Langford (1986) have collectively supported the view that the term 'ependymoblast' should be reserved for those cells that already display, at least in their early stages, the differentiating hallmark features of ependymal cells, while exhibiting, at the same time, evidence of still-persistent mitotic activity. In other words, we are dealing with a primitive neuroepithelial precursor cell that, to a large extent, is already committed to ependymal differentiation.

Tumors in man that seem to exemplify such a stage and, therefore, are believed to represent a truly embryonal form of ependymal neoplasm, have been reported as exceptional examples occurring in young children (Rubinstein, 1970, 1972a), and subsequently confirmed by others (see Liu, Boggs and Kidd, 1976; Lorentzen and Hägerstrand, 1980; Mørk and Rubinstein, 1985; Wada *et al.*, 1986; Cruz-Sanchez *et al.*, 1988a, for more cases and references). These neoplasms, which are often massive and which may or may not be demonstrably related to a ventricular cavity, tend to be more frequently supratentorial and carry a very poor prognosis. They are characterized by their high and primitive cellularity (Figs 9.168 and 9.169), including embryonal-cell

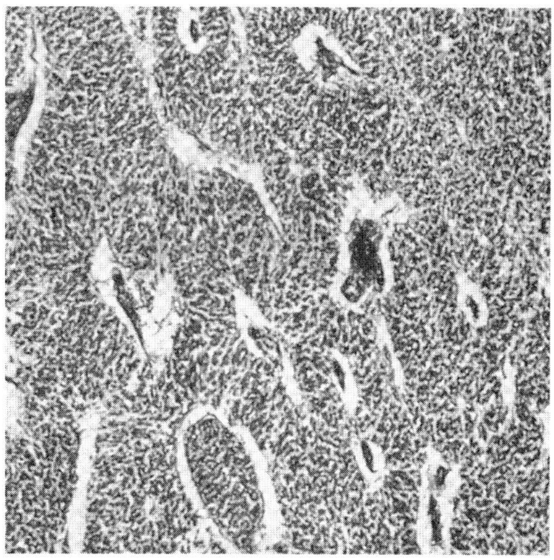

Fig. 9.168 Highly cellular cerebral ependymoblastoma showing solid anastomosing cords with a regular scanty stroma of thin-walled blood vessels. PTAH, × 65. (Reprinted from *Archives of Pathology and Laboratory Medicine*, 1970, 90, p. 35 with kind permission of the American Medical Association.)

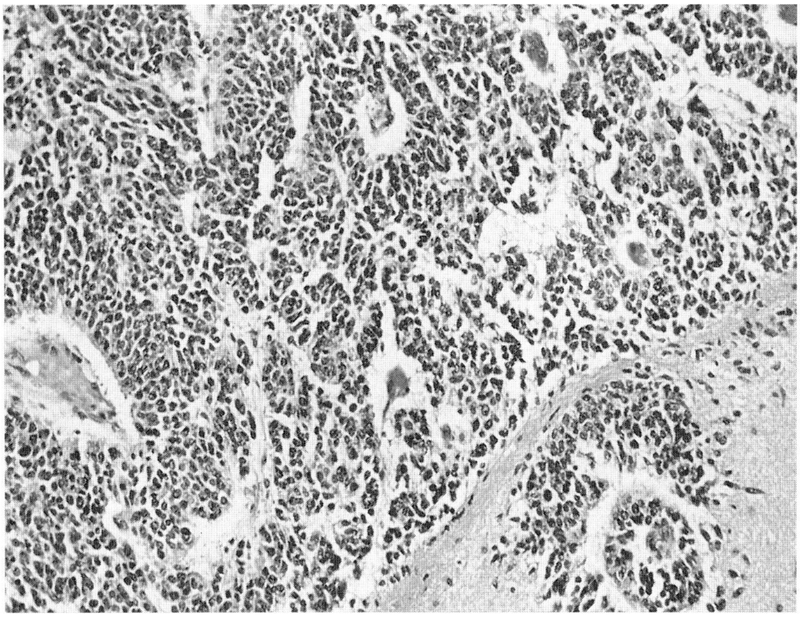

Fig. 9.169 Spinal meningeal metastasis from an ependymoblastoma originating in the fourth ventricle. Invasion of the spinal cord parenchyma (lower right) can be seen. PTAH, × 145

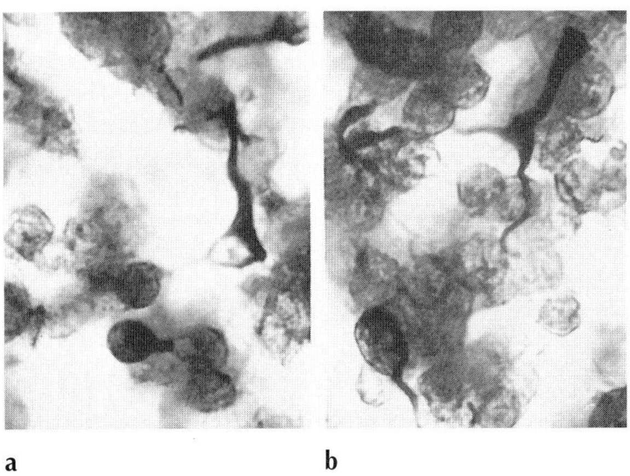

Fig. 9.170 (a and b) Same tumor as Fig. 9.168 showing uni- and multipolar spongioblasts with tortuous processes. Silver carbonate impregnation for neuroglia, × 640

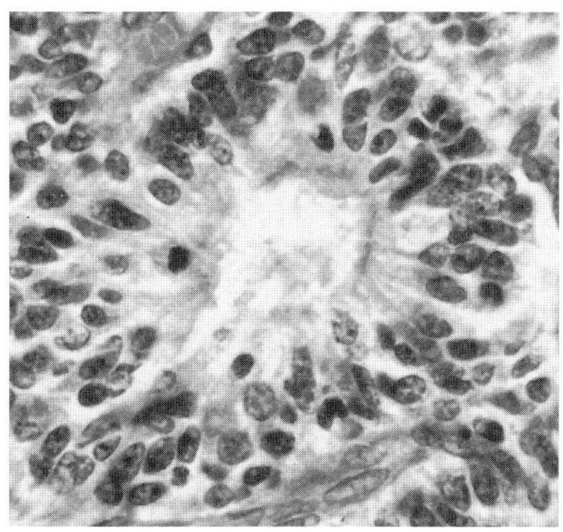

Fig. 9.171 Ependymoblastic rosette with mitotic figures. H&E, × 575

forms suggesting uni- and multipolar spongioblasts (Fig. 9.170), but diagnostically exhibit clear-cut ependymal rosettes (Fig. 9.171) and tubules (Fig. 9.172). The demonstration, by appropriate silver impregnation, of polar spongioblasts (Fig. 9.170) in the tumor may perhaps be regarded as supporting an alternative origin from an intermediate ependymoglial precursor cell (see above, p. 388).

The chief clinicopathologic aspects and histologic characteristics of 12 such examples, including those of seven previously unreported cases, have been reviewed in detail elsewhere (Mørk and Rubinstein, 1985). While it shares with the classic ependymoma the gross feature of appearing circumscribed, the ependymoblastoma differs from it by the frequency with which focal microscopic

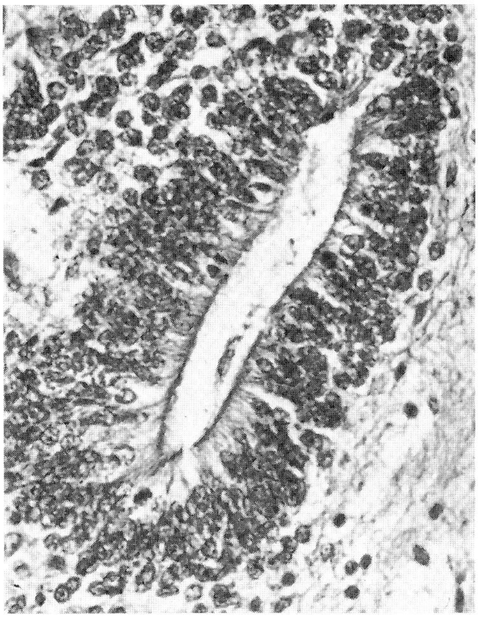

Fig. 9.172 Ependymomatous tubule at the periphery of the tumor in Fig. 9.168, demonstrating mitotic figures in juxtatubular cells. H&E, × 350. (Reprinted from *Archives of Pathology and Laboratory Medicine*, 1970, 90, p. 35 with kind permission of the American Medical Association.)

invasion and leptomeningeal involvement are demonstrable, and widespread metastases may consequently occur in the cerebrospinal subarachnoid space (Fig. 9.173), in the manner of a medulloblastoma. On the other hand, the absence of cellular pleomorphism, giant cells, multinucleation and pseudopalisades, and the scanty proliferation of endothelial-cells are characteristics that delineate this highly distinctive neoplasm from an ependymoma with secondary anaplastic change.

In the case recorded by Wada *et al.* (1986) of a 17-year-old female with extensive leptomeningeal spread, the primary site of origin is obscure, as none was found within the central neuraxis. A few examples that developed extraneural metastases have been noted (Glasauer and Yuan, 1963; Campbell *et al.*, 1984, case 20; Mørk and Rubinstein, 1985, case 8).

The electron microscopic characteristics of one such tumor, a fourth-ventricle growth infiltrating the vermis and the cerebellar hemispheres in a 4-year-old boy, have been well documented by Langford (1986). In an unpublished case, submitted to Duke University Medical Center by Azzarelli, of a massive cerebral hemispheric growth in a female infant, the electron microscopic features were again similar.

Astroblastomas

Astroblastomas have received relatively little attention since their original description by Bailey and Bucy in 1930. Because of their great rarity as a pure entity, their existence has sometimes been questioned, or they have been interpreted as a subgroup of astrocytomas. As noted on p. 334, gemistocytic astrocytomas may include astroblastic structures, but these formations are only a relatively minor element

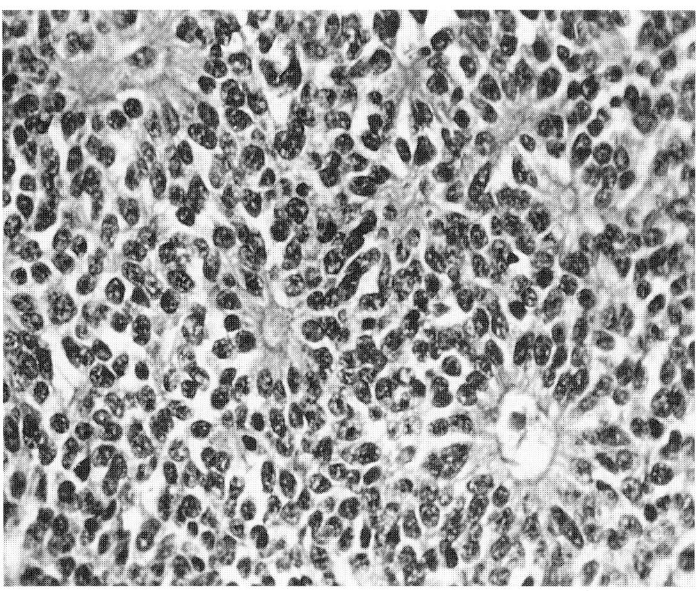

Fig. 9.173 Same tumor as Fig. 9.169, showing multiple rosettes in the leptomeningeal infiltrate. H&E, × 300

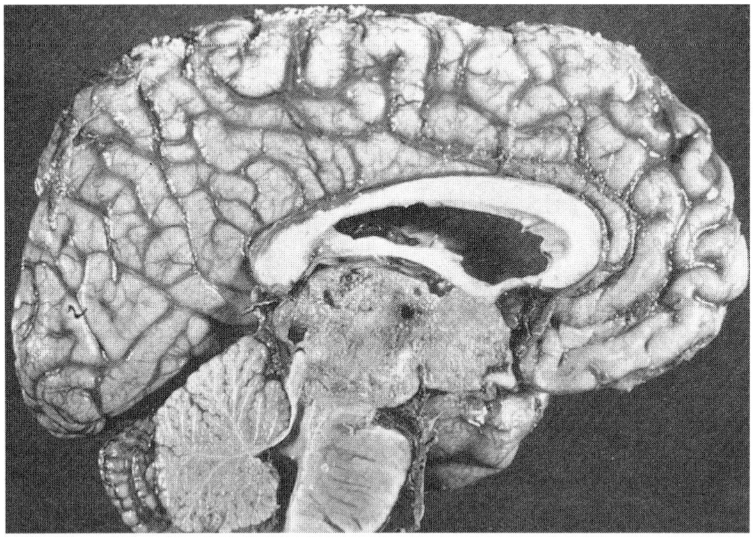

Fig. 9.174 Parapineal astroblastoma occupying the third ventricle in a 22-year-old male. (Courtesy of Dr J.H.N. Deck)

in the histologic picture. Again, areas with astroblastoma focal features may be found in anaplastic astrocytomas and in glioblastomas. The examination, then, demands that special caution be exercised when the biopsy material is limited: an extensive survey of the resected specimen is necessary before the diagnosis of astroblastoma can confidently be made.

Acceptance of this tumor as a separate, albeit exceptional, entity has rested on two bases. The first was the observation of small, clinically unsuspected examples, one being a well-defined nodule measuring 1 cm in diameter in necropsy material from the corpus callosum of a man aged 35 years, an illustration of which was published in earlier editions of this book (e.g., Russell and Rubinstein, 1977, Fig. 131). The second basis is a review of the clinicopathologic features of 23 cases, most of which were submitted for review by Rubinstein (Bonnin and Rubinstein, 1989). These experiences supported, and to some degree extended, the observations of Bailey and Bucy (1930) in that they facilitated the recognition of two histologic subtypes of astroblastoma: one in which the architectural pattern and the cytologic features were those of a relatively well-differentiated glial tumor, and one in which the astroblastic pattern was associated with the microscopic features of a more malignant glioma. The existence of these two subgroups may, to some extent, account for the variations in biologic behavior of the astroblastoma, as discussed below. The following descriptions are, therefore, based largely on the survey of Rubinstein's published material.

Following the publication of the review, and subsequent to the previous edition of this book, Rubinstein performed an exhaustive tissue culture and ultrastructural examination of two cases of astroblastoma and discovered features that suggested a similarity with, and possible origin from, the tanycyte, a transitional cell since found to be placed developmentally between the primitive glioblast and the mature ependymal lining cell (Gould, Howard and Papadaki, 1990). The concept is more fully discussed on p. 388.

Age incidence and site

Most astroblastomas are encountered in patients in the first three decades of life. Those exceptional examples arising in later life have been the highly malignant form. Sex distribution is about even. The cerebral hemispheres are most often affected, the tumor usually involving the cortex and subcortical white matter or the paraventricular region. In the latter situation, it may compress the ventricle and encroach upon it, but the growth is not primarily intraventricular. Though this sparing of the ventricular system had been seen as a feature distinguishing it from ependymoma – the type of glioma with which the astroblastoma may be most often confused – many supratentorial ependymomas are found to have no apparent connection with the lateral ventricles (Van Tassel, Lee and Bruner, 1986). Occasionally, however, as shown in Fig. 9.174, the tumor primarily occupies a ventricle. In the illustrated example, it was adjacent to, but distinct from,

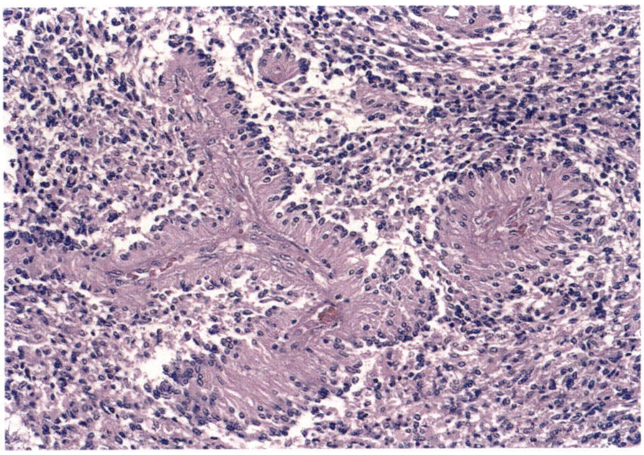

Fig. 9.175 Astroblastoma from the right frontal region in a 23-year-old woman. H&E, × 250

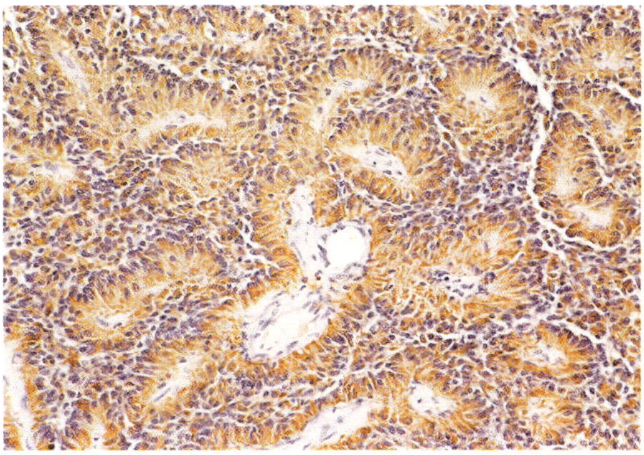

Fig. 9.176 Same case as Fig. 9.175. GFAP immunoperoxidase, × 250

the pineal gland. Occasional examples may occupy the cerebellum, where they tend to be paramedial.

Macroscopic appearance

Astroblastomas are almost always well defined (Fig. 9.174) and their cut surfaces are usually homogeneous, soft and pink-gray. Small or large cysts are frequent, and central areas of necrosis are found in the larger examples.

Microscopic appearance

The tumor is richly and evenly supplied by blood vessels that form an important element architecturally with respect to their intimate relation to the tumor cells (Figs 9.175 and 9.176). The vessel walls show conspicuous hyaline thickening. The tumor cells are thickly clustered about the vessels, giving the appearance of pseudorosettes in cross section and of uninterrupted rows where the vessels are longitudinally displayed. The nuclei are located at some distance away from the vessel, but processes of varying length and thickness extend vertically to the vessel wall and often end there as an expanded footplate. The nuclei are usually oval, often slightly irregular or notched, and contain coarse chromatin nodes, thus differing from the regular spheroidal nuclei with delicate punctate chromatin that is characteristic of ependymomas. The perikaryon is angulated, club-shaped or fusiform and, in addition to the main vascular-related process, shorter cytoplasmic processes are often fairly well developed. Cellular atypia may be present and is sometimes extensive in places, where it may be associated with multinucleation. Typically, however, mitotic figures are scanty or encountered in moderate numbers only in the histologically lower-grade variant, a feature that separates the low-grade tumor from its high-grade variant. Another feature of importance in distinguishing between the grades is the absence of vascular endothelial proliferation in the low-grade group.

In contrast to ependymomas, in which the intervascular architecture of the tumor is characteristically compact (see Fig. 9.132), the spaces lying between the pseudorosettes of astroblastomas are rarefied (Figs 9.175 and 9.176). They are occupied by scanty spindle cells or irregularly stellate cells. Many of these are probably related to vessels outside the plane of the section. Again, in contrast to the ependymomas, staining with PTAH historically reveals no or few neuroglial fibrils. In this respect, the astroblastoma illustrates the importance of the immunomorphologic expression of GFAP in a poorly fibrillated glioma, for this protein can always be demonstrated in the tumor cells, although expression may vary greatly from case to case and from field to field. In some examples or in some areas, only a small number of cells are immunopositive; in others, the immunopositive cells are frequent, being most often perivascular (Fig. 9.176). There is no correlation between the extent and distribution of tumor cell positivity for the protein and the cytologic features seen with conventional stains. The same feature has been noted by Yamashita *et al.* (1985) and by Husain and Leestma (1986). More recent studies (Cabello *et al.*, 1991; Pizer *et al.*, 1995) have shown the intense immunopositivity for vimentin, of most of the tumor cells suggesting this as a possible label of their derivation from a more primitive precursor cell. The tumor cells may also express S-100 protein, but do not express low-molecular-weight cytokeratins (e.g., CAM 5.2). The outer cytoplasmic membranes of the tumor cells are often

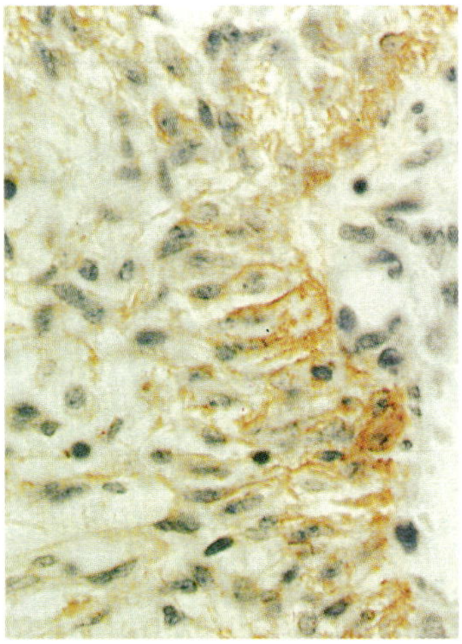

Fig. 9.177 Astroblastoma. Immunoperoxidase reaction with Leu 7 (HNK-1) monoclonal antibody, × 400

positive when immunostained with the anti-Leu 7 monoclonal antibody (Perentes and Rubinstein, 1986) (Fig. 9.177).

Necrosis may be present in the center of the tumor or as small discrete foci that may not be patently associated with malignant features in the adjacent tumor. Their significance in the biologic evolution of the growth is uncertain. In Rubinstein's experience (Bonnin and Rubinstein, 1989), they are not invariably associated with an ominous prognosis.

While the typical astroblastoma has a uniform histologic picture, some examples include, in addition, more solid or compact, nonpapillary areas with the features of astrocytoma, thus emphasizing the relationship of astroblastoma with other neoplasms of the astrocytic group. Nevertheless, despite the preponderance of the astroblastic architecture in Rubinstein's series of 23 astroblastomas

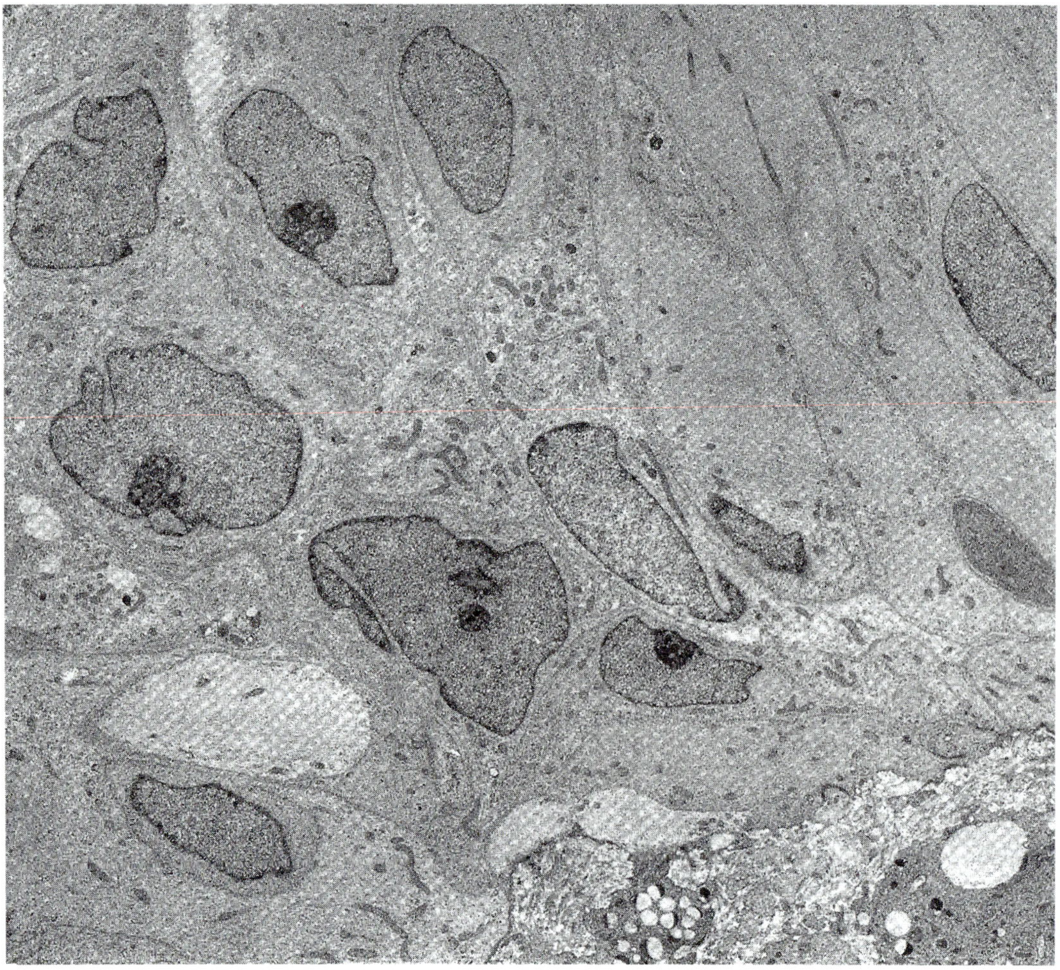

Fig. 9.178 Overview of polarized glial cells in a frontoparietal astroblastoma removed from a 9-year-old female. The cells were cultured on sponge foam for 70 days. A basal lamina (lower right) separates the cells from a degenerated capillary vessel. × 3000 (In collaboration with Dr Mary M. Herman)

(Bonnin and Rubinstein, 1989), 13 of which had long-term follow-up, almost half of the cases showed the cellular characteristics of a malignant glioma. Significant features of these cases were mitotic activity, vascular endothelial proliferation and a more irregular histologic pattern with focal blurring of the astroblastic architecture, highly compact areas with the cellular appearance of anaplastic astrocytoma, or even oligodendroglioma, and invasion into the adjacent parenchyma or leptomeninges. A further noteworthy feature of some of these examples was the presence of transitional areas of malignant gemistocytic astrocytoma. The postoperative clinical behavior of these cases has confirmed the ominous significance to be attached to their histologic aspects, for, in two of the four patients with high histologic grade tumors, conversion of the tumor into a glioblastoma was subsequently documented.

From the differential diagnostic standpoint, the most frequent type of glioma with which the well-differentiated astroblastoma is likely to be confused is an ependymoma. As can be seen from the description above, the two forms of glioma can usually be distinguished by the pattern of their histologic organization, the nuclear characteristics of the tumor cells, the thickness of their perivascular cytoplasmic processes, the presence of footplates and the extent to which the cells demonstrate glial fibril formation. The last feature is often conspicuous in ependymomas, where the perivascular cell processes usually taper to a point (see Figs 9.132 and 9.155). On the other hand, the immunohistochemical expression of GFAP is of no assistance in the differential diagnosis because the cells of both tumors will demonstrate the protein and exhibit a similar pattern of distribution. Expression of GFAP is, however, of considerable importance in helping to distinguish the astroblastoma from a papillary meningioma, another tumor with which the astroblastoma may be confused, particularly astroblastoma malignant forms.

Electron microscopy

Few astroblastomas have been studied by electron microscopy, but a detailed and exhaustive description by Rubinstein and Herman (1989) gives an excellent insight into this facet of the tumor. The resemblance to the tanycyte is justifiably emphasized. An example examined by Kubota *et al.* (1985) showed astrocytes present in different degrees of maturity and displaying large numbers of coated vesicles. Intermediate filaments were numerous in the cell processes of a typical case studied by Husain and Leestma (1986). Irregular electron-dense intracytoplasmic granular bodies closely resembling Rosenthal fibers have been noted by Hoag, Sima and Rozdilsky (1986). In one of Rubinstein's cases (Rubinstein and Herman, 1989), arising in the left frontoparietal region of a 9-year-old female and then maintained *in vitro*, the fine structural features were those of polarized glial cells (Fig. 9.178) in which the basal portions contained delicate filaments (Figs 9.179 and 9.180) and were covered by a well-defined basal lamina (Figs 9.179 and 9.180) that separated them from the capillary blood vessels. Their apical portions sometimes displayed bleb-like cytoplasmic protrusions and were capped by multiple surface microvilli with narrowing of their pedicles, giving them a purse-string appearance (Fig. 9.181). Long intercellular junctions of the zonula adherens type, interrupted by microrosettes, were also present (Fig. 9.182), but in small numbers and associated with only occasional cilia and basal bodies. A characteristic feature of the tumor cells was the presence of delicate lamella-like interdigitations, or pleatings, along some of their lateral borders (Figs 9.180 and 9.182). These appearances collectively suggest features intermediary between those of ependymal cells and astrocytes; the tumor lacked the pronounced cell surface characteristics of an ependymoma as shown in Fig. 9.139.

The features rather recalled those of tanycytes, a type of cell intrinsic to the ependyma of submammalian vertebrates, but which, in addition to the

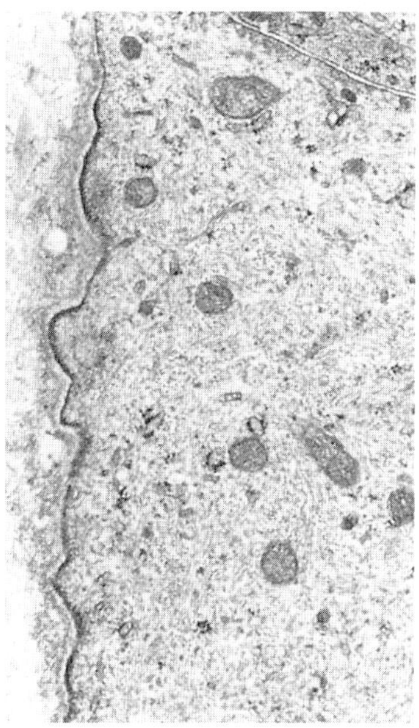

Fig. 9.179 Same tumor as Fig. 9.178. Polarized glial cells cultured on sponge foam for 2 weeks. The tumor cells are resting on a well-defined basal lamina and contain delicate filaments, × 14 000

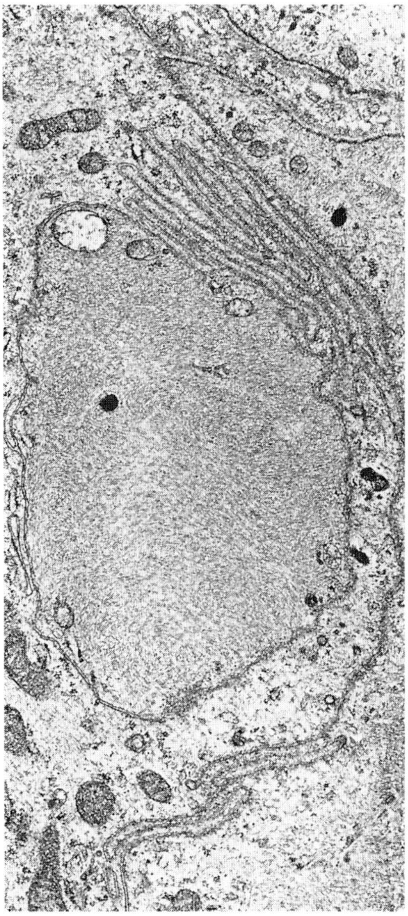

Fig. 9.180 Same tumor as Figs 9.178 and 9.179 after culture on sponge foam for 41 days. The cytoplasmic membranes are pleated along the lateral cell borders. Note the basal lamina at the top of the field. × 10 000 (Courtesy of Dr Mary M. Herman)

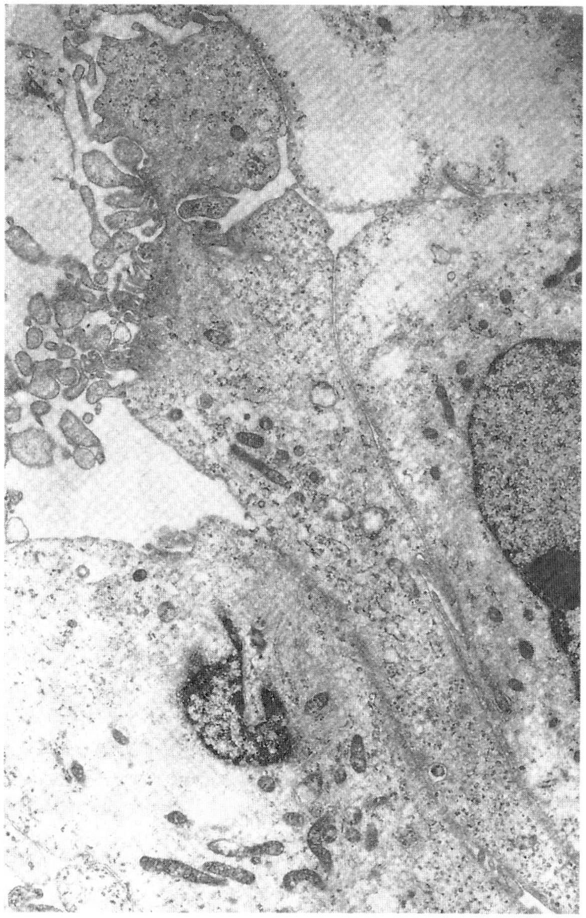

Fig. 9.181 Same case as Figs 9.178–9.180; original tumor. Note the purse-string appearance of the apical portion of a tumor cell, capped with numerous surface microvilli. × 4500

more typical epithelial ependymocytes, has also been found to be scattered along the ependymal lining of the embryonal and neonatal mammalian brain (Peters, Palay and Webster, 1976, pp. 270–4; Gould, Howard and Papadaki, 1990). Another related cell to be considered was designated an 'ependymal astrocyte' by Tennyson and Pappas (1962); this type of cell which, while displaying the same apical features as the tanycyte, differs from it by having multiple branched basal-cell processes. More recent fine structural studies on tanycytes in the adult mammalian CNS (Rafols and Goshgarian, 1985) have not maintained that distinction. In any event, it is conceivable that, in some cases, the astroblastoma may have originated from the neoplastic proliferation of this transient, or intermediate, type of glial cell, the tanycyte (Gould, Howard and Papadaki, 1990). Such a presumed cell of origin might reasonably account for the paraventricular localization of some astroblastomas and also for the great rarity of this type of glioma. Assuming that the tanycyte may represent, in the higher mammalian brain at least, only a transitory phase in central neuroepithelial ontogeny, one may also assume that the number of such replicating cells vulnerable to neoplastic transformation must be small.

Tissue culture

In vitro studies on the astroblastoma have so far been limited to the observations of one typical tumor by Costero (1962) and to one case published by Rubinstein and Herman (1989). In the case of the 9-year-old girl mentioned in the latter paper, tissue culture (on coverslips) from the primary

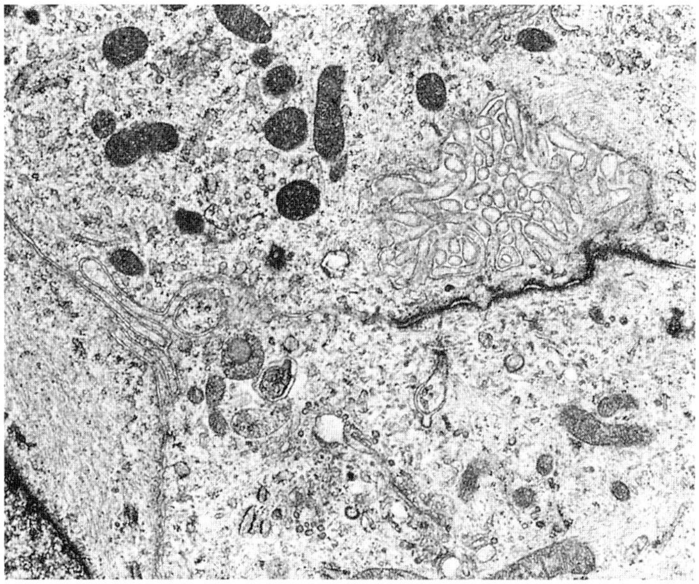

Fig. 9.182 Same culture as Fig. 9.179. Apices of tumor cells with long intercellular junctions interrupted by a microrosette. Note the interdigitations of cytoplasmic membranes at left of center. × 10 000 (In collaboration with Dr Mary M. Herman)

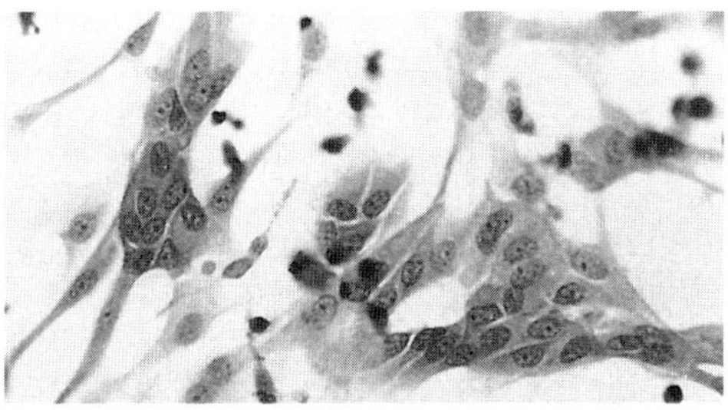

Fig. 9.183 Tissue culture, on collagen-coated coverslip, from the same astroblastoma as in Figs. 9.178–9.182. Outgrowths are apparent, after 7 days *in vitro*, of flattened epithelial-like glial cells with processes. H&E, × 300.

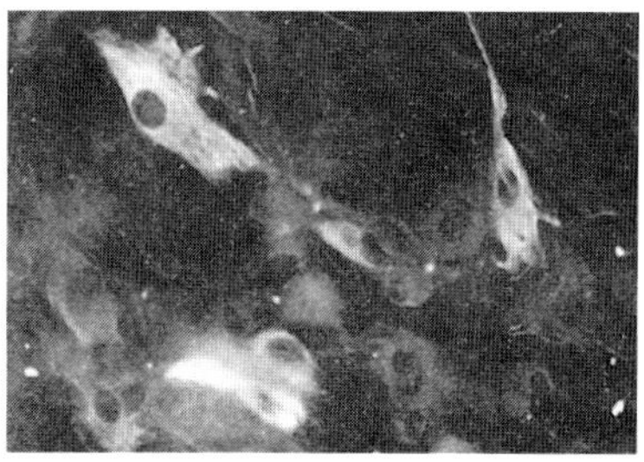

Fig. 9.184 Culture of same tumor as Fig. 9.183 after 16 days *in vitro*. GFAP indirect immunofluorescence (dilution 1:150), × 400

explants yielded outgrowths of flattened, angulated, triangular or quadrilateral cells with the epithelial features of early developing normal astrocytes *in vitro* (Fig. 9.183), but showing, by immunofluorescence, intense positivity for GFAP (Fig. 9.184). In an organ culture system, the explants preserved their perivascular papillary architecture, showed increased neuroglial fiber formation in long-standing cultures and retained their capacity for expressing GFAP. By electron microscopy, increased gliofibrillogenesis was evident in the cells of the older cultures, but some of the features seen at the apices of the cells of the original tumor, such as the long intercellular junctions of the zonula adherens type and the microrosettes, were maintained even after 8 months *in vitro*.

Biologic behavior

Quite apart from those examples that seem to represent a stage of anaplasia in astrocytomas, the natural history of the astroblastoma seems to place it between the astrocytoma and the glioblastoma. But the variability of the clinical outcome and the difficulty of separating those with a relatively more favorable evolution from those in which the course was progressive and fatal, as seen in the literature, have rendered their prognostic assessment a matter of considerable difficulty. Thus, some of the 25 cases described by Bailey and Bucy (1930) may well have been anaplastic astrocytomas, but in their case 12, for example, the patient was alive and well 7 years after the operative removal of a large solid and cystic parietal growth. In Bailey and Bucy's series, such a favorable outcome was exceptional, and the relative malignancy of the other examples in their series may well have been due to anaplasia. Similar difficulties in predicting prognosis were experienced by Elvidge, Penfield and Cone (1937), who, in their record of 13 astroblastomas (6%) in a series of 210 gliomas, found it hard to separate these tumors from astrocytoma, on the one hand, and glioblastoma, on the other. The clinicopathologic correlations that Rubinstein attempted to establish (Bonnin and Rubinstein, 1989) reinforced the suspicion that astroblastomas with histologic features indicative of anaplasia are susceptible to malignant progression to glioblastoma.

Among Rubinstein' reported cases of astroblastoma that showed relatively benign histologic features—a uniform cytologic pattern, rare mitotic figures and minimal or absent vascular endothelial proliferation—and where the subjects survived surgical resection, two patients, both of them children, were alive and well, the first after 12 years and the second after 20 years, and had no recurrences. In another case of this group, a 5-year-old girl with a cerebellar hemispheric astroblastoma experienced recurrence, with conversion to glioblastoma, 5 years after surgery. In addition, two of the patients in the other group—those harboring tumors with the high-grade histologic features mentioned above—showed progression to glioblastoma, one at 10 months and the other at 16 months after surgery, with further progression of one to a gliosarcoma. In the latter instance, the 13-year-old boy, with symptoms of the tumor predating surgical excision by at least 4 years, survived for 2½ years after the first operation. The lack of predictability of some of these tumors and the difficulty of correlating their histologic appearance with their subsequent clinical behavior are further emphasized by one case in which the morphologic picture was undoubtedly that of a malignant glioma, but the patient was known to be alive several years after the initial operation. In this case, in a 29-year-old female with a right frontal astroblastoma, multiple recurrences manifested themselves, in the area of previous craniotomy and partly beyond the site of the original tumor, after 8 years. Microscopically, the tumors were the picture of a pure astroblastoma, devoid of the large areas of anaplastic glioma and necrosis that were present in the initial growth. In a case reported by Kubota *et al.* (1985), a 30-year-old woman with a left frontoparietal astroblastoma was reported to be well and free of neurologic deficit 11 years after surgery. In a case reported by Husain and Leestma (1986), a 3-year-old girl had a clinical course extending over a 5-year period, punctuated by five surgical resections. Thus, the clinicopathologic correlates on this rare neoplasm are far from uniform.

Controversial or unresolved issues

As discussed on p. 415, useful prognostic criteria identifiable by light microscopy continue to challenge pathologists working with these posterior fossa ependymomas. Attention must now turn also to other methods and models with which to study this problem. Proliferation indices have yet to be thoroughly explored. Furthermore, the significance of finding SV40 large-T-antigen sequence homologies in ependymomas needs further validation and testing. Preliminary cytogenetic studies are beginning to uncover recurrent chromosomal abnormalities that clearly need further evaluation by the techniques of fluorescence *in situ* hybridization and comparative genomic hybridization. Xenogeneic models of human ependymomas offer the exciting potential of expanding the limited human biopsy material to provide tissues for biochemical, histochemical and chemotherapeutic analyses.

Alternatively, advances in the understanding of molecular mechanisms will increase our understanding of ependymogenesis by discovering increasingly specific characteristics of the ependymal phenotype. In this way, the embryonic cell of origin of the tanycyte and the subependymal glial cells will be discovered, and the peculiar histologic features of the astroblastoma and the myxopapillary ependymoma may be studied. Investigations into phenotypic differentiation may uncover mechanisms active in the subependymoma but not found in other ependymomas. These problems make the ependymal cell and its neoplastic counterpart areas of potentially fruitful investigation.

Glioblastomas multiforme

World Health Organization classification

In the 1993 WHO classification (Kleihues, Burger and Scheithauer, 1993), glioblastoma is considered to reside in the group of astrocytic gliomas. It includes the variants of giant-cell glioblastoma and gliosarcoma.

The currently accepted view of glioblastoma is that it is the manifestation, through a variable time span but usually within a fairly short duration, of rapidly progressive anaplasia in an astrocytoma, more rarely in an oligodendroglioma and rather often in a mixed astrocytoma–oligodendroglioma. The conceptual distinction between 'primary' and 'secondary' glioblastoma, already implicit in Scherer's observations in 1940 (Scherer, 1940a), retains some of its relevance today.

In molecular genetic terms, anaplastic progression in tumors results from successive mutations and failure of DNA to effect repair. In the course of this progression, phenotypic features appear that recapitulate, but may not be related to, stages of glial cytogenesis. Some of these were reflected in the older term 'spongioblastoma' that was given to this neoplasm. It is, however, well accepted that malignant progression is associated with a much wider range of phenotypic expression and that the latter may include the synthesis of abnormal cell products and the development of characteristics that may seem remote from the more conventional expectations of glial morphology. Clinically, although much is left to be discovered concerning critical events in the neoplastic progression of astrocytes, the continued practice of separating the anaplastic astrocytoma from the glioblastoma yields significant information.

Incidence

Some of the statistics on the relative frequency of glioblastomas among gliomas in general are discussed in the chapter on epidemiology (Chapter 1). Generally speaking, glioblastomas represent 15–20% of all intracranial tumors and account for about half the number of cerebral gliomas, but the range among different series is wide. The peak age for incidence is between 65 and 74 years (Greig *et al.*, 1990; Desmeules, Mikkelsen and Mao, 1992; Helseth, 1995; Polednak and Flannery, 1995). While decidedly rare before age 30 years, glioblastoma occurrence exempts no age, and cases may arise in childhood. Rubinstein (Russell and Rubinstein, 1989, pp. 219–47) compiled seven examples presenting within 2 months of birth (one being a gliosarcoma). Seven previously described congenital examples, arising in either a cerebral or a cerebellar hemisphere, were reviewed by Itoh *et al.* (1987) in their report of a personal case that originated in the right cerebellar hemisphere.

The sex distribution shows a preponderance of males, with the male:female distribution ranging from 2:1 to 3:2.

Association with other tumors and conditions

Rubinstein noted, at autopsy, five separate examples of glioblastoma occurring with an intracranial meningioma in a different area of the cerebrum (Russell and Rubinstein, 1989, p. 220). As both types of growth are relatively common, the association is almost certainly coincidental. The same argument is applicable to its concurrence with colloid cysts of the third ventricle, of which he described two examples, and with small pituitary adenomas. For a tabulation of reported cases of glioblastoma associated with other intracranial tumors in the same individual, the reader is referred to the review by Manuelidis and Solitare (1971).

An association of possibly greater significance is that of a glioblastoma or malignant astrocytoma with NF type 1, an association seen particularly with cerebellar astrocytomas. While only about 8% of cerebellar astrocytomas prove to be malignant in the general population, up to 50% of cerebellar astrocytomas in neurofibromatosis patients may show features of malignancy (Ilgren, Kinnier-Wilson and Stiller, 1985).

The occurrence of glioblastomas after cranial irradiation for unrelated primary tumors is rare, but several cases have been reported. The radiation doses ranged from as little as 24 Gy, given for prophylactic treatment of childhood leukemia, to 60 Gy, given for such tumors as craniopharyngioma and pituitary adenoma (Tsang *et al.*, 1993). The latency period varied from about 4 years to more than 20 years. Children irradiated for leukemia prophylaxis seemed to be especially susceptible to the development of subsequent glioblastoma. A comprehensive literature review has been presented by Shapiro, Mealey and Sartorius (1989).

Sites in the cerebrum

With glioblastoma, the white matter of the brain is characteristically involved and the distribution of the tumor is wide, arising with a site frequency in proportion to the amount of white matter present. It can generally be stated, however, that the anterior part of the brain is implicated far more frequently than the posterior and, in agreement with Zülch and Christensen (1956, pp. 1–702), the occipital lobes must be regarded as a rare site. The frontal lobes are most often involved (Fig. 9.185); in many examples, the tumor occupies more than one lobe. The deeper structures, particularly the corpus callosum, are often implicated. The 'butterfly' pattern, as seen in coronal sections, whereby a mass of growth in either cerebral hemisphere is linked to the opposite side through the corpus callosum, is highly characteristic (Fig. 186).

Various other combined sites of growth are also common, such as the temporal lobe in conjunction with the basal ganglia of the same hemisphere, and the occipital lobe with the splenium of the corpus

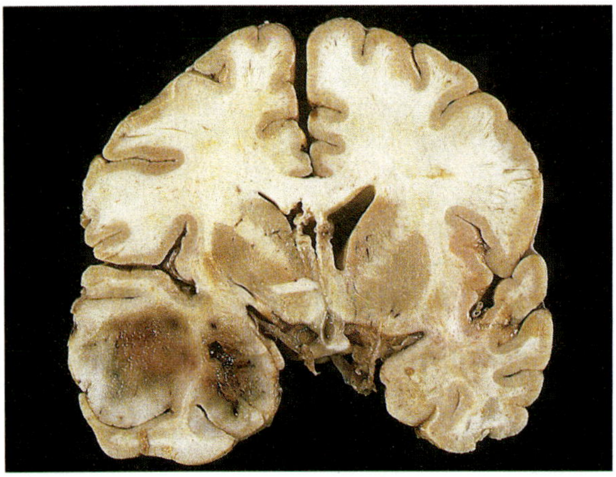

Fig. 9.185 Glioblastoma of left temporal lobe.

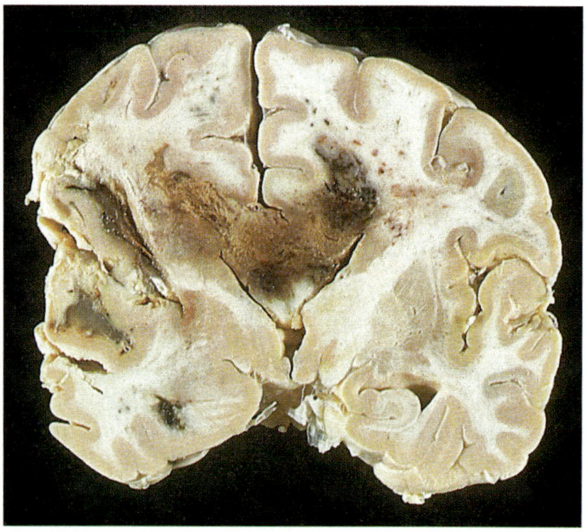

Fig. 9.186 Treated glioblastoma of the 'butterfly' type showing thickened corpus callosum with irregular extension of tumor into each frontal lobe.

callosum. Glioblastomas of the basal ganglia sometimes extend by way of the crus to involve the midbrain, or through the gray commissure to the thalamus of the opposite side.

After the frontal lobes, the temporal lobes are next in order of frequency of involvement. In contrast, Rubinstein noted that, in anaplastic astrocytomas, the temporal lobes may be relatively spared compared with other parts of the cerebrum (Russell and Rubinstein, 1989).

Other sites in the neuraxis

The more caudal parts of the brain, such as the brainstem and the cerebellum, are less often the site of glioblastomas, though pontine examples in children are well known. Mention has already been made of the occurrence of malignant astrocytomas in the cerebellum of patients with NF type 1. Though glioblastomas of the cerebellum are rare, this may be an associated site in those patients with multifocal gliomas.

The spinal cord is another site in which circumscribed glioblastomas may occasionally be encountered, usually occupying and expanding several cervical or thoracic segments. The data published by Slooff, Kernohan and MacCarty (1964, pp. 31–61) indicate that glioblastomas ('astrocytomas, grades 3 and 4') account for only 7.5% of primary spinal gliomas.

Macroscopic appearance

The affected part of the brain is expanded by a deceptively circumscribed mass, which, when restricted to a single lobe, tends to be more or less spherical. This is well displayed by the temporal lobe tumors. For the larger growths that involve several lobes or the central parts of the brain, the outlines are more irregular (Fig. 9.186). The 'butterfly' type has already been mentioned and provides an excellent example of this feature. The more superficially placed examples often penetrate the cortex, invade the adjacent leptomeninges and become attached to the dura (see p. 516). Those in the depths are apt to break through the ependyma and so pave the way to metastases via the CSF (see Figs 9.306 and 9.307). The glioblastomas involving the brainstem or the spinal cord may break through the pia into the subarachnoid space to spread and metastasize widely in the cerebrospinal pathways.

The *cut surfaces* are characteristically variegated. Opaque, creamy yellow areas resulting from necrosis or lipid change are typical and produce a mottled picture, contributed to also by recent and old hemorrhages. These are often associated with increased vascularization. Greatly thickened blood vessels may be occluded by thrombus, especially in or near the necrotic areas. Frequently, all but a peripheral rim of the tumor displays these features. The residual tissue is usually pinkish gray, often appears rather soft and granular, and merges with an irregular outer zone of firmer astrocytic growth. One or more cysts are often found; as a rule, they are small and contain clear yellow fluid or altered blood.

Several studies, including those of Burger (1983), have correlated these features with the appearances seen on CT scanning: the central areas of necrosis present as a variable, often extensive confluent region of low density, the surrounding zone of hypercellularity as a rim with marked contrast enhancement, and the outer region of peripheral tumor infiltration as a perilesional zone of low density. Systematic measurements have confirmed that the amount of viable tumor is often restricted to a narrow peripheral zone.

A feature stressed by McKeran and Thomas (1980) is the relatively extensive brain swelling and edema that may be associated with a tumor of relatively small size.

Information obtainable in the living patient by CT and MRI has intensified the importance of multifocality in glioblastomas. The problem is also relevant to the origin of tumor recurrence after apparently total resection of the localized growth.

The most reliable figures in the past have been obtained almost exclusively from postmortem studies. Scherer (1940b) claimed that as many as 20% of all cases of glioblastoma were multifocal. Such a high figure is difficult to accept. Courville (1936) found a multicentric origin in only 9.4% of his glioblastomas, and even this considerably lower incidence has not been confirmed by our experience or that of others (van Tassel, Lee and Bruner, 1988; Kyritsis *et al.*, 1993a). The descriptions of Scherer (1940b) and Courville (1936) leave open the alternative interpretations, in some of their cases, of either regional or ventricle-mediated metastases and of multiple foci of malignant progression proceeding in a diffuse astrocytoma. However, there is no doubt as to the existence of a percentage of cases in which true multicentricity can be satisfactorily established, as in the more recent well-documented studies by Barnard and Geddes (1987), van Tassel, Lee and Bruner (1988) and Kyritsis *et al.* (1993a).

Of greater significance as an expression of true multiplicity are those examples in which the tumors are widely separated, occupying different lobes or even different hemispheres. Before the routine use of sensitive radiologic imaging techniques, they were infrequent, and were described by Rubinstein (Russell and Rubinstein, 1989) in only four of a group of 173 cerebral gliomas of the astrocytic series (2.3%). This figure agreed with those subsequently published by Batzdorf and Malamud (1963) and Budka *et al.* (1980), the latter of whom reported an incidence of 3.1% of multiple tumors in 619 gliomas. Moertel, Dockerty and Baggenstoss (1961), in their analysis of necropsies at the Mayo Clinic, recorded 15 examples of multiple gliomas from a total of 305 subjects with verified tumors of this type, resulting therefore in a somewhat higher incidence of 4.9%. Using large hemispheric sections, Barnard and Geddes (1987) obtained the still appreciably higher incidence of 7.5% in 241 gliomas.

Two more recent studies, covering the period 1980–92 and using neuroradiologic imaging, showed an incidence of multiple gliomas ranging from 4.8% to 9.2% when cases of both synchronous (present at first examination) and metachronous (occurring only after treatment) tumors were included (van Tassel, Lee and Bruner 1988; Kyritsis *et al.*, 1993a). Nearly all of these cases were malignant gliomas. Only one low-grade astrocytoma was seen as multiple foci at presentation. About half the cases in each series showed multiple cerebral lesions at initial presentation. Since the incidence of multifocal malignant gliomas at first presentation seemed to be increased over the previous estimation of 1.1–2.5%, the authors hypothesize that the increased recognition may be due to improved imaging techniques. Another reason, with therapeutic implications, may be that these studies both required a tissue diagnosis of a brain tumor for treatment. In the past, the appearance of multiple lesions on radiologic imaging scans may have been presumed to represent systemic metastatic disease and have been treated as such, without biopsy. The apparent pattern of dissemination was analyzed radiologically by Kyritsis *et al.* (1993a) and found to be meningeal (57%), subependymal (24%), intraventricular (8%) and direct (11%). In 14 patients in the series (27%), however, no route of spread could be identified. Several additional isolated reports have been recently published emphasizing the occurrence of multifocal gliomas in which at least one of the foci is cerebellar (Kudo *et al.*, 1990; Salvati *et al.*, 1991; Kotwica and Papierz, 1992).

Radiographic appearance

The radiologic findings of glioblastoma multiforme reflect the heterogeneous findings seen on histopathology. Investigation by MRI demonstrates a poorly delineated mass exhibiting mixed signal intensity with areas of necrosis or cyst formation. The mass usually has low T1 signal intensity with areas of irregular, thick-walled enhancement post-contrast [Fig. 9.187(a)]. Areas of central necrosis have a decreased, or heterogeneous, enhancement pattern; intratumoral cysts do not enhance. On T2-weighted images, the mass demonstrates heterogeneous increased signal intensity, often defining the areas of cystic necrosis or cyst formation as higher T2 signal areas [Fig. 9.187(b)]. There is usually significant vasogenic edema. It may be difficult to define the margins of the mass in cases of more infiltrative tumor. Hemorrhage or blood products tend to identify anaplastic regions. Significant vasogenic edema, mass effect and/or herniation frequently accompany such an aggressive neoplasm. Spread of tumor along white matter tracks and

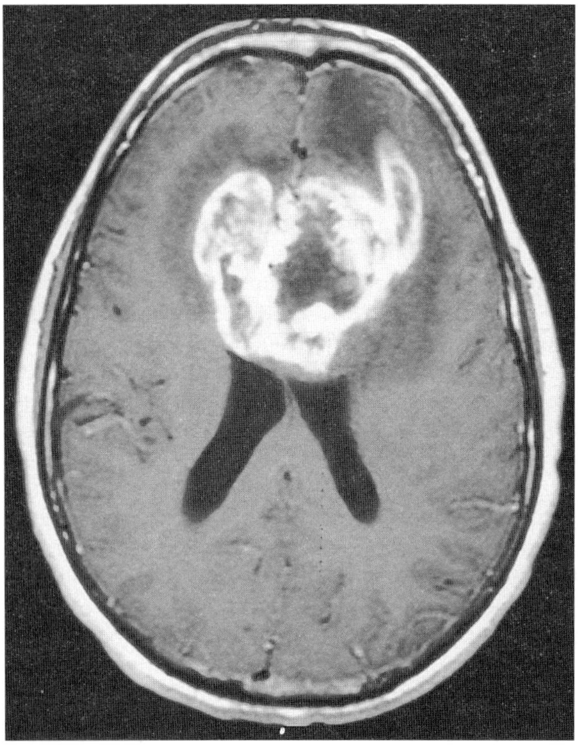

a

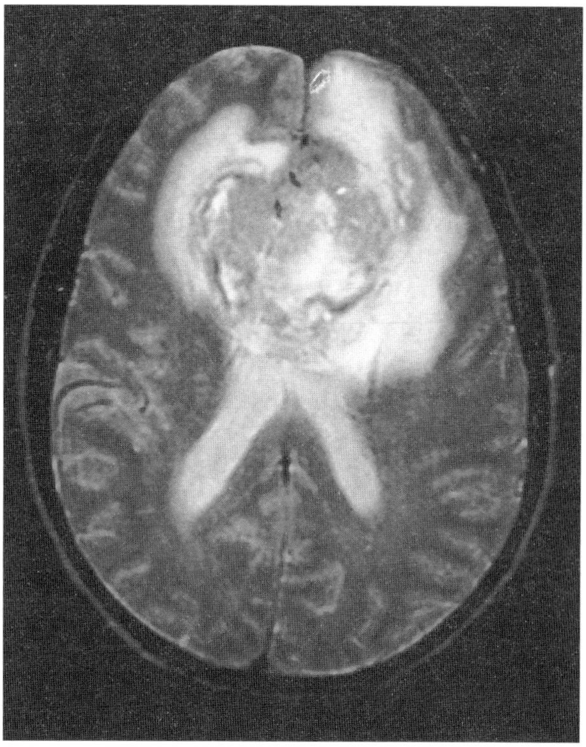

b

Fig. 9.187 Two MRIs of a 36-year-old man. (a) Axial T1-weighted postcontrast image demonstrates a large enhancing mass in both frontal lobes, with areas of cystic necrosis centrally. Noted peripherally are areas of low T1 signal indicating vasogenic edema. There is marked mass effect on both lateral ventricles. (b) Axial T2-weighted image demonstrates the complex signal intensity within the large mass. The areas of cystic necrosis demonstrate somewhat higher T2 signal. Peripherally, around the tumor, are areas of vasogenic edema. Anteriorly, two flow voids demonstrate encapsulated vessels. This appearance is typical for a large aggressive glioblastoma multiforme tumor. The dense enhancement, vasogenic edema, areas of cystic necrosis and ability to cross the corpus callosum are characteristic.

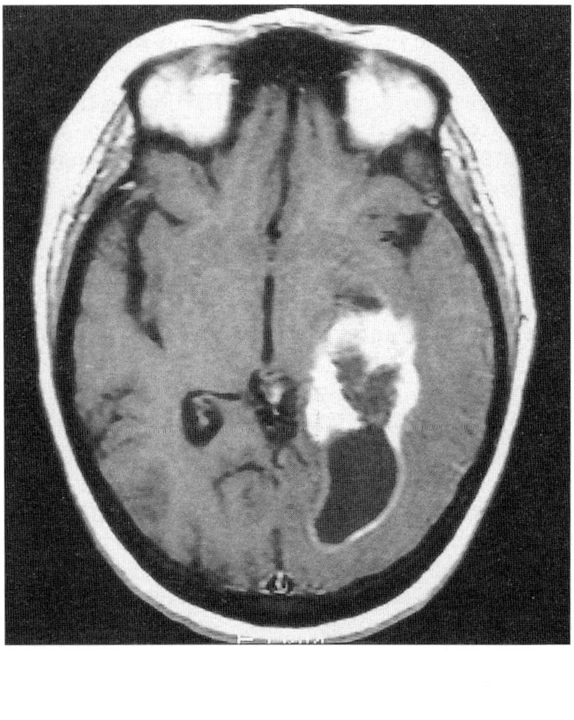

Fig. 9.188 Axial T1-weighted postcontrast MRI of a 45-year-old woman with a left periventricular and posterior basal ganglion mass. Dense, irregular enhancement is noted with a central area of necrosis. Note the abnormal enhancement around the trapped occipital horn, which is dilated. This represents subependymal extension of glioblastoma multiforme.

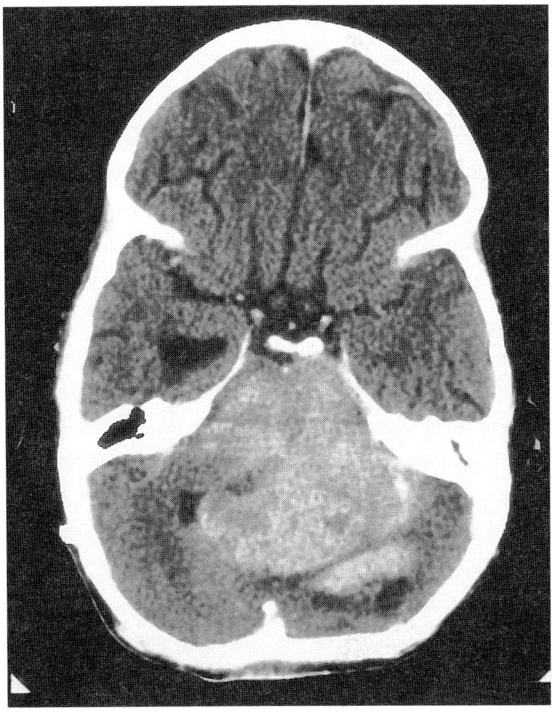

Fig. 9.189 Axial postcontrast CT image of 6-year-old girl demonstrating a very large enhancing mass in the posterior fossa. This mass involves the pons, cerebellar peduncles and much of the adjacent cerebellum. The fourth ventricle is deviated posteriorly to the right side. Cystic areas of lower density are noted within the mass, which has intense but mildly heterogeneous enhancement. There is also marked mass effect with exophytic encasement of the basilar artery by the mass. Obstructive hydrocephalus is suggested since the right temporal horn is dilated. This case represents glioblastoma multiforme involving the pons and left cerebellar peduncle.

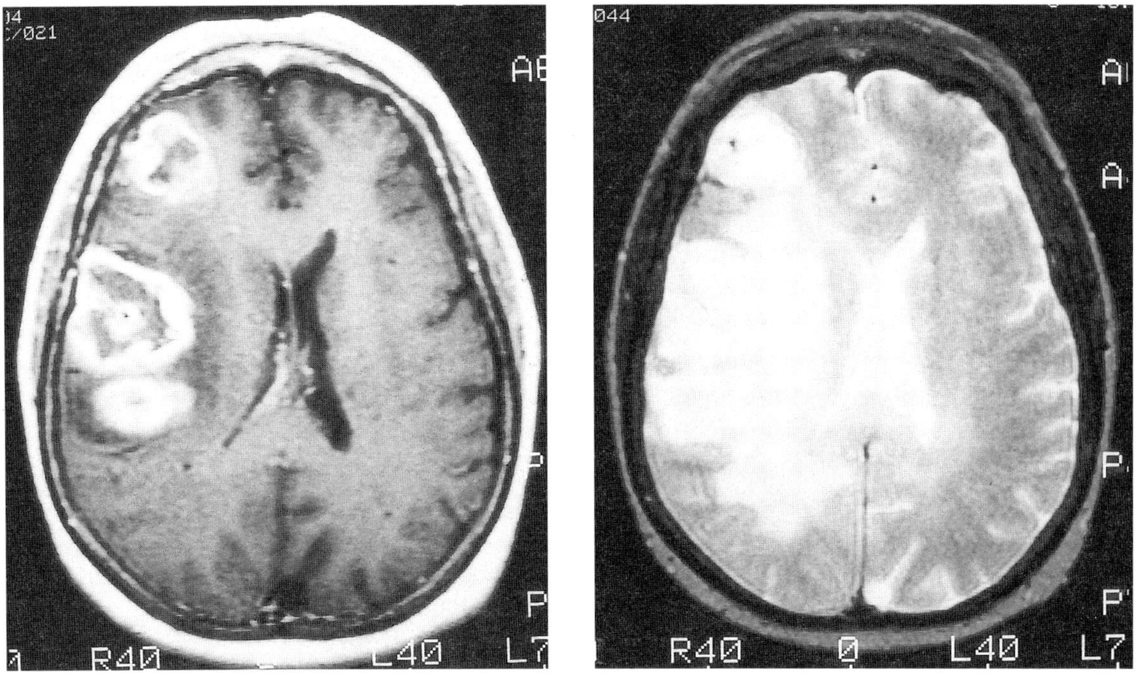

a b

Fig. 9.190 Two MRIs of a 65-year-old female. (a) Axial T1-weighted postcontrast image demonstrates three areas of enhancement in the right frontal lobe. There is surrounding low T1 signal indicating edema, and mass effect is noted on the ipsilateral lateral ventricle. The dense, irregular, thick-walled enhancement with central necrosis suggests high-grade neoplasm. (b) Axial T2-weighted image demonstrates the high T2 signal intensity surrounding the areas of enhancement. This case represents multicentric glioblastoma multiforme. The areas of high T2 signal indicate areas of vasogenic edema and infiltrating tumor along the ventricular ependyma is commonly seen (Fig. 9.188); leptomeningeal disease or CSF seeding may also occur. Extension across the corpus callosum may occur, resulting in the so-called 'butterfly' pattern (Fig. 9.187).

At CT scanning, heterogeneous density is frequently seen, with the hypercellular components being slightly dense to isodense and areas of cystic necrosis being relatively hypodense (Fig. 9.189). Enhancement with contrast is seen in most cases, defining an irregular thickened rim of the tumor. Calcification, better seen by CT, is an infrequent finding.

At angiography, most tumors are hypervascular with prominent neovascularity, tumor blush and irregular pooling of contrast. Areas of arteriovenous shunting and early draining veins are commonly seen. There may be recruitment of adjacent vessels.

Multicentric gliomas usually are found to have anaplastic features histologically. Multiple areas of abnormal enhancement frequently have connecting areas of edema or nonenhancing tumor seen at CT scanning and MRI (Fig. 190). Frequently, there is infiltrative tumor within these areas of abnormal density and signal, with subsequent breakdown of blood–brain barrier to demonstrate contrast enhancement.

Microscopic appearance

As the term 'multiforme' implies, the salient feature is the diversity of cell forms encountered. This, together with the dense cellularity of the tumor and the presence of focal necroses, often makes the diagnosis obvious at first glance.

However, the variability from field to field and between different examples within the group as a whole precludes the assimilation of the tumor into a single histologic picture. In the majority of cases, but to a variable extent, many of the fields show anaplastic astrocytic features of a gemistocytic, fibrillary or pilocytic character, as illustrated in Figs 9.2, 9.27 and 9.42. One of the hallmark features is the high density of small, poorly differentiated cells in which the picture of monomorphic anaplasia is superimposing itself upon spindle-shaped neoplastic astrocytes (Fig. 9.191). In some areas, these fusiform cells may be packed into short interwoven bundles, but they frequently and characteristically exhibit what is commonly called 'pseudopalisading' (Fig. 9.192): the cells are arranged side by side in rows and their processes are directed toward a central area of necrosis. If the necrosis is large, the pseudopalisades are long and undulating; but sometimes the focus is very small, and the palisade is more in the nature of a rosette. These elongated cells, with their fine tapering processes, previously interpreted as 'spongioblasts', are clearly neoplastic astrocytes, as they can be shown to express GFAP and to contain neuroglial fibrils (Fig. 9.193). This histologic pattern in an astrocytic neoplasm is diagnostic for glioblastoma, and its prevalence is indicated by Rubinstein's estimate of its occurrence in 83% of the tumors in this category (Russell and Rubinstein, 1989).

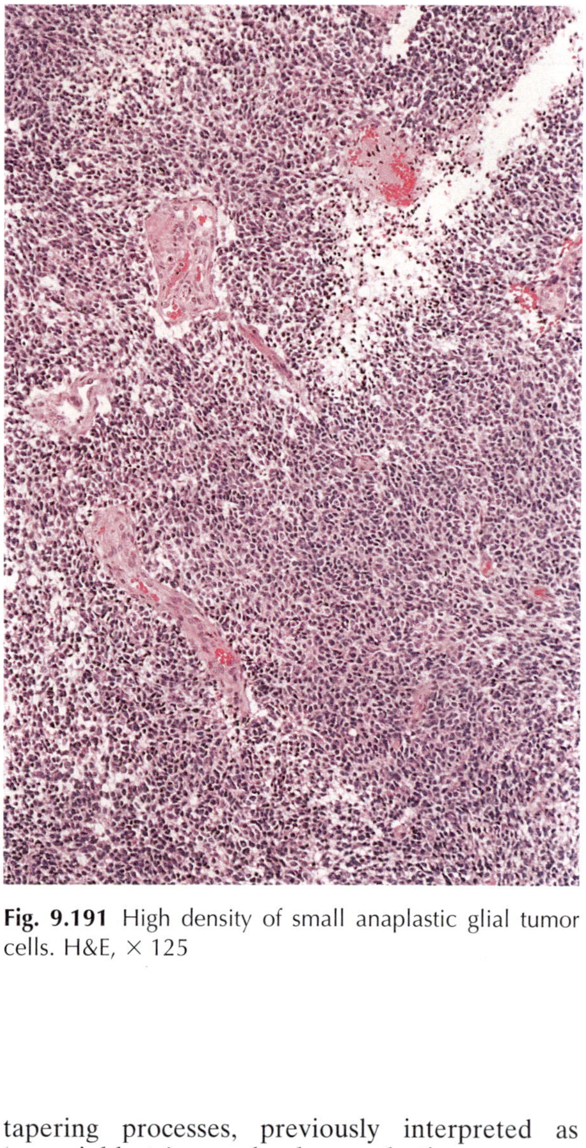

Fig. 9.191 High density of small anaplastic glial tumor cells. H&E, × 125

In other fields, the anaplastic features are expressed as a marked polymorphism of the tumor cells, including the presence of giant and multinucleated forms (Fig. 9.194). In some examples, these may be so conspicuous as to seem to dominate the picture, but, even so, they usually do not form the majority of the cells. One variant is largely composed of monster giant cells. Reactivity for GFAP, however, proves these also to have an astrocytic phenotype.

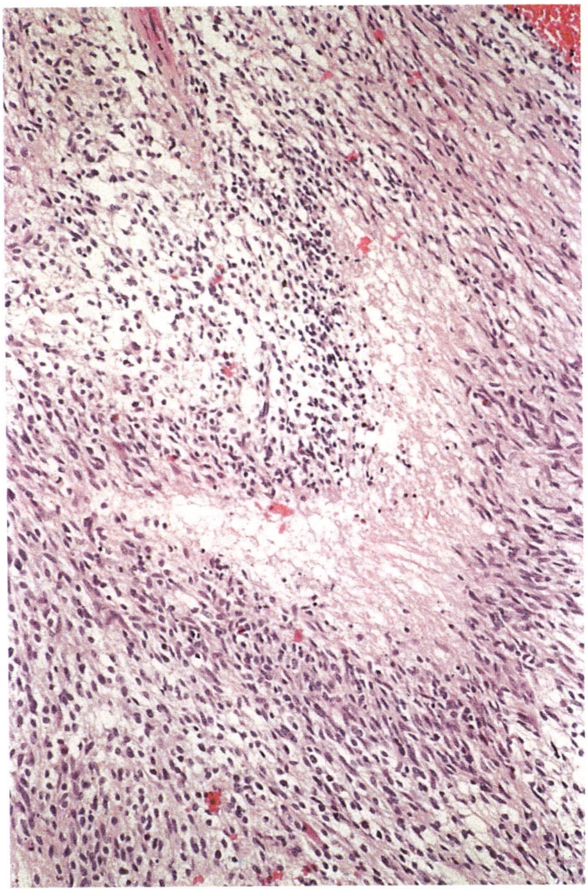

Fig. 9.192 Small tumor cells forming palisades around a necrotic central focus. H&E, × 125

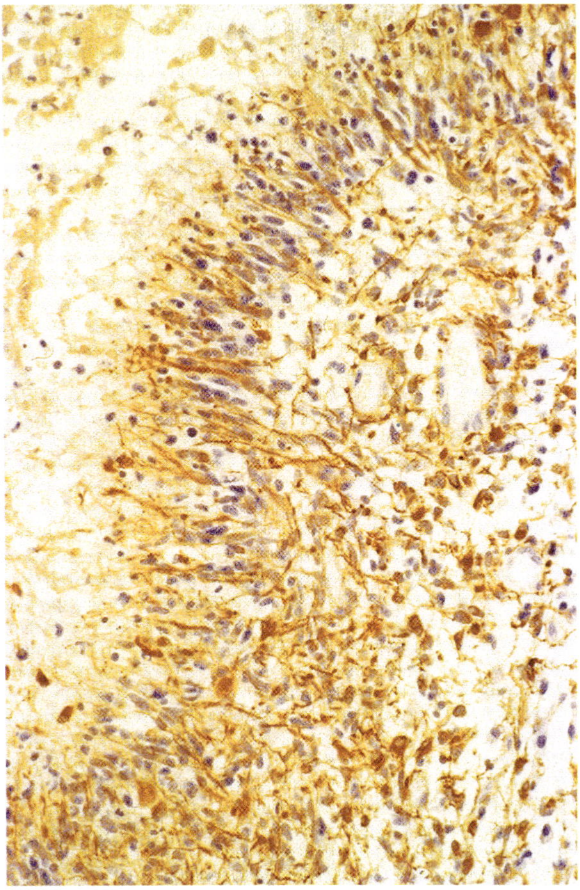

Fig. 9.193 The astrocytic character of the palisading tumor cells demonstrated by positive cytoplasmic reactivity GFAP. GFAP immunoperoxidase, × 250

Finally, the diagnostic picture must take into account the almost pathognomonic frequency of microvascular proliferation, both within and adjacent to the tumor (Fig. 9.195).

Vascular changes

These form an important and characteristic part of the microscopic picture (Barker *et al.*, 1996). Some degree of microvascular proliferation is present in 95% of glioblastomas. While almost pathognomonic for these neoplasms, it may, however, also be met in other types of glioma. In a diffuse cerebral astrocytoma, microvascular proliferation should be regarded as a sign of anaplasia. On the other hand, in a cerebellar astrocytoma, a pilocytic astrocytoma of the hypothalamic region or an oligodendroglioma, it does not, by itself, carry any premonitory significance. It is apparent in any event that this feature may, to some extent, accompany all types of intracerebral neoplasms, including metastatic carcinomas.

The proliferation affects the smallest blood vessels, mainly the capillaries, which are numerically increased. Although this microvascular proliferation has long been considered as proliferation of endothelial cells, recent immunohistologic studies have suggested a major contribution of pericytes and/or vascular smooth muscle cells (Haddad *et al.*, 1992b; Wesseling *et al.*, 1995). The vessels, some of which retain their thin-walled structure, become excessively convoluted and form masses that resemble renal glomerular tufts (Fig. 9.195). Often, these convoluted capillaries are arranged in a linear band that may extend over several low-power fields. They are then frequently aligned to large areas of necrosis, but are usually not accompanied by any regional increase in the density of the tumor cells

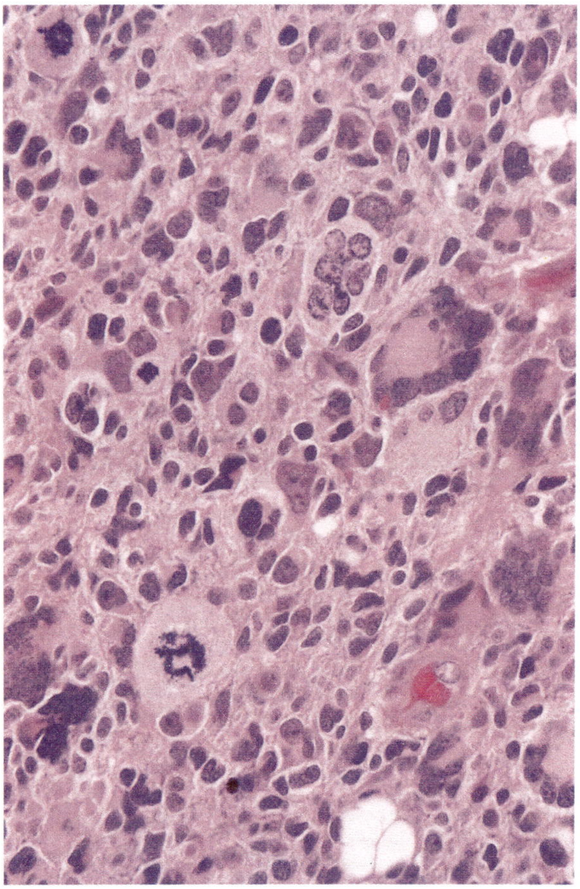

Fig. 9.194 Cellular pleomorphism, with multinucleated giant cells containing hyperchromatic irregular nuclei. H&E, × 500

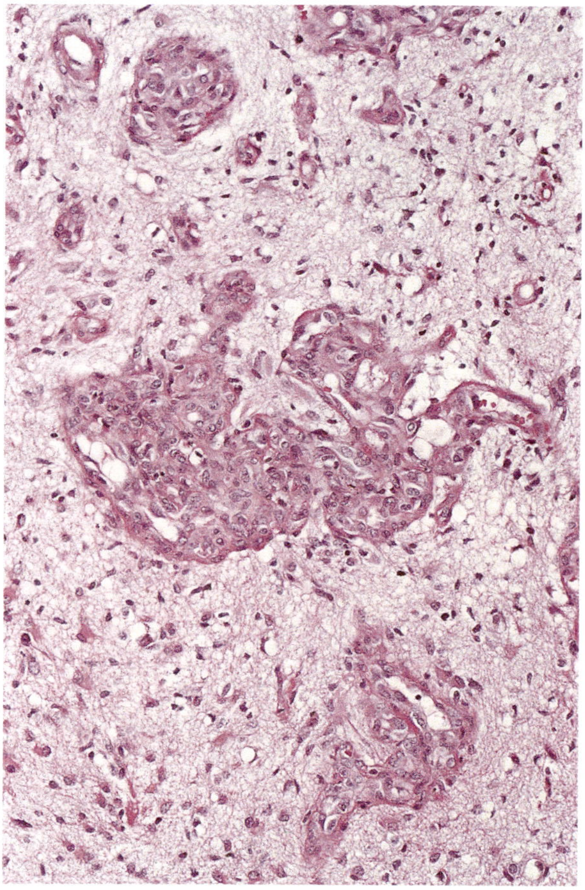

Fig. 9.195 Microvascular proliferation in brain immediately adjacent to tumor. H&E, × 250

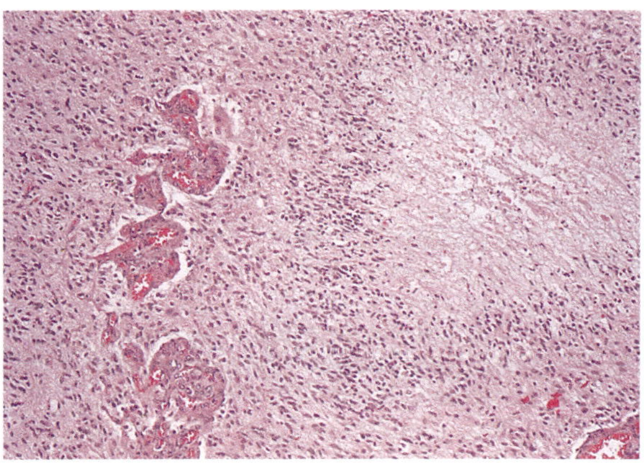

Fig. 9.196 Linear band of proliferative vessels forming an arcade associated with tumor necrosis and palisading cells. H&E, × 125

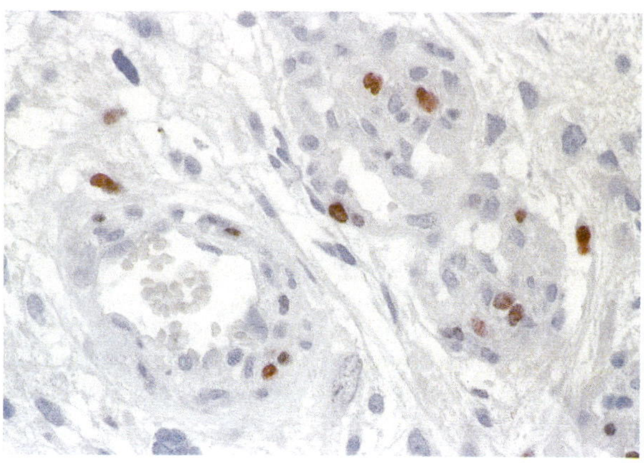

Fig. 9.197 Nuclear labeling for BrdU in the proliferating vascular cells of a glioblastoma. BrdU immunoperoxidase, × 500

(Fig. 9.196). The proliferating vascular cells are plump and often show mitotic activity. Indeed, an autoradiographic study of rat gliomas induced by an avian sarcoma virus has shown that these cells may have a higher LI of DNA synthesis than the glioma cells (Groothuis *et al.*, 1980). On the other hand, the more recent observations by Nagashima, Hoshino and Cho (1987) on human glioblastomas labeled for the S phase with a monoclonal antibody against BrdU, while indicating an appreciably higher than normal LI of 4.5% for the vascular components, showed it to be lower than that of the tumor cells themselves (9.9%) (Fig. 9.197).

With the electron microscope, this proliferation is seen to be accompanied by a reduplication of the capillary basement membrane, thus creating an abnormal perivascular space containing connective tissue fibers and cells (Luse, 1960). Focal discontinuities and reduplication of the outer basement membrane—also described by Luse and noted by Raimondi (1966)—produce a partial incorporation of the glial cells into the outer part of the blood vessel wall, a feature independently confirmed by the detailed studies of Nyström (1960) on the capillary changes in glioblastomas. Actual penetration of the vascular lumen by glial tumor cells has been claimed by some observers (Kung, Lee and Bakay, 1969), but could not be confirmed by others (Weller, Foy and Cox, 1977). Tracer studies have demonstrated various degrees of patency in the endothelial junctional complexes, and these have been held partly to account for the blood–brain barrier abnormalities found in malignant gliomas (Long, 1970).

Different mechanisms have been invoked to explain these proliferative changes. To attribute them, as argued by Storring and Duguid (1954), to intravascular thrombosis with subsequent organization and recanalization, does not adequately explain what is seen. The deposition of fibrin thrombus, completely or incompletely filling the lumen, is sometimes found in the small arteries or arterioles of glioblastomas and may be associated with fibrinoid necrosis in the walls of the vessels. Occlusion of the larger arteries leads to great collagenous thickening of their walls. Later stages in the organization of mural thrombi result in the local formation of small cushions of endothelial cells, but the appearances are readily distinguishable from the more prevalent diffuse microvascular proliferation in capillaries, the walls and lumens of which are quite free from fibrin. The two processes appear quite independent of one another; the thrombotic complications are more apt to occur in the central areas of necrosis, while microvascular proliferation may be most conspicuous near the periphery and even extend beyond the actual confines of the tumor. Many observers, including Scherer (1935b), have suggested that vascular proliferation heralds the growth of the neoplasm. A sequence depicting the progression of this feature, preceding the growth of a glioblastoma as it advances toward, and then ruptures through, the ventricular ependyma, has been illustrated elsewhere (Rubinstein, 1972b, Figs 50–53).

The phenomenon is not restricted to the growth of malignant gliomas within the central neuraxis. Rubinstein has also illustrated (Rubinstein, 1972b, Fig. 54) a marked degree of microvascular proliferation among gemistocytic astrocytes occupying a cervical lymph node in the case of a glioblastoma that metastasized extracranially (reported by Labitzke, 1962), and a similar finding was noted by Nigogosyan, De La Pava and Pickren (1962) in the pulmonary metastases of their case. It is uncertain whether the proliferating microvascular cells originated from the metastatic transfer of stromal elements from within the brain tumor, or whether they resulted from stroma-inductive properties on the part of the metastasizing glial cells on the infiltrated extraneural tissues.

The roles of various growth factors in this proliferative vascular change is a subject of intense investigation and is discussed in detail in Chapter 3.

Electron microscopy

As might be expected, the cell shape, cell size and nuclear configuration show a considerable degree of pleomorphism, stressed by many observers (Luse, 1960; Raimondi, Mullan and Evans, 1962; Raimondi, 1966; Zülch and Wechsler, 1968). A marked increase in the number of mitochondria was noted by Luse and by Raimondi; mitochondrial enlargement and the presence of highly atypical cristae have also been documented (Tani *et al.*, 1971). Intranuclear inclusions, representing cytoplasmic invaginations, are fairly common (Robertson and MacLean, 1965). Irregularly elongated or concentrically arranged, usually juxtanuclear, membranous stacks, consisting of closely apposed cisternae and possibly being of nuclear origin, have been described as present in the cytoplasm (Tani and Ametani, 1971). Luse (1960) first noted the frequency with which the cytoplasmic membrane shows plications. Scanning electron microscopy vividly documents the ruffling of the cell surface (Fig. 9.198), a feature of the malignant cell that is presumably associated with increased motility and metabolic activity of the cell membrane (see discussions by Pontén, 1975; and Collins, 1983).

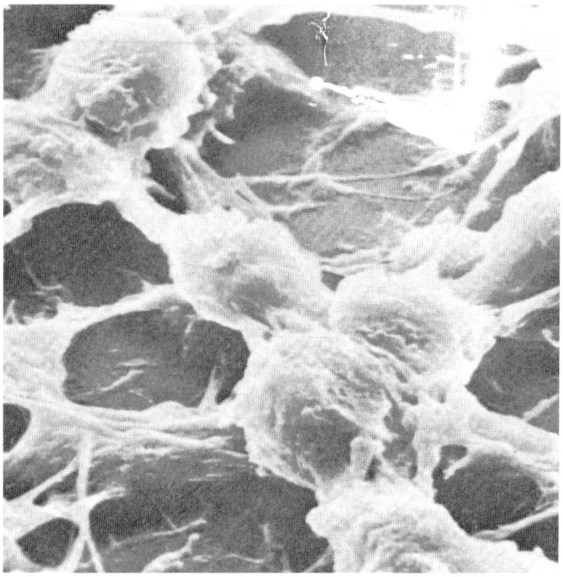

Fig. 9.198 Scanning electron micrograph of tumor cells in a glioblastoma, showing delicate ruffling of cell surfaces. × 2500 (Courtesy of Dr A. Arnold)

The presence of compact bundles of cytoplasmic filaments, measuring 8–10 nm in diameter and identifying the tumor cells as astrocytes, varies according to their degree of differentiation (Fig. 9.199). The smaller anaplastic cells tend to lack filaments.

Immunohistochemistry

The astrocytic nature of the cells can virtually always be confirmed, at least in the less anaplastic areas and often, unexpectedly, in some of the less differentiated elements, by the presence of GFAP (Fig. 9.200). There is general agreement that the number of GFAP-positive cells is inversely proportional to the anaplastic character of astrocytic neoplasms (Deck *et al.*, 1978; Eng and Rubinstein, 1978; van der Meulen, Houthoff and Ebels, 1978; Duffy *et al.*, 1980; Velasco *et al.*, 1980; Pasquier *et al.*, 1983). Phosphotungstic acid–hematoxylin staining may fail to reveal glial fibers. It does not necessarily correlate with, and has largely been supplanted by, immunostaining for GFAP (Deck

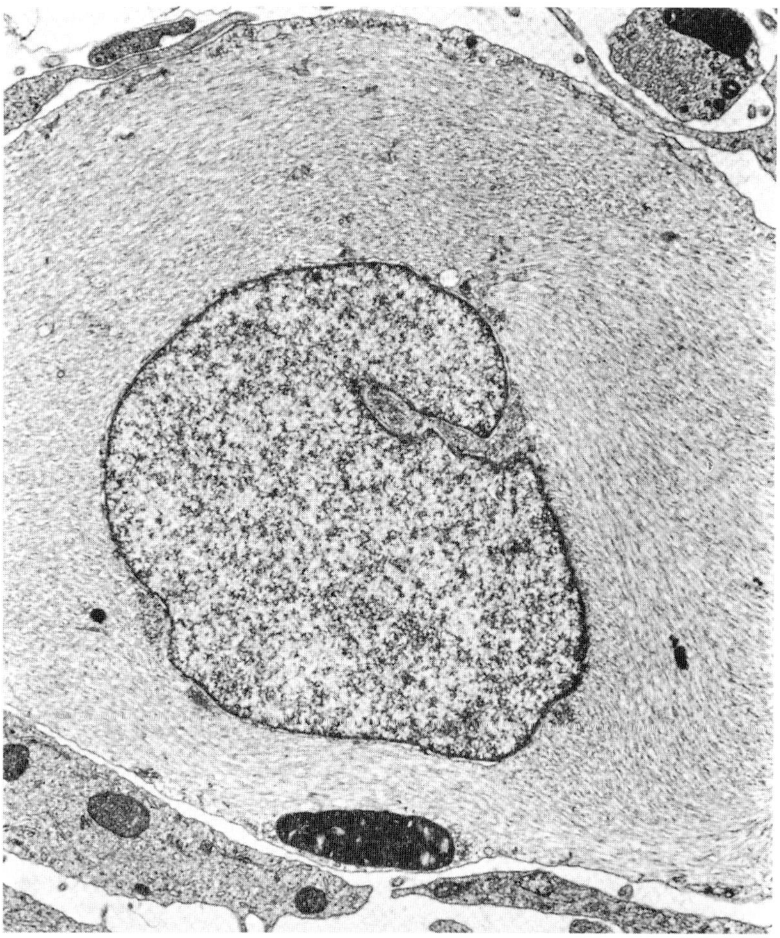

Fig. 9.199 Glioblastoma cultured for 20 days on sponge foam. The cytoplasm of the tumor cell is packed with glial filaments, which displace the other organelles to the periphery. × 16 000 (Courtesy of Dr J.C. Sipe and Dr Mary M. Herman and reprinted from the *American Journal of Pathology*, 1973, pp. 588–606, figure 6 with kind permission of the American Society for Investigative Pathology.)

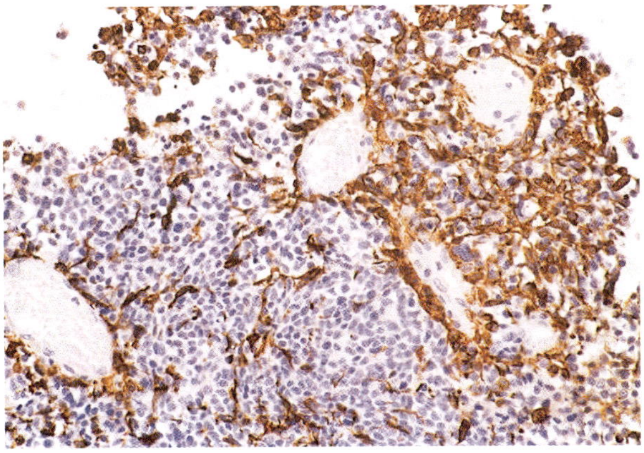

Fig. 9.200 A small-cell glioblastoma growing in the leptomeninges. This tumor retains an astrocytic phenotype demonstrated by its cytoplasmic reactivity for GFAP. GFAP immunoperoxidase, × 250

et al., 1978; De Armond, Eng and Rubinstein, 1980). The immunohistochemical detection of GFAP has, therefore, been especially valuable with respect to some of the atypical variants of glioblastoma.

Several reports have recently confirmed the expression of keratin proteins and mRNA in gliomas (Ng and Lo, 1989; Franke *et al.*, 1991; Cosgrove *et al.*, 1993; Kashima, Vinters and Campagnoni, 1995). The protein has been found by using Western blot analysis and using immunohistochemistry on frozen and paraffin-embedded tissue sections. The RNA was detected by using Northern blot analysis.

Atypical features and variants of glioblastoma

Because of the emphasis on the astrocytic origin of this neoplasm, the considerable variability of its cytologic picture has sometimes been underestimated. It is, however, readily apparent that the glioblastoma cell may show morphologic features that extend well beyond those traditionally associated with an astrocytic or even a glial cell. These atypical features may, in some cases, cause considerable diagnostic difficulties.

In some instances, as in the two examples reported by Kornfeld (1986), the tumor is largely composed of granular-appearing cells (Fig. 9.201). The recognition of these cases, termed 'granular-cell glioblastoma', depends upon the demonstration of features transitional to neoplastic astrocytes and upon the confirmation of the glial origin of the granular cells by the immunopositivity of these transitional forms for GFAP.

The same criteria are applicable to another variant, characterized by the presence of large amounts of intracellular *lipid* (Figs 9.202 and 9.203). Three instances have been described in detail (Kepes and Rubinstein, 1981). These tumors, situated deep within the brain and containing areas of necrosis, should be distinguished from the group of considerably more benign pleomorphic xanthoastrocytomas. Occasionally, a heavily lipidized glioblastoma of this kind may consist chiefly of large numbers of uni- and multinucleated giant or monster cells, as in the example reported by Gherardi *et al.* (1986). Rubinstein (Russell and Rubinstein, 1989) also described a glioblastoma in a 34-year-old woman (case submitted by Dr R. Schober), and one of us (J.M.B.) has seen a separate case in a 26-year-old woman, in which the tumor contained foci of cells that were heavily lipidized in some areas and granular in others.

Reference has already been made, in the histologic description of the classic glioblastoma, to the frequency with which small, closely packed anaplastic cells demonstrate features transitional to fusiform glial cells. Other fields may consist of *solid cellular trabeculae and clusters* of almost epithelial appearance (Fig. 9.204). The same development has been noted and illustrated by Budka, Podreka and Zaunbauer (1979) and Galloway and Roessmann (1986). When present, these features are often seen in the immediate vicinity of a rich mesenchymal stroma. A biphasic histologic pattern will then result, in which the separation of groups of apparently clear-cut, small anaplastic cells within a malignant astrocytoma may, at first, invite the suspicion of metastatic carcinoma in a glioma. However, the presence of GFAP clearly identifies these epithelial-like formations as glial. The diagnostic problem may further be compounded by the development, in these anaplastic foci, of a cribriform pattern or of trabeculae and pseudoacinar structures (Fig. 9.205) as documented by Kepes, Fulling and Garcia (1982) in five examples of mixed glioblastoma and fibrosarcoma. Rubinstein also described, in two cases (one glioblastoma and one mixed glioblastoma and fibrosarcoma), a *papillary* pattern formed by low- and medium-sized columnar cells, occasionally stratified and resting on a delicate vascular connective tissue stroma, in which the general histologic features closely resembled those of a medulloepithelioma (Mørk, Rubinstein and Kepes, 1988). Unlike those of the cerebral medulloepithelioma, however, the papillary formations contain cells that are positive for GFAP (Fig. 9.206).

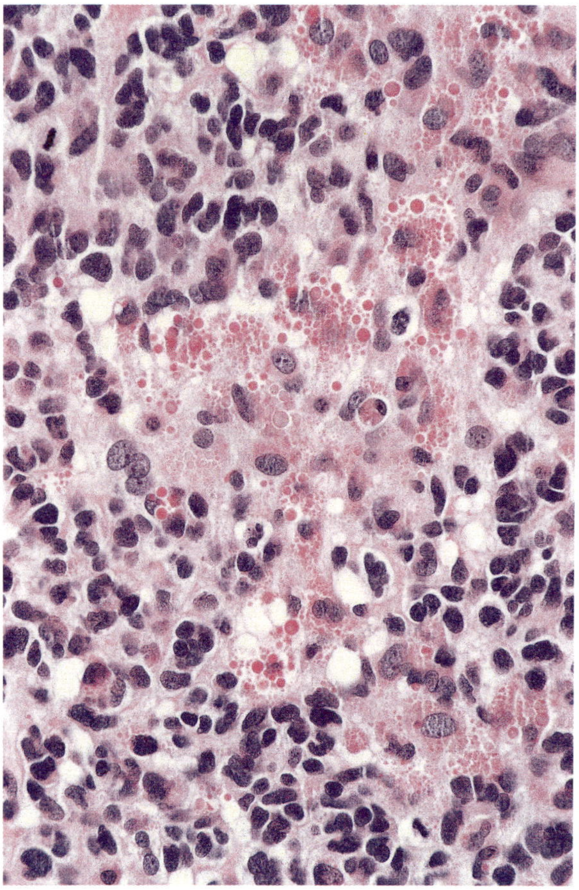

Fig. 9.201 Granular cells in a glioblastoma. H&E, × 500.

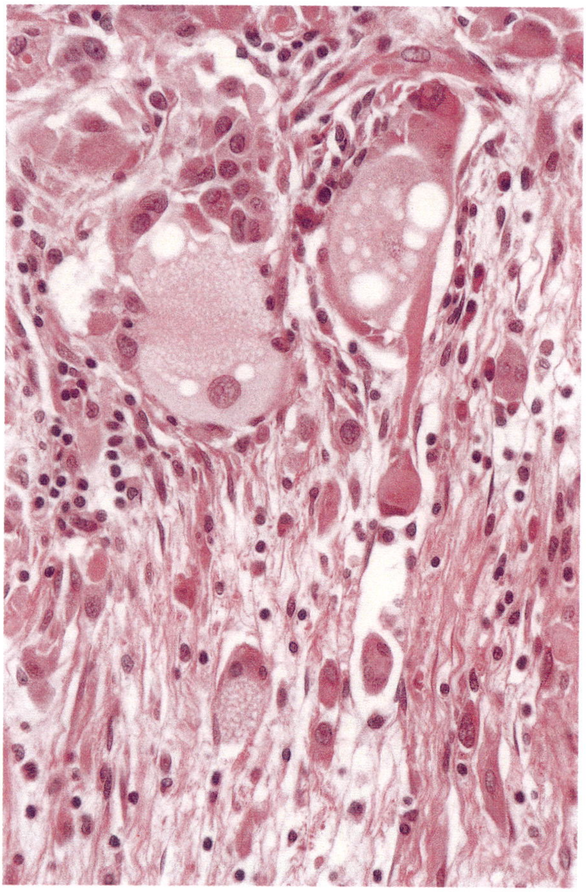

Fig. 9.202 Glioblastoma with lipidization of tumor cells. H&E, × 500

Finally, these epithelial-like foci may show, as described in six patients studied by Mørk *et al.* (1988), focal squamous changes, with keratinization and even epithelial pearl formation. These foci may also be recognized by antibodies to EMA (Fig. 9.207). In this study, immunoperoxidase stains for cytokeratins were positive in five tumors and correlated well with squamous-cell morphology (Fig. 9.208).

This development, therefore, seems to represent an extreme form of epithelial metaplasia originating in the multipotential more primitive cells of a glioblastoma. Its recognition is of importance if the misinterpretation of carcinomatous deposits in a malignant glioma, reinforced by too exclusive a reliance on the immunomorphologic demonstration of cell-related intermediate filament proteins, is to be avoided.

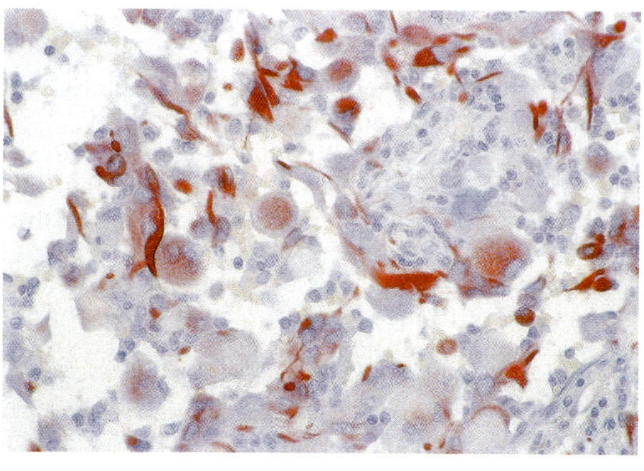

Fig. 9.203 Same case as Fig. 9.202. Positive reactivity for GFAP confirms the astrocytic character of the lipidized cells. GFAP immunoperoxidase, × 500

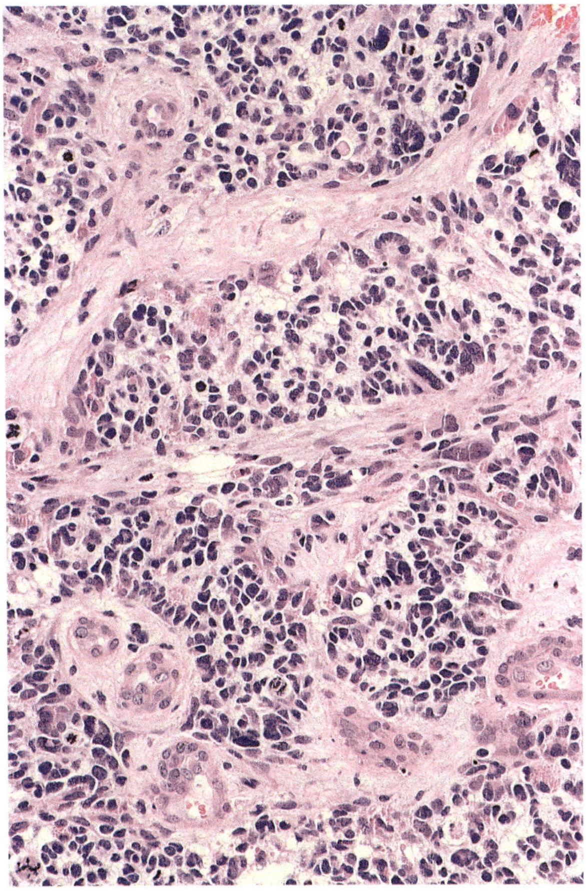

Fig. 9.204 Well-circumscribed foci of densely cellular anaplasia arranged in epithelial-like formations within a glioblastoma. H&E, × 250

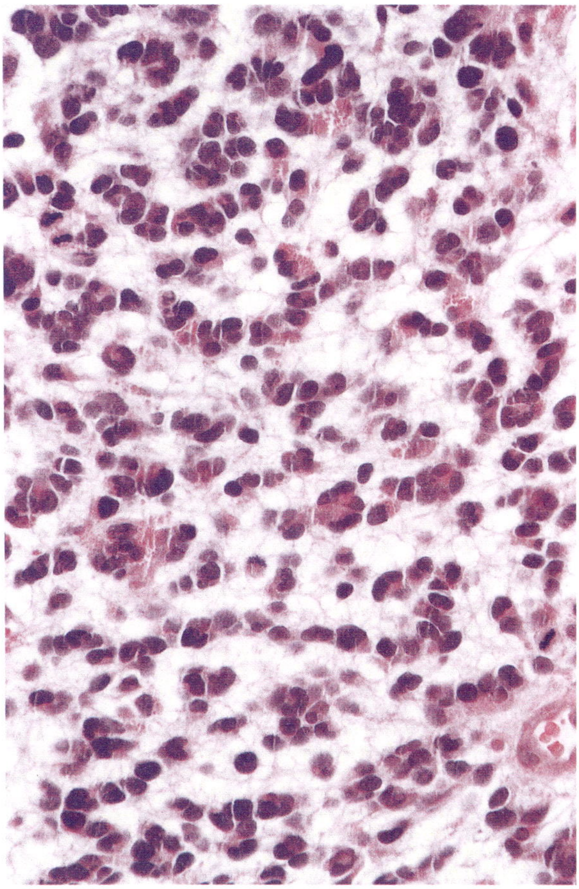

Fig. 9.205 Trabecular pattern of cell arrangement in a glioblastoma. H&E, × 500

As noted by Kepes, Fulling and Garcia (1982) and Mørk *et al.* (1988), these epithelial structures seem to be especially associated with gliosarcomas. However, they can be seen in uncomplicated glioblastomas. An additional series of lipidized and epithelial glioblastomas with an aggressive biologic behavior has been reported (Rosenblum, Erlandson and Budzilovich, 1991).

Giant-cell glioblastomas

In the description of the microscopic appearances of glioblastomas in all their variety, mention is made of multinucleated giant cells. Although these may be conspicuous in places, they usually are not numerically preponderant. Occasionally, they are a sequel of radiation therapy, in which case similar giant cells may then also be seen in more benign gliomas, but unaccompanied by other features of anaplasia.

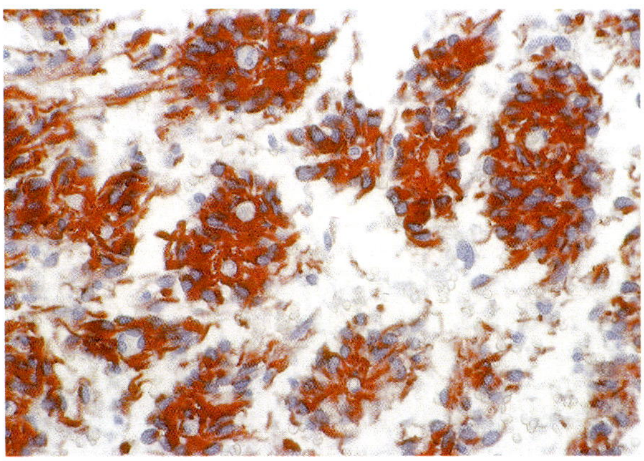

Fig. 9.206 Perivascular papillary arrangements of glioblastoma cells with strong cytoplasmic reactivity for GFAP. GFAP immunoperoxidase, × 500

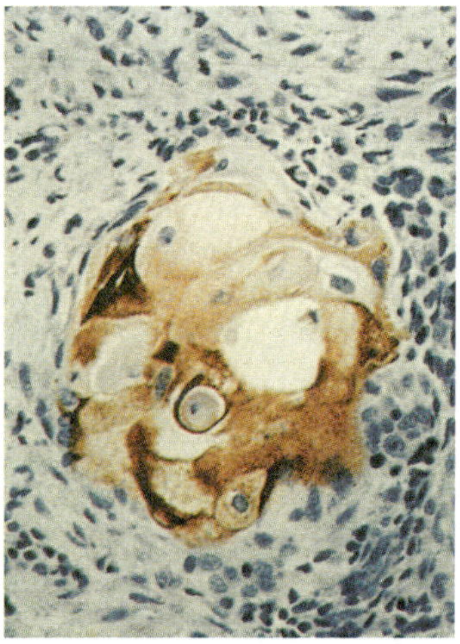

Fig. 9.207 Squamous metaplasia, with epithelial pearl formation, in the gliomatous portion of a gliosarcoma. EMA immunoperoxidase, × 240

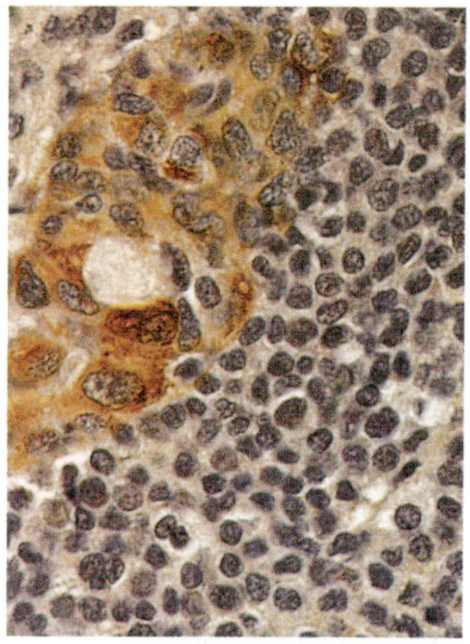

Fig. 9.208 Squamous metaplasia in anaplastic cells of a glioblastoma. Cytokeratin immunoperoxidase, × 360 (Courtesy of Dr John J. Kepes)

We are concerned here, however, with what we regard as a glioblastoma subtype: a group of rare tumors in which the component cells, as a whole, are abnormally large and include multinucleated forms of monster size. Their interpretation, provocatively discussed by Scherer (1935a), has long been controversial. They have been variously designated as ganglioglioneuroma (Schmincke, 1914; Paul, 1926), ganglioglioblastoma (Wätjen, 1930), spongioblastoma multiforme ganglioides (Foerster and Gagel, 1931), ganglioglioma (Courville, 1931), retothelial sarcoma (Foot and Cohen, 1933), spongioneuroblastoma (Globus, 1938, case 17) or malignant ganglioneuroma (Allegra and Serra, 1950). Zülch (Tönnis and Zülch, 1939) earlier regarded them as a variety of glioblastoma ('glioblastoma gigantocellulare ganglioides'), but subsequently interpreted them as 'monstrocellular sarcomas' (Zülch and Christensen, 1956, pp. 1–702) and attributed their origin to the cerebral blood vessels. Again, because of their cytology and, in particular, the ganglioid appearance of the nuclei, they have been aligned with the giant-cell tumors of tuberous sclerosis, which has been interpreted as a distinctive variety of astrocytoma. It is highly debatable that the tumors under discussion represent a malignant form of the latter, because anaplastic changes in subependymal giant-cell astrocytomas are quite exceptional.

These tumors have no preponderant site within the brain. They may occur at any age and, unlike the classic glioblastoma, are just as likely to affect the younger as the older age groups; many examples are diagnosed in patients in the first or second decade. Macroscopically, they are usually well defined, at least in places, and their cut surfaces may be more granular than are those of the typical glioblastoma. They exhibit extensive areas of necrosis and are often cystic. Foci of lipid degeneration may be conspicuous.

Microscopically, the cells are characteristically, but not invariably, arranged in perivascular pseudorosettes, these formations being separated by necrotic foci containing degenerating leukocytes. The tumor cells may also form palisades about the necroses. Cellular polymorphism is considerable, but, apart from the exaggerated monster and multinucleated forms (Fig. 9.209), the cells, as a whole, tend to be plump or pyramidal and have coarse cytoplasmic processes. Their ganglionic appearance is enhanced by the large vesicular nuclei containing conspicuous nucleoli (Fig. 9.210). Nissl bodies and neurofibrils are not demonstrable. Mitotic figures are numerous and often atypical (Fig. 9.211). In addition, there are many smaller, mainly fusiform, cells; syncytial formations are occasionally observed. In most examples, the astrocytic nature of the tumor cells is demonstrated by immunopositivity for GFAP, as documented by, in particular, Duffy *et al.* (1980). Occasionally, the giant cells may be heavily lipidized, as in the tumor described by Gherardi *et al.* (1986). Further support for the astrocytic nature of this neoplasm is provided by the presence, confirmed in several cases examined by

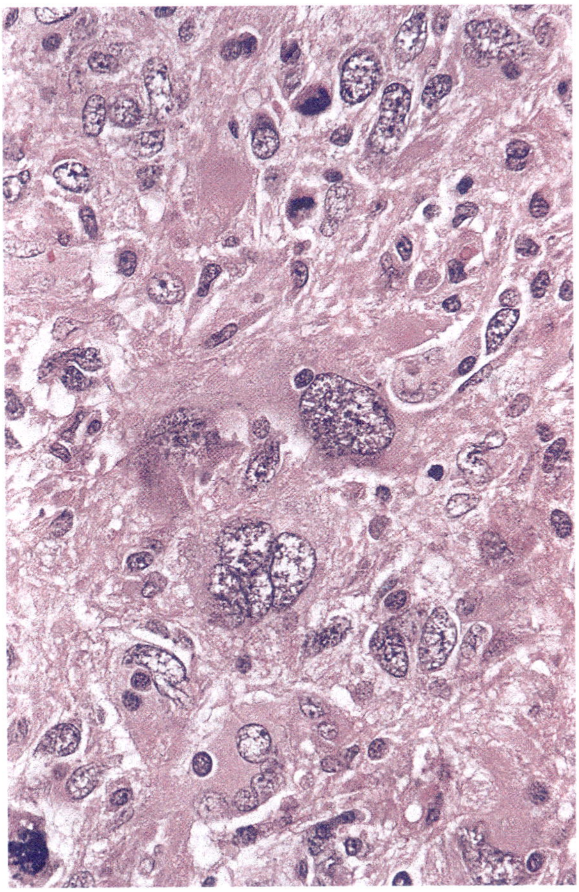

Fig. 9.209 Giant pleomorphic and multinucleated cells in a glioblastoma. H&E, × 500

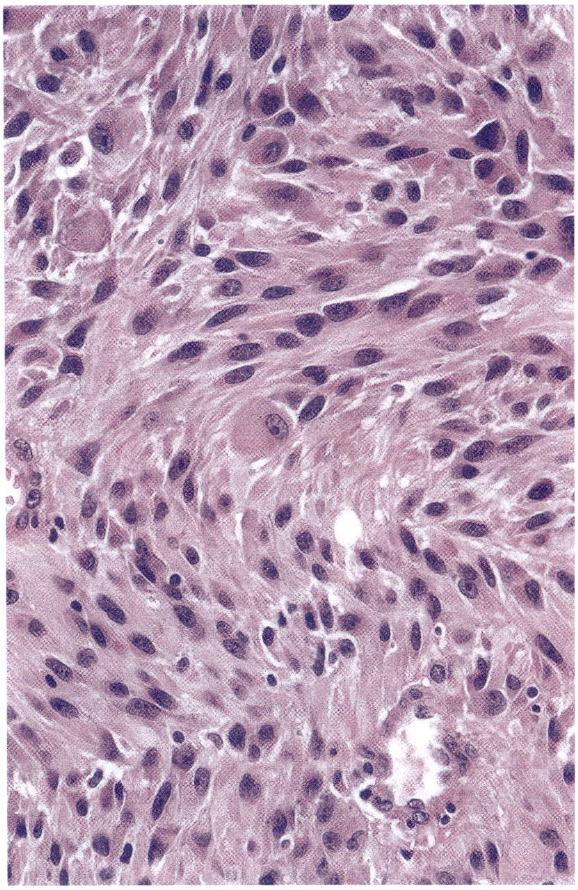

Fig. 9.210 Spindle cells and pleomorphic cells, some resembling ganglion cells, in a glioblastoma. H&E, × 500

Rubinstein, of transitions to areas of unequivocal 'ordinary' glioblastoma or to gemistocytic astrocytoma (see Rubinstein, 1972b; Figs 62 and 63, as well as the reports by Becker, Benyo and Roessmann, 1967; and Hadfield and Silverberg, 1972).

On the other hand, the development of reticulin fibrils and other connective tissue may be extensive in places, and in the past this has been used as a major argument for the interpretation of these tumors as sarcomas. The reticulin networks are usually most conspicuous in relation to the blood vessels and the margins of necrotic areas. Indeed, the supporting blood vessels may be unusually abundant, to the extent of presenting an angiomatous appearance. In general, they are thin walled, but, occasionally are thickened focally by fibrinoid material. Their lining endothelium is of the normal flattened type and microvascular proliferation is quite exceptional. The blood vessels are sometimes surrounded by cuffs of small, radiating columnar cells or spindle-shaped cells containing oval hyperchromatic nuclei. The nature of these cells is uncertain: some resemble microglia, but others appear to form transitions with the larger tumor cells. Elsewhere, there are perivascular cuffs of obvious lymphocytes and plasma cells, and lymphocytes may be found in conspicuous numbers further afield. Occasionally, however, as in the classic glioblastoma, a perivascular sarcomatous change may develop, as noted in six examples in Rubinstein's experience (Russell and Rubinstein, 1989). It is presumable in such cases that the appearances conform most to those of the tumors regarded by others as 'monstrocellular sarcomas', but the glial elements in Rubinstein's examples were always clearly recognizable.

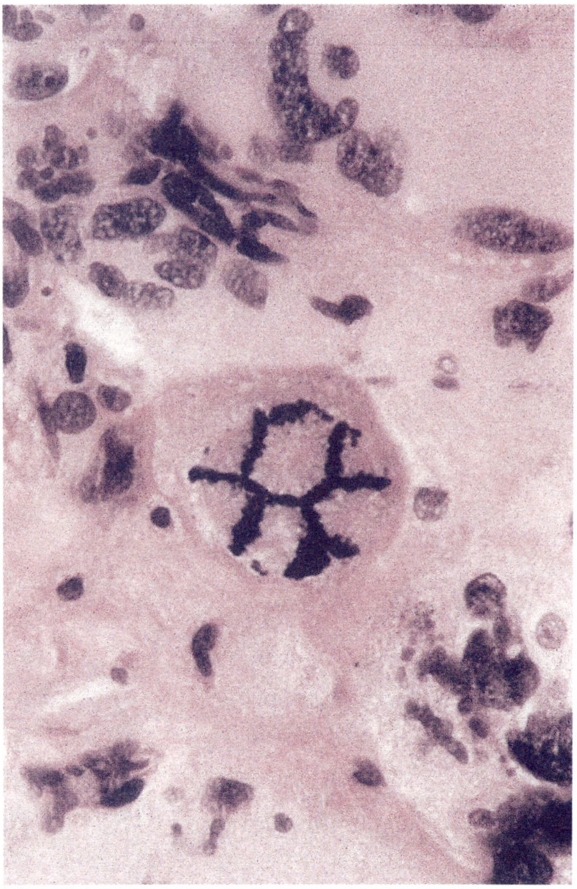

Fig. 9.211 Bizarre mitotic figure in a giant-cell glioblastoma. H&E, × 500

Despite the apparent gross circumscription of the tumor, infiltration of the adjacent brain is often evident microscopically, and the regional leptomeninges, too, are prone to invasion (Margetts and Kalyan-Raman, 1989). There are, however, clinical indications that this type of malignant glioma may carry a somewhat less sinister prognosis, perhaps because it is better outlined, than the classic glioblastoma, as confirmed by Burger and Vollmer (1980), who found that there was a positive relationship between postoperative survival of the patient and the presence of a giant-cell glioblastoma. On the other hand, there is no doubt that some of the cases originally diagnosed or subsequently reported as giant-cell glioblastomas or monstrocellular sarcomas with unusually long postoperative survival have been found, on re-evaluation, to belong to the considerably more benign group of pleomorphic xanthoastrocytomas (Kepes, Rubinstein and Eng, 1979).

Mixed gliomas and sarcomas ('gliosarcomas')

Details of this development were originally reported by Feigin and his coworkers (Feigin and Gross, 1955; Feigin *et al.*, 1958) and by Rubinstein (1956, 1964), but it is of historic interest that Stroebe (1895) initially recognized the sarcomatous changes in glioblastoma and appropriately used the term 'gliosarcoma'. A clinicopathologic review of 24 examples by Morantz, Feigin and Ransohoff (1976) drew attention to its relative frequency, which they assessed at 8% of all glioblastomas. Their account of its predilection for the temporal lobe and of its presentation as a tough, well-circumscribed lobulated mass, firmly attached to the dura, that at operation may often first be mistaken for a meningioma is fully in accord with the experience of Rubinstein (Russell and Rubinstein, 1989) (Fig. 9.212). These workers also considered that the sarcomatous change may be accompanied by a relative increase in the likelihood of remote metastases, but, except for this complication, its prognosis seems essentially no different from that of the usual glioblastoma. Some of these features have been disputed in the report of Meis, Martz and Nelson (1991) in an analysis of 26 cases of gliosarcoma retrieved from a series of 1479 glioblastomas that were part of a Radiation Therapy Oncology Group randomized clinical trial. In this study, the incidence of gliosarcomas among glioblastomas was 1.8%; these tumors had no predilection for the temporal lobe and the survival was similar to that of glioblastoma.

Although the cell of origin of the mesenchymal component is still disputed, the histologic appearance of these neoplasms is quite characteristic, featuring a marble-like intermingling of glial and mesenchymal tissue, distinctively distinguished by the immunopositivity of the former for GFAP (Duffy, Graf and Rapport, 1977; Deck *et al.*, 1978; Slowik *et al.*, 1985) (Fig. 9.213) and S-100 protein, and the absence of staining for these markers in the mesenchymal component. In addition, the histologic features of the mesenchymal tissue must permit an independent diagnosis of sarcoma to be made for this component (Fig. 9.214), ensuring that this tissue is not merely a robust reactive proliferative response to the presence of the glioma or extreme microvascular proliferation in a glioblastoma. Criteria for the diagnosis of sarcoma include high cellularity, frequent mitotic activity and the presence of atypical mitoses. The study of Meis, Martz and Nelson (1991) found the most frequent sarcoma to be malignant fibrous histiocytoma.

The perivascular arrangement of sarcoma cells is usually clearly outlined by silver impregnations for reticulin. The wealth of reticulin fibrils, with their

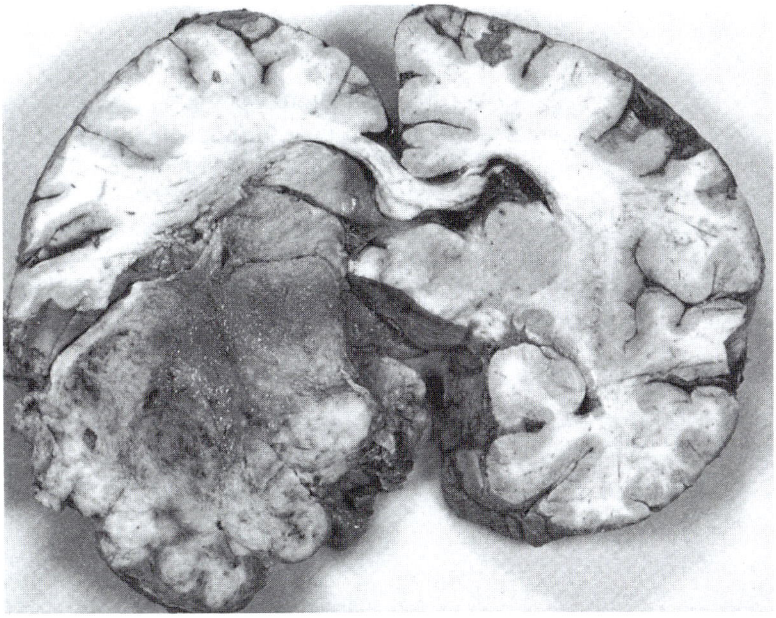

Fig. 9.212 Mixed glioblastoma and fibrosarcoma (gliosarcoma) of temporal lobe, firmly attached to the dura. (Reprinted from *Acta Neurochirurgica*, 1964, suppl. X, pp. 141–158, figure 16 with kind permission of Springer-Verlag.)

characteristic pericellular distribution and their limitation to the sarcomatous areas, provides a sharp contrast to the adjacent glioma, and immunohistochemical stains for GFAP further emphasize the distinction. Without special immunohistochemical markers, it may be difficult to definitively identify or distinguish between the two types of tissue.

The mesenchymal neoplastic tissue may, on occasion, undergo metaplasia with the production of cartilage and osteoid (Fig. 9.215), as noted by Rubinstein in eight instances (Russell and Rubinstein, 1989), and even, as an exceptional development, rhabdomyoblasts (Goldman, 1969; Barnard *et al.*, 1986). Eventually, the sarcoma may reach such massive proportions that the glioma is

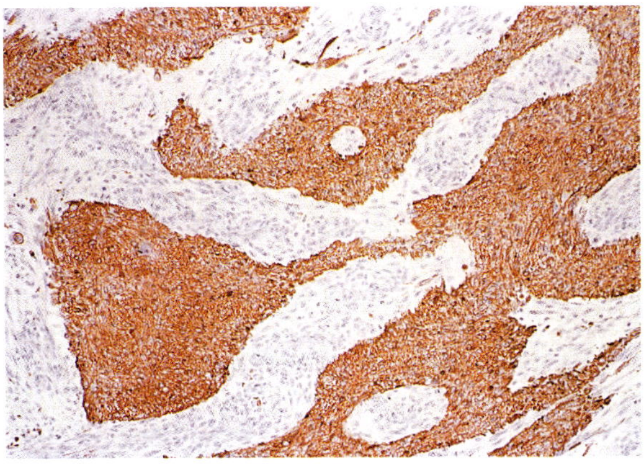

Fig. 9.213 Marbleized mixed pattern of glioma (positive) and fibrosarcoma (negative) in a gliosarcoma as demonstrated by GFAP immunostain. GFAP immunoperoxidase, × 125

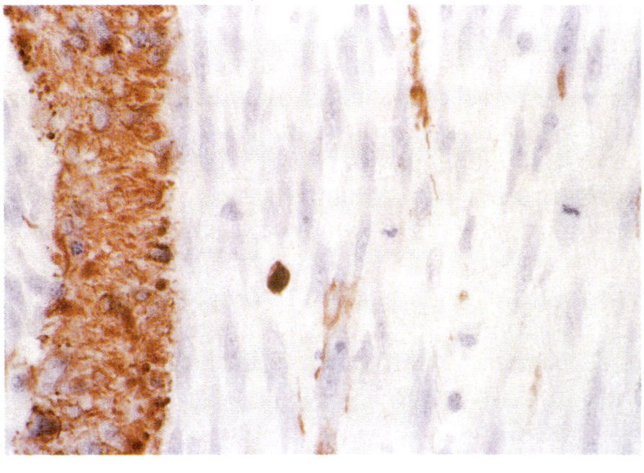

Fig. 9.214 Same case as Fig. 9.213 The sarcomatous areas must have independent features of malignancy, such as high cellularity and frequent mitoses. GFAP immunoperoxidase, × 500

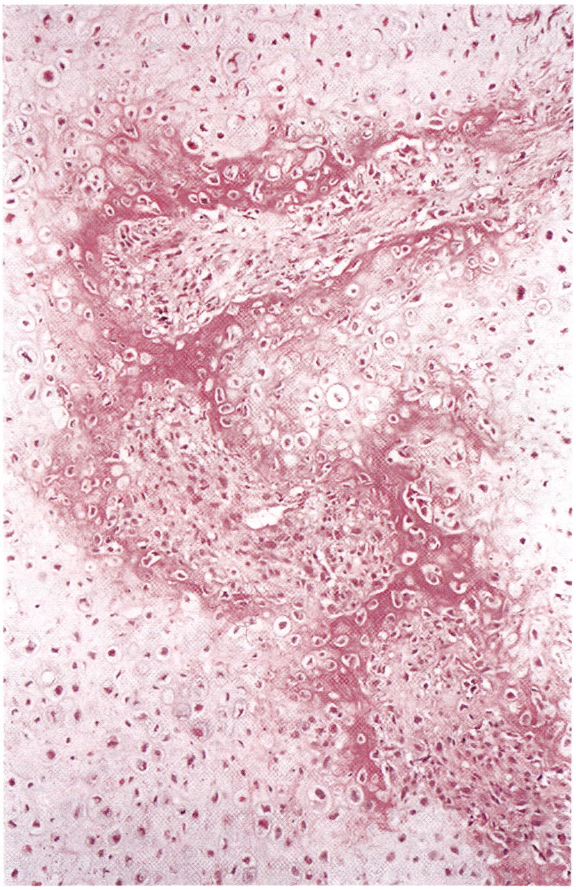

Fig. 9.215 Recurrent temporal lobe gliosarcoma in a 41-year-old woman showing areas of osteogenic sarcoma and chondrosarcoma. H&E, × 125

overshadowed. The demonstration of a gliomatous element may then no longer be possible, or may be documented only after extensive sampling. Because attachment to the dura is frequent (Fig. 9.212), difficulty may arise in deciding which of the two tissue elements is primary, since, as discussed by Rubinstein, a malignant invasive meningioma or a primary sarcoma may induce a malignant gliomatous reaction, for which the term 'sarcoglioma' has been proposed. Some of the reported cases of mixed glioma and sarcoma that include cartilaginous elements (Sarmiento *et al.*, 1979; Richman, Balis and Maniscalco, 1980) leave open either interpretation.

The presence of giant cells is usually more often related to the glial than to the sarcomatous elements. Rubinstein noted six examples of a rare feature: the giant-cell variant of glioblastoma (see below) on which a sarcomatous change, largely perivascular, was superimposed (Russell and Rubinstein, 1989). A similar development has been described by Arjona *et al.* (1977). The identification of the giant cells in these tumors may present difficulties, but the application of GFAP immunohistochemistry may be of assistance.

Electron microscopy studies of gliosarcomas include those of Peña and Felter (1973), Diaz-Flores and his coworkers (Arjona *et al.*, 1977; Diaz-Flores *et al.*, 1979) and, more recently, those of Slowik *et al.* (1985) and K.L. Ho (1990c). They essentially confirm the light microscopy distinctions between glial and mesenchymal cells, but offer varying interpretations as to the origin of the latter, some of them being endothelial, others pericytic and yet others myofibroblastic.

Immunohistochemical data using markers for endothelial cells have, therefore, not unexpectedly, yielded conflicting results. McComb *et al.* (1982) were able to obtain immunopositivity for the factor VIII/von Willebrand factor-related antigen only in the vascular endothelial cells of gliosarcomas and not in the neoplastic mesenchymal elements. They therefore suggested that the latter were derived either from nonendothelial cells or from cells that had undergone antigenic loss as a result of transformation. Schiffer *et al.* (1984) and Slowik *et al.* (1985), on the other hand, found transitional areas of immunopositivity, which confirmed that at least part of the sarcomatous components originated from vascular endothelial proliferation (Fig. 9.216). In the experience of Rubinstein, only the areas of typical angiosarcoma in gliosarcomas have been focally, but unquestionably, immunopositive for the factor VIII-related antigen (Russell and Rubinstein, 1989). Isolated cells in the sarcomatous areas have been reported to be immunopositive for laminin and fibronectin (Schiffer *et al.*, 1984) and for the *Ulex europaeus* agglutinin-1 (UEA-1) lectin (Slowik *et al.*, 1985). Kochi and Budka (1987) found the sarcoma cells to be negative for the factor VIII/von Willebrand factor-related antigen and positive for fibronectin as well as for three monohistiocytic markers—lysozyme, alpha-1-antitrypsin and alpha-1-antichymotrypsin—and concluded that the sarcomatous component in gliosarcomas was more likely to be derived from histiocytic elements in the perivascular spaces than from proliferated endothelial cells. However, the cell-type specificity of markers for histiocytes is far from established when tested in the context of neoplasms. Other studies have found immunopositivity for smooth muscle antigens in the mesenchymal component, further supporting a vascular origin, whether from smooth muscle or pericytes (Haddad *et al.*, 1992c). Recent studies,

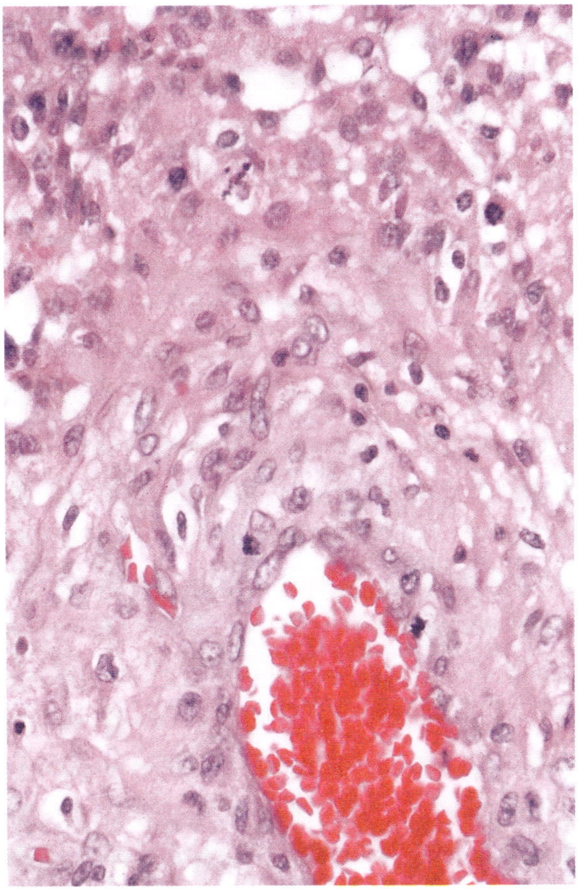

Fig. 9.216 Same case as Fig. 9.215. First resection (shown here) of temporal lobe tumor showed a glioblastoma with excessive microvascular proliferation and frequent mitotic figures in vessel walls. Recurrence 10 months later showed a gliosarcoma. H&E, × 500

however, have found similar alterations of the *TP53* gene and *TP53* protein in both the gliomatous and the sarcomatous elements of some gliosarcomas, suggesting a common origin of the two cellular components from neoplastic astrocytes (Albrecht, Connelly and Bruner, 1993; Biernat *et al.*, 1995).

Relationship of glioblastomas to anaplastic astrocytomas

Reference has already been made to the relationship that exists between glioblastomas and anaplastic astrocytomas, and the reader is referred to the section on anaplastic astrocytomas, where their incidence, gross features, microscopic features and the time factors associated with their evolution are reviewed. The problem of distinguishing between 'primary' glioblastomas and those anaplastic astrocytomas that have secondarily progressed over time to become glioblastomas has been extensively discussed (Russell and Rubinstein, 1989).

On clinical grounds, and as described by Scherer (1940a), the biologic evolution of the demonstrably anaplastic astrocytoma is often longer than that of the glioblastoma. Winger, Macdonald and Cairncross (1989) also noted that glioblastoma patients with a history of a pre-existing lower-grade glioma ('secondary' glioblastoma) appeared to have a better prognosis than those patients whose glioblastomas arose primarily. Scherer (1940a) reported that, in the latter, the clinical history was usually less than a year, whereas in the former it could be more than a year and might exceed 2 years. It is virtually impossible to make the distinction between 'primary' and 'secondary' glioblastoma by histologic examination alone. Rubinstein reported a retrospective analysis of a series of 129 necropsies examined during the period 1946–55, in which the diagnosis of cerebral glioblastoma had already been made from their microscopic appearance (Russell and Rubinstein, 1989). Despite an attempt to classify the glioblastomas as 'primary' or 'secondary', based on the presence of included lower-grade astrocytoma, the results were inconclusive.

Recognition of genetic differences among gliomas and the use of molecular genetic techniques have contributed to the present understanding and a hypothesis regarding this issue. It is well known that glioblastomas have a high frequency of amplification of the gene coding for the epidermal growth factor receptor (EGFR), ranging from 25% to 50%, and that this is a distinguishing feature from lower-grade astrocytomas, which have acquired this change in less than 10% of cases (Libermann *et al.*, 1985; A.J. Wong *et al.*, 1987; Bigner *et al.*, 1988a). In addition, a consistent loss of a portion of chromosome 10 has been seen in glioblastomas (James *et al.*, 1988; Fults *et al.*, 1992; Rasheed *et al.*, 1992; von Deimling *et al.*, 1992b). A tumor suppressor gene (*PTEN*) has recently been identified (Li *et al.*, 1997; Steck *et al.*, 1997). Its protein product, PTEN (phosphatase and tensin homolog deleted on chromosome 10; also called MMAC1, mutated in multiple advanced cancers 1), is a tyrosine phosphatase. It has also been noted that all grades of astrocytoma show a high percentage of tumors with loss of portions of chromosome 17, specifically the short arm, in a region that encodes the *TP53* tumor suppressor gene (El-Azouzi *et al.*, 1989; Fults *et al.*, 1989; von Deimling *et al.*, 1992a). Studies of the relationships among these genetic alterations have suggested that glioblastomas may be grouped into at least three subsets (von Deimling *et al.*, 1992a, 1992b, 1993; Lang *et al.*, 1994). One subset characteristically shows loss of heterozygosity for chromosome 17 without amplification of the *EGFR* gene. The second demonstrates *EGFR* gene amplification without loss of chromosome 17. These two groups account for about two thirds of glioblastomas examined, so at least one additional group without either *EGFR* amplification or chromosome 17 loss is seen. A strong correlation of chromosome 10 loss with the histologic subtype of glioblastoma showing *EGFR* amplification has been noted. These data permit the construction of a hypothetical grouping of glioblastomas into (1) those arising directly as 'primary' glioblastomas without loss of chromosome 17 or progression from lower-grade tumors and (2) those glioblastomas arising by sequential malignant progression of lower-grade astrocytomas with initial loss of heterozygosity for chromosome 17 ('secondary' glioblastomas) (Reifenberger *et al.*, 1996). Since astrocytomas with loss of heterozygosity for chromosome 17 have been reported in younger patients in some studies, and an extended survival has been reported for patients whose tumors progress from anaplastic astrocytoma to glioblastoma over those who develop glioblastoma primarily, these data regarding the genetic subsets of glioblastomas correlate with previously known clinical features (Louis, 1996; Watanabe *et al.*, 1996). The molecular genetics of gliomas is more thoroughly discussed in Chapter 2.

Agreement, however, is still not unanimous as to whether glioblastoma should be considered a separate category of malignant glioma or a progression, at least in some significant proportion of cases, from a lower-grade astrocytic glioma. The analyses of J.S. Nelson *et al.* (1983), Burger *et al.* (1985) and D.F. Nelson *et al.* (1985), using as a single clear-cut criterion the presence of focal necroses as pathognomonic for glioblastoma, found that glioblastomas and anaplastic astrocytomas display highly significant differences in the duration of their preoperative symptoms and in the length of postoperative survival of patients with these tumors. It appears from these studies that, once the anaplastic changes in an astrocytoma have progressed to the development of ominous focal necroses, the prognosis becomes that of a glioblastoma. It seems, however, that in such cases survival may sometimes extend over more than 2 years, as shown in the analysis by Jelsma and Bucy (1967), who identified eight such patients in their series. Conversely, even within the group of glioblastomas, the presence of more differentiated astrocytomatous areas may be associated with somewhat longer postoperative survival times for patients (Burger and Green, 1987).

Heterogeneity of malignant glial cell populations

The preceding pages have stressed the polymorphic character of the cells in glioblastoma, and have thus provided a morphologic basis for the current emphasis on the heterogeneity of this and other malignant neoplasms. It is widely accepted that this concept needs to be enlarged to encompass virtually all levels of structural and functional neoplastic organization, including differential growth rates; differences in surface antigens; cell anchorage properties and metastatic potential of the various cell populations; and differential sensitivity to antineoplastic agents, hormones and radiation. Regardless of the histogenesis of the tumor, increased malignancy seems to be associated with increased genetic lability, which results in a progressive increase in mutation rates so that tumor progression is accompanied by the stepwise selection of clonal sublines. Thus, phenotypic and functional heterogeneity is essentially an expression of karyotypic (or genotypic) variability. The molecular genetic investigations cited above, and the additional studies of Berkman *et al.* (1992) and Sidransky *et al.* (1992), are compelling evidence for the monoclonal origin of glioblastoma, both at the time of initial presentation and at recurrence.

Kinetics

Tumor progression in glioblastomas is linked to their proliferation kinetics. The studies by Hoshino and his collaborators (see Hoshino, 1981, for review), using autoradiography on gliomas obtained at operation from patients who were administered tritiated thymidine intravenously before surgery, have provided a valuable body of baseline data. Not unexpectedly, glioblastomas show a great deal of variation in their LI, which varies from 0% in the necrotic areas to values ranging from 5% to 16% in the viable areas (Hoshino and Wilson, 1979). These values were appreciably higher than those of well-differentiated gliomas, which showed an LI of usually less than 1%, whereas anaplastic astrocytomas had LIs of intermediate range, averaging 4% and reflecting the degree of anaplasia. Steel (1980) estimated from different published figures that the LIs of high-grade and intermediate-grade astrocytomas ranged widely, from 0.6% to 11.4%. Similar studies have suggested that the gemistocytic tumor astrocytes and the giant cells in glioblastomas may make little or no contribution to the proliferating pool.

With a double labeling technique, Hoshino *et al.* (1972) estimated that the DNA synthesis phase in the proliferating cells of glioblastomas and anaplastic astrocytomas ranges from 4 to 13 hours; Steel (1980) suggested a slightly higher value of 15 hours, in conformity with the mean values of other solid human malignancies. The tumor cell cycle times calculated by Hoshino *et al.* (1975) in three patients had a mean duration of 57 hours, but a somewhat higher mean of 75 hours was subsequently estimated after stathmokinetic analysis; this latter estimate, however, showed considerable spread from 36 to 152 hours (Hoshino and Wilson, 1979). The potential doubling times of glioblastomas and anaplastic astrocytomas have been shown, after the use of mitostatic agents *in vivo*, to have a mean of 11 to 12 days according to Hoshino, Wilson and Muraoka (1979) and were hypothesized by Steel (1980) to be approximately 10 days. Such an estimate obviously does not take into account two decisive factors: the rate of cell loss (which may affect both the proliferating and nonproliferating pools) and the existence of a large population of nondividing cells. The cell loss factor in glioblastomas has been empirically assumed to be about 85% (Hoshino *et al.*, 1972), comparable to that of other human malignancies, and a figure to be expected since spontaneous necrosis is one of their characteristic features.

The kinetics analyses of Hoshino and his colleagues, then, indicate that the rate of tumor growth correlates, not with the overall length of the tumor cell cycle or of any portion thereof, but with the size of the proliferating compartment; the major difference between gliomas of different degrees of malignancy resides in their respective *growth fractions*. This has been estimated by Hoshino and Wilson (1979) to range from 0.21 to 0.44 in glioblastomas, and from 0.14 to 0.25 in anaplastic astrocytomas.

The kinetics values discussed in the preceding paragraphs are relevant to the use of chemotherapeutic agents that may be specific to the cell cycle. They are also essential to an understanding of the growth of gliomas *in vivo* and of the role played by the instability of neoplastic cell populations in tumor progression. As pointed out by Hoshino (1984), therapeutic considerations may have to take into account the relative sizes and respective drug sensitivities of the cycling and noncycling pools, and the existence or absence of any interchange between the pools.

Another approach to glioblastoma kinetics has been through flow cytometry studies designed to measure the DNA content of single cells and to extrapolate the respective distributions of the cell cycle phases and proliferative (S phase) fraction from the data obtained after cell sorting. The technique, which relies on the quantification of fluorescence emitted by a DNA-bound dye as tumor cell nuclei rapidly flow past a high-intensity laser beam, permits the construction of peaks showing the relative frequency of cell populations with diploid and multiploid karyotypes. From those peaks may be derived the relative percentage of cells in DNA synthesis. The results of this procedure have been published by Hoshino *et al.* (1978), Lehmann and Krug (1980), Spaar *et al.* (1986), and, more recently, by Coons and Johnson (1993a) with an exhaustive examination of regional heterogeneity in gliomas. Coons and Johnson have largely confirmed that, in the more malignant gliomas, a substantial population of cells are synthesizing DNA and that a good deal of heterogeneity in the distribution of the predominant ploidy is to be found in different regions of the same tumor. It is of interest that, in malignant gliomas, aneuploidy does not always appear to be related directly to a poor biologic behavior of the tumor; thus, the small anaplastic cells in glioblastomas have been found to have a DNA content that is diploid or near-diploid, whereas anaplastic astrocytomas may show a more complex DNA distribution (Giangaspero *et al.*, 1987). Although, generally speaking, diploid neoplasms appear to be associated with a better outcome than are aneuploid neoplasms, progression from anaplastic astrocytoma to the clinically more malignant glioblastoma was not found by these workers to be paralleled by any progression of the tumor cells to increased aneuploidy. In an extensive regional analysis using flow cytometry, Coons and Johnson (1993a) found a regional heterogeneity of diploid and aneuploid patterns in all types of gliomas, including glioblastoma. This was in agreement with histologic heterogeneity in the same tumors. There was less heterogeneity in the S-phase fraction (SPF) than in ploidy, and SPF did correlate with tumor histologic grade. In an additional study, these investigators found, using multivariate analysis, independent significance of the SPF-group values with prognosis (Coons, Johnson and Pearl, 1994). Other investigators have paradoxically shown a longer patient survival for those astrocytomas with an aneuploid pattern than for those with a diploid pattern (Salmon *et al.*, 1992). These authors also correlated six DNA histogram types in a multivariate analysis, yielding significant independent prognostic information for patient survival (Salmon *et al.*, 1994).

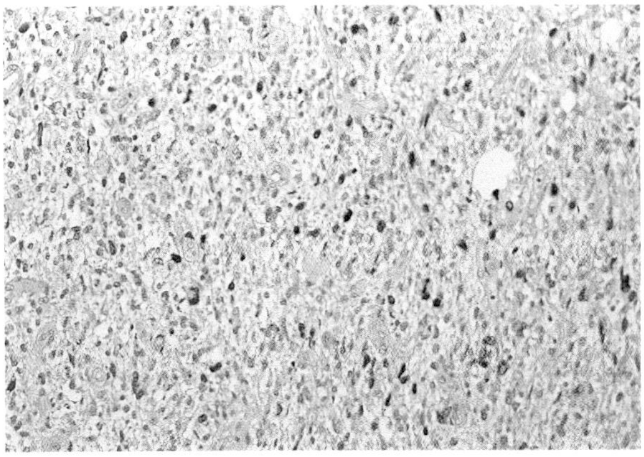

Fig. 9.217 Glioblastoma immunostained for BrdU, demonstrating nuclear positivity in cells that are in the S phase. Labeling index in this case is 11.8%. BrdU immunoperoxidase, × 250

Another method has been devised to estimate the percentage of tumor cells in the DNA synthesis phase, and several studies have been published. The method is based on the immunoperoxidase demonstration of a thymidine analog, BrdU, which is incorporated into the nuclear DNA after intravenous injection at the time of craniotomy, and is then detected, in tissue sections, in the tumor cell nuclei by means of a monoclonal antibody against BrdU (Fig. 9.217). Compared with autoradiography, the technique has the advantages of speed and of avoiding possible radiation hazard and myelotoxicity. It does require pre-operative permission of the patient and intravenous injection of a cytotoxic and potentially mutagenic agent. The results of Hoshino *et al.* (1986) indicate that the LIs provided by this procedure are similar to those obtained with the much more laborious technique of autoradiography. In multiple published reports, the BrdU LI has correlated significantly with patient survival, especially in the lower-grade and anaplastic astrocytomas. It has generally not been analyzed using multivariate statistical methods, however. It has proved to be more predictive of patient survival than is tumor histologic grading in univariate analysis of low-grade and anaplastic astrocytomas (Hoshino *et al.*, 1988, 1989). Similar results have been obtained by Yoshii *et al.* (1986), who, while confirming, as expected, that the estimate of the growth fraction correlated well with biologic malignancy, quite appropriately emphasized the fact that cell loss, which plays an important role in determining tumor growth, is not taken into account in such calculations. Thus, any estimates of cell cycle times based on those data tend to be considerably overestimated. It should also be noted that, within the glioblastoma group, the existence of any significant correlation between postoperative survival of the patient and LI of the tissue removed at surgery has not been confirmed (Bookwalter *et al.*, 1986; Hoshino *et al.*, 1993; Ritter *et al.*, 1994), so any discrepancies may be due to the heterogeneity and the genetic instability of the tumor as well as to the bias introduced by tissue selection.

Other potential indicators of proliferation have also been used in an attempt to predict the biologic behavior of gliomas more accurately than does histologic grading alone. Proliferating cell nuclear antigen (PCNA) is a 261-amino-acid nuclear protein whose synthesis correlates with DNA replication and cellular proliferation. It is present in phases of the cell cycle other than G0, but has an extended half-life (more than 20 hours); thus, its detection cannot be equated with DNA synthesis. There are several available antibodies that can be used for immunohistochemical detection of PCNA in frozen or paraffin-embedded tissue. The epitopes are, however, heavily fixation-dependent (Tahan *et al.*, 1995), even when considering the formalin-resistant epitope PC10. Preoperative treatment of patients with dexamethasone, a common situation for glioma patients, has been shown to affect the PCNA LI in meningiomas (Gottschalk *et al.*, 1992). Despite this, the PCNA LI has been correlated with tumor grade in a study of 44 diffuse fibrillary astrocytomas (Allegranza *et al.*, 1991b), but has not correlated with survival in a separate study limited to glioblastomas (Frigge *et al.*, 1992).

The monoclonal antibody Ki-67 detects a nuclear antigen that is present in proliferating cells in all cell cycle phases except G0 and can be detected immunohistochemically using frozen tissue sections. The antigen has been characterized (Gerdes *et al.*, 1991), and the antibody has been applied to brain tumors (Burger, Shibata and Kleihues, 1986). Unfortunately, the technique is severely limited by the necessity of using frozen tissue, as the morphology is less than optimal, and the tissue intended for labeling must be selected and kept frozen before the final tissue diagnosis is available. The issue of heterogeneity is a major one, since not every area of tissue is potentially available for retrospective labeling analysis. The Ki-67 LI has been shown to correlate with tumor grade (Burger, Shibata and Kleihues, 1986; Zuber, Hamou and de Tribolet, 1988; Coons and Johnson, 1993b), but no large studies of correlation with prognosis have been completed.

Even though BrdU seems to be a somewhat clinically relevant label for measuring cell proliferation in gliomas, not all patients can be intravenously injected perioperatively, a requirement for its use. The MIB-1 antibody has recently been constructed

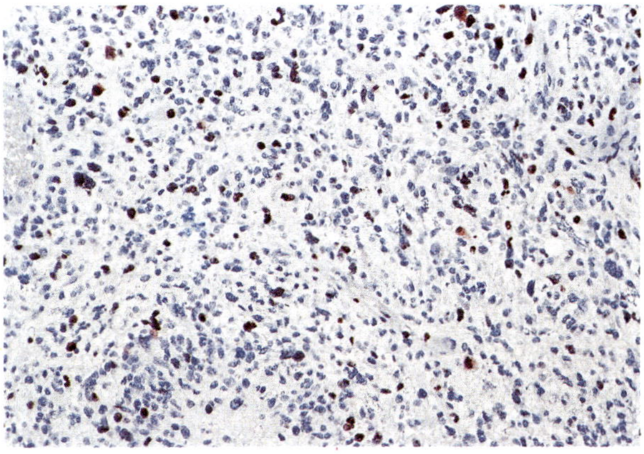

Fig. 9.218 Same case as Fig. 9.217 with staining for MIB-1 proliferation antigen and showing a similar appearance of nuclear labeling. Labeling index is 17.7%, since cells in phases other than the S phase are labeled by this marker. MIB-1 immunoperoxidase, × 250

to the Ki-67 antigen (Key *et al.*, 1993). The advantage of MIB-1 is that it can be reliably used for routinely processed brain tumor tissue that has not been handled by special methods *in vivo* or *in vitro* (Cattoretti *et al.*, 1992). It is potentially useful for labeling in every patient who has operative tissue available for diagnosis. In addition, since this is an antibody to an endogenous antigen, there is no problem with distribution after injection (Onda *et al.*, 1994b). A single study exists comparing MIB-1 with BrdU LI in a small series of glioblastomas, but MIB-1 LI has not been correlated with predictive value for survival in other types and grades of primary brain tumors (Onda *et al.*, 1994a). Because of its ease of application to routine operative specimens of brain tumors and its predicted correlation with patient survival, this proliferation marker will probably be more widely used in the near future (Fig. 9.218).

Tissue and cell culture

The descriptive approach that plays such a role in all *in vitro* work has often made it difficult to separate glioblastomas from anaplastic astrocytomas. For an account of the *in vitro* behavior of *primary explants* of glioblastomas, the reader is referred to the previously recorded observations by Russell and Rubinstein (Lumsden, 1971), where the tissue culture features of astrocytic gliomas in ascending grades of malignancy are summarized.

The characteristics of permanent or established glial cell lines, most of which have been obtained from glioblastomas, and the studies performed on those lines are reviewed on p. 180.

The applications of the organ culture method to the *in vitro* study of different glioma types have already been mentioned in the sections on astrocytomas and ependymomas. The technique greatly favors cellular differentiation. In all the glioblastomas that were successfully maintained in this manner, astrocytic differentiation, usually after 3–4 weeks *in vitro*, was invariably demonstrated by light (Rubinstein, Herman and Foley, 1973) and electron (Sipe, Herman and Rubinstein, 1973) microscopy, as illustrated in Fig. 9.199. The development of palisades, characteristic of glioblastomas *in vivo*, was not seen, but has been described in similar preparations by Saez, Campbell and Laws (1977), who also employed this approach for the qualitative evaluation of cytotoxicity *in vitro* as a possible guide to chemotherapy.

The kinetics of malignant gliomas *in vitro* have been more completely discussed in the previous edition of this text (Russell and Rubinstein, 1989).

Xenogeneic transplantation of glioblastomas

The heterologous transplantation of biopsy specimens of glioblastomas and of cell lines derived from them is considered on p. 180, together with that of astrocytic gliomas in general. Almost all the human glioma cell lines that have so far been successfully transplanted and serially passaged for several transfer generations have (with the exception of a few cerebellar medulloblastomas) been derived from glioblastomas.

Growth, spread and metastatic potential

Direct extension

Some of the features resulting from the direct spread of glioblastomas through the neural tissues have already been indicated in the description of their gross appearances, and the frequency with which superficially placed examples penetrate the adjacent meninges has been mentioned. Localized infiltration of the leptomeninges is often followed by firm union with the dura, resulting in marked fibrous connective tissue proliferation at the site of meningeal attachment. The presentation at operation may therefore be one that mimics, on first inspection, that of a meningioma. A biopsy obtained from such a superficial part of the tumor may be highly confusing because of the fibroblastic reaction originating from the leptomeninges. In some instances, the reaction is slight or even imperceptible, but, quite often, an excess of reticulin and collagen fibers is produced in response to the proliferation and infiltration of neoplastic cells. The latter are then apt to assume a spindle, or pilocytic shape; the microscopic appearances may then easily be mistaken for those of a fibrosarcoma. The

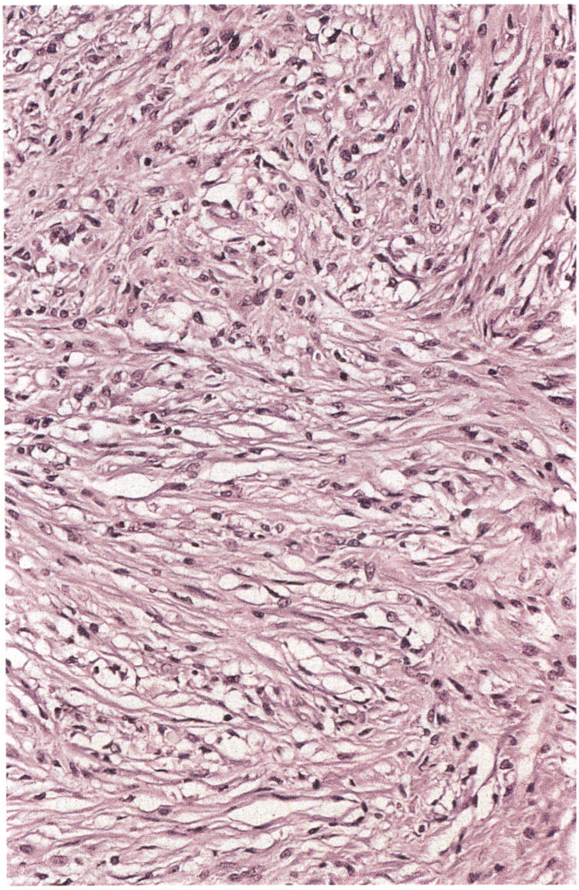

Fig. 9.219 Spindle-cell glioblastoma invading the leptomeninges. In such an instance, this tumor might be confused with fibrosarcoma. H&E, × 250

immunoperoxidase stain for GFAP is often invaluable in establishing the glial nature of the tumor (Figs 9.219 and 9.220).

The dura, in general, appears resistant to penetration by the glioblastoma: microscopically, the inner surface alone is usually infiltrated. Penetration of the lumen of an adjacent venous sinus is exceptional. When this occurs, it has been shown to be an avenue for the opening of extraneural dissemination, as demonstrated in the cases reported by Rubinstein (1967), Schuster *et al.* (1976, case 4) and Pasquier *et al.* (1980, case 2).

Likewise, direct extension to bone is an exceptional event that, when present, has been shown to herald the development of extracranial deposits. These cases fall into two categories. In the first, the tumor is superficially situated over the convexity, as illustrated in the following two examples, both involving the posterior part of the cerebrum.

The first case, submitted to Rubinstein (Russell and Rubinstein, 1989) by Dr J.H.N. Deck, was that

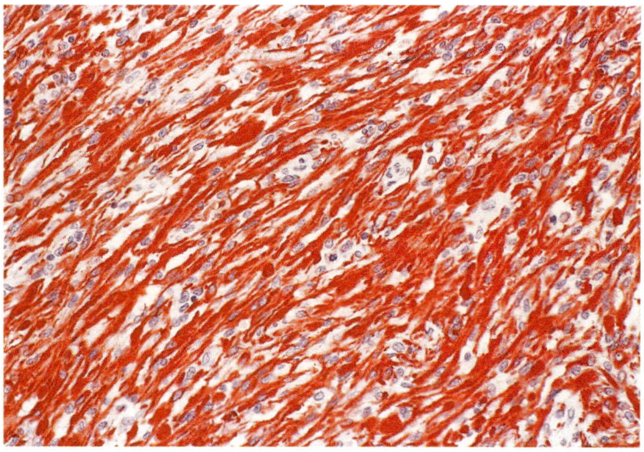

Fig. 9.220 Same case as Fig. 9.219. Immunostaining GFAP shows strong diffuse cytoplasmic reactivity, confirming this tumor as an astrocytoma rather than a fibrosarcoma. GFAP immunoperoxidase, × 250

of a 70-year-old woman who presented, first, with a painless and, later, tender, bone-invading and eroding mass located over the left occiput and histologically mimicking a sarcoma. Autopsy 6 months later revealed a large, immediately underlying occipital glioblastoma; extensive metastatic spread was found in the pericardium and the pleurae.

The other example, referred to Rubinstein by Dr S.T. Pilbeam, New South Wales, was in a girl who had a convergent left strabismus since the age of 11 months and who, at the age of 3 years, presented with a soft-tissue swelling over the occiput. Operation revealed a necrotic tumor that had eroded the bone and occupied the left occipital lobe. The patient did not survive the operation, and autopsy disclosed numerous small pulmonary pleural and parenchymatous deposits, with necrotic growth in the hilar lymph nodes. Microscopically, the cerebral tumor was a glioblastoma, with areas resembling a malignant protoplasmic astrocytoma. Permeation of small dural venules by tumor was demonstrated. Presumably, in this instance, the relatively slow growth, at an early age, of a superficial occipital glioma before union of the cranial sutures favored local extension into bone, with the spontaneous development of distant metastasis.

The exceptional character of a spontaneous transdural extension, by a malignant glioma, over the convexity of the skull is confirmed by the report of Kawano *et al.* (1977). In their case, a malignant parasagittal astrocytoma had invaded the frontoparietal dura, skull and subgaleal space, perhaps following infiltration of the pacchionian granulations. Whether this patient subsequently developed extraneural metastases is not known.

The second site of bone extension seems relatively less uncommon: it involves the medial structures of the middle fossa and is typically associated with a temporal glioblastoma. Again, such a development may pave the way for the metastasis outside the CNS. One recorded case occurred in a 26-year-old male (Liwnicz and Rubinstein, 1979, case 1). The other, submitted to Rubinstein by Dr Lucy B. Rorke, was in a 7-year-old girl with a superficial left medial temporal glioblastoma that had eroded through the greater wing of the sphenoid and the sella turcica. In this remarkable instance, the tumor had extended as a firm fibrous mass, presenting in the nasopharynx at necropsy. Distant deposits were found in the vertebral marrow, liver sinusoids, adrenal medulla and hilar lymph notes, and had studded the pleurae. However, since this patient had a left ventriculopleural anastomosis performed for the relief of hydrocephalus 7 months before death, and was found to have extensive meningeal and ventricular dissemination from the glioblastoma, tumor dissemination by way of the shunting operation appears more probable.

Infiltration of these parts of the skull may, indeed, be more frequent than these few observations would suggest when it is remembered how often herniations of cerebral cortex through the dura are to be found in the middle fossae in any sustained increase of intracranial pressure. This is confirmed by the reports of Sanerkin (1962) and Nager (1967, case 1), both of which describe the spontaneous transdural extension of temporal lobe glioblastomas with consequent invasion and destruction of the temporal bone. In Nager's case, bone destruction was massive and tumor protruded through the tympanic membrane into the external auditory canal. Also, Hoyt *et al.* (1972) have drawn attention to a similar phenomenon that may involve the anterior fossa in frontal and frontotemporal glioblastomas and result in invasion of the posterior orbital tissues, an event that recalls the sequence occasionally seen with fronto-orbital metastases from cerebellar medulloblastomas.

Ventriculoleptomeningeal spread

Neoplastic infiltration of the ependyma of the lateral and third ventricles is frequent (see Fig. 9.304). Microscopically, the neighboring ependymal cells may develop tapering fibrillated processes. Breaching of the surface epithelium, perhaps associated with focal ependymal defects resulting from obstructive hydrocephalus (Nishio *et al.*, 1982), paves the way for the dissemination of tumor cells by the CSF and the development of metastases at distant points both within the ventricular system and in the subarachnoid space (see Figs 9.305–9.307). It is possible that the frequency of this development has been underestimated in the past, as the necropsy studies published by Erlich and Davis (1978) and Nishio *et al.* (1982) appear to suggest. In autopsy specimens, deposits in the ventricular walls are recognized as rather discrete, elevated cushions of growth of variable size and number. The choroid plexuses may be involved. As a rule, these metastases seldom penetrate deeply into the adjacent tissue, and their direction of growth is mainly towards the cavity. Microscopically, as might be expected, foci of tumor cells may also be found as implantations that are too small to be seen with the naked eye.

Metastases in the leptomeninges either are nodular or form diffuse sheets of translucent grayish appearance. The latter is more frequent at the base of the brain (see Fig. 9.305) and over the cerebellar folia. Nodular growths, which may attain a considerable size, are more often found in the subarachnoid space over the dorsal aspect of the spinal cord and in the cauda equina (Fig. 9.306). They tend to be attached to the posterior roots, which become infiltrated by the tumor cells.

Extraneural deposits

As considered more fully in the last section of this chapter ('Growth and dissemination of central neuroepithelial tumors', p. 504), increasing numbers of glioblastomas with remote extraneural metastases have been reported in recent years. They now form the majority of gliomas with this complication (Smith, Hardman and Earle, 1969a; Liwnicz and Rubinstein, 1979; Pasquier *et al.*, 1980). The most frequent sites of metastasis are the lungs and lymph nodes, followed by the bones, liver and pleura (see Fig. 9.309). The development of remote deposits in cases of mixed glioblastoma and fibrosarcoma (gliosarcomas), most often in the lungs, liver and other viscera, has also been recorded (see review by Pasquier *et al.*, 1980), and it is possible that this type of tumor may be rather more often associated with this sequel than other forms of glioma (Smith, Hardman and Earle, 1969b; Cerame, Guthikonda and Kohli, 1985). Usually, both tissue elements have been identified in the deposits, but occasionally only the sarcomatous component may be present, as in two of the cases reported by Smith, Hardman and Earle (1969b) and in one seen by Rubinstein (Weaver *et al.*, 1984). For a general review of the mechanisms of metastatic extraneural spread, the avenues by which it may be opened and the relationship that this development bears to prior surgical procedures, the reader is referred to the last section of this chapter.

Recurrence: factors determining length of postoperative survival

The sinister prognosis of glioblastoma is well known, the mortality after 2 years being almost 90%, even after extensive operative removal followed by radiation therapy (Jelsma and Bucy, 1967, 1969; Leibel, Scott and Loeffler, 1994). Massive recurrence at the original site is to be anticipated, often characterized histologically by an overwhelming proliferation of small anaplastic cells, as noted by several observers (Budka, Podreka and Zaunbauer, 1979; Giangaspero and Burger, 1983; Schmitt, 1983b). Serial CT scans have confirmed that the recurrence takes place in almost all patients within a 2-cm margin of the primary site (Hochberg and Pruitt, 1980; Wallner *et al.*, 1989; Garden *et al.*, 1991; Gaspar *et al.*, 1992). Both the microscopic features of the recurrence and its localization indicate, therefore, that it results from local tumor infiltration of rapidly growing subpopulations that may have been preferentially selected on the basis of their radioresistance. These subpopulations were presumably derived from residual tumor elements whose removal even comprehensive surgical resection has not been able to achieve. Compelling evidence for this monoclonal neoplastic cell expansion, rather than continued anaplastic transformation of additional cell populations, is found in several of the molecular genetic investigations previously cited (James *et al.*, 1988; Berkman *et al.*, 1992; Sidransky *et al.*, 1992; Lang *et al.*, 1994).

Reference has already been made to the correlative studies by J.S. Nelson *et al.* (1983), Burger *et al.* (1985), D.F. Nelson *et al.* (1985) and Burger and Green (1987) on the criteria determining the postoperative behavior of glioblastomas, with emphasis on those features that distinguish glioblastomas from anaplastic astrocytomas. In addition to the presence of focal necroses, which are decisive in the prognostic assessment of glioblastomas, age is a factor of significance, with younger patients having longer postoperative survival times. This observation has been corroborated in other studies (Jelsma and Bucy, 1967; Schiffer *et al.*, 1979; McLendon *et al.*, 1985).

Finally, notice should be taken of the fact that, exceptionally, extirpation of a cerebral glioblastoma may be successful, as recorded in isolated instances (see Bucy *et al.*, 1985, for case report and literature review). Care should be taken, in this context, to avoid confusion with the pleomorphic xanthoastrocytoma, which has often in the past been misinterpreted as a giant-cell glioblastoma. Nevertheless, from the histologic studies of Rubinstein (Russell and Rubinstein, 1989, p. 247), the rare existence of classic glioblastomas in which surgical resection has been followed by many years of tumor-free survival and apparent clinical cure has been confirmed. These have included two examples referred to Rubinstein for review: one in a 43-year-old male, with a known 11-year survival from a left frontal glioblastoma; and one in a 9-year-old female, who survived 18 years after the excision of a left parietal glioblastoma.

TUMORS OF NEURONAL CELLS AND OF PRIMITIVE BIPOTENTIAL PRECURSORS

World Health Organization classification

The most recently revised WHO classification of tumors of the CNS (Kleihues, Burger and Scheithauer, 1993) categorizes the predominately neuronal tumors covered in this section thus:

1.7. Neuronal and mixed neuronal–glial tumors
- 1.7.1. Gangliocytoma
- 1.7.2. Dysplastic gangliocytomas of cerebellum (Lhermitte-Duclos)
- 1.7.3. Desmoplastic infantile ganglioglioma
- 1.7.4. Dysembryoplastic neuroepithelial tumor
- 1.7.5. Ganglioglioma
- 1.7.6. Anaplastic (malignant) ganglioglioma
- 1.7.7. Central neurocytoma

1.9. Embryonal tumors
- 1.9.1. Medulloepithelioma
- 1.9.2. Neuroblastoma
  - 1.9.2.1. Ganglioneuroblastoma
- 1.9.4. Primitive neuroectodermal tumors
  - 1.9.4.1. Medulloblastoma

  Variants:
  - 1.9.4.1.1. Desmoplastic medulloblastoma
  - 1.9.4.1.2. Medullomyoblastoma
  - 1.9.4.1.3. Melanotic medulloblastoma

The present section largely agrees with the system as put forth, with some differences. Anaplastic (malignant) ganglioglioma, characterized by a benign ganglion cell component and a proliferative glial component, is discussed along with gangliogliomas in this section. Recently, however, certain tumors have been recognized in which a malignant neuroblastic component is identified. We prefer categorizing these latter tumors as cerebral neuroblastomas with maturation. It is clear that the typical ganglioglioma shows no proliferative activity in the ganglion cell (neuronal) component; thus, in agreement with Russell and

Rubinstein (1989), we continue to categorize neuronal tumors with proliferating stem-cell components as neuroblastomas, taking the proliferative activity of the cells as proof of the presence of neuroblasts.

The concept of the PNET as put forth by Rorke (1983) and Becker and Hinton (1983) is avoided in the WHO system. Rather, the WHO system puts forth the PNET as a generic term for cerebellar medulloblastomas and for neoplasms that are morphologically indistinguishable from the medulloblastoma but are located at other sites in the CNS (Kleihues, Burger and Scheithauer, 1993). Our reasons are discussed more thoroughly on p. 480, but, in summary, we continue to support a cytogenetic basis for the categorization of tumors, an idea that the PNET system disavows.

Medulloepitheliomas

The existence of this entity, originally proposed by Bailey and Cushing (1925) as the most primitive and multipotential of the CNS neoplasms in their scheme of tumor classification, only became fully recognized after its detailed description by Treip (1957) and the subsequent publication of several confirmatory examples. All these cases fulfill the criteria initially laid down by Bailey and Cushing (1925). More than 30 tumors of this type have now been reported, the largest series to date being published from the Children's Hospital of Philadelphia (Molloy *et al.*, 1996).

Russell and Rubinstein (1989) have stated that the cerebral medulloepithelioma represents the prototype of embryonal central neuroepithelial tumors. Its hallmark features are its architectural pattern, which recapitulates that of the primitive medullary epithelium, and its capacity for multiple divergent differentiation, which in some cases may span the entire range of central neuroepithelial cytogenesis from the most embryonal to the most differentiated cell forms.

Sites

The cerebral hemispheres are most often involved and, in almost half the cases, the tumor presents in a lateral ventricle, as would be expected from its postulated origin from primitive undifferentiated matrix cells. Occasionally, however, it arises in the cerebrum, quite separately from the ependymal lining (Deck, 1969; Molloy *et al.*, 1996). It has also been reported in the posterior fossa (Best, 1974; Sato *et al.*, 1980; Bonnin *et al.*, 1984a; Molloy *et al.*, 1996). Rarer sites are the midbrain (Treip, 1957) and the cauda equina (Karch and Urich, 1972).

Associated lesions

Recorded elsewhere (Bonnin *et al.*, 1984a) is the association of a cerebellar medulloepithelioma with the development of a Wilms' tumor of the kidney. In Treip's (1957) case, the tumor was contiguous with a large meningeal hamartoma of the brainstem.

Age incidence

As expected, the cerebral medulloepithelioma is predominantly a tumor of early childhood, most cases having been reported between the ages of 6 months and 5 years. Congenital examples have been described (Treip, 1957; Sato *et al.*, 1980), as well as occasional cases presenting in the second decade (Scheithauer and Rubinstein, 1979). There seems to be no special sex predilection (Molloy *et al.*, 1996).

Macroscopic appearance

The tumors are characteristically well circumscribed, often massive, with grayish pink, soft, friable cut surfaces, usually with extensive hemorrhagic and necrotic areas (Fig. 9.221). Cystic changes may be present. Extensive local dissemination is occasionally encountered at initial presentation while diffuse dissemination is often seen at death (Molloy *et al.*, 1996).

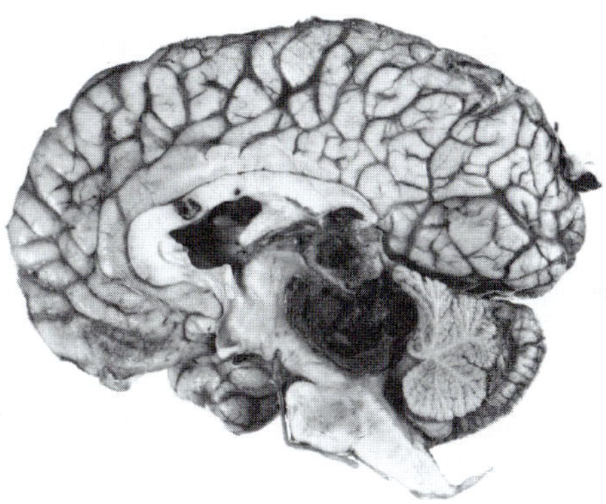

Fig. 9.221 Midsagittal section of a medulloepithelioma arising in the brainstem of a 24-year-old male who was well 10 months prior to death. The large hemorrhagic necrotic tumor mass arose in the region of the posterior third ventricle and extends posteriorly to involve the fourth ventricle/cerebellum and is eroding into the tegmentum, producing hydrocephalus.

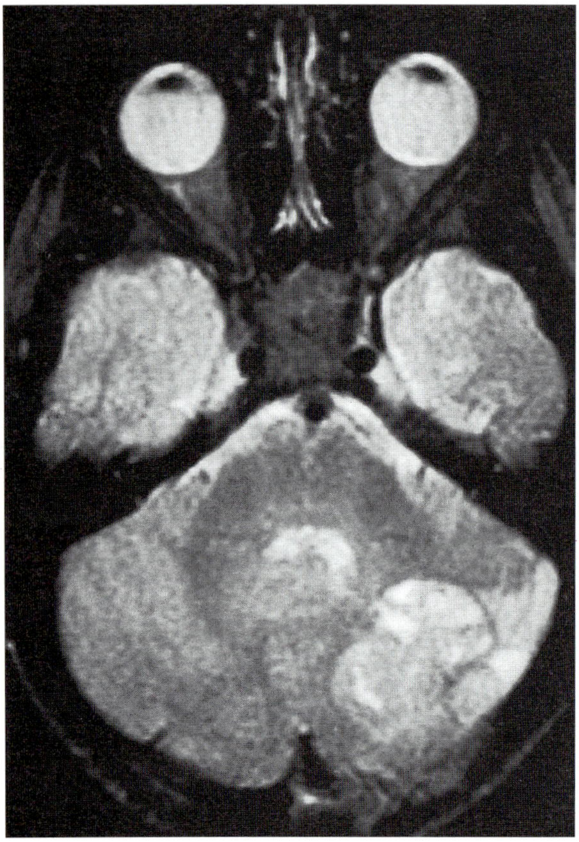

Fig. 9.222 Axial T2-weighted MRI demonstrating a large left cerebellar mass that has mild hyperintensity relative to gray matter. Small curvilinear cystic areas are identified centrally as areas of high T2 signal intensity. Minimum associated edema is present.

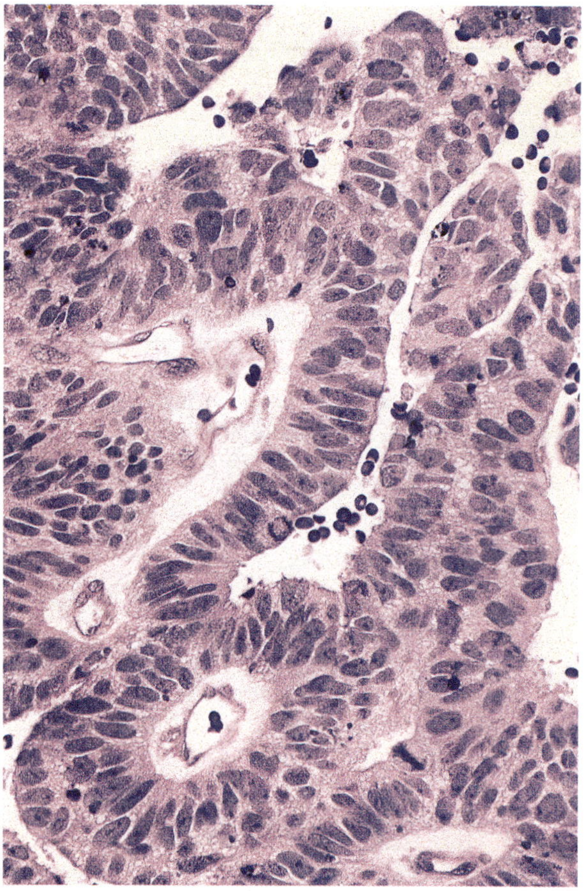

Fig. 9.223 Medulloepithelioma showing ribbons and tubules of primitive neuroepithelial cells. H&E, × 190

Radiographic appearance

The imaging appearance of medulloepithelioma reflects the large, well-defined nature of these tumors with well-circumscribed margins and apparent lobulations. The majority of the mass tends to have a mildly low T1 signal intensity relative to gray matter, and an isointense or mildly hyperintense T2 signal intensity. Frequently, there are areas of cyst formation within the mass. Areas of necrosis or hemorrhage may also develop. The tumor shows variable enhancement patterns ranging from areas of no enhancement to mild heterogeneous enhancement or nodular enhancement. There is usually only minimum surrounding edema (Fig. 9.222).

Microscopic appearance

The microscopic appearance of the medulloepithelioma is highly distinctive. The tumor displays closely aligned cells in a papillary or tubular pattern that recalls the structure of the primitive epithelium of the medullary plate and neural tube. In the more solid areas, the cells may form elongated ribbons (Fig. 9.223). Cytologically, the cells may vary from columnar to a low cuboidal shape and are devoid of cilia and blepharoplasts, thereby distinguishing them from those of a papillary ependymoma. The luminal margin of the tubules often suggests the presence of an internal limiting membranc (Fig. 9.224): This consists of an irregular eosinophilic glycogen-layer positive by PAS stain, the apices of the cells being occasionally capped by minute bleb-like structures. The presence of such an internal membrane has occasionally been questioned (Karch and Urich, 1972; Pollak and Friede, 1977): on the basis of electron microscopic observations, Pollak and Friede (1977) proposed that it may only represent an amorphous surface coating covering the neuroepithelial cells, its electron density being

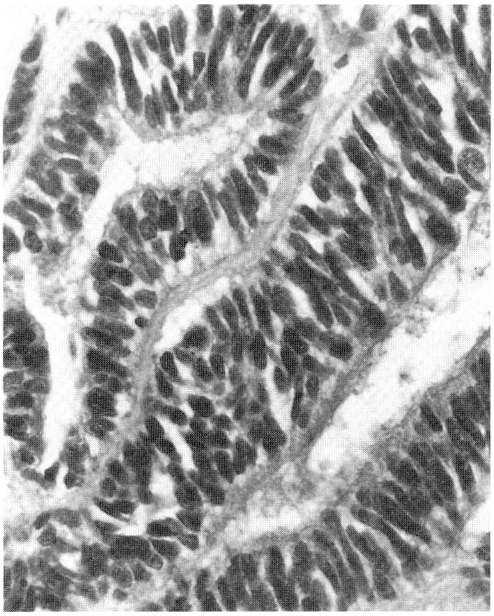

Fig. 9.224 Subcortical parietal occipital medulloepithelioma arising in a 5-year-old boy showing stratified columnar cells bordered by an internal and external limiting membrane. Note the mitotic figure (lower right) on the abluminal side of the lining cells. H&E, × 375

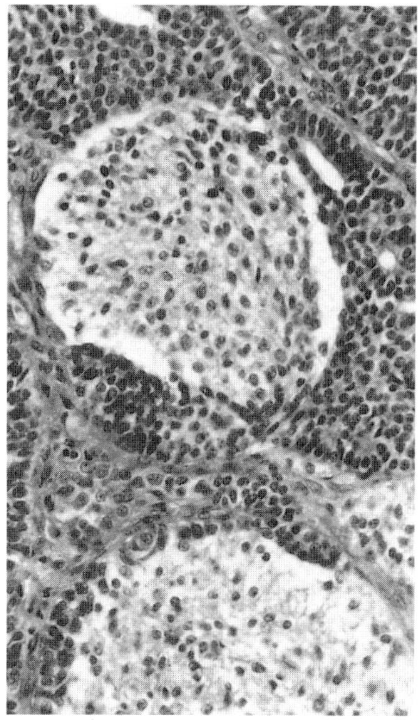

Fig. 9.225 Pale islands of cells suggestive of astrocytic differentiation in the medulloepithelioma described in Fig. 9.224. H&E, × 190

similar to that of basement membrane. Apparently, the fine structure of the neural tube shows no membrane on its inner surface (Troost, Jansen and Dingemans, 1990). On the other hand, the external limiting cell membrane (Fig. 9.224) of the epithelial tubules and ribbons is more clear cut and consists of a crisp glycogen-positive basement membrane that rests on a delicate connective tissue network containing reticulin fibrils but little collagen. The cell nuclei usually have coarse chromatin nodes and, occasionally, multiple nucleoli. Mitotic figures are numerous and most frequently found on the abluminal side of the cells lining the tubular spaces (Fig. 9.224), a feature that recalls the localization of the nuclei of the primitive ventricular cells in their mitotic phase in the early stages of central neurocytogenesis.

As noted elsewhere (pp. 000 and 000), the tubular and papillary formations of the cerebral medulloepithelioma may closely mimic the architectural pattern and cellular features of two other papillary tumors characteristically occurring in childhood and also typically involving the ventricular system or its neighborhood: a malignant choroid plexus papilloma, and a papillary teratoma predominantly composed of endodermal sinus tumor or embryonal carcinoma elements. In the medulloepithelioma, however, the pseudostratification of tall columnar cells is most distinctive and, in many cases, the correct diagnosis may be arrived at by virtue of the capacity of the tumor to exhibit differentiation in other microscopic fields.

As pointed out by numerous investigators (Treip, 1957; Russell and Rubinstein, 1989; Molloy *et al.*, 1996), a common feature is the presence of patternless sheets of tumor cells exhibiting hyperchromatic nuclei and high nuclear-to-cytoplasmic ratios. In these areas, immunochemical stains for glial or neuronal antigens may bind individual cells or, occasionally, groups of cells. Indeed, Caccamo, Herman and Rubinstein (1989) and Molloy *et al.* (1996) noted mature ganglion cells and glial cells in a minority of cases. Furthermore, the neuronal antigen, class III β-tubulin, could be detected in rare cells forming the primitive medullary tubules, indicative of early neuronal commitment. Glial differentiation may be expressed along ependymal, ependymoblastic, astrocytic (Fig. 9.225), spongioblastic, or oligodendroglial lines, or as mixtures of different glial cell types (Deck, 1969; Jellinger, 1972). The full gamut of neural cytologic types, embracing the entire spectrum from the most embryonal to the most differentiated cell forms of both glial and neuronal lineage, has been recorded in several examples (Scheithauer and Rubinstein, 1979; Sato *et al.*, 1980; Auer and Becker, 1983;

Bonnin *et al.*, 1984a; Caccamo, Herman and Rubinstein, 1989).

The *mesenchymal stromal* elements may vary greatly from case to case. In some examples, the connective tissue is tenuous; the delicate supporting blood vessels are devoid of the endothelial capillary proliferation characteristic of malignant gliomas. Other examples, as noted by Karch and Urich (1972), may display a prominent vascular and fibrous connective tissue stroma including, in one case, areas of cartilage, bone and striated muscle (Auer and Becker, 1983).

The latter feature most likely represents an instance of stromal metaplasia, a phenomenon recorded not only in embryonal tumors, but also in other neural neoplasms such as the ependymoma. Auer and Becker (1983), however, have suggested that their case should be regarded as a neoplasm of mixed mesenchymal and neuroepithelial origin and that, while not strictly a teratoma, it illustrates an example of osseous, cartilaginous and myoblastic differentiation originating from neuroectodermal tumor cell derivatives. This view gains some apparent support from other intriguing observations on the presence of striated muscle fibers in some variants of cerebellar medulloblastoma (see p. 000), of rhabdomyosarcomatous elements in some ciliary medulloepitheliomas (see p. 000), and from tissue culture studies on nitrosourea-induced neuronal and glial cell lines whose progeny has been reported to express the phenotypic and neuropharmacologic features of skeletal muscle cells (Brandt, Kimes and Klier, 1976; Lennon, Peterson and Schubert, 1979). Even more surprisingly, a cell line obtained from human malignant medulloblastoma has been reported to show striated muscle differentiation (Giangaspero *et al.*, 1992), although whether such cells were derived originally from neuroectodermal elements or from their supporting mesenchymal stroma remains open to debate. In the present context is the observation by Russell (1960), in a 23-year-old man, of striated muscle fibers in a frontal tumor that was originally designated by Davie (1932) as a medulloepithelioma and that was consequently reassigned to the teratoma group. Indeed, the precise relationship of medulloepithelioma to teratoma has been the subject of some controversy. Since both tumors share the dual features of being embryonal and multipotential, and since, as recalled above, a medulloepithelioma may occasionally be associated with another apparently independent lesion of malformative or embryonal neoplastic nature, the distinction between the two may perhaps be more semantic than conceptual. The main difference, of course, lies in the more restricted differentiating potential of the medulloepithelioma. On the other hand, neuroepithelial differentiation has been found in more than 75% of teratomas at all sites and in all the reported intracranial examples (Willis, 1971). Although it is clear that phenotypic expression is less restricted in neoplasia, the suggestion by Auer and Becker (1983) that skeletal muscle might be expressed in the primitive central medulloepithelioma raises, in any event, fascinating issues on the regulation of neoplastic neuroepithelial phenotypic expression and differentiation.

Electron microscopy

The fine structure of two cases, claimed to be medulloepithelioma, have been reported (Pollak and Friede, 1977; Troost, Jansen and Dingemans, 1990). The electron microscopic features were those of poorly differentiated cells with sparse cytoplasmic organelles, devoid of cilia or microvilli. Pollak and Friede (1977) noted an amorphous surface coating along the luminal side of the cell plasma membranes that was not seen in the other case. The basal surfaces of the epithelial cells rested on a distinct continuous, and often folded, basement membrane. In both cases were found zonulae adherentes along the lateral cell surfaces. Troost, Jansen and Dingemans (1990) noted that the capillary endothelial cells lacked fenestrations. Further electron microscopic descriptions of cerebral medulloepitheliomas are clearly needed.

Evolution and metastatic potential

As expected from their primitive cytologic features, these tumors are highly malignant. The usual survival time from the onset of symptoms is 6 months. Cerebrospinal seeding has been described (Van Epps, Samuelson and McCormick, 1967; Pollak and Friede, 1977; Molloy *et al.*, 1996) and, in the case described by Van Epps, Samuelson and McCormick (1967), extraneural metastases had developed in the regional lymph nodes following the appearance of several tumor nodules in the craniotomy scar 6 months after surgical intervention.

Medulloblastomas (including cerebellar neuroblastoma)

The prevailing name 'medulloblastoma', given by Bailey and Cushing (1925), is unfortunate because no embryonal cell has been identified as a medulloblast. However, recent evidence suggests that cells exist which can be equated with the 'indifferent cells' of Schaper (1897b) in that there is a limited potential to differentiate into neurons and glia (Valtz *et al.*, 1991). These cells were originally conceived as being undifferentiated elements of the mantle layer of the embryo that had, as yet, acquired none of the features that would permit their identification as either glia- or neuron-committed. Recent studies have shown that conditionally immortalized embryonal rat hippocampal cells, when transplanted into the cerebellum, acquire features of internal granular cells and Bergmann glia (Renfranz, Cunningham and McKay, 1991). These data are in accord with the views of Schaper (1897b) and the hypotheses of Bailey and Cushing (1925) that tumors of these cells could arise in either the cerebrum or cerebellum. It is clear, given the experimental protocol, that these implantation studies are indicative of differentiating capabilities inherent to the cell, as well as inductive influences of the recipient tissues, and they appear to support the development of mature neurons and glia from clones of immortalized cells when placed in the cerebellum.

Cytogenesis

By definition, medulloblastomas are restricted to the cerebellum. This restriction is supported by the fact that the histogenesis of the cerebellum is uniquely different from that of other parts of the central neuraxis. The origin of cerebellar medulloblastomas has, in consequence, been ascribed to three main sources. Stevenson and Echlin (1934) postulated an origin from the external granular layer (fetal granular layer of Obersteiner). This subpial layer of small primitive cells is present throughout the cerebellar cortex at birth and gradually disappears during the first year of life. The cells migrate inwards to augment the neurons of the definitive internal granular layer. They have also been regarded as the source of cortical neuroglia (Kershman, 1938; Fujita, Shimada and Nakamura, 1966; Fujita, 1967). However, more recent studies have resulted in divergent views: some have supported the early views of Ramón y Cajal (1952) that the cells of the external granular layer give rise to neurons only (Swarz and Del Cerro, 1977; Hallonet and Le Douarin, 1993), while others have indicated that Bergmann glia may also arise from the external granular layer (Renfranz, Cunningham and McKay, 1991). In fact, the histogenesis of the cerebellar cortical glia is still a matter of uncertainty (Lewis *et al.*, 1977). The Bergmann glia are generally believed to arise from the primary germinal zone (ventricular layer) of the cerebellum, an idea also supported by quail-chick chimera studies (Hallonet and Le Douarin, 1993), studies that also demonstrate that Purkinje cells arise from cells migrating radially from the primary germinal zone (ventricular layer) of the cerebellum. More importantly, these studies have resolved the origin of the external granular layer cells from the metencephalic vesicles at the 12–14 somite stage, as well as the migration pathways these cells ultimately take to arrive in the internal granular layer (Alvarado-Mallart, 1993; Hallonet and Le Douarin, 1993; Le Douarin, 1993).

The validity of extrapolating cytogenetic conclusions from histologic features in a neoplasm may have to be qualified because phenotypic expression of a neoplastic cell appears to be less restricted than that of the tissue from which it is held to arise (Brüstle and McKay, 1995). Without prejudice, therefore, to the histogenetic capabilities of the external granular layer or of other embryonal cells normally derived from the cerebellar germinative zones, the phenotypic features of the cerebellar medulloblastoma suggest that it originates from primitive neuroepithelial cells whose progeny have the capacity to express antigenic and cytologic features of either glial or neuronal lines.

In any event, many of the microscopic features of medulloblastomas can be explained by their derivation from the external granular layer or its remnants. The occasional focal persistence of cell rests from that layer has been documented by Brzustowicz and Kernohan (1952) and Yachnis, Rorke and Trojanowski (1994). Scheinker (1939) reported a medulloblastoma in a 49-year-old, which showed evidence that the fetal granular layer had persisted; furthermore, serial sectioning demonstrated a connection between the tumor and that layer. It must, however, be remembered that these surface localizations of tumor cells beneath the pia might rather be interpreted as manifestations of the subpial 'secondary structures' of neoplastic spread defined by Scherer (Rubinstein and Northfield, 1964). On the other hand, Rubinstein's study of one congenital midline cerebellar medulloblastoma appears to lend partial support to the original hypothesis of Stevenson and Echlin (1934). In that example, the fetal granular layer adjacent to the tumor showed marked neoplastic proliferations that formed an irregular sawtooth pattern extending into most of the molecular layer (Figs 9.226–9.228), and all transitions were seen between the normal external granular layer and tumor formation (Kadin, Rubinstein and Nelson, 1970). A similar pattern of diffuse cellular proliferation involving the external granular layer, mainly of the vermis (and microscopically resembling a medulloblastoma), has been recorded in a neonate by Amacher, Torres and Rittenhouse (1986).

Subsequent to the case report, Russell and Rubinstein (1989) noted two additional examples in which an abnormal, presumably neoplastic, proliferation of the fetal granular layer was purportedly associated with a tumor mass in the cerebellum.

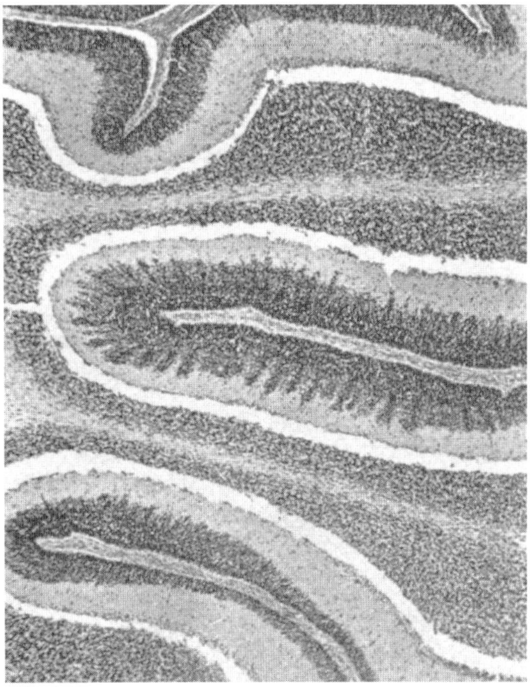

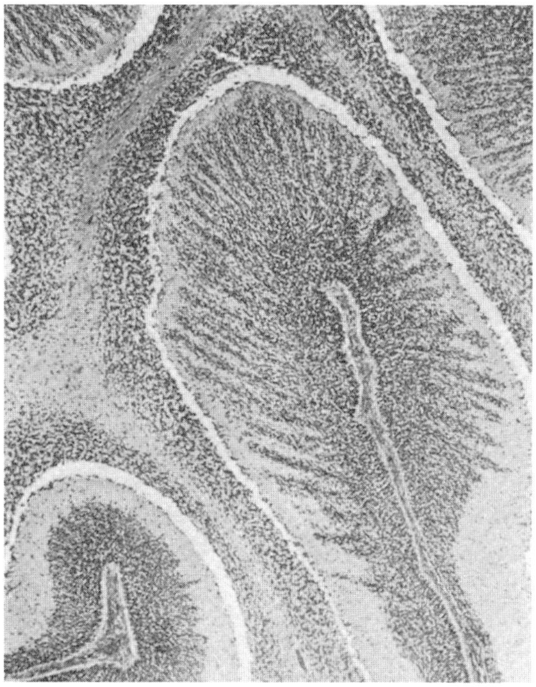

Figs 9.226 and 9.227 Sawtooth pattern of neoplastic proliferation of fetal granular layer associated with a congenital midline medulloblastoma in a premature infant. Both H&E, × 40 (From Kadin, Rubinstein and Nelson, 1970)

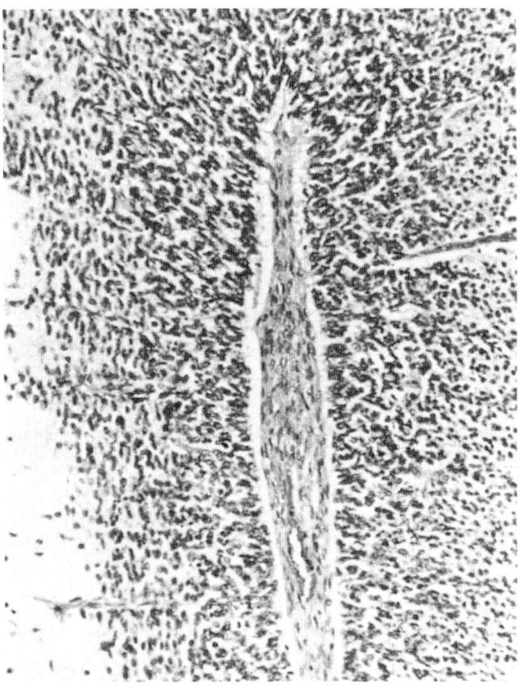

Fig. 9.228 Higher magnification of Fig. 9.227, again showing the infiltrating tumor cells perpendicular to the arachnoid. H&E, × 130

The first case was a hemispheric medulloblastoma, presumably congenital, with astrocytic cytologic features; the external granular layer was markedly thickened and merged in places with the neoplasm, with a distinct focus of cerebellar micropolygyria noted in close proximity. In Russell and Rubinstein's (1989) second case, a diffuse and mitotically active proliferation of the external granular layer was associated with excessive plication of the cortical cerebellar folia in a 7-month-old male. In this latter case, the neoplastic proliferation of both glial and neuronal elements progressed over the following 3 years into development of a deep cerebellar ganglioglioma contiguous to a diffuse cortical, relatively orderly, gangliogliomatosis. This latter component was noted to have some architectural features in common with those of the dysplastic gangliocytoma of the cerebellum (see p. 505).

Yachnis, Rorke and Trojanowski (1994) have also described abnormalities of cell migration among a variety of fetuses and infants ranging in age from 15 weeks postconception to 15 months postnatal. They noted the previously reported association of cerebellar cell migrational disturbances in patients with germline trisomy 13–15 and trisomy 18 (Norman, 1966; Warkany, Passarge and Smith,

1966; Rorke, Fogelson and Riggs, 1968). These investigators suggested that these aberrant residual germinal cells or glia may prolong the window of vulnerability to neoplastic transformation, and they demonstrated a persistently proliferating population of cells in these aggregates using an anti-PCNA antibody.

The quail-chick chimera studies cited previously appear to uphold some of Raaf and Kernohan's (1944) concepts. The latter authors attributed certain of the midline examples to nests of primitive cells in the posterior medullary velum. They based this theory upon an examination of the cerebellum in 161 embryos, fetuses and infants from 8 weeks to 5 years of age. The quail-chick chimera studies have confirmed that cells destined to form the external granular layer pass through a 'germinal bud' situated at the hind end of the posterior medullary velum. This bud normally disappears before the end of the first month of extrauterine life. Raaf and Kernohan (1944) found abnormal persistence of these cells in 23/104 cerebella in which this region was examined microscopically; the cells morphologically resembled those of medulloblastoma. Ringertz and Tola (1950), similarly, in their report of 11 cases of medulloblastoma, found that a small group (six cases) appeared to arise from the anterior medullary velum. Because cells originating in the roof of the primitive fourth ventricle migrate dorsally and laterally to form the external granular layer, it has been postulated that tumors may arise from germinative cells, or their remnants, anywhere along their migratory path. Because the migratory process normally proceeds in a lateral direction, this hypothesis may explain the relatively higher frequency of laterally situated tumors in adults (Kadin, Rubinstein and Nelson, 1970). Interestingly, these studies also indicate that some cells from the group destined to form the external granular layer may also migrate to the optic tectum, the nosologic implication being that medulloblastomas may also arise in the quadrigeminal plate.

Studies such as these implicate a mechanism for the homeobox genes, which are master control genes involved in, at least, gross organization of body parts (VandenBerg, Herman and Rubinstein, 1987). Early evidence from studies performed using mice and birds indicates that the homeobox genes *EN1, EN2, WNT1, OTX1* and *OTX2* are involved in cerebellar organization and regional specificity (Joyner *et al.*, 1991; Alvarado-Mallart, 1993; Hawkes *et al.*, 1993; Frantz *et al.*, 1994; Oberdick, 1994). Preliminary studies of homeobox gene expression in medulloblastomas support the idea that this area might be a fruitful avenue for research. Kozmik *et al.* (1995) have found *PAX5* expressed in 70% of medulloblastomas, *PAX6* in 78%, *EN1* in 57% and *EN2* in 78%. Furthermore, these authors indicate that the genes *WNT1, PAX1, PAX2* and *PAX3* were either infrequently expressed or not expressed at all. The presence of *EN1* and *EN2* gene expression was interpreted by the authors as supporting an origin from the external granular cell layer. Although raising the possibility that *PAX5* expression correlated with a blocked level of differentiation corresponding to a period when *PAX5* is expressed at the midbrain/hindbrain boundary region of the embryo (12–14 somite stage), they discounted this theory because of the lack of coexpression of *WNT1* or *PAX2* as described by Alvarado-Mallart (1993). Rather, these authors interpreted diffuse *PAX5* expression in classical medulloblastomas and absence of *PAX5* expression in the pale islands of desmoplastic medulloblastomas as correlating with a cell proliferation potential in these locations (Kozmik *et al.*, 1995).

Furthermore, the influence of cell adhesion molecules and growth factors involved in directing cell migration and maturation appear significant in this very complex system of embryogenesis (Gao, Heintz and Hatten, 1991; Aloe and Vigneti, 1992; Giordano *et al.*, 1992; Gocht *et al.*, 1992; Lagunowich, *et al.*, 1992; Hatten, 1993; Streit *et al.*, 1993; Smits *et al.*, 1996).

A third possible source of origin for the medulloblastoma, namely the internal granular neurons, has been proposed on the basis of observations on experimentally induced tumors obtained in adult mice by topical application of carcinogenic hydrocarbons (Zimmerman, 1969), and in hamsters following their inoculation at birth with the JC strain of human papovavirus (Zu Rhein and Varakis, 1979; Nagashima *et al.*, 1984). As noted in the chapters on experimentally induced neoplasms (Chapter 5), the neoplastically transformed cells in the latter case are presumably those of the external granular layer, which are still replicating at the time of inoculation of the virus, whereas, microscopically, the tumors produced seem to originate from the internal granular layer. Indeed, some authorities have, in the past, identified the medulloblastoma with the neuroblastoma and regarded this tumor as incapable of glial differentiation (Tola, 1951; Bailey, 1955, 1971). However, the tools at our disposal for phenotypic identification indicate that glial cells may be encountered in medulloblastomas. Indeed, the identification of at least some of these neoplasms as cerebellar neuroblastomas, on the basis of their electron microscopic features, can also be fully endorsed. Innovative new approaches are needed in order to reconcile these different theories of the origins, locations and histomorphologies of the medulloblastoma.

On both cytogenetic and practical grounds, therefore, we continue to endorse Rubinstein's firm insistence on maintaining a separation between the medulloblastomas and the embryonal neoplasms found elsewhere in the CNS. Developmentally, the cerebellum follows a unique scheme that includes not only an external-to-internal migratory pathway, but also, frequently, a postnatal residuum of embryonic cells. Histogenetically, the developmental pathway or pathways available to an embryonic neural cell are only grudgingly yielding clues for the construction of an embryonic paradigm (e.g., Frederiksen *et al.*, 1988; Trojanowski, Tohyama and Lee, 1992; Zimmerman *et al.*, 1994), such as that available for hematopoietic neoplasms. Epidemiologically, the cerebellum is unique in its high incidence of neoplasms that are phenotypically neuronal. Thus, the current view that the medulloblastoma is essentially a cerebellar neoplasm is retained, with the corollary that those reported as occurring primarily in other sites should be regarded with skepticism. Even with this separation, we recognize that the entity known as the medulloblastoma will be further subdivided based on such factors as degree of maturation, chromosomal abnormalities, susceptibility to treatment, length of patient survival, and other features to be disclosed by advancing knowledge (VandenBerg, Herman and Rubinstein, 1987).

Epidemiology

There is general agreement that medulloblastomas constitute 7–8% of all intracranial tumors of neuroepithelial origin (see Zülch and Christensen, 1956, pp. 118–43). Their predominance in childhood has long been recognized, accounting for up to 25% of intracranial tumors in this population, approximately equal in frequency to the cerebellar astrocytomas. In the Scandinavian countries, Clausen *et al.* (1990) have calculated a yearly incidence of 0.5 per 100 000 children. Approximately 50% occur in the first decade, having a maximal incidence at 3–5 years of age (Farwell, Dohrmann and Flannery, 1984; Clausen *et al.*, 1990) and being rare in the first year (Buetow, Smirniotopoulos and Done, 1990; Oi, Kokunai and Matsumoto, 1990). Ringertz and Tola (1950) found that 64% occurred between birth and 14 years of age, with a maximal incidence at age 5–9 years, while Farwell, Dohrmann and Flannery (1984) noted the maximal incidence at 3–9 years of age. A second peak was noted in adults ranging from 20 to 24 years of age by Ringertz and Tola (1950). Russell and Rubinstein (1989) noted, in a personal series of 55 cases, 33 examples in the first decade, 14 between the ages of 17 and 31 years, and three cases in the fifth decade.

Data pooled by Kopelson, Linggood and Kleinman (1982), from nine published series totaling almost 200 patients, suggest that about 30% of medulloblastomas occur in adults. More recently, a review of the Surveillance, Epidemiology and End Results (SEER) data, which includes 161 patients, indicates that only 32% of medulloblastomas occur in people over 10 years of age, with 31% occurring in children less than 4 years old and 36% being diagnosed in children aged between 5 and 10 years (Roberts *et al.*, 1991). Exceptional is the case, reported by Russell and Rubinstein (1989), of a 48-year-old male in whom a cerebellar medulloblastoma recurred massively, with metastatic deposits in the cervical lymph nodes, 13 years later. Zülch and Christensen (1956) mention that the oldest patient in their series was 53 years of age. Its occurrence in 73-year-olds was recorded by Kepes, Morantz and Dorzab (1987) and again by Robey *et al.* (1988), and in a 67-year-old and a 71-year-old by Cervoni *et al.* (1994b).

Racially, medulloblastomas exhibit no obvious bias, with 81.6% of the tumors in the SEER data (Roberts *et al.*, 1991) diagnosed in Caucasians and 9.6% in African-Americans. Males are generally affected more often than females by a ratio of 4:3 (57%:43% in the Connecticut data; Farwell, Dohrmann and Flannery, 1984) although the SEER data suggest a much stronger male predominance of 63–37%. Similarly, Clausen *et al.* (1990) note a 2:1 male:female ratio in the Scandinavian countries.

A seasonal fluctuation in the incidence of the tumor has been reported from Japan (Finlay, 1986), suggesting that patients with this tumor are more often born in the winter months; a similar fluctuation has apparently been noted in the incidence of congenital cerebral defects. Clausen *et al.* (1990) did not note a seasonal fluctuation in the Scandinavian countries. Farwell, Dohrmann and Flannery (1984), scrutinizing the Connecticut Tumor Registry, found an apparently excessive number of medulloblastomas in children born from 1954 to 1958; contamination with SV40 of the poliomyelitis vaccine given to the mothers at the time of pregnancy was suggested as a possible prenatal factor (but see Chapter 5, on the lack of evidence that exposure to SV40 in the neonatal period might be carcinogenic in man). The same workers also noted a relative increase in the incidence of lymphohematopoietic and CNS neoplasias in parents and siblings of children with medulloblastoma (Farwell and Flannery, 1984).

Familial cases have been described (Griepentrog and Pauly, 1957; Bickerstaff, Connolly and Woolf, 1967; Belamaric and Chau, 1969). The first of these groups of workers reported the presentation of cerebellar medulloblastoma in female identical twins at the ages of 8 and 11 weeks. In the first patient, a coincidental teratoid tumor in the chest contained microscopic foci with embryonal cells said to resemble medulloblastoma. The familial occurrence of the tumor has more recently been analyzed by Tijssen (1986), who reviewed 21 familial examples. Of these, four concerned monozygotic twins, nine recorded the occurrence of medulloblastoma in siblings and eight noted the existence of siblings with different brain tumors of which one was a medulloblastoma.

The association of medulloblastoma with certain hereditary or familial diseases, some of them autosomal dominant, others recessive, has also been documented. The most frequent of these is the nevoid basal-cell carcinoma syndrome (Neblett, Waltz and Anderson, 1971; Hawkins, Hoffman and Becker, 1979; Naguib *et al.*, 1982; Evans, Birch and Orton, 1991; Evans *et al.*, 1991; Schofield *et al.*, 1995), also known as Gorlin's syndrome (Gorlin and Goltz, 1960) and reviewed in Volume 2, p. 399. The disorder is autosomal dominant, with a high penetrance and a variable expression. Another inherited disorder with a higher than sporadic association with medulloblastoma is the familial colorectal cancer syndrome (Volume 2, p. 167).

Collectively, and in the light of other neoplastic lesions and other familial syndromes occasionally encountered in association with the tumor, it seems likely that heritable and other congenital factors (Thorne *et al.*, 1994) play a role in the genesis of some medulloblastomas, with evidence continuing to grow. Rare examples of congenital medulloblastomas have been reported (see Kayama *et al.*, 1993, for references), including the cases of Griepentrog and Pauly (1957). In addition to the previously quoted tumor in the vermis of a 13-week-old infant born 2 months prematurely (Kadin, Rubinstein and Nelson, 1970), Russell and Rubinstein (1989) noted one in a female infant aged 7 weeks; expansion of the skull was noticed 10 days after birth in this case. Jänisch *et al.* (1984), who reviewed the records from 1960 to 1979 of 55 histologically verified CNS tumors in the fetal and neonatal period, found that medulloblastomas (13 cases) constituted the largest single group. In contrast, Buetow, Smirniotopoulos and Done (1990) found only four medulloblastomas among their 45 patients with brain tumors diagnosed before 60 days of age.

Associated lesions

The coexistence of a cerebellar medulloblastoma with another tumor has also been noted. Waldbaur *et al.* (1976) reported monozygotic twins with a medulloblastoma in one and a pineoblastoma in the other. Three infants, ranging from 1 day to 12 months of age, reportedly had both a cerebellar medulloblastoma and a malignant rhabdoid tumor of the kidney (Bonnin *et al.*, 1984a). Russell and Rubinstein (1989) also previously noted the case of a 3½-year-old female who had a medulloblastoma associated with a fibrolipomatous hamartoma of the leptomeninges, focal cerebellar micropolygyria and cerebellar cortical ectopias. Medulloblastomas have also been reported to occur sporadically in patients with ataxia–telangiectasis, xeroderma pigmentosa and the blue rubber bleb nevus syndrome (see Tijssen, 1986, for references).

Macroscopic appearance

The location of medulloblastomas within the cerebellum may not be entirely random, with a midline situation being characteristic in childhood (Figs 9.229 and 9.230). In the 1989 series of Russell and Rubinstein, 67% were midcerebellar; in the series of Maraziotis *et al.* (1992) that included 29 children less than 16 years of age, 90% were in the vermis. In the series of 144 children reviewed by Park *et al.* (1983) from the Hospital for Sick Children in Toronto, 93% of medulloblastomas were situated in the cerebellar vermis. Most are posterior, encroaching on the cisterna magna as well as on the cavity of the fourth ventricle (Figs 9.229 and 9.230), but some are too extensive to permit their site of origin to be determined. A minority are laterally situated in the hemispheres, a fact long known and repeatedly confirmed (Rubinstein and Northfield 1964; Chatty and Earle, 1971; Müller, Slowik and Schröder, 1978), and are more characteristic of adult tumors (Ferrante *et al.*, 1991; Aragonés *et al.*, 1994; Carrie *et al.*, 1994; Prados *et al.*, 1995). For example, 12/17 patients older than 15 years of age, reported by Schindler and Gullotta (1983), had hemispheric tumors. In rare instances, the main mass projects into the cerebellopontine angle or may arise from the tonsil.

Medulloblastomas are soft, rather friable and moderately demarcated from the cerebellar tissues. At autopsy, their cut surfaces can be grayish white or pink, but are more often described as red or purplish when exposed at operation, and the larger examples may show central areas of necrosis; cystic foci and microcalcifications are rare (Jaffey *et al.*, 1995). The cavity of the fourth ventricle is commonly occupied by extensions of the growth (Fig. 9.230) and may be occluded; the floor of the cavity is then often infiltrated. A tongue-like process may even plug the caudal end of the aqueduct. Likewise, the cerebellar peduncles may be infiltrated and the cisterna magna filled with growth. The hemispherically situated examples in adults characteristically present as unusually clearly demarcated masses with

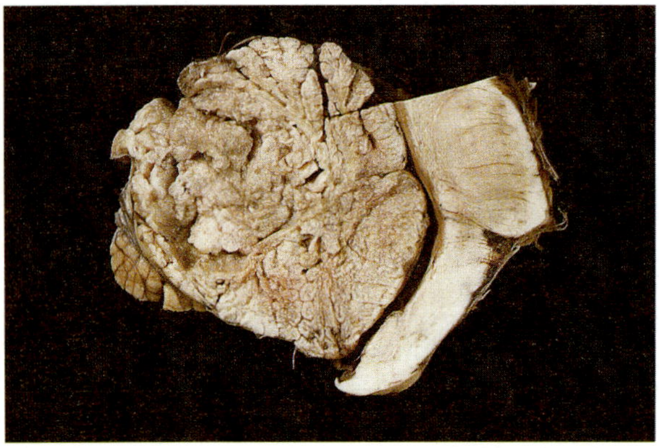

Fig. 9.229 Midline cerebellar medulloblastoma projecting into the fourth ventricle.

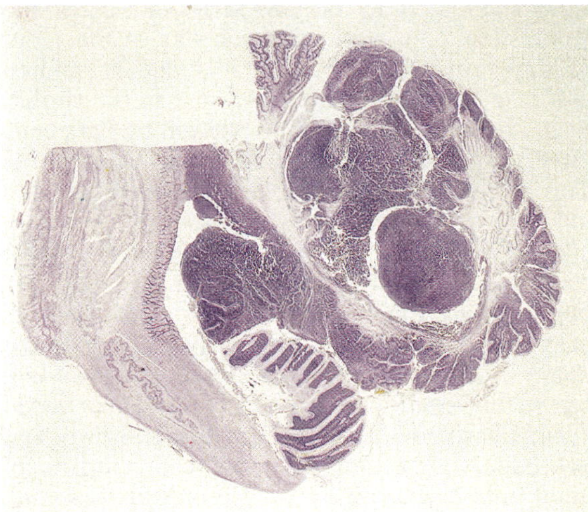

Fig. 9.230 Same case as Fig. 9.229. Midsagittal whole mount section revealing the diffuse infiltration of the cerebellar folia by medulloblastoma. Cresyl fast violet, × 1

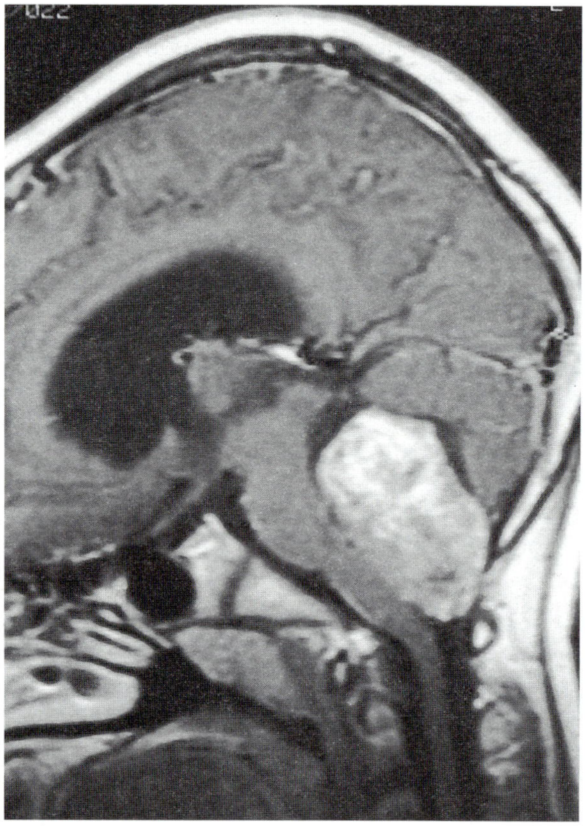

Fig. 9.231 Sagittal T1-weighted postcontrast MRI demonstrating a large mass that lies within the fourth ventricle and extends inferiorly to the foramen magnum. The brainstem is deviated anteriorly and the cerebellum is deviated posteriorly. The mass demonstrates enhancement with some heterogeneous areas. Note the enlarged lateral ventricles indicating obstructive hydrocephalus.

a smooth or slightly lobulated outline and a crisp, almost woody, consistency. They are usually found on the dorsal surface of the lobe, but are not attached to the tentorium. Occasionally, the tumor grows *en plaque* along the surface of the cerebellum.

Diffuse involvement of the regional leptomeninges, producing sheets of growth that obscure the underlying structures, is characteristic and paves the way to remote metastasis by the cerebrospinal pathway. But, the retrograde ventricular metastases, affecting particularly the floor of the third ventricle, are due to the extensions into the fourth ventricle and resulting stasis. Russell and Rubinstein (1989) noted an example in which the infundibular metastasis was larger than the primary growth. Metastases should also be sought in the leptomeninges over the cerebral convexities and in the subarachnoid space of the spinal canal, where they may either be discrete or appear as a diffuse opalescent infiltration over the posterior surface of the cord. Two notable sites of metastasis are the lumbosacral cord and the orbital surface of the frontal lobe, with secondary invasion and destruction of the cribriform plate (Rubinstein, 1959; Jereb *et al.*, 1981), a sequence of events that is altered by the optimal exposure of these regions to craniospinal radiotherapy (Donnal *et al.*, 1992).

Radiographic appearance

The imaging study of choice for evaluation of medulloblastoma is MRI. Signal intensity on T1-weighted images is usually hypointense, while

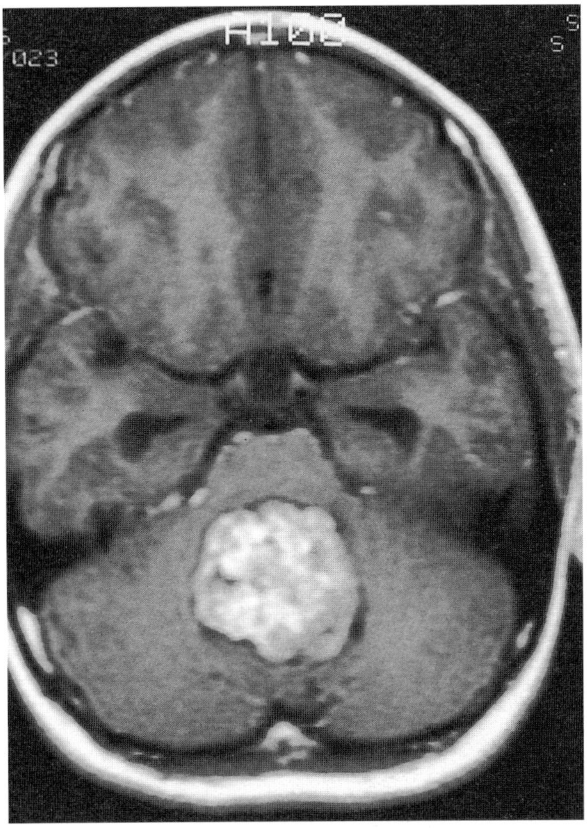

Fig. 9.232 Same as Fig. 9.231. Axial T1-weighted post-contrast image demonstrating filling of the fourth ventricles by the enhancing mass. Moderate enhancement with mild heterogeneity is noted in the tumor. This is the typical pattern of medulloblastoma as demonstrated in this 7-year-old patient. Note the temporal horn dilatation, suggesting obstructive hydrocephalus. No leptomeningeal enhancement is found in this patient.

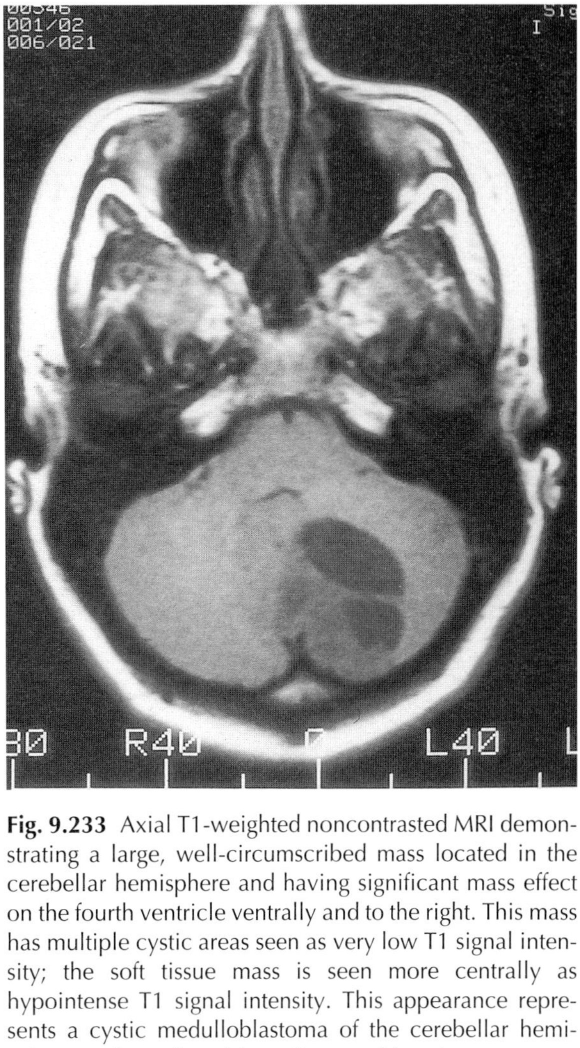

Fig. 9.233 Axial T1-weighted noncontrasted MRI demonstrating a large, well-circumscribed mass located in the cerebellar hemisphere and having significant mass effect on the fourth ventricle ventrally and to the right. This mass has multiple cystic areas seen as very low T1 signal intensity; the soft tissue mass is seen more centrally as hypointense T1 signal intensity. This appearance represents a cystic medulloblastoma of the cerebellar hemisphere and was found in a 42-year-old patient.

signal intensity on T2-weighted images is usually iso- or hyperintense. Following contrast administration, there is usually enhancement to a moderate degree. This may be homogeneous, although areas of heterogeneity are often present. Small cystic areas may be seen and, occasionally, there are areas of hemorrhage.

Masses involving the fourth ventricle compress the pons and medulla anteriorly while enlarging the fourth ventricle and deviating the cerebellum posteriorly. Obstructive hydrocephalus is commonly seen at presentation (Figs 9.231 and 9.232).

Locations outside the fourth ventricle are more commonly identified in teenagers and adults, with only one third of such cases being intraventricular. The cerebellar hemispheres are a common location. In older patients, medulloblastomas contain cystic areas in up to 80% of cases (Fig. 9.233).

The appearance of medulloblastoma on noncontrasted CT scans typically demonstrates a moderately hyperdense mass. This is due to dense cellularity and the relatively high nuclear-to-cytoplasmic ratio. Enhancement pattern on CT scanning is usually homogeneous and moderately strong. Cystic areas within the tumors are relatively common. Uncommonly, the tumor may not enhance or may show areas of hemorrhage.

It is important to evaluate the leptomeninges since up to 50% of patients develop metastatic disease. At presentation, this is seen in approximately 20% of patients. Leptomeningeal seeding to the brain or spine are common and both components of the neuraxis should be evaluated. An MRI with contrast is superior to other imaging techniques for detection of metastatic disease. With CT scanning, as demonstrated by enhanced CT images,

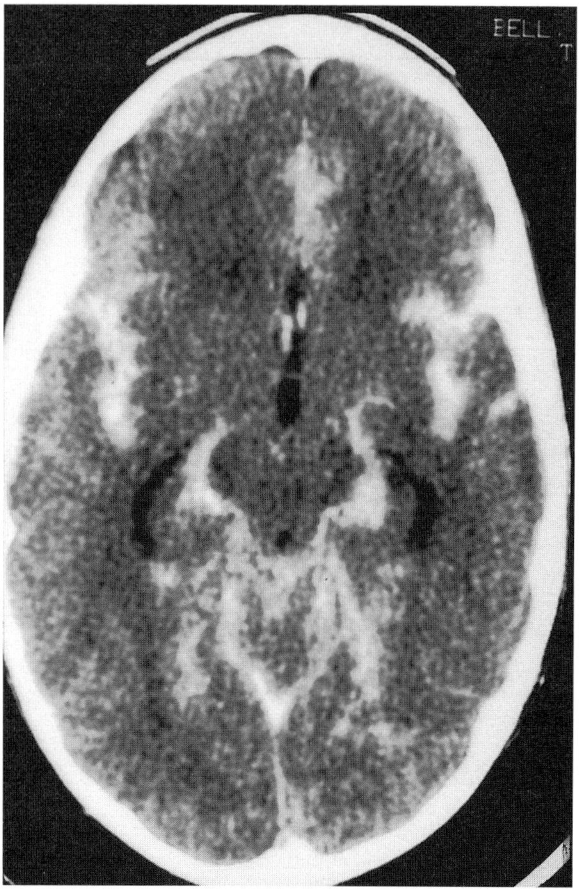

Fig. 9.234 Axial postcontrast CT demonstrating severe diffuse leptomeningeal enhancement. Leptomeningeal seeding is a common finding with medulloblastoma, although seldom to this degree. On noncontrast CT, these areas are typically of high density and may be confused with subarachnoid hemorrhage.

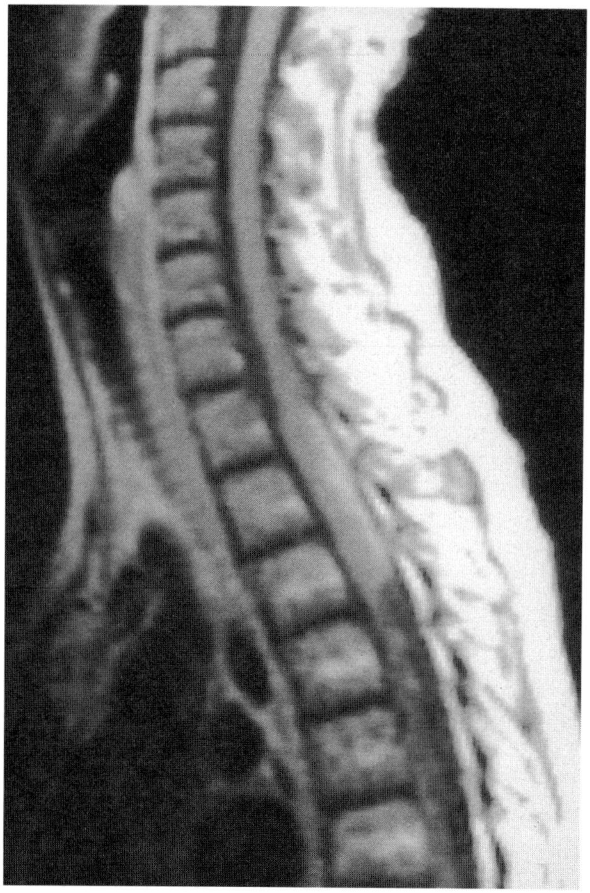

Fig. 9.235 Sagittal T1-weighted postcontrast MRI demonstrating abnormal enhancement posterior to the spinal cord at the T1–T3 level in a patient with medulloblastoma. This enhancing tumor represents spinal seeding or drop metastasis. Arachnoid seeding of tumor in the brain typically enhances with contrast and exhibits a gyriform, nodular appearance. Drop metastases in the spinal canal also usually enhance. These metastases may subsequently invade the spinal cord. Occasional metastases to the bone and extracranial sites may also occur.

the abnormal enhancement areas in the brain typically enhance with contrast and have a gyriform, nodular appearance (Fig. 9.234). Drop metastases in the spinal canal also usually enhance. These may lie in the lumbar sac along nerve roots or along the spinal cord. Occasional metastasis to the bone and extracranial sites may occur (Fig. 9.235).

Microscopic appearance

The salient feature of the medulloblastoma is its extreme cellular density. Every field is packed with small cells in which the cytoplasm is scanty and poorly defined and the nuclei round or oval, being variable in size and highly hematoxylinophilic, imparting a blue tinctorial quality to histologic sections. Mitoses are usually abundant. In many examples, there are no special architectural arrangements of the cells; they simply form irregular masses supported by a tenuous stroma of blood vessels in which endothelial proliferation is occasionally evident, a feature known as the 'classic' old diffuse pattern (Fig. 9.236).

In some examples, neuroblastic differentiation is manifested by the formation of rosettes of the Homer Wright type (Fig. 9.237). They may be limited to a small part of the tumor or may occasionally be demonstrated in large numbers within the leptomeninges. In the rosettes, the cytoplasm of

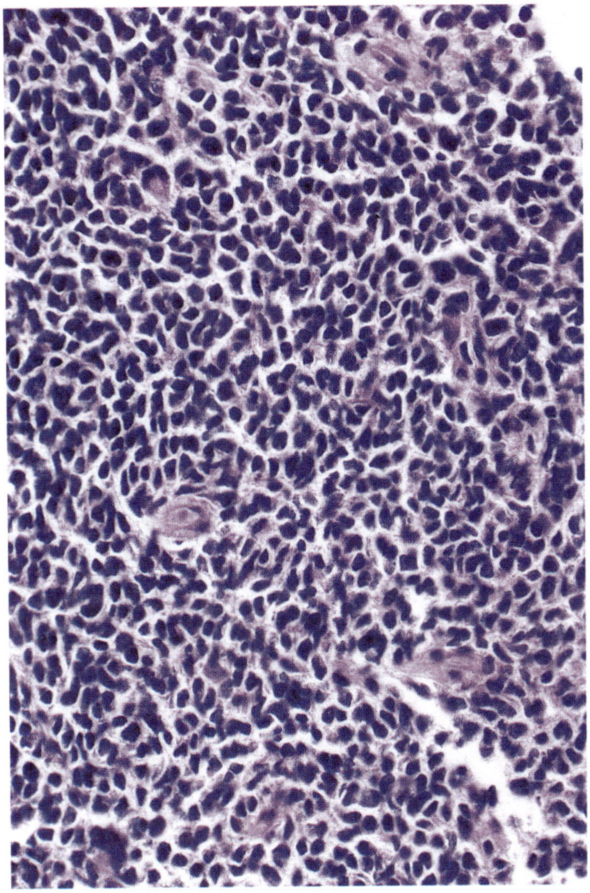

Fig. 9.236 Sheets of anaplastic cells interrupted by small vessels, which is characteristic of the classic pattern of medulloblastoma. H&E, × 100

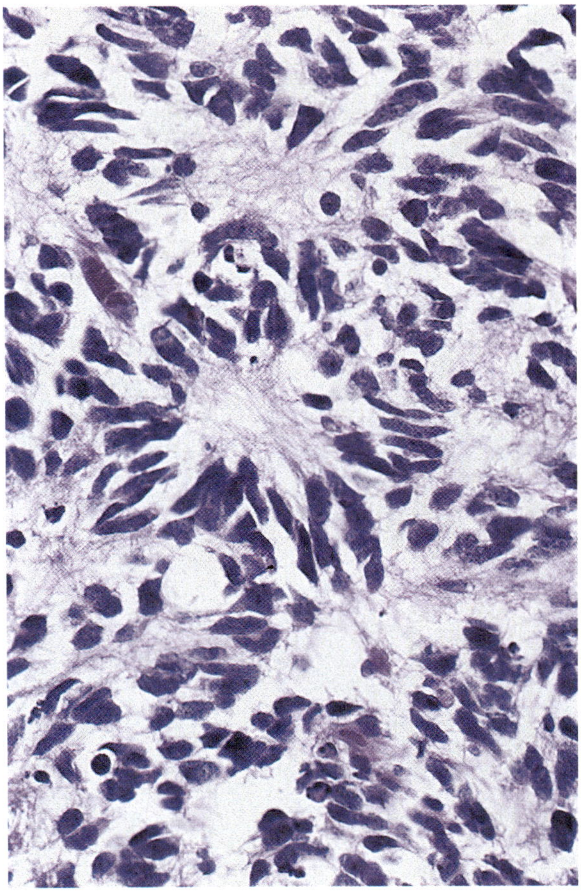

Fig. 9.237 Cerebellar medulloblastomas may occasionally exhibit conspicuous Homer Wright rosettes, a finding more typical of older patients. H&E, × 80

the tumor cells forms a carrot-shaped tapering process; the cell nuclei lie at the periphery of the rosette, the center being occupied by the converging processes. Argyrophilic neurofibrils can be demonstrated in the latter in favorable circumstances. More rarely, accentuation of this neuroblastic differentiation is found when the neuroblasts form fleurettes that are characterized by cells with elongated fibrillated processes, leashed together at one end, and nuclei with a distinct nucleolus occupying a pale nucleoplasm spraying forth on the opposite end. Even more rarely, as noted first by Orville Bailey (1955), further transitions to atypical yet mature-looking ganglion cells may be found, a feature that Rubinstein noted in only six cases, in two adults aged 21 and 29 years and in four children (Russell and Rubinstein, 1989), and Burger *et al.* (1987) noted in 3/51 childhood tumors. The appearance and distribution of these more mature cells preclude their interpretation as nonneoplastic cells of the host tissues.

When phenotypic expression is restricted to the neuronal line, the tumor might also be designated as a ganglioneuroblastoma, as in the examples described by Kuhlenbeck and Haymaker (1946, case 7) in a 22-year-old man—in whom the tumor could have arisen from a persistent remnant of the external granular layer (see p. 457)—and by Durity, Dolman and Moyes (1968) in the cerebellar hemisphere of a 3-year-old girl. The case reported by de Chadarévian *et al.* (1987), in a 2½-year-old girl with a recurrence of her tumor 4 years later, is of special interest in documenting the sequential maturation of a cerebellar neuroblastoma into a ganglioneuroma; in addition, melanosis was demonstrated in the recurrence.

On the other hand, tumors exhibiting phenotypic divergence may show, in the more mature areas, the classic features of a ganglioglioma, as in the cases published by Kane and Aronson (1967) and Warzok, Jaenisch and Lang (1983). In the tumor reported by the latter authors, and interpreted as a

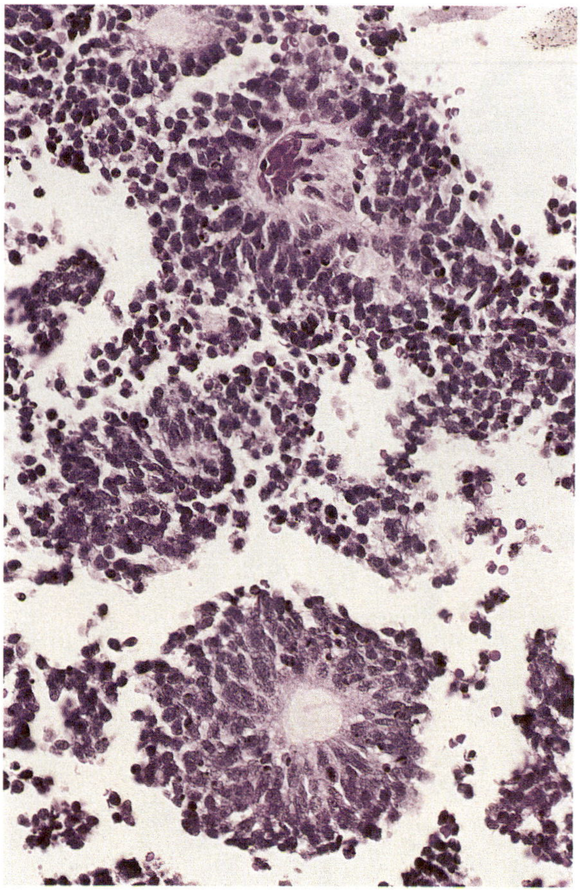

Fig. 9.238 Medulloblastoma. Vessels may occasionally exhibit conspicuous perpendicular collaring of tumor cells, which is suggestive of perivascular pseudorosettes. In some tumors, necrosis may be so conspicuous as to result in a pseudopapillary formation. H&E, × 80

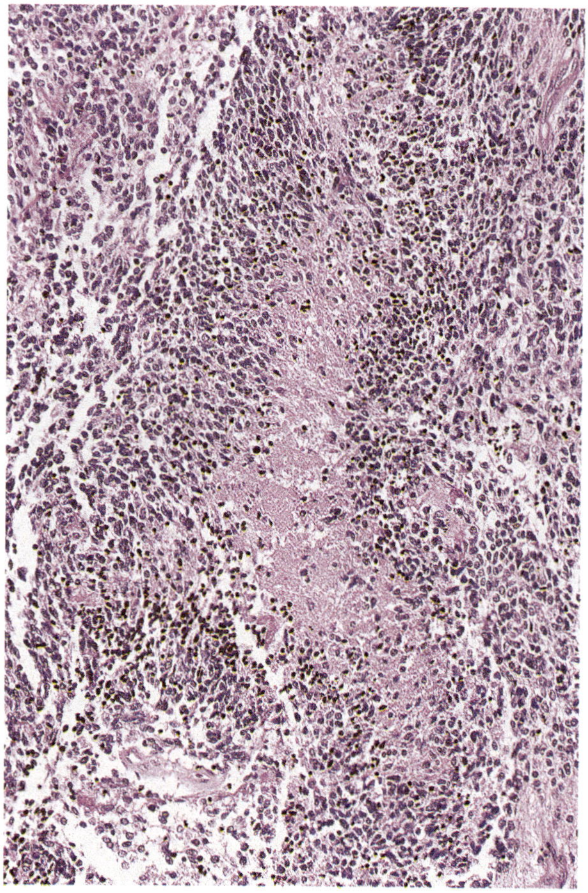

Fig. 9.239 Medulloblastoma. Focus of necrosis surrounded by pseudopalisading tumor cells is strongly reminiscent of the glioblastoma. H&E, × 50

cerebellar neuroblastoma, conversion to a ganglioglioma occurred 5 years after the original operation. Exceptionally, maturation of medulloblastoma cells into neurons has been seen in remote subarachnoid deposits with tumor cells forming Homer-Wright rosettes in a frontal metastasis, as described by Kadota, Arai and Sato (1995).

Occasionally, the tumor cells are arranged as pseudorosettes about the supporting blood vessels. This, though reminiscent of the ependymomas, is distinguished by the absence of an eosinophilic fibrillary zone separating the vessel wall from the perikaryon of the medulloblastoma cells (Ringertz and Tola, 1950). In areas of extensive necrosis, perivascular sparing may be evident, imparting a pseudopapillary appearance to the tumor (Fig. 9.238).

The features noted by Bodian and Lawson (1953), Rubinstein and Northfield (1964) and Willis (1967), of foci indistinguishable from oligodendroglioma, exhibit the immunohistochemical markers of neurons (Burger *et al.*, 1987).

There are also cases of otherwise typical medulloblastomas in which the glial features are so accentuated as to form pseudopalisades around small areas of necrosis, accompanied by vascular endothelial proliferation, producing a microscopic picture highly suggestive of a glioblastoma (Fig. 9.239). In contrast to the gliomas, however, these histologic findings impart no prognostic information in the medulloblastoma (Goldberg-Stern *et al.*, 1991). Multinucleation and giant-cell formation with bizarre pleomorphic nuclei have also been noted in a midline medulloblastoma that had recurred and had become heavily calcified 4 years after the administration of radiotherapy. These features are most consistent with radiation changes, as noted independently in a report by Oppenheimer (1969). In other cases, showing its kinship to the

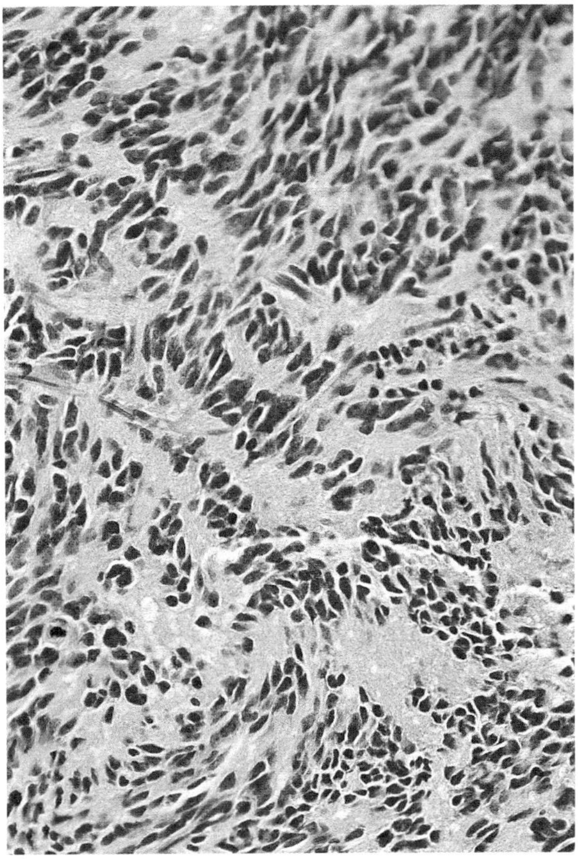

Fig. 9.240 Rhythmic palisading of tumor cells may occasionally be encountered in medulloblastomas and is more typical of older patients. H&E, × 80

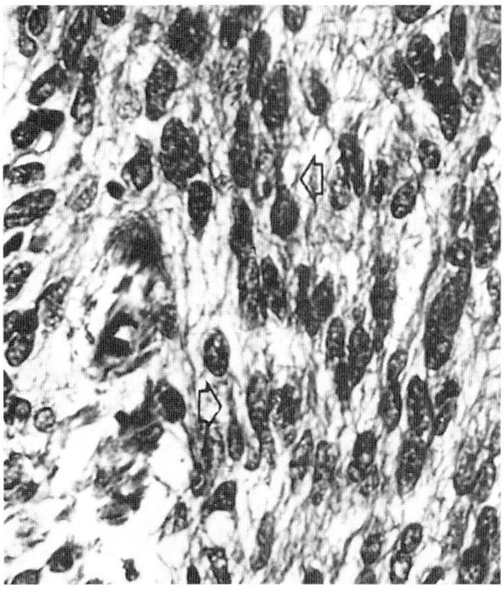

Fig. 9.241 Unipolar spongioblastic cells (arrows) in a metastasis from a cerebellar medulloblastoma that arose in the vermis of a 5-year-old girl. PTAH, × 525 (Reprinted from *Handbook of Clinical Neurology,* P.J. Vinken and G.W. Bruyn (eds), 1973, chapter 9, figure 9, with kind permission from Elsevier Science-NL, Sara Burgerhartstraat 25, 1055 KV Amsterdam, The Netherlands.)

supratentorial neuroblastic neoplasms, the occasional propensity to mimic spongioblastomas with rhythmic palisading (Fig. 9.240) may also be seen. In these neoplasms, there may be seen interlacing bundles of uni- or bipolar cells in which delicate neuroglial fibrils are demonstrable with PTAH stain (Fig. 9.241).

The phenotypic expression of astrocytic features, as suggested by Willis (1967), is exceptional, but Rubinstein noted several examples of this development, most frequently in older patients in the fourth or fifth decade. However, it is clear that Rubinstein (Russell and Rubinstein, 1989) considered the occasional propensity of medulloblastoma cells to express glial phenotypic markers to be linked to the occurrence of gliomas in medulloblastomas. Bailey and Cushing (1925) suggested that some medulloblastomas are composed largely or entirely of neuroglial cells with, exceptionally, a medulloblastoma as the end stage in the anaplastic transformation of an initially more mature astrocytic glioma. The observations of Willis (1962a), who contended that transitional features could be found linking cerebellar astrocytomas and medulloblastomas, have been supported by Rubinstein, Herman and Hanbery (1974). These authors recorded the neoplasm of a 14-year-old girl as showing a diffusely infiltrating cerebellar and brainstem astrocytoma associated with a medulloblastoma in the vermis, with transitional features between the two components. Similar cases have been described, including the recurrent bilateral cerebellar tumor removed from a 38-year-old woman as described by Müller and Schaefer (1974), a diffuse brainstem astrocytoma adjacent to a desmoplastic cerebellar medulloblastoma in an 11-year-old male as reported by Schmitt (1983a) and two examples of malignant cerebellar glioma recorded by Steinberg *et al.* (1985, cases 7 and 8). Alternatively, the somewhat similar examples reported by Barnard and Pambakian (1980) and Feigin, Epstein and Mangiardi (1983) were interpreted as exemplifying maturation of a medulloblastoma into an astrocytoma. The extreme rarity of co-occurrence of true gliomas and medulloblastomas suggests a statistical argument of collision, or synchronous, tumors. Apparently, a variety of factors are operative in the genesis of phenotypic divergence that are difficult to discern in individual cases. Even monoclonality of tumor cell populations has proven difficult to establish in any given tumor. It is becoming obvious that, like the gliomas, medulloblastomas are composed of heterogeneous tumor cell populations. Thus, maturation of some populations, induction of other transformed populations into the proliferating cell pool, and malignant progression with eventual overgrowth may be found in any one medulloblastoma's evolution and treatment. Contributions of electron microscopy, immunohistochemistry and tissue culture to the elucidation of the phenotypic capabilities of the medulloblastoma cell are reviewed below.

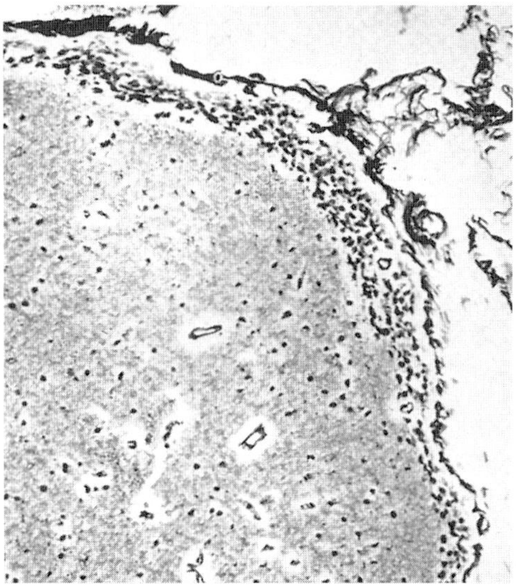

Fig. 9.242 A rim of subpial tumor mimicking the external granular layer and lying in the cerebellar cortex adjacent to a large desmoplastic medulloblastoma that originated in the vermis of a 32-year-old man. Reticulin stain, × 80 (Reprinted from *Handbook of Clinical Neurology*, P.J. Vinken and G.W. Bruyn (eds), 1973, chapter 9, figure 18, with kind permission from Elsevier Science-NL, Sara Burgerhartstraat 25, 1055 KV Amsterdam, The Netherlands.)

Alternatively, local recurrences of the primary neoplasm should be distinguished from the occasionally reported late appearance of a cerebellar astrocytoma in the same region, as in the case described by Klériga *et al.* (1978), where an 11-year-old child was apparently successfully treated for a desmoplastic medulloblastoma of the left cerebellar hemisphere at the age of 10 months; or, in the case described by Dell, Cohen and Kushner (1981), where a low-grade cerebellar astrocytoma developed in a 20-year-old woman who had been successfully treated for a midline medulloblastoma at the age of 4 years; or, more recently, in the case recorded by Schmidbauer *et al.* (1987), where a glioblastoma occurred in a 21-year-old man at the cerebellar site from which a medulloblastoma had apparently been totally excised 6 years earlier. Similarly, the Duke University experience records four patients treated for medulloblastoma who developed gliomas, all of which occurred in the radiation fields 6 or more years after their medulloblastoma diagnosis. The suspicion that the later appearance of an astrocytic glioma in these patients may have been induced by the radiation therapy that had been successfully administered to the medulloblastoma must be entertained, especially in

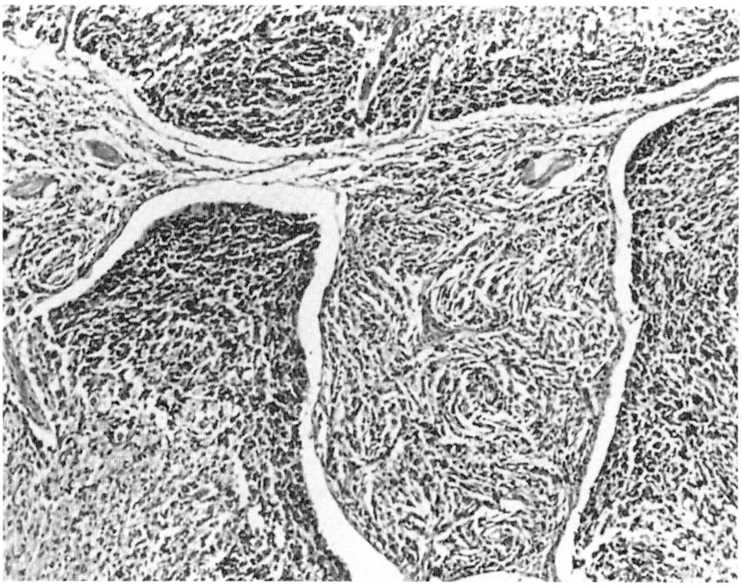

Fig. 9.243 Desmoplastic medulloblastoma arising in a 44-year-old male. The nodular tumor in the leptomeninges (center) shows a trabecular and whirled pattern and is adjacent to medulloblastoma cells heavily infiltrating the superficial molecular layer. H&E, × 70

view of the evidence that has surfaced in recent years of radiation as a neurocarcinogen. Similar suspicion is attached to the case reported by Pearl, Mirra and Miles (1980) of a left parieto-occipital glioblastoma that occurred at the age of 18 years in a patient who had been treated for a medulloblastoma 13 years previously.

Desmoplastic variant of medulloblastoma

As mentioned previously, in some medulloblastomas, most notably those found in adults, there is a conspicuous aggregation of tumor cells beneath the pia, while the subjacent cortex is undisturbed (Fig. 9.242). Moreover, the tumor cells frequently penetrate the adjacent leptomeninges (Fig. 9.243). In the latter situation, they excite a variable but often striking amount of connective tissue reaction (Fig. 9.244). The arrangements of the cells are correspondingly modified and they may form whorls or trabeculae separated by collagen strands (Figs 9.243 and 9.244), a phenomenon shared with glial neoplasms invading the leptomeninges (see p. 514). In addition, this variant of medulloblastoma, for which the term 'desmoplastic' was proposed (Rubinstein and Northfield, 1964), often displays reticulin-free pale islands of tumor haracterized by cells that demonstrate more cytoplasm contiguous to more compact, reticulin-rich cellular trabeculae (Fig. 9.245). The interpretation that the fibrous connective tissue proliferation in the subarachnoid spaces in these examples is attributable to a response by the meningeal fibroblasts to tumor invasion usually can be verified by the demonstration of two different cell populations in the meningeal infiltrates (Fig. 9.246). In contrast, the usual finding of neuronal or glial phenotypic expression confined to the cells in the pale islands suggests that other factors are operative in these neoplasms that distinguish them from the typical 'classic' medulloblastomas. The association of desmoplastic medulloblastomas with Gorlin's syndrome raises another distinguishing feature (Schofield *et al.*, 1995). It is possible that the desmoplastic variant of medulloblastoma has, in a number of cases, arisen from neoplastically transformed cells in the superficial part of the molecular layer (Figs 9.242 and 9.243), thus resulting in early invasion of the leptomeningeal spaces. It is, indeed, for this form of growth that an origin from the external granular layer or its remnants has most frequently been championed (Stevenson and Echlin, 1934; Scheinker, 1939; Kadin, Rubinstein and Nelson, 1970). Exceptionally, the proliferative leptomeninges are the seat of an intense chronic inflammatory cellular response

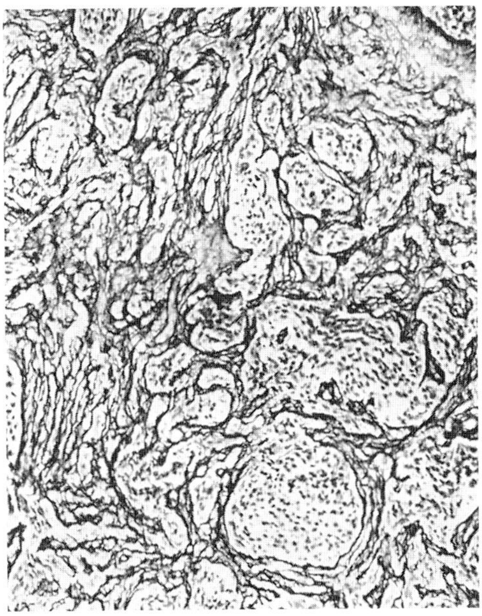

Fig. 9.244 Lateral lobe tumor arising in a 25-year-old woman. The pattern of irregular leptomeningeal infiltration shows reticulin-free islands of various sizes. Reticulin, × 95.

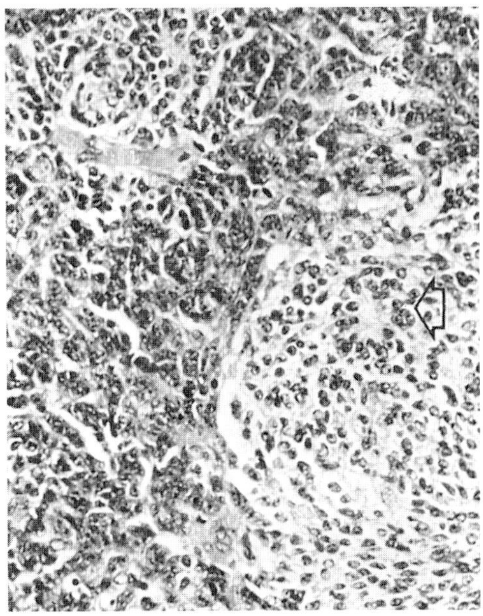

Fig. 9.245 Lighter foci (upper left and lower right) of less compact reticulin-free tumor cells, with intervening more darkly staining cells compressed by connective tissue, in a medulloblastoma originating in a 21-year-old woman. Note the rosette (arrow). H&E, × 225

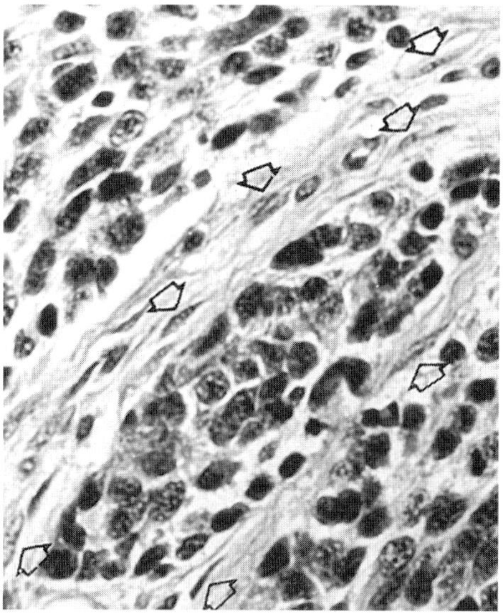

Fig. 9.246 Same case as Fig. 9.244 Groups of darkly staining medulloblastoma cells infiltrating the leptomeninges and separated by more lightly staining spindle-shaped fibroblasts (arrows). H&E, × 500 (Reprinted from *Handbook of Clinical Neurology*, P.J. Vinken and G.W. Bruyn (eds), 1973, chapter 9, figure 26, with kind permission from Elsevier Science-NL, Sara Burgerhartstraat 25, 1055 KV Amsterdam, The Netherlands.)

that may progress to the formation of lymphoid follicles with germinal centers.

Other variants of medulloblastoma

A variant of medulloblastoma containing papillary formations and bearing melanin pigment, possibly allied to or identical with the melanotic neuroectodermal tumor of infancy (see Volume 2, p. 349; also Borello and Gorlin, 1966), has been reported by Fowler and Simpson (1962) and by Rubinstein (Rubinstein and Northfield, 1964). Sung, Mastri and Segal (1973) described a tumor arising in the vermis of a 3-year-old boy that, like the two previously reported cases, spread extensively through the cerebrospinal pathways. A case communicated by Boesel, Suhan and Sayers (1978) arose in the vermis of a 4-year-old boy and was noted, by ultrastructural examination, to have the features of melanosomal melanin in the tumor cells. A further example of this curious pigmented variant has since been seen by Drut and Jones (1983) in a 7-year-old boy, and the fine structural features of a melanotic cerebellar tumor in a 3-year-old boy have, in addition, been compared with those of the human fetal pineal gland (Kinney *et al.*, 1983). The presence of melanosomes was confirmed in both situations. Any link between these tumors and pigmented pineoblastomas (Best, 1973) is unknown.

Another exceptionally rare form of medulloblastoma is one in which striated muscle cells are demonstrable ('medullomyoblastoma') (Dickson *et al.*, 1983; Smith and Davidson, 1984; Höll *et al.*, 1991; Parham *et al.*, 1992; Schiffer *et al.*, 1992). These cases straddle the somewhat ill-defined boundaries that separate primitive central neuroepithelial tumors from embryonal rhabdomyosarcomas and from teratomatous neoplasms with restricted differentiation potential, some of which may include a maldevelopmental component. They are, therefore, treated in greater detail in Volume 2, p. 323.

Lastly, a lipidized variant of medulloblastoma has been described (Budka, 1974; Chimelli, Hahn and Budka, 1991; Davis *et al.*, 1993; Ellison, Zygmunt and Weller, 1993). The significance of these variants lies in avoiding confusion with other tumors with lipoblastic or adipocytic differentiation. These tumors have been reported almost entirely in adults and apparently exhibit a highly favorable prognosis, with patient survivals of more than 5 years without further therapy recorded (Davis *et al.*, 1993; Budka and Chimelli, 1994).

Cerebellar neuroblastomas

The separation, within the category of the medulloblastomas, of a tumor that demonstrably deserves to be designated as a neuroblastoma has been well documented, on electron microscopic grounds, in reports by Shin *et al.* (1978), Hirano and Shin (1979), Yagishita *et al.* (1980, 1982), Pearl and Takei (1981) and Schofield *et al.* (1992). All examples share a number of remarkably constant microscopic features: by light microscopy, a lobulated pattern of cells with regular, delicate, round or oval nuclei of neuroblastic appearance distributed on a fine neuropil, and, by electron microscopy, abundant, closely packed neuritic cell processes containing large numbers of clear-centered vesicles, well-developed synaptic complexes and, less frequently, dense-core vesicles. These descriptions leave little room to doubt the existence of a subgroup of medulloblastomas to be clearly aligned with some of the examples of neuroblastoma that have been recorded elsewhere in the cerebral hemispheres (p. 480) and with which the cerebellar examples should, in strict logic, be integrated. There is preliminary data from the clinical point of view that patients whose tumors exhibit evidence of cerebellar neuroblastic phenotypes display a better prognosis than those with other types of medulloblastoma (Schofield *et al.*, 1992), a possibility earlier suggested by the subsequent maturation to adult ganglion cell forms reported in previous examples (Kane and Aronson, 1967; Warzok, Jaenisch and Lang, 1983; de Chadarévian *et al.*, 1987).

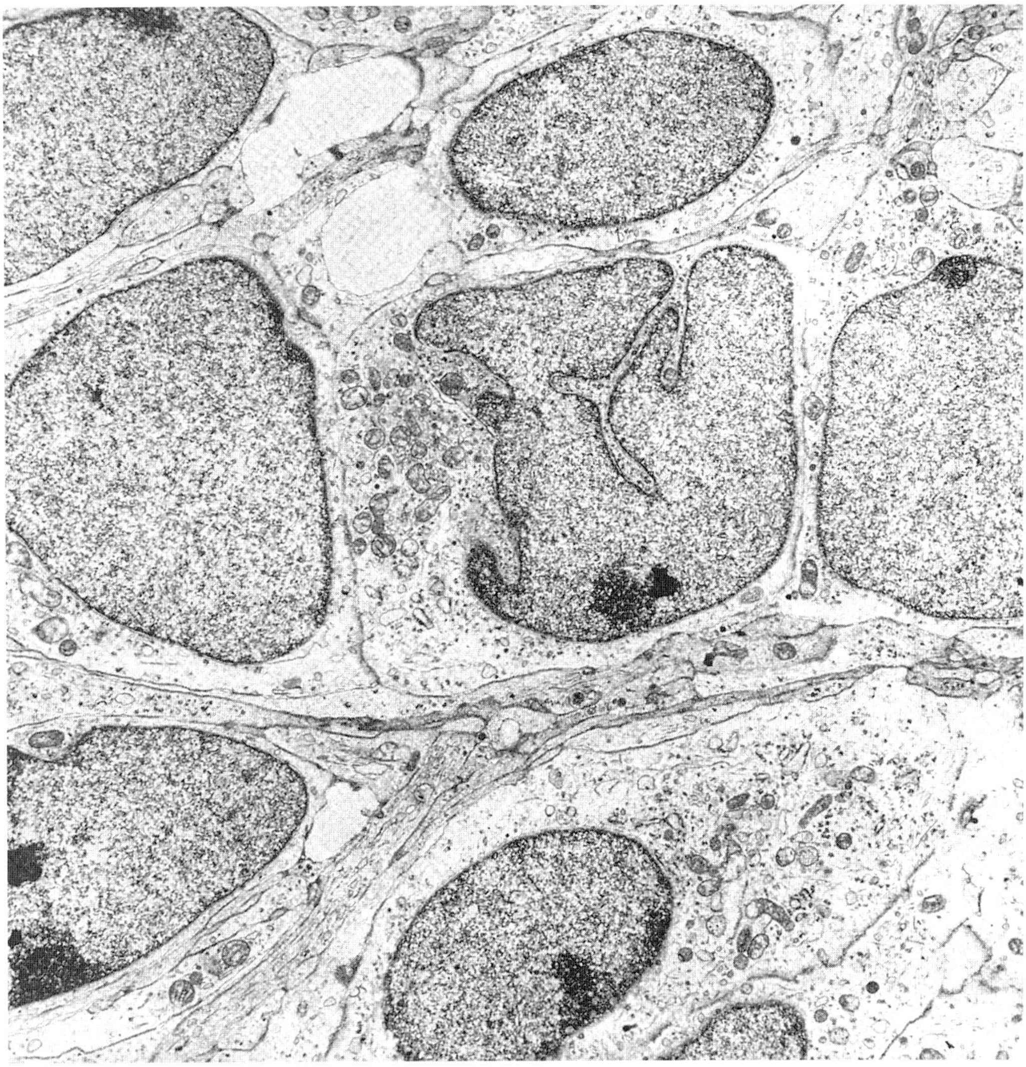

Fig. 9.247 Electron micrograph of cerebellar lobe medulloblastoma in a 2-year-old boy. These poorly differentiated, oval and polyhedral cells with scanty cytoplasm contain chiefly mitochondria and ribosomes and have few cell processes. × 5400 (Courtesy of Dr Mary M. Herman)

Electron microscopy

Most reports (Voigt, 1968; Matakas, Cervós-Navarro and Gullotta, 1970) have emphasized the lack of distinguishing cytoplasmic features in medulloblastoma tumor cells (Fig. 9.247). The presence of intercellular junctional complexes, noted in one neonatal case (Kadin, Rubinstein and Nelson, 1970) and subsequently confirmed in another example (Rubinstein, Herman and Hanbery, 1974), appears to be a relatively frequent feature (Hassoun, Hirano and Zimmerman, 1975), but its significance is hardly specific. A number of reports (Ermel and Brucher, 1974; Camins *et al.*, 1980; Azzarelli, Muller and Mirkin, 1983; Moss, 1983) have documented the occasional presence of fine structural features suggestive of neuroblastic differentiation, the most convincing of which is that of dense-core vesicles and, possibly, of rudimentary synaptic structures as in one of the cases described by Ermel and Brucher (1974). Similarly, the finding of microtubules (Katsetos, Liu and Zacks, 1988) lends support to a neuroblastic phenotype. Much more definite is the identification, as detailed above, of some medulloblastomas as undeniable neuroblastomas originating in the cerebellum.

On the other hand, the demonstration of bundles of cytoplasmic filaments measuring 8–10 nm in diameter, already noted by Raimondi, Mullan and Evans (1962), has also been confirmed by electron microscopy in occasional examples, as in the cases reported by Rubinstein, Herman and Hanbery (1974), Müller and Schaefer (1974), Camins *et al.* (1980), Moss (1983) and Katsetos, Liu and Zachs (1988). In the case described by Müller and Schaefer (1974), filament formation in the tumor cell processes was associated with the characteristic fine structural equivalent of Rosenthal fibers, suggesting an astrocytic lineage.

Immunohistochemistry

Immunohistochemical methods have been used as a means of exploring the spectrum of phenotypic expression by medulloblastomas. The demonstration, by immunoperoxidase, of GFAP in a small proportion of tumor cells has been confirmed in various general studies on the immunoreactivity of gliomas for the protein, including those by Deck *et al.* (1978), Eng and Rubinstein (1978), Velasco *et al.* (1980), Mannoji *et al.* (1981), Palmer, Kasselberg and Netsky (1981), Roessmann *et al.* (1983) and Trojanowski, Lee and Schlaepfer (1984). The view that none of the GFAP-positive cells in medulloblastomas is likely to be neoplastic (Coffin, Mukai and Dehner, 1983; Schindler and Gullotta, 1983) can be countered by the finding of GFAP-positive medulloblastoma cells infiltrating the cerebellar subarachnoid space, and by the occasional positivity of medulloblastoma cells permeating the bone marrow, when extraneural dissemination has occurred (Fig. 9.248), or the lymph nodes (Ghobrial *et al.*, 1989). The immunohistochemical studies by Herpers and Budka (1985), Kumanishi *et al.* (1985), Burger *et al.* (1987), Hayashi *et al.* (1987), Szymas *et al.* (1987), Katsetos, Liu and Zacks (1988), Katsetos *et al.* (1989) and Molenaar and Trojanowski (1994) have further documented the immunopositivity of some of the tumor cells for GFAP. Immunoreactivity of the neoplastic cells for S-100 protein has also been demonstrated (Kimura, Budka and Soler-Federsppiel, 1986; Sawa *et al.*, 1986a; Hayashi *et al.*, 1987).

Some of the cells in medulloblastomas have been found to be immunopositive when tested with immunohistochemical reagents that recognize the 68-kDa, 150-kDa and 200-kDa NFP subunits (NFP-L, NFP-M and NFP-H, respectively) (Roessmann *et al.*, 1983; Sawa *et al.*, 1986a; Katsetos *et al.*, 1991; Kleinert, 1991a, 1991b). Interestingly, Zeltzer *et al.* (1990) found that a larger proportion of medulloblastomas reacted against a MAb for the high-molecular-weight neurofilament protein (NFP-H, 15/17 tumors) than for low-molecular-weight protein (NFP-L, 1/17 tumors). Although none of 10 medulloblastomas tested by Trojanowski, Lee and Schlaepfer (1984) against a MAb to NFP showed any immunopositivity, subsequent studies revealed immunoreactivity in 16/22 medulloblastomas when the tumors were tested against fresh frozen material using additional antibodies (Gould *et al.*, 1990). Similarly, tests with antibodies against synaptophysin, a 38-kDa membrane glycoprotein of presynaptic vesicles in various neurons and neuroendocrine cells, have demonstrated immunoreactivity by both immunofluorescence and immunoperoxidase (Fig. 9.249) methods in a majority of medulloblastomas (Schwechheimer, Wiedenmann and Franke, 1987; Katsetos *et al.*, 1989, 1995; Katsetos and Burger, 1994; Harris *et al.*, 1990;

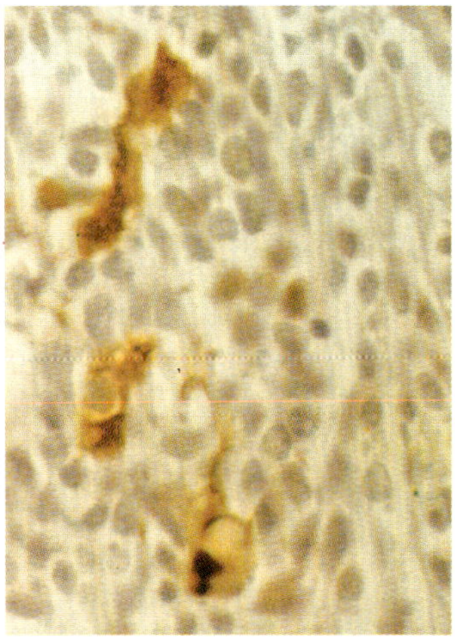

Fig. 9.248 Focal GFAP positive metastatic medulloblastoma cells in bone marrow, × 1000

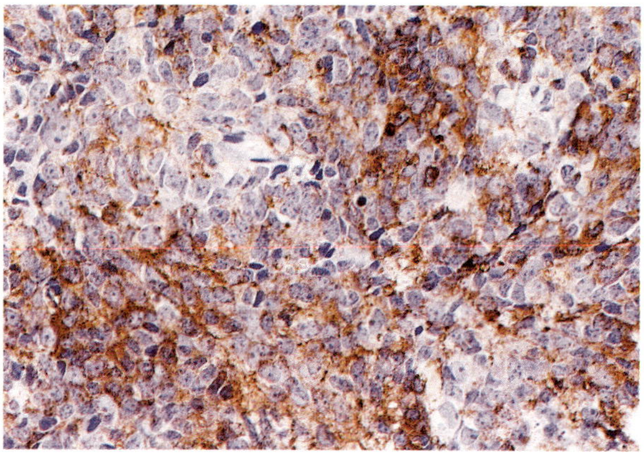

Fig. 9.249 Diffuse cytoplasmic immunoreactivity of medulloblastoma cells against synaptophysin antibody. × 132

Maraziotis *et al.*, 1992). Immunohistochemical studies against class III β-tubulin, a presumptive neuron-specific isoform of tubulin, have demonstrated immunoreactivity in a large majority of medulloblastomas (Katsetos *et al.*, 1989, 1993; Maraziotis *et al.*, 1992). Other neuronal markers that have been studied for their utility in these neoplasms include a variety of neuropeptides that were variably present in 10/22 medulloblastomas (Gould *et al.*, 1990); calcineurin, which has been found to be expressed in 7/27 medulloblastomas (Goto *et al.*, 1987); and protein gene product (PGP) 9.5, another presumed neuron-specific protein of unknown function that was identified immunohistochemically in medulloblastomas (Cruz-Sanchez *et al.*, 1989; Harris *et al.*, 1990). Smith *et al.* (1993) have identified synapsin 1, a phosphoprotein localized to the cytoplasmic surface of synaptic vesicles of neurons, in 1/11 fixed medulloblastomas. These studies reinforce the view that the tumor has the capacity for neuronal expression as well as for divergent neuronal and glial phenotypic expression.

Neuron-specific (γ-γ isoform) enolase has been shown to be frequently positive in these neoplasms (Nakajima *et al.*, 1984; Velasco, Ghobrial and Ross, 1985; Sawa *et al.*, 1986a; Burger *et al.*, 1987; Hayashi *et al.*, 1987) and was found by Burger *et al.* (1987) to be especially prominent in focal islands of relatively reduced cellularity, which are sometimes associated with neuroblastic rosettes. Velasco, Ghobrial and Ross (1985) and Burger *et al.* (1987) have interpreted these observations as primitive neuronal features. However, the deregulated expression of NSE (and its immunoreactivity) in nonneuronal tumors in areas of presumed anoxic stress must temper this observation.

On the other hand, the immunohistochemical demonstration of the photoreceptor markers retinal S-antigen (arrestin) and rod-opsin by Korf *et al.* (1987) in 9/28 cerebellar medulloblastomas, and by Jaffey *et al.* (1995) in 8/17 medulloblastomas, is of significance in reinforcing the apparent link that may exist between medulloblastoma and pineoblastoma. Perentes has reported that 8/16 cerebellar medulloblastomas tested expressed the S-antigen (Bonnin and Perentes, 1988) and Maraziotis *et al.* (1992) have described its immunoreactivity in 16 medulloblastomas, including five desmoplastic variants. Similarly, Kramm *et al.* (1991) characterized the variable expression patterns of S-antigen, rod-opsin, and 11-cis-retinal in three medulloblastomas using a variety of immunochemical techniques. Subsequently, Korf *et al.* (1992) demonstrated the presence of interphotoreceptor retinoid-binding protein (IRBP) in a medulloblastoma. Of further significance is the finding of Flexner-Wintersteiner rosettes in two cases reported by Jaffey *et al.* (1995). Further characterizing these two tumors was the presence of calcifying necrosis, a feature of retinoblastomas but not of medulloblastomas.

The NCAMs, which exist as four sialylated isoforms of molecular mass 180 kDa, 170 kDa, 145 kDa and 120 kDa, and a nonsialylated isoform of 95 kDa, have been described in medulloblastomas (Frost *et al.*, 1991; Molenaar, de Leij and Trojanowski, 1991). In Western blot studies of medulloblastoma homogenates, NCAM is identified as a smear ranging between 140 and 250 kDa, a pattern similar to that of embryonic fetal brain. The role of the various NCAM isoforms is unknown but is hypothesized to be involved in cell-cell interactions, mobility and, possibly, metastasis (Figarella-Branger, Durbec and Rougon, 1990; Frost *et al.*, 1991).

A number of MAbs that recognize membrane proteins of normal fetal and neoplastic neuroepithelial cells, including neuroblastoma cell lines, have been found to cross-react with medulloblastoma tumor cells (Coakham *et al.*, 1985; Bourne *et al.*, 1986; Zeltzer *et al.*, 1990).

Cytogenetics and molecular genetics

The cytogenetic data of medulloblastoma is critically reviewed in Chapter 2. Briefly, a small number of medulloblastomas have been karyotyped; most of them appear to be diploid, but aneuploidy has also been found (Latimer, AlSaadi and Robbins, 1987). It has been hinted that those with a diploid pattern may have a better prognosis (Neumann *et al.*, 1993), although data from flow cytometric studies have yielded conflicting results (see below). Banding analysis suggests that the chromosomal deviations are closer to those seen in peripheral neuroblastoma and retinoblastoma than in malignant gliomas, i.e., that they involve structural changes, such as deletions or unbalanced translocations, rather than gains or losses of whole chromosomes (Bigner *et al.*, 1988b). Isochromosome 17q is the most frequent chromosomal abnormality seen in medulloblastomas (Biegel *et al.*, 1989; Bigner, Mark and Bigner, 1990), a finding supported by microsatellite probe analysis (Cogen *et al.*, 1990, 1992; Cogan, 1991–92; Thomas and Raffel, 1991; Albrecht *et al.*, 1994; Batra *et al.*, 1995). In contrast, *TP53*, a tumor suppressor gene, is mutated only infrequently in medulloblastomas, implying that another tumor suppressor gene may be located on 17p distal to *TP53* on the 17p arm (Cogen *et al.*, 1990, 1992; Saylors *et al.*, 1991; Batra *et al.*, 1995). Also, double-minute chromatin bodies and homogeneously staining regions found in medulloblastomas mediate genic amplification, most commonly that of *MYC* (Bigner *et al.*, 1988b, 1990). Of some interest is the absence of the 11;22 translocation in medulloblastomas, a marker usually found in Ewing's sarcoma, the peripheral primitive neuroectodermal tumor (Jay *et al.*, 1995). Similarly negative results have been reported for *CDKN2B* and *CDKN2A*, genes often deleted in glioblastomas (Jen *et al.*, 1994). Recently, Scheurlen and Senf (1995) have found an embryonal splice variant of the *NF1* gene involving the GTPase-associated protein (GAP)-related domain. These authors note that this particular splice variant is extremely effective in suppressing $p21^{ras}$ and hypothesize that this variant may interfere with the signal transduction of $p21^{ras}$ during neuronal differentiation. Thus, these authors theorize that 'such an arrest of a $p21^{ras}$-dependent differentiation pathway may explain the persistence of primitive pluripotential neuronal cells in this tumor' (Scheurlen and Senf, 1995).

Biologic behavior, evolution, prognostic factors and recurrence

Medulloblastomas are highly malignant neoplasms, notorious for their aptitude to invade the subarachnoid space and the fourth ventricle early in their course, and to disseminate promptly through the cerebrospinal pathways. However, the application of vigorous and extensive postoperative radiation to the entire neuraxis has appreciably improved the dismal prognosis that was attached to these tumors (see Christensen and Als, 1956; Chatty and Earle, 1971; Park *et al.*, 1983; Hershatter, Halperin and Cox, 1986; Garton *et al.*, 1990; Geyer *et al.*, 1991; Halberg *et al.*, 1991; Krischer *et al.*, 1991; Packer *et al.*, 1991). The clinical series that have appeared in the last three decades (Bloom, Wallace and Henk, 1969; Marsa *et al.*, 1975; Sheline, 1975, 1977; Mealey and Hall, 1977; Hirsch *et al.*, 1979; Berry *et al.*, 1981; Chin and Maruyama, 1981, 1983; Bloom, 1982; Silverman and Simpson, 1982; Park *et al.*, 1983; Leibel and Sheline, 1987; Hubbard *et al.*, 1989; Bloom and Bessell, 1990; Garton *et al.*, 1990; Jenkin *et al.*, 1990; Hazuka *et al.*, 1992; Zerbini *et al.*, 1993; Carrie *et al.*, 1994; Frost *et al.*, 1995; Prados *et al.*, 1995; Sure *et al.*, 1995; Tinkler and Lucraft, 1995) have shown 5-year survival rates of 40–80%, and 10-year survival rates of 40–50%. From these reviews, it is also clear that improved survival rates are closely related to the extent of surgical resection of the growth and to the magnitude of the radiation dose administered. The best results have been obtained in patients who received a posterior fossa dose of 50 Gy or more after apparently total excision.

The older series by Kopelson, Linggood and Kleinman (1982), however, showed a wide range of 5- and 10-year postoperative survival figures for all patients with medulloblastomas; the more energetic radiation modalities, now currently administered to the central neuraxis, have raised the 5-year survival figure to 46% in one series (Kopelson, Linggood and Kleinman, 1983) and to 5- and 10-year survivals of 63% and 38%, respectively, in another (Hughes, 1984) and to 78% and 55%, respectively, in a third (Haie *et al.*, 1985). These figures are, therefore, broadly comparable with the 5- and 10-year survivals of 47% and 42%, respectively, in childhood medulloblastomas (Park *et al.*, 1983).

The significance of adult-onset versus childhood-onset medulloblastomas in terms of prognosis remains unclear. The tumors are laterally situated more frequently in adults (Carrie *et al.*, 1994; Becker, Becker and Sobel, 1995; Frost *et al.*, 1995; Prados *et al.*, 1995) than in children (Chatty and Earle, 1971). A lateral location appears to favor total surgical resection, although it is not the only factor, as reflected by a 49% rate of lateral tumors seen by Carrie *et al.* (1994) which compared with a total resectability rate of 66% of patients. As pointed out by Haie-Meder and Song (1995), despite a total resection rate that varies from 40% to 70% amongst adult studies, the overall survival rates do not differ significantly from the childhood studies where extent of resection is of prognostic value. The value of a surgeon's postoperative assessment of surgical resection is also less reliable than a postoperative imaging study (Gnekow *et al.*, 1991; Albright *et al.*, 1996). Regardless, it is clear that brainstem or ventricular-floor involvement and dissemination beyond posterior fossa are significant factors in both children and adults.

The prognostic significance of desmoplasia in a medulloblastoma is controversial. While some investigators have stated that patients with desmoplastic medulloblastomas live longer (Sure *et al.*, 1995), others have denied any correlation between survival and histologic type (Chatty and Earle, 1971; Park *et al.*, 1983). Sure *et al.* (1995), in support of their finding that desmoplasia is prognostic of prolonged patient survival, indicate that the definition of desmoplasia is problematic. In their study, they defined desmoplasia based on the presence of reticulin fibers in the tumor, rather than on the presence or absence of pale-staining nodules of tumor cells. Tumors with 'minimal' reticulin were considered transitional types and grouped as classic tumors.

Indeed, attempts to correlate prognosis with histologic evidence of local invasion or with features of cytologic differentiation have long been unrewarding. Spitz, Shenkin and Grant (1947), in an early analysis of 30 adult patients who had survival periods ranging from 6 months to 8 years (in the days that antedated modern radiotherapeutic approaches), found no histologic criterion by which survival could be foretold. Indeed, those with a well-demarcated tumor fared no better and no worse than those in whom the tumor was obviously infiltrating.

The evidence that neuroblastic features indicate a better prognosis than an undifferentiated tumor is less than compelling; Chatty and Earle (1971) confirm such a lack of correlation, and the more recent attempts to establish one are not convincing. Although the study of Schofield *et al.* (1992) suggests that expression of either a neuronal or glial phenotype indicates a better prognosis, the previous studies reported by Packer *et al.* (1984), Caputy *et al.* (1987) and Szymas *et al.* (1987) lead to divergent conclusions. In any event, the significance of any differences demonstrated in these endeavors seems marginal, except for the entity defined as the cerebellar neuroblastoma, which appears to have a good prognosis.

On the other hand, attempts (Kopelson, Linggood and Kleinman, 1983; Schofield *et al.*, 1992; Sure *et al.*, 1995; Albright *et al.*, 1996) to identify more general factors of statistical significance that might collectively have a bearing on prognosis have included the size and location of the tumor as estimated at the time of operation (T stage); the presence or absence of metastatic spread (M stage); and histopathologic features, such as the demonstration of necrosis, mitotic figures, desmoplasia and cytoplasmic processes. The results are statistically suggestive, although the data of Berry *et al.* (1981) and Zerbini *et al.* (1993) do not support the prognostic value of some of these factors.

Kinetics of medulloblastoma

A study by Hoshino *et al.* (1985) of four patients who had medulloblastomas and were given ^{3}H-thymidine before operation showed LIs of 11.2–14.4% in three midline examples and 8% in one lateral lobe tumor. In a study of 30 patients with medulloblastoma, Ito *et al.* (1992a) used pulse labeling with BrdU and iododeoxyuridine in a double labeling technique that allowed an estimation of S-phase duration and theoretical doubling time. This study confirmed the earlier work of Hoshino *et al.* (1985) suggesting a widely variable fraction of cells in DNA synthesis ranging from 3.9% to 38.2% with a mean LI of 11.7% [standard error (SE) 1.3%]. The S-phase duration was calculated to be 8.0 hours, and the theoretical doubling time ranged from 25 to 82 hours.

Although LIs are appreciably higher for medulloblastoma than for malignant glioma, the patient survival times vary considerably with medulloblastoma. There is little doubt that differences in survival times between medulloblastoma and malignant glioma are attributable to the considerably greater sensitivity of the former to radiotherapy. In medulloblastoma, LIs ranging from 6% to 32% have been reported with BrdU (Murovic *et al.*, 1986; Yoshii *et al.*, 1986; Ito *et al.*, 1992a). Hirakawa *et al.* (1986) estimated the observed doubling times of the tumor to range from 9 to 69 days, with rates of cell loss varying, respectively, from 74% to 97%. The total cell cycle times were calculated to range from 22 to 32 hours, with the S phase occupying approximately 26% of the total cell cycle time. Ito *et al.* (1992a), using MRI to measure observed doubling times in three cases, determined cell loss factors of 0.89, 0.86 and 0.96, suggesting an effect of therapy and programmed cell death of 1 log factor. One study indicated that a BrdU LI of greater than 20% may foretell a poor prognosis. The Ki-67 antigen also appears to be a useful target for determining cells that have begun to synthesize DNA (beyond G0; Fig. 9.250) (Deckert, Reifenberger and Wechsler, 1989; Schiffer *et al.*, 1994; 1995).

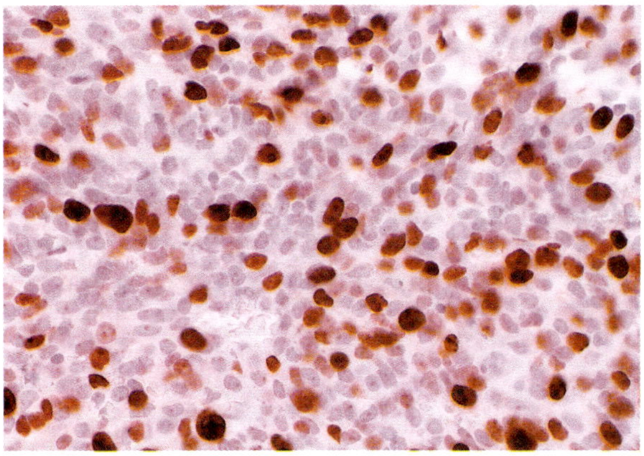

Fig. 9.250 The MIB-1 labeling of medulloblastoma. Approximately 25% of medulloblastoma tumor cell nuclei react against the monoclonal antibody MIB-1. × 132

Spectrophotometry has proven to be an effective and efficient means of identifying abnormal cellular DNA content (ploidy) in childhood solid tumors of neuronal origin by both flow cytometry and microspectrophotometry (Frederiksen, Reske-Nielsen and Bichel, 1978; Frederiksen *et al.*, 1979; Mørk and Laerum, 1980; Tomita *et al.*, 1988; Yasue *et al.*, 1989; Tomita, Das and Radkowski, 1990). Gajjar *et al.* (1993) applied flow cytometry to medulloblastomas from 30 children who were similar in age, tumor stage and extent of resection. This study suggested a significant survival advantage for children whose tumors contained only hyperdiploid cells (ploidy ranging between 1.2 and 1.8 times the normal DNA complement of surrounding lymphocytes) compared with children whose tumors contained a diploid or tetraploid stem line. Similar clinical results are noted from ploidy analyses using either microspectrophotometry (Schofield *et al.*, 1992) or flow cytometry on archival, paraffin-embedded material (Tomita *et al.*, 1988; Yasue *et al.*, 1989; Tomita, Das and Radkowski, 1990). Schofield *et al.* (1992), in the study noted above, demonstrated one advantage of microspectrophotometry when they found that patients with neoplasms exhibiting neuroblastic features, although having a diploid chromosome number, exhibited survival rates equal to patients with aneuploid neoplasms, survivals that were significantly longer than those for patients with the other diploid tumors. These investigators, apparently refining previous studies, reported that when neuroblastic neoplasms were separated from the study group, aneuploidy (hyperdiploidy) was an indicator of poor prognosis. Thus, further studies are required to investigate the interrelationship among cytologic features, phenotypic expression, aneuploidy and survival.

Kinetic analysis of tumor cell S-phase fraction by flow cytometry is obviously complicated by indigenous, benign, nonproliferating cells. It is of no surprise to find this technique to be inconclusive in this use (Yasue *et al.*, 1989). Thus, Zerbini *et al.* (1993) suggest that, when similarly treated patients are analyzed, patients with diploid or tetraploid tumors had fewer recurrences than patients with aneuploid tumors. In contrast, Gajjar *et al.* (1993) report that patients with hyperdiploid tumors survive longer than patients with diploid tumors.

The kinetic parameters of D283 Med have been evaluated after the cell line was maintained *in vitro* in an organ culture system and cumulatively labeled (Nakagawa *et al.*, 1987). The line had an *in vitro* growth fraction of 35%, with a total cell cycle time of 30 hours; the duration of the S phase was approximately 10 hours, an estimate that seems to correspond reasonably closely to those reported for medulloblastoma *in situ*.

Molecular markers

The cytogenetic finding of an isochromosome 17q in 30–50% of medulloblastomas (Biegel *et al.*, 1989; Bigner, Mark and Bigner, 1990; Vagner-Capodano *et al.*, 1994) has been exploited on a molecular basis by Cogen and colleagues (Cogen *et al.*,1990, 1992; Cogen, 1991–92), Thomas and Raffel (1991), Biegel *et al.* (1992) and Batra *et al.* (1995). Studies implicate a loss of heterozygosity (LOH) at locus 17p13 (McDonald *et al.*, 1994) that appears distinct from, and distal to, the *TP53* gene. The LOH at this locus is associated with a poor response to treatment (Cogen, 1991–92) and with a significantly shortened survival (Batra *et al.*, 1995) although the latter is controversial (Biegel *et al.*, 1997). The absence of involvement by *TP53* is further supported by several groups (Saylors *et al.*, 1991; Biegel *et al.*, 1992; Cogen *et al.*, 1992; Adesina, Nalbantoglu and Cavenee, 1994; Albrecht *et al.*, 1994; Batra *et al.*, 1995) who have found *TP53* mutations in less than 6% of medulloblastomas.

Other markers that may prove to be useful from a prognostic standpoint include the apoptosis-related gene *BCL2* (Heck, Pyle and Bruner, 1994), the transmembrane growth factor *ERBB2* (Gilbertson *et al.*, 1995) and the neurotrophin *TRKC* (Segal *et al.*, 1994). Both *MYCN* and *MYC*, while intriguing because of the frequent correlation between gene amplification and double minutes in karyotypic analysis, appear to be amplified in approximately 10% of patients, all of whom have a very poor prognosis (Batra *et al.*, 1995; Schutz *et al.*, 1996). The significance of amplification of *MYC* family genes may reside in characterizing certain medulloblastoma subsets, such as the large-cell variant of medulloblastoma (Giangaspero *et al.*, 1992).

Tumor recurrence

Tumor *recurrence* in the posterior fossa is by far the most frequent cause of clinical relapse. When it occurs in a child, it usually does so within 2 years of treatment (Torres *et al.*, 1994), especially after relatively low doses of radiation. Recurrence may take place beyond the fifth postradiation year, but such a late event is more likely to occur in adults (Hughes, 1984; Louis and Hochberg, 1990). Collins' law, which estimates the critical period of risk for the recurrence of embryonal tumors, has been found to be upheld in the overwhelming majority of medulloblastomas, the rare exceptions being usually fairly close to the limit of the risk period (Bloom, Wallace and Henk, 1969; Quest *et al.*, 1978; Bloom, 1982; Park *et al.*, 1983). Both Latchaw *et al.* (1985) and Brown *et al.* (1995) estimate that Collins' law is violated in less than 4% of medulloblastomas, while Belza *et al.* (1991) noted it held true in only 83% of cases. The clinical and biologic significance of tumor recurrence cannot be understated; Torres *et al.* (1994) found the prognosis of children with tumor recurrence to be uniformly bleak.

Cerebrospinal spread

Local leptomeningeal involvement and intraventricular extension characteristically herald the development of cerebrospinal spread (Figs 9.234

and 9.235). The *incidence* of cerebrospinal metastases varies: in clinical series, it has been reported to be in the region of 10% to 20% (Jereb, Reid and Ahuja, 1982; Park *et al.*, 1983; Flannery *et al.*, 1990), but the incidence is considerably higher in necropsy material, where metastases are noted in more than half the cases. By contrast to the frequency of subarachnoid spread, metastasis in the subdural space, presumably resulting from transgression of the arachnoid membrane by tumor, is exceptional (Koenig, 1971).

Metastatic deposits at remote sites often invade the adjacent neural tissues diffusely, either by direct extension or by way of the perivascular sheaths of perforating blood vessels (Fig. 9.251). By reason of their rapid development and size, these deposits may occasionally be chiefly responsible for neurologic signs and symptoms and may be erroneously interpreted as the primary growth when the cerebellar focus is relatively small and inconspicuous. The floor of the third ventricle and, even more so, the spinal canal at any level are noteworthy in this context. Another notable site of massive secondary tumor involvement in the supratentorial compartment is the orbital surface of the frontal lobe. Recurrences may appear in the region of the cribriform plate after apparently successful craniospinal irradiation, and this has been related to ocular shielding and thus incomplete therapy (Donnal *et al.*, 1992).

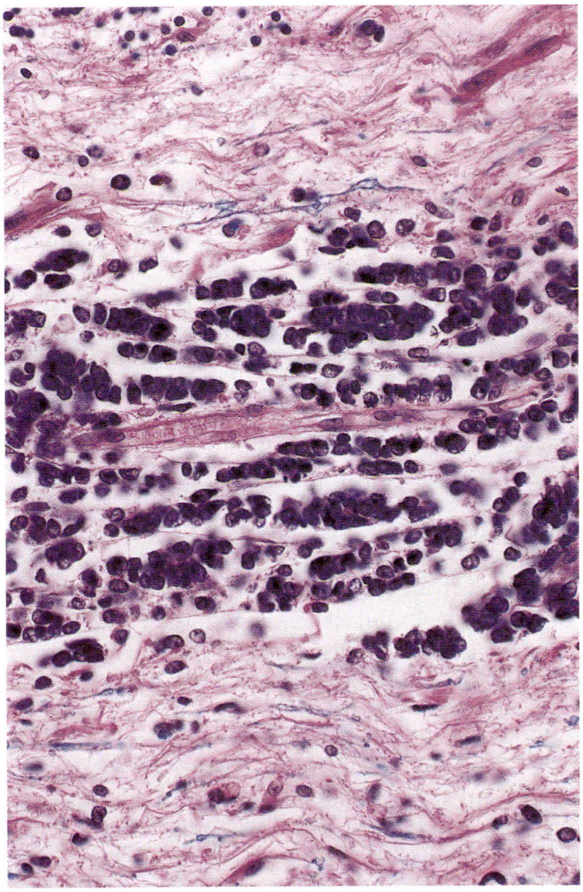

Fig. 9.251 Tumor cells extending beyond the main tumor mass by spreading along the Virchow-Robin space, both within the cerebellum as well as distally. Occasionally, this pattern may be confused with a lymphoma. H&E, × 100

Extraneural metastases

Extraneural metastatic spread has been repeatedly confirmed in the past two decades and thoroughly reviewed by Kleinman, Hochberg and Richardson (1981), Campbell *et al.* (1984) and Tarbell *et al.* (1991). The incidence of systemic deposits in patients with medulloblastoma is estimated by these workers to be around 5%, with somewhat higher incidence rates of 17% and 9% being recorded in childhood cases by, respectively, McComb, Davis and Isaacs (1981) and Park *et al.* (1983). Although Hoffman, Hendrick and Humphreys (1976) initially suggested that systemic metastases may be related to systemic shunting, Berger *et al.* (1991) have noted that shunting did not appear to be a factor in systemic dissemination. Adult cases, particularly of the desmoplastic variant, seem to have been especially associated with the development of remote systemic deposits (Rubinstein and Northfield, 1964; Kopelson, Linggood and Kleinman, 1982; Spencer *et al.*, 1984), although McComb, Davis and Isaacs (1981) could not confirm that extraneural metastases were especially frequent with the desmoplastic variant in childhood examples. The distribution of metastases does not appear to be influenced by age at diagnosis (Rochkind *et al.*, 1991). It is apparent, in any event, that medulloblastomas may show a relatively higher incidence of distant extraneural spread than the gliomas (Liwnicz and Rubinstein, 1979). Tarbell *et al.* (1991) calculated that the risk of recurrence among extracranial and intracranial relapses was equal and suggested that high-dose craniospinal irradiation had altered the pattern of relapse.

Russell and Rubinstein (1989) have previously noted extraneural metastases in 11 patients, six of whom were also recorded in detail elsewhere (Rubinstein, 1959; Rubinstein and Northfield, 1964; Liwnicz and Rubinstein, 1979; Kleinman, Hochberg and Richardson, 1981, case 2; Pollak, Miller and Vye, 1981). They noted that, in many instances, this development has followed surgical intervention for removal of the growth; but, in two published examples, the pathway of distant spread was demonstrably independent of the site of previous craniotomy, i.e., the roof of the orbit in one case (Rubinstein, 1959) and the spinal paravertebral tissues in the other (Liwnicz and Rubinstein, 1979). The spinal canal has been shown, in several instances, to be an important site of exit in medulloblastomas, paving the way for the development of more remote dissemination.

Exceptional examples of medulloblastomas initially presenting with extraneural deposits have been reported, as in the two cases in infants with cervical metastatic masses described by McComb *et al.* (1980) and in a 26-year-old woman recorded by Pollak, Miller and Vye (1981). In the latter case, the patient was thought to have leukemia because of widespread bone marrow involvement by tumor cells (Fig. 9.248); their medulloblastic nature was confirmed by the discovery of a cerebellar medulloblastoma at postmortem 13 months later. One of us (R.E.M.) has seen a similar case, submitted by Dr Ashraf Ali, of a teenage child with diffuse systemic bone marrow involvement by cells that were forming cohesive clumps on bone marrow aspiration and were immunoreactive for synaptophysin. A cerebellar tumor was also found concurrently that proved to be a medulloblastoma.

The *lymph nodes* and the *bones* (see Fig. 9.312) are the most frequent and characteristic sites of extraneural metastases (Liwnicz and Rubinstein, 1979; Kleinman, Hochberg and Richardson, 1981; Campbell *et al.*, 1984; Alwasiak *et al.*, 1991; Berger *et al.*, 1991; Rochkind *et al.*, 1991; Tarbell *et al.*, 1991; Sheikh and Kanaan, 1994). Skeletal involvement may be massive and widespread (Rubinstein and Northfield, 1964; Spencer *et al.*, 1984). Depression of bone marrow function resulting in anemia, leukopenia and thrombocytopenia, sometimes associated with myelosclerosis, may then be present: hematophagocytosis by metastatic medulloblastoma cells has been reported as an exceptional finding (Youness *et al.*, 1980). On the other hand, as noted in earlier reports (Rubinstein, 1959; Drachman, Winter and Karon, 1963), the lungs are often curiously free of tumor deposits and are affected usually in patients who have been subjected to ventriculosystemic bypass procedures (Makeever and King, 1966; Kleinman, Hochberg and Richardson, 1981), evidence indicative of a shunt-related metastasis (Berger *et al.*, 1991). The placenta is an exceptional host to metastatic disease (Brossard *et al.*, 1994).

Markers of prognostic significance: summary

In summary, the clinical data indicate that patients with tumors located in the cerebellar hemispheres have survival advantages over patients with tumors in the vermis (Rubinstein and Northfield, 1964; Chatty and Earle, 1971; Park *et al.*, 1983; Sure *et al.*, 1995), and both groups survive longer if the tumor is confined to the cerebellum without evidence of brainstem extension (Chang, Housepian and Herbert, 1969; Chatty and Earle, 1971; Kopelson, Linggood and Kleinman, 1983; Park *et al.*, 1983; Laurent, Chang and Cohen, 1985; Sure *et al.*, 1995). Similarly, patients whose tumors are situated such as to allow a gross total resection survive longer than patients whose tumors allow only a partial resection because of invasion into the brainstem or peduncles (Kopelson, Linggood and Kleinman, 1983; Park *et al.*, 1983; Laurent, Chang, Cohen, 1985; Watt and Winfield, 1987; Yasue *et al.*, 1989; Evans *et al.*, 1990; Cervoni and Cantore, 1995; Sure *et al.*, 1995; Albright *et al.*, 1996). Likewise, patients with metastatic tumor deposits have a worse prognosis than patients with tumors confined to the cerebellum (Kopelson, Linggood and Kleinman, 1983; Tomita and McLone, 1983; Berger *et al.*, 1991; Geyer *et al.*, 1992; Albright *et al.*, 1996). Finally, tumor recurrence, whether local or distant, signifies a bleak prognosis (Torres *et al.*, 1994).

Cell culture and xenograft studies

Early studies of medulloblastoma in both organ culture and short-term cell cultures were useful in characterizing the *in vitro* phenotypic features of medulloblastoma and advancing the concept of phenotypic divergence in medulloblastoma (Kersting, 1968; Liss, 1969; Lumsden, 1971, 1974; Rubinstein, Herman and Hanbery, 1974; Weichselbaum *et al.*, 1977) and are reviewed more completely in the previous edition (Russell and Rubinstein, 1989).

Reports on the characterization of permanent human medulloblastoma cell lines are increasing. The most work, to date, has been done on seven cell lines: Daoy (Jacobsen, Jenkyn and Papadimitriou, 1985), D283 Med (Friedman *et al.*, 1985), D341 Med (Friedman *et al.*, 1988), D 384 Med and D425 Med (Bigner *et al.*, 1990), and ONS-76 and ONS-81 (Tamura *et al.*, 1989). Another cell line, D458 Med, derived from a recurrence in the CSF from the patient from whom D425 Med was established, has also been reported (He *et al.*, 1991). The five 'D' (Duke) lines grow in suspension as spheroids, while Daoy, under the same conditions, grows as an adherent monolayer. Karyotypically, the Duke cell lines are near diploid, while Daoy is tetraploid. Thus, a dichotomy between the Duke lines and the adherent Daoy is immediately apparent. Furthermore, the Duke lines express synaptophysin, medium- (NFP-M) and high- (NFP-H) molecular-weight NFPs and amplified levels of c-myc protein (Bigner *et al.*, 1990), but do not express class I or II HLA antigens, Thy-1, CALLA or nerve growth factor receptor. It has been postulated that these different NFP profiles may represent stages in neuronal differentiation (Gould *et al.*, 1990; Tohyama *et al.*, 1991). Ganglioside expression was confined to those gangliosides present in normal brain and in tumors of neuroectodermal origin (neuroblastomas and melanomas) (Svennerholm, 1988), while none of the so-called glioma-associated gangliosides, 3'-isoLM1 and 3',6'-isoLD1 (Månsson *et al.*, 1986), have been found. In contrast, Daoy differs by expressing normal levels of c-myc protein (McLendon *et al.*, 1995a) and exhibiting reactivity with MAbs to HLA class I antigen, EGFR and tenascin; it does not express synaptophysin. The ONS lines reported by Tamura *et al.* (1989) also exhibit neuronal phenotypic markers. All of the medulloblastoma lines established in the Duke program have proven identities by both karyotypic and DNA fingerprint comparisons with the original tumor biopsy specimens. A primary tumor karyotype was not obtained from Daoy, and no DNA fingerprint analysis has been reported comparing the genotypic profiles of the culture with the original biopsy, thus further weakening the use of this line as proof for glial expression in medulloblastomas. Both subcutaneous and intracranial xenograft models have been established for all of the Duke cell lines. In addition, a nude rat model of intrathecal leptomeningeal dissemination has been established that allows these cultures to be used to test efficacy of therapeutic regimens.

Medulloblastomas growing as xenografts include the human medulloblastoma cell lines D283 Med, D341 Med, D384 Med and D425 Med (Friedman *et al.*, 1985, 1988), which grow both intracranial and subcutaneous in athymic mice. In D283, the intracranial but not the subcutaneous transplants show Homer Wright rosette formation. All xenografts express NSE but not GFAP or S-100 protein. All three subunits of the NFP triplet are expressed in D243 Med (Trojanowski *et al.*, 1987).

The established line Daoy, obtained from a desmoplastic medulloblastoma and less differentiated than the D283 Med, was described by Jacobsen, Jenkyn and Papadimitriou (1985). When injected intracerebrally in nude mice, however, it results in diffuse infiltration of the brain parenchyma rather than a circumscribed mass.

A pattern of rather extensive intraventricular and subarachnoid dissemination was obtained on xenogeneic transplantation of another line, D341 Med. Flow cytometric studies show NFP expression (both phosphorylated and nonphosphorylated forms of NFP-M and NFP-H) (Trojanowski, Tohyama and Lee, 1992), NSE and glutamine synthetase, but not GFAP or S-100 protein in this xenograft. Karyotypic study reveals a large number of double-minute chromatin bodies in the tumor cells consonant with its amplification (20-fold) of the *MYC* oncogene.

In addition to the heterotransplantation of the established medulloblastoma cell lines described, one tumor has also been reported by Sawa *et al.* (1986b) to have been successfully passaged in nude mice and found to maintain positivity for the 68-kDa and 160-kDa NFPs after intracerebral inoculation.

The TE-671 line, established by McAllister *et al.* (1977) and originally believed to be of medulloblastomatous origin, has proven to be a rhabdomyosarcoma line, which discrepancy accounts for the finding of acetylcholinesterase activity (Schlesinger *et al.*, 1981) and the presence of nicotinic cholinergic receptors (Syapin, Salvaterra and Engelhardt, 1982) and actin (Mørk *et al.*, 1986b).

Controversial or unresolved issues

Unresolved questions and controversies surround the topic medulloblastoma and have drawn significant interest from the brain tumor community. The issues of classification raised by Becker and Hinton (1983), Rorke (1983), and Rubinstein (Rubinstein, Herman and VandenBerg, 1984) have served to focus the debate on a cell of origin as well as on factors of maturation, differentiation, and regulation of phenotypic expression. The cytogenetic and molecular genetic work of Bigner *et al.* (1988b), Cogen (1991–92), Saylors *et al.* (1991) and Batra *et al.* (1995) have shed light on factors related to tumorigenesis and progression, particularly with regard to chromosome 17 and to oncogene amplification. The identification of inherited tumor syndromes such as Gorlin's syndrome (Gorlin, 1987; Evans, Birch and Orton, 1991; Evans *et al.*, 1991) and familial colon carcinoma syndrome (*APC* deletion), which also feature medulloblastomas as a component, will help elucidate factors involved in tumorigenesis. The significant issue raised by the PNET debate is the lack of utility provided by light microscopic examination in identifying markers of prognostic significance in medulloblastomas. The short-term goal of medulloblastoma research will be toward the characterization of such markers in order that therapy can be tailored to the tumor, minimizing the debilitating effects of therapy. Long-term goals will be twofold: one will be oriented toward the epidemiologic questions of characterizing at-risk populations and discerning factors of pathogenesis; the other will be aimed at identifying biologic factors that can be exploited for therapeutic efficacy.

Neuroblastomas

Apart from the medulloblastomas of the cerebellum, which show neuroblastic differentiation, tumors of this nature arise with great rarity in other parts of the CNS. They are appropriately termed neuroblastomas, as their primitive character aligns them with the much more common neuroblastomas of the adrenal medulla and the sympathetic ganglia.

In 1973, Hart and Earle (1973) proposed that certain supratentorial tumors of infancy, which were characterized microscopically by a high nuclear-to-cytoplasmic ratio and greater than 95% of the tumor cells lacking differentiation by light microscopy, should be classified as PNETs. The advent of immunologic reagents has subsequently aided in the characterization of many of these neoplasms, several of which are now recognized as small-cell gliomas of infancy (Friede, Janzer and Roessmann, 1982). However, cases still exist that either lack phenotypic markers for accurate characterization or that require ultrastructural analysis for classification. The vast majority of these remaining cases can be shown to exhibit features of a neuronal phenotype. Histologically, the similarities to the classic medulloblastomas were recognized by Rorke (1983) and by Becker and Hinton (1983) who proposed that the term 'primitive neuroectodermal tumor' should be used to characterize all CNS neoplasms of embryonal neuroectodermal origin, including those tumors also known as medulloepithelioma, neuroblastoma, polar spongioblastoma, pineoblastoma, ependymoblastoma, retinoblastoma and olfactory neuroblastoma. The rationale for this recharacterization was that '[f]rom a practical, histologic point of view, these tumors are often indistinguishable from one another and are best thought of as primitive neuroectodermal tumors with or without differentiating features' (Becker and Hinton, 1983). Supporters of the system noted that it also encompassed the plasticity of the neoplastically transformed embryonal neuroectodermal cell to express divergent neuroectodermal phenotypes.

Histologically, a number of factors distinguish these tumors at a light microscopic level. Flexner-Wintersteiner rosettes are common in retinoblastomas, infrequent in pineoblastomas, rare in medulloblastomas and absent in cerebral neuroblastomas. Calcification is common in retinoblastomas and cerebral neuroblastomas and absent in medulloblastomas. 'Pale islands' of tumor cells are present in up to two thirds of childhood medulloblastomas (Katsetos, Liu and Zacks, 1988) and occasionally in medulloepitheliomas, but are unheard of in cerebral neuroblastomas, retinoblastomas and pineoblastomas. True ependymal rosettes are found in the ependymoblastoma (Rubinstein, 1970; Mørk and Rubinstein, 1985) but are absent in the other neoplasms, while medullary rosettes and tubes define the medulloepithelioma.

The inherited brain tumor syndromes (discussed in Chapter 16) further subdivide these malignant embryonal tumors of neuroectodermal origin based on susceptibility of certain subtypes to the inherited neoplastic influence. For example, medulloblastomas form the spectrum of neoplasms encountered in patients with familial colonic carcinoma syndromes characterized by a deletion in the *APC* gene (Burger and Hamilton, 1995), as well as Gorlin's syndrome (Gorlin, 1987; Evans *et al.*, 1991). Retinoblastomas and pineoblastomas are the primary neoplasms found in *RB1* deletion syndrome. Similarly, molecular genetic data from sporadic tumors also exhibit changes that select out these light microscopically indistinguishable tumors. Deletions of the *RB1* gene are confined to retinoblastomas and certain pineoblastomas. Isochromosome 17q is a common karyotypic finding in medulloblastomas but is infrequent elsewhere. Given that the germline mutations characteristic of these syndromes affect every cell in the body, the implication is that the neoplastically targeted cells are uniquely dependent on the altered protein for critical control of cell cycle functions, functions that other cells apparently have alternate mechanisms of controlling. Thus, in the *RB1* deletion syndrome, only retinal cells and pineal cells exhibit a dependency on the RB1 protein, a point that also reflects on the two structures, common phylogenetic origins.

Another line of evidence involves the persistent expression of proteins in neoplasia. The Zic protein is homologous to the *Drosophila* pair-rule gene *opa*. Recent studies have shown that the expression of this protein is restricted to internal and external granular cells in mature and developing cerebella. In one study, 23/26 medulloblastomas were immunoreactive for this protein, while no other tumors exhibited reactivity, including retinoblastomas, pineoblastomas, ependymoblastomas, ganglioneuromas and glioblastomas, nor was it found in a diverse spectrum of non-CNS neoplasms (Yokota *et al.*, 1996). Although it is not clear in the original report if any other cerebellar tumors were studied, the preliminary studies suggest that this protein may be a useful marker in distinguishing medulloblastomas from other embryonal neuroectodermal tumors. Thus, as evidence continues to mount supporting distinctions in histogenesis, tumorigenesis and therapy among these malignant neuroectodermal tumors of embryonal origin, we persist in characterizing them on the basis of cytogenesis.

Cytogenesis

Development of neuroblastomas in the cerebral hemispheres may, at first glance, seem paradoxical due to the lack of proliferative activity of migrating neuroblasts implicit in current schemes of central neurocytogenesis (Fujita, 1963). The assumption that the postmitotic neuroblasts can no longer be the target of carcinogenesis duly accounts for the exceptional rarity of neuronal tumors obtained after the transplacental administration of neuro-oncogenic alkylating agents (see Chapter 5). However, primitive neuronal cells are the specific target of transformation in the rat and hamster when the human adenovirus type 12 is locally injected in the neonate (Mukai, 1976). This implies that, in these rodents at birth and shortly thereafter, there must be a turnover of cells in which the differentiating potential is restricted to the neuronal line. Presumably, this must be the case also in man if we are to explain the occurrence of the admittedly exceptional central neuroblastoma. Little information is available, however, on the postnatal sites of continuing neuronogenesis, which sites might constitute the source of these tumors. As noted and illustrated above (p. 457), the fetal external granular layer of the cerebellum, or its remnants, may represent such a source in medulloblastomas. A potential area of cortical neuronogenesis is the subpial granular layer of the cerebral hemispheres, which normally disappears by the 8th month of intrauterine life, but of which remnants have been reported in the frontal lobe 6 months after birth (Brun, 1965). Another potential site is the dentate fascia of the hippocampus, which may function as a postnatal source of small neurons in the temporal cortex (Kaplan and Hinds, 1977; Guéneau *et al.*, 1982). These possible sources are, however, entirely speculative: autoradiographic studies on the primate brain have shown that, with the possible exception – during the neonatal period – of a few granular cells in the cerebellum and hippocampus, there is no renewal of neurons after birth (Rakic, 1985).

Incidence

The rarity of cerebral neuroblastomas among brain tumors in general makes it virtually impossible to assess their frequency. Nevertheless, since the first edition of this book (Russell and Rubinstein, 1959), when Russell and Rubinstein reported on the features of two personally examined examples, the literature on these tumors has accrued considerably, largely as a result of the work of Rubinstein in bringing attention to these lesions (Horten and Rubinstein, 1976; Bennett and Rubinstein, 1984).

In 1976, Horten and Rubinstein described a personal series of 35 tumors; 12 cases from the literature, of which nine showed evidence of ganglionic maturation, were also briefly quoted (see Horten and Rubinstein, 1976, for references) although four cases were subsequently reclassified by Rubinstein as desmoplastic infantile gangliogliomas (VandenBerg *et al.*, 1987) (p. 485). Since then, new examples have been documented by others, usually as isolated case reports. They essentially confirm the pathologic features of this entity along with ultrastructural characteristics (Azzarelli *et al.*, 1977; Rhodes *et al.*, 1978; Ojeda, Jacobsen and Papadimitriou, 1980; Pearl *et al.*, 1981; Pigott *et al.*, 1990; Mondkar *et al.*, 1994; Rhodes *et al.*, 1994; Delisle *et al.*, 1995) and associated biochemical findings, such as catecholamine levels (Ahdevaara *et al.*, 1977; Azzarelli *et al.*, 1977) and, in one instance, elevated nerve growth factor in the serum (Meyer *et al.*, 1980). Bennett and Rubinstein (1984) also reported on an additional 35 examples of cerebral neuroblastoma referred for consultation, permitting a closer reassessment of their clinical evolution; this series remains the largest collection reviewed by one group. Simultaneous with this re-evaluation, a follow-up analysis of 11 examples from the University of California in San Francisco appeared (Berger *et al.*, 1983). More recently, the case reports on primitive neuronal tumors of the cerebrum have tended to emphasize their polyphenotypic character, with mixed glial and/or mesenchymal elements drawing the investigator's attention (Dastur, 1982; Gambarelli *et al.*, 1982; Gaffney *et al.*, 1985; Tang *et al.*, 1985; Jay *et al.*, 1994; Delisle, 1995).

Age and sex incidence

In the Rubinstein series (Bennett and Rubinstein, 1984), 80% of the cases occurred in the first decade, more than half within the first 5 years. Twenty-five percent of the tumors made their appearance before the age of 2 years. There was no sex predilection.

Sites

The distribution of neuroblastomas within the cerebral hemispheres corresponds to the relative size of the various lobes, the tumors occurring most frequently in the frontal and frontoparietal regions. However, while the following discussion is largely concerned with the cerebral examples, other regions of the central neuraxis may also be occasionally involved. Thus, three spinal intramedullary neuroblastomas, of which two were in children and one was in an adult, have been noted by Rubinstein (Russell and Rubinstein, 1989). Three examples arising in the cauda equina of adults have been reported by Kepes *et al.* (1985). The pons, too, may be an exceptional site (Hassin and Munch-Petersen, 1951, case 1). Neuroblastomas originating in the cerebellum prove difficult to separate from the broad and well-entrenched entity of cerebellar medulloblastomas with various degrees of neuroblastic differentiation; convenience dictates their inclusion in the latter section (p. 470). Intra-ventricular neurocytomas are discussed separately.

Macroscopic appearance

Characteristically, almost all neuroblastomas are well defined and circumscribed (Fig. 9.252). Many are unusually firm and lobulated, this being directly related to the proportion of desmoplastic stroma demonstrable histologically. The cut surfaces tend to be granular, revealing foci of hemorrhage or necrosis. Cyst formation is frequent, often accounting for the large size of the neoplasm and, according to Berger *et al.* (1983), may signify a more favorable prognosis, perhaps due to the better

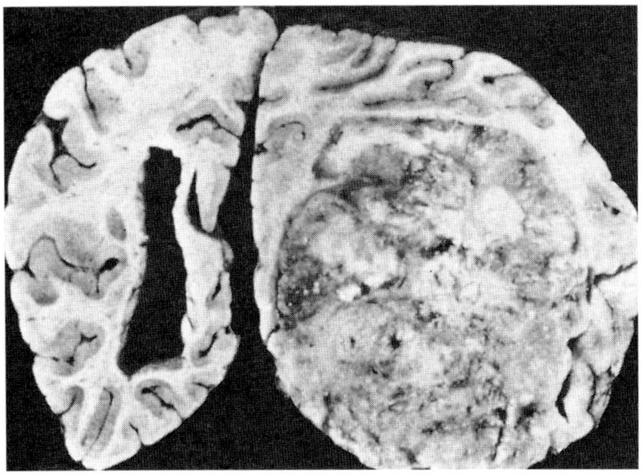

Fig. 9.252 Large well-defined occipital neuroblastoma showing a gray granular cut surface with foci of pale necrosis in a 4-year-old girl. (Courtesy of Dr J.E. Olvera Rabiela)

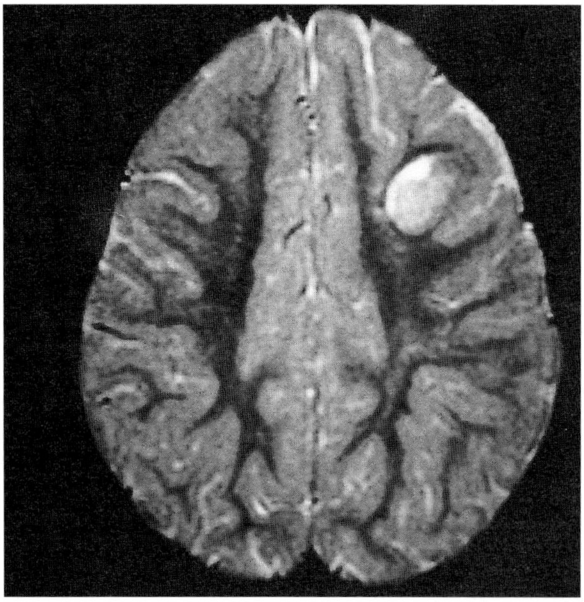

Fig. 9.253 Axial T2-weighted MRI demonstrating a mass in the left frontal lobe at the gray–white junctions. The tumor is viewed with increased T2 signal intensity and a mildly heterogeneous signal intensity. With contrast, there is mild heterogeneous enhancement. No significant vasogenic tumoral edema is identified.

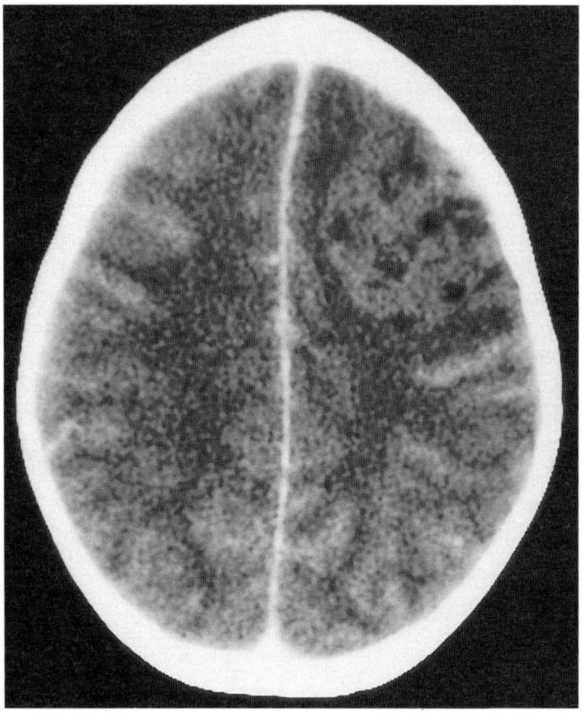

Fig. 9.254 Axial CT postcontrast image showing a left frontal intra-axial tumor that is very heterogeneous in density. No definite calcification is present. There is mild heterogeneous contrast enhancement.

opportunity for more complete surgical removal. In some cases, extensive areas of gelatinous degeneration are demonstrable.

Radiographic appearance

Primary cerebral neuroblastoma is typically a large supertentorial hemispheric mass that has well-demarcated borders and heterogeneous signal intensity. Areas of cysts, hemorrhage, calcification and necrosis are common. At MRI, these masses have variable signal intensity on both T1- and T2-weighted sequences, with enhancement patterns that are also heterogeneous (Fig. 9.253). Calcifications are easier to identify on CT evaluation (Fig. 9.254).

Microscopic appearance

The microscopic picture is one of high cellular density and shows a good deal of variation, not only within the group as a whole, but also within the individual case (Fig. 9.255). Rubinstein reports (Russell and Rubinstein, 1989) that approximately half the tumors in his series closely resemble peripheral neuroblastomas or cerebellar medulloblastomas. This pattern, designated the *classical* variant, consists of densely cellular fields of small round or oval cells with darkly staining nuclei; Homer Wright rosettes are often found therein (Fig. 9.256). Mitotic figures are numerous. A background fibrillarity produced by the tumor cells is often encountered, just as found in peripheral neuroblastomas.

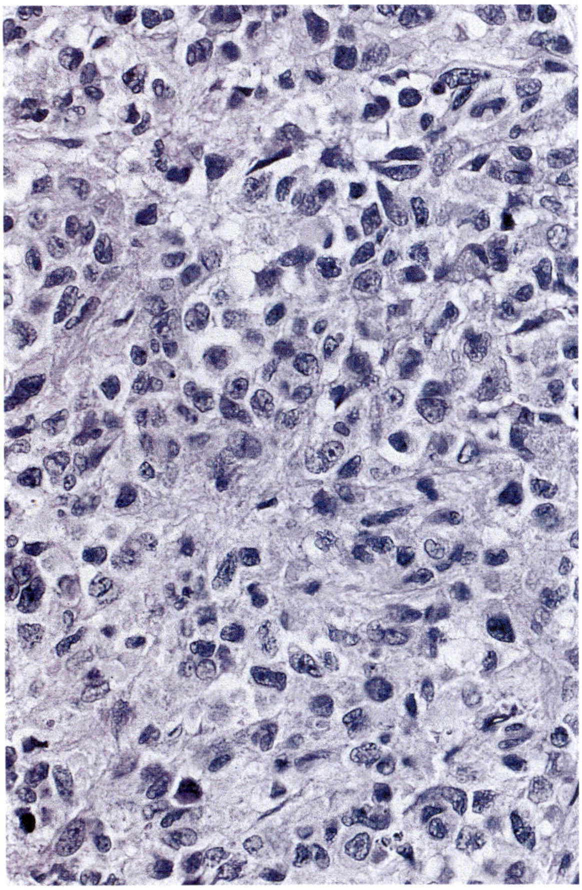

a

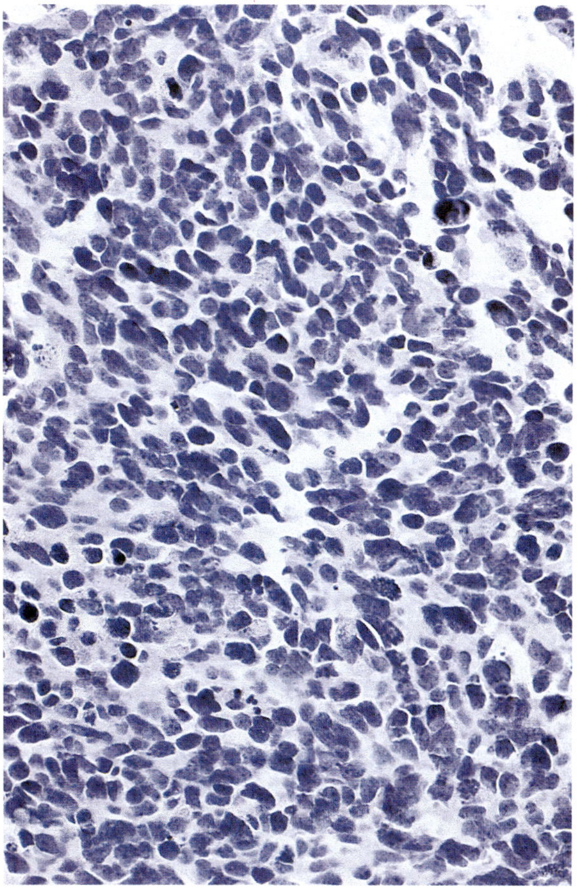

b

Fig. 9.255 Cerebral neuroblastoma. Histologically, neuroblastomas exhibit high cellular density and significant cytologic variability. This pattern may vary from (a) the open vesicular nuclei with a modest amount of fibrillar cytoplasm (H&E, × 150) to (b) small anaplastic cells reminiscent of medulloblastoma (H&E, × 100)

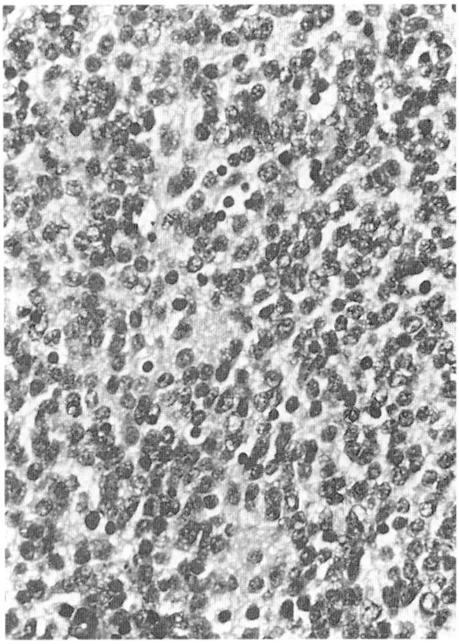

Fig. 9.256 Parieto-occipital neuroblastoma in a 9-year-old girl showing poorly defined Homer Wright rosettes. H&E, × 225

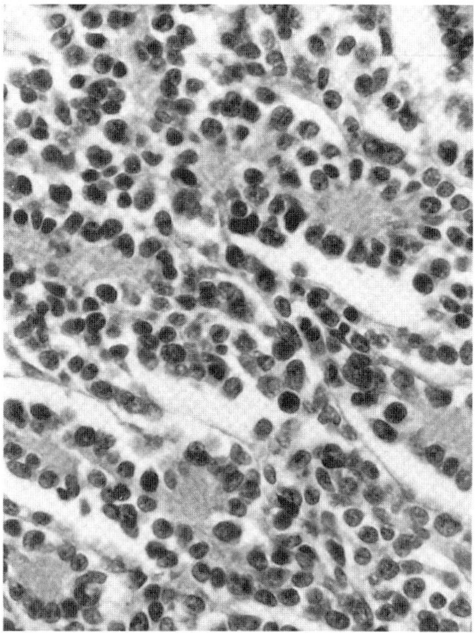

Fig. 9.257 Microscopic sections taken from the gross neuroblastoma demonstrated in Fig. 9.252. These sections reveal a streaming arrangement of tumor cells in the leptomeninges, forming Homer Wright rosettes. H&E, × 300

Tumors that do not fulfill the criteria for the *classical* neuroblastoma show, either throughout or focally, the development of a fibrous connective tissue stroma. This stroma ranges from a rather compact lobular framework, interweaving among clusters of neoplastic cells, to areas of intense fibrous proliferation running in parallel streams between them, conferring a *desmoplastic* appearance to the most extreme examples. This feature becomes especially conspicuous when the growth invades the leptomeninges. Rubinstein (Russell and Rubinstein, 1989) states that this feature, which sharply distinguishes the neuroblastomas from other primary central neuroepithelial neoplasms, suggests an unusual capacity on the part of these primitive tumor cells for stroma induction analogous to the desmoplastic medulloblastoma. Rubinstein notes (Russell and Rubinstein, 1989) that, in one example, the desmoplastic features became increasingly prominent in the recurrences, culminating in a sarcomatous transformation of the stroma, with the development of a mixed neuroblastoma–fibrosarcoma.

The desmoplastic and the classical variants of cerebral neuroblastoma are frequently bridged by *transitional* examples. Both the desmoplastic and the transitional variants often are composed of cells that are larger than those in the classical variant and have spheroidal, polygonal or pyramidal cytoplasmic outlines, clear vesiculated nuclei and small nucleoli. Homer Wright rosettes are less often demonstrable than in the classical variant, but are illustrated in Fig. 9.257 in a subarachnoid deposit from a transitional case. In some examples, the cells are noted to be arranged in irregular syncytial groups, the general appearance under low power being cribriform or microcystic in places. Even in the more desmoplastic tumors, clusters of small undifferentiated neuroblasts arranged against a delicately fibrillated neuropil may be found. Russell and Rubinstein (1989) noted that patients with the desmoplastic or the transitional variant have a somewhat lower mean age at diagnosis compared with those harboring the classical variant, but the histologic pattern is of no predictive value regarding postoperative survival (Bennett and Rubinstein, 1984).

In the absence of light or electron microscopic evidence of ganglionic differentiation, the microscopic picture may, because of the primitive character of the tumor cells and the protean appearances produced by the mesenchymal stromal response, present considerable diagnostic difficulties. The classical variant may be mistaken for an oligodendroglioma or an ependymoma. The transitional and desmoplastic variants often resemble

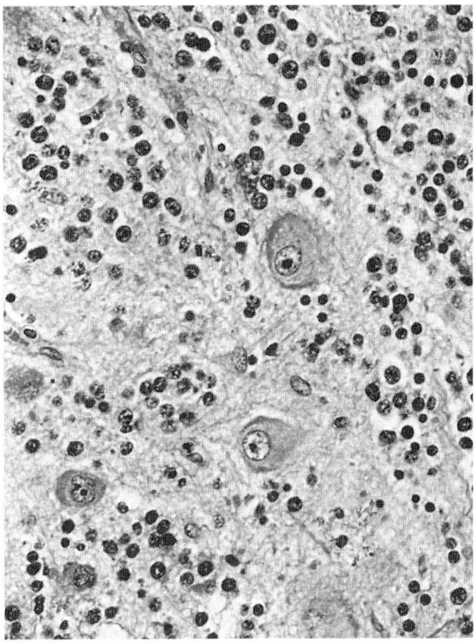

Fig. 9.258 Differentiating left frontoparietal neuroblastoma in a 5-year-old male. H&E, × 225

poorly differentiated meningeal sarcomas. Both the sarcomas and the desmoplastic neuroblastomas share a common capacity to stimulate a marked hypertrophic astrocytic reaction in the invaded brain. Indeed, malignant gliomas may occasionally be encountered (Tang *et al.*, 1985).

The tumor cells may occasionally be arranged in parallel streams and palisades, resembling the pattern seen in polar spongioblastoma (Horten and Rubinstein, 1976, case 31, Fig. 17). This feature has also been recorded by Becker and Hinton (1983, Fig. 7) as well as by Langford and Camel (1987) and Ojeda, Spagnolo and Vaughan (1987) in two cases in which the neuroblastic nature of the tumors was established by electron microscopy.

Differentiation

The demonstration, often focal only, of differentiation to more mature ganglionic forms, resulting in the picture of a ganglioneuroblastoma, provides important evidence for the inferential recognition of the less-differentiated elements as neuroblasts. Differentiation is most frequently found in the classical variant (Fig. 9.258), where it occurs in up to 50% of cases. It is encountered much less often in the desmoplastic variant, lowering the overall incidence of ganglionic differentiation to about 25% of Bennett and Rubinstein's (1984) cases. They noted that no significant age difference was found between patients harboring tumors and those without ganglionic differentiation, and no correlation could be made between postoperative survival times and the presence or absence of this feature.

It could be argued that some of the instances of differentiating cerebral neuroblastoma (Horten and Rubinstein, 1976; Jay *et al.*, 1994; McLendon *et al.*, 1996, case 2) constitute transitional links with the gangliocytomas (discussed on p. 493). This is further exemplified by the exceptional cases reported by Kernohan, Learmonth and Doyle (1932, case 1) of a 16-year-old girl with a temporoparietal tumor that recurred 6 years after enucleation; by Liss (1960) of a 31-year-old male with a right parietal mass; and by Torres *et al.* (1985) of a 3-year-old girl with a temporal tumor that recurred 9 years later. In all those cases, maturation from a neuroblastoma to a ganglioneuroma occurred after a prolonged clinical course.

Desmoplastic infantile gangliogliomas

Rubinstein's series (Horten and Rubinstein, 1976) included four examples of neuroblastoma originating in infants and presenting predominantly as extracerebral meningeal growths, resulting in a considerable degree of desmoplasia (cases 32–35); one of the tumors had previously been described by Miller and Ramsden (1966). Further study of these and seven other similar examples disclosed that the great majority display divergent differentiation along astrocytic as well as neuronal lines. Although these tumors are generally massive, they carry a favorable prognosis after complete or subtotal resection. By virtue of their characteristic histologic features, age incidence and clinical behavior, VandenBerg *et al.* (1987) point out that they seem to represent a distinct clinicopathologic entity that biologically aligns them more closely with the gangliogliomas than with the cerebral neuroblastomas (Ng, Fung and Ma, 1990; Paulus *et al.*, 1992). They are, therefore, discussed and illustrated on p. 507 under the heading 'Desmoplastic infantile gangliogliomas'.

Electron microscopy

A number of reports have documented the electron microscopic features of cerebral neuroblastomas, but their appearance is often less distinctive than is that of the cerebellar neuroblastomas (*see* p. 470). In the less-differentiated examples, the perikarya of the cells usually contain only a sparse population of cytoplasmic organelles. Among these, dense-core

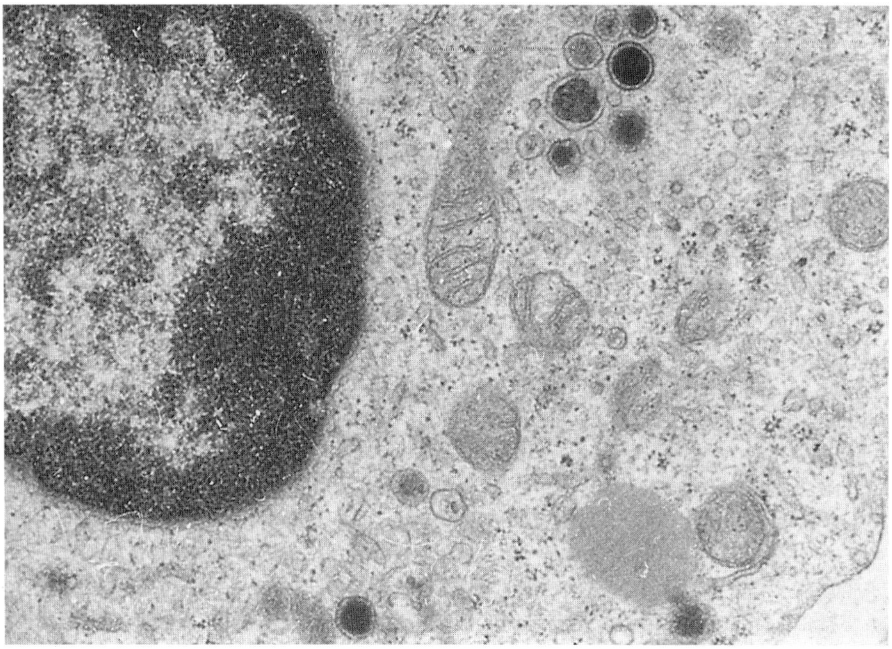

Fig. 9.259 Electron micrograph of a tumor cell from a left frontal neuroblastoma in a 4-year-old boy. Dense-core vesicles are apparent in the perikaryon, × 24 000 (From Goldammer and Goebel, 1980)

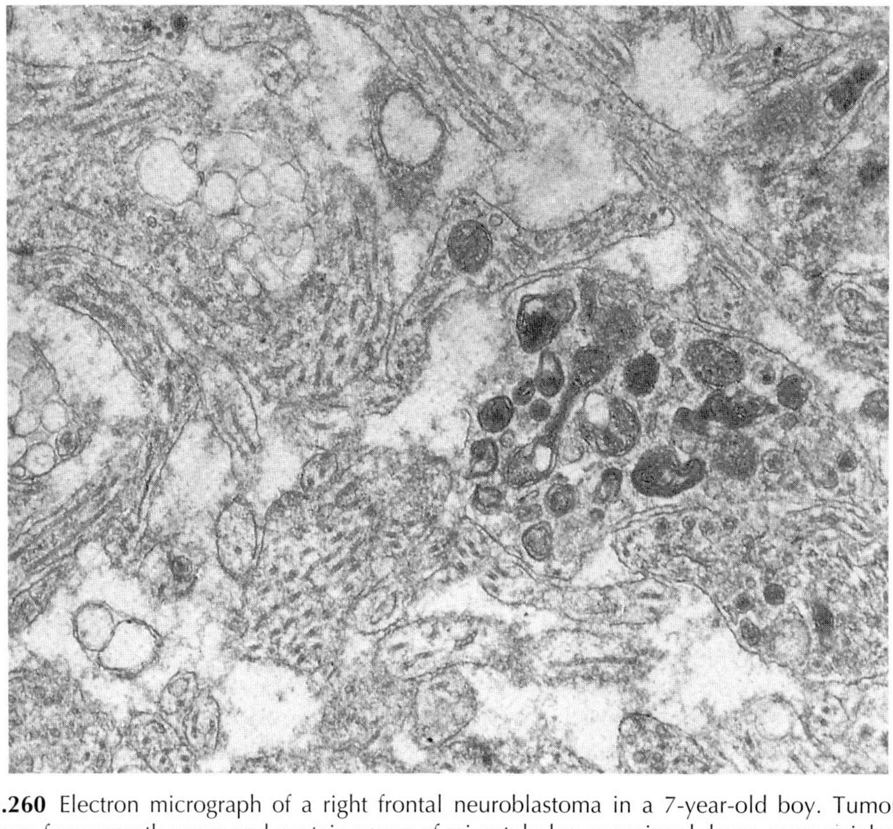

Fig. 9.260 Electron micrograph of a right frontal neuroblastoma in a 7-year-old boy. Tumor cell processes form growth cones and contain arrays of microtubules, occasional dense-core vesicles, and larger electron-dense bodies, some of which are laminated. Note the synapse in the left lower corner. × 24 000 (Courtesy of Professor H.H. Goebel)

vesicles with an outer diameter ranging from 150 nm to 400 nm and an inner core ranging from 135 nm to 250 nm may be demonstrable. They are illustrated in Fig. 9.259 taken from a left frontal neuroblastoma of the transitional variant (Horten and Rubinstein, 1976, case 22), whose electron microscopic features were subsequently reported by Goldammer and Goebel (1980). The presence of dense-core vesicles has also been noted by others (Azzarelli *et al.*, 1977; Pearl *et al.*, 1981, 1985; Gambarelli *et al.*, 1982; Hassoun *et al.*, 1982; Jerdan *et al.*, 1983; Tang *et al.*, 1985; Ojeda *et al.*, 1986; Townsend and Seaman, 1986; Nishio *et al.*, 1988; Pigott *et al.*, 1990; Delisle *et al.*, 1995) but is not invariable. These vesicles were not seen in the examples considered by Henriquez, Robertson and Marshall (1973) or by Rhodes *et al.* (1978). With increasing differentiation of the tumor, the number of dense-core vesicles increases and, when they are found in the perikaryon, these vesicles may then be associated with stacks of rough endoplasmic reticulum. The cell processes may sometimes terminate as growth cones and often contain arrays of microtubules (Figs 9.260 and 9.261). In the more differentiated examples, variable numbers of dense-core vesicles are found in the processes (Fig. 9.261). Large membrane-bound dense bodies may also be conspicuous (Fig. 9.260). The demonstration of synapses is exceptional (Figs 9.260 and 9.262) but has been documented by Ojeda and coworkers (Ojeda, Jacobsen and Papadimitriou, 1980; Ojeda *et al.*, 1986), Hassoun *et al.* (1982) and Townsend and Seaman (1986).

Rare examples have been reported of neuroblastomas with divergent cell populations as determined by ultrastructural features, including neoplasms described by Azzarelli *et al.* (1977), Dastur (1982), Gambarelli *et al.* (1982), Tang *et al.* (1985) and Delisle *et al.* (1995). In 1977, Azzarelli *et al.* described a supratentorial neuroblastoma with four distinct cell types, including neuroblasts, identified by dense-core vesicles. Similarly, Dastur, in 1982, reported four ultrastructurally distinct cell types in a neuroblastoma, including neuroblastic cells. The case of Gambarelli *et al.* (1982), which exhibited three cell types, is considered by Paulus *et al.* (1992) to be the first example of a desmoplastic supratentorial ganglioglioma.

Immunohistochemistry

With the exception of the rare examples that exhibit glial cell populations, the tumor cells in

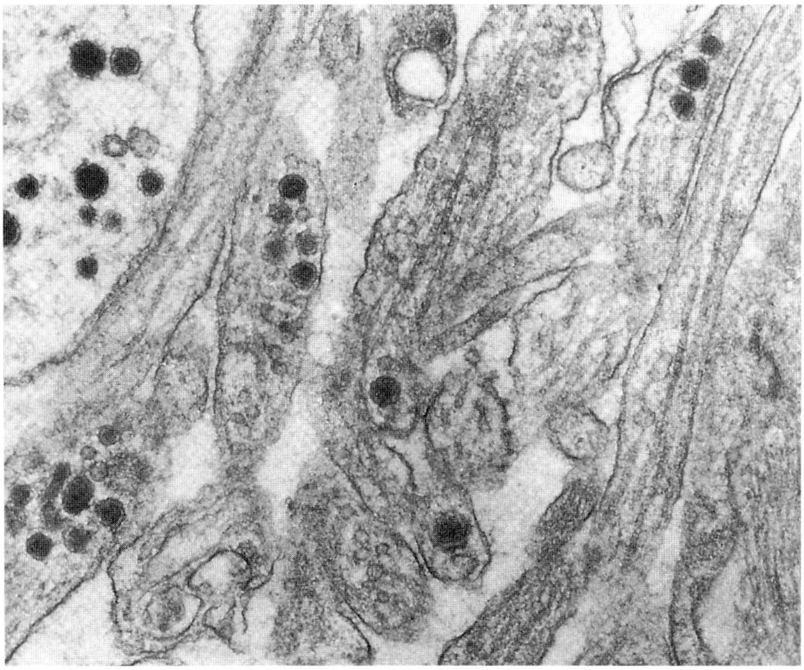

Fig. 9.261 Electron micrograph from a massive, deep, partially calcified, right frontal differentiating neuroblastoma in an 18-month-old boy. Tumor cell processes contain arrays of microtubules and dense-core vesicles. × 42 000 (Courtesy of Dr E.E. May)

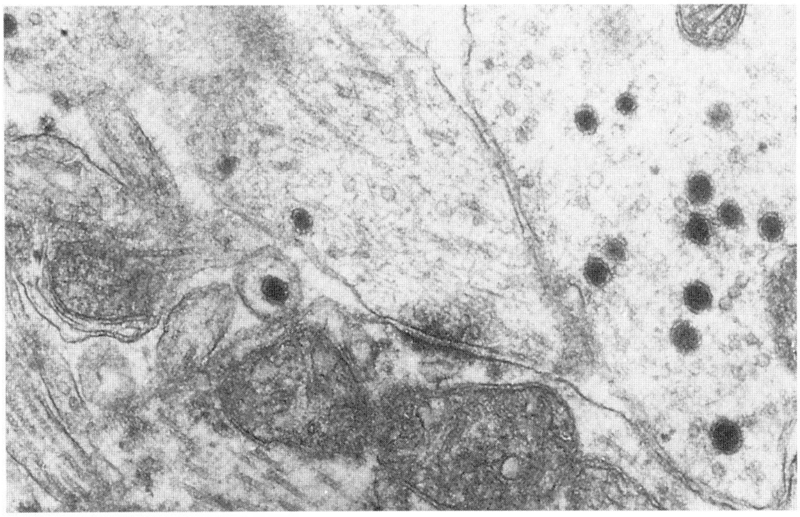

Fig. 9.262 Same case as Fig. 9.261 showing intercellular junctional complexes and suggesting an immature synapse. × 42 000 (Courtesy of Dr E.E. May)

neuroblastomas are negative for GFAP. Some examples, according to Roessmann *et al.* (1983) and Kepes *et al.* (1985), contain cells that stain for the 68-kDa subunit of neurofilaments. Several of the reports quoted above mention the positivity of tumor cells for NSE, but the inference that this immunoreaction is an indication of neuronal origin is, as we have seen, questionable. Importantly, immunohistochemical stains for synaptophysin and class III β-tubulin may be useful for the characterization of neuroblasts (Katsetos *et al.*, 1993). Older methods, such as silver impregnation stains for neurites, may also be useful; such a confirmation was possible in many examples of the Rubinstein (Horten and Rubinstein, 1976; Bennett and Rubinstein, 1984) series. Cerebral neuroblastoma cells have been shown to cross-react with MAbs raised against human fetal brain tissue; the immunoreactions, using such a panel, closely resemble those of cerebellar medulloblastoma (Coakham *et al.*, 1985). Rubinstein noted two central neurocytomas that reacted positively to anti-Leu 7 MAb, but three cerebral neuroblastomas that were negative (Perentes and Rubinstein, 1986). One of two cerebral neuroblastomas has been shown by Goto *et al.* (1987) to contain calcineurin. In their review of eight poorly differentiated supratentorial tumors, Harris *et al.* (1990) note that all stained for PGP 9.5 while none stained for GFAP, synaptophysin or neurofilament peptides.

Tissue culture

The *in vitro* growth of the cerebral neuroblastoma has so far hardly been described. Ojeda, Jacobsen and Papadimitriou (1980) reported the outgrowth and migration of cells with fine processes; after approximately 2 weeks in culture, the cells became stationary and formed a monolayer with a complex network of branching and interlacing processes. No special steps were taken to confirm the neuronal nature of the cells in the outgrowth or to exclude the alternative that they may have been surviving astrocytes obtained at the time of the explantation.

Biochemical features

In a few cases, information is available on the production, by the tumor, of catecholamines and their metabolites. Azzarelli *et al.* (1977) reported raised levels of catecholamines in the urine and CSF in an 18-month-old boy with neuroblastoma, but Ahdevaara *et al.* (1977) found these to be normal in a 13-year-old girl with such a tumor. In three of the cerebral hemispheric cases reviewed by Bennett and Rubinstein (1984), urinary excretion of catecholamines and their metabolites was found to be normal; but in a 35-year-old male with a large upper cervical intramedullary neuroblastoma, referred to Dr Rubinstein by Professor D.A. Simpson, bioassay of the tumor showed raised levels of adrenaline, noradrenaline and dopamine, and the patient had increased urinary excretion of metadrenaline and vanillylmandelic acid, which returned to normal after removal of the growth (Russell and Rubinstein, 1989).

Elevated levels of serum nerve growth factor in a 15-month-old male child who had a cystic tumor in the third ventricle and who later developed malignant cells in the spinal fluid and in the iliac crest were reported by Meyer *et al.* (1980). However, in the absence of an autopsy, the possibility of a visceral primary neuroblastoma that escaped clinical detection cannot be excluded.

Growth and biologic behavior

While in their pathologic character and degree of malignancy these neoplasms often conform to primitive gliomas, it is apparent that, in a substantial number of cases, the prognosis for long-term survival may be relatively more favorable than with other malignant central neuroepithelial tumors. The overall 3-year survival period in the Bennett and Rubinstein (1984) series of 70 cases was 60%. While long-term follow-up figures are incomplete, Rubinstein (Russell and Rubinstein, 1989) estimated that 30% or more of patients with a cerebral neuroblastoma have a 5-year postoperative survival. The figures in the smaller series of Berger *et al.* (1983) indicate postoperative survival times ranging from 4 to 9 years in eight of their 11 patients. In the Bennett and Rubinstein (1984) series, reanalyzed by Russell and Rubinstein (1989), eight patients survived 7 years after the initial diagnosis, three for more than 10 years. In the case illustrated in Fig. 9.256, of a 9-year-old girl with a right parieto-occipital tumor, the patient was known to be alive and well 13 years after her first craniotomy, despite recurrence of the tumor 2 years after the initial operation.

Recurrence is indeed a frequent sequel, in most cases occurring within the first 3 years after surgery. In some cases, however, it may be delayed, as exemplified by two patients in our series in whom it took place 5 and 7 years, respectively, after operation. With few exceptions, recurrence or death from the tumor follows Collins' law, i.e., the period of risk is a function of the initial age at diagnosis, as seems to be the case in the great majority of cerebellar medulloblastomas (see p. 000).

Tumor recurrence took place in approximately 40% of the patients who survived surgery, as analyzed by Bennett and Rubinstein (1984). A similar incidence was found by Berger *et al.* (1983). Berger *et al.* noted that all four of their patients who had a recurrence had solid tumors, whereas six of their seven patients without recurrence had tumors with a largely cystic component. About one third of the patients in the Horten and Rubinstein (1976) and the Bennett and Rubinstein (1984) series in whom the tumor recurred have survived, but they had not yet passed the 'period of risk' at the time of review.

Metastases

In addition to the risk of local recurrences, a notable development is that of metastases in the cerebrospinal pathways. This was demonstrated in 8/21 patients (Horten and Rubinstein, 1976), the number probably being an underestimate since many patients who died were not autopsied. In one patient, cerebrospinal metastases developed in the absence of previous operation.

The occurrence of *extraneural* metastases has also been reported. In a case noted by Russell and Rubinstein (1989), dissemination of distant deposits in the vertebrae and in the liver took place after two local recurrences of the growth invaded the superior sagittal sinus. Widespread cerebrospinal spread was also present. In another example noted by Bennett and Rubinstein (1984), in a 35-year-old male with a temporal lobe neuroblastoma of the transitional variant, bony metastases in the lumbar spine developed 3 years after excision of the original tumor, and additional multiple skeletal metastases made their appearance 2 years later despite vigorous treatment by chemotherapy. The patient died with multiple bony involvement 7 years after the initial operation, but no recurrent intracranial tumor was demonstrated by CT. No autopsy was performed.

Other examples recording the occurrence of extraneural metastases include a case of Sakaki *et al.* (1981) in which a 19-year-old girl developed metastatic deposits in the scalp and the cervical lymph nodes following repeated operations for a temporo-occipital neuroblastoma over a period of 10 years, and a case described by Henriquez, Robertson and Marshall (1973) in which a cerebral neuroblastoma in a 7-year-old boy metastasized spontaneously to the posterior cervical and supraclavicular lymph nodes.

In conclusion, the biologic behavior of the cerebral neuroblastoma, with its high rate of recurrence, occasionally delayed, and its sometimes protracted clinical course, often recalls in its pathologic features the evolution of the cerebellar medulloblastoma before the days of complete neuraxial radiation treatment. While no convincing objective evidence exists at this time that survival is enhanced by postoperative radiotherapy with or without adjuvant chemotherapy, Russell and Rubinstein (1989) indicated that the relative frequency of tumor metastasis raised the advisability of radiation treatment, for these neoplasms, to the entire neuraxis. Berger *et al.* (1983), on the other hand, are of the view that central neuraxial radiation should be reserved for cases in which myelography or CSF examination demonstrates evidence of tumor dissemination.

Mixed primitive neuroepithelial tumors showing bidirectional ganglionic and glial differentiation

A few isolated reports (Azzarelli *et al.*, 1977; Dastur, 1982; Gambarelli *et al.*, 1982; Tang *et al.*, 1985; Jay *et al.*, 1994; Delisle *et al.*, 1995) have documented the occasional occurrence, in very young subjects, of a tumor with the cytologic features of cerebral neuroblastoma associated with variable numbers of neoplastic glial elements, resulting in a complex neoplasm showing bidirectional neuronal and glial differentiation. The Gambarelli *et al.* (1982) case, of a 10-month-old boy, is of unusual interest in demonstrating, in addition, the presence of satellite mesenchymal cells that were interpreted as Schwann cells and enclosed nonmyelinated neurites, an observation that recalls the presence of mesenchymal cells, surrounded by a basement membrane, identified by electron microscopy in a ganglioglioma (see p. 500). The Tang *et al.* (1985) case was an example of a composite neuroblastoma and astrocytoma in which the two cell types were quite distinctive. A similar case has been noted in the Duke University archival material (submitted by Dr John Harrison; McLendon *et al.*, 1997). Feigin and Budzilovich (1974) had previously noted astrocytomatous components in two of their six cerebral neuroblastomas. Of more basic interest, cytogenetics, performed on the Delisle *et al.* (1995) case, indicates a chromosome 11 breakpoint different from that found in Ewing's sarcoma.

The possibility of demonstrating divergent differentiation by immunostaining techniques for GFAP and for the 68-kDa subunit of neurofilaments within the same tumor has been stressed by Roessmann *et al.* (1983) in their immunohistochemical study of various central neuroepithelial neoplasms of childhood. Undoubtedly, the increased use of these sensitive methods is expected to uncover a growing number of such cases. Their frequency cannot be estimated at this time, but so far they remain relatively rare. As already noted, there exists in infants a highly distinctive form of desmoplastic supratentorial neuroepithelial neoplasm that demonstrates divergent neuroepithelial differentiation and in which the desmoplastic component seems to be largely attributable to a massive participation of the leptomeningeal fibroblasts. Astrocytic differentiation is established by the presence of GFAP, and neuronal differentiation by that of neoplastic ganglion cells, of axonal processes identified by silver impregnations for neurites and by the immunomorphologic demonstration, in the tumor cells and their processes, of an antigenic determinant recognized by a MAb against the 200-kDa neurofilament triplet polypeptide. Thus the presence of neoplastic astrocytes in neuroblastomas appears exceptional. Cases of this kind will need to be carefully documented and recorded. With limited surgical biopsy specimens, interpretative problems often hinge, however, on whether the fragments are representative of the tumor as a whole and on whether they can be submitted for study by techniques more sophisticated than routine histologic stains.

The identification of distinct clinicopathologic entities is essential for the elucidation of these problems. Some workers have unfortunately attempted to resolve them by creating an overall category that, under the somewhat uninformative name 'primitive neuroectodermal tumors of childhood', appears to be made up of a collection of poorly differentiated cerebral neuroepithelial neoplasms in the young, on which the documentation is generally too incomplete to permit their assignment to a definite tumor cell type. Whether they represent a true histologic entity cannot be determined because the criteria for their definition lack precision. Some of these cases may represent small-cell infantile gliomas; the majority probably are instances of cerebral neuroblastoma, an inference that seems corroborated by the electron microscopic description of a few such examples, according to which the cytoplasm of some of the tumor cells contained dense-core vesicles (Markesbery and Challa, 1979). The impression, however, is often conveyed that this term is being indiscriminately applied to tumors on which the sampling or the information has been inadequate or on which, for technical reasons, studies have been insufficient.

Central neurocytomas

Attention has been drawn to the occurrence of lesions, presenting as intraventricular calcified neoplasms in young adults, which by light microscopy are virtually indistinguishable from oligodendrogliomas, but which by electron microscopy show evidence of neuronal differentiation, including the presence of synapses (Hassoun *et al.*, 1982; Jerdan *et al.*, 1983; Figarella-Branger *et al.*, 1992; Hara *et al.*, 1993). There is increasing evidence from the more recent reports by Pearl *et al.* (1985), Wilson, Leaffer and Kohout (1985), Ojeda *et al.* (1986), Townsend and Seaman (1986), Nishio *et al.* (1988), Figarella-Branger *et al.* (1992), Hara *et al.* (1993),

Rhodes *et al.* (1994) and Kim *et al.* (1996) that these intraventricular examples constitute a separate subset of cerebral neuroblastoma. Because of the mature character of some of their fine structural features, the term 'central neurocytoma' has been proposed for these rare tumors. Most of the so-called ependymomas of the foramen of Monro appear to fall into this category, although some true examples of this entity appear to exist (Severi *et al.*, 1989). Presenting generally in young adults but ranging in age from 6 years to 64 years, the tumors characteristically have an intraventricular location and seem to be associated with a relatively favorable course, particularly in those younger than 50 years (Figarella-Branger *et al.*, 1992).

Macroscopic appearance

The consistent intraventricular location within the septum pellucidum of the central neurocytoma and its lack of infiltrative tendencies appear to deny alternative designations of periventricular neurocytoma or interventricular neurocytoma (Hassoun *et al.*, 1993). Grossly, the tumors are soft and friable with a red or gray color. Calcification is easily found. It has been reported that the tumor easily separates from surrounding tissues, although the margin of resection was not evaluated (Figarella-Branger, 1992).

Radiographic appearance

The MRI appearance of neurocytoma is a heterogeneous signal mass that is largely isointense to brain on T1-weighted images. The T2 signal intensity is isointense to hyperintense, again with prominent areas of heterogeneous signal. Contrast enhancement is variable, and there are frequently areas of necrosis or calcification (Fig. 9.263). Imaging cannot separate this tumor from oligodendroglioma; differential diagnosis also includes pilocytic astrocytoma and ependymoma.

The CT scans demonstrate a heterogeneous mass that is iso- to slightly hyperdense. Multiple small cysts and areas of calcification are frequently seen. Contrast enhancement pattern is variable, but usually portions of the tumor will enhance to some degree. Hydrocephalus is almost always identified. There is usually an area of attachment to the superior lateral aspect of the ventricle wall.

Microscopic appearance

Microscopically, the tumor cells have been characterized as having a 'honeycomb' appearance because of their distinct polyhedral membranous outlines and central round, regular nuclei (Fig. 9.264). The cytoplasm is characterized by perinuclear eosinophilic wisps that have ragged edges related to retraction from the membranes (Fig. 9.265). Within the nucleus, a small inconspicuous nucleolus may be found. Other features that result in confusion between these tumors and the oligodendroglioma are the arcuating vascular pattern and the not infrequent granular calcifications that dot the microscopic fields. Smear preparations of the fresh tumor cells may disclose short, stubby cytoplasmic processes. Regions reminiscent of the pineocytoma may also be encountered in the histologic section when islands of tumors cells are separated by eosinophilic fibrillar regions. Occasional tumors may reveal a disturbing number of mitoses and necrotic foci, the significance of which is still debated.

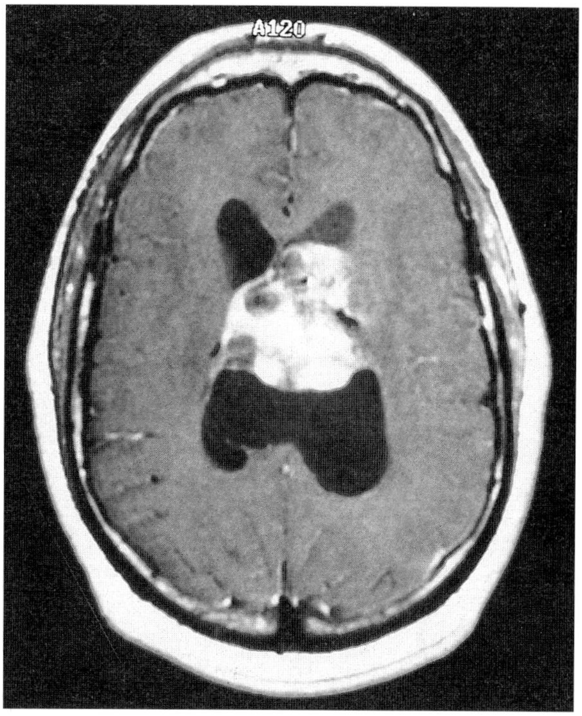

Fig. 9.263 Axial T1-weighted postcontrast MRI revealing a large enhancing tumor mass within the lateral ventricles above the level of the foramen of Monro. There are multiple areas of heterogenous enhancement with an irregular margin along the left lateral ventricle. Slight increased signal intensity of CSF within the left frontal horn may represent relative obstruction and increased protein concentration.

These tumors, when strictly defined by both intraventricular location and 'honeycomb' histologic appearance, apparently confer a uniformly good prognosis, although one report suggests that

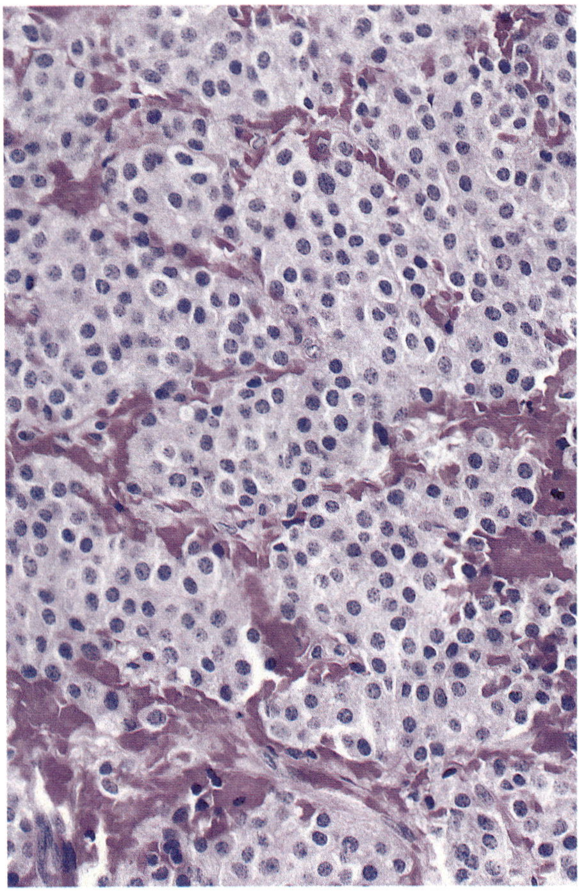

Fig. 9.264 Typical honeycomb appearance of central neurocytoma revealing a distinctive polyhedral membranous outline and central round regular nuclei. H&E, × 100

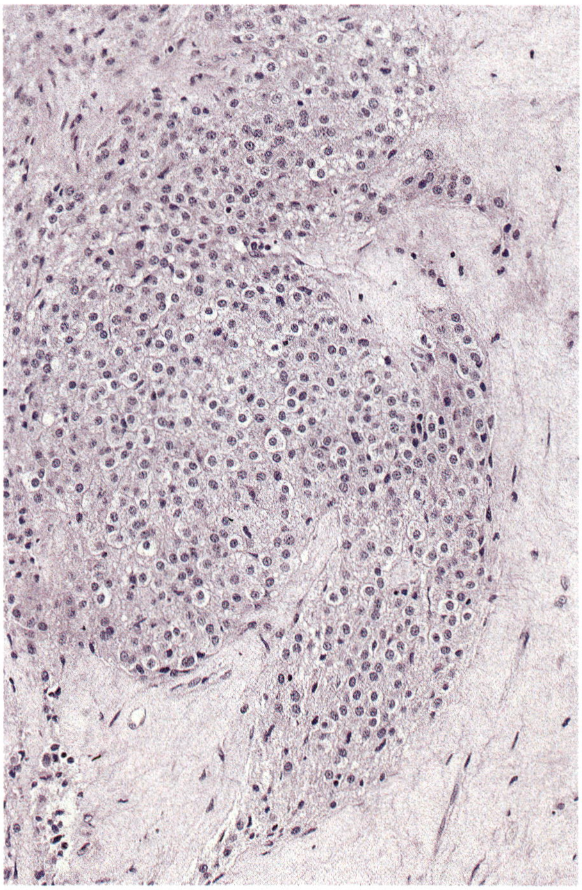

Fig. 9.265 Neurocytoma: cytoplasmic retraction results in perinuclear halos, a condition reminiscent of oligodendroglioma. H&E, × 50

a patient age of greater than 50 years has a negative influence on survival (Figarella-Branger *et al.*, 1992). Some cases reported as 'malignant neurocytic' lesions have been located outside of the ventricles and have not demonstrated the prototypic histologic appearance (Mrak, 1994). Although von Deimling *et al.* (1990) classified two neoplasms as malignant based on 'high mitotic activity, considerable vascular proliferation and tumor necrosis indicating an increased proliferative potential', no clinical follow-up has been reported. The study of Louis *et al.* (1990), moreover, suggests that, in the presence of other typical features, necrosis may not be a significant finding. Furthermore, Kim *et al.* (1996) noted that proliferation potential, as determined immunohistochemically with PCNA and cytometrically by flow cytometry, was not elevated in their two recurrences.

The recent review of Rhodes *et al.* (1994) of 135 cases of intraventricular neuronal neoplasms published since 1982 suggests the existence of three histologic patterns in these tumors. These categories include 'those tumors with a predominantly or partially honeycomb (oligodendrocytoma-like) appearance (in 100/137 patients); those tumors with differentiated neuronal features, including Homer Wright rosettes, silver-positive neurites or occasional large ganglion cells (in 24/137 patients) and undifferentiated tumors (in 13/137 patients)'. Although long-term follow-up was scanty, these investigators did support the contention of Hassoun *et al.* (1993) that the survival rate for patients whose tumors had the typical appearance and evidence of neuronal phenotype by histologic or cytochemical means was significantly better than the survival rate for differentiated or undifferentiated hemispheric neuroblastomas. Again, the corollary appears to be true: patients whose intraventricular tumors do not exhibit neuronal differentiation are subject to the same survival rate as are patients with hemispheric undifferentiated neuroblastomas (Rhodes *et al.*, 1994).

Immunohistochemistry

These tumors are nearly uniform in their expression of the synaptophysin antigen (von Deimling *et al.*, 1990; Figarella-Branger *et al.*, 1992; Hessler *et al.*, 1992; Kim *et al.*, 1996). von Deimling *et al.* (1990), in a review of 11 central neurocytomas, have noted GFAP immunoreactivity in two cases, both of which also showed synaptophysin immunoreactivity. Whether cells could coexpress both GFAP and synaptophysin was unclear (von Deimling *et al.*, 1990). Hessler *et al.* (1992) reported that their 11 tumors revealed immunoreactivity for both the class III β-tubulin antigen (using the antibody TUJ1) and type 2 MAP, staining both the cell bodies and processes. An antibody against the MAP, tau, reacted immunohistochemically with cells in 5/10 cases, while 4/10 cases reacted against a phosphorylation-dependent NFP-H antibody and 6/10 cases reacted against an antibody directed against a phosphorylation-independent NFP-H and NFP-M. Interestingly, synaptophysin was absent in 1/10 cases, although the investigators noted that an artifact of prolonged fixation could not be ruled out. Although GFAP immunoreactivity was noted in the tumor, absolute attribution to neoplastic cells could not be made (Hessler *et al.*, 1992).

Figarella-Branger *et al.* (1992) performed immunoblot analysis on two central neurocytomas for NCAM antigens and found distinct bands corresponding to molecular masses 140 and 180 kDa as well as a fuzzy band between 140 and 180 kDa. Individually, one tumor also exhibited a 120-kDa isoform, whereas the other exhibited a 210-kDa isoform.

Electron microscopy

Ultrastructural examination confirmed the presence of neurosecretory granules in all cases (Louis *et al.*, 1990; Figarella-Branger *et al.*, 1992; Hessler *et al.*, 1992). Parallel tubular arrays that have been described in the tumor cells have been shown, by ultrastructural immunomicroscopy in four cases, to label with antibodies to class III β-tubulin and MAP2 (Hessler *et al.*, 1992). As noted above, synapses are a common finding (Hassoun *et al.*, 1982; Jerdan *et al.*, 1983; Figarella-Branger *et al.*, 1992; Hara *et al.*, 1993).

Molecular genetics

Information on cytogenetics, ploidy analysis and gene expression in central neurocytomas is scanty. Cerdá-Nicolás *et al.* (1993) have karyotyped one tumor and found it to be 46, XY, but they also noted various anomalies in rare metaphases, including –17 in three metaphases.

Kim *et al.* (1996) performed ploidy analysis by flow cytometry on 10 cases and found all to be diploid. They also noted a mean proliferation index of 7.8% (range 5.1–9.6%).

Cytogenesis

von Deimling *et al.* (1990) have fixed the cell of origin for neurocytomas as being the subependymal plate of the lateral ventricles. In contrast to the malignant embryonal tumors found in the pediatric population that Rorke (1983) suggests are derived from the embryonal subependymal matrix zones at all levels of the nervous system, these investigators believe the neurocytoma originates from the remnants of a persistent postnatal cell population.

Associated lesions

The association of an intraventricular neuroblastoma with von Hippel-Lindau's disease has been reported (Pearl *et al.*, 1981) as has the association of cerebral ganglioglioma with NF type 1 (Parizel *et al.*, 1991). Both incidents are considered coincidental.

Ganglioneuromas (gangliocytomas) and gangliogliomas

The existence of pure central *ganglioneuromas*, or *gangliocytomas*, i.e., tumors composed predominantly of mature gangliocytes of distinctive appearance supported by a stroma of spindle-shaped glial cells and containing calcospherites, has long been recognized. The concept of mixed neurogliogenic tumors, or *gangliogliomas*, in which adult ganglion cells and relatively mature glial tumor cells participate together, dates more precisely from the observations of Courville (1930, 1931; Courville and Anderson, 1941), Wolf and Morton (1937) and Bailey and Beiser (1947). Considering the group of differentiated ganglion cell tumors of the CNS as a whole, it is apparent that there are varying degrees of neoplastic evolution in the glial component. This variability makes the clear-cut separation of the gangliocytomas from the gangliogliomas difficult. Thus, at one end of the scale is found a tumor in which mature, often dysmorphic neurons are the most conspicuous elements. These ganglionic neurons are associated with stromal glial cells that are relatively scanty and show little or no evidence of proliferation. At the other end, there is a tumor that, at first glance under the microscope, appears to be a densely fibrillar, collagenized glioma with a ganglionic element that is relatively unobtrusive. The two extremes are, therefore, bridged by histologic variations that, moreover, may coexist within the same specimen. This variability acquires significance when the biologic potential of gangliogliomas is assessed. Thus, there is epidemiologic evidence (see p. 503) that when they undergo anaplastic change, as in exceptional circumstances, it is the glial and not the neuronal element that bears the change. Neoplasms with both ganglion cells and malignant neuroblastic populations obviously exist but have been classified in this book as, and are discussed as, central neuroblastomas with maturation (p. 490). Both the gangliocytomas and the gangliogliomas share, however, common characteristics in respect to their incidence, site of election, macroscopic features and, as a rule, biologic behavior. They will, therefore, be considered together.

As a preliminary, it is necessary to examine the *morphologic criteria appropriate to their diagnosis*. This review is desirable because of the frequent admission, in this group of tumors, of debatable examples, variously designated as ganglioneuromas, ganglioblastomas, spongioneuroblastomas, etc., which are almost certainly variants of glioblastoma. The almost invariable inclusion in successive reviews of these controversial examples has had the result of vitiating some of the epidemiologic conclusions that have been drawn in respect to the age incidence of ganglion cell tumors and their distribution within the CNS. Contrary to the claim by Globus (1938), according to whom the supratentorial 'glioneuromas' and 'spongioneuroblastomas' constitute a little more than 12% of the total number of supratentorial tumors of neuroectodermal derivation, the view of Bailey and Beiser (1947) that genuine ganglion cell tumors of the CNS are relatively exceptional must clearly be endorsed. This conclusion is further reinforced by the relatively small numbers of cases in reported series on gangliogliomas that have appeared recently (Mickle, 1992; Celli *et al.*, 1993; Morris *et al.*, 1993).

The diagnostic problems presented by the identification of central ganglionic tumors are as follows:

1. The recognition of ganglion cells The older descriptions make apparent that reliance was too often placed on the nuclear characteristics of the tumor cells. The result was that elements with large vesiculated nuclei and conspicuous nucleoli were often mistaken for neoplastic neurons. This mistake is especially obvious in gliomas containing cells that display prominent ganglionic features, as in the subependymal giant-cell astrocytomas typically associated with tuberous sclerosis (Volume 2, p. 390) and in some of the giant-cell glioblastomas (p. 440). The cells of those tumors characteristically lack both Nissl bodies and neurofibrils demonstrable with either silver impregnation methods specific for neurites or with immunohistochemical methods for synaptophysin or neurofilaments. In addition, the large ganglioid elements in giant-cell glioblastomas often display numerous mitotic figures and monstrous-cell forms, which strongly argue against their identification as differentiated neurons.

Blind reliance on some techniques, including both histochemical techniques such as the Nissl and PTAH stains and immunohistochemical stains such as NSE, is to be discouraged. The Nissl and PTAH stains may result in false positives because of the nucleolar component staining to mimic small nerve cell nuclei (Bailey and Beiser, 1947), as in those of the granular cortex: the NSE stains because of the deregulated expression of enolase in neoplastic glial cells (Vinores *et al.*, 1984). These mistakes are further compounded in some gliomas by the growing zones of astrocytomas in which may be found small clusters of cells around blood vessels and pre-existing neurons [Scherer's (1936) perivascular and perineuronal structures]: these morphologic mimics recall the small collections of ganglion cell precursor cells ('Bildungsnester') that have been encountered in genuine ganglioneuromas.

Ultrastructural features, including neuritic cell processes occupied by microtubules, intracellular dense-core and clear-centered vesicles and synaptic complexes, offer definite corroboration of their ganglionic nature.

2. The neoplastic nature of the ganglion cells demonstrable in the tumor The determination that the ganglion cells identified in a tumor are neoplastic rather than innocent bystanders engulfed, without their destruction, by the encroachment of a diffusely infiltrating astrocytoma is a diagnostic problem that has long been recognized (Cox, 1933; Scherer, 1936). Likewise, the presence, in a tumor, of myelinated or nonmyelinated nerve fibers must be interpreted with caution because of the frequency with which they are found to be preserved in astrocytic gliomas. Histologic, biologic and cytologic evidence must be sought in the recognition of the neoplastic character of the ganglion cells. Histology allows the identification of neurons that are clearly heterotopic, such as in the white matter, the cortical molecular layer (in which case, axis cylinders may sometimes be demonstrated in the adjacent leptomeninges) or in subarachnoid or intraventricular locations. Biologically, the distribution of the neurons belies a neoplastic process, with ganglion cells found arranged in irregular groupings among which transitional forms may be traced from the less to the more differentiated gangliocytes (a distribution that contrasts with the even spacing of isolated mature nerve cells included in infiltrating cortical astrocytomas). Cytologically, neoplastic neurons often have bizarre, dysmorphic forms varying in sizes and shapes, and abnormal orientation or branching of their axonal or dendritic processes. They are not uncommonly binucleated. With regard to this latter feature, however, Courville (1956) drew attention to the presence of multinucleated nerve cells as a reactive phenomenon at the edges of infiltrating gliomas; their sole presence, therefore, is not necessarily indicative of their neoplastic nature.

3. The identification of gangliocytic precursor cells
The existence of neuroblasts in mature ganglion cell tumors is controversial. The inference that the cells with small spherical nuclei containing a delicate chromatin network, often found in these tumors, constitute ganglion cell precursors, though occasionally corroborated by silver impregnations specific for neurites, is more often denied by lymphocyte markers. Routine staining techniques alone, as repeatedly stressed by previous observers, are unreliable for the identification of these cells. The presence of cellular clusters, in which transitional forms from less differentiated to more mature neurons are closely intermingled, gives indirect support for the identification of the less differentiated cells as neuroblasts. Immunohistochemical techniques and electron microscopy provide the most definitive evidence, so far, for the identification of these otherwise poorly differentiated cells.

A number of excellent series on ganglion cell neoplasms have been published, including Russell and Rubinstein's (1989) personal collection of 120 unequivocal ganglion cell tumors of the CNS (gangliocytomas and gangliogliomas), reviewed in the previous edition of this book. The features to be described are largely based on the Russell and Rubinstein (1989) data supplemented by the studies of Courville (1930; Courville and Anderson, 1941), Wolf and Morton (1937), Silver *et al.* (1991), Mickle (1992), Celli *et al.* (1993), Krouwer *et al.* (1993), Wolf *et al.* (1994), Zentner *et al.* (1994), Khajavi *et al.*, 1995 and Prayson, Khajavi and Comair (1995), all of whom are essentially in agreement.

Incidence

These neoplasms occur most frequently in children and young adults: about 80% of the cases in most series present under the age of 30 years. It is, therefore, not surprising that the incidence of ganglion cell tumors is greater in pediatric clinical material: their frequency in children has been estimated to be around 4–4.5% of all CNS tumors (Sutton *et al.*, 1983), although some series derived from epileptic patients indicate an incidence as high as 38% (Morris *et al.*, 1993). Approximately 10% of the patients are in the early months of life, their symptoms often dating from birth and attributable either to a massive tumor or to an extensive diffuse cortical lesion in which a combination of maldevelopmental and neoplastic features were evidently to be traced to fetal life. Such an example is illustrated in Figs 9.266 and 9.267 from a large frontoparietal

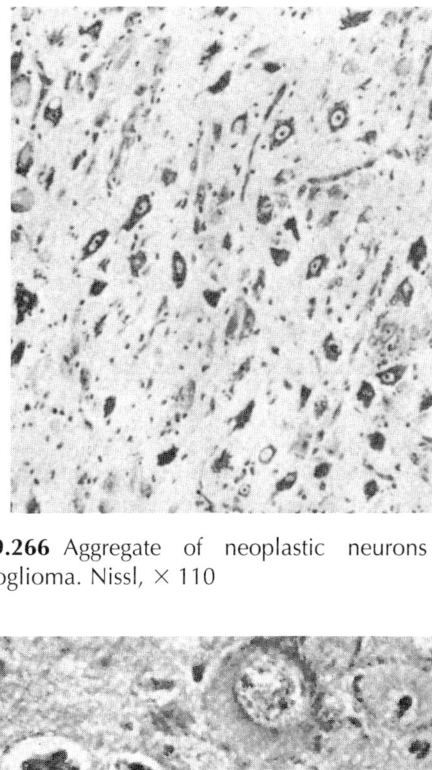

Fig. 9.266 Aggregate of neoplastic neurons in a ganglioglioma. Nissl, × 110

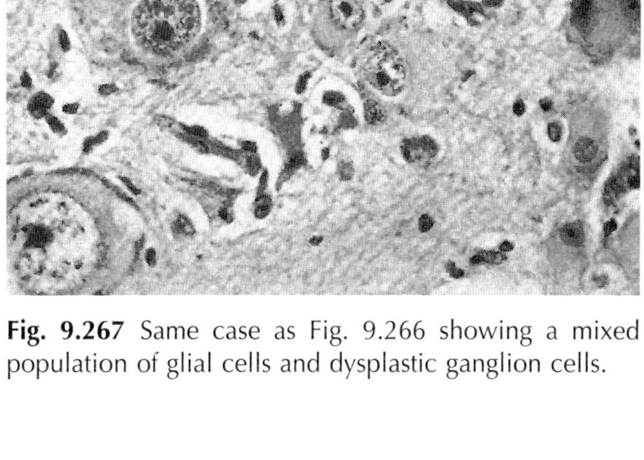

Fig. 9.267 Same case as Fig. 9.266 showing a mixed population of glial cells and dysplastic ganglion cells.

ganglioglioma in a 2-month-old infant who had symptoms from birth. However, no age seems to be exempt: Rubinstein's oldest patient was a 70-year-old male reported to be alive and well 6 years after removal of the tumor. Even in adult cases, a characteristic history of long-standing epileptic seizures, sometimes associated with mental retardation, often suggests that the neoplasm had its onset in early life. The sex ratio suggests a male predominance of about 3:2, although a female predominance has been reported in one series (Celli *et al.*, 1993).

Sites

By far the most frequent site is the *temporal lobe*, which accounts for about 30% of the cases. No area in the CNS, however, appears to be exempt. Notable situations are the floor of the third ventricle, when signs may be referable to pituitary deficiency (Alpers and Grant, 1931), hypothalamic compromise, such as precocious puberty (Horrax and Bailey, 1928, case 3), or diabetes insipidus (Doyle and Kernohan, 1931); any of the intraventricular cavities; the basal ganglia (Fujimura *et al.*, 1995); and the brainstem (Richmond *et al.*, 1966; Garcia, McGarry and Collada, 1984; Hirose *et al.*, 1992; Karamitopoulou *et al.*, 1995). Uncommon sites, each accounting for less than 10% of the cases, include the cerebellum (Furie *et al.*, 1993; Handa, Yamagami and Furuta, 1994; Blatt *et al.*, 1995), the pineal gland (Hunt and Johnson, 1989; Tokoro *et al.*, 1993; M.D. Johnson *et al.*, 1995) and the spinal cord (Kernohan, Learmonth and Doyle, 1932, cases 8 and 9; Bevilacqua and Sarnelli, 1979; Miller, Towfighi and Page, 1990; Hirose *et al.*, 1992; Wacker *et al.*, 1992). Occasionally, the lesion in the spinal cord may be unusually extensive and its entire length may be almost completely involved.

Some forms of ganglion cell tumors are treated separately as variants: they include the highly characteristic dysplastic gangliocytomas of the cerebellum (of Lhermitte-Duclos, p. 505), the intrasellar ganglioneuromas associated with clinical evidence of active pituitary secretion (p. 504), the distinctive desmoplastic infantile gangliogliomas (p. 507) and the dysembryoplastic neuroepithelial tumor (p. 509). The special type of mixed paraganglioma and gangliocytoma that originates in the cauda equina and that may, in a number of cases, be found to arise from the conus medullaris or the filum terminale is discussed in Chapter 20 (p. 551).

Multiplicity and associated lesions

Ganglion cell tumors of the CNS are usually single, but multiple neoplasms have occasionally been recorded (Bielschowsky, 1925). As discussed below, the mode of development and the growth characteristics of this group of tumors often suggest a hamartomatous origin. That an association with ectopic lesions or other congenital anomalies may occasionally be discovered, either in the same vicinity or more remotely situated, is not surprising. In about 5% of cases reported from the Russell and Rubinstein (1989) series, anomalies of a congenital nature were present: Down's syndrome, partial agenesis of the corpus callosum, orofaciodigital synostosis, leptomeningeal glioneuronal ectopias, cerebellar micropolygyria (in two cases of cerebellar ganglioglioma) and glioneuronal ectopias of the temporal cortex (in a hippocampal ganglioglioma). Previously referred to (p. 458) is the remarkable example in which a deep cerebellar ganglioglioma contiguous with a diffuse gangliogliomatosis of the cerebellar cortex had been associated with an abnormal proliferation of the fetal external granular layer demonstrated at an earlier stage of brain development. The significance of this finding seems to be more coincidental than causative, given the recently demonstrated origin of Purkinje cells from periventricular matrix cells versus the origin of internal granular cells from the external granular cells. However, aberrant maturation from external granule cell descendants cannot be ruled out (i.e., medulloblastoma with maturation), particularly given the findings of Wacker *et al.* (1992) of loss of heterozygosity in the chromosomal 17p arm in a cerebellar tumor with diffuse leptomeningeal dissemination, a finding occasionally noted in aggressive medulloblastomas (see Chapter 2). Molecular events influencing the development of gangliocytomas are gradually being revealed. For instance, Menchine *et al.* (1995) have noted abnormal expression of tuberous sclerosis genes in sporadic gangliogliomas of the cerebrum. Similarly, a strong association exists between Cowden's syndrome (multiple hamartomas syndrome) and dysplastic gangliocytomas of the cerebellum (Lhermitte-Duclos syndrome) (Chapter 16, p. 401).

An association of gangliogliomas (or histologically comparable neoplasms of a different designation) with tuberous sclerosis has also been claimed, but the presence of unequivocal neuronal elements participating in a cerebral tumor associated with typical tuberous sclerosis seems to be exceptional (Ferraro and Doolittle, 1936; Nakamura and Becker, 1983, case 7). The lesions recorded, respectively, by Jervis (1954) as 'spongioneuroblastoma' and by Davis and Nelson (1961) as unilateral ganglioglioma, in cases interpreted as *formes frustes* of the disease, are unquestionably composed of mixed, abnormal neuronal and glial cells, but Russell and Rubinstein (1989) stated that these cases appear to represent examples of massive congenital hemispheric gangliogliomas with very wide distribution, even reaching to the basal ganglia. A somewhat similar instance of a diffuse unilateral gangliocytic hamartoblastoma in a 42-day-old female, but in which glial cells were not involved, was reported by Dom and Brucher (1969). All these cases seem to have features in common with the tumor illustrated in Figs 9.266 and 9.267, of which Russell and Rubinstein (1989) noted six virtually identical examples, almost all of which had their clinical onset at or soon after birth and who were operated on within the first few months of life. The microscopic picture of these large, sometimes very extensive tumors reportedly suggested morphologic similarities with the cortical lesions of tuberous sclerosis, but the other stigmata of the disease may be lacking. Although the lesion, in some of these instances, implicated the larger part of a cerebral hemisphere, and its hamartomatous nature was, therefore, unmistakable, Russell and Rubinstein (1989) point out that it should be distinguished from the classic tuber of tuberous sclerosis. The question of the neuronal nature of the subependymal giant-cell tumors associated with tuberous sclerosis has already been discussed (Chapter 16, p. 390).

Macroscopic appearance

With the exception of some of the massive congenital hemispheric lesions, presenting in infants soon after birth, that may be diffuse, these tumors are usually small, firm and well circumscribed, with gray, finely granular cut surfaces. They are often cystic. Small focal calcifications are frequent. Occasionally, the tumor consists of a mural nodule attached to the wall of a single large cyst. Diffuse spread of a cerebral ganglioglioma, particularly in an older patient, is almost always referable to the astrocytic component of the neoplasm; case 7 of Kernohan, Learmonth and Doyle (1932), a very diffuse gangliocytoma that occupied the right parietal lobe of a 39-year-old woman, is exceptional.

Radiographic appearance

Gangliogliomas are well evaluated by MRI. These masses tend to present in children and young adults who have seizures, and the tumors typically involve the temporal lobe or, less likely, the frontal lobe. At MRI, the mass is usually of low T1 signal intensity and high T2 signal intensity. Commonly, there is a cyst within the mass (Fig. 9.268). The enhancement pattern is variable, but an area of intense nodular enhancement in the solid portion of the tumor is commonly seen (Fig. 9.269). A rim enhancement pattern may also

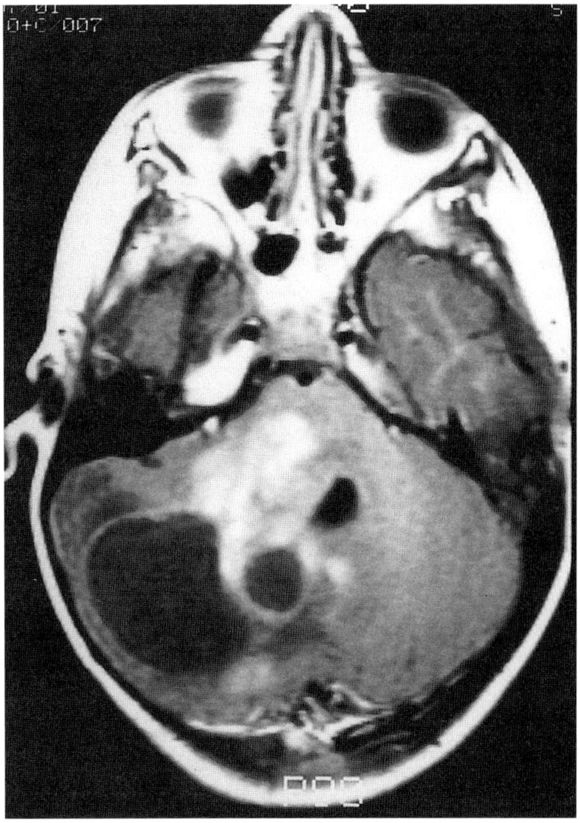

Fig. 9.268 Axial T1-weighted postcontrast MRI of a gangliocytoma demonstrating an ill-defined mass of the right cerebellar peduncle and hemisphere. The mass has multiple cystic components peripherally and ill-defined moderate enhancement more centrally, extending to the pons. The fourth ventricle is deviated to the left. The mass is large in size relative to the overall degree of mass effect on the cerebellum. The T2 signal intensity in this patient was increased throughout the general area of the tumor with marked increased T2 signal intensity of the cystic component.

occur. At CT scanning, calcification within the mural nodule may be seen. If the tumor is located superficially, there may be erosive changes of the adjacent calvarium (Zentner *et al.*, 1994).

Microscopic appearance

Microscopic appearance may vary considerably according to the extent to which neuronal and glial elements participate in the neoplastic process. The *pure gangliocytoma* is a poorly to moderately cellular tumor in which numerous cells of manifestly neuronal origin, albeit dysmorphic appearance, are instantly recognized. Many, as in Fig. 9.266, are well differentiated, but abnormal and bizarre forms

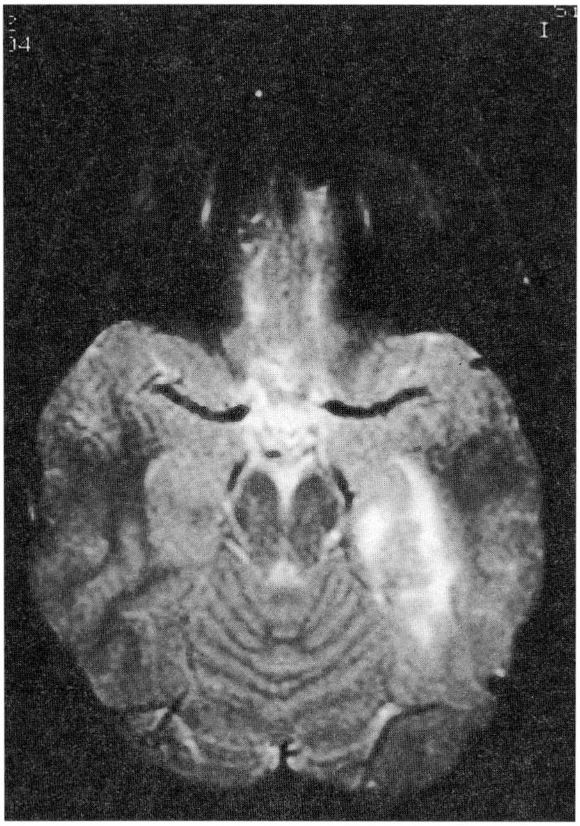

Fig. 9.269 Axial T2-weighted MRI of a ganglioglioma. Abnormal T2 signal intensity is seen in the medial left temporal lobe. This extends along the hippocampus, and there is a well-defined cystic area along the medial aspect of the mass. Typically, on contrasted images, gangliogliomas reveal a nodular homogeneous intense enhancement.

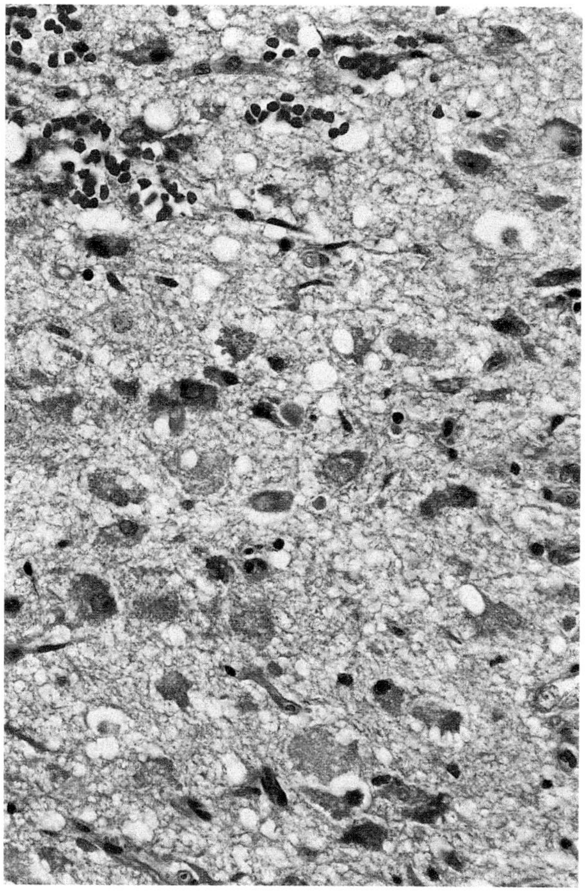

Fig. 9.271 Dysmorphic ganglion cells, which may be characterized by irregular orientation and anomalous processes with an early branching. H&E, × 100

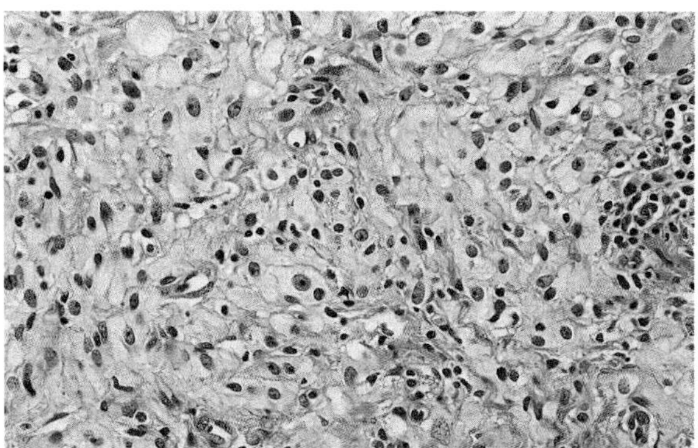

Fig. 9.270 Ganglion cell tumor. Occasional ganglion cell tumors will reveal a profusion of neuronal cells that vary markedly in size and cytologic features. H&E, × 100

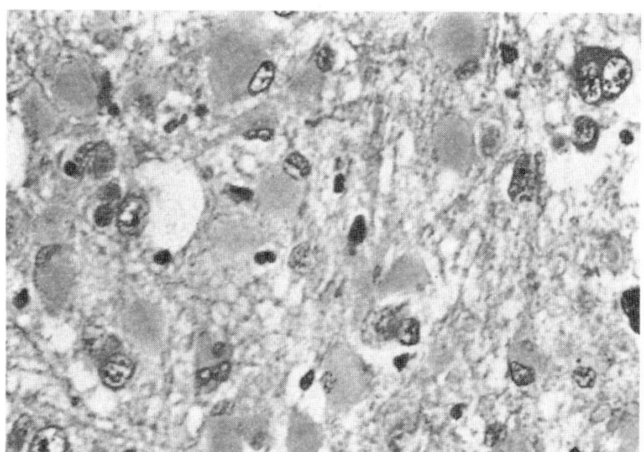

Fig. 9.272 Ganglioglioma with gemistocytic astrocytes and two binucleated neurons. H&E, × 330

varying greatly in size and in shape, including giant and quite small cells, are found in abundance (Figs 9.267, 9.270 and 9.271). The neurons are often irregularly oriented and exhibit anomalous processes with early branching. Multinucleate, especially binucleate, forms are frequent (Fig. 9.272), but mitotic figures are never seen. The Nissl substance is often well formed but somewhat irregular. With Bielschowsky's silver techniques, neurofibrils, leashes of axis cylinders and irregularly coursing, tortuous neuritic processes are demonstrable: these conspicuous and varied morphologic anomalies clearly distinguish them from the pre-existing neurites that can be found in infiltrating astrocytomas. Silver impregnations and immunoperoxidase stains for NFPs and for synaptophysin also help to identify scattered neuroblasts. The distribution of the neoplastic nerve cells often varies throughout the tumor: the cells may form closely packed clusters ('Bildungsnester'), especially in the neighborhood of blood vessels.

Whereas, in the pure gangliocytomas, the glial element consists of a scanty stroma of spindle cells, in *gangliogliomas*, astrocytes of a neoplastic nature clearly proliferate. Here, the first impression is often, in fact, that of either a pilocytic astrocytoma or a fibrillary astrocytoma, and it is only on closer examination that neoplastic nerve cells with the cytologic characteristics described above are revealed (Fig. 9.273). At the other end of the scale, these cells may be so scanty amidst the gliomatous masses that only the realization of their ectopic situation will prompt the correct diagnosis. Personal observations are in agreement with the analysis of Wolf and Morton (1937) that, in the group as a whole, the intermediate forms are the most frequently encountered, i.e., gangliogliomas in which neuronal and glial elements are intermingled in approximately equal proportions. Perivascular lymphocytic infiltrates are so much more common in ganglion cell tumors than in gliomas as to make the search for ganglion cells justifiable in any low-grade glial tumor with significant lymphoid infiltrates (Figs 9.270 and 9.273).

In gangliogliomas, the glial component shows, as a rule, though not always, a degree of cellular differentiation parallel to the neuronal component and, therefore, exhibits the features of an *astrocytoma*. Although these tumors usually show rather sparse uni- and bipolar pilocytic cells, plump gemistocytic astrocytes may also be seen (Fig. 9.272). In some examples, cellular features closely resemble those of an *oligodendroglioma* (Allegranza *et al.*, 1990), but cells with these features may be difficult to distinguish from small granular neurons and could even be neurons of the character found in the central neurocytoma (Yamamoto *et al.*, 1996).

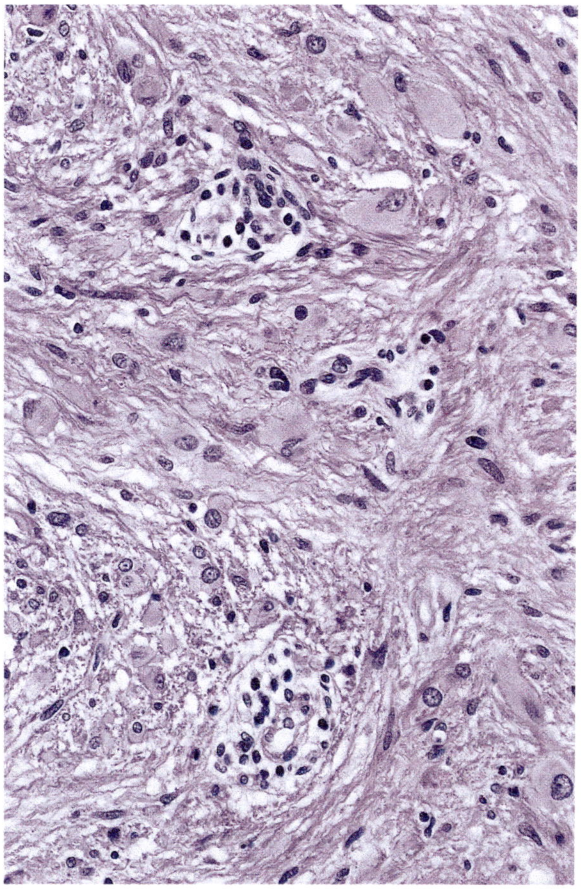

Fig. 9.273 Ganglioglioma exhibiting predominantly bipolar astrocytes in a fascicular arrangement in which the ganglion cell component is less conspicuous. H&E, × 100

Rosenthal fibers and eosinophilic granular bodies may be encountered in some densely cellular tumors exhibiting nuclear pleomorphism, and these may be a useful clue in directing one toward a lower grade of astrocytic neoplasia.

Calcospherites are frequently found in the walls of the intrinsic blood vessels and sometimes in the adjacent nonneoplastic brain tissue. In some cases, the *connective tissue stroma* is particularly abundant (Fig. 9.274) and forms a thick interlacing meshwork in the midst of which large ganglion cells are arranged either singly or in small groups. This conspicuous fibrovascular stroma is characteristically confined to the gangliocytic component of gangliogliomas and is lacking in those areas that are formed solely by glial elements. The massive congenital cortical gangliogliomas of infants, already referred to above, do not contain such a connective tissue stroma.

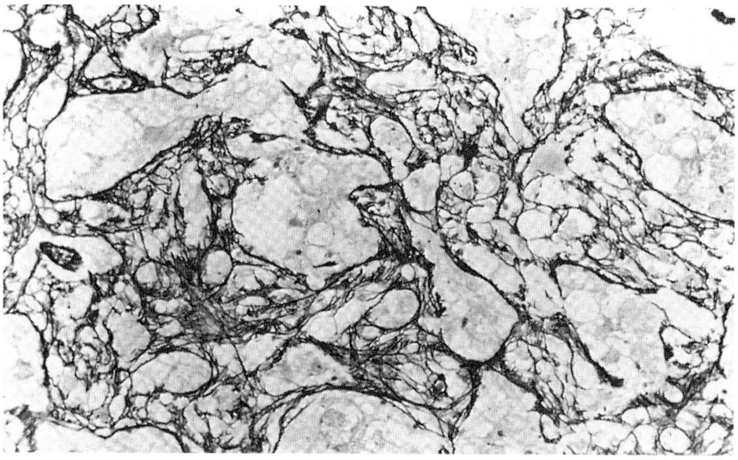

Fig. 9.274 Abundant network of reticulin fibers surrounding ganglion cells. Reticulin, × 120

When the tumor is adjacent to or invades the leptomeninges, infiltration of the pia-arachnoid by argyrophilic neurites may be conspicuous.

Cytogenetics and molecular analysis

Cytogenetic analyses of gangliogliomas are largely lacking. Ploidy analysis, as determined by flow cytometry, is available on two cases, one of which revealed a significant aneuploid population (Bowles *et al.*, 1988) that was said to be predictive of an anaplastic population, the other of which was diploid (Jay *et al.*, 1995) but was found in an obviously malignant neoplasm. Ploidy analysis of benign ganglion cell tumors is also lacking, most likely based on the assumption that such a study would find uniform diploidy.

Electron microscopy

Studies of a ganglioneuroma (Robertson, Hendry and Vogel, 1964) and gangliogliomas (Rubinstein and Herman, 1972; Miller, Lang and Epstein, 1993) disclose, as a notable feature, the presence of dense-core vesicles in the neuronal cytoplasm and cell processes. The vesicles in the latter case measure from 125 nm to 180 nm in diameter (Fig. 9.275). Synaptic contacts between the tumor cells and adjacent processes are also demonstrable and explain the dense synaptophysin immunoreactivity seen around the ganglion cells (Miller, Lang and Epstein, 1993) (Figs 9.276 and 9.277). Another feature is the presence of concentrically laminated bodies (Fig. 9.278) resembling those reported in experimental axonal reaction and degeneration, some of which could represent degenerative changes in the dense-core vesicles. In gangliogliomas, the astrocytic nature of the tumor cells is confirmed by the presence of glial filaments, with which intensely osmiophilic dense bodies, representing the electron microscopic equivalent of Rosenthal fibers, sometimes merge. A third cell type, believed to be mesenchymal, is also found adjacent to abundant collagen fibrils and surrounding the convoluted basement membrane material; Rubinstein and Herman (1972) opined that this cell is presumably responsible for the rich connective tissue stroma often characteristic of the ganglion cell neoplasms in the CNS. In both of these tumor types, the morphologic features suggest to the authors a possible relationship with nerve cell tumors originating from autonomic nervous tissue, a relationship also suggested (p. 504 and Chapter 15, p. 342) by the resemblance of the cells of a ganglionic hamartoma of the tuber cinereum to those in sympathetic ganglia. The speculation that the material visualized in the dense-core vesicles bears any relationship to catecholamines finds support in the immunohistochemical demonstration by Kawai *et al.* (1987) of tyrosine hydroxylase, a rate-limiting enzyme of catecholamine synthesis, in the neurons of a parietal ganglioglioma in a 2-year-old girl.

The neurons of gangliogliomas have occasionally been reported to show the intracellular alterations characteristic of generalized ganglion cell degeneration or of disorders due to abnormal storage. These changes have included the development of neurofibrillary tangles with the accumulation of paired helical filaments (Oberc-Greenwood *et al.*, 1984; Soffer, Umansky and Goldman, 1995), and the presence of membranous cytoplasmic bodies, curvilinear bodies and zebra bodies (Itoh, Yagishita and Chiba, 1987; Takahashi *et al.*, 1987) resembling those seen in gangliosidosis; branched tubular

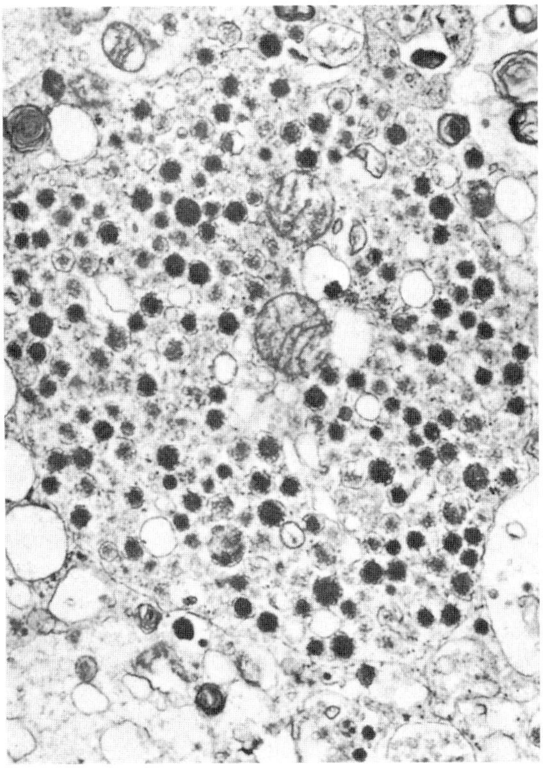

Fig. 9.275 Electron micrograph showing a temporal lobe ganglioglioma with numerous dense-core vesicles and two mitochondria in a nonmyelinated nerve process. × 15 900

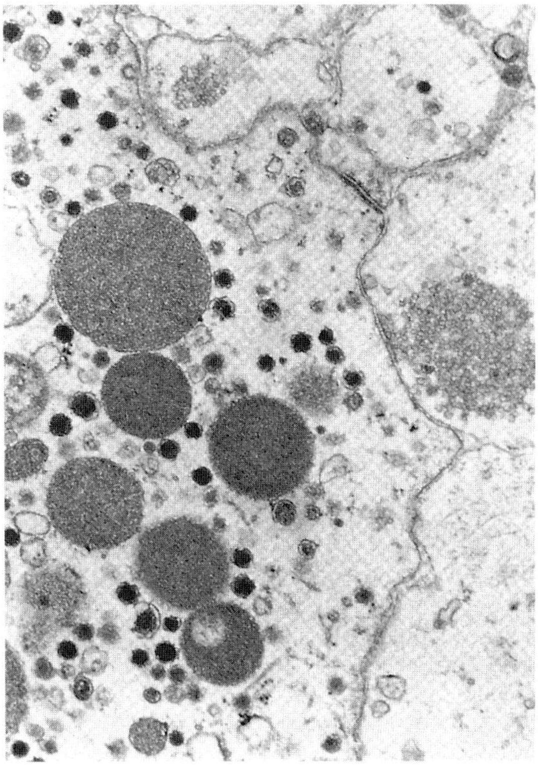

Fig. 9.276 Same case as Fig. 9.275 showing numerous dense-core vesicles and large membrane-bound autophagic vacuoles in the perikaryon of a tumor cell. Note the axosomatic synapse in the right middle field. × 17 300 (Reprinted from *Recent Advances in Neuropathology*, 1979, figure 8.7a, with kind permission of Churchill Livingstone.)

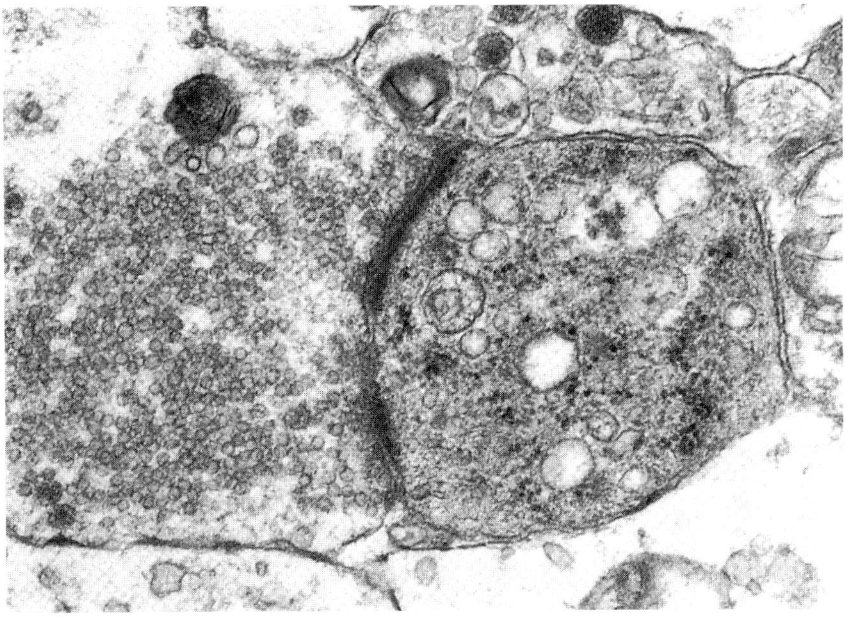

Fig. 9.277 Same case as Fig. 9.275. Axodendritic synapse with occasional dense-core vesicles (lower left) among the clear-centered synaptic vesicles. × 37 400 (Reprinted from *Recent Advances in Neuropathology*, 1979, figure 8.7b courtesy of Churchill Livingstone with the permission of Dr Mary M. Herman)

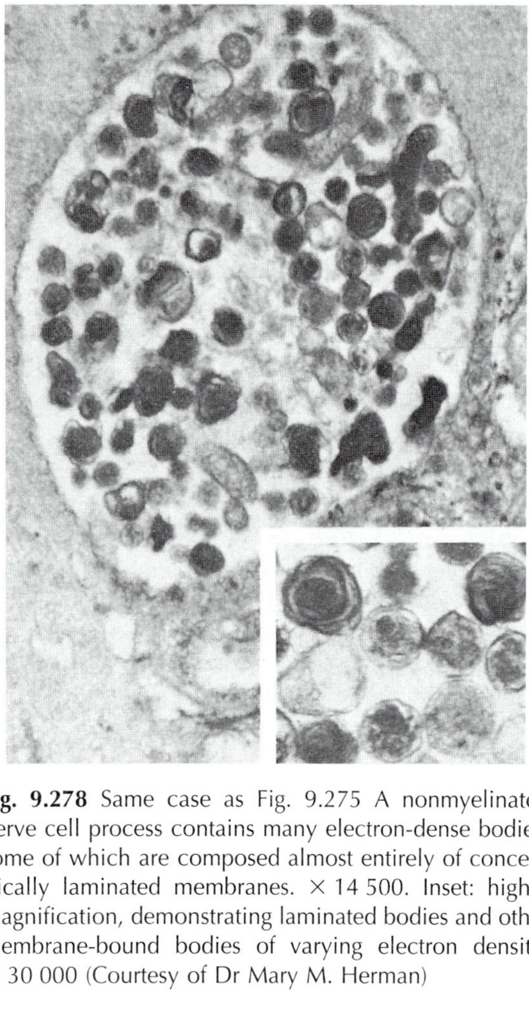

Fig. 9.278 Same case as Fig. 9.275 A nonmyelinated nerve cell process contains many electron-dense bodies, some of which are composed almost entirely of concentrically laminated membranes. × 14 500. Inset: higher magnification, demonstrating laminated bodies and other membrane-bound bodies of varying electron density. × 30 000 (Courtesy of Dr Mary M. Herman)

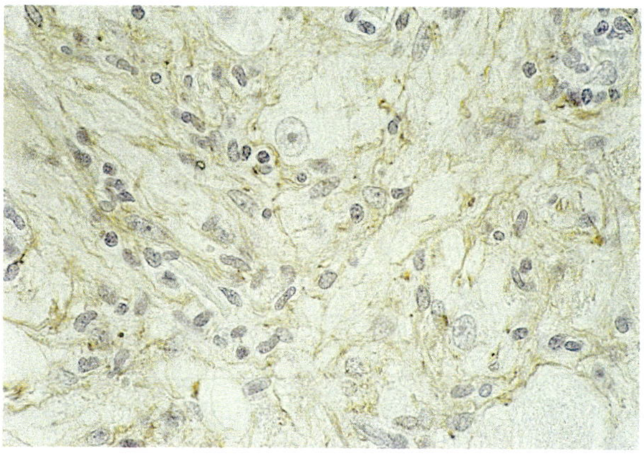

Fig. 9.279 An immunohistochemical stain for GFAP surrounds and highlights the nonreactive ganglion cell. × 520

structures (Ito, Yamashita and Chiba, 1987) similar to those seen in infantile neuraxonal dystrophy; and, in the distended neurites, Hirano and Lafora bodies (Takahashi *et al.*, 1987). The significance of these alterations in relation to any metabolic change postulated to occur in neoplastic ganglion cells is unclear.

Immunohistochemistry

As expected, the glial elements in gangliogliomas typically demonstrate the presence of GFAP, thus permitting their easy distinction from the neuronal component. A puzzling observation, however, is the apparent lack of concordance in the immunopositivity for GFAP of cells that in routine stains would be immediately interpreted as astrocytic, and the apparent presence of the protein in cells that display cellular features more characteristic of neurons, a feature reminiscent of the large cells found in the cortical lesions and 'candle gutterings' of tuberous sclerosis. The more typical ganglion cells, however, are GFAP-negative (Fig. 9.279). Paradoxically, immunostaining for GFAP may be used to highlight ganglion cells by their absence of staining amidst a background of strongly immunoreactive glial cells involved in this neoplasm. By contrast, ganglion cells have been shown to be immunopositive for NFP with either polyvalent antisera (Roessmann *et al.*, 1983) or MAbs (Trojanowski, Lee and Schlaepfer, 1984). Furthermore, one study on a tumor exhibiting paired helical filaments has shown the filaments to exhibit immunoreactivity against antibodies to phosphorylated neurofilaments, paired helical filament/tau protein, and ubiquitin, indicating the presence of both normal and abnormal structural proteins (Soffer, Umansky and Goldman, 1995). The ganglionic elements of two gangliogliomas have been shown to contain calcineurin (Goto *et al.*, 1987).

We have already mentioned above the finding by Kawai *et al.* (1987) of tyrosine hydroxylase in the neurons of a ganglioglioma. Azzarelli, Luerssen and Wolfe (1991) have described tyrosine hydroxylase immunoreactivity in an 8-year-old boy who had severe systemic hypertension during resection of the tumor, reminiscent of the hypertensive episodes during resections of pheochromocytomas. Diepholder *et al.* (1991), however, found immunoreactivity for tyrosine hydroxylase and dopamine β-hydroxylase in only 1/13 gangliogliomas. Regulatory peptides similar to those found in peripheral neuronal neoplasms have also been found by Giangaspero *et al.* (1985) in central ganglion cell tumors: the peptides have included VIP (vasoactive intestinal polypeptide) in 8/19 such neoplasms and neurotensin in 2/19. Although proliferation indices, as determined for gangliogliomas by flow cytometry, are largely lacking, data acquired from immunohistochemical means are becoming available. The most popular method, because of its ease of application, uses the Ki-67/MIB-1 antigen as a target. Two studies have shown evidence that ganglion cells do not proliferate, with only the glial component exhibiting labeled nuclei (Wolf *et al.*, 1994; Prayson, Khajavi and Comair, 1995). Similarly, BrdU incorporation studies indicate low LIs for the ganglion cell component (Krouwer *et al.*, 1993). Standard histopathologic grading schemes for astrocytes appear to correlate well with the astrocytic LIs determined by both MIB-1 and BrdU. Krouwer *et al.* (1993) and Prayson, Khajavi and Comair (1995) indicate that elevated astrocytic LIs (<1%) are found in those tumors exhibiting astrocytic components characterized by nuclear pleomorphism, vascular proliferation and/or necrosis with pseudopalisading.

Immunohistochemical studies for the p53 antigen by Wolf *et al.* (1994) did not reveal the protein in any of the tumors. This finding is considered to be indicative of a normal p53 status.

Clinical evolution

Their slow growth, well-differentiated cellular features, and usually small size and good demarcation, which permits surgical resection with favorable location, are all factors that counsel a relatively good prognosis for ganglion cell tumors in the great majority of cases. Long postoperative survival periods have been confirmed in clinical series, such as those reported by Johannsson, Rekate and Roessmann (1981), Kalyan-Raman and Olivero (1987), Silver *et al.* (1991); Celli *et al.* (1993); Krouwer *et al.* (1993); Lang *et al.* (1993) and Zentner *et al.* (1994). Johannsson, Rekate and Roessmann (1981) were unable to relate the biologic behavior of their cases to any obvious histologic parameters, such as the degree of cell density, cellular pleomorphism, the presence of vascular proliferation or of local meningeal invasion, or the demonstration of necrosis or hemorrhage; a similar lack of histologic correlation was noted in both the series of Kalyan-Raman and Olivero (1987) and in the series of Miller and collaborators (Lang *et al.*, 1993; Miller, Lang and Epstein, 1993). In contrast, Krouwer *et al.* (1993) found the features of glioblastoma to be predictive only of recurrence and not survival. Adequate documentation of long postoperative follow-up of 20 years or more remains, however, exceptional. Noteworthy is the case recorded by Serebrin and Robertson (1984) of the indolent progressive growth of a ganglioneuroma that arose in the pituitary fossa, and the personal example recorded by Russell and Rubinstein (1962), referred to in further detail below, of a ganglioglioma that originated in the lateral ventricle of a 26-year-old woman and that was followed for 25 years. Similarly, Davidson, Graham and Carey (1992) note the history of an untreated ganglioglioma diagnosed 10 years before death and associated with a 46-year history of neurologic symptoms.

The vast majority of gangliogliomas are found during radiographic studies for epilepsy, particularly in children (Chamberlain and Press, 1990; Tampieri *et al.*, 1991; Mickle, 1992; Otsubo *et al.*, 1992; Smith *et al.*, 1992; Celli *et al.*, 1993; Morris *et al.*, 1993; Zentner *et al.*, 1994). Indeed, the characteristic history is that of a young adult with a longstanding history of epilepsy. Although the majority of gangliogliomas are found in the temporal lobes, gangliogliomas of the spinal cord and medulla are more commonly found in children, most likely related to an earlier evaluation than those patients with seizures (Albright and Byrd, 1980).

Complete resection appears to produce long-term recurrence-free survival (Haddad *et al.*, 1992a; Zentner *et al.*, 1994). Complete seizure relief is obtained with resection in up to 80% of patients and >75% reduction in seizure activity is found in the vast majority of the remainder (Zentner *et al.*, 1994). Postoperative radiotherapy is largely avoided (Garrido *et al.*, 1978; Johannsson, Rekate and Roessmann, 1981; Sutton *et al.*, 1983; Zentner *et al.*, 1994), although Mickle (1992) states otherwise for incomplete resections. The utility of radiation therapy and/or chemotherapy in anaplastic gangliogliomas has not been studied and prospective studies will be difficult given the lack of consensus on the histopathologic criteria for diagnosing these lesions (Zentner *et al.*, 1994).

Malignant forms

While a malignant change in gangliogliomas is rare, the incidence reported by Russell and Rubinstein (1989), amounting to about 10% of cases, is probably an excessive estimate in view of the selective nature of the material referred for consultation. Most of the examples in the older literature that report on presumed neuronal tumors having malignant features variously designate the tumors as malignant ganglioneuromas, ganglioblastomas and ganglioneuroblastomas, but these examples do not seem to be gangliogliomas and probably belong to the variety of pseudoganglionic giant-cell glioblastoma described elsewhere (p. 440).

Acceptable instances of ganglion cell tumors with biologic and histologic evidence of malignant transformation include those reported by Kernohan,

Learmonth and Doyle (1932, case 3); Tönnis and Zülch (1939, case 4; see also Zülch and Christensen, 1956, pp. 381–99) and Sasaki *et al.* (1996). In the present context, however, we should distinguish between the anaplastic changes occurring in an originally benign, well-differentiated ganglioglioma and the type of ganglion cell tumor, described in greater detail on p. 000, in which the more actively growing cell populations are clearly of neuroblastic character. This latter neoplasm may be more convincingly interpreted as cerebral neuroblastoma with maturation. The case described by Jay *et al.* (1994) appears to fall into this latter category, along with the cases we (McLendon *et al.*, 1997) have described.

If the latter cases with malignant neuronal and/or glial populations are clearly separated from those under present discussion, malignant change occurring in a ganglioglioma is restricted to the glial element, in agreement with the propensity of glial tumors to undergo anaplasia in the course of their evolution. This change is further consistent with the postmitotic state of the involved neurons. Russell and Rubinstein (1989) reported their experience in ten cases and confirmed, in all examples, that the anaplastic evolution of the tumor proceeds in the direction of a glioblastoma. Although too few cases have been accumulated to characterize an age incidence, Russell and Rubinstein (1989) noted that almost all cases were found in the younger age groups. Even infantile cases have been reported (Hall, Yunis and Albright, 1986). Examples include those in the report of Bowles *et al.* (1988) of malignant glial features and an aneuploid DNA histogram by flow cytometry, and that recorded by Christensen (1971) of a neoplasm exhibiting anaplastic progression. One of the patients of Kalyan-Raman and Olivero (1987) developed a glioblastoma 5 years after resection of a ganglioglioma, and one of the patients reported by Krouwer *et al.* (1993) died at 65 weeks postsurgery. Similarly, Sasaki *et al.* (1996) reported a 26-year-old man who initially presented with a ganglioglioma that exhibited 'atypical' glial cells and who died 9 years later of a malignant glioma.

A striking demonstration that this evolution may occur after a considerably protracted period of time is provided by a case reported in greater detail elsewhere (Russell and Rubinstein, 1962). In this example, the patient survived for 25 years after the partial removal of a ganglioglioma from the lateral wall of the left frontal horn; clinical evidence of a recurrence became manifest in the last 2 years of this period. The recurrence proved to be a massive anaplastic astrocytoma traversing the length of the corpus callosum and fanning out into both occipital lobes. Posteriorly, its appearances were those of a glioblastoma; anteriorly, the lateral part of the growth was well demarcated and principally composed of ganglion cells. Since the latter were restricted to this relatively small area of the neoplasm, it is clear that the fatal outcome was entirely due to a malignant change in the glial component. Allegranza *et al.* (1990) have also reported the exceptional case [reviewed by Rubinstein (Russell and Rubinstein, 1989)] of an anaplastic ganglioglioma, arising in an adult, in which the malignant component was entirely composed of a malignant oligodendroglioma.

Metastases

Metastatic involvement in the CNS is exceptional. Russell and Rubinstein (1989) have noted one case in which a recurrent lower thoracic tumor developed in a 13-year-old boy known to have had a primary temporal lobe ganglioglioma. A similar evolution also seems to have occurred in the case ambiguously characterized by Wahl and Dillard (1972) as an example of multiple ganglioneuromas: i.e., a ganglion cell tumor of the temporal lobe, in a 15-year-old boy, that was associated with multiple cerebrospinal subarachnoid tumors of similar histology, accompanied by a marked desmoplastic reaction in the leptomeninges. The case described by Karamitopoulou *et al.* (1995) appears to represent a ganglioglioma that spread locally, but extensively, to involve the meningeal surfaces of the brainstem and the fourth ventricle in a man with a 16-year history of neurologic symptoms. Zentner *et al.* (1994) record drop metastases to the spinal cord in one of their 51 patients studied.

Special variants of gangliocytomas and gangliogliomas

Intrasellar, endocrinologically active gangliocytoma

Attention has been drawn, in recent years, to the intriguing incidence of ganglion cells in the pituitary fossa, often, but not invariably, associated with clinical features indicative of increased pituitary activity (see Towfighi *et al.*, 1996, for report of three cases and review of 32 previously published examples). As pointed out by Towfighi, these tumors have been called, alternatively, ganglioneuroma, ganglioneuroma and adenoma, gangliocytoma, gangliocytoma with adenoma, neurosecretory ganglion cell choristoma, pituitary adenoma with neuronal choristoma, hypothalamic neuronal hamartoma with pituitary adenoma, and hypothalamic gangliocytoma. In most of the patients in whom endocrine features were present, these consisted of acromegaly or, less frequently, the effects of prolactinemia or of Cushing's disease. In some examples, as reported by Rhodes *et al.* (1982), Burchiel, Shaw and Kelly (1983) and Scheithauer *et al.* (1983), the endocrine symptoms have been attributable to the association of this lesion with a functional pituitary adenoma. Some of the ganglion cells have been shown to be immunoreactive for somatostatin, whereas other cells, presumably of adenohypophyseal origin, were found by immunoperoxidase to contain growth hormone, prolactin, ACTH, β-endorphin, VIP, vasopressin and neurophysin (Kamel, Horoupian and Silverberg, 1989; Puchner *et al.*, 1993). Furthermore, these ganglion cells were shown to be immunoreactive for NFP, synaptophysin and NSE (Li *et al.*, 1989; Horvath *et al.*, 1994).

It has been hypothesized that displaced hypothalamic neurons in the pituitary fossa might produce a growth hormone-releasing factor that would stimulate the proliferation of a hormonally active adenoma. Alternatively, the ganglion cells themselves could be the target of growth- and differentiation-stimulating factors induced by adenohypophyseal cells. In favor of the former hypothesis is the association, reported by Scheithauer *et al.* (1983) in one of their two cases, of a large hypothalamic neuronal hamartoma, similar to those described on p. 000, with a small separate growth hormone-secreting pituitary adenoma. A similar line of argument would account for the intrasellar gangliocytomas associated with Cushing's disease, one of which, reported by Asa *et al.* (1984), demonstrated ACTH-releasing hormone in the neuronal cell bodies as well as hyperplasia of ACTH- and β-endorphin-containing cells of the adjacent pituitary elements.

Dysplastic gangliocytomas of the cerebellum (Lhermitte-Duclos disease)

This curious but well-documented lesion, which combines the features of a congenital malformation, a simple hypertrophy and a tumor affecting the cerebellum, has been repeatedly described in detail under various designations, including dysplastic gangliocytoma, Purkinjeoma (Christensen, 1937), gangliomatosis of the cerebellum, diffuse hypertrophy of the cerebellar cortex and, perhaps its best known appellation, Lhermitte-Duclos disease. Patients with this tumor may exhibit ataxia, mild mental retardation and a self-limited seizure disorder (Eng *et al.*, 1994). The Russell and Rubinstein (1989) series included 10 such cases, usually originating in young adults in the second or third decade, with a marked preponderance of males. Exceptional examples have been reported as a congenital lesion (Roessmann and Wongmongkolrit, 1984). An association with Cowden's syndrome is well established (Padberg *et al.*, 1991; Albrecht *et al.*, 1992; Williams *et al.*, 1992; Rimbau and Isamat, 1994; Vinchon *et al.*, 1994; Vital *et al.*, 1994; Wells *et al.*, 1994) and is discussed in Chapter 16. The condition is characterized by loss of the normal cortical architecture

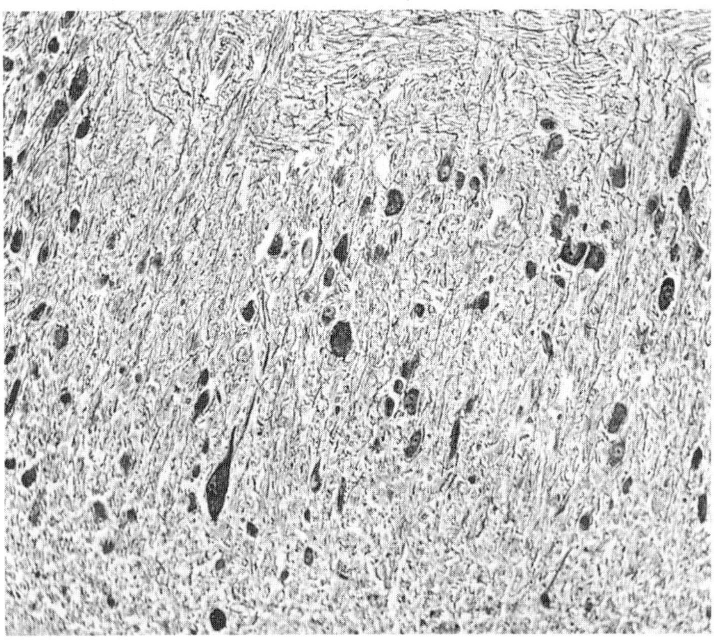

Fig. 9.280 Dysplastic gangliocytoma of the cerebellum. Luxol fast blue–Bodian silver impregnation, × 115

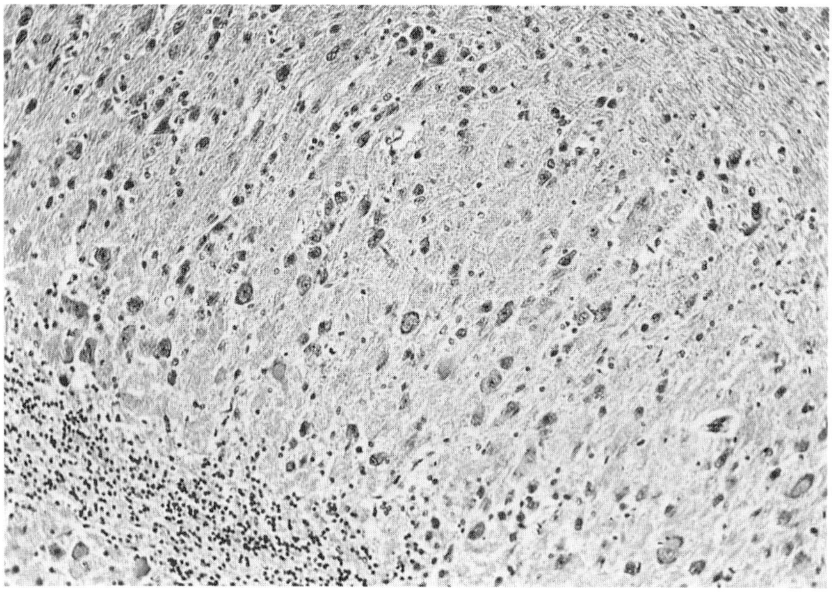

Fig. 9.281 Same case as Fig. 9.280. Abundant abnormal neurons are present, many of which bear a resemblance to Purkinje cells. H&E, × 115

and thickening of the folia over a limited area. On microscopic examination, the folia seem to be composed of an outer layer of well-developed radial and more superficially distributed parallel myelinated nerve fibers (Fig. 9.280), and an inner layer containing many abnormal neurons, some of which bear a superficial resemblance to Purkinje cells (Fig. 9.281). The digitate white matter is either absent or greatly reduced. Authoritative studies of this disease include that of Oppenheimer (1955), and that of Ambler, Pogacar and Sidman (1969) who reviewed 34 previously published cases and reported the first familial examples, in a mother and son.

Most observers who have studied these tumors agree that the histologic features are best explained by viewing the apparently neoplastic nerve cells as substantially enlarged granular neurons in which the axons, normally directed towards the pial surface, may show abnormal myelination. Golgi and electron microscopic studies (Pritchett and King, 1978; Ferrer, Isamat and Acebes, 1979; Reznik and Schoenen, 1983) have essentially supported that interpretation. An interesting speculation about the pathogenesis of the lesion, discussed at length by Hallervorden (1959), is that the hypertrophy of the internal granular neurons could be an acquired compensatory phenomenon incurred by those granular cells that were derived from the primitive ventricular neuroepithelium, secondary to focal absence or maldevelopment of part of the fetal external granular layer. Such a hypothesis is based on the theory, championed by the German school of neuroembryology, that the internal granular neurons have a dual source of origin, a view that is not, however, accepted by other authorities.

A further complication in our understanding of Lhermitte-Duclos disease has been added by the immunohistochemical study of Shiurba *et al.* (1988), which has shown that some of the larger abnormal neurons have a number of features in common with those of Purkinje cells: namely, they are recognized by the pan-T-cell antibody, anti-Leu 4; they are surrounded by axosomatic synapses visualized by the antisynaptic vesicle glycoprotein antibody, SV2; and they contain both nonphosphorylated and phosphorylated neurofilament epitopes. The condition may, therefore, represent a complex hamartoma of cytologically heterogeneous character rather than a simple hypertrophy of the granular neurons. In any event, further support for its hamartomatous basis is provided by its known association with other congenital malformations, including, in some cases, megalencephaly. Notable examples include also that described by Carbone, Brihaye and Drochmans (1955), in which the lesion was associated with a parieto-occipital glioblastoma; cases that may be considered exceptions to a hamartomatous origin include those described by Christian (1961) in which the condition was marked by a slow clinical evolution extending over a period of 29 years; by Stapleton, Wilkins and Bell (1992) in which the tumor recurred in the cerebellum 20 years after resection, presenting the second time

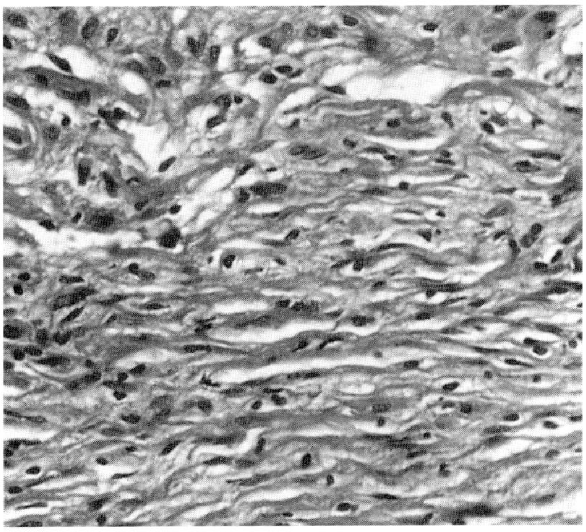

Fig. 9.282 Left parietal tumor in a 10-month-old male. The marked desmoplastic appearance is produced by fibroblastic proliferation in the leptomeninges. H&E, × 250

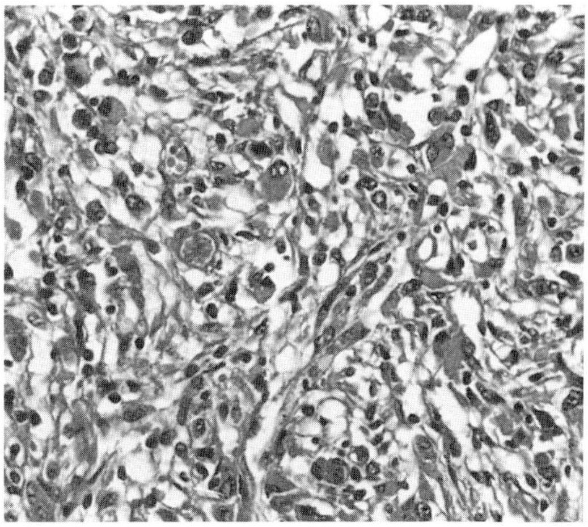

Fig. 9.283 Desmoplastic portion of a right parietal tumor in an 11-month-old boy. Large pleomorphic neuroepithelial cells are admixed with fibroblasts. H&E, × 250

with subarachnoid hemorrhage; by Banerjee and Gleadhill (1979) of a tumor that recurred 11 years after surgery; and by Marano, Johnson and Spetzler (1988) of a case recurring three times over a period of 4 years.

Desmoplastic infantile gangliogliomas

Under this not entirely satisfactory term are grouped a number of highly characteristic supratentorial neuroepithelial neoplasms presenting clinically as large cystic masses in infancy, often within 4 months of age, almost all at less than 18 months of age, and most frequently involving the frontal and parietal regions (VandenBerg *et al.*, 1987; de Chadarévian, Pattisapu and Faerber, 1990; Ng, Fung and Ma, 1990; Paulus *et al.*, 1992; Rushing, Rorke and Sutton, 1993; Taguchi *et al.*, 1993; Duffner *et al.*, 1994; Sperner *et al.*, 1994). Since VandenBerg's study (VandenBerg *et al.*, 1987), the tumor has come to be recognized by the existence of an extensive desmoplastic component that is associated with a predominantly leptomeningeal direction of growth (Fig. 9.282). The fibroblastic elements are, however, admixed with variable numbers of pleomorphic neuroepithelial cells (Fig. 9.283), and divergent differentiation along astrocytic and neuronal lines can be demonstrated in the great majority of examples when immunohistochemical techniques and silver impregnations for neurites are applied. Astrocytic differentiation can be established in all such tumors by the presence of GFAP (Fig. 9.284). Immunoperoxidase preparations using a MAb against the 200-kDa NFP confirms the presence of neuritic differentiation (Fig. 9.285), which in some cases is further documented

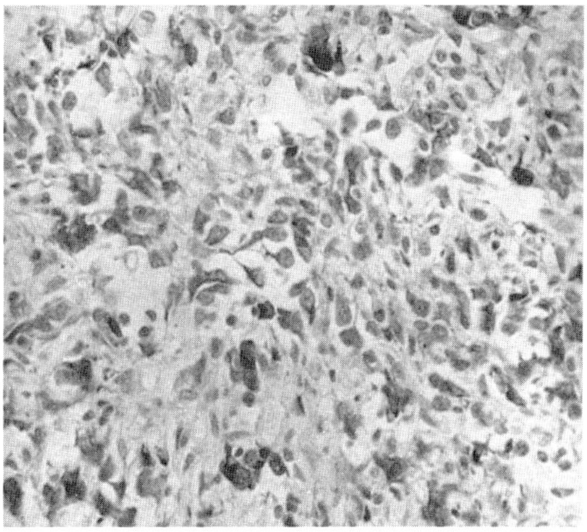

Fig. 9.284 Same case as Fig. 9.283 from a similar field. Numerous GFAP-positive tumor cells are seen. GFAP immunoperoxidase, × 250

by Bielschowsky silver impregnations. In a number of tumors, mature ganglion cells are present (Fig. 9.286). A frequent histologic feature is the demonstration of islands of reactive neuroglia encompassed in the desmoplastic growth (Figs 9.285 and 9.287). By electron microscopy, the neoplastic glial elements display a pericytoplasmic basal lamina characteristic of subpial cerebral astrocytes (VandenBerg *et al.*, 1987; Ng, Fung and Ma, 1990).

Four tumors included in the VandenBerg *et al.* (1987) study were previously, on the basis of their neuritic differentiation, included in the report of

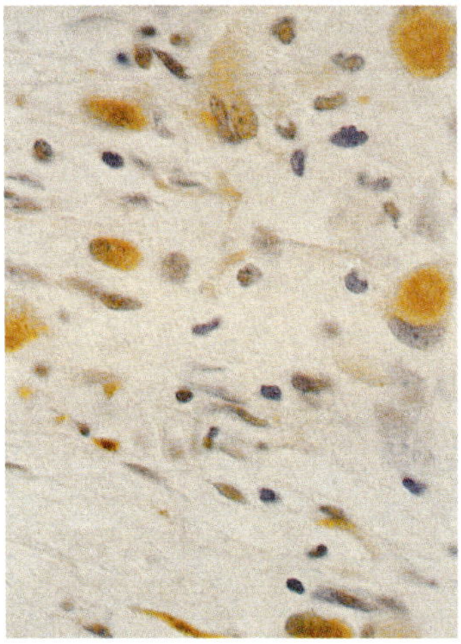

Fig. 9.285 Neuronal cells are readily highlighted by an immunoperoxidase reaction for the 200-kDa NFP in desmoplastic infantile ganglioglioma. NFP immunoperoxidase, × 360

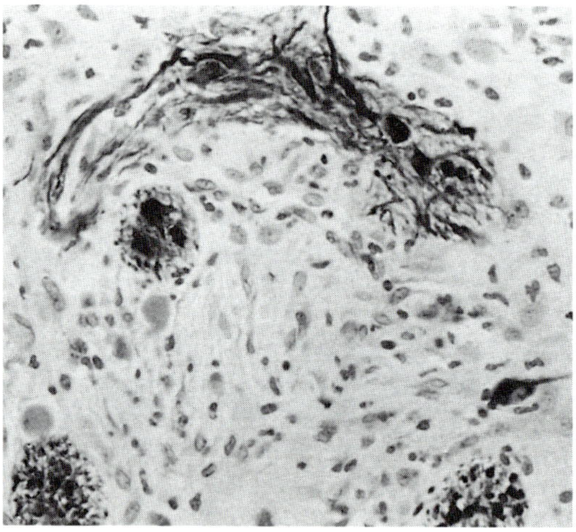

Fig. 9.287 Right frontoparietal tumor in a 4-month-old girl. Islands of GFAP-positive reactive gliosis are seen in this desmoplastic tumor. Note a GFAP-positive tumor cell near the right margin. GFAP immunoperoxisase, × 250.

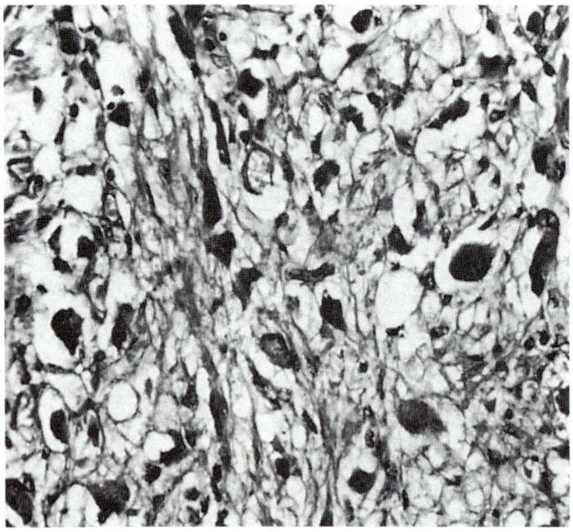

Fig. 9.286 Same case as Fig. 9.283 Mature ganglion cells are found amidst a fibrous connective tissue. Bielschowsky silver impregnation, × 225

Horten and Rubinstein as examples of desmoplastic cerebral neuroblastomas in infants (Horten and Rubinstein, 1976, cases 32–35). It is likely that the cases of superficial cerebral astrocytoma, characterized by a similarly intense desmoplasia and restricted to infants (described by Taratuto *et al.*, 1984) (see p. 359), are instances of the same or a closely related entity, except for the fact that, in the cases of Taratuto *et al.*, only astrocytic differentiation was documented. In the Horten and Rubinstein (1976) series, not every tumor showed divergent differentiation, but restriction to the astrocytic line was exceptional. Similarly, the cases described by Dastur (1982) and Gambarelli *et al.* (1982) may represent early examples of this tumor.

More recently, superficial cerebral and cerebellar tumors have been described, in older patients (15–25 years old), in which large plump xanthomatous astrocytes are found embedded in dense collagenized fibrous connective tissue alongside ganglion-type neurons (Furuta *et al.*, 1992; Lindboe, Cappelen and Kepes, 1992; Kuchelmeister *et al.*, 1995; Kordek *et al.*, 1995). While some authors put forth the tumors as noninfantile variants of desmoplastic gangliogliomas (Kuchelmeister *et al.*, 1995), the pattern emerging from the recent literature appears to support the contention of Lindboe, Cappelen and Kepes (1992) that the tumor is a ganglioglioma with pleomorphic xanthoastrocytoma as a glial component. It is unlikely that this tumor is the end result of an untreated desmoplastic infantile ganglioglioma, given the very large size of the latter at diagnosis.

Histologically, these tumors may appear ominous, exhibiting marked cellularity focally, and mitotic activity. Indeed, a recent report from the Pediatric Oncology Group indicates that four cases of this tumor had originally been diagnosed as grade 3 astrocytoma, malignant meningioma, leptomeningeal fibrosarcoma, and gliosarcoma (Duffner *et al.*, 1994). Despite their voluminous size, desmoplastic infantile gangliogliomas have been successfully resected (complete or subtotal resection) and the patients have followed a favorable clinical course, extending in some cases over several years of tumor-free survival. From the morphologic and biologic points of view, therefore, this group of tumors represents a distinct entity in which the massive size of the growths points to their pre- or perinatal development and for which histologic recognition as a special form of embryonal CNS neoplasm is predictive of a favorable prognosis.

Dysembryoplastic neuroepithelial tumors

The dysembryoplastic neuroepithelial tumor (DNT) is a recently described entity of which little is known. Best described as a tumor, for its mass produces a grossly and radiographically identifiable lesion, its neoplastic character is not understood. Its propensity to be associated with cortical migrational abnormalities, and its multilobular architecture, led some investigators (Burger and Scheithauer, 1994) to classify the lesion as 'quasi-hamartomatous'. The tumor has drawn considerable attention for its temporal lobe location, resulting in its clinical association with epilepsy, most notably partial complex seizures.

In reviews of case material submitted from epilepsy patients, Wolf *et al.* (1995) identified DNTs in 11–43 patients. These DNTs were described as multilobulated tumors varying in size from 0.5 to 15 mm and predominately located in the cortex. Similarly, the material that formed the seminal report on this entity (Daumas-Duport *et al.*, 1988a) revealed a common spectrum of gross anatomic findings, including a cortical location and a multinodular architecture usually associated with cortical disorganization.

Histologically, the lobules that characterize DNTs are formed from small round oligodendroglial-like cells that are associated with an

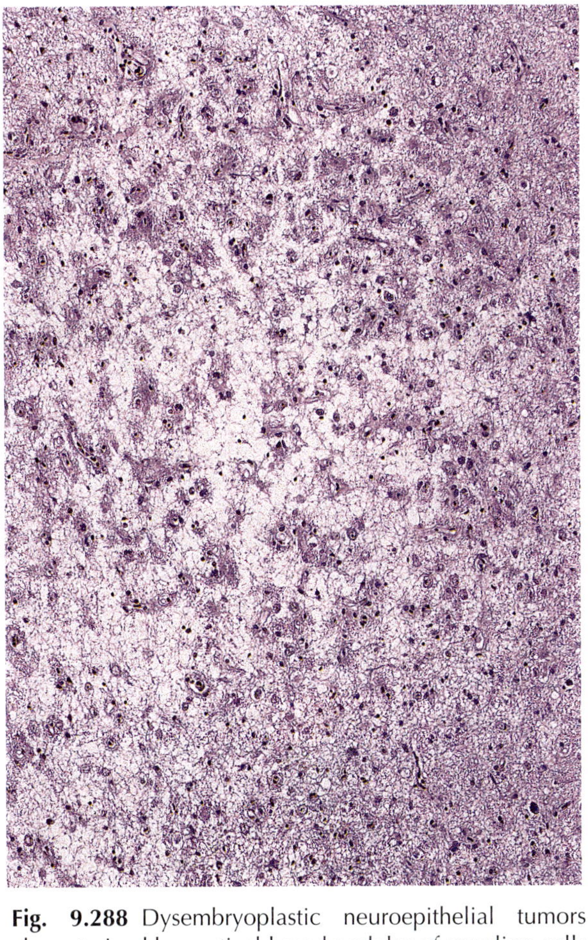

Fig. 9.288 Dysembryoplastic neuroepithelial tumors characterized by cortical-based nodules of ganglion cells and oligodendroglial cells. H&E, × 33

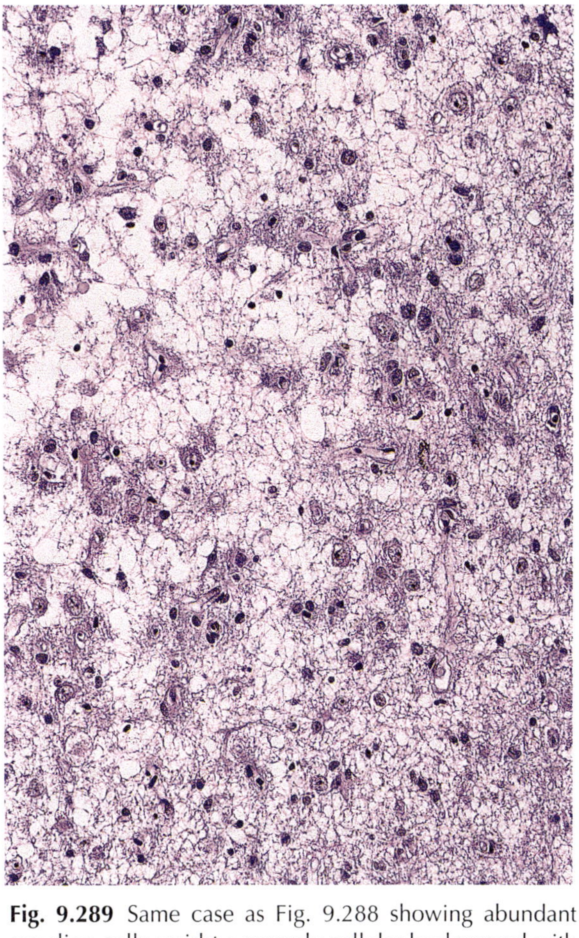

Fig. 9.289 Same case as Fig. 9.288 showing abundant ganglion cells amidst a sparsely cellular background with occasional small round oligodendroglial cells. This tumor lacks the specific glioneuronal elements of oligodendroglial cells aligned along linear processes. H&E, × 66

abundant mucinous background, producing a microcystic appearance, highlightable with an Alcian blue stain. The small round cells can assume a variety of appearances within the mucin, but generally are aligned along the side of an eosinophilic structure, occasionally seen to be vascularized. The significance of this pattern appears to represent an extreme form of 'secondary structure' (as originally defined by Scherer, 1936) in which the oligodendroglia-like cells are closely aligned to axons – axons that apparently belong to the neurons 'floating' in the mucinous material. This finding has been termed a 'specific glioneuronal element' by Daumas-Duport (1993) and is used by her to confirm the diagnosis of DNT. In one review, however, she points out that the specific glioneuronal element will be found in only half of the cases that she categorizes as DNT (Figs 9.288 and 9.289). Among those lesions that exhibit the 'specific element', a spectrum of cells and histologic morphologies may also be encountered, including pilocytic astrocytes, fibrillar astrocytes, sheets of oligodendroglia, eosinophilic granular bodies and punctate microcalcifications. Mitotic activity may also be encountered and, as reported by several investigators (Daumas-Duport, 1993; Hirose *et al.*, 1994; Taratuto *et al.*, 1995), can be quite brisk and associated with a high LI for the proliferation-related antigens, MIB-1 and Ki-67. However, to date, this feature has not been associated with clinical malignancy.

Immunohistochemistry

The oligodendroglial nature of the small round cells is largely confirmed by their reactivity for S-100 protein and lack of reactivity for synaptophysin and the neurofilament peptides. The MAb TUJ-1, which reacts with class III β-tubulin, also occasionally stains these cells, as do anti-GFAP antibodies (Hirose *et al.*, 1994). Antibodies to NSE have not been shown to bind these cells (Daumas-Duport, 1993).

The neuronal cells react with TUJ-1, synaptophysin and the neurofilaments (Hirose *et al.*, 1994). That some small round oligodendroglial-like cells react with these antibodies suggest that some of these cells may be neurons. Regardless, as pointed out by Hirose *et al.* (1994), their identification in a tumor, with otherwise typical glial features, may tip the investigator to the diagnosis of DNT.

Histogenesis

The divergent population of cells represented in the DNT suggests progenitor cells capable of glial or neuronal phenotypical maturation. The association of this tumor with neuronal migrational abnormalities has suggested the possibility of an origin in the subpial, or external, granular layer. Remnants of the subpial granular layer have been found in the temporal and frontal lobes of otherwise normal infants coming to autopsy (Brun, 1965); these locations correlate with the sites of this tumor. A key issue in ontogeny is the relationship of the small oligodendroglial-like cell, which expresses neuronal markers, with the mature neurons in the tumor.

Origin and mode of development of ganglion cell tumors

The histogenesis of some of the ganglion cell tumors originating in the temporal lobe is open to speculation. A possibility arises that the subgranular zone of the dentate gyrus might function, in the mammalian brain, as a source of continuing cytogenesis for granular neurons after birth (Guéneau *et al.*, 1982). In the primate brain, however, neuronogenesis in the fascia dentata has been shown to taper off within the first 2 months of postnatal life (Rakic and Nowakowski, 1981). As already mentioned (p. 481), there is no evidence that further generation of ganglion cells takes place after that time (Rakic, 1985). Thus, the characteristics of this neoplasm, including: (1) its slow and protracted clinical evolution; (2) its sporadic manifestation as a massive congenital lesion in which a marked malformative component is evidently present in the area of the brain that it occupies; and (3) its occasional association with structural congenital anomalies involving the CNS, emphasize the close relationship that exists, in this overall group, between malformation and new growth. By the time these tumors are surgically excised, clear morphologic evidence that the neoplastic nerve cells were derived from more primitive forms is usually inconspicuous: typical neuroblastic rosettes are generally absent, and individual neuroblasts may not be identified with certainty. Examples in which more primitive cellular areas are easily demonstrated, which Russell and Rubinstein (1989) preferred to interpret as central neuroblastomas with maturation (Hall, Yunis and Albright, 1986), are in the minority: they are discussed in greater detail in the section on cerebral neuroblastomas (p. 490). Analogous to the peripheral ganglioneuroma, the histologic picture in a central ganglioneuroma or ganglioglioma is the end result of the maturation process and terminal differentiation incurred by the progeny of an initially more primitive neuroblastic population. The clinical and biologic evolution certainly suggest a neoplasm in which the growth fraction of the neoplastic neuronal cells is very low. Furthermore, the larger proportion of the daughter cells generated in the mitotically active pool appear to lose the capacity to re-enter the cycle as they undergo gangliocytic differentiation. Thus, the natural progression of the ganglion element is towards increasing maturation and, eventually, growth arrest. In contrast, the glial element in gangliogliomas does not necessarily follow a similar pathway of differentiation. Although no studies are extant on the proliferating population of cells, anaplastic change of the glial cell population should result in the tumor assuming a malignant progression. Malignant progression is, fortunately, a rare event and, when it does occur, it is usually found after a protracted clinical course.

The malformative element in ganglion cell tumors of the CNS is also suggested by their occasional development in the white matter, where neoplastic proliferation of the neurons could have occurred in sites harboring ectopic gray matter islands. Such islands, nest-like but not neoplastic, are indeed sporadically encountered as incidental findings in the white matter of otherwise normal brains. Similar foci of ectopic cortex have also been found in relation to the hypothalamus (Chapter 15, p. 342); hence, tumors assumed to arise at the site of such rests might plausibly be classified as hamartomas. Support for the hamartomatous origin of some of the gangliogliomas involving the temporal lobe is provided by the study of Cavanagh (1958) on eight cases of temporal lobe epilepsy in which small microscopic nodular lesions, some of which were of maldevelopmental nature and others of which showed early evidence of neoplastic transformation, were reasonably assumed to have been present for many years and may have originated in early childhood. Two of these cases were examples of early gangliogliomas in the para-amygdaloid region.

In the previous edition of this book, Russell and Rubinstein (1989) related the incidental finding of a small circumscribed nodule projecting from the tuber cinereum in a 34-year-old woman dying of generalized sarcoidosis. The nodule contained many abnormal giant neurons—often exhibiting grotesque shapes, cytoplasmic vacuoles and multinucleation—mingled with irregular, sometimes very large, reniform glial nuclei reminiscent of Alzheimer glia. A Bielschowsky impregnation revealed a rich network of unusually coarse and obviously abnormal nerve fibers and of irregular circumvoluted ganglionic processes with bulbous expansions, mixed with many finer neurofibrils and uni- and bipolar neuroblasts. The ectopic nature of this nodule is suggested by the marked resemblance of its nerve cells to the multidendritic neurons found in sympathetic ganglia and in pathologically altered sensory cerebrospinal ganglia (de Castro, 1932). Russell and Rubinstein (1989) reported that, in one example, the satellite cells that normally line the connective tissue enclosing the ganglia were replaced by a stroma of glial elements that were themselves the seat of pathologic changes. Such a nodule can, therefore, reasonably be interpreted as a link between a simple ectopic hamartoma of the hypothalamus (Chapter 15, p. 342), on the one hand, and a fully developed ganglioglioma of the floor of the third ventricle, on the other. Also included in the same category is the minute tumor observed as an incidental finding by Courville (1930, case 2) in an exactly similar location.

Nevertheless, to regard all ganglion cell tumors simply as malformations, as some authors have done (e.g., Schär and Christensen, 1939), is certainly questionable. The behavior of these tumors, as has been shown, is often that of true neoplasms.

Growth and dissemination of central neuroepithelial tumors

To a large extent, the patterns of growth and dissemination of primary central neuroepithelial tumors, especially the gliomas, are determined not only by the intrinsic malignancy of the tumor cells themselves, but also by their topographic relationship to the central neural parenchyma; by their capacity to transgress the pia, with consequent invasion of the perivascular and leptomeningeal spaces, or to breach the ependyma—resulting in ventricular and meningeal metastases; by the absence of a lymphatic system draining the CNS; and by the relative resistance of the parenchymal blood vessels to glioma cell invasion. It is convenient to consider these developments under three main headings: (1) local spread, (2) metastasis by way of the CSF and (3) remote metastases.

LOCAL SPREAD

Generally speaking, all neuroepithelial tumors originating from the central neuraxis are diffuse in the sense that they have no capsule. At one end of the spectrum, the ependymomas, pineocytomas and choroid plexus papillomas are generally well defined, with the exception of their malignant counterparts; growth takes place by expansion rather than by infiltration. Others, such as the oligodendrogliomas, cerebellar astrocytomas, cerebral neuroblastomas and some examples of glioblastoma, appear fairly well circumscribed to the naked eye, but microscopically display various degrees of peripheral infiltration, often greater than might have been suspected (Coakley *et al.*, 1995).

However, this zone of infiltration may be comparatively narrow. In some instances, especially in the glioblastomas, the margin of the growth may be accentuated by a zone of central necrosis, but, microscopically, this does not limit the glioma, for infiltrating tumor cells are invariably found beyond this zone (Kelly *et al.*, 1987).

At the other end of the spectrum are the diffusely infiltrating gliomas: cerebral and brainstem astrocytomas, gliomas of the anterior optic pathways and gliomatosis cerebri. The process whereby the greater part of the cerebral hemispheres and, in some cases, other regions of the central neuraxis, as well, come to be occupied by such a homogeneous tumor (see Figs 9.39 and 9.41) is quite enigmatic. In those examples in which only a part of one cerebral hemisphere is involved, it seems reasonable that progressive centrifugal growth and infiltration have taken place from a single focus. Although not entirely conclusive, a recent clonal analysis of multiple separate foci in each of 12 malignant gliomas suggests that these tumors are indeed monoclonal, and that even extensively infiltrating examples arise from migration of tumor cells (Kattar *et al.*, 1996).

Much more is known of the subsequent stages of growth and spread within the CNS parenchyma. The careful and still relevant studies of Scherer (1938, 1940a) are of importance in this context for, as he pointed out, a variety of *secondary structures* can be detected beyond the confines of the main tumor that seem to herald the growing margins of the neoplasm. These secondary structures, for details of which the reader should consult Scherer's papers, include cellular aggregates about neurons, blood vessels and in the subpial marginal zone of the cortex (see Figs 9.25, 9.26 and 9.39). The last is rather common and, as Scherer has stated, is sometimes seen in conjunction with subcortical astrocytomas when the intervening cortex is not obviously infiltrated. An analogous concentration of tumor cells in the subependymal neuroglia is more rarely encountered. Scherer's perivascular secondary structures are aggregates outside the Virchow-Robin spaces and are usually confined to the gray matter. Perineuronal, perivascular and surface aggregates are often concomitant.

In the cerebral white matter, especially the corona radiata and the internal capsule, further concentrations of tumor cells have been described and illustrated by Scherer as being in alignment with the nerve fiber tracts (see Fig. 9.290). These varieties of his 'secondary structures' may be peri- or intrafascicular according to the degree of penetration of the nerve bundles. They are less frequent than the previous examples and provide an excellent demonstration of the adaptation of tumor growth to the tissues of the host (Fig. 9.291).

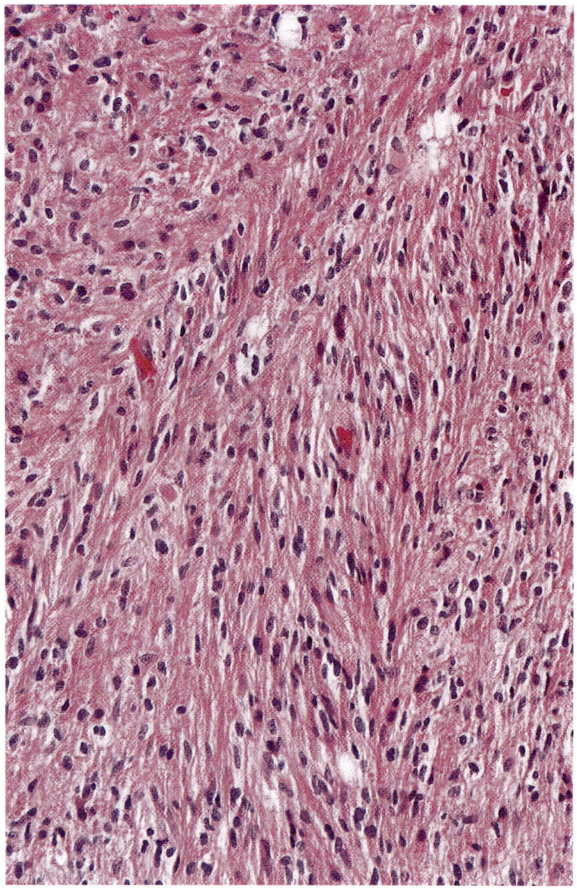

Fig. 9.290 Anaplastic astrocytoma assuming pilocytic character in splenium of the corpus callosum. H&E, × 250

As already recounted (p. 329), these various cellular aggregates were interpreted by Scherer as manifestations of early anaplasia. On cytologic grounds, there is support for his argument, but this should perhaps be confined to the perineuronal, perivascular and surface formations. In connection with these foci of increased cellularity, especially those occurring along the subpial interfaces, it is important to note that, whereas Scherer specifically drew attention to their presence in infiltrating cerebral astrocytomas, they may also be found in oligodendrogliomas and cerebellar medulloblastomas. Their presence in oligodendrogliomas tends to support the interpretation that they are a preferential site in the migration of neoplastic cells.

In many gliomas, especially glioblastomas, the border of the tumor may be more clearly defined in certain parts than in others (Fig. 9.292). As Scherer (1940b) pointed out, some of the glioblastomas in

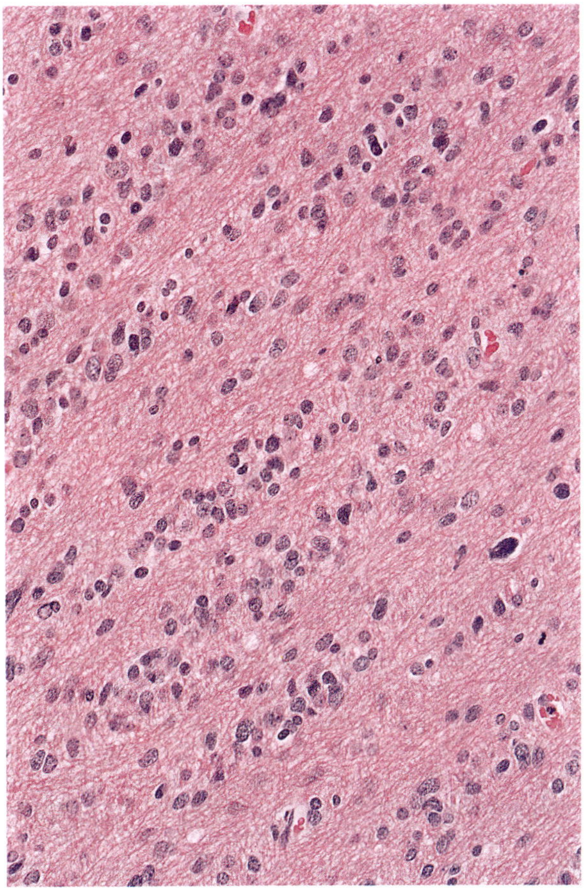

Fig. 9.291 Intrafascicular secondary structure in an anaplastic astrocytoma infiltrating the corpus callosum. H&E, × 250

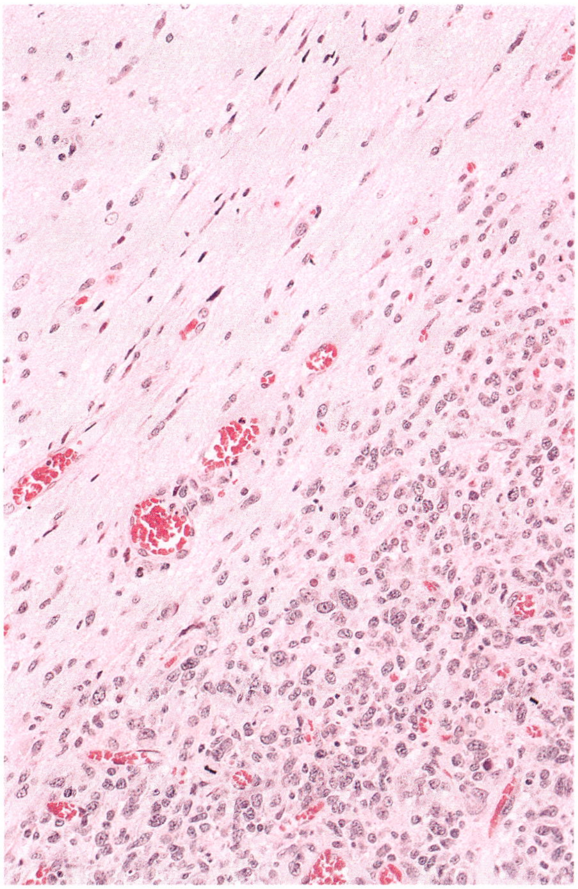

Fig. 9.292 Deceptively well-defined edge of a glioblastoma with the surrounding brain. H&E, × 250

the subcortical white matter may be sharply limited by the cortex and do not invade it; or they may spread more diffusely in the white matter, throwing out digitate processes into the central parts of the adjacent convolutions. They may similarly respect the gray matter of the basal ganglia.

Diffuse growth is a characteristic of most cerebral astrocytomas and has already been emphasized (pp. 325 and 331). The most extreme example of this is gliomatosis cerebri.

The role of the extracellular matrix is becoming paramount in the investigation of glioma invasion. Studies have implicated the serine proteases, their inhibitors, the integrins, and cell motility in glioma migration and grades of malignancy (Gladson and Cheresh, 1991; Rao *et al.*, 1993; De Clerck *et al.*, 1994; Mohanam *et al.*, 1994; Giese *et al.*, 1995; Paulus and Tonn, 1995). The failure to invade basement membranes and vascular walls may involve the different matrix components of gliomas and the absence of appropriate degradative substances in the glioma cellular repertoire.

The monoclonal origin of gliomas can be reconciled with the apparent multicentricity of some of these tumors and the diffuse nature of gliomatosis cerebri if we accept the current postulate that neoplastic transformation results from a progressive series of multiple step-like mutational events (Vogelstein and Kinzler, 1993). Should the first of these events be initiated in a single clone of the still mitotically active neuroepithelial cells before the end of their migration in the CNS, then it is quite conceivable that, after one or more stages of latency, the subsequent events necessary for tumor promotion will involve the multiple and distantly separated descendants of the originally targeted cells. The topographic separation of the cell progeny within the brain would then result in apparent glioma multicentricity, in distinct multiple gliomas, or even in extremely diffuse forms of glioma.

In the process of direct spread through the CNS, the cells of a glioma penetrate the neural parenchyma, and the cell bodies of the host tissues, both glial and neuronal, are incorporated in the margins of the tumor. The host cells may later be destroyed, although in some instances, notably in the diffuse cerebral astrocytomas, they remain preserved. Entrapped normal neurons can often be identified, even relatively deeply, within a glioma. Permeation of the lumen of blood vessels, including the capillaries, is, for practical purposes, never found as long as the tumor remains confined to the neural parenchyma (Bernstein and Woodard, 1995). This is evidently a major reason why remote extraneural metastases occur only in rare circumstances. Although glioma cells are prone to invade the superficial pia mater, they relatively seldom transgress the outer border of the perivascular spaces. When invasion of the Virchow-Robin spaces occurs, the affected blood vessels are generally those within the confines of the tumor. The cells show little tendency to spread further afield, nor do they breach the walls of the encircled blood vessels. It is still not clear why the cells of some gliomas, and not of others, are able to break through the pia–glial membrane of the perivascular spaces. This feature is not necessarily an expression of increased malignancy as judged by the usual cytologic criteria, for it can be seen in benign cerebellar and low-grade cerebral astrocytomas. However, those examples in which it is most often found have been diffuse astrocytomas with foci of anaplasia, and these tumors have also displayed a marked tendency to invade the leptomeninges. In the example illustrated in Fig. 9.293, a cuff of tumor lies outside the pia–glial membrane, from which bridges can be traced into the infiltrated Virchow-Robin spaces, with local interruption of the limiting reticulin partition.

Another exceptional form of astrocytic glioma is one in which the growth consists of a diffuse neoplastic proliferation, either subpial or subependymal, without any well-defined tumor mass. Microscopically, one or more small foci of glioblastoma may be demonstrable. A feature of these two variants is their respective aptitude for early invasion of the subarachnoid spaces or ventricular cavities. Examples of the first category may be mistaken for cases of primary leptomeningeal gliomatosis.

Local meningeal spread

Any glioma presenting at the surface of the brain is likely to invade the adjacent leptomeninges (Fig. 9.294). This feature bears little relation to the intrinsic histologic malignancy of the tumor. The cerebellar astrocytomas are particularly prone to this development, which, however, does not seem to affect their biologic behavior (Figs 9.295 and 9.296). Indeed, Herpers, Budka and McCormick (1984) have drawn attention to the apparently greater degree of differentiation to be noted even in anaplastic astrocytic tumor cells when they invade the meninges or the connective tissues, as shown by their relatively increased amounts of GFAP compared with the main body of the neoplasm (Fig. 9.297). The immunoreactivity of the tumor cells for GFAP is also often increased in the perivascular zones, and it is therefore possible that, in some way, contact with mesenchymal tissues is a factor that may induce the increased production of GFAP by

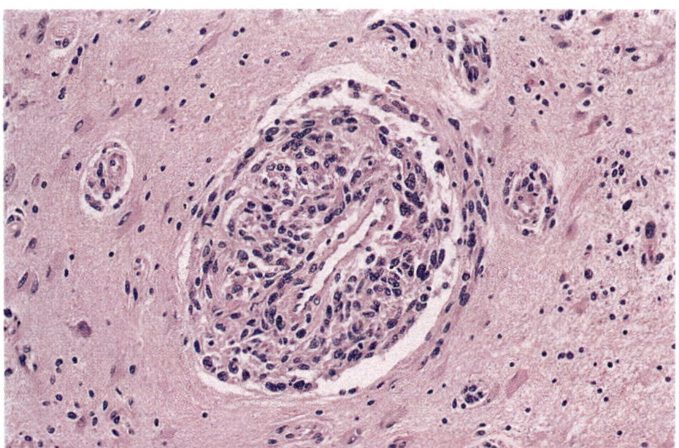

Fig. 9.293 Tumor cells of anaplastic astrocytoma filling the Virchow-Robin space and extending to form an outer, perivascular zone. H&E, × 250

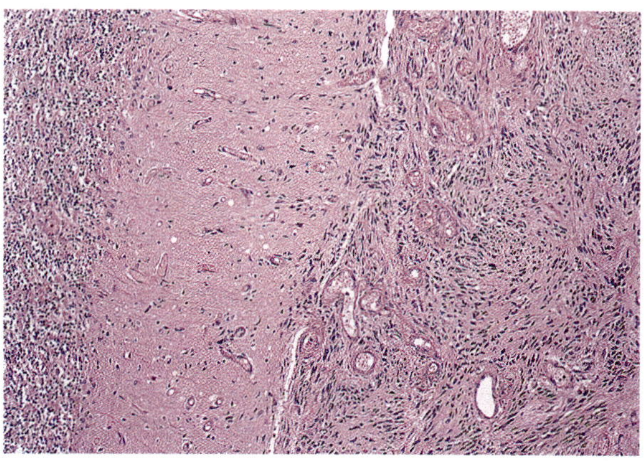

Fig. 9.294 Invasion of the cerebellar leptomeninges by tumor cells of a glioblastoma. H&E, × 125

glial tumor cells. The hypothesis gains support from the experimental work of Rutka *et al.* (1987, 1988), who found that cultures from an anaplastic glioma cell line became more differentiated and increased their GFAP production 20-fold when they were grown on an extracellular matrix enriched with laminin, fibronectin, types I and IV collagen and procollagen III. Glioma cell proliferation was also

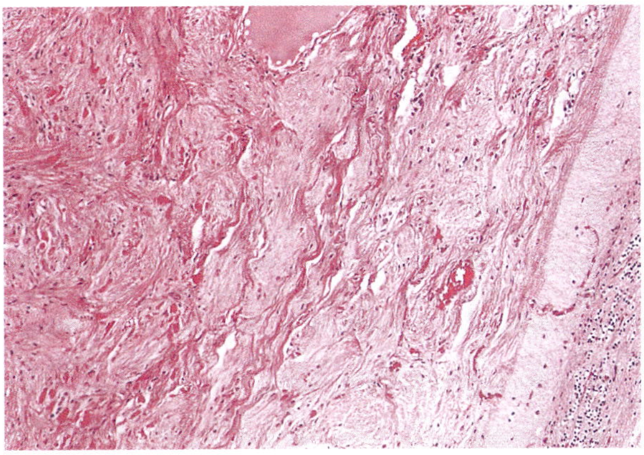

a

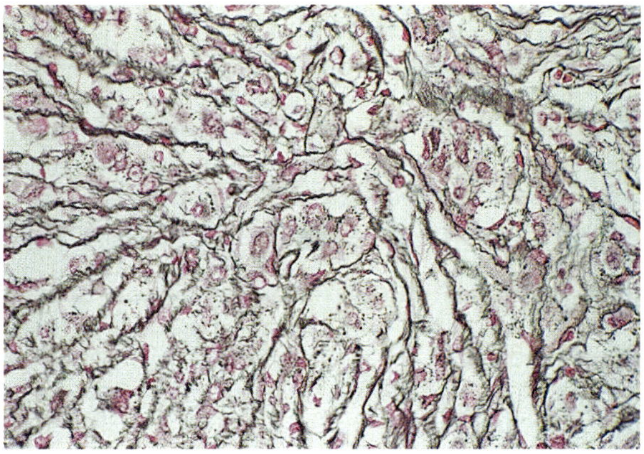

b

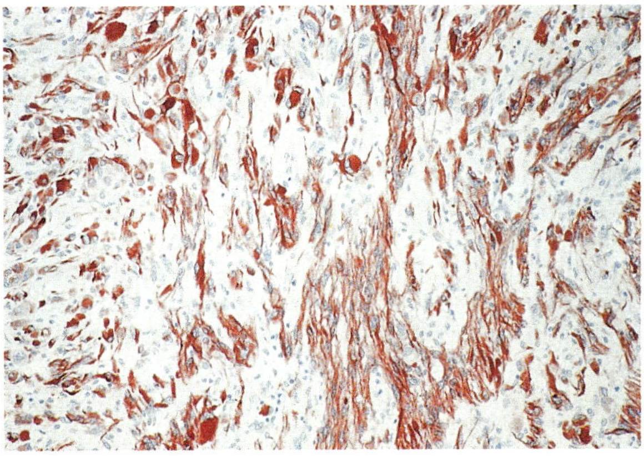

c

Fig. 9.295 (a) Cerebellar astrocytoma invading the subarachnoid space. H&E, × 125. (b) Same tumor. Leptomeningeal reticulin fibers intimately related to invading astrocytoma, highlighted by stain for reticulin. Reticulin stain, × 275 (c) Same tumor. Leptomeningeal invasion by cerebellar astrocytoma. Positive reactivity for GFAP in tumor cells with absence of reaction in intervening leptomeningeal collagen and fibroblasts. GFAP immunoperoxidase and hematoxylin, × 125

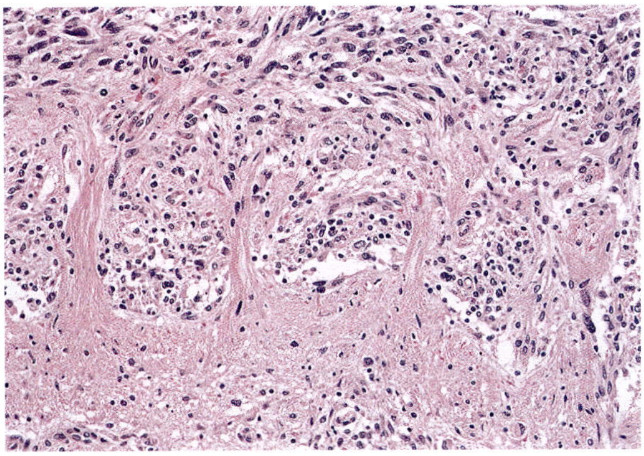

Fig. 9.296 Reinvasion of astrocytoma of temporal lobe from leptomeninges into brain. H&E, × 250

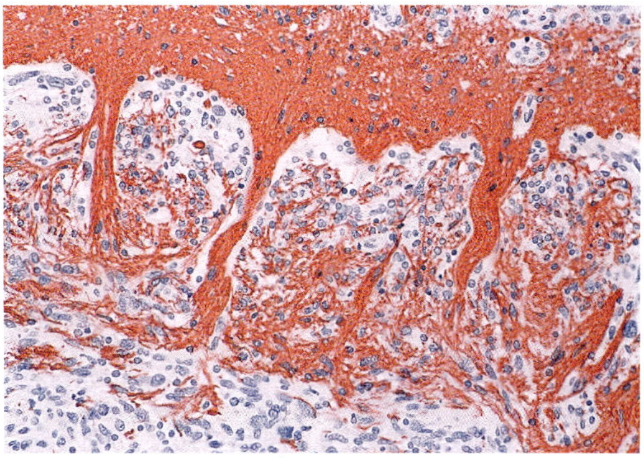

Fig. 9.297 Immunoperoxidase stain for GFAP emphasizes dense fibrillarity of astrocytoma reinvading brain. GFAP immunoperoxidase and hematoxylin, × 250

inhibited. On the other hand, the cerebellar medulloblastoma provides an example of the reverse phenomenon, namely one in which local meningeal infiltration accompanies extreme malignancy and constitutes one of the factors leading to cerebrospinal metastases.

In the progress of local leptomeningeal spread, the surface of the brain, at points beyond the confines of the primary growth, may be reinvaded by a reversal of the process (Fig. 9.298). Secondary reinvasion, with the resulting production of an apparently separate focus of tumor, has been observed in several examples of glioblastoma multiforme as a sequel to infiltration of the leptomeninges (Figs 9.296 and 9.297).

Neoplastic infiltration of the pia mater in the depths of a sulcus is rather readily followed by invasion of the cortex of the opposite convolution (Fig. 9.298). Re-entry of tumor cells into the brain tissue may accompany the perforating vessels, but this process is more often independent of these vessels and takes the form of an irregular subpial zone with finger-like projections into the deeper tissues (Figs. 9.296 and 9.297).

Both the glioblastomas and anaplastic astrocytomas may proceed further to gain an attachment to the adjacent dura mater. This union, although usually firm, does not lead to any alteration of the stout collagenous layers of the dura and, microscopically, infiltration by tumor cells accompanied by a fibroblastic and capillary proliferation is confined to the thin inner layer. In conformity with this, the optic nerve gliomas, as already noted (p. 367), have a remarkable tendency to infiltrate and expand the sheath of Schwalbe, but do not penetrate the dura (see Fig. 9.84).

As related elsewhere (p. 450), the extension of a glioblastoma into the lumen of a large dural venous sinus is exceptional (Kleinschmidt-Demasters, 1996). Rubinstein (1959) reported a case of cerebellar medulloblastoma with extracranial metastases, in which microscopic invasion of several dural veins from a large retro-orbital deposit was clearly demonstrated. A similar phenomenon has been noted to occur, in the lower spinal dura, in two cases of malignant metastasizing brainstem glioma, by Kepes *et al.* (1976). Direct spontaneous transdural extension by a glioblastoma or an anaplastic astrocytoma is exceptional (Kawano *et al.*, 1977; Shuangshoti, Kasantikul and Suwanwela, 1987).

Reactive proliferation is also found, in variable degrees, where the leptomeninges are invaded by tumor cells. As a result, the latter become subdivided into groups through the multiplication of benign fibroblasts that deposit a network of reticulin and collagen fibers [Fig. 9.295(b)]. The extent and density of the fibers vary greatly from case to case and doubtless are an expression of the age of the lesion. Yet it is surprising, in view of the acknowledged malignancy and rapid growth of the medulloblastomas, that the density of the collagen may, in some examples, be greater than that seen in many of the cerebellar astrocytomas. Curious linear and whorled patterns result from the alignment of the tumor cells with the interfibrillary spaces (Fig. 9.299) and these patterns are characteristic of the desmoplastic variant of medulloblastoma, considered in greater detail on p. 469. A similar picture may also be found in invasive cerebral glioblastomas, although a sparser network of delicate reticulin is more usual [Figs. 9.295(a) and (b)]. A differential diagnostic problem may indeed

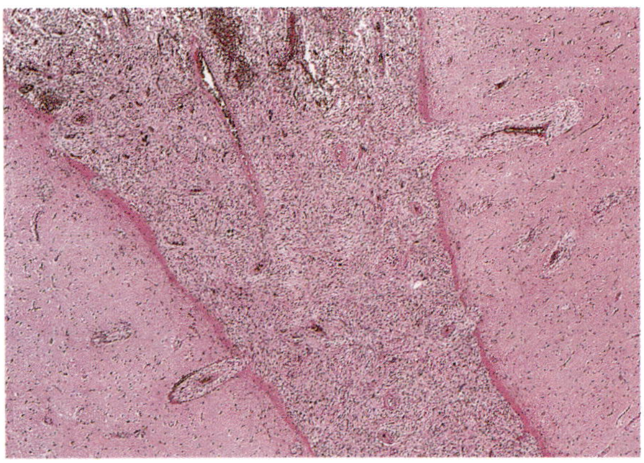

Fig. 9.298 Sulcus filled with leptomeningeal tumor. Both sides of the sulcus show reinvasion along perivascular spaces. H&E, × 50

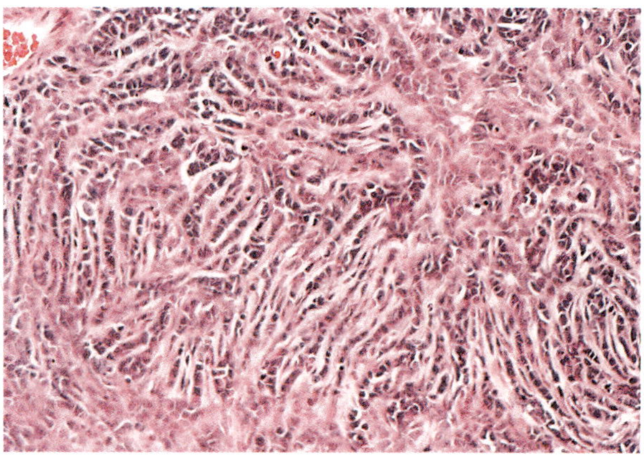

Fig. 9.299 Infiltration of the leptomeninges by medulloblastoma. H&E, × 250

be raised in those examples of cerebral astrocytoma that present largely as exophytic (i.e., apparently extracerebral) growths, where the shape of the tumor cells (Fig. 9.300) and the abundance of the intercellular reticulin network evoked by these cells may, at first, invite the interpretation of a meningioma; it is in such cases that the demonstration of GFAP in the cells occupying the leptomeninges is of considerable assistance in establishing the diagnosis.

The CNS provides several examples of such exophytic growths in which the extent of intraparenchymal tumor involvement may be relatively slight or even minimal. These include the optic nerve gliomas, the desmoplastic medulloblastomas of adolescents and young adults, the pleomorphic xanthoastrocytomas and the desmoplastic infantile gangliogliomas. Many examples of so-called 'primary leptomeningeal astrocytoma' may be superficial gliomas in which a narrow zone of neoplastic proliferation in the superficial part of the cortical molecular layer has escaped detection. In other instances, the primary site remains undiscovered until autopsy (Davila *et al.*, 1993).

The conspicuous proliferation of connective tissue elements that accompanies subarachnoid invasion by glial tumor cells may not remain confined to the meninges, but, in many glioblastomas of the cerebral convexities, tends to spread into the subjacent tumor. The superficial parts of the latter can, therefore, as indicated on p. 428, macroscopically mimic a meningioma, especially when firm adhesion to the dura has been established. The deposition of reticulin and collagen fibers in the zone of attachment toughens the consistency of the tumor, and the sampling of tissue from this region for diagnostic biopsy should therefore be avoided due to the confusing microscopic appearances. The latter may become even more difficult when, as occasionally happens, the proliferating meningeal cells have themselves acquired neoplastic features, with the production of a mixed glioblastoma and sarcoma. This event is, however, distinctly rare, and Rubinstein mentions only one such case (Russell and Rubinstein, 1989, p. 430).

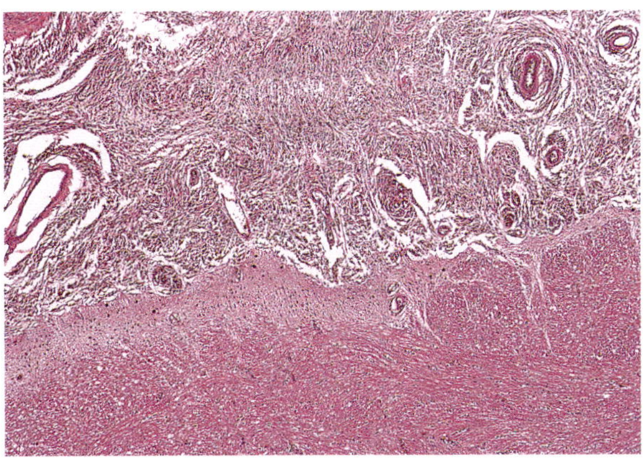

Fig. 9.300 Primary leptomeningeal astrocytoma in a 54-year-old man. No evidence of a parenchymal component was discovered with MRI of the craniospinal axis. H&E, × 50

Local ependymal spread

Replacement of the ependyma of the ventricular system by growth also results from the direct spread of infiltrating gliomas (see Fig. 9.301). Before the surface is reached, the local ependymal cells often acquire long fibrillated processes (p. 451), concomitant with the development of immunopositivity for GFAP. In some situations the encroachment of the tumor may obstruct the flow of CSF and lead

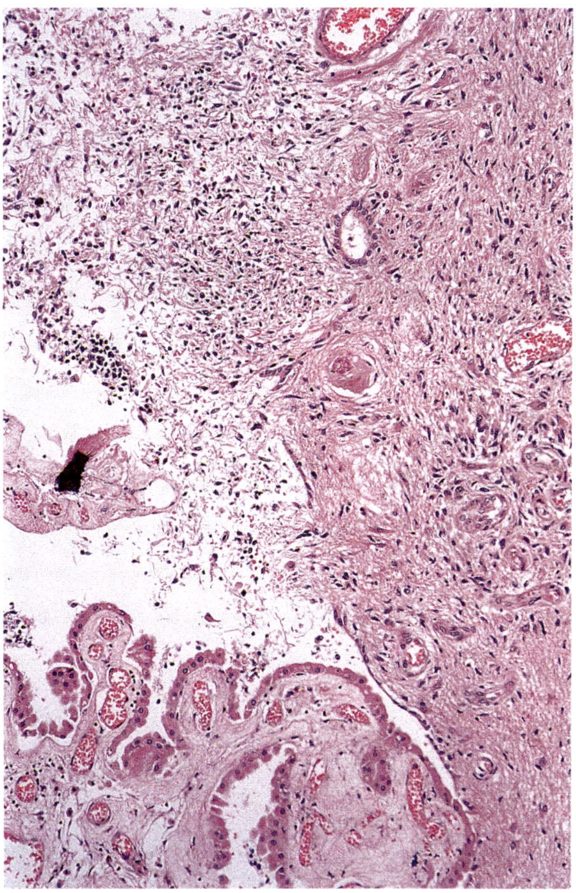

Fig. 9.301 Glioblastoma invading the ventricle with penetration of the ependymal layer. H&E, × 125

to internal hydrocephalus; e.g., astrocytomas of the quadrigeminal plate and the medulloblastomas that occlude the fourth ventricle.

An important consequence of ependymal infiltration is the development of metastases via the CSF.

METASTASIS BY THE CEREBROSPINAL FLUID

When the ependymal epithelium is breached, the way is clear for the shedding of tumor cells into the ventricular fluid (Fig. 9.302). Many of these cells are probably not viable, as shown by the autoradiographic studies by Shinozaki (1981) on the labeling indices of clusters of ventricular and subependymal tumor cells induced in the rat by the human adenovirus type 12. Presumably, such degenerated and dead cells are phagocytosed by the arachnoidal cells. However, it is well recognized that some of the viable tumor cells that have penetrated beyond the ependyma and been carried by the CSF can become sequestered and attached at distant points, either ependymal or leptomeningeal, and here proliferate to form true metastases.

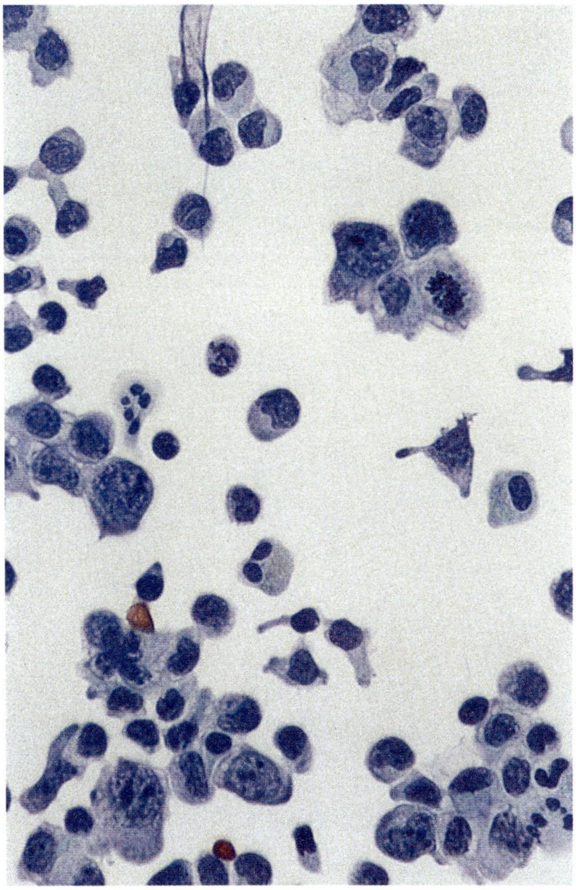

Fig. 9.302 Tumor cells of anaplastic astrocytoma in CSF. Papanicolaou stain, × 500

Secondary deposits can arise in the ependyma or the leptomeninges, or both together, or consecutively. Their incidence in those sites, when the factors favorable to metastasis are present, cannot be predicted in the individual case, but both the older observations in this regard (Cairns and Russell, 1931) and the more recent analyses by Erlich and Davis (1978), Yung, Horten and Shapiro (1980), Friede, Janzer and Roessmann (1982), Nishio *et al.* (1982), Kandt *et al.* (1984), Awad, Bay and Rogers (1986), Onda *et al.*, (1989), Vertosick and Selker (1990) and Grabb, Albright and Pang (1992) all indicate that cerebrospinal metastases from gliomas of different types are more common than is generally realized. In their large series of supratentorial glioblastomas or other anaplastic gliomas from the neuro-oncology service of the University of California in San Francisco, Choucair *et al.* (1986) estimated the development of cerebrospinal metastases to occur in 5–9% of the patients. In general, this is seen as a relatively late complication (Vertosick and Selker, 1990; Schwaninger *et al.*, 1992). It might be surmised that with intraventricular growths, ependymal metastases would predominate numerically. But this is seldom true and, indeed, the metastases may be wholly meningeal. It is apparent that the healthy, intact and ciliated ependymal surface does not readily permit the attachment of loosely circulating tumor cells. However, in the presence of obstructive hydrocephalus, the factors of stagnation and damage to the ependyma are more favorable to implantation. This is well exemplified by occlusive medulloblastomas in the fourth ventricle when the soft, friable character of the tumor supplies the additional conditions that are needed (Cairns and Russell, 1931). Likewise, Nishio *et al.* (1982) have stressed that local ependymal defects—which, while present also in normal brains, occur more often and more widely in obstructive hydrocephalus—will favor the implantation and growth of ventricular deposits. Another factor that may be more significant than the intrinsic benign or malignant character of the primary tumor is its texture, which partly depends on the degree of adhesiveness between the tumor cells. This is illustrated not only by the metastatic tendencies of medulloblastomas (Jennings *et al.*, 1993), but also in some examples of oligodendroglioma (Pitt *et al.*, 1992). The firm and circumscribed ependymomas arising in the region of the fourth ventricle show little tendency to metastasize, although the conditions are, in all other respects, highly favorable. The problem is further complicated by the fact that successful implantation of tumor cells that have seeded in the cerebrospinal pathways may be promoted or modified by other factors that are still poorly understood. Thus, attempts to correlate the clinical incidence of tumor cell dispersion in the CSF with the satellite colony-forming ability of tumors *in vitro* on the basis of reduced cellular adhesiveness have not been conclusive (Batzdorf and Gold, 1974). Even clinically and histologically low-grade supratentorial astrocytomas or benign cerebellar pilocytic astrocytomas can demonstrate diffuse or nodular CSF dissemination (Mishima *et al.*, 1992; Pollack *et al.*, 1994; Gajjar *et al.*, 1995). This does not preclude long-term survival for these patients since some of these disseminated deposits show low proliferative rates and may not grow demonstrably over time.

It might, again, be anticipated that when the primary tumor impinges directly on the basal cisterns or on the adjacent leptomeninges, the way would be paved for meningeal metastasis, with relative sparing of the ventricular ependyma. Although this is the sequel in some cases, it is also true that ventricular metastases may be found. The ebb and flow in the circulation of the CSF has long been known to permit the ascent of particulate matter from the meninges to the ventricles, even when the pathways are anatomically normal, e.g., in the early stages of purulent leptomeningitis (Cairns and Russell, 1946). In a case previously reported by Russell (1949), miliary nodules of metastatic glioma were found in the walls of the fourth, and a few in the third, ventricles as the result of leptomeningeal spread from an intramedullary oligodendroglioma of the cervical cord. Since any diffuse cellular infiltration of the basal meninges will produce internal hydrocephalus in proportion to its density and duration, this development will further facilitate the ascent of tumor cells to the ventricles from an extracerebral neoplasm. It is therefore appropriate to mention here the importance of examining the spinal cord whenever gliomatosis of the cerebral leptomeninges cannot clearly be accounted for and to recall that a malignant spinal intramedullary glioma may be a primary source of intracranial subarachnoid and ventricular seeding (Mallory, 1908; Eade and Urich, 1971).

A number of well-documented cases of primary leptomeningeal gliomatosis have now been reported, both in the brain and in the spinal cord (Ramsay, Goshko and Nag, 1990; Giordana *et al.*, 1995). They may be of either astrocytic or oligodendroglial morphology (Chen, MacDonald and Ramsay 1995; Rogers *et al.*, 1995) (see p. 514).

Several publications (Eden, 1938; O'Connell, 1946; Andrews *et al.*, 1978; Maria *et al.*, 1986; Johnson and Schwarz, 1987) have established the capacity of tumors arising in the caudal segments of the spinal cord and even of the conus medullaris, as recorded of an astrocytoma at this site by Perese, Slepian and Nigogosyan (1959), to metastasize via the CSF to the intracranial cavity (Fig. 9.303).

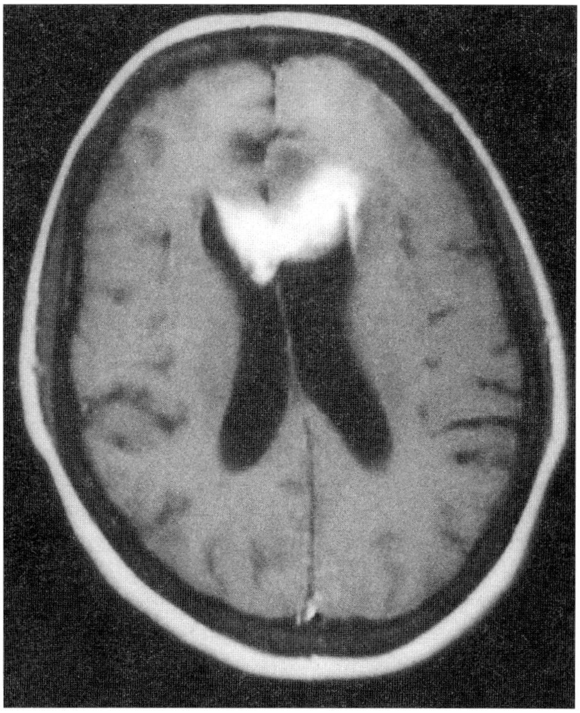

Fig. 9.303 An MRI of supratentorial spread of primary spinal cord glioblastoma. This 30-year-old woman was diagnosed with a thoracic spinal cord glioblastoma 5 months before this scan showed periventricular enhancing tumor in the brain.

Finally, we should note that such an ascending mode of spread is not necessarily restricted to histologically malignant gliomas. Rubinstein and Logan (1970) reported the development of a metastatic fourth-ventricle deposit 6 years after incomplete surgical removal of a slowly growing papillary ependymoma of the cauda equina.

Sites involved and macroscopic appearance

Ependyma

In some examples of cerebral glioblastoma, the ventricular ependyma may be profusely peppered with minute nodular metastases, an appearance that earned the title of *ependymitis blastomatosa*

(Hasenjäger, 1938). More often, the deposits are confined to recesses where the eddying of the CSF helps the deposition of cells. The ventricular horns and the supraoptic and infundibular recesses of the third ventricle are common sites.

The metastases are readily recognized as dome-shaped nodules, often with smooth surfaces, that project from the ependyma. Those derived from medulloblastomas are more soft and friable; they may be confluent, especially in the walls of the third ventricle, and, through direct invasion, structures such as the fornix and the septum pellucidum may be extensively destroyed. In examples where the basal leptomeninges are extensively infiltrated, it should be recalled that the central parts of the brain can also be reached following invasion of the tela choroidea.

The degree to which ependymal implantations lead to neoplastic infiltration of the subjacent tissues varies greatly. It is often slight, with the proliferating cells rather heaped on the surface. But, in glioblastomas (Fig. 9.304), and occasionally in medulloblastomas, an active and massive invasion of the brain parenchyma may follow, superficially mimicking the appearances of a multifocal glioma. In rare cases, the ependymal spread may be in the nature of a continuous film over the ventricular surface, as in the metastasizing oligodendrogliomas reported by Blumenfeld and Gardner (1945), where the tumor formed a gelatinous and hemorrhagic lining throughout the ventricles. Finally, in some instances, the ventricular metastases may form a remarkably thick confluent coat of creamy gelatinous tissue that completely replaces the ependymal and subependymal layers and narrows the ventricular cavities, as illustrated in Fig. 9.304, from a left thalamic glioblastoma that had ruptured into the temporal horn.

Meninges

Metastatic deposits of gliomas have a predilection for the basal leptomeninges of the brain and the dorsal aspect of the spinal cord. The factors governing their distribution are the normal flow of the CSF, the existence of recesses in the subarachnoid space where the tumor cells can gain a foothold and, to some extent, the influence of gravity.

Brain

Cells reaching the basal leptomeninges by way of the foramina of Luschka and Magendie are likely to be caught up in the meshes adjacent to the basal cisterns and, in parts where these are related to the nerve roots, often in the cerebellopontine angles. Nodular deposits on these roots are common. Even

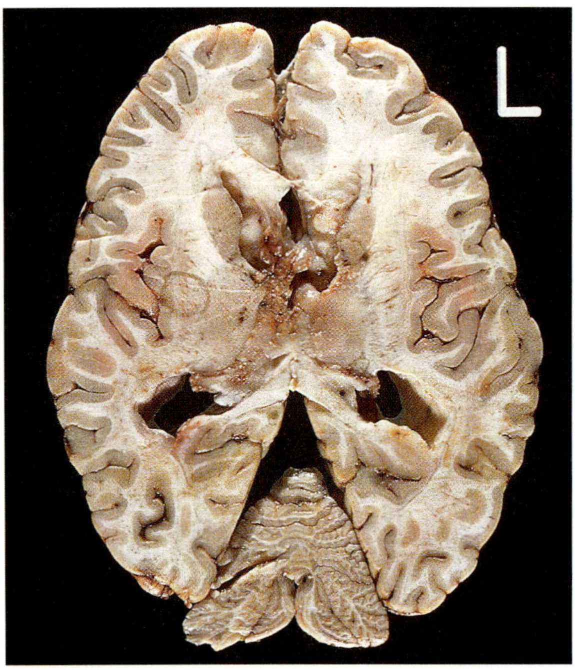

Fig. 9.304 Thick coating of tumor in a patient with a left thalamic glioblastoma after rupture into the ventricular system.

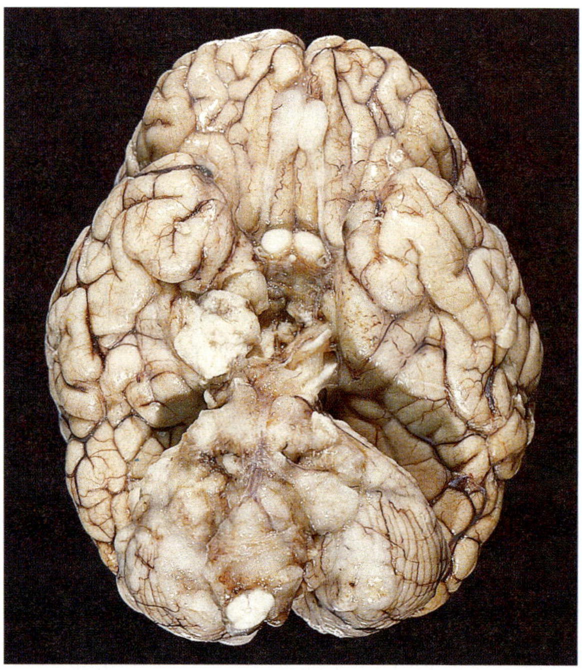

Fig. 9.305 Same case as Fig. 9.304. Extensive cerebrospinal dissemination of glioblastoma. The basal aspects of the brainstem are covered by tumor.

more common is the formation of diffuse sheets of growth beneath the arachnoid membrane that obscure the main blood vessels and other structures. The appearances vary from a faint opalescence to thick layers of dense opacity, as demonstrated over the floor of the third ventricle and the basal aspect of the brainstem in Fig. 9.305. These formations are due to the direct spread of growth from metastatic foci, and some of them are, presumably, the result of the confluence of initially separate deposits. With medulloblastomas or other tumors, such as malignant brainstem astrocytomas, that impinge directly upon the basal cisterns, it is often impossible to determine how much of the meningeal growth is due to direct spread from the primary neoplasm; the same is true of retinoblastomas that extend back to the optic chiasm. But, often, leptomeningeal dissemination presents, in addition, as more discrete foci of subarachnoid growth scattered over the cerebral and cerebellar convexities. They are identified as flat areas of variable opacity, obscuring the subjacent sulci and blood vessels. On sectioning, the growth is seen to penetrate into the sulci, causing adhesion of the opposing convolutions.

Microscopically, there is a leptomeningeal reaction, as already described in the local spread of primary gliomas, which varies with the duration of the condition. The propensity of the proliferating tumor cells to reinvade the brain varies widely and, to some extent, is proportionate to the rapidity of the growth and to the intrinsic malignancy of the tumor. Extensive reinvasion may be anticipated in many of the medulloblastomas, the more malignant of the metastasizing oligodendrogliomas and in some examples of glioblastoma. It has also been seen in retinoblastoma (Cairns and Russell, 1931, case 2). The cerebral surface may then be penetrated in an irregular manner over wide areas, and tongues of cells originating from these penetrations may extend into the deeper layers. In some cases, invasion appears restricted to the adventitial sheaths of the perforating blood vessels and to the immediately adjacent neural tissue (Fig. 9.296). Although, as indicated above, such behavior is especially associated with the more malignant gliomas, reinvasion of the neural parenchyma by a histologically benign metastasizing astrocytoma may also occur.

Spinal cord

Spinal subarachnoid spread usually accompanies cerebral meningeal metastasis; in some instances, the cord is selectively involved. Evidence should be sought especially on the dorsal aspect, and all levels down to the tip of the cauda equina need to be scrutinized because metastasis may be restricted to the extreme caudal end. The predominance of deposits in this part of the neuraxis is due to the effect of gravity.

The manifestations are either *diffuse* or *nodular*. In the most extreme examples, the whole of the cord and its roots are obscured by a continuous mass of tumor that distends the arachnoid membrane and is of maximal thickness dorsally; the nerve roots may appear considerably thickened and enveloped by the confluent growth (Fig. 9.306). Much of this may be due to direct spread when secondary to a medulloblastoma of the posterior vermis. Yet, in these cases, it is not infrequently found that the layer of growth is interrupted at one or more points, especially in the upper thoracic segments, and it is then evident that the process of diffuse secondary spread is a combination of multiple focal metastases and tertiary direct spread from these deposits.

Patches of diffuse spread may also be combined with more discrete nodules of growth. The latter are often situated on the posterior roots, either at their

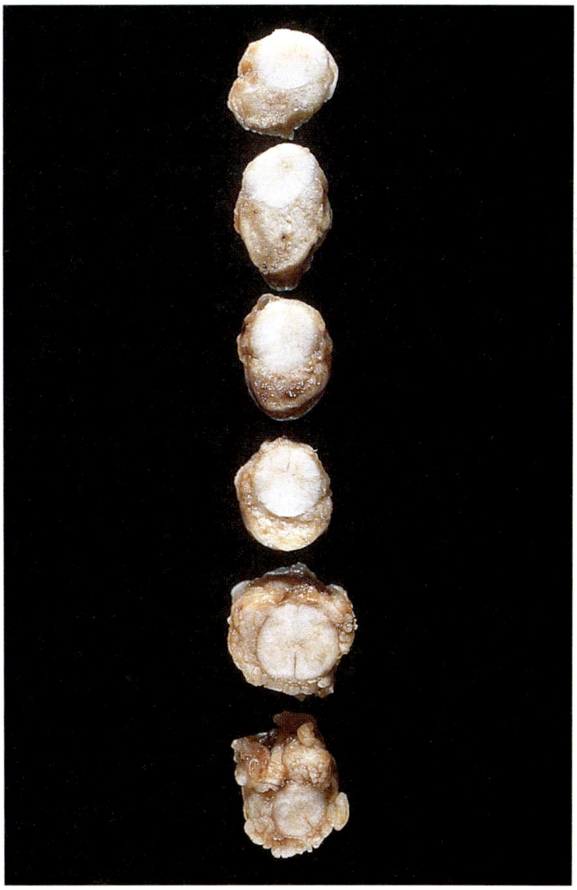

Fig. 9.306 Same case as Fig. 9.304. Diffuse metastatic glioblastoma coating the spinal cord and nerve roots.

junction with the spinal cord or at the point where they pass outwards through the arachnoid membrane. They also favor the roots of the cauda equina, which are then matted together by the growth. Although, in general, these nodules are seldom more than a few millimeters in diameter, they occasionally attain a sufficient size to cause neurologic symptoms and may then dominate the clinical picture. A series of 18 cases in which spinal metastases were the clinical mode of presentation, and which included 11 medulloblastomas, 3 glioblastomas and 2 anaplastic astrocytomas, was recorded from the files of the Armed Forces Institute of Pathology by Pezeshkpour, Henry and Armbrustmacher (1984). A recent series of note is that of 11 patients, described by Vertosick and Selker (1990), with spread of supratentorial glioblastoma to the brainstem and spinal cord. The patients in this series had a mean age of 38.5 years. An additional case of an intramedullary spinal cord metastasis from a supratentorial glioblastoma in the absence of diffuse CSF dissemination is described by Hamilton, Tranmer and Hagen (1993). There was no evidence of supratentorial recurrence at the time.

The *cellular morphology* of these metastases bears a general resemblance to the parent growth (Fig. 9.302), but the architectural features of the latter may be lost. Thus, the rosettes of retinoblastomas and medulloblastomas are seldom found in the metastases. In the glioblastomas, the metastatic foci may display a greater degree of histologic anaplasia than the primary growth. For example, a cerebral tumor may be largely of pilocytic character due to the penetration by the cells of the nerve fiber bundles of the white matter. But, the spinal metastases may display extreme cellular polymorphism, including many multinucleated giant cells. On the other hand, the metastases in glioblastomas may appear more astrocytic and differentiated than the parent tumor (Cairns and Russell, 1931, case 6). It is as though the conditions of growth in the subarachnoid space and the liberation of the neoplastic cells from environmental restrictions within the cerebrum allow a fuller display of the cells' morphologic potentialities, perhaps analogous with the behavior of such cells in tissue culture.

Reinvasion of the spinal cord with consequent destruction is variable, but is rarely conspicuous in glioblastomas, although it may be severe in medulloblastomas. The spinal nerve roots, on the other hand, are seldom spared (Fig. 9.307), even by tumors of relatively slower progression, if the metastatic growth happens to be of a diffuse character.

A further sequel of cerebrospinal spread is that it may open a secondary pathway for dissemination outside the central neuraxis: this may take place

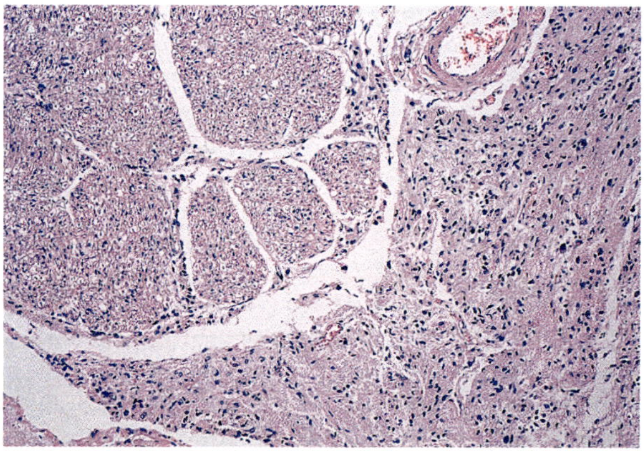

Fig. 9.307 Metastatic glioblastoma infiltrating the spinal leptomeninges and nerve roots. H&E, × 125

after local bony destruction that follows the development of metastatic deposits in the cauda equina or over the orbital aspect of the frontal lobes, as in medulloblastomas, or through neoplastic permeation of the spinal nerve roots as they egress from their meningeal sleeves, or as a consequence of direct dural transgression by intrathecal metastatic growth, with secondary invasion of the epidural space. Matsumoto *et al.* (1987) recorded the unusual development of a sacral epidural metastasis from a mixed cerebral astrocytoma and oligodendroglioma, but in which neither myelography nor examination of the spinal fluid provided any evidence of intradural tumor. In this case, therefore, hematogenous metastasis to the perineurial tissue or to the epidural space was postulated to have occurred, although no evidence in favor of such a hypothesis was available.

REMOTE METASTASES

The development of extraneural metastases in malignant gliomas, a rare event, has been extensively documented over the past four decades, and some of Rubinstein's observations have been related in earlier editions of this book (Russell and Rubinstein, 1977, 341–5). General reviews that provide clinical and other details of large series of cases include those of Smith, Hardman and Earle (1969a), who analyzed a series of 35 cases from the files of the Armed Forces Institute of Pathology that comprised 23 glioblastomas and 8 medulloblastomas; of Pasquier *et al.* (1980), who reviewed the clinicopathologic aspects of 72 reported cases of glioblastoma and malignant astrocytoma; of Kleinman, Hochberg and Richardson (1981), who systematically listed the clinical and pathologic features of 103 recorded examples of cerebellar medulloblastoma; and of Liwnicz and Rubinstein (1979), who more specifically directed their attention to the pathways of spread leading to distant dissemination and to the relationship that can be established between the sites of exit of the primary growths or their intra-axial metastases, on the one hand, and the site of original tumor resection, on the other. This section is organized to examine the anatomic factors that pave the way for such a complication, its relationship to previous craniectomy procedures and to the artificial opening of routes of spread by diversionary shunting operations, the different types and frequency of tumors with which it is associated, and the topographic distribution of the deposits in relation to the respective glioma types. Additional details will be found in the relevant sections of the text where the metastatic behavior of the various forms of central neuroepithelial tumor is reviewed.

Factors contributing to the production of extraneural metastases

The increased recording of this occurrence in the past 20 years, now estimated to approach 20–25 cases per 5-year period (Cerame, Guthikonda and Kohli, 1985), may partly reflect the overall improved survival rate of patients with malignant gliomas who have been treated by surgical resection and radiation therapy. However, as noted elsewhere (Liwnicz and Rubinstein, 1979), with the exception of a small number of patients with lower spinal ependymomas, usually of the myxopapillary variant, there is no definitive evidence that this sequel is associated with longer postoperative survival times in any specific type of glioma.

It is quite apparent that it is the acquired capacity of the glial tumor cells to permeate the blood vessels once they infiltrate the tissues outside the leptomeninges that probably constitutes the first step by which they are given access to, and are subsequently permitted to be maintained in, the extraneural tissues once they have become blood borne. Since glioblastoma cells have been demonstrated to have no propensity for intravasation into blood vessels (Bernstein and Woodard, 1995), the event that usually plays the major role in opening such an access is previous, sometimes repeated, *craniotomy*, leading to direct invasion of the extrameningeal tissues by the recurrent growth either at the craniectomy site or in some other region of the central neuraxis. Many of the earlier case reports point to the massive extracranial eruption of the tumor through the surgical defect as a preliminary to direct access to the lymphatics and to the blood vasculature outside the CNS.

Sites of tumor egress and pathways of extraneural spread

In several examples, there was involvement of the *cervical lymph nodes*, often secondary to nodular deposits in the scalp at the site of craniotomy and, presumably, resulting from local lymphatic permeation. Some of these lymph nodes have been the first sign of metastasis. Cases have been diagnosed by fine-needle aspiration cytology with immunohistologic confirmation (Gonzalez-Campora *et al.*, 1993). This was the sequence in the oligodendrogliomas reported by James and Pagel (1951) and by Cappelaere *et al.* (1972, cases 2 and 3), in the metastasizing ependymomas recorded by Maass (1954) and by Wen and Barrows (1957), and in the glioblastomas and anaplastic astrocytomas described by Labitzke (1962), Pasquier *et al.* (1980, cases 1 and 2) and Hoffman *et al.* (1981). On the other hand, as documented in several reports (see discussion in Rubinstein, 1967, for references), an equally important avenue has been shown to be opened in operated gliomas as a consequence of *venous permeation*, demonstrable either in a major dural sinus or in the smaller meningeal veins at the primary site, or in the distant metastases—usually the lungs. It is obvious, then, that surgical intervention will, in a number of instances, provide the path of entry for tumor cells into the systemic circulation, but the extent to which entry actually results in significant transport of viable neoplastic cells through the bloodstream is unclear. Claims that tumor cells can be demonstrated in the circulation at the time of, or immediately after, craniotomy have so far remained unconfirmed. What can be stated, however, is that the histologic demonstration of venous permeation by a glioma, while an exceptionally rare observation, should be regarded as a foreboding of distant dissemination. In summary, then, the classic well-established pathway of tumor exit that paves the way to remote spread is direct transdural extension into the soft tissues at the site of repeated operations, with demonstrable permeation of the veins by tumor cells in the immediately adjacent extracerebral sites.

There is also evidence that the pathway of entry of the tumor into the extrameningeal tissues may be unrelated to the actual craniectomy site. Notable in this context is the likelihood of the floor of the *middle fossa* to be the site of egress by tumor cells in cerebral glioblastomas, typically after temporal craniotomy, secondary to invasion and consequent destruction of the medial temporal bone (Liwnicz and Rubinstein, 1979, case 1; Pasquier *et al.*, 1980, case 2). As discussed in Chapter 18, p. 463, a determining factor in this development may be herniation of the cerebral cortex through the dura of the

Table 9.3 Sites of exit of tumor from the central neuraxis in 85 gliomas with extraneural metastases

Site of exit of glioma	Astrocytoma	Oligodendroglioma	Ependymoma	Glioblastoma	Medulloblastoma
Cranial convexity	5	3	10	8	0
Anterior fossa floor	1	0	0	3	1
Middle fossa floor	1	0	1	7	2
Posterior fossa	0	0	0	1	6
Spinal canal	2	1	6	1	6
Shunt	1	0	0	4	6
Unknown site	1	1	1	1	5

middle fossa as a result of continuously increased intracranial pressure, to which may be added herniation into the extradural spaces via the exits of the intracranial blood vessels and cranial nerve roots.

Another notable site of exit of tumor from the central neuraxis prior to the formation of extraneural deposits, in medulloblastoma this time, is the *vertebral column*, where it may follow invasion of the paravertebral tissues and retroperitoneal spaces by spinal arachnoid metastases (Liwnicz and Rubinstein, 1979, case 3; Jamjoom *et al.*, 1989). Again, in previously treated medulloblastomas that subsequently metastasized through the CSF, egress of the tumor cells may follow erosion of the floor of the *anterior fossa*, resulting in penetration of the orbital roof and ethmoid sinuses; this may be associated with neoplastic permeation of the frontal dural veins (Rubinstein, 1959). Liwnicz and Rubinstein (1979) analyzed a series of 85 reported cases with extraneural dissemination in which the sites of exit of tumor from the neuraxis had been documented. The findings are summarized in Table 9.3.

After excluding, from the cases collated above, the 11 examples with metastases reported till then to have developed after shunting procedures, and nine cases in which the sites of tumor exit could not be determined, they were able to assess, in the 65 remaining patients, the relationship between the site of egress of the glioma from the neuraxis and the original site of operation. As Fig. 9.308 indicates, with the exception of the gliomas originating in the posterior fossa, extrameningeal tumor extension at a site remote from the operative flap is at least as common as direct extension from the region of the flap itself. In summary, then, the mechanism paving the way to remote spread in many of those cases is spontaneous transdural extension either in the base of the skull or in the spinal canal at a site remote from prior operation. The obvious conclusion is that it is not so much the craniotomy itself that technically opens the immediate route for further spread as the late indirect sequel of the operation, as a result of which the survival of the patient is prolonged and the glioma cells are eventually permitted to gain access to extrameningeal sites wherever tumor recurrence takes place.

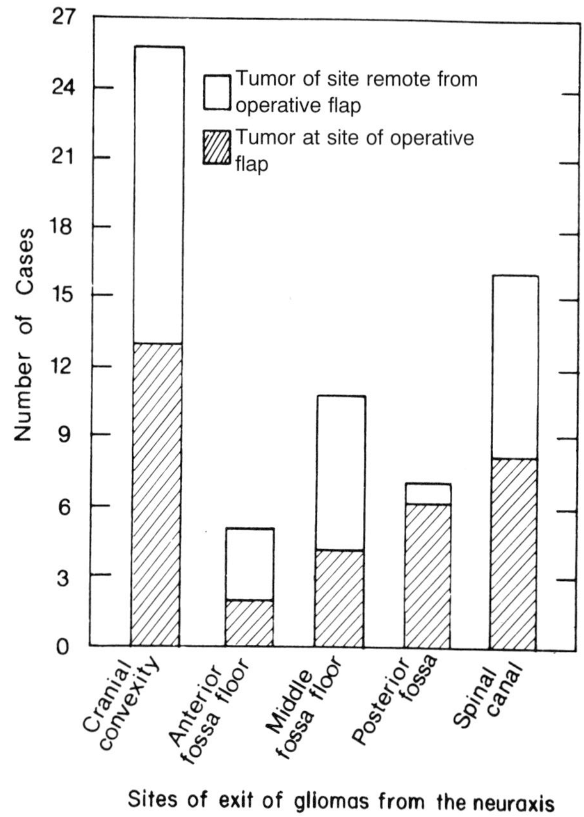

Fig. 9.308 Relationship between the glioma sites of exit from the central neuraxis and the original sites of operation in 65 reported cases. (From Liwnicz and Rubinstein, 1979, and reprinted from *Human Pathology*, 1979, pp. 453–467, figure 11, with kind permission of W.B. Saunders Company.)

Diversionary shunting procedures

Shunting procedures (ventriculopleural, ventriculoperitoneal, ventriculocaval or ventriculoatrial) for the relief of obstructive hydrocephalus in intracranial gliomas have been shown to be a notable potential route for tumor dissemination. Unlike the examples of extracranial spread following craniotomy, a prerequisite is the development of cerebrospinal metastases from the primary growth (Newton, Rosenblum and Walker, 1992). These authors reported two cases of peritoneal seeding of posterior fossa glioblastomas through ventriculoperitoneal shunts. The patients also had leptomeningeal gliomatosis involving the spinal cord and the base of the brain. In patients in whom a ventriculopleural shunt was implanted, the clinical presentation may be that of a massive terminal pleural effusion, as in the examples reported by Brust, Moiel and Rosenberg (1968), by Wakamatsu *et al.* (1971) and in the case described on p. 451.

As shown in Table 9.3, this development has most often been documented in medulloblastomas (see also Kleinman, Hochberg and Richardson, 1981; Hoffman and Duffner, 1985, Tables 2 and 3; Jamjoom *et al.*, 1993). After 41 decompressive ventriculoperitoneal shunting operations performed by Hoffman, Hendrick and Humphreys (1976) for cerebellar medulloblastoma, six of the patients eventually succumbed with systemic metastases, and in four of these the distribution of the metastatic spread, combined with the absence of local tumor recurrence and the initial presence of abdominal clinical manifestations, clearly implicated the shunt as the route of dissemination: in all four patients, the peritoneal surfaces were coated with medulloblastoma deposits. Bone marrow metastases were also found in all of these four patients. The high incidence of medulloblastoma in this category reflects both the frequency with which it metastasizes in the cerebrospinal pathways and the selection of these patients for such bypass operations: about one quarter of the patients with extraneural metastatic medulloblastoma (and one third of the childhood patients) had a diversionary systemic cerebrospinal shunt, according to Hoffman and Duffner (1985), who suggested that, if possible, preoperative diversionary procedures should be avoided or that an internal shunt should be placed to prevent the need for systemic diversion of the CSF. In patients in whom hydrocephalus progresses despite surgical resection of the tumor, they advocate that a filtering device be incorporated into the shunt.

Development of extraneural metastases prior to, or in the absence of, cranial surgery

The literature of recent years has recorded an increasing number of cases of malignant glioma in which extraneural metastases developed either prior to, or in the absence of, cranial surgical intervention. In some of these cases, as in the examples reported by Rubinstein (1967), Anzil (1970) and Shuangshoti, Kasantikul and Suwanwela (1987), and in the case briefly described on p. 450, transdural invasion had demonstrably taken place, with consequent permeation of the dural veins or sinuses by the growth. In several cases, spontaneous distant metastases also occurred (Brew and Garrick, 1987; Shuangshoti, Kasantikul and Suwanwela, 1987).

More exceptional have been the examples of spontaneously occurring metastases in which vascular permeation by neoplastic cells was demonstrated within the primary tumor: therefore, in its intrinsic vasculature. Such cases have been reported (Hulbanni and Goodman, 1976; Choi, Holt and McDonald, 1981; Ojeda and Sterrett, 1984), thus adding further support to the argument that the ability of the tumor cells to transgress the walls of the vasculature at the primary site is the most important of the sequential steps needed for the successful blood-borne dissemination of malignant gliomas and the development of overt metastatic deposits.

In other, again rare, instances, the presence of a cervical lymph node metastasis has been the first manifestation of an intracerebral neoplasm, as reported by Henriquez, Robertson and Marshall (1973) in a 7-year-old boy with a cerebral neuroblastoma, and by Dolman (1974) in a 35-year-old woman with a glioblastoma. Even more exceptional was the case of a 26-year-old woman who first presented with multiple osseous involvement by tumor cells (Fig. 9.248), originally interpreted as a myelosclerosis associated with an aleukemic leukemia, and who was found at necropsy to harbor a clinically silent cerebellar medulloblastoma (Pollak, Miller and Vye, 1981). Notable also is the case reported by Brander and Turner (1975), in which a mixed oligodendroglioma and astrocytoma had been clinically present for 12 years before the spontaneous development of multiple pleural metastases. Gamis *et al.* (1990) described an 11-year-old girl who exhibited diffuse osteoblastic metastases at presentation with a glioblastoma.

Glioma types associated with extraneural metastases

Many of the early acceptable examples of gliomas with extraneural metastases were ependymomas, in which slow growth, repeated recurrences, prolonged survival and multiple operations were important contributory factors to this complication. It is now clear that all forms of glioma are liable to metastasize outside the CNS, the most frequently recorded being the glioblastomas and malignant

Table 9.4 Incidence of types of glioma with extraneural metastases (116 cases) compared with an unselected series of gliomas examined at necropsy

Glioma type	Relative incidence of type of glioma with extraneural metastases (%; 116 cases)	Relative incidence of glioma in London Hospital necropsy series 1928–39, 1946–55 (%; 496 cases)
Malignant astrocytoma	10.3	21.3
Oligodendroglioma	5.2	5.0
Ependymoma	16.4	6.2
Glioblastoma multiforme	41.4	57.3
Medulloblastoma	26.7	6.2

astrocytomas (Pasquier *et al.*, 1980), followed by the cerebellar medulloblastomas (Kleinman, Hochberg and Richardson, 1981). Liwnicz and Rubinstein (1979) tabulated, among the 116 acceptable reported examples, 50 glioblastomas, 32 medulloblastomas, 17 ependymomas, 10 malignant astrocytomas and 7 oligodendrogliomas. An appreciable number of further cases have since been described. In Table 9.4, the incidence of the different types of glioma listed in that review as having developed extraneural metastases is compared with the necropsy figures of 496 uncomplicated gliomas recorded in two nonconsecutive decades in the pathology department of The London Hospital. In the Liwnicz and Rubinstein series, the preponderance of metastasizing glioblastomas reflects their high degree of malignancy and is in agreement with that of the glioblastomas in the unselected (London Hospital) necropsy series. The unusually high incidence of metastasizing medulloblastomas is probably due to the prolonged survival of these patients after vigorous postoperative treatment with craniospinal irradiation, to selective case reporting and perhaps to the greater likelihood of obtaining postmortem examinations on pediatric patients. Prolonged survival time presumably plays a significant role in the relatively high proportion of metastasizing ependymomas in this series, particularly in patients with spinal cord ependymomas of the myxopapillary variant, in whom the total length of clinical history may range from 10 to 30 years (see p. 416).

Sites of extraneural metastases

The distribution of distant metastases according to the various types of glioma in the 116 cases reviewed is shown in Fig. 9.309. The apparent selectivity of some of the extraneural tissues for the development of deposits from certain glioma cell types has been repeatedly documented: the lungs and lymph nodes in glioblastomas and ependymomas; and the bones and lymph nodes in cerebellar medulloblastomas. The relative sparing of the lungs in medulloblastomas, although not absolute, has often been noted (Rubinstein, 1959; Drachman, Winter and Karon, 1963), but, as pointed out by Kleinman, Hochberg and Richardson (1981), this apparent resistance no longer holds in patients in whom ventriculoatrial shunts have been performed. More cases of osseous metastases in glioblastoma or astrocytoma have been published recently (Lo Russo *et al.*, 1988; Gamis *et al.*, 1990; Lampl *et al.*, 1990; Myers, Egelhoff and Myers, 1990; Longee *et al.*, 1991; Chestnut *et al.*, 1993). A case of liver metastasis of glioblastoma, preceding any surgical intervention, has also been confirmed (Leifer *et al.*, 1989). The causes of this pattern of relatively selective distribution according to glioma cell type are not known.

Other factors that may play a role in the development of extraneural metastases

The anatomic observations and inferences discussed in the preceding paragraphs go some way towards explaining some of the mechanisms underlying the process of extraneural metastatic tumor formation in malignant gliomas. Liwnicz and Rubinstein (1979) argued that, in certain circumstances and in varying degrees that may depend on their structural features, glioma cells have the capacity to perform all the steps that have been deemed necessary for the development of metastasizing neoplasms of nonneural origin: detachment of single tumor cells from the primary growth, migration to blood vessel boundaries, penetration of the vascular walls at the primary site, dissemination via the systemic circulation, arrest within a distant target organ, egress through the vascular walls of the target organ into its stroma, formation of micrometastases (i.e., implantations of tumor cells without stroma formation) and, finally, inducement of a vascular neogenesis in association with

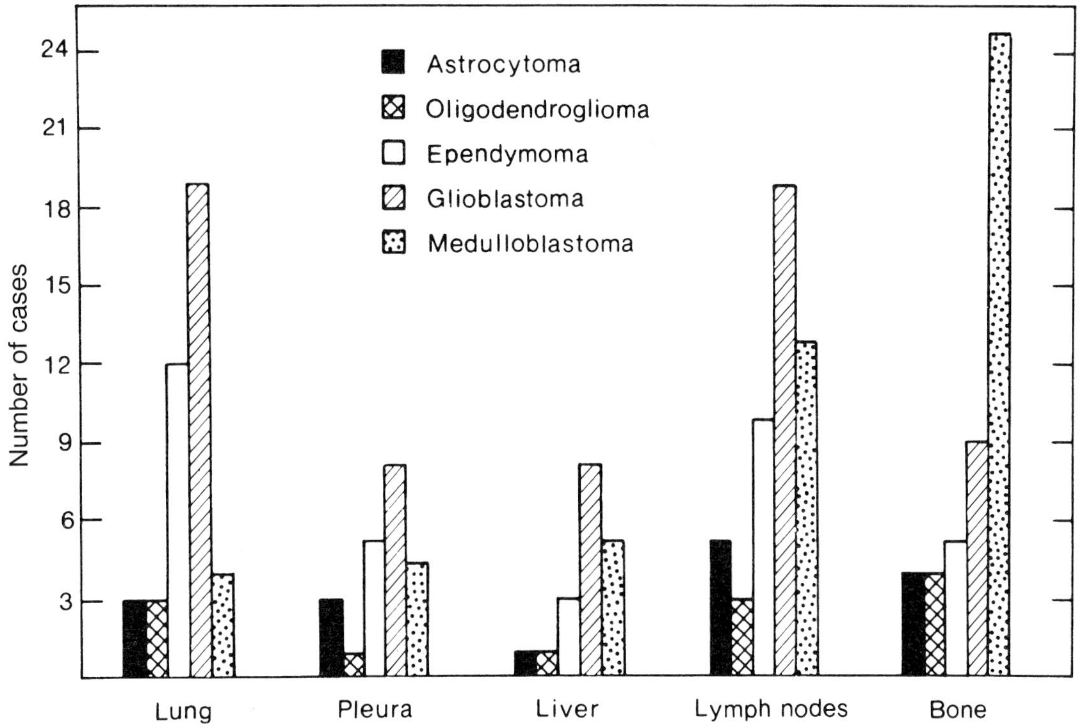

Fig. 9.309 Distribution of extraneural metastases according to the type of glioma in 116 reported cases. (From Liwnicz and Rubinstein, 1979, and reprinted from *Human Pathology*, 1979, pp. 453–467, figure 12, with kind permission of W.B. Saunders Company.)

overt metastatic tumor formation. Yet the capacity of glioma cells to perform these consecutive steps does not explain the rarity of this development when contrasted to the behavior of primary extracranial malignant neoplasms, or the peculiar features that it displays when it occurs. While, as documented above, mechanical access to the lymphatic system or to the blood vessels must play a decisive role in the process, the rarity of that sequence is intriguing considering the frequency with which access to the blood vessels must be gained in the course of surgery. The failure of some human glioma cell lines to express CD15, a selectin that functions as a ligand for endothelial adhesion, has been postulated as precluding the adhesion of circulating glioma cells to systemic endothelium (Martin *et al.*, 1995). It has also been postulated that, since the CNS lacks a connective tissue stroma, gliomas can grow and spread easily in their primary environment, so that subpopulations capable of metastasis are not selected, as putatively occurs with systemic tumors (Pansera and Pansera, 1992). Also, when distant dissemination occurs, secondary foci, with the notable exception of those that may result from shunting procedures, tend to be scanty, and their distribution often selective of other organ systems, suggesting that additional factors must prevent the successful growth of central neuroepithelial tumors in remote sites. The affinity of certain sites for the development of metastatic deposits from different glioma cell types has been summarized. The claims that tumor cells can often be demonstrated in the circulation at the time of craniotomy, or immediately thereafter, have not been convincingly demonstrated. While in many instances the development of metastatic deposits seems to have followed penetration of the veins by tumor cells, it is curious that such a phenomenon should more often be demonstrable in the extrameningeal and extracranial tissues than within the brain tumor itself. While it has been reported that the direct injection, into the caudal vein of mice, of homogenates from experimentally induced gliomas will promote the growth of glial tumors in the liver, kidneys, spleen and lungs (Zimmerman, 1957), this is by no means an almost invariable sequel, in contrast to the effect of cell suspensions prepared from highly metastasizing experimental tumors, such as the rabbit Brown-Pearce and V_2 carcinomas. Likewise, the intravenous injection of different human´ and animal glioma lines into athymic nude mice results in an incidence of metastatic tumors—most often pulmonary, and much less commonly renal or hepatic—that varies according to the tumor line employed (Mandybur, Liwnicz and Wechsler, 1984).

Relevant to this problem are the reports that experimental transplants of gliomas to the anterior chamber of the eye were not followed by metastasis (Freeman and Zimmerman, 1944), and that, after 32 days the intracerebral implantation of the Brown-Pearce carcinoma in rabbits failed, to produce extraneural deposits (Shivas, 1959). However, the latter experiments were refuted by Greene and Harvey (1964a), who transplanted visceral tissues from brain tumor-bearing hamsters and rabbits into normal syngeneic animals and subsequently obtained tumor growth in the tissue transplants in all instances. Further experiments by Greene and Harvey (1964b) confirmed that this sequence of events may also take place after heterologous transplantation. In experiments reported by Vecht *et al.* (1981), cells derived from rat malignant astrocytomas, obtained by the intramuscular administration of ethylnitrosourea, were intracerebrally injected into syngeneic animals and produced metastases in largest numbers in the cervical lymph nodes, followed by the lungs. This development seemed statistically related to the progression of local extracerebral outgrowths from the intracerebrally implanted tumor cells and to the presence of diffuse leptomeningeal spread. These experiments essentially confirm the already numerous observations from human pathology that relate the development of remote metastases to the invasion of lymphatic channels and blood vessels once the tumor cells have transgressed the boundaries of the CNS; they do not add further information on the part played by any other factor that would determine the successful development of gliomatous deposits in extraneural sites or that could influence host–tumor cell relationships. Some of these, possibly related to the endothelial binding capacity of tumor cells, have been suggested by Greene and Harvey (1964b). Experimental *in vitro* studies on the ability of different tumor cell types to adhere to endothelial cells have demonstrated that glioma cells may show preferential adhesion to cerebral capillary endothelium (Alby and Auerbach, 1984). While such experiments do not throw any obvious light on the mechanisms of extraneural metastasis in gliomas, they indicate that differences expressed at the surface of endothelial cells may be recognized by neoplastic glial cells (Martin *et al.*, 1995).

A factor that would also influence the detection of remote metastases might well be the cytokinetics of glioma growth. This as provocatively recalled by Alvord (1976), might result, in the majority of cases, in the demise of the patient from his space-occupying lesion before visceral deposits have reached a size large enough for their detection—a point already established experimentally by the transplantation work of Greene and Harvey (1964b).

References

Aarabi, B., Long, D.M. and Miller, N.R. (1978) Enlarging optic chiasmal glioma with stable visual acuity. *Surgical Neurology* **10**, 175–7.

Adesina, A.M., Nalbantoglu, J. and Cavenee, W.K. (1994) *p53* Gene mutation and *mdm2* gene amplification are uncommon in medulloblastoma. *Cancer Research* **54**, 5649–51.

Aebi, M. and Kraus-Ruppert, R. (1978) Oligodendroglioma with a twenty-two year history. Clinicopathological case report. *Journal of Neurology* **219**, 139–44.

Afra, D., Müller, W., Slowik, F. and Firsching, R. (1986) Supratentorial lobar pilocytic astrocytomas: report of 45 operated cases, including 9 recurrences. *Acta Neurochirurgica* **81**, 90–3.

Ahdevaara, P., Kalimo, H., Törmä, T. and Haltia, M. (1977) Differentiating intracerebral neuroblastoma. Report of a case and review of the literature. *Cancer* **40**, 784–8.

Albrecht, S., Connelly, J.H. and Bruner, J.M. (1993) Distribution of p53 protein expression in gliosarcomas: an immunohistochemical study. *Acta Neuropathologica* **85**, 222–6.

Albrecht, S., Haber, R.M., Goodman, J.C. and Duvic, M. (1992) Cowden syndrome and Lhermitte-Duclos disease. *Cancer* **70**, 869–76.

Albrecht, S., von Deimling, A., Pietsch, T., Giangaspero, F., Brandner, S., Kleihues, P. and Wiestler, O.D. (1994) Microsatellite analysis of loss of heterozygosity on chromosomes 9q, 11p and 17p in medulloblastomas. *Neuropathology and Applied Neurobiology* **20**, 74–81.

Albright, A.L., Price, R.A. and Guthkelch, A.N. (1983) Brain stem gliomas of children. A clinicopathological study. *Cancer* **52**, 2313–19.

——(1985) Diencephalic gliomas of children. A clinicopathologic study. *Cancer* **55**, 2789–93.

Albright, A.L., Guthkelch, A.N., Packer, R.J., Price, R.A. and Rorke, L.B. (1986) Prognostic factors in pediatric brain-stem gliomas. *Journal of Neurosurgery* **65**, 751–5.

Albright, A.L., Wisoff, J.H., Zeltzer, P.M., Boyett, J.M., Rorke, L.B. and Stanley, P. (1996) Effects of medulloblastoma resections on outcome in children: a report from the Children's Cancer Group. *Neurosurgery* **38**, 265–71.

Albright, L. and Byrd, R.P. (1980) Ganglioglioma of the entire spinal cord. *Child's Brain* **6**, 274–80.

Alby, L. and Auerbach, R. (1984) Differential adhesion of tumor cells to capillary endothelial cells *in vitro*. *Proceedings of the National Academy of Sciences U.S.A.* **81**, 5739–43.

Alitalo, K., Bornstein, P., Vaheri, A. and Sage, H. (1983) Biosynthesis of an unusual collagen type by human astrocytoma cells in vitro. *Journal of Biological Chemistry* **258**, 2653–61.

Allegra, S. and Serra, P. (1950) Ganglioneuroma recidivante maligno del cervello. *Rivista di Patologia Nervosa e Mentale* **71**, 94–108.

Allegranza, A., Pileri, S., Frank, G. and Ferracini, R. (1990) Cerebral ganglioglioma with anaplastic oligodendroglial component. *Histopathology* **17**, 439–41.

Allegranza, A., Ferraresi, S., Bruzzone, M. and Giombini, S. (1991a) Cerebromeningothelial pleomorphic xanthoastrocytoma. Report on four cases: clinical, radiologic and pathological features. (Including a case with malignant evolution). *Neurosurgical Review* **14**, 43–9.

Allegranza, A., Girlando, S., Arrigoni, G.L., Veronese, S., Mauri, F.A., Gambacorta, M., Pollo, B., Palma, P.D. and Barbareschi, M. (1991b) Proliferating cell nuclear antigen expression in central nervous system neoplasms. *Virchows Archiv A, Pathological Anatomy and Histopathology* **419**, 417–23.

Aloe, L. and Vigneti, E. (1992) *In vivo* and *in vitro* NGF studies on developing cerebellar cells. *Neuroreport* **3**, 279–82.

Alpers, B.J. and Grant, F.C. (1931) The ganglioneuromas of the central nervous system. *Archives of Neurology and Psychiatry* **26**, 501–23.

Alpers, C.E., Davis, R.L. and Wilson, C.B. (1982) Persistence and late malignant transformation of childhood cerebellar astrocytoma. *Journal of Neurosurgery* **57**, 548–51.

Alvarado-Mallart, R.-M. (1993) Fate and potentialities of the avian mesencephalic/metencephalic neuroepithelium. *Journal of Neurobiology* **24**, 1341–55.

Alvisi, C., Cerisoli, M. and Maccheroni, M.E. (1985) Long-term results of surgically treated brainstem gliomas. *Acta Neurochirurgica* **76**, 12–17.

Alvord, E.C. Jr (1976) Why do gliomas not metastasize? *Archives of Neurology* **33**, 73–5.

Alvord, E.C. Jr and Lofton, S. (1988) Gliomas of the optic nerve or chiasm. Outcome by patients' age, tumor site, and treatment. *Journal of Neurosurgery* **68**, 85–98.

al-Wahhabi, B., Choudhury, A.R., Chaudhri, K.A., Haleem, A. and Sharif, H. (1992) Multicentric glioma of the spinal cord. *British Journal of Neurosurgery* **6**, 495–9.

Alwasiak, J., Mirecka, B., Wozniak, L. and Liberski, P.P. (1991) Neuroblastic differentiation of metastases of medulloblastoma to extracranial lymph node: an ultrastructural study. *Ultrastructural Pathology* **15**, 647–54.

Amacher, A.L., Torres, Q.U. and Rittenhouse, S. (1986) Congenital medulloblastoma: an inquiry into origins. *Child's Nervous System* **2**, 262–5.

Ambler, M., Pogacar, S. and Sidman, R. (1969) Lhermitte-Duclos disease (granule cell hypertrophy of the cerebellum). Pathological analysis of the first familial cases. *Journal of Neuropathology and Experimental Neurology* **28**, 622–47.

Andrews, A.A., Enriques, L., Renaudin, J. and Tomiyasu, U. (1978) Spinal intramedullary glioblastoma with intracranial seeding. *Archives of Neurology* **35**, 244–5.

Angevine, J.B. Jr, Bodian, D., Coulombre, A.J., Edds, M.V. Jr, Hamburger, V., Jacobson, M., Lyser, K.M., Prestige, M.C., Sidman, R.L., Varon, S. and Weiss, P.A. (1970) Embryonic vertebrate central nervous system: revised terminology. *Anatomical Record* **166**, 257–62.

Antanitus, D.S., Choi, B.H. and Lapham, L.W. (1976) The demonstration of glial fibrillary acidic protein in the cerebrum of the human fetus by indirect immunofluorescence. *Brain Research* **103**, 613–16.

Anzil, A.P. (1970) Glioblastoma multiforme with extracranial metastases in the absence of previous craniotomy. *Journal of Neurosurgery* **33**, 88–94.

Aragonés, M.P., Magallón, R., Piqueras, C., Ley, L., Vaquero, J. and Bravo, G. (1994) Medulloblastoma in adulthood: prognostic factors influencing survival and recurrence. *Acta Neurochirurgica* **127**, 65–8.

Arenella, L.S. and Herndon, R.M. (1984) Mature oligodendrocytes. Division following experimental demyelination in adult animals. *Archives of Neurology* **41**, 1162–5.

Arjona, V., Aneiros, J., Linares, J., Aguilar, D. and Diaz-Flores, L. (1977) Sarcomatoid transformation of the vascular walls in giant cell glioblastoma. *Morfologia Normal y Patológica* **1**, 319–34.

Armington, W.G., Osborn, A.G., Cubberley, D.A., Harnsberger, H.R., Boyer, R., Naidich, T.P. and Sherry, R.G. (1985) Supratentorial ependymoma: CT appearance. *Radiology* **157**, 367–72.

Artigas, J., Cervos-Navarro, J., Iglesias, J.R. and Erhardt, G. (1985) Gliomatosis cerebri: clinical and histological findings. *Clinical Neuropathology* **4**, 135–48.

Asa, S.L., Kovacs, K., Tindall, G.T., Barrow, D.L., Horvath, E. and Vecsei, P. (1984) Cushing's disease associated with an intrasellar gangliocytoma producing corticotrophin-releasing factor. *Annals of Internal Medicine* **101**, 789–93.

Asai, A., Hoshino, T., Edwards, M.S.B. and Davis, R.L. (1992) Predicting the recurrence of ependymomas from the bromodeoxyuridine labeling index. *Child's Nervous System* **8**, 273–8.

Auer, R.N. and Becker, L.E. (1983) Cerebral medulloepithelioma with bone, cartilage, and striated muscle. Light microscopic and immunohistochemical study. *Journal of Neuropathology and Experimental Neurology* **42**, 256–67.

Awad, I., Bay, J.W. and Rogers, L. (1986) Leptomeningeal metastasis from supratentorial malignant gliomas. *Neurosurgery* **19**, 247–51.

Azzarelli, B., Luerssen, T.G. and Wolfe, T.M. (1991) Intramedullary secretory gangliocytoma. *Acta Neuropathologica* **82**, 402–7.

Azzarelli, B., Muller, J. and Mirkin, L.D. (1983) Medulloblastoma (?) with epithelioid features. *Acta Neuropathologica* **61**, 109–15.

Azzarelli, B., Rekate, H.L. and Roessmann, U. (1977) Subependymoma. A case report with ultrastructural study. *Acta Neuropathologica* **40**, 279–82.

Azzarelli, B., Richards, D.E., Anton, A.H. and Roessmann, U. (1977) Central neuroblastoma. Electron microscopic observations and catecholamine determinations. *Journal of Neuropathology and Experimental Neurology* **36**, 384–97.

Bailey, O.T. (1955) On the histogenesis of certain tumors of the medulloblastoma group. In *Proceedings of the 2nd International Congress of Neuropathology*. (London) Amsterdam: Excerpta Medica, Part I, 239–41.

——(1971) Medulloblastoma. In Minckler, J. (ed.), *Pathology of the nervous system*, Vol. 2. New York: McGraw-Hill, 2071–81.

Bailey, P. (1927) Further remarks concerning tumors of the glioma group. *Bulletin of the Johns Hopkins Hospital* **40**, 354–89.

Bailey, P. and Beiser, H. (1947) Concerning gangliogliomas of the brain. *Journal of Neuropathology and Experimental Neurology* **6**, 24–34.

Bailey, P. and Bucy, P.C. (1929) Oligodendrogliomas of the brain. *Journal of Pathology and Bacteriology* **32**, 735–51.

——(1930) Astroblastomas of the brain. *Acta Psychiatrica et Neurologica Scandinavica* **5**, 439–61.

Bailey, P. and Cushing, H. (1925) Medulloblastoma cerebelli: a common type of midcerebellar glioma of childhood. *Archives of Neurology and Psychiatry* **14**, 192–224.

——(1926) *A classification of tumors of the glioma group*. Philadelphia: Lippincott.

Bailey, P. and Eisenhardt, L. (1932) Spongioblastomas of the brain. *Journal of Comparative Neurology* **56**, 391–430.

Balko, M.G., Blisard, K.S. and Samaha, F.J. (1992) Oligodendroglial gliomatosis cerebri. *Human Pathology* **23**, 706–7.

Baloyannis, S. (1981) The fine structure of the isomorphic oligodendroglioma. *Anticancer Research* **1**, 243–8.

Banerjee, A.K. and Gleadhill, C.A. (1979) Lhermitte-Duclos disease (diffuse cerebellar hypertrophy). Prolonged post-operative survival. *Irish Journal of Medical Science* **148**, 97–9.

Bardosi, A., Dimitri, T. and Gabius, H.J. (1988) Endogenous carbohydrate-binding proteins in oligodendrogliomas. A histochemical study. *Acta Neuropathologica* **76**, 55–61.

Barker, F.G. II, Davis, R.L., Chang, S.M. and Prados, M.D. (1996) Necrosis as a prognostic factor in glioblastoma multiforme. *Cancer* **77**, 1161–6.

Barnard, R.O. (1968) The development of malignancy in oligodendrogliomas. *Journal of Pathology and Bacteriology* **96**, 113–23.

Barnard, R.O. and Geddes, J.F. (1987) The incidence of multifocal cerebral gliomas. A histologic study of large hemisphere sections. *Cancer* **60**, 1519–31.

Barnard, R.O. and Pambakian, H. (1980) Astrocytic differentiation in medulloblastoma. *Journal of Neurology, Neurosurgery and Psychiatry* **43**, 1041–4.

Barnard, R.O. and Scott, T. (1980) A note on the nature of eosinophilic granular bodies in astrocytic gliomas. *Acta Neuropathologica* **50**, 245–7.

Barnard, R.O., Bradford, R., Scott, T. and Thomas, D.G. (1986) Gliomyosarcoma. Report of a case of rhabdomyosarcoma arising in a malignant glioma. *Acta Neuropathologica* **69**, 23–7.

Barone, B.M. and Elvidge, A.R. (1970) Ependymomas. A clinical survey. *Journal of Neurosurgery* **33**, 428–38.

Batra, S.K., McLendon, R.E., Koo, J.S., Castelino-Prabhu, S., Fuchs, H.E., Krischer, J.P., Friedman, H.S., Bigner, D.D. and Bigner, S.H. (1995) Prognostic implications of chromosome 17p deletions in human medulloblastomas. *Journal of Neuro-Oncology* **24**, 39–45.

Batzdorf, U. and Gold, V. (1974) Dispersion of central nervous system tumors. Correlation between clinical aspects and tissue culture studies. *Journal of Neurosurgery* **41**, 691–8.

Batzdorf, U. and Malamud, N. (1963) The problem of multicentric gliomas. *Journal of Neurosurgery* **20**, 122–36.

Beck, D.J.K. and Russell, D.S. (1942) Oligodendrogliomatosis of the cerebrospinal pathway. *Brain* **65**, 352–72.

Becker, D.P., Benyo, R. and Roessmann, U. (1967) Glial origin of monstrocellular tumor. Case report of prolonged survival. *Journal of Neurosurgery* **26**, 72–7.

Becker, L.E. and Hinton, D. (1983) Primitive neuroectodermal tumors of the central nervous system. *Human Pathology* **14**, 538–50.

Becker, R.L., Becker, A.D. and Sobel, D.F. (1995) Adult medulloblastoma: review of 13 cases with emphasis on MRI. *Neuroradiology* **37**, 104–8.

Belamaric, J. and Chau, A.S. (1969) Medulloblastoma in newborn sisters. Report of two cases. *Journal of Neurosurgery* **30**, 76–9.

Bell, D.A., Woodruff, J.M. and Scully, R.E. (1984) Ependymoma of the broad ligament. A report of two cases. *American Journal of Surgical Pathology* **8**, 203–9.

Belza, M.G., Donaldson, S.S., Steinberg, G.K., Cox, R.S. and Cogen, P.H. (1991) Medulloblastoma: freedom from relapse longer than 8 years—a therapeutic cure? *Journal of Neurosurgery* **75**, 575–82.

Bennett, J.P. Jr and Rubinstein, L.J. (1984) The biological behavior of primary cerebral neuroblastoma: a reappraisal of the clinical course in a series of 70 cases. *Annals of Neurology* **16**, 21–7.

Berger, M.S., Edwards, M.S.B., Wara, W.M., Levin, V.A. and Wilson, C.B. (1983) Primary cerebral neuroblastoma. Long-term follow-up review and therapeutic guidelines. *Journal of Neurosurgery* **59**, 418–23.

Berger, M.S., Baumeister, B., Geyer, J.R., Milstein, J., Kanev, P.M. and LeRoux, P.D. (1991) The risks of metastases from shunting in children with primary central nervous system tumors. *Journal of Neurosurgery* **74**, 872–7.

Bergin, D.J., Johnson, T.E., Spencer, W.H. and McCord, C.D. (1988) Ganglioglioma of the optic nerve. *American Journal of Ophthalmology* **105**, 146–9.

Bergsagel, D.J., Finegold, M.J., Butel, J.S., Kupsky, W.J. and Garcea, R.L. (1992) DNA sequences similar to those of simian virus 40 in ependymomas and choroid plexus tumors of childhood. *New England Journal of Medicine* **326**, 988–93.

Berkman, R.A., Clark, W.C., Saxena, A., Robertson, J.T., Oldfield, E.H. and Ali, I.U. (1992) Clonal composition of glioblastoma multiforme. *Journal of Neurosurgery* **77**, 432–7.

Bernell, W.R., Kepes, J.J. and Seitz, E.P. (1972) Late malignant recurrence of childhood cerebellar astrocytoma. Report of 2 cases. *Journal of Neurosurgery* **37**, 470–4.

Bernstein, J.J. and Woodard, C.A. (1995) Glioblastoma cells do not intravasate into blood vessels. *Neurosurgery* **36**, 124–32.

Bernstein, M., Hoffman, H.J., Halliday, W.C., Hendrick, E.B. and Humphreys, R.P. (1984) Thalamic tumors in children. Long-term follow-up and treatment guidelines. *Journal of Neurosurgery* **61**, 649–56.

Berry, M.P., Jenkin, R.D.T., Keen, C.W., Nair, B.D. and Simpson, W.J. (1981) Radiation treatment for medulloblastoma. A 21-year review. *Journal of Neurosurgery* **55**, 43–51.

Best, P.V. (1963) Intracranial oligodendrogliomatosis. *Journal of Neurology, Neurosurgery and Psychiatry* **26**, 249–56.

——(1973) A medulloblastoma-like tumour with melanin formation. *Journal of Pathology* **110**, 109–11.

——(1974) Posterior fossa medulloepithelioma. *Journal of the Neurological Sciences* **22**, 511–18.

Bevilacqua, G. and Sarnelli, R. (1979) Ganglioglioma of the spinal cord. A case with a long survival. *Acta Neuropathologica* **48**, 239–42.

Bickerstaff, E.R., Connolly, R.C. and Woolf, A.L. (1967) Cerebellar medulloblastoma occurring in brothers. *Acta Neuropathologica* **8**, 104–7.

Biegel, J.A., Rorke, L.B., Packer, R.J., Sutton, L.N., Schut, L., Bonner, K. and Emanuel, B.S. (1989) Isochromosome 17q in primitive neuroectodermal tumors of the central nervous system. *Genes, Chromosomes and Cancer* **1**, 139–47.

Biegel, J.A., Burk, C.D., Barr, F.G. and Emanuel, B.S. (1992) Evidence for a 17p tumor related locus distinct from p53 in pediatric primitive neuroectodermal tumors. *Cancer Research* **52**, 3391–5.

Biegel J.A., Janss, A. J., Raffel, C., Sutton, L., Rorke, L.B., Harper, J.M. and Phillips, P.C. (1997) Prognostic significance of chromosome 17p deletions in childhood primitive neuroectodermal tumors (medulloblastomas) of the central nervous system. *Clinical Cancer Research* **3**, 473–8.

Bielschowsky, M. (1925) Das multiple Ganglioneurom des Gehirns und seine Entstehung. *Journal für Psychologie und Neurologie* **32**, 1–20.

Biernat, W., Aguzzi A., Sure, U., Grant, J.W., Kleihues, P. and Hegi, M.E. (1995) Identical mutations of the *p53* tumor suppressor gene in the gliomatous and the sarcomatous components of gliosarcomas suggest a common origin from glial cells. *Journal of Neuropathology and Experimental Neurology* **54**, 651–6.

Bignami, A. and Dahl, D. (1974) Astrocyte-specific protein and neuroglial differentiation. An immunofluorescence study with antibodies to the glial fibrillary acidic protein. *Journal of Comparative Neurology* **153**, 27–38.

Bignami, A., Raju, T. and Dahl, D. (1982) Localisation of vimentin, the nonspecific intermediate filament protein in embryonal glia and in early differentiating neurons: *in vivo* and *in vitro* immunofluorescence study of the rat embryo with vimentin and neurofilament antisera. *Developmental Biology* **91**, 286–95.

Bignami, A., Eng, L.F., Dahl, D. and Uyeda, C.T. (1972) Localization of the glial fibrillary acidic protein in astrocytes by immunofluorescence. *Brain Research* **43**, 429–35.

Bigner, S.H., Mark, J. and Bigner, D.D. (1990) Cytogenetics of human brain tumors. *Cancer Genetics and Cytogenetics* **47**, 141–54.

Bigner, S.H., Burger, P.C., Wong, A.J., Werner, M.H., Hamilton, S.R., Muhlbaier, L.H., Vogelstein, B. and Bigner, D.D. (1988a) Gene amplification in malignant human gliomas: clinical and histopathologic aspects. *Journal of Neuropathology and Experimental Neurology* **47**, 191–205.

Bigner, S.H., Mark, J., Friedman, H.S., Biegel, J.A. and Bigner, D.D. (1988b) Structural chromosomal abnormalities in human medulloblastoma. *Cancer Genetics and Cytogenetics* **30**, 91–101.

Bigner, S.H., Friedman, H.S., Vogelstein, B., Oakes, W.J. and Bigner, D.D. (1990) Amplification of the c-*myc* gene in human medulloblastoma cell lines and xenografts. *Cancer Research* **50**, 2347–50.

Bjørklund, H., Eriksdotter-Nilsson, M., Dahl, D. and Olson, L. (1984) Astrocytes in smears of CNS tissues as visualized by GFA and vimentin immunofluorescence. *Medical Biology* **62**, 38–48.

Blatt, G.L., Ahuja, A., Miller, L.L, Ostrow, P.T. and Soloniuk, D.S. (1995) Cerebellomedullary ganglioglioma: CT and MR findings. *AJNR. American Journal of Neuroradiology* **16**, 790–2.

Blatt, J., Jaffe, R., Deutsch, M. and Adkins, J.C. (1986) Neurofibromatosis and childhood tumors. *Cancer* **57**, 1225–9.

Bloom, H.J.G. (1982) Intracranial tumors: response and resistance to therapeutic endeavors, 1970–1980. *International Journal of Radiation Oncology, Biology and Physics* **8**, 1083–1113.

Bloom, H.J.G. and Bessell, E.M. (1990) Medulloblastoma in adults: a review of 47 patients treated between 1952 and 1981. *International Journal of Radiation Oncology, Biology and Physics* **18**, 763–72.

Bloom, H J.G., Wallace, E.N.K. and Henk, J.M. (1969) The treatment and prognosis of medulloblastoma in children. A study of 82 verified cases. *American Journal of Roentgenology, Radium Therapy and Nuclear Medicine* **105**, 43–62.

Blumenfeld, C.M. and Gardner, W.J. (1945) Disseminated oligodendroglioma. *Archives of Neurology and Psychiatry* **54**, 274–9.

Bodian, M. and Lawson, D. (1953) The intracranial neoplastic diseases of childhood. A description of their natural history based on a clinico-pathological study of 129 cases. *British Journal of Surgery* **40**, 368–92.

Boesel, C.P., Suhan, J.P. and Sayers, M.P. (1978) Melanotic medulloblastoma. Report of a case with ultrastructural findings. *Journal of Neuropathology and Experimental Neurology* **37**, 531–43.

Bonnin, J.M. and Perentes, E. (1988) Retinal S-antigen immunoreactivity in medulloblastomas. *Acta Neuropathologica* **76**, 204–7.

Bonnin, J.M. and Rubinstein, L.J. (1989) Astroblastomas: a pathological study of 23 tumors, with a postoperative follow-up in 13 patients. *Neurosurgery* **25**, 6–13.

Bonnin, J.M., Peña, C.E. and Rubinstein, L.J. (1983) Mixed capillary hemangioblastoma and glioma. A redefinition of the angioglioma. *Journal of Neuropathology and Experimental Neurology* **42**, 504–16.

Bonnin, J.M., Rubinstein, L.J., Palmer, N.F. and Beckwith, J.B. (1984a) The association of embryonal tumors originating in the kidney and in the brain. A report of seven cases. *Cancer* **54**, 2137–46.

Bonnin, J.M., Rubinstein, L.J., Papasozomenos, S.Ch. and Marangos, P.J. (1984b) Subependymal giant cell astrocytoma. Significance and possible cytogenic implications of an immunohistochemical study. *Acta Neuropathologica* **62**, 185–93.

Bookwalter, J.W. III, Selker, R.G., Schiffer, L., Randall, M., Iannuzzi, D. and Kristofik, M. (1986) Brain-tumor cell kinetics correlated with survival. *Journal of Neurosurgery* **65**, 795–8.

Borello, E.D. and Gorlin, R.J. (1966) Melanotic neuroectodermal tumor of infancy—a neoplasm of neural crest origin. Report of a case associated with high urinary excretion of vanilmandelic acid. *Cancer* **19**, 196–206.

Borit, A. and Richardson, E.P. Jr (1982) The biological and clinical behaviour of pilocytic astrocytomas of the optic pathways. *Brain* **105**, 161–87.

Bourlond, J., Bourlond, A. and Rousseau, C. (1994) Retrolumbar subcutaneous ependymoma and giant bathing-trunk nevocellular nevus. *International Journal of Dermatology* **33**, 488–92.

Bourne, S.P., Coakham, H.B., Kemshead, J.T., Brownell, B., Allan, P.M. and Davies, A.G. (1986) The role of monoclonal antibodies in the diagnosis and characterization of medulloblastoma. In Zeltzer, P.M. and Pochedly, C. (eds), *Medulloblastomas in children: new concepts in tumor biology, diagnosis and treatment.* New York: Praeger, 87–103.

Bowles, A.P., Pantazis, C.G., Allen, M.B. Jr, Martinez, J. and Allsbrook, W.C. Jr (1988) Ganglioglioma, a malignant tumor? Correlation with flow deoxyribonucleic acid cytometric analysis. *Neurosurgery* **23**, 376–81.

Boykin, F.C., Cowen, D., Iannucci, C.A.J. and Wolf, A. (1954) Subependymal glomerate astrocytomas. *Journal of Neuropathology and Experimental Neurology* **13**, 30–49.

Brander, W.L. and Turner, D.R. (1975) Extracranial metastases from a glioma in the absence of surgical intervention. *Journal of Neurology, Neurosurgery and Psychiatry* **38**, 1133–5.

Brandt, B.L., Kimes, B.W. and Klier, F.G. (1976) Development of a clonal myogenic cell line with unusual biochemical properties. *Journal of Cellular Physiology* **88**, 255–75.

Brenner, M. (1994) Structure and regulation of the *GFAP* gene. *Brain Pathology* **4**, 245–57.

Brenner, M., Kisseberth, W.C., Su, Y., Besnard, F. and Messing, A. (1994) GFAP promoter directs astrocyte-specific expression in transgenic mice. *Journal of Neuroscience* **14**, 1030–7.

Brett, M. and Weller, R.O. (1978) Intracellular serum proteins in cerebral gliomas and metastatic tumours. An immunoperoxidase study. *Neuropathology and Applied Neurobiology* **4**, 263–72.

Brew, B.J. and Garrick, R. (1987) Gliomas presenting outside the central nervous system. *Clinical and Experimental Neurology* **23**, 111–17.

Brightman, M.W. and Palay, S.L. (1963) The fine structure of ependyma in the brain of the rat. *Journal of Cell Biology* **19**, 415–39.

Brossard, J., Abish, S., Bernstein, M.L., Baruchel, S., Kovacs, L. and Pollack, R. (1994) Maternal malignancy involving the products of conception: a report of malignant melanoma and medulloblastoma. *American Journal of Pediatric Hematology/Oncology* **16**, 380–3.

Brown, W.D., Tavaré, C.J., Sobel, E.L. and Gilles, F.H. (1995) Medulloblastoma and Collins' law: a critical review of the concept of a period of risk for tumor recurrence and patient survival. *Neurosurgery* **36**, 691–7.

Bruggers, C.S., Friedman, H.S., Phillips, P.C., Wiener, M.D., Hockenberger, B., Oakes, W.J. and Buckley, E.G. (1991) Leptomeningeal dissemination of optic pathway gliomas in three children. *American Journal of Ophthalmology* **111**, 719–23.

Brun, A. (1965) The subpial granular layer of the foetal cerebral cortex in man. Its ontogeny and significance in congenital cortical malformations. *Acta Pathologica et Microbiologica Scandinavica* (**Suppl. 179**).

Bruner, J.M. (1987) Oligodendroglioma: diagnosis and prognosis. *Seminars in Diagnostic Pathology* **4**, 251–61.

Brust, J.C.M., Moiel, R.H. and Rosenberg, R.N. (1968) Glial tumor metastases through a ventriculopleural shunt. Resultant massive pleural effusion. *Archives of Neurology* **18**, 649–53.

Brüstle, O. and McKay, R.D.G. (1995) The neuroepithelial stem cell concept: implications for neuro-oncology. *Journal of Neuro-Oncology* **24**, 57–9.

Brzustowicz, R.J. and Kernohan, J.W. (1952) Cell rests in the region of the fourth ventricle. II. Histologic and embryologic consideration. *Archives of Neurology and Psychiatry* **67**, 592–611.

Bucy, P.C. and Gustafson, W.A. (1939) Structure, nature and classification of cerebellar astrocytomas. *American Journal of Cancer* **35**, 327–53.

Bucy, P.C., Oberhill, H.R., Siqueira, E.B., Zimmerman, H.M. and Jelsma, R.K. (1985) Cerebral glioblastomas can be cured. *Neurosurgery* **16**, 714–17.

Budka, H. (1974) Intracranial lipomatous hamartomas (intracranial 'lipomas'). A study of 13 cases including combinations with medulloblastoma, colloid and epidermoid cysts, angiomatosis and other malformations. *Acta Neuropathologica* **28**, 205–22.

——(1975) Partially resected and irradiated cerebellar astrocytoma of childhood: malignant evolution after 28 years. *Acta Neurochirurgica* **32**, 139–46.

Budka, H. and Chimelli, L. (1994) Lipomatous medulloblastoma in adults: a new tumor type with possible favorable prognosis. *Human Pathology* **25**, 730–1.

Budka, H. and Sunder-Plassmann, M. (1980) Benign mixed glial-mesenchymal tumour ('glio-fibroma') of the spinal cord. *Acta Neurochirurgica* **55**, 141–5.

Budka, H. and Wöber, G. (1974) Primary glioblastoma of the cerebellum. Report of a case associated with multifocal dysplastic glial changes. *Acta Neurochirurgica* **31**, 115–21.

Budka, H., Podreka, I. and Zaunbauer, F. (1979) Overgrowth of a primitive cell population in operated recurrent gliomas: the possible role of chemo- and radiotherapy. In Paoletti, P., Walker, M.D., Butti, G. and Knerich, R. (eds), *Multidisciplinary aspects of brain tumor therapy.* Amsterdam: Elsevier/North-Holland Biomedical Press, 357–62.

Budka, H., Podreka, I., Reisner, Th. and Zeiler, K. (1980) Diagnostic and pathomorphological aspects of glioma multiplicity. *Neurosurgical Review* **3**, 233–41.

Buetow, P.C., Smirniotopoulos, J.G. and Done, S. (1990) Congenital brain tumors: a review of 45 cases. *AJNR. American Journal of Neuroradiology* **11**, 793–9.

Bullard, D.E., Rawlings, C.E. III, Phillips, B., Cox, E.B., Schold, S.C., Burger, P. and Halperin, E.C. (1987) Oligodendroglioma. An analysis of the value of radiation therapy. *Cancer* **60**, 2179–88.

Bullon, M.M., Alvarez-Gago, T., Fernandez-Ruiz, B. and Aguirre, C. (1984) Glial fibrillary acidic protein (GFAP) in spinal cord of postnatal rat. An immunoperoxidase study in semithin sections. *Brain Research* **316**, 129–33.

Burchiel, K.J., Shaw, C.-M. and Kelly, W.A. (1983) A mixed functional microadenoma and ganglioneuroma of the pituitary fossa. *Journal of Neurosurgery* **58**, 416–20.

Burger, P.C. (1983) Pathologic anatomy and CT correlations in the glioblastoma multiforme. *Applied Neurophysiology* **46**, 180–7.

Burger, P.C. and Fuller, G.N. (1991) Pathology—trends and pitfalls in histologic diagnosis, immunopathology, and applications of oncogene research. *Neurologic Clinics of North America* **9**, 249–71.

Burger, P.C. and Green, S.B. (1987) Patient age, histologic features, and length of survival in patients with glioblastoma multiforme. *Cancer* **59**, 1617–25.

Burger, P.C. and Hamilton, S.R. (1995) Brain tumors in Turcot syndrome. *Journal of Neuropathology and Experimental Neurology* **54** (Suppl.), 425.

Burger, P.C. and Scheithauer, B.W. (1994) *Tumors of the central nervous system*. Atlas of tumor pathology, third series, fascicle 10. Washington, D.C.: Armed Forces Institute of Pathology.

Burger, P.C. and Vogel, F.S. (1982) *Surgical pathology of the nervous system and its coverings*. Second edition. New York: Churchill Livingstone, 193–437.

Burger, P.C. and Vollmer, R.T. (1980) Histologic factors of prognostic significance in the glioblastoma multiforme. *Cancer* **46**, 1179–86.

Burger, P.C., Scheithauer, B.W. and Vogel, F.S. (1991) *Surgical pathology of the nervous system and its coverings*. Third edition. New York: Churchill Livingstone.

Burger, P.C., Shibata, T. and Kleihues, P. (1986) The use of the monoclonal antibody Ki-67 in the identification of proliferating cells: application to surgical neuropathology. *American Journal of Surgical Pathology* **10**, 611–17.

Burger, P.C., Vogel, F.S., Green, S.B. and Strike, T.A. (1985) Glioblastoma multiforme and anaplastic astrocytoma. Pathologic criteria and prognostic implications. *Cancer* **56**, 1106–11.

Burger, P.C., Grahmann, F.C., Bliestle, A. and Kleihues, P. (1987) Differentiation in the medulloblastoma. A histological and immunohistochemical study. *Acta Neuropathologica* **73**, 115–23.

Burnstine, M.A., Levin, L.A., Louis, D.N., Hedley-Whyte, E.T., Kupsky, W.J., Doepner, D. and Albert, D.M. (1993) Nucleolar organizer regions in optic gliomas. *Brain* **116**, 1465–76.

Cabello, A., Madero, S., Castresana, A. and Diaz-Lobato, R. (1991) Astroblastoma. Electron microscopy and immunohistochemical findings: case report. *Surgical Neurology* **35**, 116–21.

Caccamo, D.V., Herman, M.M. and Rubinstein, L.J. (1989) An immunohistochemical study of the primitive and maturing elements of human cerebral medulloepitheliomas. *Acta Neuropathologica* **79**, 248–54.

Caine, G.D., Weller, R.O., Davis, B.E. and Cox, S. (1980) Mechanisms of uptake and the fate of serum proteins and horseradish peroxidase in cultured human glioma cells. A light- and electron-immunocytochemical study. *Acta Neuropathologica* **52**, 169–77.

Cairncross, J.G. and Macdonald, D.R. (1988) Successful chemotherapy for recurrent malignant oligodendroglioma. *Annals of Neurology* **23**, 360–4.

Cairns, H. and Russell, D.S. (1931) Intracranial and spinal metastases in gliomas of the brain. *Brain* **54**, 377–420.

——(1946) Cerebral arteritis and phlebitis in pneumococcal meningitis. *Journal of Pathology and Bacteriology* **58**, 649–65.

Camins, M.B., Cravioto, H.M., Epstein, F. and Ransohoff, J. (1980) Medulloblastoma: an ultrastructural study—evidence for astrocytic and neuronal differentiation. *Neurosurgery* **6**, 398–411.

Campbell, A.N., Chan, H.S.L., Becker, L.E., Daneman, A., Park, T.S. and Hoffman, H.J. (1984) Extracranial metastases in childhood primary intracranial tumors. A report of 21 cases and review of the literature. *Cancer* **53**, 974–81.

Canti, R.G., Bland, J.O.W. and Russell, D.S. (1937) Tissue culture in gliomata. Cinematograph demonstration. *Research Publications—Association for Research in Nervous and Mental Disease* **16**, 1–24.

Cappelaere, P., Clay, A., Adenis, L., Demaille, A. and Laine, E. (1972) Les métastases des tumeurs cérébrales primitives en dehors du névraxe. A propos de trois observations. *Bulletin du Cancer* **59**, 235–54.

Caputy, A.J., McCullough, D.C., Manz, H.J., Patterson, K. and Hammock, M.K. (1987) A review of the factors influencing the prognosis of medulloblastoma. The importance of cell differentiation. *Journal of Neurosurgery* **66**, 80–7.

Carbone, R., Brihaye, J. and Drochmans, P. (1955) Spongioblastome pariéto-occipital et gangliocytome dysplasique du cervelet chez le même malade. *Acta Neurologica et Psychatrica Belgica* **55**, 568–80.

Carrie, C., Lasset, C., Alapetite, C., Haie-Meder, C., Hoffstetter, S., Demaille, M.-C., Kerr, C., Wagner, J.-P., Lagrange, J.-L., Maire, J.-P., Seng, S.-H., Man, Y.O.C.T.K., Murraciole, X. and Pinto, N. (1994) Multivariate analysis of prognostic factors in adult patients with medulloblastoma. *Cancer* **74**, 2352–60.

Cattoretti, G., Becker, M.H.G., Key, G., Duchrow, M., Schlüter, C., Galle, J. and Gerdes J. (1992) Monoclonal antibodies against recombinant parts of the Ki-67 antigen (MIB 1 and MIB 3) detect proliferating cells in microwave-processed formalin-fixed paraffin sections. *Journal of Pathology* **168**, 357–63.

Cavanagh, J.B. (1958) On certain small tumours encountered in the temporal lobe. *Brain* **81**, 389–405.

Celli, P., Cervoni, L. and Cantore, G. (1993) Ependymoma of the filum terminale: treatment and prognostic factors in a series of 28 cases. *Acta Neurochirurgica* **124**, 99–103.

Celli, P., Scarpinati, M., Nardacci, B., Cervoni, L. and Cantore, G.P. (1993) Gangliogliomas of the cerebral hemispheres. Report of 14 cases with long-term follow-up and review of the literature. *Acta Neurochirurgica* **125**, 52–7.

Cerame, M.A., Guthikonda, M. and Kohli, C.M. (1985) Extraneural metastases in gliosarcoma: a case report and review of the literature. *Neurosurgery* **17**, 413–18.

Cerda-Nicolas, M. and Kepes, J.J. (1993) Gliofibromas (including malignant forms), and gliosarcomas: a comparative study and review of the literature. *Acta Neuropathologica* **85**, 349–61.

Cerdá-Nicolás, M., López-Ginés, C., Peydro-Olaya, A. and Llombart-Bosch, A. (1993) Central neurocytoma: a cytogenetic case study. *Cancer Genetics and Cytogenetics* **65**, 173–4.

Ceriani, R.L., Thompson, K., Peterson, J.A. and Abraham, S. (1977) Surface differentiation antigen of human mammary epithelial cells carried on the human milk fat globule. *Proceedings of the National Academy of Sciences U.S.A.* **74**, 582–6.

Cervoni, L. and Cantore, G. (1995) Medulloblastoma in pediatric age: a single-institution review of prognostic factors. *Child's Nervous System* **11**, 80–5.

Cervoni, L., Celli, P., Fortuna, A. and Cantore, G. (1994a) Recurrence of spinal ependymoma. Risk factors and long-term survival. *Spine* **19**, 2838–41.

Cervoni, L., Maleci, A., Salvati, M., Delfini, R. and Cantore, G. (1994b) Medulloblastoma in late adults: report of two cases and critical review of the literature. *Journal of Neuro-Oncology* **19**, 169–73.

Cervós-Navarro, J., Artigas, J., Aruffo, C. and Iglesias, J. (1987) The fine structure of gliomatosis cerebri. *Virchows Archiv A, Pathological Anatomy and Histopathology* **411**, 93–8.

Chamberlain, M.C. and Press, G.A. (1990) Temporal lobe ganglioglioma in refractory epilepsy: CT and MR in three cases. *Journal of Neuro-Oncology* **9**, 81–7.

Chan, H.S.L., Becker, L.E., Hoffman, H.J., Humphreys, R.P., Hendrick, E.B., Fitz, C.R. and Chuang, S.H. (1984) Myxopapillary ependymoma of the filum terminale and cauda equina in childhood: report of seven cases and review of the literature. *Neurosurgery* **14**, 204–10.

Chang, C.H., Housepian, E.M. and Herbert, C. Jr (1969) An operative staging system and a megavoltage radiotherapeutic technic for cerebellar medulloblastomas. *Radiology* **93**, 1351–9.

Chason, J.L. (1956) Subependymal mixed gliomas. *Journal of Neuropathology and Experimental Neurology* **15**, 461–70.

Chatty, E.M. and Earle, K.M. (1971) Medulloblastoma. A report of 201 cases with emphasis on the relationship of histologic variants to survival. *Cancer* **28**, 977–83.

Chen, R., Macdonald, D.R. and Ramsay, D.A. (1995) Primary diffuse leptomeningeal oligodendroglioma: case report. *Journal of Neurosurgery* **83**, 724–8.

Chestnut, R.M., Abitbol, J.J., Chamberlain, M. and Marshall, L.F. (1993) Vertebral collapse with quadraparesis due to metastatic glioblastoma multiforme: case report and review of the literature. *Journal of Neuro-Oncology* **16**, 135–40.

Chilton, J., Caughron, M.R. and Kepes, J.J. (1990) Ganglioglioma of the optic chiasm: case report and review of the literature. *Neurosurgery* **26**, 1042–5.

Chimelli, L., Hahn, M.D. and Budka, H. (1991) Lipomatous differentiation in a medulloblastoma. *Acta Neuropathologica* **81**, 471–3.

Chin, H.W. and Maruyama, Y. (1981) Results of radiation treatment of cerebellar medulloblastoma. *International Journal of Radiation Oncology, Biology and Physics* **7**, 737–42.

——(1983) Early response and long-term results in the radiotherapy of childhood medulloblastoma. *Journal of Neuro-Oncology* **1**, 53–9.

Chin, H.W., Hazel, J.J., Kim, T.H. and Webster, J.H. (1980) Oligodendrogliomas. I. A clinical study of cerebral oligodendrogliomas. *Cancer* **45**, 1458–66.

Chin, H.W., Maruyama, Y., Tibbs, P., Markesbery, W. and Young, B. (1984) Cerebellar glioblastoma in childhood. *Journal of Neuro-Oncology* **2**, 79–84.

Chiu, J.K., Woo, S.Y., Ater, J., Connelly, J., Bruner, J.M., Maor, M.H., van Eys, J., Oswald, M.J. and Shallenberger, R. (1992) Intracranial ependymoma in children: analysis of prognostic factors. *Journal of Neuro-Oncology* **13**, 283–90.

Choi, B.H. (1981) Radial glia of developing human fetal spinal cord: Golgi, immunohistochemical and electron microscopic study. *Brain Research* **227**, 249–67.

——(1986) Glial fibrillary acidic protein in radial glia of early human fetal cerebrum: a light and electron microscopic immunoperoxidase study. *Journal of Neuropathology and Experimental Neurology* **45**, 408–18.

Choi, B.H. and Kim, R.C. (1984) Expression of glial fibrillary acidic protein in immature oligodendroglia. *Science* **223**, 407–9.

——(1985) Expression of glial fibrillary acidic protein by immature oligodendroglia and its implications. *Journal of Neuroimmunology* **8**, 215–35.

Choi, B.H. and Lapham, L.W. (1978) Radial glia in the human fetal cerebrum: a combined Golgi, immunofluorescent and electron microscopic study. *Brain Research* **148**, 295–311.

——(1980) Evolution of Bergmann glia in developing human fetal cerebellum: a Golgi, electron microscopic and immunofluorescent study. *Brain Research* **190**, 369–83.

Choi, B.H., Holt, J.T. and McDonald, J.V. (1981) Occult malignant astrocytoma of pons with extracranial metastasis to bone prior to craniotomy. *Acta Neuropathologica* **54**, 269–73.

Choi, B.H., Kim, R.C. and Lapham, L.W. (1983) Do radial glia give rise to both astroglial and oligodendroglial cells? *Brain Research* **284**, 119–35.

Choucair, A.K., Levin, V.A., Gutin, P.H., Davis, R.L., Silver, P., Edwards, M.S.B. and Wilson, C.B. (1986) Development of multiple lesions during radiation therapy and chemotherapy in patients with gliomas. *Journal of Neurosurgery* **65**, 654–8.

Christensen, E. (1937) Über Ganglienzellgeschwülste in Gehirn. *Virchows Archiv für Pathologische Anatomie und Physiologie* **300**, 567–81.

——(1971) Nerve cell tumors (central and peripheral). In Minckler, J. (ed.), *Pathology of the nervous system*, Vol. 2. New York: McGraw-Hill, 2081–114.

Christensen, E. and Als, E. (1956) Medulloblastomas. *Acta Psychiatrica et Neurologica Scandinavica Supplementum* **108**, 87–99.

Christensen, E. and Andersen, S.R. (1952) Primary tumors of optic nerve and chiasm. *Acta Psychiatrica et Neurologica Scandinavica* **27**, 5–16.

Christian, H.J. (1961) So-called 'gangliocytoma' of the cerebellum. *Journal of Neurosurgery* **18**, 125–8.

Clarenbach, P., Kleihues, P., Metzel, E. and Dichgans, J. (1979) Simultaneous clinical manifestation of subependymoma of the fourth ventricle in identical twins. *Journal of Neurosurgery* **50**, 655–9.

Clark, G.B., Henry, J.M. and McKeever, P.E. (1985) Cerebral pilocytic astrocytoma. *Cancer* **56**, 1128–33.

Clausen, N., Garwics, S., Glomstein, A., Jonmundsson, G., Kruus, S. and Yssing, M. (1990) Medulloblastoma in Nordic children. I. Incidence and mortality. *Acta Paediatrica Scandinavica Supplement* **371**, 5–11.

Coakham, H.B., Garson, J.A., Allan, P.M., Harper, E.I., Brownell, B., Kemshead, J.T. and Lane, E.B. (1985) Immunohistological diagnosis of central nervous system tumours using a monoclonal antibody panel. *Journal of Clinical Pathology* **38**, 165–73.

Coakley, K.J., Huston, J. III, Scheithauer, B.W., Forbes, G. and Kelly, P.J. (1995) Pilocytic astrocytomas: well demarcated magnetic resonance appearance despite frequent infiltration histologically. *Mayo Clinic Proceedings* **70**, 747–51.

Coffin, C.M., Mukai, K. and Dehner, L.P. (1983) Glial differentiation in medulloblastomas. Histogenetic insight, glial reaction, or invasion of brain? *American Journal of Surgical Pathology* **7**, 555–65.

Coffin, C.M., Swanson, P.E., Wick, M.R. and Dehner, L.P. (1993) An immunohistochemical comparison of chordoma with renal cell carcinoma, colorectal adenocarcinoma, and myxopapillary ependymoma: a potential diagnostic dilemma in the diminutive biopsy. *Modern Pathology* **6**, 531–8.

Cogan, D.G., Poppen, J.L. and Hicks, S.P. (1961) Ganglioneuroma of chiasm and optic nerves. *Archives of Ophthalmology* **65**, 481–2.

Cogen, P.H. (1991–92) Prognostic significance of molecular genetic markers in childhood brain tumors. *Pediatric Neurosurgery* **17**, 245–50.

Cogen, P.H., Daneshvar, L., Metzger, A.K. and Edwards, M.S.B. (1990) Deletion mapping of the medulloblastoma locus on chromosome 17p. *Genomics* **8**, 279–85.

Cogen, P.H., Daneshvar, L., Metzger, A.K., Duyk, G., Edwards, M.S.B. and Sheffield, V.C. (1992) Involvement of multiple chromosome 17p loci in medulloblastoma tumorigenesis. *American Journal of Human Genetics* **50**, 584–9.

Cohen, A.R., Wisoff, J.H., Allen, J.C. and Epstein, F. (1989) Malignant astrocytomas of the spinal cord. *Journal of Neurosurgery* **70**, 50–4.

Cohen, M. (1919) Primary intradural tumor of the orbital portion of the optic nerve. *Archives of Ophthalmology* **48**, 19–22.

Cohen, M.E., Duffner, P.K., Heffner, R.R., Lacey, D.J. and Brecher, M. (1986) Prognostic factors in brainstem gliomas. *Neurology* **36**, 602–5.

Collins, V.P. (1983) Cultured human glial and glioma cells. *International Review of Experimental Pathology* **24**, 135–202.

Cooling, R.J. and Wright, J.E. (1979) Arachnoid hyperplasia in optic nerve glioma: confusion with orbital meningioma. *British Journal of Ophthalmology* **63**, 596–9.

Coons, S.W. and Johnson, P.C. (1993a) Regional heterogeneity in the DNA content of human gliomas. *Cancer* **72**, 3052–60.

——(1993b) Regional heterogeneity in the proliferative activity of human gliomas as measured by the Ki-67 labeling index. *Journal of Neuropathology and Experimental Neurology* **52**, 609–18.

——(1996) Ki-67/MIB-1 labeling index predicts patient survival in low grade and anaplastic astrocytomas. *Journal of Neuropathology and Experimental Neurology* **55**, 665A.

Coons, S.W., Johnson, P.C. and Pearl, D.K. (1994) Prognostic significance of flow cytometry deoxyribonucleic acid analysis of human astrocytomas. *Neurosurgery* **35**, 119–26.

Cosgrove, M.M., Rich, K.A., Kunin, S.A., Sherrod, A.E. and Martin, S.E. (1993) Keratin intermediate filament expression in astrocytic neoplasms: analysis by immunohistochemistry, Western blot, and Northern hybridization. *Modern Pathology* **6**, 342–7.

Costero, I. (1962) Pathology of glial neoplasms. In Fields, W.S. and Sharkey, P.C. (eds), *The biology and treatment of intracranial tumors*. Springfield, Ill.: Charles C. Thomas, 178–217.

Couch, J.R. and Weiss, S.A. (1974) Gliomatosis cerebri. Report of four cases and review of the literature. *Neurology* **24**, 504–11.

Courville, C.B. (1930) Ganglioglioma. Tumor of the central nervous system: review of the literature and report of two cases. *Archives of Neurology and Psychiatry* **24**, 439–91.

——(1931) Gangliogliomas. A further report with special reference to those occurring in the temporal lobe. *Archives of Neurology and Psychiatry* **25**, 307–26.

——(1936) Multiple primary tumors of the brain. Review of the literature and report of 21 cases. *American Journal of Cancer* **26**, 703–31.

——(1956) Multinucleation of cortical nerve cells at margin of malignant glioma. Its possible significance with respect to the neoplastic development of gangliogliomas. *Journal of Neuropathology and Experimental Neurology* **15**, 369–76.

Courville, C.B. and Anderson, F.M. (1941) Neurogliogenic tumors of the central nervous system. *Bulletin of the Los Angeles Neurological Society* **6**, 154–76.

Courville, C.B. and Broussalian, S.L. (1961) Plastic ependymomas of the lateral recess. Report of eight verified cases. *Journal of Neurosurgery* **18**, 792–9.

Cox, L.B. (1933) The cytology of the glioma group; with special reference to the inclusion of cells derived from the invaded tissue. *American Journal of Pathology* **9**, 839–907.

Craig, W.M. and Kernohan, J.W. (1938) Tumors of the fourth ventricle. *Journal of the American Medical Association* **111**, 2370–7.

Crotty, T.B., Hooker, R.P., Swensen, S.J., Scheithauer, B.W. and Myers, J.L. (1992) Primary malignant ependymoma of the lung. *Mayo Clinic Proceedings* **67**, 373–8.

Cruz-Sanchez, F.F., Haustein, J., Rossi, M.L., Cervos-Navarro, J. and Hughes, J.T. (1988a) Ependymoblastoma: a histological, immunohistological and ultrastructural study of five cases. *Histopathology* **12**, 17–27.

Cruz-Sanchez, F.F., Iglesias, J.R., Rossi, M.L., Cervos-Navarro, J., Figols, J. and Haustein, J. (1988b) Histologic characterization of 41 ependymomas with the help of a personal computer. *Cancer* **62**, 150–62.

Cruz-Sanchez, F.F., Rossi, M.L., Hughes, J.T., Esiri, M.M. and Coakham, H.B. (1989) Medulloblastoma. An immunohistological study of 50 cases. *Acta Neuropathologica* **79**, 205–10.

Cruz-Sanchez, F.F., Rossi M.L., Buller J.R., Carboni P. Jr, Fineron P.W. and Coakham H.B. (1991) Oligodendrogliomas: a clinical, histological, immunocytochemical and lectin-binding study. *Histopathology* **19**, 361–7.

Cutarelli, P.E., Roessmann, U.R., Miller, R.H., Specht, C.S. and Grossniklaus, H.E. (1991) Immunohistochemical properties of human optic nerve glioma. Evidence of type 1 astrocyte origin. *Investigative Ophthalmology and Visual Science* **32**, 2521–4.

Dahl, D. (1981) The vimentin-GFA protein transition in rat neuroglia cytoskeleton occurs at the time of myelination. *Journal of Neuroscience Research* **6**, 741–8.

Dahl, D. and Bignami, A. (1983) The glial fibrillary acidic protein and astrocytic 10–nanometer filaments. In Lajtha, A. (ed.), *Handbook of neurochemistry*, Vol. 5. New York: Plenum Press, 127–51.

Dastur, D.K. (1982) Cerebral ganglioglioneuroblastoma: an unusual brain tumour of the neuron series. *Journal of Neurology, Neurosurgery and Psychiatry* **45**, 139–42.

Daumas-Duport, C. (1993) Dysembryoplastic neuroepithelial tumours. *Brain Pathology* **3**, 283–95.

Daumas-Duport, C., Scheithauer, B.W., Chodkiewicz, J.-P., Laws, E.R. Jr and Vedrenne, C. (1988a) Dysembryoplastic neuroepithelial tumor: a surgically curable tumor of young patients with intractable partial seizures. *Neurosurgery* **23**, 545–56.

Daumas-Duport, C., Scheithauer, B.W., O'Fallon, J. and Kelly, P. (1988b) Grading of astrocytomas. A simple and reproducible method. *Cancer* **62**, 2152–65.

Davidson, L.A., Graham, D.I. and Carey, F.A. (1992) Chronic neurological dysfunction attributable to a ganglioglioma. *Histopathology* **21**, 275–8.

Davie, T.B. (1932) Medullo-epitheliomas of the brain and retina. *Journal of Pathology and Bacteriology* **35**, 359–66.

Davila, G., Duyckaerts, C., Lazareth, J.P., Poisson, M. and Delattre, J.Y. (1993) Diffuse primary leptomeningeal gliomatosis. *Journal of Neuro-Oncology* **15**, 45–9.

Davis, D.G., Wilson, D., Schmitz, M. and Markesbery, W.R. (1993) Lipidized medulloblastoma in adults. *Human Pathology* **24**, 990–5.

Davis, F.A. (1940) Primary tumors of the optic nerve (a phenomenon of Recklinghausen's disease): a clinical and pathologic study with a report of five cases and a review of the literature. *Archives of Ophthalmology* **23**, 735–821 and 957–1022.

Davis, L., Martin, J., Goldstein, S.L. and Ashkenazy, M. (1949) A study of 211 patients with verified glioblastoma multiforme. *Journal of Neurosurgery* **6**, 33–44.

Davis, R.L. (1971) Astrocytomas. In Minckler, J. (ed.), *Pathology of the nervous system*, Vol. 2. New York: McGraw-Hill, 2007–26.

Davis, R.L. and Nelson, E. (1961) Unilateral ganglioglioma in a tubero-sclerotic brain. *Journal of Neuropathology and Experimental Neurology* **20**, 571–81.

De Armond, S.J., Eng, L.F. and Rubinstein, L.J. (1980) The application of glial fibrillary acidic (GFA) protein immunohistochemistry in neurooncology. A progress report. *Pathology Research and Practice* **168**, 374–94.

de Castro, F. (1932) Sensory ganglia of the cranial and spinal nerves. Normal and pathological. In Penfield, W. (ed.), *Cytology and cellular pathology of the nervous system*, Vol. 1. New York: Hafner, 91–143.

de Chadarévian, J.-P. and Hollenberg, R.D. (1979) Subependymal giant cell tumor of tuberose sclerosis. A light and ultrastructural study. *Journal of Neuropathology and Experimental Neurology* **38**, 419–33.

de Chadarévian, J.-P., Pattisapu, J.V. and Faerber, E.N. (1990) Desmoplastic cerebral astrocytoma of infancy. Light microscopy, immunocytochemistry, and ultrastructure. *Cancer* **66**, 173–9.

de Chadarévian, J.-P., Montes, J.L., O'Gorman, A.M. and Freeman, C.R. (1987) Maturation of cerebellar neuroblastoma into ganglioneuroma with melanosis. A histologic, immunocytochemical, and ultrastructural study. *Cancer* **59**, 69–76.

Deck, J.H.N. (1969) Cerebral medulloepithelioma with maturation into ependymal cells and ganglion cells. *Journal of Neuropathology and Experimental Neurology* **28**, 442–54.

Deck, J.H.N., Ramjohn, S. and Dardick, I. (1990) 'Anemone' cell (villiform) tumor of the brain. *Ultrastructural Pathology* **14**, 87–94.

Deck, J.H.N., Eng, L.F., Bigbee, J. and Woodcock, S.M. (1978) The role of glial fibrillary acidic protein in the diagnosis of central nervous system tumors. *Acta Neuropathologica* **42**, 183–90.

Deckert, M., Reifenberger, G. and Wechsler, W. (1989) Determination of the proliferative potential of human brain tumors using the monoclonal antibody Ki-67. *Journal of Cancer Research and Clinical Oncology* **115**, 179–88.

De Clerck, Y.A., Shimada, H., Gonzalez-Gomez, I. and Raffel, C. (1994) Tumoral invasion in the central nervous system. *Journal of Neuro-Oncology* **18**, 111–21.

de la Monte, S. (1989) Uniform lineage of oligodendrogliomas. *American Journal of Pathology* **135**, 529–40.

Deliganis, A.V., Geyer, J.R. and Berger, M.S. (1996) Prognostic significance of type 1 neurofibromatosis

(von Recklinghausen disease) in childhood optic glioma. *Neurosurgery* **38**, 1114–19.
Delisle, M.B., Dastugue, N., Uro, E., Montmayeur, F., Boetto, S., Graber, D. and Hassoun, J. (1995) Mixed desmoplastic primitive neuroepithelial tumor of infancy: a light microscopic, immunocytochemical, ultrastructural and genetic study. *Acta Neuropathologica* **89**, 99–104.
Dell, S., Cohen, M. and Kushner, M. (1981) Period of risk hypothesis after prophylactic radiotherapy. *Child's Brain* **8**, 372–81.
del Rio-Hortega, P. (1944) Contribucion al conocimiento citologico de los oligodendrogliomas. *Archivos de Histologia Normal y Patológica* **2**, 266–7.
Desmeules, M., Mikkelsen, T. and Mao, Y. (1992) Increasing incidence of primary malignant brain tumors: influence of diagnostic methods. *Journal of the National Cancer Institute* **84**, 442–5.
de Vitry, F., Picart, R., Jacque, C. and Tixier-Vidal, A. (1981) Glial fibrillary acidic protein. A cellular marker of tanycytes in the mouse hypothalamus. *Developmental Neuroscience* **4**, 457–60.
Diaz-Flores, L., Caballero, T., Sanchez, G., Aguilar, D. and Martos, S. (1979) Nature and histogenesis of the sarcomatous component in mixed sarcoma-glioma forms. *Morfología Normal y Patológica* **3**, 253–66.
Dickson, D.W., Hart, M.N., Menezes, A. and Cancilla, P.A. (1983) Medulloblastoma with glial and rhabdomyoblastic differentiation. A myoglobin and glial fibrillary acidic protein immunohistochemical and ultrastructural study. *Journal of Neuropathology and Experimental Neurology* **42**, 639–47.
Diepholder, H.M., Schwechheimer, K., Mohadjer, M., Knoth, R. and Volk, B. (1991) A clinicopathologic and immunomorphologic study of 13 cases of ganglioglioma. *Cancer* **68**, 2192–201.
Dohrmann, G.J., Farwell, J.R. and Flannery J.T. (1976) Glioblastoma multiforme in children. *Journal of Neurosurgery* **44**, 442–8.
Dolman, C.L. (1974) Lymph node metastasis as first manifestation of glioblastoma. *Journal of Neurosurgery* **41**, 607–9.
——(1989) Glial fibrillary acidic protein and cartilage. *Acta Neuropathologica* **79**, 101–3.
Dom, R. and Brucher, J.-M. (1969) Hamartoblastome (gangliocytome diffus) unilatéral de l'écorce cérébrale associé à une dégénérescence soudanophile de la substance blanche du côté opposé. *Revue Neurologique* **120**, 307–18.
Donnal, J., Halperin, E.C., Friedman, H.S. and Boyko, O.B. (1992) Subfrontal recurrence of medulloblastoma. *AJNR. American Journal of Neuroradiology* **13**, 1617–18.
Doyle, J.B. and Kernohan, J.W. (1931) Ganglioneuroma of third ventricle with diabetes insipidus and hypopituitarism. *Journal of Nervous and Mental Disease* **73**, 55–61.
Drachman, D.A., Winter, T.S. III and Karon, M. (1963) Medulloblastoma with extracranial metastases. *Archives of Neurology* **9**, 518–30.
Drut, R. and Jones, M.C. (1983) Melanotic medulloblastoma of infancy. A case report with immunohistochemical study and literature review. *Morfología Normal y Patológica* **7**, 53–62.
Duffell, D., Farber, L., Chou, S., Hartmann, J.F. and Nelson, E. (1963) Electron microscopic observations on astrocytomas. *American Journal of Pathology* **43**, 539–54.
Duffner, P.K., Cohen, M.E., Myers, M.H. and Heise, H.W. (1986) Survival of children with brain tumours: SEER program, 1973–1980. *Neurology* **36**, 597–601.
Duffner, P.K., Burger, P.C., Cohen, M.E., Sanford, R.A., Krischer, J.P., Elterman, R., Aronin, P.A., Pullen, J., Horowitz, M.E., Parent, A., Martin, P. and Kun, L.E. (1994) Desmoplastic infantile gangliogliomas: an approach to therapy. *Neurosurgery* **34**, 583–9.
Duffy, P.E., Graf, L. and Rapport, M.M. (1977) Identification of glial fibrillary acidic protein by immunoperoxidase method in human brain tumors. *Journal of Neuropathology and Experimental Neurology* **36**, 645–52.
Duffy, P.E., Graf, L., Huang, Y.-Y. and Rapport, M.M. (1979) Glial fibrillary acidic protein in ependymomas and other brain tumors. Distribution, diagnostic criteria, and relation to formation of processes. *Journal of the Neurological Sciences* **40**, 133–46.
Duffy, P.E., Huang, Y.-Y., Rapport, M.M. and Graf, L. (1980) Glial fibrillary acidic protein in giant cell tumors of brain and other gliomas. A possible relationship to malignancy, differentiation, and pleomorphism of glia. *Acta Neuropathologica* **52**, 51–7.
Duggan, M.A., Hugh, J., Nation, J.G., Robertson, D.I. and Stuart, G.C.E. (1989) Ependymoma of the uterosacral ligament. *Cancer* **64**, 2565–71.
Dunn, D.W. and Purvin, V. (1990) Optic pathway gliomas in neurofibromatosis. *Developmental Medicine and Child Neurology* **32**, 820–31.
Durity, F.A., Dolman, C.L. and Moyes, P.D. (1968) Ganglioneuroblastoma of the cerebellum. Case report. *Journal of Neurosurgery* **28**, 270–3.
Dutton, J.J. (1991) Optic nerve gliomas and meningiomas. *Neurologic Clinics of North America* **9**, 163–77.
Eade, O.E. and Urich, H. (1971) Metastasising gliomas in young subjects. *Journal of Pathology* **103**, 245–56.
Earnest, F. III, Kernohan, J.W. and Craig, W.McK. (1950) Oligodendrogliomas. Review of 200 cases. *Archives of Neurology and Psychiatry* **63**, 964–76.
Eden, K.C. (1938) Dissemination of glioma of spinal cord in leptomeninges. *Brain* **61**, 298–310.
El-Azouzi, M., Chung, R.Y., Farmer, G.E., Martuza, R.L., Black, P.McL., Rouleau, G.A., Hettlich, C., Hedley-Whyte, E.T., Zervas, N.T., Panagopoulos, K., Nakamura, Y., Gusella, J.F. and Seizinger, B.R. (1989) Loss of distinct regions on the short arm of chromosome 17 associated with tumorigenesis of human astrocytomas. *Proceedings of the National Academy of Sciences U.S.A.* **86**, 7186–90.
Ellison, D.W., Zygmunt, S.C. and Weller, R.O. (1993) Neurocytoma/lipoma (neurolipocytoma) of the cerebellum. *Neuropathology and Applied Neurobiology* **19**, 95–8.
Elvidge, A., Penfield, W. and Cone, W. (1937) The gliomas of the central nervous system. A study of two hundred and ten verified cases. In *Tumors of the nervous system. An investigation of the most recent*

advances. Association for Research in Nervous and Mental Disease, Vol. 16. Baltimore, Md.: Williams & Wilkins, 107–81.

Elvidge, A.R. (1968) Long-term survival in the astrocytoma series. *Journal of Neurosurgery* **28**, 399–404.

Elvidge, A.R. and Martinez-Coll, A. (1956) Long-term follow-up of 106 cases of astrocytoma. *Journal of Neurosurgery* **13**, 318–31.

Eng, C., Murday, V., Seal, S., Mohammed, S., Hodgson, S.V., Chaudary, M.A., Fentiman, I.S., Ponder, B.A.J. and Eeles, R.A. (1994) Cowden syndrome and Lhermitte-Duclos disease in a family: a single genetic syndrome with pleiotrophy? *Journal of Medical Genetics* 458–61.

Eng, L.F. and DeArmond, S.J. (1983) Immunochemistry of the glial fibrillary acidic protein. In Zimmerman, H.M. (ed.), *Progress in neuropathology*, Vol. 5. New York: Raven Press, 19–39.

Eng, L.F. and Rubinstein, L.J. (1978) Contribution of immunohistochemistry to diagnostic problems of human cerebral tumors. *Journal of Histochemistry and Cytochemistry* **26**, 513–22.

Eng, L.F., D'Amelio, F.E. and Smith M.E. (1989) Dissociation of GFAP intermediate filaments in EAE: observations in the lumbar spinal cord. *Glia* **2**, 308–17.

Eng, L.F., Vanderhaeghen, J.J., Bignami, A. and Gerstl, B. (1971) An acidic protein isolated from fibrous astrocytes. *Brain Research* **28**, 351–4.

Epstein, F. and McCleary, E.L. (1986) Intrinsic brainstem tumors of childhood: surgical indications. *Journal of Neurosurgery* **64**, 11–15.

Epstein, F.J. and Farmer, J.-P. (1993) Brain-stem glioma growth patterns. *Journal of Neurosurgery* **78**, 408–12.

Epstein, F.J. and Wisoff, J.H. (1990) Surgical management of brain stem tumors in childhood and adolescence. *Neurosurgery Clinics of North America* **1**, 111–21.

Epstein, F.J., Farmer, J.-P. and Freed, D. (1992) Adult intramedullary astrocytomas of the spinal cord. *Journal of Neurosurgery* **77**, 355–9.

Erdelyi, E., VandenBerg, S.R., Raese, J., Barchas, J.D., Rubinstein, L.J. and Herman, M.M. (1981) Neural differentiation in the OTT-6050 mouse teratoma. Enzymatic and immunofluorescence characteristics of a tumor fraction showing melanogenesis in neuroepithelial cells. *Virchows Archiv A, Pathological Anatomy and Histology* **393**, 27–37.

Erlich, S.S. and Davis, R.L. (1978) Spinal subarachnoid metastases from primary intracranial glioblastoma multiforme. *Cancer* **42**, 2854–64.

Ermel, A.E. and Brucher, J.M. (1974) Arguments ultrastructuraux en faveur de l'appartenance du medulloblastome à la lighee neuronale. *Acta Neurologica Belgica* **74**, 208–20.

Ernestus, R.I., Wilcke, O. and Schröder, R. (1991) Supratentorial ependymomas in childhood: clinicopathological findings and prognosis. *Acta Neurochirurgica* **111**, 96–102.

Escalona-Zapata, J. (1981) Uncommon oligodendrogliomas. *Acta Neuropathologica* (Suppl. 7), 94–6.

Escalona-Zapata, J. and Diez-Nau, M.D. (1981) Distinctive growth patterns between cerebral and cerebellar astrocytomas—a tissue culture study. *Histopathology* **5**, 639–50.

Evans, A.E., Jenkin, R.D.T., Sposto, R., Ortega, J.A., Wilson, C.B., Wara, W., Ertel, I.J., Kramer, S., Chang, C.H., Leikin, S.L. and Hammond, G.D. (1990) The treatment of medulloblastoma. Results of a prospective randomized trial of radiation therapy with and without CCNU, vincristine, and prednisone. *Journal of Neurosurgery* **72**, 572–82.

Evans, D.G.R., Birch, J.M. and Orton, C.I. (1991) Brain tumours and the occurrence of severe invasive basal cell carcinoma in first degree relatives with Gorlin syndrome. *British Journal of Neurosurgery* **5**, 643–6.

Evans, D.G.R., Farndon, P.A., Burnell, L.D., Gattamaneni, H.R. and Birch, J.M. (1991) The incidence of Gorlin syndrome in 173 consecutive cases of medulloblastoma. *British Journal of Cancer* **64**, 959–61.

Farwell, J. and Flannery, J.T. (1984) Cancer in relatives of children with central-nervous-system neoplasms. *New England Journal of Medicine* **311**, 749–53.

Farwell, J.R., Dohrmann, G.J. and Flannery, J.T. (1984) Medulloblastoma in childhood: an epidemiological study. *Journal of Neurosurgery* **61**, 657–64.

Favier, J., Pizzolato, G.P. and Berney, J. (1985) Oligodendroglial tumors in childhood. *Child's Nervous System* **1**, 33–8.

Feigin, I. and Budzilovich, G.N. (1974) Tumors of neurons and their precursors. *Journal of Neuropathology and Experimental Neurology* **33**, 483–506.

Feigin, I. and Volk, B.W. (1951) Malignant ependymoma infiltrating scalp. *Archives of Pathology* **51**, 466–71.

Feigin, I., Epstein, F. and Mangiardi, J. (1983) Extensive advanced maturation of medulloblastoma to astrocytoma and ependymoma. *Journal of Neuro-Oncology* **1**, 95–108.

Feigin, I., Ransohoff, J. and Lieberman, A. (1976) Sarcoma arising in oligodendroglioma of the brain. *Journal of Neuropathology and Experimental Neurology* **35**, 679–84.

Feigin, I., Allen, L.B., Lipkin, L. and Gross, S.W. (1958) The endothelial hyperplasia of the cerebral blood vessels with brain tumors, and its sarcomatous transformation. *Cancer* **11**, 264–77.

Feigin, I.H. and Gross, S.W. (1955) Sarcoma arising in glioblastoma of brain. *American Journal of Pathology* **31**, 633–53.

Fenstermaker, R.A., Ganz, E. and Roessmann, U. (1989) Giant invasive intracerebral dermoid tumor with subependymoma-like reaction: case report. *Neurosurgery* **4**, 646–8.

Ferrante, L., Mastronardi, L., Celli, P., Acqui, M., Cervoni, L. and Fortuna, A. (1991) Medulloblastoma in adulthood. *Journal of Neurosurgical Sciences* **35**, 23–30.

Ferrante, L., Mastronardi, L., Celli, P., Lunardi, P., Acqui, M. and Fortuna, A. (1992) Intramedullary spinal cord ependymomas–a study of 45 cases with long-term follow-up. *Acta Neurochirurgica* **119**, 74–9.

Ferrante, L., Mastronardi, L., Schettini, G., Lunardi, P. and Fortuna, A. (1994) Fourth ventricle ependymomas. A study of 20 cases with survival analysis. *Acta Neurochirurgica* **131**, 67–74.

Ferraro, A. and Doolittle, G.J. (1936) Tuberous sclerosis (diffuse neurospongioblastosis). *Psychiatric Quarterly* **10**, 365–416.

Ferrer, I., Isamat, F. and Acebes, J. (1979) A Golgi and electron microscopic study of a dysplastic gangliocytoma of the cerebellum. *Acta Neuropathologica* **47**, 163–5.

Ferry, D.J., Hardman, J.M. and Earle, K.M. (1969) Syringomyelia and intramedullary neoplasms. *Medical Annals of the District of Columbia* **38**, 363–5.

Figarella-Branger, D.F., Durbec, P.L. and Rougon, G.N. (1990) Differential spectrum of expression of neural cell adhesion molecule isoforms and L1 adhesion molecules on human neuroectodermal tumors. *Cancer Research* **50**, 6364–70.

Figarella-Branger, D., Gambarelli, D., Dollo, C., Devictor, B., Perez-Castillo, A.M., Genitori, L., Lena, G., Choux, M. and Pellissier, J.F. (1991) Infratentorial ependymomas of childhood. Correlation between histological features, immunohistological phenotype, silver nucleolar organizer region staining values and post-operative survival in 16 cases. *Acta Neuropathologica* **82**, 208–16.

Figarella-Branger, D., Pellissier, J.F., Daumas-Duport, C., Delisle, M.B., Pasquier, B., Parent, M., Gambarelli, D., Rougon, G. and Hassoun, J. (1992) Central neurocytomas. Critical evaluation of a small-cell neuronal tumor. *American Journal of Surgical Pathology* **16**, 97–109.

Figols, J., Iglesias-Rozas, J.R. and Kazner, E. (1985) Myelin basic protein (MBP) in human gliomas: a study of twenty-five cases. *Clinical Neuropathology* **4**, 116–20.

Finlay, J.L. (1986) Natural history and epidemiology of medulloblastoma. In Zeltzer, P.M. and Pochedly, C. (eds), *Medulloblastomas in children. New concepts in tumor biology, diagnosis and treatment.* New York: Praeger, 22–36.

Fischer, E.G., Sotrel, A. and Welch, K. (1982) Cerebral hemangioma with glial neoplasia (angioglioma?). Report of two cases. *Journal of Neurosurgery* **56**, 430–4.

Fitzgibbons, P.L., Turner, R.R., Appley, A.J., Bishop, P.C., Nichols, P.W., Epstein, A.L., Apuzzo, M.L. and Chandrasoma, P.T. (1988) Flow cytometric DNA and nuclear antigen content in astrocytic neoplasms. *American Journal of Clinical Pathology* **89**, 640–4.

Flament-Durand, J. and Brion, J.P. (1985) Tanycytes: morphology and functions. A review. *International Review of Cytology* **96**, 121–55.

Flannery, A.M., Tomita, T., Radkowski, M. and McLone, D.G. (1990) Medulloblastomas in childhood: postsurgical evaluation with myelography and cerebrospinal fluid cytology. *Journal of Neuro-Oncology* **8**, 149–51.

Foerster, O. and Gagel, O. (1931) Ein Fall von sog. Gliom des Nervus opticus—Spongioblastoma multiforme ganglioides. *Zeitschrift für die gesamte Neurologie und Psychiatrie* **136**, 335–66.

Fokes, E.C. Jr and Earle, K.M. (1969) Ependymomas: clinical and pathological aspects. *Journal of Neurosurgery* **30**, 585–94.

Foot, N.C. and Cohen, S. (1933) Report of a case of retotheliosarcoma (reticulo-sarcoma) of the cerebral hemisphere. *American Journal of Pathology* **9**, 123–32.

Forsyth, P.A., Shaw, E.G., Scheithauer, B.W., O'Fallon, J.R., Layton, D.D. Jr and Katzman, J.A. (1993) Supratentorial pilocytic astrocytomas. A clinicopathologic, prognostic, and flow cytometric study of 51 patients. *Cancer* **72**, 1335–42.

Fortuna, A., Celli, P. and Palma, L. (1980) Oligodendrogliomas of the spinal cord. *Acta Neurochirurgica* **52**, 305–29.

Fowler, M. and Simpson, D.A. (1962) A malignant melanin-forming tumour of the cerebellum. *Journal of Pathology and Bacteriology* **84**, 307–11.

Franke, F.E., Schachenmayr, W., Osborn, M. and Altmannsberger, M. (1991) Unexpected immunoreactivities of intermediate filament antibodies in human brain and brain tumors. *American Journal of Pathology* **139**, 67–79.

Frantz, G.D., Weimann, J.M., Levin, M.E. and McConnell, S.K. (1994) Otx1 and Otx2 define layers and regions in developing cerebral cortex and cerebellum. *Journal of Neuroscience* **14**, 5725–40.

Frederiksen, K., Jat, P.S., Valtz, N., Levy, D. and McKay, R. (1988) Immortalization of precursor cells from the mammalian CNS. *Neuron* **1**, 439–48.

Frederiksen, P., Reske-Nielsen, E. and Bichel, P. (1978) Flow cytometry in tumours of the brain. *Acta Neuropathologica* **41**, 179–83.

Frederiksen, P., Knudsen, V., Reske-Nielsen, E. and Bichel, P. (1979) Flow cytometric DNA analysis in human medulloblastomas. In Paoletti, P., Walker, M.D., Butti, G. and Knerich, R. (eds), *Multidisciplinary aspects of brain tumor therapy*. Amsterdam: Elsevier/North-Holland Biomedical Press, 363–7.

Freeman, D. and Zimmerman, H.M. (1944) Experimental brain tumors: behavior in intraocular transplants. *Cancer Research* **4**, 273–8.

Freeman, L. and Feigin, I. (1963) Oligodendroglioma with 35–year survival. *Journal of Neurosurgery* **20**, 363–5.

French, J.D. and Bucy, P.C. (1948) Tumors of the septum pellucidum. *Journal of Neurosurgery* **5**, 433–49.

Friede, R.L. (1978) Gliofibroma. A peculiar neoplasia of collagen forming glia-like cells. *Journal of Neuropathology and Experimental Neurology* **37**, 300–13.

Friede, R.L. and Pollak, A. (1978) The cytogenic basis for classifying ependymomas. *Journal of Neuropathology and Experimental Neurology* **37**, 103–18.

Friede, R.L., Janzer, R.C. and Roessmann, U. (1982) Infantile small cell gliomas. *Acta Neuropathologica* **57**, 103–10.

Friedman, H.S., Burger, P.C., Bigner, S.H., Trojanowski, J.Q., Wikstrand, C.J., Halperin, E.C. and Bigner, D.D. (1985) Establishment and characterization of the human medulloblastoma cell line and transplantable xenograft D283 Med. *Journal of Neuropathology and Experimental Neurology* **44**, 592–605.

Friedman, H.S., Burger, P.C., Bigner, S.H., Trojanowski, J.Q., Brodeur, G.M., He, X., Wikstrand, C.J., Kurtzberg, J., Berens, M.E., Halperin, E.C. and Bigner, D.D. (1988) Phenotypic and genotypic analysis of a human medulloblastoma cell line and transplantable xenograft (D341 Med) demonstrating amplification of c-*myc*. *American Journal of Pathology* **130**, 472–84.

Frigge, C., Reifenberger, G., Vogeley, K.T., Messing, M., Roosen, N. and Wechsler, W. (1992) Immunohistochemical demonstration of proliferating cell nuclear antigen in glioblastomas—pronounced heterogeneity and lack of prognostic significance. *Journal of Cancer Research and Clinical Oncology* **118**, 289–95.

Frost, G., Patel, K., Bourne, S., Coakham, H.B. and Kemshead, J.T. (1991) Expression of alternative isoforms of the neural cell adhesion molecule (NCAM) on normal brain and a variety of brain tumours. *Neuropathology and Applied Neurobiology* **17**, 207–17.

Frost, P.J., Laperriere, N.J., Wong, C.S., Milosevic, M.F., Simpson, W.J.S. and Pintilie, M. (1995) Medulloblastoma in adults. *International Journal of Radiation Oncology, Biology and Physics* **32**, 951–7.

Fu, Y.-S., Chen, A.T.L., Kay, S. and Young, H.F. (1974) Is subependymoma (subependymal glomerate astrocytoma) an astrocytoma or ependymoma? A comparative ultrastructural and tissue culture study. *Cancer* **34**, 1992–2008.

Fujimura, M., Kayama, T., Kumabe, T. and Yoshimoto, T. (1995) Ganglioglioma in the basal ganglia totally resected by a trans-distal Sylvian approach. *Tohoku Journal of Experimental Medicine* **175**, 211–18.

Fujita, S. (1963) The matrix cell and cytogenesis in the developing central nervous system. *Journal of Comparative Neurology* **120**, 37–42.

——(1967) Quantitative analysis of cell proliferation and differentiation in the cortex of the postnatal mouse cerebellum. *Journal of Cell Biology* **32**, 277–87.

Fujita, S., Shimada, N. and Nakamura, T. (1966) H^3-thymidine autoradiographic studies on the cell proliferation and differentiation in the external and internal granular layers of the mouse cerebellum. *Journal of Comparative Neurology* **128**, 191–208.

Fulling, K.H. and Garcia, D.M. (1985) Anaplastic astrocytoma of the adult cerebrum. Prognostic value of histologic features. *Cancer* **55**, 928–31.

Fulling, K.H. and Nelson, J.S. (1984) Cerebral astrocytic neoplasms in the adult: contribution of histologic examination to the assessment of prognosis. *Seminars in Diagnostic Pathology* **1**, 152–63.

Fults, D., Tippets, R.H., Thomas, G.A., Nakamura, Y, and White. R. (1989) Loss of heterozygosity for loci on chromosome 17p in human malignant astrocytoma. *Cancer Research* **49**, 6572–7.

Fults, D., Brockmeyer, D., Tullous, M.W., Pedone, C.A. and Cawthon, R.M. (1992) *p53* mutation and loss of heterozygosity on chromosomes 17 and 10 during human astrocytoma progression. *Cancer Research* **52**, 674–9.

Furie, D.M., Felsberg, G.J., Tien, R.D., Friedman, H.S., Fuchs, H. and McLendon, R. (1993) MRI of gangliocytoma of cerebellum and spinal cord. *Journal of Computer Assisted Tomography* **17**, 488–91.

Furness, P.N., Lowe, J. and Tarrant, G.S. (1990) Subepithelial basement membrane deposition and intermediate filament expression in choroid plexus neoplasms and ependymomas. *Histopathology* **16**, 251–5.

Furuta, A., Takahashi, H., Ikuta, F., Onda, K., Takeda, N. and Tanaka, R. (1992) Temporal lobe tumor demonstrating ganglioglioma and pleomorphic xanthoastrocytoma components. Case report. *Journal of Neurosurgery* **77**, 143–7.

Gaffney, C.C., Sloane, J.P., Bradley, N.J. and Bloom, H.J.G. (1985) Primitive neuroectodermal tumours of the cerebrum. Pathology and treatment. *Journal of Neuro-Oncology* **3**, 23–33.

Gajjar, A., Bhargava, R., Jenkins, J.J., Heideman, R., Sanford, R.A., Langston, J.W., Walter, A.W., Kuttesch, J.F., Muhlbauer, M. and Kun, L.E. (1995) Low-grade astrocytoma with neuraxis dissemination at diagnosis. *Journal of Neurosurgery* **83**, 67–71.

Gajjar, A.J., Heideman, R.L., Douglass, E.C., Kun, L.E., Kovnar, E.H., Sanford, R.A., Fairclough, D.L., Ayers, D. and Look, A.T. (1993) Relation of tumor-cell ploidy to survival in children with medulloblastoma. *Journal of Clinical Oncology* **11**, 2211–17.

Galea, E., Dupouey, P. and Feinstein, D.L. (1995) Glial fibrillary acidic protein mRNA isotypes: expression *in vitro* and *in vivo*. *Journal of Neuroscience Research* **41**, 452–61.

Galloway, P.G. and Roessmann, U. (1986) Anaplastic astrocytoma mimicking metastatic carcinoma. *American Journal of Surgical Pathology* **10**, 728–32.

Galou, M., Pournin, S., Ensergueix, D., Ridet, J.L., Tchelingerian, J.L., Lossouarn, L., Privat, A., Babinet, C. and Dupouey, P. (1994) Normal and pathological expression of GFAP promoter elements in transgenic mice. *Glia* **12**, 281–93.

Gambarelli, D., Hassoun, J., Choux, M. and Toga, M. (1982) Complex cerebral tumor with evidence of neuronal, glial and Schwann cell differentiation: a histologic, immunocytochemical and ultrastructural study. *Cancer* **49**, 1420–8.

Gamis, A.S., Egelhoff, J., Roloson, G., Young, J., Woods, G.M., Newman, R. and Freeman, A.I. (1990) Diffuse bony metastases at presentation in a child with glioblastoma multiforme. A case report. *Cancer* **66**, 180–4.

Gao, W.-Q., Heintz, N. and Hatten, M.E. (1991) Cerebellar granule cell neurogenesis is regulated by cell-cell interactions in vitro. *Neuron* **6**, 705–15.

Garcia, C.A., McGarry, P.A. and Collada, M. (1984) Ganglioglioma of the brain stem. Case report. *Journal of Neurosurgery* **60**, 431–4.

Garcia, D.M. and Fulling, K.H. (1985) Juvenile pilocytic astrocytoma of the cerebrum in adults. A distinctive neoplasm with favorable prognosis. *Journal of Neurosurgery* **63**, 382–6.

Garcia, D.M., Fulling, K.H. and Marks, J.E. (1985) The value of radiation therapy in addition to surgery for astrocytomas of the adult cerebrum. *Cancer* **55**, 919–27.

Garcia, J.H. and Lemmi, H. (1970) Ultrastructure of oligodendroglioma of the spinal cord. *American Journal of Clinical Pathology* **54**, 757–65.

Garcia-Bengochea, F. and Collins, G.H. (1969) Monstrocellular sarcoma of the brain: 6-year post-operative survival. *Journal of Neurosurgery* **31**, 686–9.

Garden, A.S., Maor, M.H., Yung, W.K.A., Bruner, J.M., Woo, S.Y., Moser, R.P. and Lee Y.Y. (1991) Outcome and patterns of failure following limited-volume irradiation for malignant astrocytomas. *Radiotherapy and Oncology* **20**, 99–110.

Garner, A. and Klintworth, G.K. (1994a) Tumors of the orbit, optic nerve and lacrimal sac. In Garner, A. and Klintworth, G.K. (eds), *Pathobiology of ocular disease. A dynamic approach*, Part B. Second edition. New York: Marcel Dekker, 1523–606.

——(eds) (1994b) *Pathobiology of ocular disease. A dynamic approach*. Second edition. New York: Marcel Dekker.

Garrido, E., Becker, L.F., Hoffman, H.J., Hendrick, E.B. and Humphreys, R. (1978) Gangliogliomas in children. A clinicopathological study. *Child's Brain* **4**, 339–46.

Garton, G.R., Schomberg, P.J., Scheithauer, B.W., Shaw, E.G., Blackwell, C.R., Laws, E.R.Jr and Earle, J.D. (1990) Medulloblastoma—prognostic factors and outcome of treatment: review of the Mayo Clinic experience. *Mayo Clinic Proceedings* **65**, 1077–86.

Gaspar, L.E., Fisher, B.J., MacDonald, D.R., Le Ber, D.V., Halperin, E.C., Schold, S.C. Jr and Cairncross, J.G. (1992) Supratentorial malignant glioma: patterns of recurrence and implications for external beam local treatment. *International Journal of Radiation Oncology, Biology and Physics* **24**, 55–7.

Georges, P.M., Notermann, J. and Flament-Durand, J. (1983) Glioblastoma in childhood. *Journal of Neuro-Oncology* **1**, 275–8.

Gerdes, J., Li, L., Schlueter, C., Duchrow, M., Wohlenberg, C., Gerlach, C., Stahmer, I., Kloth, S., Brandt, E. and Flad, H.-D. (1991) Immunobiochemical and molecular biologic characterization of the cell proliferation-associated nuclear antigen that is defined by monoclonal antibody Ki-67. *American Journal of Pathology* **138**, 867–73.

Geyer, J.R., Schofield, D., Berger, M. and Milstein, J. (1992) Differentiation of a primitive neuroectodermal tumor into a benign ganglioglioma. *Journal of Neuro-Oncology* **14**, 237–41.

Geyer, R., Levy, M., Berger, M.S., Milstein, J., Griffin, B. and Bleyer, W.A. (1991) Infants with medulloblastoma: a single institution review of survival. *Neurosurgery* **29**, 707–11.

Gherardi, R., Baudrimont, M., Nguyen, J.P., Gaston, A., Cesaro, P., Degos, J.D., Caron, J.P. and Poirier, J. (1986) Monstrocellular heavily lipidized malignant glioma. *Acta Neuropathologica* **69**, 28–32.

Ghobrial, M., Velasco, M., Ross, E. and Gonzalez, J. (1989) Astrocytic differentiation in metastatic medulloblastoma. *Laboratory Investigation* **60**, 33A.

Giangaspero, F. and Burger, P.C. (1983) Correlations between cytologic composition and biologic behavior in the glioblastoma multiforme. A postmortem study of 50 cases. *Cancer* **52**, 2320–33.

Giangaspero, F., Burger, P.C., Budwit, D.A., Usellini, L. and Mancini, A.M. (1985) Regulatory peptides in neuronal neoplasms of the central nervous system. *Clinical Neuropathology* **4**, 111–15.

Giangaspero, F., Chieco, P., Lisignoli, G. and Burger, P.C. (1987) Comparison of cytologic composition with microfluorometric DNA analysis of the glioblastoma multiforme and anaplastic astrocytoma. *Cancer* **60**, 59–65.

Giangaspero, F., Rigobello, L., Badiali, M., Loda, M., Andreini, L., Basso, G., Zorzi, F. and Montaldi, A. (1992) Large-cell medulloblastomas. A distinct variant with highly aggressive behavior. *American Journal of Surgical Pathology* **16**, 687–93.

Giannini, C., Scheithauer, B.W., Burger, P.C., Christensen, M.R., Wollan, P.C., Sebo, T.J., Forsyth, P.A. and Hayostek, C.J. (1996) The MIB-1 LI in pilocytic and diffuse astrocytomas. *Journal of Neuropathology and Experimental Neurology* **55**, 605A.

Giese, A., Loo, M.A., Rief, M.D., Tran, N. and Berens, M.E. (1995) Substrates for astrocytoma invasion. *Neurosurgery* **37**, 294–302.

Gilbertson, R.J., Pearson, A.D.J., Perry, R.H., Jaros, E. and Kelly, P.J. (1995) Prognostic significance of the c-*erb*B-2 oncogene product in childhood medulloblastoma. *British Journal of Cancer* **71**, 473–7.

Giordana, M.T., Bradac, G.B., Pagni, C.A., Marino, S. and Attanasio, A. (1995) Primary diffuse leptomeningeal gliomatosis with anaplastic features. *Acta Neurochirurgica* **132**, 154–9.

Giordano, S., Sherman, L., Lyman, W. and Morrison, R. (1992) Multiple molecular weight forms of basic fibroblast growth factor are developmentally regulated in the central nervous system. *Developmental Biology* **152**, 293–303.

Gjerris, F. and Klinken, L. (1978) Long-term prognosis in children with benign cerebellar astrocytoma. *Journal of Neurosurgery* **49**, 179–84.

Gladson, C.L. and Cheresh, D.A. (1991) Glioblastoma expression of vitronectin and the alpha v beta 3 integrin. Adhesion mechanism for transformed glial cells. *Journal of Clinical Investigation* **88**, 1924–32.

Glasauer, F.E. and Yuan, R.H.P. (1963) Intracranial tumors with extracranial metastases. *Journal of Neurosurgery* **20**, 474–93.

Glass, J., Hochberg, F.H., Gruber M.L., Louis D.N., Smith D. and Rattner, B. (1992) The treatment of oligodendrogliomas and mixed oligodendroglioma-astrocytomas with PCV chemotherapy. *Journal of Neurosurgery* **76**, 741–5.

Glasser, R., Rojiani, A.M., Mickle, J.P. and Eskin, T.A. (1995) Delayed occurrence of cerebellar pleomorphic xanthoastrocytoma after supratentorial pleomorphic xanthoastrocytoma removal. Case report. *Journal of Neurosurgery* **82**, 116–18.

Globus, J.H. (1938) Glioneuroma and spongioneuroblastoma, forms of primary neuroectodermal tumors of the brain. *American Journal of Cancer* **32**, 163–220.

Gnekow, A.K., Bailey, C., Michaelis, J., Wellek, S. and Kleihues, P. (1991) SIOP/GPO medulloblastoma trial II. Med 84: annual status report. *Medical and Pediatric Oncology* **19**, 435.

Gocht, A., Zeunert, G., Laas, R. and Löhler, J. (1992) The carbohydrate epitope 3-fucosyl-*N*-acetyllactosamine is developmentally regulated in the human cerebellum. *Anatomy and Embryology* **186**, 543–56.

Goebel, H.H. and Cravioto, H. (1972) Ultrastructure of human and experimental ependymomas. *Journal of Neuropathology and Experimental Neurology* **31**, 54–71.

Goldammer, D. and Goebel, H.H. (1980) Dense core vesicles in the desmoplastic variant of cerebral neuroblastoma. *Acta Neuropathologica* **50**, 81–3.

Goldberg-Stern, H., Gadoth, N., Stern, S., Cohen, I.J., Zaizov, R. and Sandbank, U. (1991) The prognostic significance of glial fibrillary acidic protein staining in medulloblastoma. *Cancer* **68**, 568–73.

Goldman, R.L. (1969) Gliomyosarcoma of the cerebrum. Report of a unique case. *American Journal of Clinical Pathology* **52**, 741–4.

Goldwein, J.W., Glauser, T.A., Packer, R.J., Finlay, J.L., Sutton, L.N., Curran, W.J., Laehy, J.M., Rorke, L.B., Schut, L. and D'Angio, G.J. (1990) Recurrent intracranial ependymomas in children. Survival, patterns of failure, and prognostic factors. *Cancer* **66**, 557–63.

Goldwein, J.W., Corn, B.W., Finlay, J.L., Packer, R.J., Rorke, L.B. and Schut, L. (1991) Is craniospinal irradiation required to cure children with malignant (anaplastic) intracranial ependymomas? *Cancer* **67**, 2766–71.

Gomez, J.G., Garcia, J.H. and Colon, L.E. (1985) A variant of cerebral glioma called pleomorphic xanthoastrocytoma: case report. *Neurosurgery* **16**, 703–6.

Gonzalez-Campora, R., Otal-Salaverri, C., Vazquez-Ramirez, F., Salguero-Villadiego, M. and Galera-Davidson, H. (1993) Metastatic glioblastoma multiforme in cervical lymph nodes. Report of a case with diagnosis by fine needle aspiration. *Acta Cytologica* **37**, 938–42.

Gorlin, R.J. (1987) Nevoid basal-cell carcinoma syndrome. *Medicine* **66**, 98–113.

Gorlin, R.J. and Goltz, R.W. (1960) Multiple nevoid basal-cell epithelioma, jaw cysts and bifid rib. A syndrome. *New England Journal of Medicine* **262**, 908–12.

Goto, S., Matsukado, Y., Mihara, Y., Inoue, N. and Miyamoto, E. (1987) An immunocytochemical demonstration of calcineurin in human nerve cell tumors. A comparison with neuron-specific enolase and glial fibrillary acidic protein. *Cancer* **60**, 2948–57.

Gottesman, M., Laufer, H. and Patel, M. (1991) Gliomatosis cerebri: a case report. *Clinical Neuropathology* **10**, 303–5.

Gottschalk, J., Goebel, S.,Jautzke, G., Martin, H., Zimmer, C., Märzheuser-Brands, S. and Cervós-Navarro, J. (1992) Influence of preoperative dexamethasone therapy on proliferating cell nuclear antigen (PCNA) expression in comparison to other parameters in meningiomas. *Histology and Histopathology* **7**, 653–61.

Gould, S.J. and Howard, S. (1987) An immunohistochemical study of the germinal layer in the late gestation human fetal brain. *Neuropathology and Applied Neurobiology* **13**, 421–37.

——(1988) Glial differentiation in the germinal layer of fetal and preterm infant brain: an immunocytochemical study. *Pediatric Pathology* **8**, 25–36.

Gould, S.J., Howard, S. and Papadaki, L. (1990) The development of ependyma in the human fetal brain: an immunohistological and electron microscopic study. *Brain Research. Developmental Brain Research* **55**, 255–67.

Gould, V.E., Jansson, D.S., Molenaar, W.M., Rorke, L.B., Trojanowski, J.Q., Lee, V.M.Y., Packer, R.J. and Franke, W.W. (1990) Primitive neuroectodermal tumors of the central nervous system. Patterns of expression of neuroendocrine markers, and all classes of intermediate filament proteins. *Laboratory Investigation* **62**, 498–509.

Grabb, P.A., Albright, A.L. and Pang, D. (1992) Dissemination of supratentorial malignant gliomas via the cerebrospinal fluid in children. *Neurosurgery* **30**, 64–71.

Grant, J.W. and Gallagher, P.J. (1986) Pleomorphic xanthoastrocytoma. Immunohistochemical methods for differentiation from fibrous histiocytomas with similar morphology. *American Journal of Surgical Pathology* **10**, 336–41.

Grcevic, N. and Yates, P.O. (1957) Rosenthal fibres in tumours of the central nervous system. *Journal of Pathology and Bacteriology* **73**, 467–72.

Greene, H.S.N. and Harvey, E.K. (1964a) Metastasis from the brain. *Cancer Research* **24**, 1021–7.

——(1964b) Metastases of heterologously transplanted tumors. *Cancer Research* **24**, 1678–87.

Greig, N.H., Ries, L.G., Yancik, R. and Rapoport, S.I. (1990) Increasing annual incidence of primary malignant brain tumors in the elderly. *Journal of the National Cancer Institute* **82**, 1621–4.

Griepentrog, F. and Pauly, H. (1957) Intra- und extrakranielle, frühmanifeste Medulloblastome bei erbgleichen Zwillingen. *Zentralblatt Für Neurochirurgie* **17**, 129–41.

Griffin, C.A., Long, P.P., Carson, B.S. and Brem, H. (1992) Chromosome abnormalities in low-grade central nervous system tumors. *Cancer Genetics and Cytogenetics* **60**, 67–73.

Gritzman, M.C.D., Snyckers, F.D. and Proctor, N.S.F. (1983) Ganglioglioma of the optic nerve. A case report. *South African Medical Journal* **63**, 863–5.

Groothuis, D.R., Fischer, J.M., Vick, N.A. and Bigner, D.D. (1980) Experimental gliomas: an autoradiographic study of the endothelial component. *Neurology* **30**, 297–301.

Guccion, J.G. and Saini, N. (1991) Ependymoma: ultrastructural studies of two cases. *Ultrastructural Pathology* **15**, 159–66.

Guéneau, G., Privat, A., Drouet, J. and Court, L. (1982) Subgranular zone of the dentate gyrus of young rabbits as a secondary matrix. A high-resolution autoradiographic study. *Developmental Neuroscience* **5**, 345–58.

Guerrieri, C. and Jarlsfelt, I. (1993) Ependymoma of the ovary. A case report with immunohistochemical, ultrastructural, and DNA cytometric findings, as well as histogenetic considerations. *American Journal of Surgical Pathology* **17**, 623–32.

Guha, A., Resch, L. and Tator, C.H. (1989) Subependymoma of the thoracolumbar cord. *Journal of Neurosurgery* **71**, 781–7.

Gullotta, F. (1995) La genesi formale delle fibre di Rosenthal. *Acta Neurologica* **20**, 704.

Gullotta, F. and Fliedner, E. (1972) Spongioblastomas, astrocytomas and Rosenthal fibers. Ultra-structural, tissue culture and enzyme histochemical investigations. *Acta Neuropathologica* **22**, 68–78.

Gupta, R.K. and Pratap, D. (1992) Metastasising congenital subcutaneous sacrococcygeal ependymoma. *Indian Journal of Cancer* **29**, 76–81.

Haddad, S.F., Moore, S.A., Menezes, A.H. and VanGilder, J.C. (1992a) Ganglioglioma: 13 years of experience. *Neurosurgery* **31**, 171–8.

Haddad, S.F., Moore, S.A., Schelper, R.L. and Goeken, J.A. (1992b) Vascular smooth muscle hyperplasia underlies the formation of glomeruloid vascular structures of glioblastoma multiforme. *Journal of Neuropathology and Experimental Neurology* **51**, 488–92.

——(1992c) Smooth muscle can comprise the sarcomatous component of gliosarcomas. *Journal of Neuropathology and Experimental Neurology* **51**, 493–8.

Hadfield, M.G. and Silverberg, S.G. (1972) Light and electron microscopy of giant-cell glioblastoma. *Cancer* **30**, 989–96.

Hahn, J.S., Bejar, R. and Gladson, C.L. (1991) Neonatal subependymal giant cell astrocytoma associated with tuberous sclerosis: MRI, CT and ultrasound correlation. *Neurology* **41**, 124–8.

Haie, C., Schlienger, M., Constans, J.P., Meder, J.F., Reynaud, A. and Ghenim, C. (1985) Results of radiation treatment of medulloblastoma in adults. *International Journal of Radiation Oncology, Biology and Physics* **11**, 2051–6.

Haie-Meder, C. and Song, P.Y. (1995) Medulloblastoma: differences in adults and children—regarding Frost *et al., IJROBP* 32:951–957; 1995 and Prados *et al., IJROBP* 32:1145–1152; 1995. *International Journal of Radiation Oncology, Biology and Physics* **32**, 1255–7.

Hajos, F. and Basco, E. (1984) The surface-contact glia. *Advances in Anatomy, Embryology and Cell Biology* **84**, 1–79.

Halberg, F.E., Wara, W.M., Fippin, L.F., Edwards, M.S.B., Levin, V.A., Davis, R.L., Prados, M.B., and Wilson, C.B. (1991) Low-dose craniospinal radiation therapy for medulloblastoma. *International Journal of Radiation Oncology, Biology and Physics* **20**, 651–4.

Hall, W.A., Yunis, E.J. and Albright, A.L. (1986) Anaplastic ganglioglioma in an infant: case report and review of the literature. *Neurosurgery* **19**, 1016–20.

Hallervorden, J. (1959) Über die Hamartome (Ganglioneurome) des Kleinhirns. *Deutsche Zeitschrift für Nervenheilkunde* **179**, 531–63.

——(1961) The development of the myelin sheath and Rosenthal fibers. *Deutsche Zeitschrift für Nervenheilkunde* **181**, 547–80.

Hallonet, M.E.R. and Le Douarin, N.M. (1993) Tracing neuroepithelial cells of the mesencephalic and metencephalic alar plates during cerebellar ontogeny in quail-chick chimaeras. *European Journal of Neuroscience* **5**, 1145–55.

Halmagyi, G.M., Bignold, L.P. and Allsop, J.L. (1979) Recurrent subependymal giant-cell astrocytoma in the absence of tuberous sclerosis. *Journal of Neurosurgery* **50**, 106–9.

Hamilton, M.G., Tranmer, B.I. and Hagen, N.A. (1993) Supratentorial glioblastoma with spinal cord intramedullary metastasis. *Canadian Journal of Neurological Sciences* **20**, 65–8.

Handa, H., Yamagami, T. and Furuta, M. (1994) An adult patient with cerebellar ganglioglioma. *Journal of Neuro-Oncology* **18**, 183–9.

Hara, A., Araki, Y., Shinoda, J., Hirayama, H., Niikawa, S., Sakai, N. and Yamada, H. (1993) Central neurocytoma: proliferative assessment by nucleolar organizer region staining. *Surgical Neurology* **39**, 343–7.

Harper, C.G. and Stewart-Wynne, E.G. (1978) Malignant optic gliomas in adults. *Archives of Neurology* **35**, 731–5.

Harris, M.D., Moore, I.E., Steart, P.V. and Weller, R.O. (1990) Protein gene product (PGP) 9.5 as a reliable marker in primitive neuroectodermal tumours—an immunohistochemical study of 21 childhood cases. *Histopathology* **16**, 271–7.

Hart, M.N. and Earle, K.M. (1973) Primitive neuroectodermal tumors of the brain in children. *Cancer* **32**, 890–7.

Hasenjäger, T. (1938) Über die Ausbreitung ventrikelnaher Gliosarkome auf dem Wege des innern Liquors (Ependymitis blastomatosa). *Zeitschrift für die Gesamte Neurologie und Psychiatrie* **161**, 153–9.

Hassin, G.B. and Munch-Petersen, C.J. (1951) Central neurogenic tumors (neuroblastoma and ganglioneuroma). A pathologic study of two cases. *Journal of Neuropathology and Clinical Neurology* **1**, 63–80.

Hassoun, J., Hirano, A. and Zimmerman, H.N. (1975) Fine structure of intercellular junctions and blood vessels in medulloblastomas. *Acta Neuropathologica* **33**, 67–78.

Hassoun, J., Gambarelli, D., Grisoli, F., Pellet, W., Salamon, G., Pellissier, J.F. and Toga, M. (1982) Central neurocytoma. An electron-microscopic study of two cases. *Acta Neuropathologica* **56**, 151–6.

Hassoun, J., Söylemezoglu, F., Gambarelli, D., Figarella-Branger, D., von Ammon, K. and Kleihues, P. (1993) Central neurocytoma: a synopsis of clinical and histological features. *Brain Pathology* **3**, 297–306.

Hatten, M.E. (1993) The role of migration in central nervous system neuronal development. *Current Opinion in Neurobiology* **3**, 38–44.

Haustein, J., Cruz-Sanchez, F. and Cervós-Navarro, J. (1988) On the ultrastructure of ependymomas—a semiquantitative analysis of diagnostic criteria in 21 cases with special reference to glycogen as a marker. *Neurosurgical Review* **11**, 67–76.

Hawkes, R., Blyth, S., Chockkan, V., Tano, D., Ji, Z. and Mascher, C. (1993) Structural and molecular compartmentation in the cerebellum. *Canadian Journal of Neurological Sciences* **20**, S29–S35.

Hawkins, J.C. III, Hoffman, H.J. and Becker, L.E. (1979) Multiple nevoid basal-cell carcinoma syndrome (Gorlin's syndrome): possible confusion with metastatic medulloblastoma. *Journal of Neurosurgery* **50**, 100–2.

Hayashi, K., Notoi, M., Nose, S., Horie, Y., Akagi, T., Ogawa, K., Taguchi, K., Nizobuchi, K. and Nishimoto, A. (1987) An immunohistochemical study on the distribution of glial fibrillary acidic protein, S-100 protein, neuron-specific enolase, and neurofilament in medulloblastomas. *Acta Pathologica Japonica* **37**, 85–96.

Hayostek, C.J., Shaw, E.G., Scheithauer, B., O'Fallon, J.R., Weiland, T.L., Schomberg, P.J., Kelly, P.J. and Hu, T.C. (1993) Astrocytomas of the cerebellum. A comparative clinicopathologic study of pilocytic and diffuse astrocytomas. *Cancer* **72**, 856–69.

Hazuka, M.B., DeBiose, D.A., Henderson, R.H., and Kinzie, J.J. (1992) Survival results in adult patients treated for medulloblastoma. *Cancer* **69**, 2143–8.

He, X., Wikstrand, C.J., Friedman, H.S., Bigner, S.H., Pleasure, S., Trojanowski, J.Q. and Bigner, D.D. (1991) Differentiation characteristics of newly established medulloblastoma cell lines (D384 Med, D425 Med, and D458 Med) and their transplantable xenografts. *Laboratory Investigation* **64**, 833–43.

Heck, K., Pyle, P. and Bruner, J.M. (1994) *Bcl-2* expression in cerebellar medulloblastomas. (Abstract) *Brain Pathology* **4**, 430A.

Helseth, A. (1995) The incidence of primary central nervous system neoplasms before and after computerized tomography availability. *Journal of Neurosurgery* **83**, 999–1003.

Henriquez, A.S., Robertson, D.M. and Marshall, W.J.S. (1973) Primary neuroblastoma of the central nervous system with spontaneous extracranial metastases. *Journal of Neurosurgery* **38**, 226–31.

Henschen, F. (1955) Tumoren des Zentralnervensystems und seiner Hüllen. In Lubarsch, O., Henke, F. and Roüssle, R. (eds), *Handbuch der Speziellen Pathologischen Anatomie und Histologie*, Vol. 13, Part 3. Berlin: Springer, 413–37.

Herman, M.M., Sipe, J.C., Rubinstein, L.J., VandenBerg, S.R., Spence, A.M. and Vraa-Jensen, J. (1975) An experimental mouse testicular teratoma as a model for neuroepithelial neoplasia and differentiation. II. Electron microscopy. *American Journal of Pathology* **81**, 421–44.

Herndon, R.M., Rubinstein, L.J., Freeman, J.M. and Mathieson, G. (1970) Light and electron microscopic observations on Rosenthal fibers in Alexander's disease and in multiple sclerosis. *Journal of Neuropathology and Experimental Neurology* **29**, 524–51.

Herpers, M.J.H.M. and Budka, H. (1984) Glial fibrillary acidic protein (GFAP) in oligodendroglial tumours: gliofibrillary oligodendroglioma and transitional oligoastrocytoma as subtypes of oligodendroglioma. *Acta Neuropathologica* **64**, 265–72.

——(1985) Primitive neuroectodermal tumors including the medulloblastoma: glial differentiation signaled by immunoreactivity for GFAP is restricted to the pure desmoplastic medulloblastoma ('arachnoidal sarcoma of the cerebellum'). *Clinical Neuropathology* **4**, 12–18.

Herpers, M.J.H.M., Budka, H. and McCormick, D. (1984) Production of glial fibrillary acidic protein (GFAP) by neoplastic cells: adaptation to the microenvironment. *Acta Neuropathologica* **64**, 333–8.

Herpers, M.J.H.M., Freling, G. and Beuls, E.A.M. (1994) Pleomorphic xanthoastrocytoma in the spinal cord. Case report. *Journal of Neurosurgery* **80**, 564–9.

Herpers, M.J.H M., Ramaekers, F.C.S., Aldeweireldt, J., Moesker, O. and Slooff, J. (1986) Co-expression of glial fibrillary acidic protein (GFAP) and vimentin-type intermediate filaments in human astrocytomas. *Acta Neuropathologica* **70**, 333–9.

Hershatter, B.W., Halperin, E.C. and Cox, E.B. (1986) Medulloblastoma: the Duke University Medical Center experience. *International Journal of Radiation Oncology, Biology and Physics* **12**, 1771–7.

Hessler, R.B., Lopes, M.B., Frankfurter, A., Reidy, J. and VandenBerg, S.R. (1992) Cytoskeletal immunohistochemistry of central neurocytomas. *American Journal of Surgical Pathology* **16**, 1031–8.

Heyderman, E., Steele, K. and Ormerod, M.G. (1979) A new antigen on the epithelial membrane: its immunoperoxidase localization in normal and neoplastic tissue. *Journal of Clinical Pathology* **32**, 35–9.

Hirakawa, K., Suzuki, K., Ueda, S. and Handa, J. (1986) Fetal origin of the medulloblastoma: evidence from growth analysis of two cases. *Acta Neuropathologica* **70**, 227–34.

Hirano, A. and Shin, W.Y. (1979) Unattached presynaptic terminals in a cerebellar neuroblastoma in the human. *Neuropathology and Applied Neurobiology* **5**, 63–70.

Hirato, J., Nagayata, Y. and Ogawa, A. (1994) Expression of non-glial intermediate proteins in gliomas. *Clinical Neuropathology* **13**, 1–11.

Hirose, T., Kannuki, S., Nishida, K., Matsumoto, K., Sano, T. and Hizawa, K. (1992) Anaplastic ganglioglioma of the brain stem demonstrating active neurosecretory features of neoplastic neuronal cells. *Acta Neuropathologica* **83**, 365–70.

Hirose, T., Scheithauer, B.W., Lopes, M.B.S. and VandenBerg, S.R. (1994) Dysembryoplastic neuroepithelial tumor (DNT): an immunohistochemical and ultrastructural study. *Journal of Neuropathology and Experimental Neurology* **53**, 184–95.

Hirsch, J.F., Renier, D., Czernichow, P., Benveniste, L. and Pierre-Kahn, A. (1979) Medulloblastoma in childhood. Survival and functional results. *Acta Neurochirurgica* **48**, 1–15.

Ho, K.C., Meyer, G., Caya, J., Tieu, T.M. and Prentiss, A. (1987) Craniopharyngioma and 'reactive' subependymoma of the third ventricle. *Clinical Neuropathology* **6**, 12–15.

Ho, K.L. (1982) Tumors of the cerebral aqueduct. *Cancer* **48**, 154–62.

——(1983) Concurrence of subependymoma and heterotopic leptomeningeal neuroglial tissue. *Archives of Pathology and Laboratory Medicine* **107**, 136–40.

——(1986) Abnormal cilia in a fourth ventricular ependymoma. *Acta Neuropathologica* **70**, 30–7.

——(1990a) Microtubular aggregates within rough endoplasmic reticulum in myxopapillary ependymoma of the filum terminale. *Archives of Pathology and Laboratory Medicine* **114**, 956–60.

——(1990b) Intercellular septate-like junction of neoplastic cells in myxopapillary ependymoma of the filum terminale. *Acta Neuropathologica* **79**, 432–7.

——(1990c) Histogenesis of sarcomatous component of the gliosarcoma: an ultrastructural study. *Acta Neuropathologica* **81**, 178–88.

Hoag, G., Sima, A.A.F. and Rozdilsky, B. (1986) Astroblastoma revisited: a report of three cases. *Acta Neuropathologica* **70**, 10–16.

Hochberg, F.H. and Pruitt, A. (1980) Assumptions in the radiotherapy of glioblastoma. *Neurology* **30**, 907–11.

Hockfield, S. and McKay, R.D. (1985) Identification of major cell classes in the developing mammalian nervous system. *Journal of Neuroscience* **5**, 3310–28.

Hoffman, H.J. and Duffner, P.K. (1985) Extraneural metastases of central nervous system tumors. *Cancer* **56**, 1778–82.

Hoffman, H.J., Hendrick, E.B. and Humphreys, R.P. (1976) Metastasis via ventriculoperitoneal shunt in patients with medulloblastoma. *Journal of Neurosurgery* **44**, 562–6.

Hoffman, H.J., Becker, L.E., Jenkin, D., Chuang, S.H. and Munro, I.R. (1981) Extraneural metastases of a cerebral astrocytoma. *Canadian Journal of Neurological Sciences* **8**, 115–19.

Hoffman, H.J., Humphreys, R.P., Drake, J.M., Rutka, J.T., Becker, L.E., Jenkin, D. and Greenberg, M. (1993) Optic pathway/hypothalamic gliomas: a dilemma in management. *Pediatric Neurosurgery* **19**, 186–95.

Höll, T., Kleihues, P., Yasargil, M.G. and Wiestler, O.D. (1991) Cerebellar medullomyoblastoma with advanced neuronal differentiation and hamartomatous component. *Acta Neuropathologica* **82**, 408–13.

Horoupian, D.S., Kress, Y., Yen, S.-H. and Gaskin, F. (1982) Nickel-induced changes and reappraisal of Rosenthal fibers in focal CNS lesions. *Journal of Neuropathology and Experimental Neurology* **41**, 664–75.

Horowitz, M.E., Parham, D.M., Douglass, E.C., Kun, L.E., Houghton, J.A. and Houghton, P.J. (1987) Development and characterization of human ependymoma xenograft HxBr5. *Cancer Research* **47**, 499–504.

Horrax, G. and Bailey, P. (1928) Pineal pathology; further studies. *Archives of Neurology and Psychiatry* **19**, 394–414.

Horten, B.C. and Rubinstein, L.J. (1976) Primary cerebral neuroblastoma. A clinicopathological study of 35 cases. *Brain* **99**, 735–56.

Horvath, E., Kovacs, K., Scheithauer, B.W., Lloyd, R.V. and Smyth, H.S. (1994) Pituitary adenoma with neuronal choristoma (PANCH): composite lesion or lineage infidelity? *Ultrastructural Pathology* **18**, 565–74.

Horwich, A. and Bloom, H.J.G. (1985) Optic gliomas: radiation therapy and prognosis. *International Journal of Radiation Oncology, Biology and Physics* **11**, 1067–79.

Hoshino, T. (1981) Cellular aspects of human brain tumors (gliomas). In Fedoroff, S. and Hertz, L. (eds), *Advances in cellular neurobiology*, Vol. 2. New York: Academic Press, 167–204.

——(1984) A commentary on the biology and growth kinetics of low-grade and high-grade gliomas. *Journal of Neurosurgery* **61**, 895–900.

Hoshino, T. and Wilson, C.B. (1979) Cell kinetic analyses of human malignant brain tumors (gliomas). *Cancer* **44**, 956–62.

Hoshino, T., Wilson, C.B. and Ellis, W.G. (1975) Gemistocytic astrocytes in gliomas. An autoradiographic study. *Journal of Neuropathology and Experimental Neurology* **34**, 263–81.

Hoshino, T., Wilson, C.B. and Muraoka, I. (1979) The stathmokinetic (mitostatic) effect of vincristine and vinblastine on human gliomas. *Acta Neuropathologica* **47**, 21–5.

Hoshino, T., Barker, M., Wilson, C.B., Boldrey, E.B. and Fewer, D. (1972) Cell kinetics of human gliomas. *Journal of Neurosurgery* **37**, 15–26.

Hoshino, T., Wilson, C.B., Rosenblum, M.L. and Barker, M. (1975) Chemotherapeutic implications of growth fraction and cell cycle time in glioblastomas. *Journal of Neurosurgery* **43**, 127–35.

Hoshino, T., Nomura, K., Wilson, C.B., Knebel, K.D. and Gray, J.W. (1978) The distribution of nuclear DNA from human brain-tumor cells. Flow cytometric studies. *Journal of Neurosurgery* **49**, 13–21.

Hoshino, T., Kobayashi, S., Townsend, J.J.I. and Wilson, C.B. (1985) A cell kinetic study on medulloblastomas. *Cancer* **55**, 1711–13.

Hoshino, T., Nagashima, T., Murovic, J.A., Wilson, C.B., Edwards, M.S.B., Gutin, P.H., Davis, R.L. and DeArmond, S.J. (1986) *In situ* cell kinetic studies on human neuroectodermal tumors with bromodeoxyuridine labeling. *Journal of Neurosurgery* **64**, 453–9.

Hoshino, T., Rodriguez, L.A., Cho, K.G., Lee, K.S., Wilson, C.B., Edwards, M.S.B., Levin, V.A. and Davis, R.L. (1988) Prognostic implications of the proliferative potential of low-grade astrocytomas. *Journal of Neurosurgery* **69**, 839–42.

Hoshino, T., Prados, M., Wilson, C.B., Cho, K.G., Lee, K.-S. and Davis, R.L. (1989) Prognostic implications of the bromodeoxyuridine labeling index of human gliomas. *Journal of Neurosurgery* **71**, 335–41.

Hoshino, T., Ahn, D., Prados, M.D., Lamborn, K. and Wilson, C.B. (1993) Prognostic significance of the proliferative potential of intracranial gliomas measured by bromodeoxyuridine labeling. *International Journal of Cancer* **53**, 550–5.

Hossmann, K.-A. and Wechsler, W. (1965) Zur Feinstruktur menschlicher Spongioblastome. *Deutsche Zeitschrift für Nervenheilkunde* **187**, 327–51.

——(1971) Ultrastructural cytopathology of human cerebral gliomas. *Oncology* **25**, 455–80.

Hoyt, W.F. and Baghdassarian, S.A. (1969) Optic glioma of childhood. *British Journal of Ophthalmology* **53**, 793–8.

Hoyt, W.F., Piovanetti, E., Malamud, N. and Wilson, C.B. (1972) Cranio-orbital involvement in glioblastoma multiforme. *Neurochirurgia* **15**, 1–8.

Hoyt, W.F., Meshel, L.G., Lessell, S., Schatz, N.J. and Suckling, R.D. (1973) Malignant optic glioma of adulthood. *Brain* **96**, 121–32.

Hubbard, J.L., Scheithauer, B.W., Kispert, D.B., Carpenter, S.M., Wick, M.R. and Laws, E.R. Jr (1989) Adult cerebellar medulloblastomas: the pathological, radiographic, and clinical disease spectrum. *Journal of Neurosurgery* **70**, 536–44.

Hughes, P.G. (1984) Cerebellar medulloblastoma in adults. *Journal of Neurosurgery* **60**, 994–7.

Hulbanni, S. and Goodman, P.A. (1976) Glioblastoma multiforme with extraneural metastases in the absence of previous surgery. *Cancer* **37**, 1577–83.

Hunt, S.J. and Johnson, P.C. (1989) Melanotic ganglioglioma of the pineal region. *Acta Neuropathologica* **79**, 222–5.

Hurst, R.W., Newman, S.A. and Cail, W.S. (1988) Multifocal intracranial MR abnormalities in neurofibromatosis. *American Journal of Neuroradiology* **9**, 293–6.

Husain, A.N. and Leestma, J.E. (1986) Cerebral astroblastoma: immunohistochemical and ultrastructural features. *Journal of Neurosurgery* **64**, 657–61.

Iglesias, J.R., Richardson, E.P. Jr, Collia, F., Santos, A., Garcia, M.C. and Redondo, C. (1984) Prenatal intramedullary gliofibroma. A light and electron microscope study. *Acta Neuropathologica* **62**, 230–4.

Ikezaki, K., Matsushima, T., Inoue, T., Yokoyama, N., Kaneko, Y. and Fukui, M. (1993) Correlation of microanatomical localization with postoperative survival in posterior fossa ependymomas. *Neurosurgery* **32**, 38–44.

Ilgren, E.B. and Stiller, C.A. (1987) Cerebellar astrocytomas. Clinical characteristics and prognostic indices. *Journal of Neuro-Oncology* **4**, 293–308.

Ilgren, E.B., Kinnier-Wilson, L.M. and Stiller, C.A. (1985) Gliomas in neurofibromatosis: a series of 89 cases with evidence for enhanced malignancy in associated cerebellar astrocytomas. *Pathology Annual* **20** (Part 1), 331–58.

Imes, R.K. and Hoyt, W.F. (1986) Childhood chiasmal gliomas: update on the fate of patients in the 1969 San Francisco study. *British Journal of Ophthalmology* **70**, 179–82.

——(1991) Magnetic resonance imaging signs of optic nerve gliomas in neurofibromatosis 1. *American Journal of Ophthalmology* **111**, 729–34.

Iqbal, Z. and Sutcliffe, J.C. (1994) Subependymoma of the lateral ventricle: case report and literature review. *British Journal of Neurosurgery* **8**, 83–5.

Ito, S., Hoshino, T., Prados, M.D. and Edwards, M.S.B. (1992a) Cell kinetics of medulloblastomas. *Cancer* **70**, 671–8.

Ito, S., Hoshino, T., Shibuya, M., Prados, M.D., Edwards, M.S.B. and Davis, R.L. (1992b) Proliferative characteristics of juvenile pilocytic astrocytomas determined by bromodeoxyuridine labeling. *Neurosurgery* **31**, 413–19.

Ito, S., Chandler, K.L., Prados, M.D., Lamborn, K., Wynne, J., Malec, M.K., Wilson, C.B., Davis, R.L. and Hoshino, T. (1994) Proliferative potential and prognostic evaluation of low-grade astrocytomas. *Journal of Neuro-Oncology* **19**, 1–9.

Itoh, Y., Yagishita, S. and Chiba, Y. (1987) Cerebral gangliocytoma. An ultrastructural study. *Acta Neuropathologica* **74**, 169–78.

Itoh, Y., Kowada, M., Mineura, K. and Kojima, H. (1987) Congenital glioblastoma of the cerebellum with cytofluorometric deoxyribonucleic acid analysis. *Surgical Neurology* **27**, 163–7.

Itoyama, Y., Sternberger, N.H., Kies, M.W., Cohen, S.R., Richardson, E.P. Jr and Webster, H. de F. (1980) Immunocytochemical method to identify myelin basic protein in oligodendroglia and myelin sheaths of the human nervous system. *Annals of Neurology* **7**, 157–66.

Iwaki, T., Fukui, M., Kondo, A., Matushima, T. and Takeshita, I. (1987) Epithelial properties of pleomorphic xanthoastrocytomas determined by ultrastructural and immunohistochemical studies. *Acta Neuropathologica* **74**, 142–50.

Jacobsen, P.F. and Papadimitriou, J.M. (1989) Mesenchymal differentiation of cell lines obtained from human gliomas inoculated into nude mice. *Cancer* **63**, 682–92.

Jacobsen, P.F., Jenkyn, D.J. and Papadimitriou, J.M. (1985) Establishment of a human medulloblastoma cell line and its heterotransplantation into nude mice. *Journal of Neuropathology and Experimental Neurology* **44**, 472–85.

Jaffey, P.B., To, G.T., Xu, H.-J., Hu, S.-X., Benedict, W.F., Donoso, L.A. and Campbell, G.A. (1995) Retinoblastoma-like phenotype expressed in medulloblastomas. *Journal of Neuropathology and Experimental Neurology* **54**, 664–72.

James, C.D., Carlbom, E., Dumanski, J.P., Hansen, M., Nordenskjold, M., Collins, V.P. and Cavenee, W.K. (1988) Clonal genomic alterations in glioma malignancy stages. *Cancer Research* **48**, 5546–51.

James, C.D., He, J., Carlbom, E., Mikkelsen, T., Ridderheim, P.-A., Cavenee, W.K. and Collins, V.P. (1990) Loss of genetic information in central nervous system tumors common to children and young adults. *Genes, Chromosomes and Cancer* **2**, 94–102.

James, T.G.I. and Pagel, W. (1951) Oligodendroglioma with extracranial metastases. *British Journal of Surgery* **39**, 56–65.

Jamjoom, Z.A., Jamjoom, A.B., Sulaiman, A.H., Naim-Ur-Rahman and al Rabiaa, A. (1993) Systemic metastasis of medulloblastoma through ventriculoperitoneal shunt: report of a case and critical analysis of the literature. *Surgical Neurology* **40**, 403–10.

Jamjoom, Z.B., el Saghir, N.S., Sadiq, S., Malabarey, T. and al-Khudairy, N.N. (1989) Direct spread of medulloblastoma in adjacent extrameningeal tissues. *Acta Neurochirurgica* **97**, 171–6.

Jänisch, W., Haas, J.F., Schreiber, D. and Gerlach, H. (1984) Primary central nervous system tumors in stillborns and infants. Epidemiological considerations. *Journal of Neuro-Oncology* **2**, 113–16.

Janss, A.J., Gundy, R., Cnaan, A., Savino, P.J., Packer, R.J., Zackai, E.H., Goldwein, J.W., Sutton, L.N., Radcliffe, J., Molloy, P.T., Phillips, P.C. and Lange, B.J. (1995) Optic pathway and hypothalamic/chiasmatic gliomas in children younger than age 5 years with a 6-year follow-up. *Cancer* **75**, 1051–9.

Jay, V., Squire, J., Becker, L.E. and Humphreys, R. (1994) Malignant transformation in a ganglioglioma with anaplastic neuronal and astrocytic components. *Cancer* **73**, 2862–8.

Jay, V., Pienkowska, M., Becker, L. and Zielenska, M. (1995) Primitive neuroectodermal tumors of the cerebrum and cerebellum: absence of t(11;22) translocation by RT-PCR analysis. *Modern Pathology* **8**, 488–91.

Jelenik, J., Smirniotopoulos, J.G., Parisi, J.E. and Kanzer, M. (1990) Lateral ventricular neoplasms of the brain: differential diagnosis based on clinical, CT and MR findings. *American Journal of Neuroradiology* **11**, 567–74.

Jellinger, K. (1972) Cerebral medulloepithelioma. *Acta Neuropathologica* **22**, 95–101.

Jellinger, K. and Seitelberger, F. (1970) Zur Neuropathologie der Hirngeschwülste im Kindesalter. *Wiener Medizinische Wochenschrift* **120**, 855–61.

Jellinger, K., Minauf, M. and Salzer-Kuntschik, M. (1969) Oligodendroglioma with extraneural metastases. *Journal of Neurology, Neurosurgery and Psychiatry* **32**, 249–53.

Jelsma, R. and Bucy, P.C. (1967) The treatment of glioblastoma multiforme of the brain. *Journal of Neurosurgery* **27**, 388–400.

——(1969) Glioblastoma multiforme. Its treatment and some factors affecting survival. *Archives of Neurology* **20**, 161–71.

Jen, J., Harper, J.W., Bigner, S.H., Bigner, D.D., Papadopoulos, N., Markowitz, S., Willson, J.K.V., Kinzler, K.W. and Vogelstein, B. (1994) Deletion of *p16* and *p15* genes in brain tumors. *Cancer Research* **54**, 6353–8.

Jenkin, D., Goddard, K., Armstrong, D., Becker, L., Berry, M., Chan, H., Doherty, M., Greenberg, M., Hendrick, B., Hoffman, H., Humphreys, R., Sonley, M., Weitzman, S. and Zipursky, A. (1990) Posterior fossa medulloblastoma in childhood: treatment results and a proposal for a new staging system. *International Journal of Radiation Oncology, Biology and Physics* **19**, 265–74.

Jenkin, D., Angyalfi, S., Becker, L., Berry, M., Buncic, R., Chan, H., Doherty, M., Drake, J., Greenberg, M., Hendrick, B., Hoffman, H., Humphreys, R. and Weitzman, S. (1993) Optic glioma in children: surveillance, resection, or irradiation? *International Journal of Radiation Oncology, Biology and Physics* **25**, 215–25.

Jenkin, R.D.T., Boesel, C., Ertel, I., Evans, A., Hittle, R., Ortega, J., Sposto, R., Wara, W., Wilson, C., Anderson, J., Leikin, S. and Hammond, G.D. (1987) Brain-stem tumors in childhood: a prospective randomized trial of irradiation with and without adjuvant CCNU, VCR, and prednisone. A report of the Children's Cancer Study Group. *Journal of Neurosurgery* **66**, 227–33.

Jennings, M.T., Slatkin, N., D'Angelo, M., Ketonen, L., Johnson, M.D., Rosenblum, M., Creasy, J., Tulipan, N. and Walker, R. (1993) Neoplastic meningitis as the presentation of occult primitive neuroectodermal tumors. *Journal of Child Neurology* **8**, 306–12.

Jennings, M.T., Frenchman, M., Shehab, T., Johnson, M.D., Creasy, J., La Porte, K. and Dettbarn, W.D. (1995) Gliomatosis cerebri presenting as intractable epilepsy during early childhood. *Journal of Child Neurology* **10**, 37–45.

Jerdan, M.S., White, C.L. III, Solomon, D., Scheithauer, B.W. and Clark, A.W. (1983) Differentiated cerebral neuroblastoma in adults. *Journal of Neuropathology and Experimental Neurology* **42**, 305.

Jereb, B., Reid, A. and Ahuja, R.K. (1982) Patterns of failure in patients with medulloblastoma. *Cancer* **50**, 2941–7.

Jereb, B., Sundaresan, N., Horten, B., Reid, A. and Galicich, J.H. (1981) Supratentorial recurrences in medulloblastoma. *Cancer* **47**, 806–9.

Jervis, G.A. (1954) Spongioneuroblastoma and tuberous sclerosis. *Journal of Neuropathology and Experimental Neurology* **13**, 105–16.

Johannsson, J.H., Rekate, H.L. and Roessmann, U. (1981) Gangliogliomas: pathological and clinical correlation. *Journal of Neurosurgery* **54**, 58–63.

Johnson, D.L. and Schwarz, S. (1987) Intracranial metastases from malignant spinal-cord astrocytoma. *Journal of Neurosurgery* **66**, 621–5.

Johnson, M.D., Jennings, M.T., Lavin, P., Creasy, J.L. and Maciunas, R.J. (1995) Ganglioglioma of the pineal gland: clinical and radiographic response to stereotactic radiosurgical ablation. *Journal of Child Neurology* **10**, 247–9.

Johnson, W.B., Ruppe, M.D., Rockenstein, E.M., Price, J., Sarthy, V.P., Verderber, L.C. and Mucke, L. (1995) Indicator expression directed by regulatory sequences of the glial fibrillary acidic protein (GFAP) gene: *in vivo* comparison of distinct GFAP-lacZ transgenes. *Glia* **13**, 174–84.

Joyner, A.L., Herrup, K., Auerbach, B.A., Davis, C.A. and Rossant, J. (1991) Subtle cerebellar phenotype in mice homozygous for a targeted deletion of the *En-2* homeobox. *Science* **251**, 1239–43.

Kadin, M.E., Rubinstein, L.J. and Nelson, J.S. (1970) Neonatal cerebellar medulloblastoma originating from the fetal external granular layer. *Journal of Neuropathology and Experimental Neurology* **29**, 583–600.

Kadota, Y., Arai, H. and Sato, K. (1995) Neural differentiation and maturation in metastatic medulloblastoma. Case report. *Neurologia Medico-Chirurgica* **35**, 32–5.

Kalyan-Raman, U.P. and Olivero, W.C. (1987) Ganglioglioma: a correlative clinicopathological and radiological study of ten surgically treated cases with follow-up. *Neurosurgery* **20**, 428–33.

Kamel, O.W., Horoupian, D.S. and Silverberg, G.D. (1989) Mixed gangliocytoma-adenoma: a distinct neuroendocrine tumor of the pituitary fossa. *Human Pathology* **20**, 1198–203.

Kamitani, H., Masuzawa, H., Sato, J. and Okada, M. (1986) Ultrastructure of concentric laminations in primary human brain tumors. *Acta Neuropathologica* **71**, 83–7.

Kanamori, M., Shibuya, M., Yoshida, J., Takayasu, M. and Kageyama, N. (1985) Long-term follow-up of patients with optic glioma. *Child's Nervous System* **1**, 272–8.

Kandt, R.S., Shinnar, S., D'Souza, B.J., Singer, H.S., Wharam, M.D. and Gupta, P.K. (1984) Cerebrospinal metastases in malignant childhood astrocytomas. *Journal of Neuro-Oncology* **2**, 123–8.

Kane, W. and Aronson, S.M. (1967) Gangliogliomatous maturation in cerebellar medulloblastoma. *Acta Neuropathologica* **9**, 273–9.

Kaneko, Y., Takeshita, I., Matsushima, T., Iwaki, T., Tashima, T. and Fukui, M. (1990) Immunohistochemical study of ependymal neoplasms: histological subtypes and glial and epithelial characteristics. *Virchows Archiv A, Pathological Anatomy and Histopathology* **417**, 97–103.

Kaplan, M.S. and Hinds, J.W. (1977) Neurogenesis in the adult rat: electron microscopic analysis of light radioautographs. *Science* **197**, 1092–4.

Karamitopoulou, E., Perentes, E., Probst, A. and Wegmann, W. (1995) Ganglioglioma of the brain stem: neurological dysfunction of 16-year duration. *Clinical Neuropathology* **14**, 162–8.

Karch, S.B. and Urich, H. (1972) Medulloepithelioma: definition of an entity. *Journal of Neuropathology and Experimental Neurology* **31**, 27–53.

Kashima, T., Vinters H.V. and Campagnoni, A.T. (1995) Unexpected expression of intermediate filament protein genes in human oligodendroglioma cell lines. *Journal of Neuropathology and Experimental Neurology* **54**, 23–31.

Kashima, T., Tiu, S.N., Merrill, J.E., Vinters, H.V., Dawson, G. and Campagnoni, A.T. (1993) Expression of oligodendrocyte-associated genes in cell lines derived from human gliomas and neuroblastomas. *Cancer Research* **53**, 170–5.

Kasper, M., Perry, G. and Stosiek, P. (1991) Cytokeratin expression in human spinal meninges and ependymal cells. *Journal für Hirnforschung* **32**, 19–25.

Katsetos, C.D. and Burger, P.C. (1994) Medulloblastoma. *Seminars in Diagnostic Pathology* **11**, 85–97.

Katsetos, C.D. and Krishna, L. (1994) Lobar pilocytic astrocytomas of the cerebral hemispheres: I. Diagnosis and nosology. *Clinical Neuropathology* **13**, 295–305.

Katsetos, C.D., Liu, H.M. and Zacks, S.I. (1988) Immunohistochemical and ultrastructural observations on Homer-Wright (neuroblastic) rosettes and the 'pale islands' of human cerebellar medulloblastomas. *Human Pathology* **19**, 1219–27.

Katsetos, C.D., Herman, M.M., Frankfurter, A., Gass, P., Collins, V.P., Walker, C.C., Rosenberg, S., Barnard, R.O. and Rubinstein, L.J. (1989) Cerebellar desmoplastic medulloblastomas. A further immunohistochemical characterization of the reticulin-free pale islands. *Archives of Pathology and Laboratory Medicine* **113**, 1019–29.

Katsetos, C.D., Herman, M.M., Frankfurter, A., Uffer, S., Perentes, E. and Rubinstein, L.J. (1991) Neuron-associated class III β-tubulin isotype, microtubule-associated protein **2**, and synaptophysin in human retinoblastomas *in situ*. *Laboratory Investigation* **64**, 45–54.

Katsetos, C.D., Frankfurter, A., Christakos, S., Mancall, E.L., Vlachos, I.N. and Urich, H. (1993) Differential localization of class III β-tubulin isotype and calbindin-D_{28k} defines distinct neuronal types in the developing human cerebellar cortex. *Journal of Neuropathology and Experimental Neurology* **52**, 655–66.

Katsetos, C.D., Krishna, L., Friedberg, E., Reidy, J., Karkevelas, G. and Savory, J. (1994) Lobar pilocytic astrocytomas of the cerebral hemispheres: II. Pathobiology—morphogenesis of the eosinophilic granular bodies. *Clinical Neuropathology* **13**, 306–14.

Katsetos, C.D., Krishna, L., Frankfurter, A., Karkavelas, G., Wolfe, D.E., Valsamis, M.P., Schiffer, D., Vlachos, I.N. and Urich, H. (1995) A cytomorphological scheme of differentiating neuronal phenotypes in cerebellar medulloblastomas based on immunolocalization of class III β-tubulin isotype (βIII) and proliferating cell nuclear antigen (PCNA)/cyclin. *Clinical Neuropathology* **14**, 72–80.

Kattar, M.M., Kupsky, W.J., Shimoyama, R.K., Vo, T.D. and Sarkar, F.H. (1996) Clonal analysis of malignant gliomas in postmortem brains. (Abstract) *Laboratory Investigation* **74**, 140A.

Kawai, K., Takahashi, H., Ikuta, F., Tanimura, K., Honda, Y. and Yamazaki, H. (1987) The occurrence of catecholamine neurons in a parietal lobe ganglioglioma. *Cancer* **60**, 1532–6.

Kawano, N., Yada, K. and Yagishita, S. (1989) Clear cell ependymoma. A histological variant with diagnostic implications. *Virchows Archiv A, Pathological Anatomy and Histopathology* **415**, 467–72.

Kawano, N., Yada, K., Ogawa, Y. and Sasaki, K. (1977) Spontaneous transdural extension of malignant astrocytoma. *Journal of Neurosurgery* **47**, 766–70.

Kawano, N., Yada, K., Aihara, M. and Yagishita, S. (1983) Oligodendroglioma-like cells (clear cells) in ependymoma. *Acta Neuropathologica* **62**, 141–4.

Kayama, T., Yoshimoto, T., Shimizu, H. and Sakurai, Y. (1993) Neonatal medulloblastoma. *Journal of Neuro-Oncology* **15**, 157–63.

Kazim, M., Kennerdell, J.S., Maroon, J., Rothfus, W. and Marquardt, M. (1992) Choristoma of the optic nerve and chiasm. *Archives of Ophthalmology* **110**, 236–8.

Kehler, U., Arnold, H. and Muller, H. (1990) Long-term follow-up of infratentorial pilocytic astrocytomas. *Neurosurgical Review* **13**, 315–20.

Kelly, P.J., Daumas-Duport, C., Scheithauer, B.W., Kall, B.A. and Kispert, D.B. (1987) Stereotactic histologic correlations of computed tomography- and magnetic resonance imaging-defined abnormalities in patients with glial neoplasms. *Mayo Clinic Proceedings* **62**, 450–9.

Kepes, J.J. (1993) Pleomorphic xanthoastrocytoma: the birth of a diagnosis and concept. *Brain Pathology* **3**, 269–74.

Kepes, J.J. and Perentes, E. (1988) Glial fibrillary acidic protein in chondrocytes of elastic cartilage in the human epiglottis: an immunohistochemical study with polyvalent and monoclonal antibodies. *Anatomical Record* **220**, 296–9.

Kepes, J.J. and Rubinstein, L.J. (1981) Malignant gliomas with heavily lipidized (foamy) tumor cells: a report of three cases with immunoperoxidase study. *Cancer* **47**, 2451–9.

Kepes, J.J., Fulling, K.H. and Carcia, J.H. (1982) The clinical significance of 'adenoid' formations of neoplastic astrocytes, imitating metastatic carcinoma, in gliosarcomas. A review of five cases. *Clinical Neuropathology* **1**, 139–50.

Kepes, J.J., Kepes, M. and Slowik, F. (1973) Fibrous xanthomas and xanthosarcomas of the meninges and the brain. *Acta Neuropathologica* **23**, 187–99.

Kepes, J.J., Morantz, R.A. and Dorzab, W.E. (1987) Cerebellar medulloblastoma in a 73-year-old woman. *Neurosurgery* **21**, 81–3.

Kepes, J.J., Rubinstein, L.J. and Chiang, H. (1984) The role of astrocytes in the formation of cartilage in gliomas. An immunohistochemical study of four cases. *American Journal of Pathology* **117**, 471–83.

Kepes, J.J., Rubinstein, L.J. and Eng, L.F. (1979) Pleomorphic xanthoastrocytoma: a distinctive meningocerebral glioma of young subjects with relatively favorable prognosis. A study of 12 cases. *Cancer* **44**, 1839–52.

Kepes, J.J., Striebinger, C.M., Brackett, C.E. and Kishore, P. (1976) Gliomas (astrocytomas) of the brain-stem with spinal intra- and extradural metastases: report of three cases. *Journal of Neurology, Neurosurgery and Psychiatry* **39**, 66–76.

Kepes, J.J., Belton, K., Roessmann, U. and Ketcherside, W.J. (1985) Primitive neuroectodermal tumors of the cauda equina in adults with no detectable primary intracranial neoplasm—three case studies. *Clinical Neuropathology* **4**, 1–11.

Kepes, J.J., Rubinstein, L.J., Ansbacher, L. and Schreiber, D.J. (1989) Histopathological features of a recurrent pleomorphic xanthoastrocytoma: further corroboration of the glial nature of this neoplasm. A study of 3 cases. *Acta Neuropathologica* **78**, 585–93.

Kernohan, J.W. (1932) Primary tumors of the spinal cord and intradural filum terminale. In Penfield, W. (ed.), *Cytology and cellular pathology of the nervous system*, Vol. 3. New York: Hoeber, 993–1025.

——(1971) Oligodendrogliomas. In Minckler, J. (ed.), *Pathology of the nervous system*, Vol. 2. New York: McGraw-Hill, 1993–2007.

Kernohan, J.W. and Fletcher-Kernohan, E.M. (1937) Ependymomas. Study of 109 cases. *Research Publications—Association for Research in Nervous and Mental Disease* **16**, 182–209.

Kernohan, J.W. and Sayre, G.P. (1952) *Tumors of the central nervous system.* Atlas of tumor pathology, section X, fascicle 35. Washington, DC: Armed Forces Institute of Pathology.

Kernohan, J.W., Learmonth, J.R. and Doyle, J.B. (1932) Neuroblastomas and gangliocytomas of the central nervous system. *Brain* **55**, 287–310.

Kernohan, J.W., Mabon, R.F., Svien, H.J. and Adson, A.W. (1949) Symposium on a new and simplified concept of gliomas. A simplified classification of gliomas. *Proceedings of the Mayo Clinic* **24**, 71–5.

Kershman, J. (1938) The medulloblast and the medulloblastoma; a study of human embryos. *Archives of Neurology and Psychiatry* **40**, 937–67.

Kersting, G. (1968) Tissue culture of human gliomas. In Krayenbühl, H., Maspes, P.E. and Sweet, W.H. (eds), *Progress in neurological surgery*, Vol. 2. Basel: Karger, 165–202.

Key, G., Becker, M.H.G., Baron, B., Duchrow, M., Schlüter, C., Flad, H.-D. and Gerdes, J. (1993) New Ki-67-equivalent murine monoclonal antibodies (MIB 1–3) generated against bacterially expressed parts of the Ki-67 cDNA containing three 62 base pair repetitive elements encoding for the Ki-67 epitope. *Laboratory Investigation* **68**, 629–36.

Khajavi, K., Comair, Y.G., Prayson, R.A., Wyllie, E., Palmer, J., Estes, M.L. and Hahn, J.F. (1995) Childhood ganglioglioma and medically intractable epilepsy. *Pediatric Neurosurgery* **22**, 181–8.

Kim, D.G., Han, M.H., Lee, S.H., Chi, J.G., Cho, K.J., Kim, J.H., Choi, K.S. and Han, D.H. (1993) MRI of intracranial subependymoma: report of a case. *Neuroradiology* **35**, 185–6.

Kim, D.G., Kim, J.S., Chi, J.G., Park, S.H., Jung, H.-W., Choi, K.S. and Han, D.H. (1996) Central neurocytoma: proliferative potential and biological behavior. *Journal of Neurosurgery* **84**, 742–7.

Kim, T.S., Halliday, A.L., Hedley-Whyte, E.T. and Convery, K. (1991) Correlates of survival and the Daumas-Duport grading system for astrocytomas. *Journal of Neurosurgery* **74**, 27–37.

Kimura, T., Budka, H. and Soler-Federsppiel, S. (1986) An immunocytochemical comparison of the glia-associated proteins glial fibrillary acidic protein (GFAP) and S-100 protein (S100P) in human brain tumours. *Clinical Neuropathology* **5**, 21–7.

King, P., Cooper, P.N. and Malcolm, A.J. (1993) Soft tissue ependymoma: a report of three cases. *Histopathology* **22**, 394–6.

Kinney, H.C., Sotrel, A., Alberti, O. and Driscoll, S.G. (1983) A comparative ultrastructural study of a midline melanotic brain tumor and human fetal pineal gland. *Laboratory Investgation* **48**, 8P-9P.

Kleihues, P., Burger, P.C. and Scheithauer, B.W. (1993) *Histological typing of tumours of the central nervous system.* Second edition. WHO international histological classification of tumours. New York: Springer-Verlag.

Kleinert, R. (1991a) Immunohistochemical characterization of primitive neuroectodermal tumors and their possible relationship to the stepwise ontogenetic development of the central nervous system. 1. Ontogenetic studies. *Acta Neuropathologica* **82**, 502–7.

——(1991b) Immunohistochemical characterization of primitive neuroectodermal tumors and their possible relationship to the stepwise ontogenetic development of the central nervous system. 2. Tumor studies. *Acta Neuropathologica* **82**, 508–15.

Kleinman, G.M., Hochberg, F.H. and Richardson, E.P. Jr (1981) Systemic metastases from medulloblastoma: report of two cases and review of the literature. *Cancer* **48**, 2296–309.

Kleinman, G.M., Schoene, W.C., Walshe, T.M. III and Richardson, E.P. Jr (1978) Malignant transformation in benign cerebellar astrocytoma. *Journal of Neurosurgery* **49**, 111–18.

Kleinschmidt-Demasters, B.K. (1996) Diffuse bone marrow metastases from glioblastoma multiforme: the role of dural invasion. *Human Pathology* **27**, 197–202.

Klériga, E., Sher, J.H., Nallainthan, S.-K., Stein, S.C. and Sacher, M. (1978) Development of cerebellar malignant astrocytoma at site of a medulloblastoma treated 11 years earlier. *Journal of Neurosurgery* **49**, 445–9.

Klotz, C., Bordes, N., Laine, M.C., Sandoz, D. and Bormens, M. (1986) A protein of 175,000 daltons associated with striated rootlets in ciliated epithelia as revealed by a monoclonal antibody. *Cell Motility and the Cytoskeleton* **6**, 56–67.

Kobayashi, S., Mori, H., Ikeuchi, S. and Takakura, K. (1990) Immunohistochemical study on Rosenthal fibers in gliomas using anti-GFAP and anti-ubiquitin antibodies. *No to Shinkei* **42**, 59–64.

Kochi, N. and Budka, H. (1987) Contribution of histiocytic cells to sarcomatous development of the gliosarcoma. An immunohistochemical study. *Acta Neuropathologica* **73**, 124–30.

Koenig, C.N. (1971) Subdural spread of medulloblastoma: case report. *Journal of Neurology, Neurosurgery and Psychiatry* **34**, 436–8.

Kopelson, G., Linggood, R.M. and Kleinman, G.M. (1982) Medulloblastoma in adults: improved survival with supervoltage radiation therapy. *Cancer* **49**, 1334–7.

——(1983) Medulloblastoma. The identification of prognostic subgroups and implications for multimodality management. *Cancer* **51**, 312–19.

Kordek, R., Biernat, W., Sapieja, W., Alwasiak, J. and Liberski, P.P. (1995) Pleomorphic xanthoastrocytoma with a gangliogliomatous component: an immunohistochemical and ultrastructural study. *Acta Neuropathologica* **89**, 194–7.

Korf, H.-W., Czerwionka, M., Reiner, J., Schachenmayr, W., Schalken, J.J., de Grip, W. and Gery, I. (1987) Immunocytochemical evidence of molecular photoreceptor markers in cerebellar medulloblastomas. *Cancer* **60**, 1763–6.

Korf, H.-W., Korf, B., Schachenmayr, W., Chader, G.J. and Wiggert, B. (1992) Immunocytochemical demonstration of interphotoreceptor retinoid-binding protein in cerebellar medulloblastoma. *Acta Neuropathologica* **83**, 482–7.

Kornfeld, M. (1986) Granular cell glioblastoma: a malignant granular cell neoplasm of astrocytic origin. *Journal of Neuropathology and Experimental Neurology* **45**, 447–62.

Koslow, S.A., Claassen, D., Hirsch, W.L. and Jungreis, C.A. (1992) Gliomatosis cerebri: a case report with autopsy correlation. *Neuroradiology* **34**, 331–3.

Kotwica, Z. and Papierz, W. (1992) Cerebral and cerebellar glial tumors in the same individual. *Neurosurgery* **30**, 439–41.

Kozmik, Z., Sure, U., Rüedi, D., Busslinger, M. and Aguzzi, A. (1995) Deregulated expression of PAX5 in medulloblastoma. *Proceedings of the National Academy of Sciences U.S.A.* **92**, 5709–13.

Kramm, C.M., Korf, H.-W., Czerwionka, M., Schachenmayr, W. and de Grip, W.J. (1991) Photoreceptor differentiation in cerebellar medulloblastoma: evidence for a functional photopigment and authentic S-antigen (arrestin). *Acta Neuropathologica* **81**, 296–302.

Krischer, J.P., Ragab, A.H., Kun, L., Kim, T.H., Laurent, J.P., Boyett, J.M., Cornell, C.J., Link, M., Luthy, A.R. and Camitta, B. (1991) Nitrogen mustard, vincristine, procarbazine, and prednisone as adjuvant chemotherapy in the treatment of medulloblastoma. A Pediatric Oncology Group study. *Journal of Neurosurgery* **74**, 905–9.

Kros, J.M., de Jong, A.A. and van der Kwast, Th.H. (1992) Ultrastructural characterization of transitional cells in oligodendrogliomas. *Journal of Neuropathology and Experimental Neurology* **51**, 186–93.

Kros, J.M., Vecht, C.J. and Stefanko, S.Z. (1991) The pleomorphic xanthoastrocytoma and its differential diagnosis. *Human Pathology* **22**, 1128–35.

Kros, J.M., Van Eden, C.G., Stefanko, S.Z., Waayer-Van Batenburg, M. and van der Kwast, Th.H. (1990) Prognostic implications of glial fibrillary acidic protein containing cell types in oligodendrogliomas. *Cancer* **66**, 1204–12.

Krouwer, H.G.J. and Prados, M.D. (1995) Infiltrative astrocytomas of the thalamus. *Journal of Neurosurgery* **82**, 548–57.

Krouwer, H.G.J., Davis, R.L., Silver, P. and Prados, M. (1991) Gemistocytic astrocytomas: a reappraisal. *Journal of Neurosurgery* **74**, 399–406.

Krouwer, H.G.J., Davis, R.L., McDermott, M.W., Hoshino, T. and Prados, M.D. (1993) Gangliogliomas: a clinicopathological study of 25 cases and review of the literature. *Journal of Neuro-Oncology* **17**, 139–54.

Kubota, T., Hirano, A., Sato, K. and Yamamoto, S. (1985) The fine structure of astroblastoma. *Cancer* **55**, 745–50.

Kubota, T., Ishise, J., Yamashima, T. and Yamamoto, S. (1986) Abnormal cilia in a malignant ependymoma. *Acta Neuropathologica* **71**, 100–5.

Kuchelmeister, K., Demirel, T., Schlörer, E., Bergmann, M. and Gullotta, F. (1995) Dysembryoplastic neuroepithelial tumour of the cerebellum. *Acta Neuropathologica* **89**, 385–90.

Kudo, H., Tanaka, M., Uri, S., Suzuki, H., Tamaki, N. and Matsumoto, S. (1990) Multicentric glioblastoma multiforme occurring in the supra- and the infratentorial regions – case report. *Neurologia Medico-Chirurgica* **30**, 334–8.

Kuenzle, B.C., Weissert, M., Roulet, E., Bode, H., Schefer, S., Huisman, T., Landau, K. and Boltshauser, E. (1994) Follow-up of optic pathway gliomas in children with neurofibromatosis type 1. *Neuropediatrics* **25**, 295–300.

Kuhajda, F.P., Mendelsohn, G., Taxy, J.B. and Long, D.M. (1981) Pleomorphic xanthoastrocytoma: report of a case with light and electron microscopy. *Ultrastructural Pathology* **2**, 25–32.

Kuhlenbeck, N. and Haymaker, W. (1946) Neuroectodermal tumors containing neoplastic neuronal elements; ganglioneuroma, spongioneuroblastoma and glioneuroma, with a clinicopathologic report of eleven cases and a discussion of their origin and classification. *Military Surgeon* **99**, 273–92.

Kumanishi, T., Watabe, K. and Washiyama, K. (1985) An immunohistochemical study of aldolase C in normal nervous tissues. *Acta Neuropathologica* **67**, 309–14.

Kumanishi, T., Washiyama, K., Watabe, K. and Sekiguchi, K. (1985) Glial fibrillary acidic protein in medulloblastomas. *Acta Neuropathologica* **67**, 1–5.

Kumanishi, T., Usui, H,. Ichikawa, T., Nishiyama, A., Katagiri, T., Abe, S., Yoshida, Y., Washiyama, K., Kuwano, R. and Sakimura, K. (1992) Human glial fibrillary acidic protein (GFAP): molecular cloning of the complete cDNA sequence and chromosomal localization (chromosome 17) of the *GFAP* gene. *Acta Neuropathologica* **83**, 569–78.

Kummer, R.V., Volk, B. and Dorndorf, W. (1977) Extraneural metastasierendes Oligodendrogliom. *Archiv für Psychiatrie und Nervenkrankheiten* **223**, 287–93.

Kung, P.C., Lee, J.C. and Bakay, L. (1969) Vascular invasion by glioma cells in man: an electron microscopic study. *Journal of Neurosurgery* **31**, 339–45.

Kusaka, H., Hirano, A., Bornstein, M.B. and Raine, C.S. (1985) Basal lamina formation by astrocytes in organotypic cultures of mouse spinal cord tissue. *Journal of Neuropathology and Experimental Neurology* **44**, 295–303.

Kyritsis, A.P., Levin, V.A., Yung, W.K.A. and Leeds, N.E. (1993a) Imaging patterns of multifocal gliomas. *European Journal of Radiology* **16**, 163–70.

Kyritsis, A.P., Yung, W.K., Bruner, J., Gleason, M.J. and Levin, V.A. (1993b) The treatment of anaplastic oligodendrogliomas and mixed gliomas. *Neurosurgery* **32**, 365–70.

Labitzke, H.G. (1962) Glioblastoma multiforme with remote extracranial metastases. *Archives of Pathology* **73**, 223–9.

Lagunowich, L.A., Schneider, J.C., Chasen, S. and Grunwald, G.B. (1992) Immunohistochemical and biochemical analysis of *N*-cadherin expression during CNS development. *Journal of Neuroscience Research* **32**, 202–8.

Lampl, Y., Eshel, Y., Gilad, R. and Sarova-Pinchas, I. (1990) Glioblastoma multiforme with bone metastases and cauda equina syndrome. *Journal of Neuro-Oncology* **8**, 167–72.

Landry, C.F., Ivy, G.O. and Brown, I.R. (1990) Developmental expression of glial fibrillary acidic protein mRNA in the rat brain analyzed by *in situ* hybridization. *Journal of Neuroscience Research* **25**, 194–203.

Lang, F.F., Epstein, F.J., Ransohoff, J., Allen, J.C., Wisoff, J., Abbott, R. and Miller, D.C. (1993) Central nervous system gangliogliomas. Part 2: Clinical outcome. *Journal of Neurosurgery* **79**, 867–73.

Lang, F.F., Miller, D.C., Koslow, M. and Newcomb, E.W. (1994) Pathways leading to glioblastoma multiforme: a molecular analysis of genetic alterations in 65 astrocytic tumors. *Journal of Neurosurgery* **81**, 427–36.

Langford, L.A. (1986) The ultrastructure of the ependymoblastoma. *Acta Neuropathologica* **71**, 136–41.

Langford, L.A. and Camel, M.H. (1987) Palisading pattern in cerebral neuroblastoma mimicking the primitive polar spongioblastoma. An ultrastructural study. *Acta Neuropathologica* **73**, 153–9.

Lash, J.W. (1968) Somitic mesenchyme and its response to cartilage induction. In Fleischmajer, R. and Billingham, R.E. (eds), *Epithelial-mesenchymal interactions*. Baltimore: Williams & Wilkins, 165–72.

Latchaw, J.P., Hahn, J.F., Moylan, D.J., Humphries, R. and Mealey, J. Jr (1985) Medulloblastoma. Period of risk reviewed. *Cancer* **55**, 186–9.

Latimer, F.R., AlSaadi, A.A. and Robbins, T.O. (1987) Cytogenetic studies of human brain tumors and their clinical significance. I. Medulloblastoma. *Journal of Neuro-Oncology* **4**, 287–91.

Laurent, J.P., Chang, C.H. and Cohen, M.E. (1985) A classification system for primitive neuroectodermal tumors (medulloblastoma) of the posterior fossa. *Cancer* **56**, 1807–9.

Laws, E.R. Jr, Taylor, W.F., Clifton, M.B. and Okazaki, H. (1984) Neurosurgical management of low-grade astrocytoma of the cerebral hemispheres. *Journal of Neurosurgery* **61**, 665–73.

Le Douarin, N.M. (1993) Embryonic neural chimaeras in the study of brain development. *Trends in Neurosciences* **16**, 64–72.

Lee, K.S., Angelo, J.N., McWhorter, J.M. and Davis, C.H. Jr (1987) Symptomatic subependymomas of the cervical spinal cord. Report of two cases. *Journal of Neurosurgery* **67**, 128–31.

Lehmann, J. and Krug, H. (1980) Flow-through fluorocytophotometry of different brain tumours. *Acta Neuropathologica* **49**, 123–32.

Leibel, S.A. and Sheline, G.E. (1987) Radiation therapy for neoplasms of the brain. *Journal of Neurosurgery* **66**, 1–22.

Leibel, S.A., Scott, C.B. and Loeffler, J.S. (1994) Contemporary approaches to the treatment of malignant gliomas with radiation therapy. *Seminars in Oncology* **21**, 198–219.

Leibel, S.A., Sheline, G.E., Wara, W.M., Boldrey, E.B. and Nielsen, S.L. (1975) The role of radiation therapy in the treatment of astrocytomas. *Cancer* **35**, 1551–7.

Leifer, D., Moore, T., Ukena, T., Wilner, D., Thor, A. and Hedley-Whyte, E.T. (1989) Multifocal glioblastoma with liver metastases in the absence of surgery: case report. *Journal of Neurosurgery* **71**, 772–6.

Lendahl, U., Zimmerman, L.B. and McKay, R.D.G. (1990) CNS stem cells express a new class of intermediate filament protein. *Cell* **60**, 585–95.

Lennon, V.A., Peterson, S. and Schubert, D. (1979) Neurectoderm markers retained in phenotypical skeletal muscle cells arising from a glial cell line. *Nature* **281**, 586–8.

Levitt, P. and Rakic, P. (1980) Immunoperoxidase localization of glial fibrillary acidic protein in radial glial cells and astrocytes of the developing rhesus monkey brain. *Journal of Comparative Neurology* **193**, 815–40.

Levitt, P., Cooper, M.L. and Rakic, P. (1981) Coexistence of neuronal and glial precursor cells in the cerebral ventricular zone of the fetal monkey: an ultrastructural immunoperoxidase analysis. *Journal of Neuroscience* **1**, 27–39.

Levy, L.F. and Elvidge, A.R. (1956) Astrocytoma of brain and spinal cord. Review of 176 cases. *Journal of Neurosurgery* **13**, 413–43.

Lewis, P.D., Fülöp, Z., Hajós, F., Balázs, R. and Woodhams, P.L. (1977) Neuroglia in the internal granular layer of the developing rat cerebellar cortex. *Neuropathology and Applied Neurobiology* **3**, 183–90.

Lewis, R.A., Gerson, L.P., Axelson, K.A., Riccardi, V.M. and Whitford, R.P. (1984) von Recklinghausen neurofibromatosis. II. Incidence of optic gliomata. *Ophthalmology* **91**, 929–35.

Li, J., Yen, C., Liaw, D., Podsypanina, K., Bose, S., Wang, S.I., Puc, J., Miliaresis, C., Rodgers, L., McCombie, R., Bigner, S.H., Giovanella, B.C., Ittman, M., Tycko, B., Hibshoosh, H., Wigler, M.H. and Parsons, R. (1997) *PTEN*, a putative protein tyrosine phosphatase gene mutated in human brain, breast, and prostate cancer. *Science* **275**, 1943–7.

Li, J.Y., Racadot, O., Kujas, M., Kouadri, M., Peillon, F. and Racadot, J. (1989) Immunocytochemistry of four mixed pituitary adenomas and intrasellar gangliocytomas associated with different clinical syndromes: acromegaly, amenorrhea-galactorrhea, Cushing's disease and isolated tumoral syndrome. *Acta Neuropathologica* **77**, 320–8.

Libermann, T.A., Nusbaum, H.R., Razon, N., Kris, R., Lax, I., Soreq, H., Whittle, N., Waterfield, M.D., Ullrich, A. and Schlessinger, J. (1985) Amplification, enhanced expression and possible rearrangement of

EGF receptor gene in primary human brain tumours of glial origin. *Nature* **313**, 144–7.

Liesi, P., Dahl, D. and Vaheri, A. (1983) Laminin is produced by early rat astrocytes in primary culture. *Journal of Cell Biology* **96**, 920–4.

Liesi, P., Kaakkola, S., Dahl, D. and Vaheri, A. (1984) Laminin is induced in astrocytes of adult brain in injury. *EMBO Journal* **3**, 683–6.

Lindboe, C.F., Cappelen, J. and Kepes, J.J. (1992) Pleomorphic xanthoastrocytoma as a component of a cerebellar ganglioglioma: case report. *Neurosurgery* **31**, 353–5.

Lindegaard, K.-F., Mørk, S.J., Eide, G.E., Halvorsen, T.B., Hatlevoll, R., Solgaard, T., Dahl, O. and Ganz, J. (1987) Statistical analysis of clinicopathological features, radiotherapy, and survival in 170 cases of oligodendroglioma. *Journal of Neurosurgery* **67**, 224–30.

Liss, L. (1960) Neuroblastoma (malignant gangliocytoma) of the parietal lobe. *Journal of Neurosurgery* **17**, 529–36.

——(1961) The oligodendrogliomas. A comparative study with tissue culture and silver-carbonate techniques. *Journal of Neuropathology and Experimental Neurology* **20**, 582–92.

——(1969) Glial and parenchymal neoplasms in tissue culture. In Scharenberg, K. and Liss, L. (eds), *Neuroectodermal tumors of the central and peripheral nervous system.* Baltimore: Williams & Wilkins, 183–215.

Listernick, R., Charrow, J., Greenwald, M. and Mets, M. (1994) Natural history of optic pathway tumors in children with neurofibromatosis type 1: a longitudinal study. *Journal of Pediatrics* **125**, 63–6.

Liu, H.M., Boggs, J. and Kidd, J. (1976) Ependymomas of childhood. I. Histological survey and clinicopathological correlation. *Child's Brain* **2**, 92–110.

Liwnicz, B.H. and Rubinstein, L.J. (1979) The pathways of extraneural spread in metastasizing gliomas. A report of three cases and critical review of the literature. *Human Pathology* **10**, 453–67.

Liwnicz, B.H., Wu, S.Z. and Tew, J.M. Jr (1987) The relationship between the capillary structure and hemorrhage in gliomas. *Journal of Neurosurgery* **66**, 536–41.

Lombardi, D., Scheithauer, B.W., Meyer, F.B., Forbes, G.S., Shaw, E.G., Gibney, D.J. and Katzmann, J.A. (1991a) Symptomatic subependymoma: a clinicopathologic and flow cytometric study. *Journal of Neurosurgery* **75**, 583–8.

Lombardi, D., Scheithauer, B.W., Piepgras, D., Meyer, F.B. and Forbes, G.S. (1991b) 'Angioglioma' and the arteriovenous malformation-glioma association. *Journal of Neurosurgery* **75**, 589–96.

Long, D.M. (1970) Capillary ultrastructure and the blood-brain barrier in human malignant brain tumors. *Journal of Neurosurgery* **32**, 127–44.

Longee, D.C., Friedman, H.S., Phillips, P.C., Burger, P.C., Oakes, W.J., Heffez, D., Wharam, M., Strauss, L., Fuller, G.N. and Schold, S.C. (1991) Osteoblastic metastases from astrocyomas: a report of two cases. *Medical and Pediatric Oncology* **19**, 318–24.

Lorentzen, M. and Hägerstrand, I. (1980) Congenital ependymoblastoma. *Acta Neuropathologica* **49**, 71–4.

Lo Russo, P.M., Tapazoglou, E., Zarbo, R.J., Cullis, P.A., Austin, D. and Al-Sarraf, M. (1988) Intracranial astrocytoma with diffuse bone marrow metastasis: a case report and review of the literature. *Journal of Neuro-Oncology* **6**, 53–9.

Louis, D.N. (1996) Clinicopathologic-genetic subsets of glioblastoma multiforme: from both sides now. *Brain Pathology* **6**, 223–4.

Louis, D.N. and Gusella, J.F. (1995) A tiger behind many doors: multiple genetic pathways to malignant glioma. *Trends in Genetics* **11**, 412–15.

Louis, D.N. and Hochberg, F.H. (1990) Cerebral primitive neuroectodermal tumor in an adult, with spinal cord metastasis after 18-year dormancy. *Journal of Neuro-Oncology* **9**, 77–80.

Louis, D.N., Hedley-Whyte, E.T. and Martuza, R.L. (1989) Sarcomatous proliferation of the vasculature in a subependymoma. *Acta Neuropathologica* **78**, 332–5.

Louis, D.N., Swearingen, B., Linggood, R.M., Dickersin, G.R., Kretschmar, C., Bhan, A.K. and Hedley-Whyte, E.T. (1990) Central nervous system neurocytoma and neuroblastoma in adults—report of eight cases. *Journal of Neuro-Oncology* **9**, 231–8.

Louis, D.N., Edgerton, S., Thor, A.D. and Hedley-Whyte, E.T. (1991) Proliferating cell nuclear antigen and Ki-67 immunohistochemistry in brain tumors: a comparative study. *Acta Neuropathologica* **81**, 675–9.

Louis, D.N., von Deimling, A., Dickersin, G.R., Dooling, E.C. and Seizinger, B.R. (1992) Desmoplastic cerebral astrocytomas of infancy: a histopathologic, immunohistochemical, ultrastructural, and molecular genetic study. *Human Pathology* **23**, 1402–9.

Lowes, M., Bojsen-Moller, M., Vorre, P. and Hedegaard, O. (1978) An evaluation of gliomas of the anterior visual pathways. A 10-year survey. *Acta Neurochirurgica* **43**, 201–16.

Lu, W.Y., Goldman, M., Young, B. and Davis, D.G. (1993) Optic nerve ganglioglioma. Case report. *Journal of Neurosurgery* **78**, 979–82.

Ludwin, S.K. (1984) Proliferation of mature oligodendrocytes after trauma to the central nervous system. *Nature* **308**, 274–5.

Lumsden, C.E. (1971) The study by tissue culture of tumours of the nervous system. In Russell, D.S. and Rubinstein, L.J. (eds), *Pathology of tumours of the nervous system.* Third edition. London: Edward Arnold, 334–420.

——(1974) Tissue culture of brain tumours. In Vinken, P.J. and Bruyn, G.W. (eds), *Handbook of clinical neurology*, Vol. 17. Amsterdam: North-Holland Publishing, 42–103.

Lunsford, L.D., Somaza, S., Kondziolka, D. and Flickinger, J.C. (1995) Survival after stereotactic biopsy and irradiation of cerebral nonanaplastic, nonpilocytic astrocytoma. *Journal of Neurosurgery* **82**, 523–9.

Luse, S.A. (1960) Electron microscopic studies in brain tumors. *Neurology* **10**, 881–905.

Lyons, M.K. and Kelly, P.J. (1991) Posterior fossa ependymomas: report of 30 cases and review of the literature. *Neurosurgery* **28**, 659–65.

Maass, L. (1954) Occipital ependymoma with extracranial metastases. *Journal of Neurosurgery* **11**, 413–21.

Macaulay, R.J.B., Jay, V., Hoffman, H.J. and Becker, L.E. (1993) Increased mitotic activity as a negative prognostic indicator in pleomorphic xanthoastrocytoma. Case report. *Journal of Neurosurgery* **79**, 761–8.

Mackay, R.P. (1935) Ependymoblastoma in the fourth ventricle with new bone formation. *Archives of Neurology and Psychiatry* **34**, 844–53.

Makeever, L.C. and King, J.D. (1966) Medulloblastoma with extracranial metastasis through a ventriculovenous shunt. Report of a case and review of the literature. *American Journal of Clinical Pathology* **46**, 245–9.

Mallory, F.B. (1908) The results of the application of special histological methods with the study of tumors. *Journal of Experimental Medicine* **10**, 575–93.

Mandybur, T.I., Liwnicz, B.H. and Wechsler, W. (1984) Disseminated (metastatic) tumors in nude mice produced by intravenous injection of cells of human and nonhuman neurogenic tumor lines. *Acta Neuropathologica* **63**, 203–9.

Mannoji, H. and Becker, L.E. (1988) Ependymal and choroid plexus tumors: cytokeratin and glial fibrillary acidic protein expression. *Cancer* **61**, 1377–85.

Mannoji, H., Takeshita, I., Fukui, M., Ohta, M. and Kitamura, K. (1981) Glial fibrillary acidic protein in medulloblastoma. *Acta Neuropathologica* **55**, 63–9.

Månsson, J.E., Fredman, P., Bigner, D.D., Molin, K., Rosengren, B., Friedman, H.S. and Svennerholm, L. (1986) Characterization of new gangliosides of the lactotetraose series in murine xenografts in a human glioma cell line. *FEBS Letters* **201**, 109–13.

Manuelidis, E.E. and Solitare, G.B. (1971) Glioblastoma multiforme. In Minckler, J. (ed.) *Pathology of the nervous system*, Vol. 2, New York: McGraw-Hill, 2026–71.

Manuelidis, L., Yu, R.K. and Manuelidis, E.E. (1977) Ganglioside content and pattern in human gliomas in culture: correlation of morphological changes with altered gangliosides. *Acta Neuropathology (Berlin)* **38**, 129–35.

Marano, S.R., Johnson, P.C. and Spetzler, R.F. (1988) Recurrent Lhermitte-Duclos disease in a child. Case report. *Journal of Neurosurgery* **69**, 599–603.

Maraziotis, T., Perentes, E., Karamitopoulou, E., Nakagawa, Y., Gessaga, E.C., Probst, A. and Frankfurter, A. (1992) Neuron-associated class III β-tubulin isotype, retinal S-antigen, synaptophysin, and glial fibrillary acidic protein in human medulloblastomas: a clinicopathological analysis of 36 cases. *Acta Neuropathologica* **84**, 355–63.

Marchese, M.J. and Chang, C.H. (1990) Malignant astrocytic gliomas in children. *Cancer* **65**, 2771–8.

Margetts, J.C. and Kalyan-Raman, U.P. (1989) Giant-celled glioblastoma of brain. A clinico-pathological and radiological study of ten cases (including immunohistochemistry and ultrastructure). *Cancer* **63**, 524–31.

Maria, B.L., Cafferty, L.L., Singer, H.S., Epstein, J.I. and Carson, B.S. (1986) Diffuse leptomeningeal seeding from a malignant spinal cord astrocytoma in a child with neurofibromatosis. *Journal of Neuro-Oncology* **4**, 159–63.

Markesbery, W.R. and Challa, V.R. (1979) Electron microscopic findings in primitive neuroectodermal tumors of the cerebrum. *Cancer* **44**, 141–7.

Markwalder, T.-M., Huber, P., Markwalder, R.V. and Seiler, R.W. (1979) Primary intraventricular oligodendrogliomas. *Surgical Neurology* **11**, 25–8.

Marsa, G.W., Probert, J.C., Rubinstein, L.J. and Bagshaw, M.A. (1973) Radiation therapy in the treatment of childhood astrocytic gliomas. *Cancer* **32**, 646–55.

Marsa, G.W., Goffinet, D.R., Rubinstein, L.I. and Bagshaw, M.A. (1975) Megavoltage irradiation in the treatment of gliomas of the brain and spinal cord. *Cancer* **36**, 1681–9.

Martin, K., Akinwunmi, J., Rooprai, H.K., Kennedy, A.J., Linke, A., Ognjenovic, N. and Pilkington, G.J. (1995) Nonexpression of CD15 by neoplastic glia: a barrier to metastasis? *Anticancer Research* **15**, 1159–66.

Maruyama, R., Koga, K., Nakahara, T., Kishida, K. and Nabeshima, K. (1992) Cerebral myxopapillary ependymoma. *Human Pathology* **23**, 960–2.

Matakas, F., Cervós-Navarro, I. and Gullotta, F. (1970) The ultrastructure of medulloblastomas. *Acta Neuropathologica* **16**, 271–84.

Mathews, T. and Moossy, J. (1974) Gliomas containing bone and cartilage. *Journal of Neuropathology and Experimental Neurology* **33**, 456–71.

Matsumoto, J.Y., O'Neill, B.P., Piepgras, D.G. and Scheithauer, B. (1987) Metastatic malignant glioma with resultant extradural compression of a sacral nerve root. *Journal of Neuro-Oncology* **4**, 227–31.

Matsumura, A., Hori, A. and Spoerri, O. (1988) Spinal subependymoma presenting as an extramedullary tumor: case report. *Neurosurgery* **23**, 115–17.

Mavroudis, C., Townsend, J.J. and Wilson, C.B. (1977) A metastasizing ependymoma of the cauda equina. *Journal of Neurosurgery* **47**, 771–5.

May, P.L., Blaser, S.I., Hoffman, H.J., Humphreys, R.P. and Harwood-Nash, D.C. (1991) Benign intrinsic tectal 'tumors' in children. *Journal of Neurosurgery* **74**, 867–71.

McAllister, R.M., Isaacs, H., Rongey, R., Peer, M., Au, W., Soukup, S.W. and Gardner, M.B. (1977) Establishment of a human medulloblastoma cell line. *International Journal of Cancer* **10**, 206–12.

McCloskey, J.J., Parker, J.C. Jr, Brooks, W.H. and Blacker, H.M. (1976) Melanin as a component of cerebral gliomas. The melanotic cerebral ependymoma. *Cancer* **37**, 2373–9.

McComb, I.G., Davis, R.L. and Isaacs, H. Jr (1981) Extraneural metastatic medulloblastoma during childhood. *Neurosurgery* **9**, 548–51.

McComb, I.G., Davis, R.L., Isaacs, H. Jr and Landing, B.H. (1980) Medulloblastoma presenting as neck tumors in 2 infants. *Annals of Neurology* **7**, 113–17.

McComb, R.D., Jones, T.R., Pizzo, S.V. and Bigner, D.D. (1982) Immunohistochemical detection of factor VIII/von Willebrand factor in hyperplastic endothelial cells in glioblastoma multiforme and mixed gliomasarcoma. *Journal of Neuropathology and Experimental Neurology* **41**, 479–89.

McCormack, B.M., Miller, D.C., Budzilovich, G.N., Voorhees, G.J. and Ransohoff, J. (1992) Treatment and survival of low-grade astrocytoma in adults—1977–1988. *Neurosurgery* **31**, 636–42.

McCowage, G., Tien, R., McLendon, R., Felsberg, G., Fuchs, H., Graham, M.L., Kurtzberg, J., Moghrabi, A., Ferrell, L., Kerby, T., Duncan-Brown, M., Stewart, E., Robertson, P.L., Colvin, O.M., Golembe, B., Bigner, D.D. and Friedman, H.S. (1996) Successful treatment of childhood pilocytic astrocytomas metastatic to the leptomeninges with high-dose cyclophosphamide. *Medical and Pediatric Oncology* **27**, 32–9.

McDonald, J.D., Daneshvar, L., Willert, J.R., Matsumura, K., Waldman, F. and Cogen, P.H. (1994) Physical mapping of chromosome 17p13.3 in the region of a putative tumor suppressor gene important in medulloblastoma. *Genomics* **23**, 229–32.

McDonnell, P. and Miller, N.R. (1983) Chiasmatic and hypothalamic extension of optic nerve glioma. *Archives of Ophthalmology* **101**, 1412–15.

McKeran, R.O. and Thomas, D.G.T. (1980) The clinical study of gliomas. In Thomas, D.G.T. and Graham, D.I. (eds), *Brain tumours. Scientific basis, clinical investigation and current therapy*. London: Butterworth, 194–230.

McLendon, R.E., Bruner, J.M., Friedman, H.S., Brown, M.T., Bigner, D.D., Rasheed, B.K.A. and Bigner, S.H. (1996) Asynchronous primary brain tumors. (Abstract) *Journal of Neuro-Oncology* **28**, 99.

McLendon, R.E. and Bigner, D.D. (1994) Immunohistochemistry of the glial fibrillary acidic protein: basic and applied considerations. *Brain Pathology* **4**, 221–8.

McLendon, R.E., Robinson, J.S. Jr, Chambers, D.B., Gfufferman, S. and Burger, P.C. (1985) The glioblastoma multiforme in Georgia, 1977–1981. *Cancer* **56**, 894–7.

McLendon, R.E., Burger, P.C., Pegram, C.N., Eng, L.F. and Bigner, D.D. (1986) The immunohistochemical application of three anti-GFAP monoclonal antibodies to formalin-fixed, paraffin-embedded, normal and neoplastic brain tissues. *Journal of Neuropathology and Experimental Neurology* **45**, 692–703.

McLendon, R.E., Batra, S.K., Friedman, H.S., Rasheed, B.K.A., Bigner, D.D. and Bigner, S.H.(1995a) C-*MYC* amplification in medulloblastoma biopsies (Bxs) and xenografts (Xgs). (Abstract) *Journal of Neuro-Oncology* **24**, 134.

McLendon, R.E., Fung, K.-M., Bentley, R.C., Rasheed, B.K.A., Trojanowski, J.Q., Bigner, S.H., Bigner, D.D. and Friedman, H.S. (1995b) Production and characterization of two ependymoma xenografts. *Journal of Neuropathology and Experimental Neurology* **55**, 540–8.

McLendon, R.E., Bentley, R.C., Parisi, J.E., Tien, R.D., Harrison, J.C., Tarbell, N.J., Billitt, A.L., Gualtieri, R.J. and Friedman, H.S. (1997) Malignant supratentorial glial-neuronal neoplasms: report of two cases and review of the literature. *Archives of Pathology and Laboratory Medicine* **121**, 485–92.

Mealey, I. Jr and Hall, P.V. (1977) Medulloblastoma in children. Survival and treatment. *Journal of Neurosurgery* **46**, 56–64.

Meis, J.M., Martz, K.L and Nelson, J.S. (1991) Mixed glioblastoma multiforme and sarcoma. A clinicopathologic study of 26 radiation therapy oncology group cases. *Cancer* **67**, 2342–9.

Menchine, M., Mischel, P.S., Jimenez, J. and Vinters, H.V. (1995) TSC2 mRNA is a developmentally regulated pyramidal cell marker which is overexpressed in cytomegalic neurons of tuberous sclerosis, cortical dysplasia, and ganglioglioma. (Abstract) *Journal of Neuropathology and Experimental Neurology* **54**, 413.

Mercuri, S., Russo, A. and Palma, L. (1981) Hemispheric supratentorial astrocytomas in children. Longterm results in 29 cases. *Journal of Neurosurgery* **55**, 170–3.

Metzger, A.K., Sheffield, V.C., Duyk, G., Daneshvar, L., Edwards, M.S.B. and Cogen, P.H. (1991) Identification of a germ-line mutation in the p53 gene in a patient with an intracranial ependymoma. *Proceedings of the National Academy of Sciences U.S.A.* **88**, 7825–9.

Meyer, W.J., Schochet, S.S., Perez-Polo, J.R., Werrbach-Perez, K., Davis, A. and Haggard, M.E. (1980) Cerebral neuroblastoma with elevated nerve growth factor. *Bulletin du Cancer* **67**, 333–6.

Mickle, J.P. (1992) Ganglioglioma in children. A review of 32 cases at the University of Florida. *Pediatric Neurosurgery* **18**, 310–14.

Miettinen, M., Clark, R. and Virtanen, I. (1986) Intermediate filament proteins in choroid plexus and ependyma and their tumors. *American Journal of Pathology* **123**, 231–40.

Migheli, A. and Mocellini, C. (1990) Ultrastructural immunocytochemistry in glial tumors. *Journal of Neurosurgical Science* **34**, 219–22.

Miller, A.A. and Ramsden, F. (1966) A cerebral neuroblastoma with unusual fibrous tissue reaction. *Journal of Neuropathology and Experimental Neurology* **25**, 328–40.

Miller, C. (1968) The ultrastructure of the conus medullaris and filum terminale. *Journal of Comparative Neurology* **132**, 547–66.

Miller, D.C., Lang, F.F. and Epstein, F.J. (1993) Central nervous system gangliogliomas. *Journal of Neurosurgery* **79**, 859–66.

Miller, G., Towfighi, J. and Page, R.B. (1990) Spinal cord ganglioglioma presenting as hydrocephalus. *Journal of Neuro-Oncology* **9**, 147–52.

Min, K.-W. and Scheithauer, B.W. (1994) Oligodendroglioma: the ultrastructural spectrum. *Ultrastructural Pathology* **18**, 47–60.

Minehan, K.J., Shaw, E.G., Scheithauer, B.W., Davis, D.L. and Onofrio, B.M. (1995) Spinal cord astrocytoma: pathological and treatment considerations. *Journal of Neurosurgery* **83**, 590–5.

Mishima, K., Nakamura, M., Nakamura, H., Nakamura, O., Funata, N. and Shitara, N. (1992) Leptomeningeal dissemination of cerebellar pilocytic astrocytoma. Case report. *Journal of Neurosurgery* **77**, 788–91.

Miyake, E. (1979) Establishment of a human oligodendroglial cell line. *Acta Neuropathologica* **46**, 51–5.

Moertel, C.G., Dockerty, M.B. and Baggenstoss, A.H. (1961) Multiple primary malignant neoplasms. III. Tumors of multicentric origin. *Cancer* **14**, 238–48.

Moghrabi, A., Friedman, H.S., Burger, P.C., Tien, R. and Oakes, W.J. (1993) Carboplatin treatment of progressive optic pathway gliomas to delay radiotherapy. *Journal of Neurosurgery* **79**, 223–7.

Mohanam, S., Sawaya, R.E., Yamamoto, M., Bruner, J.M., Nicolson, G.L. and Rao, J.S. (1994) Proteolysis and invasiveness of brain tumors: role of urokinase-type plasminogen activator receptor. *Journal of Neuro-Oncology* **22**, 153–60.

Molenaar, W.M. and Trojanowski, J.Q. (1994) Primitive neuroectodermal tumors of the central nervous system in childhood: tumor biological aspects. *Critical Reviews in Oncology-Hematology* **17**, 1–25.

Molenaar, W.M., de Leij, L. and Trojanowski, J.Q. (1991) Neuroectodermal tumors of the peripheral and the central nervous system share neuroendocrine N-CAM-related antigens with small cell lung carinomas. *Acta Neuropathologica* **83**, 46–54.

Molloy, P.T., Yachnis, A.T., Rorke, L.B., Dattilo, J.J., Needle, M.N., Millar, W.S., Goldwein, J.W., Sutton, L.N. and Phillips, P.C. (1996) Central nervous system medulloepithelioma: a series of eight cases including two arising in the pons. *Journal of Neurosurgery* **84**, 430–6.

Mondkar, J., Kalgutkar, A., Nalavade, Y. and Fernandez, A. (1994) Congenital primary cerebral neuroblastoma. *Indian Pediatrics* **31**, 698–702.

Morantz, R.A., Feigin, I. and Ransohoff, J. III (1976) Clinical and pathological study of 24 cases of gliosarcoma. *Journal of Neurosurgery* **45**, 398–408.

Mørk, S.J. and Laerum, O.D. (1980) Modal DNA content of human intracranial neoplasms studied by flow cytometry. *Journal of Neurosurgery* **53**, 198–204.

Mørk, S.J. and Løken, A.C. (1977) Ependymoma. A follow-up study of 101 cases. *Cancer* **40**, 907–15.

Mørk, S.J. and Rubinstein, L.J. (1985) Ependymoblastoma. A reappraisal of a rare embryonal tumor. *Cancer* **55**, 1536–42.

Mørk, S.J., Risberg, G. and Krogness, K. (1980) Anaplastic ependymoma of the spinal cord. *Neuropathology and Applied Neurobiology* **6**, 307–11.

Mørk, S.J., Rubinstein, L.J. and Kepes, J.J. (1988) Patterns of epithelial metaplasia in malignant gliomas. I. Papillary formations mimicking medulloepithelioma. *Journal of Neuropathology and Experimental Neurology* **47**, 93–100.

Mørk, S.J., Lindegaard, K.-F., Halvorsen, T.B., Lehmann, E.H., Solgaard, T., Hatlevoli, R., Harvei, S. and Ganz, J. (1985) Oligodendroglioma: incidence and biological behavior in a defined population. *Journal of Neurosurgery* **63**, 881–9.

Mørk, S.J., Halvorsen, T.B., Lindegaard, K.-F. and Eide, G.E. (1986a) Oligodendroglioma. Histologic evaluation and prognosis. *Journal of Neuropathology and Experimental Neurology* **45**, 65–78.

Mørk, S.J., May, E.E., Papasozomenos, S.Ch. and Vinores, S.A. (1986b) Characteristics of human medulloblastoma cell line TE-671 under different growth conditions *in vitro*: a morphological and immunohistochemical study. *Neuropathology and Applied Neurobiology* **11**, 277–89.

Mørk, S.J., Rubinstein, L.J., Kepes, J.J., Perentes, E. and Uphoff, D.F. (1988) Patterns of epithelial metaplasia in malignant gliomas. II. Squamous differentiation of epithelial-like foci in gliosarcomas and glioblastomas. *Journal of Neuropathology and Experimental Neurology* **47**, 101–18.

Morris, H.H., Estes, M.L., Gilmore, R., Van Ness, P.C., Barnett, G.H. and Turnbull, J. (1993) Chronic intractable epilepsy as the only symptom of primary brain tumor. *Epilepsia* **34**, 1038–43.

Moser, F.G., Tuvia, J., LaSalla, P. and Llana, J. (1992) Ependymoma of the spinal nerve root: case report. *Neurosurgery* **31**, 962–4.

Moss, T.H. (1983) Evidence for differentiation in medulloblastomas appearing primitive on light microscopy: an ultrastructural study. *Histopathology* **7**, 919–30.

Motoi, M., Yoshino, T., Hayashi, K., Nose, S., Horie, Y. and Ogawa, K. (1985) Immunohistochemical studies on human brain tumors using anti-Leu 7 monoclonal antibody in paraffin-embedded specimens. *Acta Neuropathologica* **66**, 75–7.

Mrak, R.E. (1994) Malignant neurocytic tumor. *Human Pathology* **25**, 747–52.

Mücke, L., Oldstone, M.B.A., Morris, J.C. and Nerenberg, M.I. (1991) Rapid activation of astrocyte-specific expression of GFAP-lacZ transgene by focal injury. *The New Biologist* **3**, 465–74.

Mukai, N. (1976) Human adenovirus-induced embryonic neuronal tumor phenotype in rodents. In Zimmerman, H.M. (ed.), *Progress in neuropathology*, Vol. 3. New York: Grune & Stratton, 89–128.

Müller, W. and Schaefer, H.E. (1974) Beitrag zur morphologischen Onkotypie des Medulloblastoms. *Acta Neuropathologica* **30**, 51–61.

Müller, W., Afra, D. and Schröder, R. (1977a) Supratentorial recurrences of gliomas. Morphological studies in relation to time intervals with astrocytomas. *Acta Neurochirurgica* **37**, 75–91.

——(1977b) Supratentorial recurrences of gliomas. Morphological studies in relation to time intervals with oligodendrogliomas. *Acta Neurochirurgica* **39**, 15–25.

Müller, W., Slowik, F. and Schröder, R. (1978) Studies on the biology of medulloblastoma. *Advances in Neurosurgery* **5**, 232–5.

Muñoz-Garcia, D. and Ludwin, S.K. (1985) Intermediate glial cells and reactive astrocytes revisited. A study in organotypic tissue culture. *Journal of Neuroimmunology* **8**, 237–54.

Murovic, J.A., Nagashima, T., Hoshino, T., Edwards, M.S.B. and Davis, R.L. (1986) Pediatric central nervous system tumors: a cell kinetic study with bromodeoxyuridine. *Neurosurgery* **19**, 900–4.

Myers, T., Egelhoff, J. and Myers, M. (1990) Giloblastoma multiforme presenting as osteoblastic metastatic disease: case report and review of the literature. *American Journal of Neuroradiology* **11**, 802–3.

Nagashima, K., Yasui, K., Kimura, J., Washizu, M., Yatnaguchi, K. and Mori, W. (1984) Induction of brain tumors by a newly isolated JC virus (Tokyo-t strain). *American Journal of Pathology* **116**, 455–63.

Nagashima, T., Hoshino, T. and Cho, K.G. (1987) Proliferative potential of vascular components in human glioblastoma multiforme. *Acta Neuropathologica* **73**, 301–5.

Nagashima, T., DeArmond, S.J., Murovic, J. and Hoshino, T. (1985) Immunocytochemical demonstration of S-phase cells by anti-bromodeoxyuridine monoclonal antibody in human brain tumor tissues. *Acta Neuropathologica* **67**, 155–9.

Nager, G.T. (1967) Gliomas involving the temporal bone. Clinical and pathological aspects. *Laryngoscope* **77**, 454–88.

Naguib, M.G., Sung, J.H., Erickson, D.L., Gold, L.H.A. and Seljeskog, E.L. (1982) Central nervous system involvement in the nevoid basal cell carcinoma syndrome: case report and review of the literature. *Neurosurgery* **11**, 52–6.

Nakagawa, Y., Perentes, E. and Rubinstein, L.J. (1986) Immunohistochemical characterization of oligodendrogliomas: an analysis of multiple markers. *Acta Neuropathologica* **72**, 15–22.

——(1987) Non-specificity of anti-carbonic anhydrase C antibody as a marker in human neurooncology. *Journal of Neuropathology and Experimental Neurology* **46**, 451–60.

Nakagawa, Y., Herman, M.M., Boyd, J.C. and Rubinstein, L.J. (1987) Kinetics of the human medulloblastoma cell line, D283 Med, maintained in an organ culture system. Autoradiographic study after cumulative labelling *in vitro*: similarities to the kinetics of human medulloblastoma *in situ*. *Neuropathology and Applied Neurobiology* **13**, 439–50.

Nakajima, T., Kameya, T., Tsumuraya, M., Shimosato, Y. and Kato, K. (1984) Enolase distribution in human brain tumors, retinoblastomas and pituitary adenomas. *Brain Research* **308**, 215–22.

Nakamura, Y. and Becker, L.E. (1983) Subependymal giant-cell tumor: astrocytic or neuronal? *Acta Neuropathologica* **60**, 271–7.

Nakamura, Y., Becker, L.E. and Marks, A. (1983) Distribution of immunoreactive S-100 protein in pediatric brain tumors. *Journal of Neuropathology and Experimental Neurology* **42**, 136–45.

Nakopoulou, L., Kerezoudi, E., Thomaides, T. and Litsios, B. (1990) An immunocytochemical comparison of glial fibrillary acidic protein, S-100p and vimentin in human glial tumors. *Journal of Neuro-Oncology* **8**, 33–40.

NASGOG (North American Study Group for Optic Glioma) (1989) Tumor spread in unilateral optic glioma. Study Report No. 2. *Neurofibromatosis* **2**, 195–203.

Neblett, C.R., Waltz, T.A. and Anderson, D.E. (1971) Neurological involvement in the nevoid basal cell carcinoma syndrome. *Journal of Neurosurgery* **35**, 577–84.

Nelson, D.F., Nelson, J.S., Davis, D.R., Chang, C.H., Griffin, T.W. and Pajak, T.F. (1985) Survival and prognosis of patients with astrocytoma with atypical or anaplastic features. *Journal of Neuro-Oncology* **3**, 99–103.

Nelson, J.S., Tsukada, Y., Schoenfeld, D., Fulling, K., Lamarche, J. and Peress, N. (1983) Necrosis as a prognostic criterion in malignant supratentorial, astrocytic gliomas. *Cancer* **52**, 550–4.

Neumann, E., Kalousek, D.K., Norman, M.G., Steinbok, P., Cochrane, D.D., and Goddard, K. (1993) Cytogenetic analysis of 109 pediatric central nervous system tumors. *Cancer Genetics and Cytogenetics* **71**, 40–9.

Nevin, S. (1938) Gliomatosis cerebri. *Brain* **61**, 170–91.

Newton, H.B., Henson, J. and Walker, R.W. (1992) Extraneural metastases in ependymoma. *Journal of Neuro-Oncology* **14**, 135–42.

Newton, H.B., Rosenblum, M.K. and Walker, R.W. (1992) Extraneural metastases of infratentorial glioblastoma multiforme to the peritoneal cavity. *Cancer* **69**, 2149–53.

Ng, H.K and Lo, S.T. (1989) Cytokeratin immunoreactivity in gliomas. *Histopathology* **14**, 359–68.

Ng, T.H.K., Fung, C.F. and Ma, L.T. (1990) The pathological spectrum of desmoplastic infantile gangliogliomas. *Histopathology* **16**, 235–41.

Nigogosyan, G., De La Pava, S. and Pickren, J.W. (1962) Brain tumor with extracranial metastases. Report of two cases. *Archives of Neurology* **6**, 300–6.

Nijjar, T.S., Simpson, W.J., Gadalla, T. and McCartney, M. (1993) Oligodendroglioma. The Princess Margaret Hospital experience (1958–1984). *Cancer* **71**, 4002–6.

Nishio, S., Korosue, K., Tateishi, J., Fukui, M. and Kitamura, K. (1982) Ventricular and subarachnoid seeding of intracranial tumors of neuroectodermal origin. A study of 26 consecutive autopsy cases with reference to focal ependymal defect. *Clinical Neuropathology* **1**, 83–91.

Nishio, S., Tashima, T., Takeshita, I. and Fukui, M. (1988) Intraventricular neurocytoma: clinicopathological features of six cases. *Journal of Neurosurgery* **68**, 665–70.

Nishizaki, T., Orita, T., Abiko, S., Aoki, H. and Ito, H. (1990) Subependymal giant cell astrocytoma associated with tuberous sclerosis: with special reference to cell kinetic studies–case report. *Neurologia Medico-Chirurgica (Tokyo)* **30**, 695–7.

Norman, R.M. (1966) Neuropathological findings in trisomies 13–15 and 17–18 with special reference to the cerebellum. *Developmental Medicine and Child Neurology* **8**, 170–7.

Nyström, S. (1960) Pathological changes in blood vessels of human glioblastoma multiforme. *Acta Pathologica et Microbiologica Scandinavica* **49** (suppl. 137).

Obana, W.G., Cogen, P.H., Davis, R.L. and Edwards, M.S.B. (1991) Metastatic juvenile pilocytic astrocytoma. *Journal of Neurosurgery* **75**, 972–5.

Oberc-Greenwood, M.A., McKeever, P.E., Kornblith, P.L. and Smith, B.H. (1984) A human ganglioglioma containing paired helical filaments. *Human Pathology* **15**, 834–8.

Oberdick, J. (1994) Evidence for a genetically encoded map of functional development in the cerebellum. *Histochemistry* **102**, 1–14.

O'Connell, J.E.A. (1946) Subarachnoid dissemination of spinal tumours. *Journal of Neurology, Neurosurgery and Psychiatry* **9**, 55–62.

Ogawa, H., Sato, Y., Takeshita, I., Tateishi, J. and Kitamura, K. (1985) Transient expression of glial fibrillary acidic protein in developing oligodendrocytes in vitro. *Brain Research* **350**, 133–41.

Oi, S., Kokunai, T. and Matsumoto, S. (1990) Congenital brain tumors in Japan (ISPN Cooperative Study): specific clinical features in neonates. *Child's Nervous System* **6**, 86–91.

Oikawa, S., Sakamoto, K. and Kobayashi, N. (1994) A neonatal huge subependymal giant cell astrocytoma: case report. *Neurosurgery* **35**, 748–50.

Ojeda, V.J. and Sterrett, G.F. (1984) Cerebral gliosarcoma, pulmonary adenoid-cystic carcinoma, and pulmonary metastatic gliosarcoma: report of an untreated case. *Pathology* **16**, 217–21.

Ojeda, V.J., Jacobsen, P.F. and Papadimitriou, J.M. (1980) Primary cerebral neuroblastoma. Case report with light microscopy, tissue culture and electron microscopy study. *Pathology* **12**, 269–74.

Ojeda, V.J., Spagnolo, D.V. and Vaughan, R.J. (1987) Palisades in primary cerebral neuroblastoma simulating so-called polar spongioblastoma. A light and electron microscopical study of an adult case. *American Journal of Surgical Pathology* **11**, 316–22.

Ojeda, V.J., Stokes, B.A.R., Lee, M.A., Thomas, G.W., Papadimitriou, J.M., Cala, L.A., Stevens, S.M.B. and O'Neill, P. (1986) Primary cerebral neuroblastomas. A clinicopathological study of one adolescent and five adult patients. *Pathology* **18**, 41–9.

Onda, K., Tanaka, R., Takahashi, H., Takeda, N. and Ikuta, F. (1989) Cerebral glioblastoma with cerebrospinal fluid dissemination: a clinicopathological study of 14 cases examined by complete autopsy. *Neurosurgery* **25**, 533–40.

Onda, K., Davis, R.L., Shibuya, M., Wilson, C.B. and Hoshino, T. (1994a) Correlation between the bromodeoxyuridine labeling index and the MIB-1 and Ki-67 proliferating cell indices in cerebral gliomas. *Cancer* **74**, 1921–6.

Onda, K., Davis, R.L., Wilson, C.B. and Hoshino, T. (1994b) Regional differences in bromodeoxyuridine uptake, expression of Ki-67 protein, and nucleolar organizer region counts in glioblastoma multiforme. *Acta Neuropathologica* **87**, 586–93.

Oppenheimer, D.R. (1955) A benign 'tumour' of the cerebellum. Report on two cases of diffuse hypertrophy of the cerebellar cortex with a review of nine previously reported cases. *Journal of Neurology, Neurosurgery and Psychiatry* **18**, 199–213.

——(1969) The effect of irradiation on a medulloblastoma. *Journal of Neurology, Neurosurgery and Psychiatry* **32**, 94–8.

Ortiz de Zarate, J.C. (1954) Sur la neurofibromatose centrale de Recklinghausen dans ses relations avec les gliomes du nerf optique. *Acta Neurologica Belgica* **54**, 716–32.

O'Sullivan, C., Jenkin, D., Doherty, M.A., Hoffman, H.J. and Greenberg, M.L. (1994) Spinal cord tumors in children: long-term results of combined surgical and radiation treatment. *Journal of Neurosurgery* **81**, 507–12.

Otsubo, H., Hoffman, H.J., Humphreys, R.P., Hendrick, E.B., Drake, J.M., Hwang, P.A., Becker, L.E. and Chuang, S.H. (1992) Detection and management of gangliogliomas in children. *Surgical Neurology* **38**, 371–8.

Packer, R.J., Allen, J., Nielsen, S., Petito, C., Deck, M. and Jereb, B. (1983) Brainstem glioma: clinical manifestations of meningeal gliomatosis. *Annals of Neurology* **14**, 177–82.

Packer, R.J., Sutton, L.N., Rorke, L.B., Littman, P.A., Sposto, R., Rosenstock, J.G., Bruce, D.A. and Schut, L. (1984) Prognostic importance of cellular differentiation in medulloblastoma of childhood. *Journal of Neurosurgery* **62**, 296–301.

Packer, R.J., Sutton, L.N., Goldwein, J.W., Perilongo, G., Bunin, G., Ryan, J., Cohen, B.H., D'Angio, G., Kramer, E.D., Zimmerman, R.A., Rorke, L.B., Evans, A.E. and Schut, L. (1991) Improved survival with the use of adjuvant chemotherapy in the treatment of medulloblastoma. *Journal of Neurosurgery* **74**, 433–40.

Padberg, G.W., Schot, J.D.L., Vielvoye, G.J., Bots, G.A.M. and de Beer, F.C. (1991) Lhermitte-Duclos disease and Cowden disease: a single phakomatosis. *Annals of Neurology* **29**, 517–23.

Pagni, C.A., Giordana, M.T. and Canavero, S. (1991) Benign recurrence of a pilocytic cerebellar astrocytoma 36 years after radical removal: case report. *Neurosurgery* **28**, 606–9.

Pagni, C.A., Canavero, S., Giordana, M.T., Mascalchi, M. and Arnetolli, G. (1991) Spinal intramedullary subependymomas: case report and review of the literature. *Neurosurgery* **30**, 115–17.

Palma, L. and Guidetti, B. (1985) Cystic pilocytic astrocytomas of the cerebral hemispheres. Surgical experience with 51 cases and long-term results. *Journal of Neurosurgery* **62**, 811–15.

Palma, L., Maleci, A., Di Lorenzo, N. and Lauro, G.M. (1985) Pleomorphic xanthoastrocytoma with 18-year survival. *Journal of Neurosurgery* **63**, 808–10.

Palmer, J.O., Kasselberg, A.G. and Netsky, M.G. (1981) Differentiation of medulloblastoma. Studies including immunohistochemical localization of glial fibrillary acidic protein. *Journal of Neurosurgery* **55**, 161–9.

Pansera, F. and Pansera, E. (1992) An explanation for the rarity of extraaxial metastases in brain tumors. *Medical Hypotheses* **39**, 88–9.

Papadopoulos, D.P., Giri, S. and Evans, R.G. (1990) Prognostic factors and management of intracranial ependymomas. *Anticancer Research* **10**, 689–92.

Parham, D.M., Dias, P., Kelly, D.R., Rutledge, J.C. and Houghton, P. (1992) Desmin positivity in primitive neuroectodermal tumors of childhood. *American Journal of Surgical Pathology* **16**, 483–92.

Parizel, P.M., Martin, J.-J., Van Vyve, M., van den Hauwe, L. and De Schepper, A.M. (1991) Cerebral ganglioglioma and neurofibromatosis type I. *Neuroradiology* **33**, 357–9.

Park, T.S., Hoffman, H.J., Hendrick, E.B., Humphreys, R.P. and Becker, L.E. (1983) Medulloblastoma: clinical presentation and management. Experience at the Hospital for Sick Children, Toronto, 1950–1980. *Journal of Neurosurgery* **58**, 543–52.

Pasquier, B., Couderc, P., Pasquier, D., Panh, M.H. and N'Golet, A. (1978) Sarcoma arising in oligodendroglioma of the brain. A case with intramedullary and subarachnoid spinal metastases. *Cancer* **42**, 2753–8.

Pasquier, B., Pasquier, D., N'Golet, A., Panh, M.H. and Couderc, P. (1980) Extraneural metastases of astrocytomas and glioblastomas. Clinicopathological study of two cases and review of literature. *Cancer* **45**, 112–25.

Pasquier, B., Lachard, A., Pasquier, D., Couderc, P., Delpech, B. and Courel, M.-N. (1983) Protéine gliofibrillaire acide (GFA) et tumeurs nerveuses centrales.

Étude immunohistochimique d'une série de 207 cas. *Annales de Pathologie* **3**, 127–35.

Pasquier, B., Kojder, I., Labat, F., Keddari, E., Pasquier, D., Stoebner, P., Barge, M., Delpech, B. and Couderc, P. (1985) Le xanthoastrocytome du sujet jeune. Revue de la littérature à propos de deux observations d'évolution discordante. *Annales de Pathologie* **5**, 29–43.

Patterson, R.H. Jr, Campbell, W.G. Jr and Parsons, H. (1961) Ependymoma of the cauda equina with multiple visceral metastases. *Journal of Neurosurgery* **18**, 145–50.

Paul, F. (1926) Beitrag zur Histopathologie der Ganglioglioneurome des Zentralnervensystems. *Beiträge zur Pathologischen Anatomie und zur Allgemeinen Pathologie* **75**, 221–8.

Paulus, W. and Tonn, J.C. (1995) Interactions of glioma cells and extracellular matrix. *Journal of Neuro-Oncology* **24**, 87–91.

Paulus, W., Schlote, W., Perentes, E., Jacobi, G., Warmuth-Metz, M. and Roggendorf, W. (1992) Desmoplastic supratentorial neuroepithelial tumours of infancy. *Histopathology* **21**, 439.

Pearl, G.S. and Takei, Y. (1981) Cerebellar 'neuroblastoma': nosology as it relates to medulloblastoma. *Cancer* **47**, 772–9.

Pearl, G.S., Mirra, S.S. and Miles, M.L. (1980) Glioblastoma multiforme occurring 13 years after treatment of a medulloblastoma. *Neurosurgery* **6**, 546–51.

Pearl, G.S., Takei, Y., Stefanis, G.S. and Hoffman, J.C. (1981) Intraventricular neuroblastoma in a patient with Von Hippel-Lindau's disease. Light and electron microscopic study. *Acta Neuropathologica* **53**, 253–6.

Pearl, G.S., Takei, Y., Bakay, R.A.E. and Davis, P. (1985) Intraventricular primary cerebral neuroblastomas in adults: report of three cases. *Neurosurgery* **16**, 847–9.

Pelc, S., Brihaye, J., Périer, O., Heimann, R. and Balériaux, D. (1977) Temporal lobe oligodendroglioma developing from infancy into adulthood. *Annals of Neurology* **2**, 537–40.

Peña, C.E. and Felter, R. (1973) Ultrastructure of a composite glioma-sarcoma of the brain. *Acta Neuropathologica* **23**, 90–4.

Perentes, E. and Rubinstein, L.J. (1986) Immunohistochemical recognition of human neuroepithelial tumours by anti-Leu 7 (HNK-1) monoclonal antibody. *Acta Neuropathologica* **69**, 227–33.

Perese, D.M., Slepian, A. and Nigogosyan, G. (1959) Postoperative dissemination of astrocytoma of the spinal cord along the ventricles of the brain. *Journal of Neurosurgery* **16**, 114–19.

Perry, R.E. Jr (1957) Extracranial metastasis in a case of intracranial ependymoma. *Archives of Pathology* **64**, 337–41.

Peters, A., Palay, S.L. and Webster, H. de F. (1976) *The fine structure of the nervous system: the neurons and supporting cells*. Philadelphia: W.B. Saunders.

Petronio, J., Edwards, M.S.B., Prados, M., Freyberger, S., Rabbitt, J., Silver, P. and Levin, V.A. (1991) Management of chiasmal and hypothalamic gliomas of infancy and childhood with chemotherapy. *Journal of Neurosurgery* **74**, 701–8.

Pettinato, G., De Chiara, A., Insabato, L., Ferbo, U., Di Blasi, A. and Marino, M.G. (1989) Reactive glioma in intracranial sarcoma ('sarcoglioma'). Histology, electron microscopy and immunohistochemistry of two additional cases. *Applied Pathology* **7**, 192–200.

Pezeshkpour, G.H., Henry, J.M. and Armbrustmacher, V.W. (1984) Spinal metastases. A rare mode of presentation of brain tumors. *Cancer* **54**, 353–6.

Philippon, J.H., Clemenceau, S.H., Fauchon, F.H. and Foncin, J.F. (1993) Supratentorial low-grade astrocytomas in adults. *Neurosurgery* **32**, 554–9.

Pigott, T.J., Punt, J.A., Lowe, J.S., Henderson, M.J., Beck, A. and Gray, T. (1990) The clinical, radiological and histopathological features of cerebral primitive neuroectodermal tumours. *British Journal of Neurosurgery* **4**, 287–97.

Pilkington, G.J. and Lantos, P.L. (1982) The role of glutamine synthetase in the diagnosis of cerebral tumours. *Neuropathology and Applied Neurobiology* **8**, 227–36.

Pitt, M.A., Jones, A.W., Reeve, R.S. and Cowie, R.A. (1992) Oligodendroglioma of the fourth ventricle with intracranial and spinal oligodendrogliomatosis: a case report. *British Journal of Neurosurgery* **6**, 371–4.

Pixley, S.K.R. and de Vellis, J. (1984) Transition between immature radial glia and mature astrocytes studied with a monoclonal antibody to vimentin. *Brain Research* **317**, 201–9.

Pizer, B.L., Moss, T., Oakhill, A., Webb, D. and Coakham, H.B. (1995) Congenital astroblastoma: an immunohistochemical study. Case report. *Journal of Neurosurgery* **83**, 550–5.

Polednak, A.P. and Flannery, J.T. (1995) Brain, other central nervous system, and eye cancer. *Cancer* **75** (Suppl.), 330–7.

Pollack, I.F., Hoffman, H.J., Humphreys, R.P. and Becker, L.E. (1993) The long-term outcome after surgical treatment of dorsally exophytic brain-stem gliomas. *Journal of Neurosurgery* **78**, 859–63.

Pollack, I.F., Hurtt, M., Pang, D. and Albright, A.L. (1994) Dissemination of low grade intracranial astrocytomas in children. *Cancer* **73**, 2869–78.

Pollack, I.F., Claassen, D., al-Shboul, Q., Janosky, J.E. and Deutsch, M. (1995) Low-grade gliomas of the cerebral hemispheres in children. An analysis of 71 cases. *Journal of Neurosurgery* **82**, 537–47.

Pollak, A. and Friede, R.L. (1977) Fine structure of medulloepithelioma. *Journal of Neuropathology and Experimental Neurology* **36**, 712–25.

Pollak, E.R., Miller, H.J. and Vye, M.V. (1981) Medulloblastoma presenting as leukemia. *American Journal of Clinical Pathology* **76**, 98–103.

Pontén, J. (1975) Neoplastic human glia cells in culture. In Fogh, J. (ed.) *Human tumor cells in vitro*. New York: Plenum Press, 175–206.

Poser, C.M. (1956) *The relationship between syringomyelia and neoplasm*. Springfield, III.: Charles C. Thomas.

Post, G.R. and Dawson, G. (1992) Characterization of a cell line from a human oligodendroglioma. *Molecular and Chemical Neuropathology* **16**, 303–17.

Powell, S.Z., Yachnis, A.T., Rorke, L.B., Rojiani, A.M. and Eskin, T.A. (1996) Divergent differentiation in pleomorphic xanthoastrocytoma. Evidence for a neuronal element and possible relation to ganglion cell tumors. *American Journal of Surgical Pathology* **20**, 80–5.

Prados, M.D., Warnick, R.E., Wara, W.M., Larson, D.A., Lamborn, K. and Wilson, C.B. (1995) Medulloblastoma in adults. *International Journal of Radiation Oncology, Biology and Physics* **32**, 1145–52.

Prayson, R.A. and Estes, M.L. (1995) Protoplasmic astrocytoma. A clinicopathologic study of 16 tumors. *American Journal of Clinical Pathology* **103**, 705–9.

Prayson, R.A., Khajavi, K. and Comair, Y.G. (1995) Cortical architectural abnormalities and MIB1 immunoreactivity in gangliogliomas: a study of 60 patients with intracranial tumors. *Journal of Neuropathology and Experimental Neurology* **54**, 513–20.

Pritchett, P.S. and King, T.I. (1978) Dysplastic gangliocytoma of the cerebellum-an ultrastructural study. *Acta Neuropathologica* **42**, 1–5.

Puchner, M.J.A., Lüdecke, D.K., Valdueza, J.M., Saeger, W., Willig, R.P., Stalla, G.K. and Odink, R.J. (1993) Cushing's disease in a child caused by a corticotropin-releasing hormone-secreting intrasellar gangliocytoma associated with an adrenocorticotropic hormone-secreting pituitary adenoma. *Neurosurgery* **33**, 920–5.

Quest, D.O., Brisman, R., Antunes, J.L. and Housepian, E.M. (1978) Period of risk for recurrence in medulloblastoma. *Journal of Neurosurgery* **48**, 159–63.

Raaf, J. and Kernohan, J.W. (1944) Relation of abnormal collections of cells in posterior medullary velum of the cerebellum to origin of medulloblastoma. *Archives of Neurology and Psychiatry* **52**, 163–9.

Raff, M.C., Abney, E.A. and Fok-Seang, J. (1985) Reconstitution of a developmental clock in vitro: a critical role for astrocytes in the timing of oligodendrocyte differentiation. *Cell* **42**, 61–9.

Rafols, J.A. and Goshgarian, H.G. (1985) Spinal tanycytes in the adult rat: a correlative Golgi gold-toning study. *Anatomical Record* **211**, 75–86.

Raimondi, A.J. (1966) Ultrastructure and the biology of human brain tumors. In Krayenbühl, H., Maspes, P.E. and Sweet, W.H. (eds), *Progress in neurological surgery*, Vol. 1. Basel: Karger, 1–63.

Raimondi, A.J., Mullan, S. and Evans, J.P. (1962) Human brain tumors. An electron-microscope study. *Journal of Neurosurgery* **19**, 731–53.

Rakic, P. (1985) Limits of neurogenesis in primates. *Science* **227**, 1054–6.

Rakic, P. and Nowakowski, R.S. (1981) The time of origin of neurons in the hippocampal region of the rhesus monkey. *Journal of Comparative Neurology* **196**, 99–128.

Ramón y Cajal, S. (1952) *Histologie du système nerveux de l'homme et des vertébrés*, Vol. 1. Madrid: Consejo Superior de Investigaciones Científicas, Instituto Ramón y Cajal.

Ramsay, D.A., Goshko, V. and Nag, S. (1990) Primary spinal leptomeningeal astrocytoma. *Acta Neuropathologica* **80**, 338–41.

Ransom, D.T., Ritland, S.R., Kimmel, D.W., Moertel, C.A., Dahl, R.J., Scheithauer, B.W., Kelly, P.J. and Jenkins, R.B. (1992) Cytogenetic and loss of heterozygosity studies in ependymomas, pilocytic astrocytomas, and oligodendrogliomas. *Genes, Chromosomes and Cancer* **5**, 348–56.

Rao, J.S., Steck, P.A., Tofilon, P., Boyd, D., Ali-Osman, F., Stetler-Stevenson, W.G., Liotta L.A. and Sawaya, R. (1993) Role of plasminogen activator and of 92-KDa type IV collagenase in glioblastoma invasion using an in vitro matrigel model. *Journal of Neuro-Oncology* **18**, 129–38.

Rasheed, B.K., Fuller, G.N., Friedman, A.H., Bigner, D.D. and Bigner, S.H. (1992) Loss of heterozygosity for 10q loci in human gliomas. *Genes, Chromosomes and Cancer* **5**, 75–82.

Ravens, J.R., Adamkiewicz, L.L. and Groff, R.A. (1955) Cytology and cellular pathology of oligodendrogliomas of the brain. *Journal of Neuropathology and Experimental Neurology* **14**, 142–84.

Rawlings, C.E. III, Giangaspero, F., Burger, P.C. and Bullard, D.E. (1988) Ependymomas: a clinicopathologic study. *Surgical Neurology* **29**, 271–81.

Rawlinson, D.G., Herman, M.M. and Rubinstein, L.J. (1973) The fine structure of a myxopapillary ependymoma of the filum terminale. *Acta Neuropathologica* **25**, 1–13.

Rawlinson, D.G., Rubinstein, L.J. and Herman, M.M. (1974) *In vitro* characteristics of a myxopapillary ependymoma of the filum terminale maintained in tissue and organ culture systems. Light and electron microscopic observations. *Acta Neuropathologica* **27**, 185–200.

Reese, A.B. (1956) *Tumors of the eye and adnexa*. Atlas of tumor pathology, section X, fascicle 38. Washington, D.C.: Armed Forces Institute of Pathology.

——(1976) *Tumors of the eye*. Third edition. Hagerstown, Md.: Harper & Row.

Reeves, S.A., Helman, L.J., Allison, A. and Israel, M.A. (1989) Molecular cloning and primary structure of human glial fibrillary acidic protein. *Proceedings of the National Academy of Sciences U.S.A.* **86**, 5178–82.

Reifenberger, J., Ring, G.U., Gies, U., Cobbers, J.M.J.L., Oberstraß, J., Han, H.-X., Niederacher, D., Wechsler, W. and Reifenberger, G. (1996) Analysis of *p53* mutations and epidermal growth factor receptor amplification in recurrent gliomas with malignant progression. *Journal of Neuropathology and Experimental Neurology* **55**, 822–31.

Reimer, R. and Onofrio, B.M. (1985) Astrocytomas of the spinal cord in children and adolescents. *Journal of Neurosurgery* **63**, 669–75.

Renaudin, J.W., DiTullio, M.V. and Brown, W.J. (1979) Seeding of intracranial ependymomas in children. *Child's Brain* **5**, 408–12.

Renfranz, P.J., Cunningham, M.G. and McKay, R.D.G. (1991) Region-specific differentiation of the hippocampal stem cell line HiB5 upon implantation into the developing mammalian brain. *Cell* **66**, 713–29.

Reyes-Mugica, M., Chou, P.M. and Myint, M.M. (1994) Ependymomas in children: histologic and DNA-flow cytometric study. *Pediatric Pathology* **14**, 453–66.

Reznik, M. and Schoenen, J. (1983) Lhermitte-Duclos disease. *Acta Neuropathologica* **59**, 88–94.

Rhodes, R.H., Davis, R.L., Kassel, S.H. and Clague, B.H. (1978) Primary cerebral neuroblastoma: a light and electron microscopic study. *Acta Neuropathologica* **41**, 119–24.

Rhodes, R.H., Dusseau, J.J., Boyd, A.S. Jr and Knigge, K.M. (1982) Intrasellar neural-adenohypophyseal choristoma. A morphological and immunocytochemical study. *Journal of Neuropathology and Experimental Neurology* **41**, 267–80.

Rhodes, R.H., Cole, M., Takaoka, Y., Roessmann, U., Cotes, E.E. and Simon, J. (1994) Intraventricular cerebral neuroblastoma. Analysis of subtypes and comparison with hemispheric neuroblastoma. *Archives of Pathology and Laboratory Medicine* **118**, 897–911.

Ribadeau-Dumas, J.L., Poirier, J. and Escourolle, R. (1973) Étude ultrastructurale des lésions cérébrales de la sclérose tubéreuse de Bourneville. *Acta Neuropathologica* **25**, 259–70.

Richman, A.V., Balis, G.A. and Maniscalco, J.E. (1980) Primary intracerebral tumor with mixed chondrosarcoma and glioblastoma ——gliosarcoma or sarcoglioma? *Journal of Neuropathology and Experimental Neurology* **39**, 329–35.

Richmond, J.G., Cunningham, D.L., Fuste, F.G. and Erickson, C.C. (1966) Ganglioglioma of the brain stem. *American Journal of Clinical Pathology* **45**, 692–6.

Rimbau, J. and Isamat, F. (1994) Dysplastic gangliocytoma of the cerebellum (Lhermitte-Duclos disease) and its relation to the multiple hamartoma syndrome (Cowden disease). *Journal of Neuro-Oncology* **18**, 191–8.

Ringertz, N. (1950) Grading of gliomas. *Acta Pathologica et Microbiologica Scandinavica* **27**, 51–64.

Ringertz, N. and Nordenstam, H. (1951) Cerebellar astrocytoma. *Journal of Neuropathology and Experimental Neurology* **10**, 343–67.

Ringertz, N. and Reymond, A. (1949) Ependymomas and choroid plexus papillomas. *Journal of Neuropathology and Experimental Neurology* **8**, 355–80.

Ringertz, N. and Tola, J.H. (1950) Medulloblastoma. *Journal of Neuropathology and Experimental Neurology* **9**, 354–72.

Ritter, A.M., Sawaya, R., Hess, K.R., Levin, V.A. and Bruner, J.M. (1994) Prognostic significance of bromodeoxyuridine labeling in primary and recurrent glioblastoma multiforme. *Neurosurgery* **35**, 192–8.

Roberts, M. and German, W.J. (1966) A long term study of patients with oligodendrogliomas. Follow-up of 50 cases, including Dr Harvey Cushing's series. *Journal of Neurosurgery* **24**, 697–700.

Roberts, R.O., Lynch, C.F., Jones, M.P. and Hart, M.N. (1991) Medulloblastoma: a population-based study of 532 cases. *Journal of Neuropathology and Experimental Neurology* **50**, 134–44.

Robertson, D.M. and MacLean, J.D. (1965) Nuclear inclusions in malignant gliomas. *Archives of Neurology* **13**, 287–96.

Robertson, D.M. and Vogel, F.S. (1962) Concentric lamination of glial processes in oligodendrogliomas. *Journal of Cell Biology* **15**, 313–34.

Robertson, D.M., Hendry, W.S. and Vogel, F.S. (1964) Central ganglioneuroma: a case study using electron microscopy. *Journal of Neuropathology and Experimental Neurology* **23**, 692–705.

Robey, S.S., Olson, J.L., Brem, H. and Epstein, J.I. (1988) Posterior fossa neuroblastoma occurring in an elderly man. *Human Pathology* **19**, 365–7.

Rochkind, S., Blatt, I., Sadeh, M. and Goldhammer, Y. (1991) Extracranial metastases of medulloblastoma in adults: literature review. *Journal of Neurology, Neurosurgery and Psychiatry* **54**, 80–6.

Rodriguez, L.A., Edwards, M.S.B. and Levin, V.A. (1990) Management of hypothalamic gliomas in children: an analysis of 33 cases. *Neurosurgery* **26**, 242–7.

Roeder, M.B., Jinkins, J.R. and Bazan, C. (1994) Subependymoma of filum terminale: MR appearance. *Journal of Computer Assisted Tomography* **18**, 129–30.

Roessmann, U. and Wongmongkolrit, T. (1984) Dysplastic gangliocytoma of cerebellum in a newborn. *Journal of Neurosurgery* **60**, 845–7.

Roessmann, U., Velasco, M.E., Sindely, S.D. and Gambetti, P. (1980) Glial fibrillary acidic protein (GFAP) in ependymal cells during development. An immunocytochemical study. *Brain Research* **200**, 13–21.

Roessmann, U., Velasco, M.E., Gambetti, P. and Autilio-Gambetti, L. (1983) Neuronal and astrocytic differentiation in human neuroepithelial neoplasms. An immunohistochemical study. *Journal of Neuropathology and Experimental Neurology* **42**, 113–21.

Rogatto, S.R., Casartelli, C., Rainho, C.A. and Barbieri-Neto, J. (1993) Chromosomes in the genesis and progression of ependymomas. *Cancer Genetics and Cytogenetics* **69**, 146–52.

Rogers, L.R., Estes, M.L., Rosenbloom, S.A. and Harrold, L. (1995) Primary leptomeningeal oligdendroglioma: case report. *Neurosurgery* **36**, 166–9.

Rorke, L.B. (1983) Presidential address. The cerebellar medulloblastoma and its relationship to primitive neuroectodermal tumors. *Journal of Neuropathology and Experimental Neurology* **42**, 1–15.

Rorke, L.B., Fogelson, M.H. and Riggs, H.E. (1968) Cerebellar heterotopia in infancy. *Developmental Medicine and Child Neurology* **10**, 644–50.

Rosenblum, M.K., Erlandson, R.A. and Budzilovich, G.N. (1991) The lipid-rich epithelioid glioblastoma. *American Journal of Surgical Pathology* **15**, 925–34.

Rosenblum, M.K., Erlandson, R.A., Aleksic, S.N. and Budzilovich, G.N. (1990) Melanotic ependymoma and subependymoma. *American Journal of Surgical Pathology* **14**, 729–36.

Rosenblum, M.L. and Gerosa, M.A. (1984) Stem cell sensitivity. *Progress in Experimental Tumor Research* **28**, 1–17.

Rosenblum, M.L., Vasquez, D.A., Hoshino, T. and Wilson, C.B. (1978) Development of a clonogenic cell assay for human brain tumors. *Cancer* **41**, 2305–14.

Ross, D.A., McKeever, P.E., Sandler, H.M. and Muraszko, K.M. (1993) Myxopapillary ependymoma. *Cancer* **71**, 3114–18.

Ross, G.W. and Rubinstein, L.J. (1989) Lack of histopathological correlation of malignant ependymomas with postoperative survival. *Journal of Neurosurgery* **70**, 31–6.

Ross, I.B., Robitaille, Y., Villemure, J.G. and Tampieri, D. (1991) Diagnosis and management of gliomatosis cerebri: recent trends. *Surgical Neurology* **36**, 431–40.

Rossi, L.N., Pastorino, G., Scotti, G., Gazocchi, M., Maninetti, M.M., Zanolini, C. and Chiodi, A. (1994)

Early diagnosis of optic glioma in children with neurofibromatosis type 1. *Child's Nervous System* **10**, 426–9.
Rossitch, E. Jr, Zeidman, S.M., Burger, P.C., Curnes, J.T., Harsh, C., Anscher, M. and Oakes, W.J. (1990) Clinical and pathological analysis of spinal cord astrocytomas in children. *Neurosurgery* **27**, 193–6.
Rubinstein, L.J. (1956) The development of contiguous sarcomatous and gliomatous tissue in intracranial tumours. *Journal of Pathology and Bacteriology* **71**, 441–59.
——(1959) Extracranial metastases in cerebellar medulloblastoma. *Journal of Pathology and Bacteriology* **78**, 187–95.
——(1963) Tumeurs et hamartomes dans la neurofibromatose centrale. In Michaux, L. and Feld, M. (eds), *Les phakomatoses cérébrales*. Paris: SPEI Editeurs, 427–51.
——(1964) Morphological problems of brain tumors with mixed cell populations. *Acta Neurochirurgica* (Suppl. X), 141.
——(1967) Development of extracranial metastases from a malignant astrocytoma in the absence of previous craniotomy. *Journal of Neurosurgery* **26**, 542–7.
——(1970) The definition of the ependymoblastoma. *Archives of Pathology* **90**, 35–45.
——(1972a) Cytogenesis and differentiation of primitive central neuroepithelial tumors. *Journal of Neuropathology and Experimental Neurology* **31**, 7–26.
——(1972b) *Tumors of the central nervous system*. Atlas of tumor pathology, second series, fascicle 6, Washington, D.C.: Armed Forces Institute of Pathology.
——(1985) Embryonal central neuroepithelial tumors and their differentiating potential. A cytogenetic view of a complex neuro-oncological problem. *Journal of Neurosurgery* **62**, 795–805.
——(1988) Pathological features of optic nerve and chiasmatic gliomas. *Neurofibromatosis* **1**, 152–8.
Rubinstein, L.J. and Herman, M.M. (1972) A light- and electron-microscopic study of a temporal-lobe ganglioglioma. *Journal of the Neurological Sciences* **16**, 27–48.
——(1989) The astroblastoma and its possible cytogenic relationship to the tanycyte. An electron microscopic, immunohistochemical, tissue- and organ-culture study. *Acta Neuropathologica* **78**, 472–83.
Rubinstein, L.J. and Logan, W.J. (1970) Extraneural metastases in ependymoma of the cauda equina. *Journal of Neurology, Neurosurgery and Psychiatry* **33**, 763–70.
Rubinstein, L J. and Northfield, D.W.C. (1964) The medulloblastoma and the so-called 'arachnoidal cerebellar sarcoma'. A critical re-examination of a nosological problem. *Brain* **87**, 379–412.
Rubinstein, L.J., Herman, M.M. and Foley, V.L. (1973) *In vitro* characteristics of human glioblastomas maintained in organ culture systems. Light microscopy observations. *American Journal of Pathology* **71**, 61–80.
Rubinstein, L.J., Herman, M.M. and Hanbery, J.W. (1974) The relationship between differentiating medulloblastoma and dedifferentiating diffuse cerebellar astrocytoma. Light, electron microscopic, tissue, and organ culture observations. *Cancer* **33**, 675–90.
Rubinstein, L.J., Herman, M.M. and VandenBerg, S.R. (1984) Differentiation and anaplasia in central neuroepithelial tumors. *Progress in Experimental Tumor Research* **27**, 32–48.
Rubio, M.-P., Correa, K.M., Ramesh, V., MacCollin, M.M., Jacoby, L.B., von Deimling, A., Gusella, J.F. and Louis, D.N. (1994) Analysis of the neurofibromatosis 2 gene in human ependymomas and astrocytomas. *Cancer Research* **54**, 45–7.
Rushing, E.J., Rorke, L.B. and Sutton, L. (1993) Problems in the nosology of desmoplastic tumors of childhood. *Pediatric Neurosurgery* **19**, 57–62.
Russell, D.S. (1949) *Observations on the pathology of hydrocephalus*. Special report series 265, Medical Research Council. London: Her Majesty's Stationary Office, 112–13.
——(1960) A note on cerebral medullo-epitheliomas. *Journal of Pathology and Bacteriology* **79**, 403–4.
Russell, D.S. and Bland, J.O.W. (1933) Study of gliomas by method of tissue culture. *Journal of Pathology and Bacteriology* **36**, 273–83.
Russell, D.S. and Rubinstein, L.J. (1959) *Pathology of tumours of the nervous system*. London: Edward Arnold.
——(1962) Ganglioglioma: a case with long history and malignant evolution. *Journal of Neuropathology and Experimental Neurology* **21**, 185–93.
——(1977) *Pathology of tumours of the nervous system*. Fourth edition. London: Edward Arnold.
——(1989) *Pathology of tumours of the nervous system*. Fifth edition. London: Edward Arnold.
Rutka, J.T. and Smith, S.L. (1993) Transfection of human astrocytoma cells with glial fibrillary acidic protein complementary DNA: analysis of expression, proliferation, and tumorigenicity. *Cancer Research* **53**, 3624–31.
Rutka, J.T., Giblin, J.R., Apodaca, G., DeArmond, S.J., Stern, R. and Rosenblum, M.L. (1987) Inhibition of growth and induction of differentiation in a malignant human glioma cell line by normal leptomeningeal extracellular matrix proteins. *Cancer Research* **47**, 3515–22.
Rutka, J.T., Apodaca, G., Stern, R. and Rosenblum, M. (1988) The extracellular matrix of the central and peripheral nervous systems: structure and function. *Journal of Neurosurgery* **69**, 155–70.
Ryken, T.C., Robinson, R.A. and VanGilder, J.C. (1994) Familial occurrence of subependymoma. Report of two cases. *Journal of Neurosurgery* **80**, 1108–11.
Sadun, F., Hinton, D.R. and Sadun, A.A. (1996) Rapid growth of an optic nerve ganglioglioma in a patient with neurofibromatosis 1. *Ophthalmology* **103**, 794–9.
Saez, R.J., Campbell, R.J. and Laws, E.R. Jr (1977) Chemotherapeutic trials on human malignant astrocytomas in organ culture. *Journal of Neurosurgery* **46**, 320–7.
Sainati, L. Montaldi, A., Putti, M.C., Giangaspero, F., Rigobello, L., Stella, M., Zanesco, L. and Basso, G. (1992) Cytogenetic t(11;17)(q13;q21) in a pediatric ependymoma. Is 11q13 a recurring breakpoint in ependymomas? *Cancer Genetics and Cytogenetics* **59**, 213–16.

Sakaki, S., Mori, Y., Motozaki, T., Nakagawa, K. and Matsuoka, K. (1981) A cerebral neuroblastoma with extracranial metastases. *Surgical Neurology* **16**, 53–9.

Salmon I. and Kiss R. (1993) Relationship between proliferative activity and ploidy level in a series of 530 human brain tumors, including astrocytomas, meningiomas, schwannomas, and metastases. *Human Pathology* **24**, 329–35.

Salmon, I., Kiss, R., Dewitte, O., Gras, T., Pasteels, J.-L., Brotchi, J. and Flament-Durand, J. (1992) Histopathologic grading and DNA ploidy in relation to survival among 206 adult astrocytic tumor patients. *Cancer* **70**, 538–46.

Salmon, I., Kruczynski, A., Camby, I., Levivier, M., Pasteels, J.-L., Brotchi, J. and Kiss, R. (1993) DNA histogram typing in a series of 707 tumors of the central peripheral nervous system. *American Journal of Surgical Pathology* **17**, 1020–8.

Salmon, I., Dewitte, O., Pasteels, J.-L., Flament-Durand, J., Brotchi, J., Vereerstraeten, P. and Kiss, R. (1994) Prognostic scoring in adult astrocytic tumors using patient age, histopathological grade, and DNA histogram type. *Journal of Neurosurgery* **80**, 877–83.

Salvati, M., Oppido, P.A., Artizzu, S., Fiorenza F., Puzzilli F. and Orlando E.R. (1991) Multicentric gliomas. Report of seven cases. *Tumori* **77**, 518–22.

Salvati, M., Raco, A., Artico, M., Artizzu, S. and Ciappetta, P. (1992) Subependymoma of the spinal cord. Case report and review of the literature. *Neurosurgical Review* **15**, 65–9.

Samii, M. and Klekamp, J. (1994) Surgical results of 100 intramedullary tumors in relation to accompanying syringomyelia. *Neurosurgery* **35**, 865–73.

Sanerkin, N.G. (1962) Transdural spread of glioblastoma multiforme. *Journal of Pathology and Bacteriology* **84**, 228–33.

Sara, A., Bruner, J.M. and Mackay, B. (1994) Ultrastructure of ependymoma. *Ultrastructural Pathology* **18**, 33–42.

Sarmiento, J., Ferrer, I., Pons, L. and Ferrer, E. (1979) Cerebral mixed tumour: osteo-chondrosarcoma–glioblastoma multiforme. *Acta Neurochirurgica* **50**, 335–41.

Sarnat, H.B. (1995) Ependymal reactions to injury. *Journal of Neuropathology and Experimental Neurology* **54**, 1–15.

Sasaki, A., Hirato, J., Nakazato, Y., Tamura, M. and Kadowaki, H. (1996) Recurrent anaplastic ganglioglioma: pathological characterization of tumor cells. *Journal of Neurosurgery* **84**, 1055–9.

Sato, H., Ohmura, K., Mizushima, M., Ito, J. and Kuyama, H. (1983) Myxopapillary ependymoma of the lateral ventricle. A study on the mechanism of its stromal myxoid change. *Acta Pathologica Japonica* **33**, 1017–25.

Sato, T., Shimoda, A., Takahashi, T., Daita, G., Goto, S., Takamura, H. and Hirama, M. (1980) Congenital cerebellar neuroepithelial tumor with multiple divergent differentiations. *Acta Neuropathologica* **50**, 143–6.

Savard, M.L. and Gilchrist D.M. (1989) Ependymomas in two sisters and a maternal male cousin with mosaicism with monosomy 22 in tumour. *Pediatric Neuroscience* **15**, 80–4.

Sawa, H., Takeshita, I., Kuramitsu, M., Mannoji, H., Machi, T., Fukui, M. and Kitamura, K. (1986a) Neuronal and glial proteins in medulloblastomas. I. Immunohistochemical study. *Anticancer Research* **6**, 905–10.

Sawa, H., Takeshita, I., Kuramitsu, M., Egami, H., Fukui, M. and Sato, Y. (1986b) Neuronal and glial proteins in medulloblastomas. II. Heterotransplantation of human medulloblastoma. *Anticancer Research* **6**, 911–16.

Sawyer, J.R., Sammartino, G., Husain, M., Boop, F.A. and Chadduck, W.M. (1994) Chromosome aberrations in four ependymomas. *Cancer Genetics and Cytogenetics* **74**, 132–8.

Saylors, R.L. III, Sidransky, D., Friedman, H.S., Bigner, S.H., Bigner, D.D., Vogelstein, B. and Brodeur, G.M. (1991) Infrequent p53 gene mutations in medulloblastomas. *Cancer Research* **51**, 4721–3.

Scarpelli, M., Montironi, R., Ansuini, G., Pisani, E., Rychlicki, F., Papo, I. and Mariuzzi, G.M. (1987) The value of morphometry in prediction of survival in oligodendrogliomas. *Clinical Neuropathology* **6**, 155–9.

Schaper, A. (1897a) The earliest differentiation in the central nervous system of vertebrates. *Science* **5**, 430–1.

——(1897b) Die frühesten Differenzirungsvorgärge im centralnervensystems. *Archiv für Entwizkelungsmechanile* **5**, 81–130.

Schär, W. and Christensen, E. (1939) Missbildungstumoren des Grosshirnes. *Zentralblatt für Neurochirurgie* **3**, 142–54.

Scheinker, I.M. (1939) Zur frage der pathogenese und pathologie der medulloblastome. *Monatsschrift für Psychiatrie und Neurologie* **101**, 103–13.

Scheinker, I.M. (1945) Subependymoma (a newly recognized tumor of subependymal derivation). *Journal of Neurosurgery* **2**, 232–40.

Scheithauer, B.W. (1978) Symptomatic subependymoma. Report of 21 cases with review of the literature. *Journal of Neurosurgery* **49**, 689–96.

Scheithauer, B.W. and Bruner, J.M. (1987) The ultrastructural spectrum of astrocytic neoplasms. *Ultrastructural Pathology* **11**, 535–81.

Scheithauer, B.W. and Rubinstein, L.J. (1979) Cerebral medulloepithelioma. Report of a case with multiple divergent neuroepithelial differentiation. *Child's Brain* **5**, 62–71.

Scheithauer, B.W., Kovacs, K., Randall, R.V., Horvath, E., Okazaki, H. and Laws, E.R. Jr (1983) Hypothalamic neuronal hamartoma and adenohypophyseal neuronal choristoma: their association with growth hormone adenoma of the pituitary gland. *Journal of Neuropathology and Experimental Neurology* **42**, 648–63.

Scherer, H.-J. (1935a) Gliomstudien: II. Über die Grenzen der Zelldiagnostik in Gehirngeschwülsten, dargestellt am Beispiel des 'Glioblastoma multiforme ganglioides.' *Virchows Archiv* **294**,795–822.

——(1935b) Gliomstudien: III. Angioplastische Gliome. *Virchows Archiv* **294**, 823–63.

Scherer, H.J. (1936) Étude sur les gliomes (comportement des différents gliomes vis-à-vis des cellules ganglionnaires). *Bulletin de l'Association Française pour l'Étude du Cancer* **25**, 470–93.

——(1938) Structural development in gliomas. *American Journal of Cancer* **34**, 333–51.

——(1940a) Cerebral astrocytomas and their derivatives. *American Journal of Cancer* **40**, 159–97.

——(1940b) The forms of growth in gliomas and their practical significance. *Brain* **63**, 1–35.

Scheurlen, W.G. and Senf, L. (1995) Analysis of the gap-related domain of the neurofibromatosis type 1 (NF1) gene in childhood brain tumors. *International Journal of Cancer* **64**, 234–8.

Schiffer, D., Cavicchioli, D., Giordana, M.T., Palmtucci, L. and Piazza, A. (1979) Analysis of some factors affecting survival in malignant gliomas. *Tumori* **65**, 119–25.

Schiffer, D., Giordana, M.T., Mauro, A. and Migheli, A. (1984) GFAP, F VIII/RAg, laminin, and fibronectin in gliosarcomas: an immunohistochemical study. *Acta Neuropathologica* **63**, 108–16.

Schiffer, D., Giordana, M.T., Mauro, A., Migheli, A., Germano, I. and Giaccone, G. (1986) Immunohistochemical demonstration of vimentin in human cerebral tumors. *Acta Neuropathologica* **70**, 209–19.

Schiffer, D., Chiò, A., Giordana, M.T., Leone, M. and Soffietti, R. (1988) Prognostic value of histologic factors in adult cerebral astrocytoma. *Cancer* **61**, 1386–93.

Schiffer, D., Chiò, A., Cravioto, H., Giordana, M.T., Migheli, A., Soffietti, R. and Vigliani, M.C. (1991a) Ependymoma: internal correlations among pathological signs: the anaplastic variant. *Neurosurgery* **29**, 206–10.

Schiffer, D., Chiò, A., Giordana, M.T., Migheli, A., Palma, L., Pollo, B., Soffietti, R. and Tribolo, A. (1991b) Histologic prognostic factors in ependymoma. *Child's Nervous System* **7**, 177–82.

Schiffer, D., Giordana, M.T., Pezzotta, S., Pezzulo, T. and Vigliani, M.C. (1992) Medullomyoblastoma: report of two cases. *Child's Nervous System* **8**, 268–72.

Schiffer, D., Cravioto, G., Giordana, M.T., Mighelli, A., Pezzulo, T. and Vigliani, M.C. (1993) Is polar spongioblastoma a tumor entity? *Journal of Neurosurgery* **78**, 587–91.

Schiffer, D., Cavalla, P., Chiò, A., Giordana, M.T., Marino, S., Mauro, A. and Migheli, A. (1994) Tumor cell proliferation and apoptosis in medulloblastoma. *Acta Neuropathologica* **87**, 362–70.

Schiffer, D., Cavalla, P., Migheli, A., Chiò, A., Giordana, M.T., Marino, S. and Attanasio, A. (1995) Apoptosis and cell proliferation in human neuroepithelial tumors. *Neuroscience Letters* **195**, 81–4.

Schindler, E. and Gullotta, F. (1983) Glial fibrillary acidic protein in medulloblastomas and other embryonic CNS tumours of children. *Virchows Archiv A, Pathological Anatomy and Histopathology* **398**, 263–75.

Schlesinger, H.R., Rorke, L., Jamieson, R. and Hummeler, K. (1981) Neuronal properties of neuroectodermal tumors *in vitro*. *Cancer Research* **41**, 2573–5.

Schlote, W. (1966) Rosenthalsche Fasern' und Spongioblasten im Zentralnervensystem. Elektronenmikroskopische Untersuchungen. Bedeutung der Rosenthalschen Fasern'. *Beiträge zur Pathologischen Anatomie und zur Allgemeinen Pathologie* **133**, 461–80.

Schmechel, D.E. and Rakic, P. (1979a) Arrested proliferation of radial glial cells during midgestation in rhesus monkey. *Nature* **277**, 303–5.

——(1979b) A Golgi study of radial glial cells in developing monkey telencephalon: morphogenesis and transformation into astrocytes. *Anatomical Embryology* **156**, 115–52.

Schmidbauer, M., Budka, H., Bruckner, R. and Vorkapic, P. (1987) Glioblastoma developing at the site of a cerebellar medulloblastoma treated 6 years earlier. *Journal of Neurosurgery* **67**, 915–18.

Schmincke, A. (1914) Ein Ganglioglioneurom des Grosshirns. *Verhandlungen der Deutschen Pathologischen Gesellschaft* **17**, 537–43.

Schmitt, H.P. (1983a) Rapid anaplastic transformation of gliomas in childhood. *Neuropediatrics* **14**, 137–43.

——(1983b) Rapid anaplastic transformation in gliomas of adulthood. 'Selection' in neuro-oncogenesis. *Pathology Research and Practice* **176**, 313–23.

Schneider, J.H. Jr, Raffel, C. and McComb, J.G. (1992) Benign cerebellar astrocytomas of childhood. *Neurosurgery* **30**, 58–63.

Schnitzer, J., Franke, W.W. and Schachner, M. (1981) Immunocytochemical demonstration of vimentin in astrocytes and ependymal cells of developing and adult mouse nervous system. *Journal of Cell Biology* **90**, 435–47.

Schofield, D., West, D.C., Anthony, D.C., Marshal, R. and Sklar, J. (1995) Correlation of loss of heterozygosity at chromosome 9q with histological subtype in medulloblastomas. *American Journal of Pathology* **146**, 472–80.

Schofield, D.E., Yunis, E.J., Geyer, J.R., Albright, A.L., Berger, M.S. and Taylor, S.R. (1992) DNA content and other prognostic features in childhood medulloblastoma. Proposal of a scoring system. *Cancer* **69**, 1307–14.

Schröder, R., Ploner, C. and Ernestus, R.-I. (1993) The growth potential of ependymomas with varying grades of malignancy measured by the Ki-67 labelling index and mitotic index. *Neurosurgery Review* **16**, 145–50.

Schuier, F. (1976) Is there an anaplastic type of oligodendroglioma? A case report. *Journal of Neurology* **213**, 263–7.

Schuster, H., Jellinger, K., Gund, A. and Regele, H. (1976) Extracranial metastases of anaplastic cerebral gliomas. *Acta Neurochirurgica* **35**, 247–59.

Schutz, B.R., Scheurlen, W., Krauss, J., Dumanoir, S., Joos, S., Bentz, M. and Lichter, P. (1996) Mapping of chromosomal gains and losses in primitive neuroectodermal tumors by comparative genomic hybridization. *Genes, Chromosomes and Cancer* **16**, 196–203.

Schwaninger, M., Patt, S., Henningsen, P. and Schmidt, D. (1992) Spinal canal metastases: a late complication of glioblastoma. *Journal of Neuro-Oncology* **12**, 93–8.

Schwartz, A.M. and Ghatak, N.R. (1990) Malignant transformation of benign cerebellar astrocytoma. *Cancer* **65**, 333–6.

Schwechheimer, K., Wiedenmann, B. and Franke, W.W. (1987) Synaptophysin: a reliable marker for medulloblastomas. *Virchows Archiv A, Pathological Anatomy and Histopathology* **411**, 53–9.

Segal, R.A., Goumnerova, L.C., Kwon, Y.K., Stiles, C.D. and Pomeroy, S.L. (1994) Expression of the neurotrophin receptor TrkC is linked to a favorable outcome in medulloblastoma. *Proceedings of the National Academy of Sciences U.S.A.* **91**, 12867–71.

Selvaggi, S.M. (1992) Cytologic features of malignant ovarian monodermal teratoma with an ependymal component in peritoneal washings. *International Journal of Gynecology and Pathology* **11**, 299–303.

Serebrin, R. and Robertson, D.M. (1984) Ganglioneuroma arising in the pituitary fossa: a twenty year follow up. *Journal of Neurology, Neurosurgery and Psychiatry* **47**, 97–8.

Severi, B., Govoni, E., Laschi, R., Poletti, V., Manetto, V. and Ferracini R. (1989) Ependymoma of the foramen of Monro: ultrastructural characterization. *Ultrastructural Pathology* **13**, 35–42.

Shapiro, S., Mealey, J. Jr and Sartorius, C. (1989) Radiation-induced intracranial malignant gliomas. *Journal of Neurosurgery* **71**, 77–82.

Sharma, A. (1991) Myxopapillary ependymomas arising from nerve roots of the spinal cord. *Journal of Neurology, Neurosurgery and Psychiatry* **54**, 563–4.

Shaw, E.G., Scheithauer, B.W. and O'Fallon, J.R. (1993) Management of supratentorial low-grade gliomas. *Oncology* **7**, 97–111.

Shaw, E.G., Scheithauer, B.W., O'Fallon, J.R., Tazelaar, H.D. and Davis, D.H. (1992) Oligodendrogliomas: the Mayo Clinic experience. *Journal of Neurosurgery* **76**, 428–34.

Sheikh, B. and Kanaan, I. (1994) Lymph node metastasis in medulloblastoma. *Pediatric Neurosurgery* **20**, 269–71.

Sheline, G.E. (1975) Radiation therapy of tumors of the central nervous system in childhood. *Cancer* **35**, 957–64.

——(1977) Radiation therapy of brain tumors. *Cancer* **39**, 873–81.

Shenkin, H.A., Grant, F.C. and Drew, J.H. (1947) Postoperative period of survival of patients with oligodendroglioma of brain. *Archives of Neurology and Psychiatry* **58**, 710–15.

Shepherd, C.W., Scheithauer. B.W., Gomez, M.R., Altermatt, H.J. and Katzmann, J.A. (1991) Subependymal giant cell astrocytoma: a clinical, pathological, and flow cytometric study. *Neurosurgery* **28**, 864–8.

Sherbaniuk, R.W. and Shnitka, T.K. (1956) Metastasizing intracranial ependymoma. *American Journal of Pathology* **32**, 53–62.

Shin, W.-Y., Laufer, H., Lee, Y.-C., Aftalion, B., Hirano, A. and Zimmerman, H.M. (1978) Fine structure of a cerebellar neuroblastoma. *Acta Neuropathologica* **42**, 11–13.

Shinozaki, Y. (1981) Distribution and life history of rat brain tumors induced by human adenovirus type 12 in their early stages of the oncogenesis. *Pathology Research and Practice* **172**, 330–48.

Shiurba, R.A., Gessaga, E.C., Eng, L.F., Sternberger, L.A., Sternberger, N.H. and Urich, H. (1988) Lhermitte-Duclos disease: an immunohistochemical study of the cerebellar cortex. *Acta Neuropathologica* **75**, 474–80.

Shivas, A.A. (1959) The behaviour of Brown-Pearce carcinoma implanted in rabbit brain. *Journal of Pathology and Bacteriology* **78**, 81–6.

Shuangshoti, S., Kasantikul, V. and Suwanwela, N. (1987) Spontaneous penetration of dura mater and bone by glioblastoma multiforme. *Journal of Surgical Oncology* **36**, 36–44.

Shuman, R.M., Alvord, E.C. and Leech, R.W. (1975) The biology of childhood ependymomas. *Archives of Neurology* **32**, 731–9.

Sidransky, D., Mikkelsen, T., Schwechheimer, K., Rosenblum, M.L., Cavanee, W. and Vogelstein, B. (1992) Clonal expansion of *p53* mutant cells is associated with brain tumour progression. *Nature* **355**, 846–7.

Silver, J.M., Rawlings, C.E. III, Rossitch, E. Jr, Zeidman, S.M. and Friedman A.H. (1991) Ganglioglioma: a clinical study with long-term follow-up. *Surgical Neurology* **35**, 261–6.

Silverberg, G.D. (1971) Simple cysts of the cerebellum. *Journal of Neurosurgery* **35**, 320–7.

Silverman, C.L. and Simpson, J.R. (1982) Cerebellar medulloblastoma: the importance of posterior fossa dose to survival and patterns of failure. *International Journal of Radiation Oncology, Biology and Physics* **8**, 1869–76.

Sima, A.A.F. and Robertson, D.M. (1979) Subependymal giant-cell astrocytoma. Case report with ultrastructural study. *Journal of Neurosurgery* **50**, 240–5.

Sinson, G., Sutton, L.N., Yachnis, A.T., Duhaime, A.-C. and Schut, L. (1994) Subependymal giant cell astrocytomas in children. *Pediatric Neurosurgery* **20**, 233–9.

Sipe, J.C., Herman, M.M. and Rubinstein, L.J. (1973) Electron microscopic observations on human glioblastomas and astrocytomas maintained in organ culture systems. *American Journal of Pathology* **73**, 589–606.

Sipe, J.C., Rubinstein, L.J., Herman, M.M. and Bignami, A. (1974) Ethylnitrosourea induced astrocytomas: morphologic observations on rat tumors maintained in tissue and organ culture systems. *Laboratory Investigation* **31**, 571–9.

Siqueira, E.B. and Bucy, P.C. (1966) Chondroma arising within a mixed glioma. *Journal of Neuropathology and Experimental Neurology* **25**, 667–73.

Slooff, J.L., Kernohan, J.W. and MacCarty, C.S. (1964) *Primary intramedullary tumors of the spinal cord and filum terminale.* Philadelphia: Saunders.

Slowik, F., Jellinger, K., Gaszó, L. and Fischer, J. (1985) Gliosarcomas: histological, immunohistochemical, ultrastructural, and tissue culture studies. *Acta Neuropathologica* **67**, 201–10.

Smith, B. and Butler, M. (1973) Acid mucopolysaccharides in tumours of the myelin sheath cells, the oligodendroglioma and the neurilemmoma. *Acta Neuropathologica* **23**, 181–5.

Smith, D.A. and Lantos, P.L. (1985) Immunocytochemistry of cerebellar astrocytomas: with a special note on Rosenthal fibres. *Acta Neuropathologica* **66**, 155–9.

Smith, D.R., Hardman, J.M. and Earle, K.M. (1969a) Metastasizing neuroectodermal tumors of the central nervous system. *Journal of Neurosurgery* **31**, 50–8.

——(1969b) Contiguous glioblastoma multiforme and fibrosarcoma with extracranial metastasis. *Cancer* **24**, 270–6.

Smith, M.T., Ludwig, C.L., Godfrey, A.D. and Armbrustmacher, V.W. (1983) Grading of oligodendrogliomas. *Cancer* **52**, 2107–14.

Smith, N.M., Carli, M.M., Hanieh, A., Clark, B., Bourne, A.J. and Byard, R.W. (1992) Gangliogliomas in childhood. *Child's Nervous System* **8**, 258–62.

Smith, T.W. and Davidson, R.I. (1984) Medullomyoblastoma. A histologic, immunohistochemical, and ultrastructural study. *Cancer* **54**, 323–32.

Smith, T.W., Nikulasson, S., De Girolami, U. and De Gennaro, L.J. (1993) Immunohistochemistry of synapsin I and synaptophysin in human nervous system and neuroendocrine tumors. Applications in diagnostic neuro-oncology. *Clinical Neuropathology* **12**, 335–42.

Smits, A., van Grieken, D., Hartman, M., Lendahl, U., Funa, K. and Nistér, M. (1996) Coexpression of platelet-derived growth factor α and β receptors on medulloblastomas and other primitive neuroectodermal tumors is consistent with an immature stem cell and neuronal derivation. *Laboratory Investigation* **74**, 188–98.

Soeur, M., Monseu, G., Ketelbant, P. and Flament-Durand, J. (1979) Intramedullary ependymoma producing collagen. *Acta Neuropathologica* **47**, 159–60.

Soffer, D., Umansky, F. and Goldman, J.E. (1995) Ganglioglioma with neurofibrillary tangles (NFTs): neoplastic NFTs share antigenic determinants with NFTs of Alzheimer's disease. *Acta Neuropathologica* **89**, 451–3.

Soffietti, R., Chiò, A., Giordana, M.T., Vasario, E. and Schiffer, D. (1989) Prognostic factors in well-differentiated cerebral astrocytomas in the adult. *Neurosurgery* **24**, 686–92.

Sonneland, P.R.L., Scheithauer, B.W. and Onofrio, B.M. (1985) Myxopapillary ependymoma. A clinicopathologic and immunocytochemical study of 77 cases. *Cancer* **56**, 883–93.

Spaar, F.W., Blech, M. and Ahyai, A. (1986) DNA-flow fluorescence-cytometry of ependymomas. Report on ten surgically removed tumours. *Acta Neuropathologica* **69**, 153–60.

Spaar, F.W., Ahyai, A., Spaar, U., Gazso, L. and Zimmermann, A. (1986) Flow-cytophotometry of nuclear DNA in biopsies of 45 human gliomas and after primary culture *in vitro*. *Clinical Neuropathology* **5**, 157–75.

Spataro, J. and Sacks, O. (1968) Oligodendroglioma with remote metastases. *Journal of Neurosurgery* **28**, 373–9.

Specht, C.S., Smith, T.W., DeGirolami, U. and Price, J.M. (1986) Myxopapillary ependymoma of the filum terminale. A light and electron microscopic study. *Cancer* **58**, 310–17.

Spencer, C.D., Weiss, R.B., Van Eys, J., Cohen, P. and Edwards, B. (1984) Medulloblastoma metastatic to the marrow. Report of four cases and review of the literature. *Journal of Neuro-Oncology* **2**, 223–35.

Spencer, W.H. and Borit, A. (1967) Diffuse hyperplasia of the optic nerve in von Recklinghausen's disease. *American Journal of Ophthalmology* **64**, 638–42.

Sperner, J., Gottschalk, J., Neumann, K., Schörner, W., Lanksch, W.R. and Scheffner, D. (1994) Clinical, radiological and histological findings in desmoplastic infantile ganglioglioma. *Child's Nervous System* **10**, 458–63.

Spitz, E.B., Shenkin, H.A. and Grant, F.C. (1947) Cerebellar medulloblastoma in adults. *Archives of Neurology and Psychiatry* **57**, 417–22.

Spoor, T.C., Kennerdell, J.S., Martinez, A.J. and Zorub, D. (1980) Malignant gliomas of the optic nerve pathways. *American Journal of Ophthalmology* **89**, 284–92.

Spoto, G.P., Press, G.A., Hesselink, J.R. and Solomon, M. (1990) Intracranial ependymoma and subependymoma: MR manifestations. *American Journal of Neuroradiology* **11**, 83–91.

Stapleton, S.R., Wilkins, P.R. and Bell, B.A. (1992) Recurrent dysplastic cerebellar gangliocytoma (Lhermitte-Duclos disease) presenting with subarachnoid haemorrhage. *British Journal of Neurosurgery* **6**, 153–6.

Steck, P.A., Pershouse, M.A., Jasser, S.A., Yung, W.K.A., Lin, H., Ligon, A.H., Langford, L.A., Baumgard, M.L., Hattier, T., Davis, T., Frye, C., Hu, R., Swedlund, B., Teng, D.H.F. and Tavtigian, S.V. (1997) Identification of a candidate tumour suppressor gene, *MMAC1*, at chromosome 10q23.3 that is mutated in multiple advanced cancers. *Nature Genetics* **15**, 356–62.

Steel, G.G. (1980) Growth kinetics of brain tumours. In Thomas, D.G.T. and Graham, D.I. (eds), *Brain tumours. Scientific basis, clinical investigation and current therapy*. London: Butterworth, 10–20.

Stefansson, K. and Wollmann, R. (1980) Distribution of glial fibrillary acidic protein in central nervous system lesions of tuberous sclerosis. *Acta Neuropathologica* **52**, 135–40.

——(1981) Distribution of the neuronal specific protein, 14–3–2, in central nervous system lesions of tuberous sclerosis. *Acta Neuropathologica* **53**, 113–17.

Steinberg, G.K., Shuer, L.M., Conley, F.K. and Hanbery, J.W. (1985) Evolution and outcome in malignant astroglial neoplasms of the cerebellum. *Journal of Neurosurgery* **62**, 9–17.

Stern, J., Jakobiec, F.A. and Housepian, E.M. (1980) The architecture of optic nerve gliomas with and without neurofibromatosis. *Archives of Ophthalmology* **98**, 505–11.

Sternberger, N.H., del Cerro, C., Kies, M.W. and Herndon, R.M. (1985) Immunocytochemistry of myelin basic proteins in adult rat oligodendroglia. *Journal of Neuroimmunology* **7**, 355–63.

Stevenson, L. and Echlin, F. (1934) Nature and origin of some tumors of the cerebellum (medulloblastoma). *Archives of Neurology and Psychiatry* **31**, 93–109.

Storring, F.K. and Duguid, J.B. (1954) The vascular formations in glioblastoma. *Journal of Pathology and Bacteriology* **68**, 231–3.

Stratton, M.R., Darling, J., Lantos, P.L., Cooper, C.S. and Reeves, B.R. (1989) Cytogenetic abnormalities in human ependymomas. *International Journal of Cancer* **44**, 579–81.

Streit, A., Nolte, C., Rásony, T. and Schachner, M. (1993) Interaction of astrochondrin with extracellular matrix components and its involvement in astrocyte process formation and cerebellar granule cell migration. *Journal of Cell Biology* **120**, 799–814.

Stroebe, H. (1895) Ueber Entstehung und Bau der Gehirngliome. *Beiträge zur Pathologischen Anatomie und zur Allgemeinen Pathologie* **18**, 405–86.

Stroink, A.R., Hoffman, H.J., Hendrick, E.B. and Humphreys, R.P. (1986) Diagnosis and management of pediatric brain-stem gliomas. *Journal of Neurosurgery* **65**, 745–50.

Strøm, E.H. and Skullerud, K. (1983) Pleomorphic xanthoastrocytoma: report of 5 cases. *Clinical Neuropathology* **2**, 188–91.

Sugita, Y., Kepes, J.J., Shigemori, M., Kuramoto, S., Reifenberger, G., Kiwit, J.C.W. and Wechsler, W. (1990) Pleomorphic xanthoastrocytoma with desmoplastic reaction: angiomatous variant. Report of two cases. *Clinical Neuropathology* **9**, 271–8.

Sung, J.H., Mastri, A.R. and Segal, E.L. (1973) Melanotic medulloblastoma of the cerebellum. Report of a case. *Journal of Neuropathology and Experimental Neurology* **32**, 437–45.

Sure, U., Berghorn, W.J., Bertalanffy, H., Wakabayashi, T., Yoshida, J., Sugita, K. and Seeger, W. (1995) Staging, scoring and grading of medulloblastoma. A postoperative prognosis predicting system based on the cases of a single institute. *Acta Neurochirurgica* **132**, 59–65.

Sutton, L.N., Packer, R.J., Rorke, L.B., Bruce, D.A. and Schut, L. (1983) Cerebral gangliogliomas during childhood. *Neurosurgery* **13**, 124–8.

Sutton, L.N., Goldwein, J., Perilongo, G., Lang, B., Schut, L., Rorke, L. and Packer, R. (1990–91) Prognostic factors in childhood ependymomas. *Pediatric Neurosurgery* **16**, 57–65.

Sutton, L.N., Molloy, P.T., Sernyak, H., Goldwein, J., Phillips, P.L., Rorke, L.B., Moshang, T. Jr, Lange, B. and Packer, R.J. (1995) Long-term outcome of hypothalamic/chiasmatic astrocytomas in children treated with conservative surgery. *Journal of Neurosurgery* **83**, 583–9.

Svennerholm, L. (1988) Immunological and tumoral aspects of gangliosides. In Ledeen, R.W., Hogan, E.L., Tettamanti, G., Yates, A.J. and Yu, R.K. (eds), *New trends in ganglioside research: neurochemical and neuroregenerative aspects*. Fidia Research Series, Vol. 14. Padova: Liviana Press, 135–50.

Svien, H.J., Mabon, R.F., Kernohan, J.W. and Adson, A.W. (1949) Symposium on a new and simplified concept of gliomas. *Proceedings of the Staff Meetings of the Mayo Clinic* **24**, 54–64.

Svien, H.J., Mabon, R.F., Kernohan, J.W. and Craig, W.M. (1953) Ependymoma of brain: pathologic aspects. *Neurology* **3**, 1–15.

Swarz, J.R. and Del Cerro, M. (1977) Lack of evidence for glial cells originating from the external granular layer in mouse cerebellum. *Journal of Neurocytology* **6**, 241–50.

Syapin, P.J., Salvaterra, P.M. and Engelhardt, J.K. (1982) Neuronal-like features of TE671 cells: presence of a functional nicotinic cholinergic receptor. *Brain Research* **231**, 365–77.

Szymas, J., Biczysko, W., Gabryel, P. and Morkowski, S. (1987) Medulloblastoma: histological evaluation and prognosis. A clinical, immunohistochemical and electron microscopic study. *Child's Nervous System* **3**, 74–80.

Tabuchi, K., Moriya, Y., Furuta, T., Ohnishi, R. and Nishimoto, A. (1982) S-100 protein in human glial tumours. Qualitative and quantitative studies. *Acta Neurochirurgica* **65**, 239–51.

Taguchi, Y., Sakurai, T., Takamori, I., Sekino, H. and Tadokoro, M. (1993) Desmoplastic infantile ganglioglioma with extraparenchymatous cyst – case report. *Neurologia Medico-Chirurgica (Tokyo)* **33**, 177–80.

Tahan, S.R., Wei, Y., Ling, P. and Bistrian, B.R. (1995) Influence of formalin fixation time and tissue processing method on immunoreactivity of monoclonal antibody PC10 for proliferating cell nuclear antigen. *Modern Pathology* **8**, 177–82.

Takahashi, H., Ikuta, F., Tsuchida, T. and Tanaka, R. (1987) Ultrastructural alterations of neuronal cells in a brain stem ganglioglioma. *Acta Neuropathologica* **74**, 307–12.

Takei, Y., Mirra, S.S. and Miles, M.L. (1976) Eosinophilic granular cells in oligodendrogliomas. An ultrastructural study. *Cancer* **38**, 1968–76.

Tampieri, D., Moumdjian, R., Melanson, D. and Ethier, R. (1991) Intracerebral gangliogliomas in patients with partial complex seizures: CT and MR imaging findings. *AJNR. American Journal of Neuroradiology* **12**, 749–55.

Tamura, K., Shimizu, K., Yamada, M., Okamoto, Y., Matsui, Y., Park, K.C., Mabuchi, E., Moriuchi, S. and Mogami, H. (1989) Expression of major histocompatibility complex on human medulloblastoma cells with neuronal differentiation. *Cancer Research* **49**, 5380–4.

Tang, T.T., Harb, J.M., Mork, S.J. and Sty, J.R. (1985) Composite cerebral neuroblastoma and astrocytoma. A mixed central neuroepithelial tumor. *Cancer* **56**, 1404–12.

Tani, E. and Ametani, T. (1971) Membranous stacks in human glioblastoma multiforme. *Acta Neuropathologica* **18**, 248–56.

Tani, E. and Higashi, N. (1972) Intercellular junctions in human ependymomas. *Acta Neuropathologica* **22**, 295–304.

Tani, E., Yamashita, J., Takeuchi, J. and Handa, H. (1969) Polygonal crystalline structures and crystalline aggregates of cylindrical particles in human glioma. *Acta Neuropathologica* **13**, 324–37.

Tani, E., Ametani, T., Higashi, N. and Fujihara, E. (1971) Atypical cristae in mitochondria of human glioblastoma multiforme cells. *Journal of Ultrastructure Research* **36**, 211–21.

Taratuto, A.L., Monges, J., Lylyk, P. and Leiguarda, R. (1984) Superficial cerebral astrocytoma attached to dura. Report of six cases in infants. *Cancer* **54**, 2505–12.

Taratuto, A.L., Pomata, H., Sevlever, G., Gallo, G. and Monges, J. (1995) Dysembryoplastic neuroepithelial tumor: morphological, immunocytochemical, and deoxyribonucleic acid analyses in a pediatric series. *Neurosurgery* **36**, 474–81.

Tarbell, N.J., Loeffler, J.S., Silver, B., Lynch, E., Lavally, B.L., Kupsky, W.J., Scott, R.M. and Sallan, S.E. (1991) The change in patterns of relapse in medulloblastoma. *Cancer* **68**, 1600–4.

Tarlov, I.M. (1938) The structure of the filum terminale. *Archives of Neurology and Psychiatry* **40**, 1–17.

Tarlov, I.M. and Davidoff, L.M. (1946) Subarachnoid and ventricular implants in ependymal and other gliomas. *Journal of Neuropathology and Experimental Neurology* **5**, 213–24.

Tennyson, V.M. and Pappas, G.D. (1962) An electron microscope study of ependymal cells of the fetal, early postnatal and adult rabbit. *Zeitschrift für Zellforschung und Mikroskopische Anatomie* **56**, 595–618.

Thiel, G., Losanowa, T., Kintzel, D., Nisch, G., Martin, H., Vorpahl, K., and Witkowski, R. (1992) Karyotypes in 90 human gliomas. *Cancer Genetics and Cytogenetics* **58**, 109–20.

Thomas, G.A. and Raffel, C. (1991) Loss of heterozygosity on 6q, 16q, and 17p in human central nervous system primitive neuroectodermal tumors. *Cancer Research* **51**, 639–43.

Thorne, R.N., Pearson, A.D.J., Nicoll, J.A.R., Coakham, H.B., Oakhill, A., Mott, M.G. and Foreman, N.K. (1994) Decline in incidence of medulloblastoma in children. *Cancer* **74**, 3240–4.

Tijssen, C.C. (1986) Genetic factors and family studies in medulloblastoma. In Zeltzer, P.M. and Pochedly, C. (eds), *Medulloblastomas in children. New concepts in tumor biology, diagnosis and treatment.* New York: Praeger, 61–75.

Tinkler, D. and Lucraft, H.H. (1995) An audit of craniospinal irradiation for medulloblastoma in Newcastle 1970–1992. *Clinical Oncology* **7**, 179–83.

Tohyama, T., Lee, V.M., Rorke, L.B. and Trojanowski, J.Q. (1991) Molecular milestones that signal axonal maturation and the commitment of human spinal cord precursor cells to the neuronal or glial phenotype in development. *Journal of Comparative Neurology* **310**, 285–99.

Tohyama, T., Lee, V.M., Rorke, L.B., Marvin, M., McKay, R.D. and Trojanowski, J.Q. (1992) Nestin expression in embryonic human neuroepithelium and in human neuroepithelial tumor cells. *Laboratory Investigation* **66**, 303–13.

Tokoro, K., Chiba, Y., Ohtani, T., Abe, H. and Yagishita, S. (1993) Pineal ganglioglioma in a patient with familial basal ganglia calcification and elevated serum α-fetoprotein: case report. *Neurosurgery* **33**, 506–11.

Tola, J.S. (1951) The histopathological and biological characteristics of the primary neoplasms of the cerebellum and the fourth ventricle, with some aspects of their clinical picture, diagnosis, and treatment (on the basis of 71 verified cases). *Acta Chirurgica Scandinavica* (Suppl.), 164.

Tomita, T. and McLone, D.G. (1983) Spontaneous seeding of medulloblastoma: results of cerebrospinal fluid cytology and arachnoid biopsy from the cisterna magna. *Neurosurgery* **12**, 265–7.

Tomita, T., Das, L. and Radkowski, M.A. (1990) Bone metastases of medulloblastoma in childhood; correlation with flow cytometric DNA analysis. *Journal of Neuro-Oncology* **8**, 113–20.

Tomita, T., McLone, D.G. and Naidich, T.P. (1984) Brain stem gliomas in childhood. Rational approach and treatment. *Journal of Neuro-Oncology* **2**, 117–22.

Tomita, T., Yasue, M., Engelhard, H.H., McLone, D.G., Gonzalez-Crussi, F. and Bauer, K.D. (1988) Flow cytometric DNA analysis of medulloblastoma. Prognostic implication of aneuploidy. *Cancer* **61**, 744–9.

Tomlinson, F.H., Scheithauer, B.W., Kelly, P.J. and Forbes, G.S. (1991) Subependymoma with rhabdomyosarcomatous differentiation: report of a case and literature review. *Neurosurgery* **28**, 761–8.

Tomlinson, F.H., Scheithauer, B.W., Hayostek, C.H., Parisi, J.E., Meyer, F.B., Shaw, E.G., Weliand, T.L., Katzmann, J.A. and Jack, C.R. Jr (1994) The significance of atypia and histologic malignancy in pilocytic astrocytoma of the cerebellum: a clinicopathologic and flow cytometric study. *Journal of Child Neurology* **9**, 301–10.

Tönnis, W. and Zülch, K.J. (1939) Intrakranielle Ganglienzellgeschwülste (mit ausführlicher Beschreibung einer einhertlichen Gruppe im Grosshirn). *Zentralblatt für Neurochirurgie* **4**, 273–307.

Torres, C.F., Rebsamen, S., Silber, J.H., Sutton, L.N., Bilaniuk, L.T., Zimmerman, R.A., Goldwein, J.W., Phillips, P.C. and Lange, B.J. (1994) Surveillance scanning of children with medulloblastoma. *New England Journal of Medicine* **330**, 892–5.

Torres, L.F., Grant, N., Harding, B.N. and Scaravilli, F. (1985) Intracerebral neuroblastoma. Report of a case with neuronal maturation and long survival. *Acta Neuropathologica* **68**, 110–14.

Towfighi, J., Salam, M.M., McLendon, R.E., Powers, S. and Page, R.B. (1996) Ganglion cell-containing tumors of the pituitary gland. *Archives of Pathology and Laboratory Medicine* **120**, 369–77.

Townsend, J.J. and Seaman, J.P. (1986) Central neurocytoma–a rare benign intraventricular tumor. *Acta Neuropathologica* **71**, 167–70.

Treip, C.S. (1957) A congenital medulloepithelioma of the midbrain. *Journal of Pathology and Bacteriology* **74**, 357–63.

Trojanowski, J.Q., Lee, V.M.-Y. and Schlaepfer, W.W. (1984) An immunohistochemical study of human central and peripheral nervous system tumors, using monoclonal antibodies against neurofilaments and glial filaments. *Human Pathology* **15**, 248–57.

Trojanowski, J.Q., Tohyama, T. and Lee, V.M.-Y. (1992) Medulloblastomas and related primitive neuroectodermal brain tumors of childhood recapitulate molecular milestones in the maturation of neuroblasts. *Molecular and Chemical Neuropathology* **17**, 121–35.

Trojanowski, J.Q., Friedman, H.S., Burger, P.C. and Bigner, D.D. (1987) A rapidly dividing human medulloblastoma cell line (D283 MED) expresses all three neurofilament subunits. *American Journal of Pathology* **126**, 358–63.

Trombley, I.K. and Mirra, S.S. (1981) Ultrastructure of tuberous sclerosis: cortical tuber and subependymal tumor. *Annals of Neurology* **9**, 174–81.

Troost, D., Jansen, G.H. and Dingemans, K.P. (1990) Cerebral medulloepithelioma ——electron microscopy and immunohistochemistry. *Acta Neuropathologica* **80**, 103–7.

Tsang, R.W., Laperriere, N.J., Simpson, W.J., Brierley, J., Panzarella, T. and Smyth, H.S. (1993) Glioma arising after radiation therapy for pituitary adenoma. A report of four patients and estimation of risk. *Cancer* **72**, 2227–33.

Tsuchida, T., Shimbo, Y., Fukuda, M., Takeda, N., Tanaka, R. and Ikuta, F. (1985) Computed tomographic and histopathological studies of pontine glioma. *Child's Nervous System* **1**, 223–9.

Twiss, J.L., Anderson, L.J. and Horoupian, D.S. (1993) Globular glial fibrillary acidic protein-reactive cytoplasmic inclusions in ependymoma: an immunoelectron-microscopic study. *Acta Neuropathologica* **85**, 658–62.

Uematsu, Y., Rojas-Corona, R.R., Llena, J.F. and Hirano, A. (1989) Distribution of epithelial membrane antigen in normal and neoplastic human ependyma. *Acta Neuropathologica* **78**, 325–8.

Vagner-Capodano, A.M., Zattara-Cannoni, H., Gambarelli, D., Gentet, J.C., Genitori, L., Lena, G., Graziani, N., Raybaud, C., Choux, M. and Grisoli, F. (1994) Detection of i(17q) chromosome by fluorescent *in situ* hybridization (FISH) with interphase nuclei in medulloblastoma. *Cancer Genetics and Cytogenetics* **78**, 1–6.

Valtz, N.L.M., Hayes, T.E., Norregaard, T., Liu, S. and McKay, R.D.G. (1991) An embryonic origin for medulloblastoma. *New Biologist* **3**, 364–71.

VandenBerg, S.R. (1993) Desmoplastic infantile ganglioglioma and desmoplastic cerebral astrocytoma of infancy. *Brain Pathology* **3**, 275–81.

VandenBerg, S.R., Herman, M.M. and Rubinstein, L.J. (1987) Embryonal central neuroepithelial tumors: current concepts and future challenges. *Cancer and Metastasis Reviews* **5**, 343–64.

VandenBerg, S.R., Hess, J.R., Herman, M.M., DeArmond, S.J., Halks-Miller, M. and Rubinstein, L.J. (1981) Neural differentiation in the OTT-6050 mouse teratoma. Production of a tumor fraction showing melanogenesis in neuroepithelial cells after centrifugal elutriation. *Virchows Archiv A, Pathological Anatomy and Histology* **392**, 295–308.

VandenBerg, S.R., May, E.E., Rubinstein, L.J., Herman, M.M., Perentes, E., Vinores, S.A., Collins, V.P. and Park, T.S. (1987) Desmoplastic supratentorial neuroepithelial tumors of infancy with divergent differentiation potential (desmoplastic infantile gangliogliomas). Report on 11 cases of a distinctive embryonal tumor with favorable prognosis. *Journal of Neurosurgery* **66**, 58–71.

van der Meulen, J.D.M., Houthoff, H.J. and Ebels, E.J. (1978) Glial fibrillary acidic protein in human gliomas. *Neuropathology and Applied Neurobiology* **4**, 177–90.

Vandevelde, M., Fankhauser, R. and Luginbühl, H. (1985) Immunocytochemical studies in canine neuroectodermal brain tumors. *Acta Neuropathologica* **66**, 111–16.

Van Epps, R.R., Samuelson, D.R. and McCormick, W.F. (1967) Cerebral medulloepithelioma. Case report. *Journal of Neurosurgery* **27**, 568–73.

van Tassel, P., Lee, Y.-Y. and Bruner, J.M. (1986) Supratentorial ependymomas: computed tomographic and pathologic correlations. *Journal of Computed Tomography* **10**, 157–65.

——(1988) Synchronous and metachronous malignant gliomas: CT findings. *AJNR. American Journal of Neuroradiology* **9**, 725–32.

Vaquero, J., Herrero, J., Cabezudo, J.M. and Leunda, G. (1980) Symptomatic subependymomas of the lateral ventricles. *Acta Neurochirurgica* **53**, 99–105.

Vassallo, M. and Allen, S. (1995) An unusual cause of dementia. *Postgraduate Medical Journal* **71**, 483–4.

Vecht, Ch.J., van Zwieten, M.J., Maat, B. and van Bekkum, D.W. (1981) Metastasis from the brain of transplanted *N*-ethyl-*N*-nitrosourea-induced central nervous system tumors in rats. *European Journal of Cancer* **17**, 703–10.

Velasco, M.E., Ghobrial, M.W. and Ross, E.R. (1985) Neuron-specific enolase and neurofilament protein as markers of differentiation in medulloblastoma. *Surgical Neurology* **23**, 177–82.

Velasco, M.E., Dahl, D., Roessmann, U. and Gambetti, P. (1980) Immunohistochemical localization of glial fibrillary acidic protein in human glial neoplasms. *Cancer* **45**, 484–94.

Verhoeff, F.H. (1932) Tumors of the optic nerve. In Penfield, W. (ed.), *Cytology and cellular pathology of the nervous system*, Vol. 3. New York: Hafner, 1027–40.

Veronina, A.S. and Preobrazhensky, A.A. (1994) Developmental expression of glial fibrillary acidic protein gene in human embryos. *Neuroscience Letters* **174**, 198–200.

Versari, P., Talamonti, G., D'Aliberti, G., Fontana, R., Columbo, N. and Casadei, G. (1994) Leptomeningeal dissemination of juvenile pilocytic astrocytoma: case report. *Surgical Neurology* **41**, 318–21.

Vertosick, F.T. Jr and Selker, R.G. (1990) Brain stem and spinal metastases of supratentorial glioblastoma multiforme: a clinical series. *Neurosurgery* **27**, 516–22.

Vertosick, F.T. Jr, Selker, R.G. and Arena, V.C. (1991) Survival of patients with well-differentiated astrocytomas diagnosed in the era of computed tomography. *Neurosurgery* **28**, 496–501.

Vinchon, M., Blond, S., Lejeune, J.P., Krivosik, I., Fossati, P., Assaker, R. and Christiaens, J.L. (1994) Association of Lhermitte-Duclos and Cowden disease: report of a new case and review of the literature. *Journal of Neurology, Neurosurgery and Psychiatry* **57**, 699–704.

Vinores, S.A., Bonnin, J.M., Rubinstein, L.J. and Marangos, P.J. (1984) Immunohistochemical demonstration of neuron-specific enolase in neoplasms of the CNS and other tissues. *Archives of Pathology and Laboratory Medicine* **108**, 536–40.

Vital, A., Vital, C., Martin-Negrier, M.L., McGrogan, G., Bioulac, P., Trojani, M., Loiseau, H. and Rougier, A. (1994) Lhermitte-Duclos type cerebellum hamartoma and Cowden disease. *Clinical Neuropathology* **13**, 229–31.

Vogelstein, B. and Kinzler, K.W. (1993) The multistep nature of cancer. *Trends in Genetics* **9**, 138–41.

Voigt, W.-H. (1968) Elektronenmikroskopische Beobachtungen an menschlichen Medulloblastomen. *Deutsche Zeitschrift für Nervenheilkunde* **192**, 290–309.

Voldby, B. (1974) Disseminated, mucin-producing oligodendrogliomas. Report of 2 cases. *Acta Neurochirurgica* **30**, 299–307.

von Deimling, A., Janzer, R., Kleihues, P. and Wiestler, O.D. (1990) Patterns of differentiation in central neurocytoma. An immunohistochemical study of eleven biopsies. *Acta Neuropathologica* **79**, 473–9.

von Deimling, A., Eibl, R.H., Ohgaki, H., Louis, D.N., von Ammon, K., Petersen, I., Kleihues, P., Chung, R.Y., Wiestler, O.D. and Seizinger, B.R. (1992a) *p53* mutations are associated with 17p allelic loss in grade II and grade III astrocytoma. *Cancer Research* **52**, 2987–90.

von Deimling, A., Louis, D.N., von Ammon, K., Petersen, I., Hoell, T., Chung, R.Y., Martuza, R.L., Schoenfeld, D.A., Yasargil, M.G., Wiestler, O.D. and Seizinger, B.R. (1992b) Association of epidermal growth factor receptor gene amplification with loss of chromosome 10 in human glioblastoma multiforme. *Journal of Neurosurgery* **77**, 295–301.

von Deimling, A., von Ammon, K., Schoenfeld, D., Wiestler, O.D., Seizinger, B.R. and Louis D.N. (1993) Subsets of glioblastoma multiforme defined by molecular genetic analysis. *Brain Pathology* **3**, 19–26.

Vraa-Jensen, J., Herman, M.M., Rubinstein, L.J. and Bignami, A. (1976) *In vitro* characteristics of a fourth ventricle ependymoma maintained in organ culture systems: light and electron microscopic observations. *Neuropathology and Applied Neurobiology* **2**, 349–64.

Wacker, M.R., Cogen, P.H., Etzell, J.E., Daneshvar, L., Davis, R.L. and Prados, M.D. (1992) Diffuse leptomeningeal involvement by a ganglioglioma in a child. Case report. *Journal of Neurosurgery* **77**, 302–6.

Wada, C., Kurata, A., Hirose, R., Tazaki, Y., Kan, S., Ishihara, Y. and Kameya, T. (1986) Primary leptomeningeal ependymoblastoma. *Journal of Neurosurgery* **64**, 968–73.

Wahl, R.W. and Dillard, S.H. Jr (1972) Multiple ganglioneuromas of the central nervous system. *Archives of Pathology* **94**, 158–64.

Wakamatsu, T., Matsuo, T., Kawano, S., Teramoto, S. and Matsumura, H. (1971) Glioblastoma with extracranial metastases through ventriculo-pleural shunt. *Journal of Neurosurgery* **34**, 697–701.

Waldbaur, H., Gottschaldt, M., Schmidt, H. and Neuhäuser, G. (1976) Medulloblastom des Kleinhirns und Pineoblastom bei eineiigen Zwillingen. *Klinishe Pädiatrie* **188**, 366–71.

Waldron, J.N., Laperriere, N.J., Jaakkimainen, L., Simpson, W.J., Payne, D., Milosevic, M. and Wong, C.S. (1993) Spinal cord ependymomas: a retrospective analysis of 59 cases. *International Journal of Radiation Oncology, Biology and Physics* **27**, 223–9.

Wallner, K.E., Gonzales, M. and Sheline, G.E. (1988) Treatment of oligodendrogliomas with or without postoperative irradiation. *Journal of Neurosurgery* **68**, 684–8.

Wallner, K.E., Galicich, J.H., Krol, G., Arbit, E. and Malkin, M.G. (1989) Patterns of failure following treatment for glioblastoma multiforme and anaplastic astrocytoma. *International Journal of Radiation Oncology, Biology and Physics* **16**, 1405–9.

Walter, G.F. (1978) Kleinhirnastrocytome und Opticusgliome—eine vergleichende feinstrukturelle Untersuchung. *Virchows Archiv A, Pathological Anatomy and Histology* **380**, 59–79.

Warkany, J., Passarge, E. and Smith, L.B. (1966) Congenital malformations in autosomal trisomy syndromes. *American Journal of Diseases of Children* **112**, 502–17.

Warnick, R.E., Raisanen, J., Adornato, B.T., Prados, M.D., Davis, R.L., Larson, D.A. and Gutin, P.H. (1993) Intracranial myxopapillary ependymoma: case report. *Journal of Neuro-Oncology* **15**, 251–6.

Warzok, R., Jaenisch, W. and Lang, G. (1983) Morphology and biology of cerebellar neuroblastomas. *Journal of Neuro-Oncology* **1**, 373–9.

Watanabe, K., Tachibana, O., Sato, K., Yonekawa, Y., Kleihues, P. and Ohgaki, H. (1996) Overexpression of the EGF receptor and *p53* mutations are mutually exclusive in the evolution of primary and secondary glioblastoma. *Brain Pathology* **6**, 217–22.

Wätjen, J. (1930) Ein Ganglioglioneurom des Zentralnervensystems. *Virchows Archiv* **277**, 441–65.

Watt, T.J. and Winfield, J.A. (1987) Analyzing factors influencing medulloblastoma prognosis. *Journal of Neurosurgery* **67**, 471–2.

Weaver, D., VandenBerg, S.R., Park, T.S. and Jane, J.A. (1984) Selective peripancreatic sarcoma metastases from primary gliosarcoma. *Journal of Neurosurgery* **61**, 599–601.

Webb, J.H., Craig, W.McK. and Kernohan, J.W. (1953) Intraspinal neoplasms in the cervical region. *Journal of Neurosurgery* **10**, 360–6.

Wechsler, W. (1966) Electron microscopy of the cytodifferentiation in the developing brain of chick embryos. In Hassler, R. and Stephan, H. (eds), *Evolution of the forebrain. Phylogenesis and ontogenesis of the forebrain.* Stuttgart: Georg Thieme, 213–24.

Weichselbaum, R.R., Liszczak, T.M., Phillips, J.P., Little, J.B., Epstein, J. and Kornblith, P.L. (1977) Characterization and radiobiologic parameters of medulloblastoma *in vitro*. *Cancer* **40**, 1087–96.

Weir, B. and Elvidge, A.R. (1968) Oligodendrogliomas. An analysis of 63 cases. *Journal of Neurosurgery* **29**, 500–5.

Weiss, L. (1955) A metastasizing ependymoma of the cauda equina. *Cancer* **8**, 161–71.

Weiss, L., Sagerman, R.H., King, G.A., Chung, C.T. and Dubowy, R.L. (1987) Controversy in the management of optic nerve glioma. *Cancer* **59**, 1000–4.

Weldon-Linne, C.M., Victor, T.A., Groothuis, D.R. and Vick, N.A. (1983) Pleomorphic xanthoastrocytoma. Ultrastructural and immunohistochemical study of a case with a rapidly fatal outcome following surgery. *Cancer* **52**, 2055–63.

Weller, R.O., Foy, M. and Cox, S. (1977) The development and ultrastructure of the microvasculature in malignant gliomas. *Neuropathology and Applied Neurobiology* **3**, 307–22.

Wells, G.R., Lasner, T.M., Yousem, D.M. and Zager, E.L. (1994) Lhermitte-Duclos disease and Cowden's syndrome in an adolescent patient. Case report. *Journal of Neurosurgery* **81**, 133–6.

Wen, B.-C., Hussey, D.H., Hitchon, P.W., Schelper, R.L., Vigliotti, A.P., Doornbos, J.F. and VanGilder, J.C. (1991) The role of radiation therapy in the management of ependymomas of the spinal cord. *International*

Journal of Radiation Oncology, Biology and Physics **20**, 781–6.

Wen, H.-L. and Barrows, L.J. (1957) Ependymoma with extracranial metastases. (Abstract) *Journal of Neuropathology and Experimental Neurology* **16**, 112.

Weremowicz, S., Kupsky, W.J., Morton, C.C. and Fletcher, J.A. (1992) Cytogenetic evidence for a chromosome 22 tumor suppressor gene in ependymoma. *Cancer Genetics and Cytogenetics* **61**, 193–6.

Wernicke, C., Thiel, G., Lozanova, T., Vogel, S., Kintzel, D., Janisch, W., Lehmann, K. and Witkowski, R. (1995) Involvement of chromosome 22 in ependymomas. *Cancer Genetics and Cytogenetics* **79**, 173–6.

Wesseling, P., Schlingemann, R.O., Rietveld, F.J., Link, M., Burger, P.C. and Ruiter, D.J. (1995) Early and extensive contribution of pericytes/vascular smooth muscle cells to microvascular proliferation in glioblastoma multiforme: an immuno-light and immunoelectron microscopy study. *Journal of Neuropathology and Experimental Neurology* **54**, 304–10.

Wight, D.G.D., Holley, K.J. and Finbow, J.A.H. (1973) Metastasizing ependymoma of the cauda equina. *Journal of Clinical Pathology* **26**, 929–35.

Williams, D.W. III, Elster, A.D., Ginsberg, L.E. and Stanton, C. (1992) Recurrent Lhermitte-Duclos disease: report of two cases and association with Cowden's disease. *AJNR. Amercian Journal of Neuroradiology* **13**, 287–90.

Willis, R.A. (1958) *The borderland of embryology and pathology*. London: Butterworth.

——(1962a) *The pathology of the tumours of children*. Edinburgh: Oliver & Boyd.

——(1962b) *The borderland of embryology and pathology*. Second edition. London: Butterworth.

——(1967) *Pathology of tumours*. Fourth edition. London: Butterworth.

——(1971) Nervous tissue in teratomas. In Minckler, J. (ed.), *Pathology of the nervous system*, Vol. 2. New York: McGraw-Hill, 1937–43.

Wilson, A.J., Leaffer, D.H. and Kohout, N.D. (1985) Differentiated cerebral neuroblastoma: a tumor in need of discovery. *Human Pathology* **16**, 647–9.

Wilson, W.B., Feinsod, M., Hoyt, W.F. and Nielsen, S.L. (1976) Malignant evolution of childhood chiasmal pilocytic astrocytoma. *Neurology* **26**, 322–5.

Winger, M.J., Macdonald, D.R. and Cairncross, J.G. (1989) Supratentorial anaplastic gliomas in adults. The prognostic importance of extent of resection and prior low-grade glioma. *Journal of Neurosurgery* **71**, 487–93.

Wolf, A. and Morton, B.F. (1937) Ganglion cell tumors of the central nervous system. *Bulletin of the Neurologic Institute of New York* **6**, 453–88.

Wolf, H.K., Müller, M.B., Spänle, M., Zentner, J., Schramm, J. and Wiestler, O.D. (1994) Ganglioglioma: a detailed histopathological and immunohistochemical analysis of 61 cases. *Acta Neuropathologica* **88**, 166–73.

Wolf, H.K., Wellmer, J., Müller, M.B., Wiestler, O.D., Hufnagel, A. and Pietsch, T. (1995) Glioneuronal malformative lesions and dysembryoplastic neuroepithelial tumors in patients with chronic pharmacoresistant epilepsies. *Journal of Neuropathology and Experimental Neurology* **54**, 245–54.

Wolff, M., Santiago, H. and Duby, M.M. (1972) Delayed distant metastasis from a subcutaneous sacrococcygeal ependymoma. Case report, with tissue culture, ultrastructural observations, and review of the literature. *Cancer* **30**, 1046–67.

Wong, A.J., Bigner, S.H., Bigner D.D., Kinzler, K.W., Hamilton, S.R. and Vogelstein, B. (1987) Increased expression of the epidermal growth factor receptor gene in malignant gliomas is invariably associated with gene amplification. *Proceedings of the National Academy of Sciences of the U.S.A.* **84**, 6899–903.

Wong, J.Y.C., Uhl, V., Wara, W.M. and Sheline, G.E. (1987) Optic gliomas. A reanalysis of the University of California, San Francisco experience. *Cancer* **60**, 1847–55.

Wright, J.E., McDonald, W.I. and Call, N.B. (1980) Management of optic nerve gliomas. *British Journal of Ophthalmology* **64**, 545–52.

Wright, J.E., McNab, A.A. and McDonald, W.I. (1989) Optic nerve glioma and the management of optic nerve tumours in the young. *British Journal of Ophthalmology* **73**, 967–74.

Wulc, A.E., Bergin, D.J., Barnes, D., Scaravilli, F., Wright, J.E. and McDonald, W.I. (1989) Orbital optic nerve glioma in adult life. *Archives of Ophthalmology* **107**, 1013–16.

Yachnis, A.T., Rorke, L.B. and Trojanowski, J.Q. (1994) Cerebellar dysplasias in humans: development and possible relationship to glial and primitive neuroectodermal tumors of the cerebellar vermis. *Journal of Neuropathology and Experimental Neurology* **53**, 61–71

Yagishita, S., Itoh, Y., Chiba, Y., Yamashita, T., Nakazima, F. and Kuwabara, T. (1980) Cerebellar neuroblastoma. A light and ultrastructural study. *Acta Neuropathologica* **50**, 139–42.

Yagishita, S., Itoh, Y., Chiba, Y. and Kuwana, N. (1982) Morphological investigations on cerebellar 'neuroblastoma' group. *Acta Neuropathologica* **56**, 22–8.

Yamamoto, T., Komori, T., Shibata, N., Toyoda, C. and Kobayashi, M. (1996) Multifocal neurocytoma/gangliocytoma with extensive leptomeningeal dissemination in the brain and spinal cord. *American Journal of Surgical Pathology* **20**, 363–70.

Yamashita, J., Handa, H., Yamagami, T. and Haebara, H. (1985) Astroblastoma of pure type. *Surgical Neurology* **24**, 218–22.

Yanoff, M., Davis, R.L. and Zimmerman, L.E. (1978) Juvenile pilocytic astrocytoma ('glioma') of optic nerve: clinicopathologic study of sixty-three cases. In Jakobiec, F.A. (ed.), *Ocular and adnexal tumors*. Birmingham, Ala.: Aesculapius, 685–707.

Yasue, M., Tomita, T., Engelhard, H., Gonzalez-Crussi, F., McLone, D.G. and Bauer, K.D. (1989) Prognostic importance of DNA ploidy in medulloblastoma of childhood. *Journal of Neurosurgery* **70**, 385–91.

Yokota, N., Aruga, J., Takai, S., Yamada, K., Hamazaki, M., Iwase, T., Sugimura, H. and Mikoshiba, K. (1996) Predominant expression of human Zic in cerebellar granule cell lineage and medulloblastoma. *Cancer Research* **56**, 377–83.

Yoshii, Y., Maki, Y., Tsuboi, K., Tomono, Y., Nakagawa, K. and Hoshino, T. (1986) Estimation of growth fraction with bromodeoxyuridine in human central nervous system tumors. *Journal of Neurosurgery* **65**, 659–63.

Youness, E., Barlogie, B., Ahearn, M. and Trujillo, J.M. (1980) Tumor cell phagocytosis. Its occurrence in a patient with medulloblastoma. *Archives of Pathology and Laboratory Medicine* **104**, 651–3.

Yung, W.A., Horten, B.C. and Shapiro, W.R. (1980) Meningeal gliomatosis: a review of 12 cases. *Annals of Neurology* **8**, 605–8.

Yung, W.-K.A., Luna, M. and Borit, A. (1985) Vimentin and glial fibrillary acidic protein in human brain tumors. *Journal of Neuro-Oncology* **3**, 35.

Yung, W.K. (1989) *In vitro* chemosensitivity testing and its clinical application in human gliomas. *Neurosurgery Review* **12**, 197–203.

Zeltzer, P.M., Bodey, B., Marlin, A. and Kemshead, J. (1990) Immunophenotype profile of childhood medulloblastomas and supratentorial primitive neuroectodermal tumors using 16 monoclonal antibodies. *Cancer* **66**, 273–83.

Zentner, J., Wolf, H.K., Ostertun, B., Hufnagel, A., Campos, M.G., Solymosi, L. and Schramm, J. (1994) Gangliogliomas: clinical, radiological, and histopathological findings in 51 patients. *Journal of Neurology, Neurosurgery, and Psychiatry* **57**, 1497–502.

Zerbini, C., Gelber, R.D., Weinberg, D., Sallan, S.E., Barnes, P., Kupsky, W., Scott, R.M. and Tarbell, N.J. (1993) Prognostic factors in medulloblastoma, including DNA ploidy. *Journal of Clinical Oncology* **11**, 616–22.

Zerlin, M., Levison, S.W. and Goldman, J.E. (1995) Early patterns of migration, morphogenesis, and intermediate filament expression of subventricular zone cells in the postnatal rat forebrain. *Journal of Neuroscience* **15**, 7238–49.

Zimmerman, H.M. (1957) The natural history of intracranial neoplasms, with special reference to the gliomas. *American Journal of Surgery* **93**, 913–24.

——(1969) Brain tumors: their incidence and classification in man and their experimental production. *Annals of the New York Academy of Sciences* **159**, art. **2**, 337–59.

Zimmerman, L., Lendahl, U., Cunningham, M., McKay, R., Parr, B., Gavin, B., Mann, J., Vassileva, G. and McMahon, A. (1994) Independent regulatory elements in the nestin gene direct transgene expression to neural stem cells or muscle precursors. *Neuron* **12**, 11–24.

Zimmerman, L.E., Arkfeld, D.L., Schenken, J.B., Arkfeld, D.F. and Maris, P.J.G. (1983) A rare choristoma of the optic nerve and chiasm. *Archives of Ophthalmology* **101**, 766–70.

Zuber, P., Hamou, M.-F. and de Tribolet, N. (1988) Identification of proliferating cells in human gliomas using the monoclonal antibody Ki-67. *Neurosurgery* **22**, 364–8.

Zülch, K.J. (1957) *Brain tumors. their biology and pathology.* New York: Springer.

——(1979) *Histological typing of tumours of the central nervous system.* International histological classification of tumours 21. Geneva: World Health Organization, 19–20.

——(1986) *Brain tumors: their biology and pathology.* Third edition. Berlin: Springer-Verlag.

Zülch, K.J. and Christensen, E. (1956) *Pathologische anatomie der raumbeengenden intrakraniellen prozesse.* Handbuch der neurochirurgie **3**, Olivecrona, H. and Tönnis, W. (series eds). Berlin: Springer-Verlag.

Zülch, K.J. and Wechsler, W. (1968) Pathology and classification of gliomas. In Krayenbühl, H., Maspes, P.E. and Sweet, W.H. (eds), *Progress in neurological surgery*, Vol. 2. Basel: Karger, 1–84.

Zuppan, C.W., Mierau, G.W. and Weeks, D.A. (1994) Ependymoma with signet-ring cells. *Ultrastructural Pathology* **18**, 43–6.

Zu Rhein, G.M. and Varakis, J.N. (1979) Perinatal induction of medulloblastomas in Syrian golden hamsters by a human polyoma virus (JC). *National Cancer Institute Monographs* **51**, 205–8.

Index

Entries appearing in Volume 1 are indicated by the numeral I; those in Volume 2, by the numeral II.